Skeletal Injury in the Child

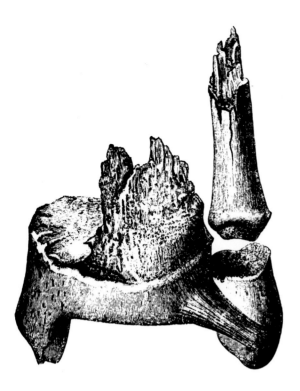

Skeletal

My Arm

This is strange . . .
I can't say it,
S'traction?
It makes your arm get better.
It holds your arm so it heals
     quicker
It feels funny
It's hard to get dressed
               change the sheets
               color
               eat.
                    By CARRIE S.

*This poem was written by a seven-year-old girl as she lay in
Dunlop's traction for a severe supracondylar humeral fracture.*

Injury in the Child

JOHN A. OGDEN, M.D.

Professor of Surgery and Pediatrics, and Chief of Orthopaedics
Chief of Children's Orthopaedics
Director, Skeletal Growth and Development Laboratory
Yale University School of Medicine
New Haven, Connecticut

LEA & FEBIGER • 1982 • PHILADELPHIA

Lᴇᴀ & Fᴇʙɪɢᴇʀ
600 Washington Square
Philadelphia, PA 19106
USA

Library of Congress Cataloging in Publication Data

Ogden, John A. (John Anthony)
 Skeletal injury in the child.

 Bibliography: p.
 Includes index.
 1. Pediatric orthopedia. 2. Fractures in children. 3. Children—
Wounds and injuries. I. Title. [DNLM: 1. Bone development.
2. Fractures—In infancy and childhood. 3. Bone and bones—
Injuries. WE 200 O34s]
 RD732.3.C48O36 1982   617′.3   81-8384
 ISBN 0-8121-0809-4   AACR2

PRINTED IN THE UNITED STATES OF AMERICA

Print Number   2   1

To Dali.
To my parents.
To the children, who will
inherit the universe.

Preface

INJURY and the subsequent reparative response of the developing skeleton are frequently disparate from the mature skeleton. This book is an outgrowth of a desire to attain a morphologic understanding of the nuances of pediatric orthopaedic trauma. As clinicians we all have a tendency to focus on specific injuries, often ignoring trauma mechanisms and the relevance of underlying anatomy to both the initial injury and long term consequences.

This book introduces the principles of diagnosis and treatment of fractures in children in a manner that first establishes a solid foundation of anatomy and pathomechanics on which treatment principles are based. Developmental anatomy is an overlooked facet of children's injuries, primarily because of the paucity of morphologic material available for use as source material. The unique opportunity to include the resources of the Skeletal Growth and Development Study Unit at Yale University allowed the inclusion of much material. In particular, I have attempted to translate the anatomic details into a form that will have practical value. I feel that the emphasis on normal structure and function and the mechanisms of response to trauma are essential to good clinical practice.

Decision making in orthopaedics is experience dependent, in that it requires a proper mental set for what is normal for the given anatomic part at a particular age. Because of the lack of available anatomic material, the orthopaedist must rely on whatever resources he can muster for normal references for most of development. One can more readily accept the importance and significance of basic anatomic developmental changes if these are presented in close relationship to current clinical situations in which the information is necessary.

This volume is primarily a clinical textbook, although discussions encompass aspects of skeletal developmental biology, particularly the response to trauma. My hope is that this book provides the medical student, the resident, and the practicing physician with a logical and progressive plan of approach to children's fractures that allows for the ready storage, retrieval, and utilization of knowledge concerning each of the specific regions of injury. Since the study of orthopaedics must be a lifelong process, this book is intended to serve both as an introduction to the study of skeletal injury, as well as a basic text for continuing study. Hopefully, it will also have import to pediatricians, general practitioners, and radiologists. The orientation is to furnish a reference book that comprehensively covers the field of musculoskeletal trauma in the child, and provides adequate information for both the specialist as well as the resident physician.

I have tried to develop a text for the teaching of basic and applied anatomy, mechanisms, concepts, and principles that are applicable to each area of injury in the pediatric patient. The factual and patient material has been carefully selected to support an understanding of these concepts and principles. In doing so I have attempted to integrate a scientific basis with the art of medicine. The test of the value of this book will be its effectiveness in stimulating further insight into the diagnosis and care of patients who face a lifetime of challenge. If this has been achieved, the work will have been worth the effort.

JOHN A. OGDEN, M.D.

Sachem's Head, Connecticut
New Haven, Connecticut

Acknowledgments

THERE are a great many individuals who generously contributed time and talent to this undertaking. This book is a synthesis of their labors and mine. Many of the cases have been contributed by fellow faculty members, residents, and orthopaedists throughout the world. I cannot name everyone, but I certainly do express my deep and sincere appreciation to each of them.

Although gratitude must be expressed to many people, I must particularly thank Dr. Wayne O. Southwick. Many years ago he had the insight to induce me to consider orthopaedics as a career. Throughout my training and subsequent affiliation on the Yale faculty, he has stimulated and encouraged my pursuits in pediatric orthopaedics and skeletal development. He has done so unselfishly and with an unceasing desire to see that each of us in the Yale program attained his maximum potential. I owe him an inexpressible debt of gratitude, and hope that this volume serves as an additional tribute to what he has given me.

Much of the morphologic research that has served as the basis for each chapter has been supported by several organizations. The Crippled Children's Aid Society has been a constant source of assistance to our Section as they have sought to continue the work and memory of Carl Henze, M.D., an early New Haven orthopaedist with a deep interest in the problems of crippled children. The Easter Seal Research Foundation and Ohse Foundation have each supplied support for the initial morphologic studies. The National Institutes of Health have given generous support to my desire to make developmental anatomy relevant to childhood trauma and disease (Grants R01-HD-10854 and K04-AM-00300). Some of the relevant animal studies have received support from the National Oceanographic and Atmospheric Administration. A Berg Fellowship through the Orthopaedic Research and Education Foundation allowed me a unique opportunity to study epiphyseal injuries in Finland with Anders Langenskiöld and pediatric orthopaedics at Oxford with Edgar Sommerville.

The photographic illustrations represent the constant efforts of Patricia Cosgrove, Mary Bronson, Gertrude Chaplin, John Braslin, and Sarah Whitaker. Processing and roentgenography of the anatomic specimens have been ingeniously accomplished by Gerald Conlogue.

Finally, I must thank Joanne Ciresi, Mary Villano, Susan Murphy, Suzanne Barnett, and Patti Milot for their unceasing efforts in typing the many drafts that went into the production of this book.

J. A. O.

Contents

Skeletal Injury in the Child

1

General Principles

Childhood injuries are a problem not only for treating physicians, but also for the entire community, and they rightfully may be considered a phase of public health education. Accidents are the leading cause of death, as well as an outstanding cause of permanent disability, among children older than one year of age. Skeletal injuries account for 10 to 15% of childhood injuries.[1] In patients with multisystem injuries, particularly if life-threatening, the tendency is to assign a low priority to fracture care, a factor which may lead to skeletal growth deformity. Adequate fracture care must be an integral part of both the emergency and the subsequent care of any multiply-injured child.[2,3]

Fractures involving the developing skeleton may be significantly different during any of the stages of chondro-osseous maturation, as well as during the stage of skeletal maturity (adulthood). Any physician treating skeletal injuries in children must be familiar with the probable mechanism of injury, the cause and long term biologic response of the injured part (particularly when a growth mechanism is involved), and the appropriate guidelines for treatment of the specific injury. These patients have all of their productive years ahead of them, and they must be treated with skills based upon experience and detailed knowledge of the capacities of repair and remodeling. If a physician relies upon principles of treatment applicable to injuries of mature bone, errors in judgement and technique may manifest themselves in permanent defects.

Basic Differences

Patient history

Unlike histories taken from conversant adults, historical details of actual injuries to children often are totally lacking, erroneous, or purposely deceptive. This is particularly true of the ''battered child.'' Frequently, no responsible person has seen the accident. The child's account may be oversimplified, halting, or incomplete. Knowing how the injury occurred often enables the physician to anticipate the full extent of the injury, including important associated injuries. Because appropriate treatment is accomplished more satisfactorily when one has some knowledge of the mechanism

of injury, the variable lack of historical data on childhood injuries requires that particular significance be attached to the physical examination, which must thoroughly assess the type of deformity, location, degree of concomitant soft tissue swelling, and integrity of innervation and circulation.

Parents

An adequate discussion with the parents is as important as the actual treatment of their child's fracture. It is essential to establish both a good doctor/child-patient relationship as well as a satisfactory doctor/parent relationship, since the latter may be instrumental in carrying out essentials of care. Elucidate the troublesome areas of diagnosis and treatment in words they can comprehend, and be absolutely certain that they do understand. Always prepare the parents for acute care as well as for potential chronic or long term problems. Discuss the possibilities of limping, loss of full range of motion, nerve injury, loss of reduction after initial treatment, and the need for re-manipulation, and emphasize the need for adequate follow-up care, which extends in many cases until skeletal maturity is attained. Proper follow-up care is probably the most difficult factor to gain compliance with, especially after the child appears outwardly normal, but it is probably the most important factor in anticipating and diagnosing problems of premature growth arrest in their early stages. During a growth spurt, seemingly minor problems may rapidly assume major importance, especially when dealing with growth mechanism injuries.

Special features

Several factors make fractures of the immature skeleton different from those of the mature skeleton. Among these are: (1) fractures are more common and more likely to occur following seemingly minimal trauma; (2) the periosteum is thicker, stronger, and more biologically active; (3) diagnosis presents special problems, in particular, the variable radiolucency of the epiphyses; (4) spontaneous correction occurs in certain, *but not all*, residual angular deformities; (5) complications are different; (6) different methods of treatment receive different emphasis; and (7) joint injuries, dislocations, or ligamentous disruptions are much less common.

3

Further major differences include the following: (1) Injuries may involve specific growth regions such as the physis or epiphyseal ossification center and lead to significant acute and/or chronic disturbances of growth. (2) Normal processes of bone remodeling in the diaphysis and metaphysis (particularly the latter) of a growing child will longitudinally realign many initially malunited fragments, making absolutely accurate anatomic reductions somewhat less important in a child than in an adult.[4,5] However, this tends to be an abused aspect of the treatment of children's fractures. Accurate anatomic reduction should be attempted whenever possible. (3) Fractures stimulate longitudinal growth by increasing blood supply to the metaphysis, physis, and epiphysis, and, at least as shown by experimental evidence, by circumferentially disrupting the periosteum and its tethering (restraint) mechanism on rates of longitudinal growth of the physis.[6] Therefore, some degree of overriding with bayonet (side-to-side) apposition may be acceptable in certain age groups and may even be desirable, particularly in fractures of the femur. (4) Bone healing is much more rapid in childhood because of the thickened, extremely osteogenic periosteum and the abundant blood supply to this region. The younger the child, the more rapid the union. The dependence of healing capacity on age is significant. Age affects the rates of skeletal healing more than it does any other tissue in the body. At birth, fracture healing is remarkably rapid, but becomes progressively less rapid during childhood and adolescence. The healing of a fracture of the femoral shaft in a newborn infant may take only 3 weeks, whereas 20 weeks is not an uncommon length in a young adult. The rate of healing in the bone is probably closely related to the osteogenic activity of the periosteum and endosteum. Nonunion usually does not occur in children. (5) It is necessary to follow the child until skeletal maturity in order to obtain meaningful conclusions. This applies to any study of the long term consequences of fractures in children. The tendency to cease follow-up care 6 to 12 months after the injury may result in subsequent presentation of significant growth deformities and irate parents.

Effect of age

Every age group from infancy to adolescence has its typical injury patterns. Children also have certain typical reactions to an injury, such as a pseudoparalysis of the newborn infant in response to a fracture of the upper extremity. Knowledge of these factors, when considered along with the mechanism of trauma, is often helpful in making a diagnosis and rendering treatment. During periods of rapid growth, children may twist or strain, a behavior which hardly seems to merit consideration by either the parent or the physician. However, this may cause chondro-osseous injury, particularly of the tibia, which is susceptible to spiral fracture in children between the ages of two and five (the so-called "toddler's" fracture).

Iqbal[7] showed that upper limb fractures in children were seven times more common than lower limb fractures, and that the incidence of fractures was much higher in the preschool period. The only fractures showing a major variation from this pattern were forearm fractures, which showed a progressive increase with age, attaining a maximum frequency in the prepubescent period, and dropping sharply in incidence after age 19. In contrast, clavicular fractures were most marked in infancy and preschool, and dropped off significantly in the school years.

The site, frequency, and nature of traumatic bone lesions are all conditioned by the age of the patient. The fetal bones, effectively protected from external trauma by the amniotic fluid and thick uterine wall, rarely are traumatized (see Chap. 8). However, chronic intrauterine stresses operating on a fetus that is in a faulty position may cause changes in the shape of fetal bones and joints, causing such postural disorders as prenatal bowing of the long bones, club feet, and hip dysplasia. Even severe local deformities, especially to the mandible, facial, and skull bones, and possibly even some types of tibial pseudarthrosis can occur.[8,9] During the birth process, and more frequently in breech deliveries, a wide variety of traumatic lesions may be incurred, including fractures of the shafts and epiphyseal cartilages. The most common obstetric fractures are those involving the skull and clavicles.[10]

During the first year, fractures are relatively rare. Multiple, severe fractures may develop, however, and may be the first indication of metabolic disorders or skeletal dysplasia (e.g., hypophosphatasia; osteogenesis imperfecta). Sides of cribs are sources of injuries to the bones of the legs and arms of infants. Most willful assaults on children occur during the first two years of life and cause the clinical syndrome of "battered child." From age two on, particularly from the time the child starts to walk, the most commonly fractured bone is the radius. The high incidence of this fracture continues and increases into adolescence, although the pattern appears to change from fractures of the shaft and distal metaphysis to fractures of the distal epiphyseal plate. Fractures of the phalanges and metacarpals are also common in the first two years while the child is learning to walk.[11] Toddler's fracture of the distal half of the tibia is common during the second to fifth years. Throughout childhood, fractures of the clavicle are common. At all ages, the automobile is the principal crippler of children, causing severe skeletal abnormalities. However, the serious hazards of snowmobiles, power lawn mowers, trail bikes, and other powered, small vehicles are becoming increasingly evident. Even nonpowered "vehicles" such as skateboards are becoming an increasingly significant cause of childhood and adolescent fractures.

The age at which growth ceases varies greatly and depends on multiple factors. The skeletal age is the determining factor when considering the effect of trauma on the growing skeleton. Trauma, mechanisms, and fracture types become different. Ligament injuries and joint dislocation become more common with the attainment of skeletal maturity.

Activity levels

Children tend to approach life at a more active level than adults. This must be considered in any treatment. Once pain subsides, the child tends to forget that an extremity is injured, and quickly will go back to normal levels of activity, which may not be conducive to fracture healing, and which may damage immobilization devices. Childhood is also a time of emphasis on competitive sports, often with a greater drive coming from the parents than from the child. Organized sports involving younger children predispose the improperly conditioned child to injury.[12-14] Furthermore, children often will try to get back into these programs as quickly as possible after the injury, often before complete healing. The additional stress from a parent to get the child back on the playing field makes medical care of these children even more difficult.

Biologic Differences

Many, if not all, of the aforementioned differences between the traumatized skeletons of an adult and a child relate to the fact that the child's skeletal elements are in a more dynamic, constantly changing growth mode, whereas the adult skeleton has ceased elongation and apposition, and is principally (and more slowly) remodeling the established elements in accord with stress responses (i.e., forming increasing patterns of secondary and tertiary osteons). The major differences between childhood and adult skeletal trauma relate to three categories: anatomy, physiology, and biomechanics.

Anatomy

Because of endochondral ossification, the chondroosseous epiphyses of children are variably radiolucent, making roentgenographic evaluation difficult, if not impossible, unless specific, usually invasive procedures (e.g., arthrography) are used. Skeletal injury sometimes must be inferred on the basis of clinical judgement, for roentgenographic substantiation may not be immediately possible, although subsequently, new bone formation may make the diagnosis certain. The physis is constantly changing, both with active longitudinal and diametric growth and in its mechanical relation to other components. Modes of failure thus vary with the degree of chondro-osseous maturation. The periosteum also differs in a child, being thicker, more readily elevated from the diaphyseal and metaphyseal bone (as by a subperiosteal fracture hematoma), less readily completely disrupted, and exhibiting greater osteogenic potential.

Schenk[15] showed that the following properties of the developing skeleton are immensely important to fracture healing: (1) there is a pronounced reaction of periosteum and endosteum that is significant in the correction of longitudinal deformities; (2) the vascular pattern of cortical bone and its microscopic structure, as well as the vascular supply of the growth plate, assume great importance in specific fractures. This involvement of the growth plate and growing articular cartilage in angular deformities is important to certain fracture concepts.

Developing bone begins with fewer lamellar components and a relatively greater porosity than mature bone. Within any given anatomic region of a bone, changes occur with age, with the natural sequence beginning with increased lamellar bone in the diaphysis. There are also relative differences in the various regions within a given bone that predispose certain regions to fracture over others. These differences in microscopic and macroscopic architecture also affect the process of fracture healing, which is different in the more dense, lamellar bone of the diaphysis, as compared to the spongy, trabecular bone of the metaphysis or epiphysis.

Physiology

The skeleton is undergoing active, frequently rapid, growth and remodeling. Therefore, fractures usually heal rapidly; nonunion is rare; overgrowth may occur; and certain angular deformities may correct totally. However, damage to the capacity of the bone to accomplish these physiologic functions may impair subsequent growth and development in several ways. Various portions of the longitudinal bones respond differently to hormones, mechanical factors, vascular changes, and trauma.

Biomechanics

The major changes undergone by developing bone are increases in the density of the cortex, particularly in the diaphysis but also in the metaphysis, and changes in the proportions of trabecular (endosteal) and cortical bone in the diaphysis, metaphysis, and epiphysis. The porosity, in cross section, of a child's bone is much greater than that of an adult's, and this may play a role in stopping fracture propagation, much as a hole drilled in glass at the end of a crack may prevent a crack from continuing. This factor undoubtedly is important, since comminuted fractures are uncommon in children. The increased amount of bone in the epiphyseal ossification center undoubtedly alters the stress/strain response pattern of the epiphysis, and it is likely that establishment of the subchondral plate over the physis alters its response to fracture.[16] Adult bone usually fails in tension, whereas a child's bone may fail in either tension or compression.

Patterns of Injury

Satisfactory treatment necessitates an understanding of what comprises each specific fracture. In essence, a fracture may be defined as a disruption of the normal continuity of the bone and/or cartilage. The disruption may or may not cause a break in the continuity of the cortical bone, a factor that can occur in children when the cortical bone, because of a greater capacity for plastic deformation prior to failure, buckles rather than breaks. This represents compression, rather than tension, failure of bone, and can only occur in children. Tensile failure, which certainly may occur in children and is the prevailing mode of failure in adults, leads to a break in structural continuity of the bone.

Each fracture needs to be described adequately.[12,17] Such a description should include: (1) the anatomic location of the fracture; (2) the type of fracture; and (3) the physical changes caused by and associated with the fracture.

Anatomic location

Terminology should locate the lesion accurately, and becomes important for comparative treatment studies. As will be seen in the clinical section, slight differences in anatomic locale of the fracture in children may have a major impact on acute treatment and potential long term problems. These definitions are illustrated in Figure 1-1:

Diaphyseal. Involvement of the central shaft of a longitudinal bone, which is usually composed of mature, lamellar bone.

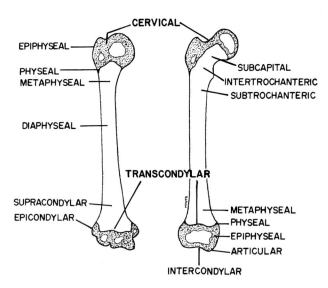

FIG. 1-1. Schematic of humerus (left) and femur (right) from a ten-year-old boy showing various anatomic locations and definitions. See text for details.

Metaphyseal. Involvement of the flaring ends of the central shaft of a longitudinal bone. The metaphyses are usually comprised of extensive endosteal trabecular bone and cortical immature fiber bone, both of which predispose the metaphyses to the torus type of fracture.

Physeal. Involvement of the endochondral growth mechanism. These fractures are discussed in detail in Chapter 4.

Epiphyseal. Involvement of the chondro-osseous end of a long bone. It is important to realize that the epiphysis may be injured only in the cartilaginous portion, which makes diagnosis extremely difficult. Again, these fractures are discussed in more detail in Chapter 4.

Articular. Involvement of the epiphyseal region that has formed the joint surface. The injury may be part of a more extensive epiphyseal injury, or it may be localized. In the latter case, the fragment may include only articular cartilage and juxtaposed, undifferentiated hyaline cartilage, or both subchondral bone and cartilage.

Epicondylar. Involvement of regions of the bone, especially around the elbow, that serve as major muscle attachments and have extensions of the physis and epiphysis.

Subcapital. Involvement just below the epiphyses of certain bones such as the proximal femur or radius.

Cervical (or Neck). Involvement along the neck of a specific bone, such as the proximal humerus or femur.

Supracondylar. Involvement above the level of the condyles and epicondyles (e.g., distal humerus).

Transcondylar. Located across the condyles, usually this is a physeal fracture of the distal humerus or femur.

Intercondylar (Intraepiphyseal). Involvement of the epiphysis, with fracture separating the normal condylar anatomic relationships.

Malleolar. Involvement of the distal regions of the fibula and tibia. Because of anatomic differences, there are significant differences in the fracture patterns of the medial and lateral malleoli.

Type of fracture

This method of description must be based on appropriate roentgenograms of the injury. The basic types, shown in Figure 1-2, are as follows:

A, Longitudinal. The fracture line follows the longitudinal axis of the diaphysis.

B, Transverse. The fracture line is at a right angle to the longitudinal axis.

C, Oblique. The fracture line is variably angled relative to the longitudinal axis, usually about 30 to 45°.

D, Spiral. The fracture line is oblique and encircles a portion of the shaft.

E, Impacted. This is a compression type injury in which the cortical and trabecular bone of each side of the fracture are crushed.

F, Comminuted. The fracture line propagates in several directions, creating multiple, variable-sized fragments. This is an uncommon type of fracture in infants and young children, but becomes more common in adolescence, particularly in the tibia.

G, Bowing. The bone is deformed beyond its capacity for full elastic recoil into permanent plastic deformation (see Chap. 2). The younger the child, the more likely it is that this type of skeletal injury will occur. It is particularly common in the fibula and the ulna, both of which may bow while the paired bone (i.e., tibia or radius) fractures. This permanent deformation may limit the reducibility of the fractured bone of the pair.

H, Greenstick. This is a common injury in children. The bone is completely fractured, with a portion of the cortex and periosteum remaining intact on the compression side. Since this intact cortical bone is usually plastically deformed (bowed), an angular deformity is common, which necessitates conversion to a complete fracture by reversal of the deformity.

I, Torus. This is an impacted injury occurring in childhood. Because of the differing response of the metaphyseal bone to a compression load, the bone buckles, rather than fracturing completely, and a relatively stable injury is created. This type of fracture primarily affects developing metaphyseal bone.

Physical change

While the aforementioned terms have been primarily descriptive, the following terms describe conditions that are of practical importance clinically. These terms indicate not only the nature of the clinical problem, but also the general type of treatment that will be required:

Extent. The fracture may be incomplete, in which case some of the cortex is intact, or it may be complete, in which case the fracture line crosses the entire circumference. Further, the fracture line may be simple (a single fracture line), segmental (separate fracture lines isolating a segment of bone), or comminuted (multiple fracture lines with multiple fragments).

Relationship of Fracture Fragments to Each Other (Fig. 1-3). These relationships define a deformity as it exists during the roentgenographic evaluation. However, because of elastic recoil, especially in children, these relationships may not represent the full extent of deformity present at the time of

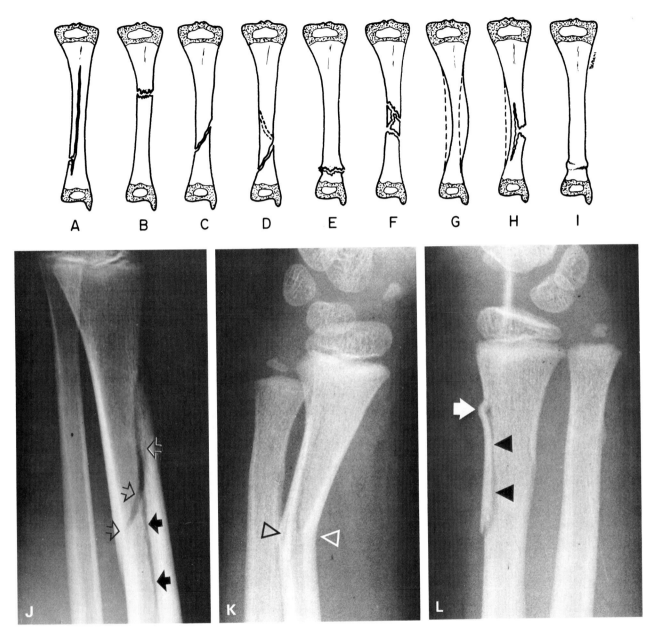

FIG. 1-2. *A–I,* Schematic of tibia from a three-year-old girl showing various types of fractures: *A,* longitudinal; *B,* transverse; *C,* oblique; *D,* spiral; *E,* impacted; *F,* comminuted; *G,* bowing (plastic deformation); *H,* greenstick; and *I,* torus. See text for details. *J–L,* Roentgenograms showing typical fracture patterns: *J,* Combination longitudinal (closed arrows) and spiral (open arrows) fracture. This is a pattern of "comminution" in the more resilient immature skeleton. *K,* Lateral view of radial and ulnar fractures in a six-year-old boy. The fracture of the radius shows an intact dorsal cortex (white arrow) and a fractured volar cortex (black arrow), a characteristic greenstick injury. The fracture is also angulated because of plastic deformation of the dorsal cortex. A significant ulnar injury is not evident in this projection. *L,* AP view of the same fracture. This view looks very different, with no angulation, a torus ulnar fracture, and a longitudinal fracture of the cortex (black arrows), which separates it from the endosteal bone and terminates in a torus injury (white arrow).

injury. The fracture may appear undisplaced or displaced, in which case the distal fragment is shifted away from its usual relationship to the proximal fragment. This shift may assume several types of deformation, which may be present singly or in any combination. These are: (1) sideways shift, (2) angulation, (3) overriding, (4) distraction, (5) impaction, and (6) rotation. The most important to correct are angular and ro-tational deformities. While the former will often correct spontaneously, though unpredictably, the latter will not cor-rect, and must be adequately treated initially, or they may require subsequent derotational osteotomy. As long as the reduction emphasizes restoration of longitudinal and rota-tional alignment, sideways shifts and overriding may be ac-ceptable.

Relationship of fracture to external environment. Basically, a fracture is either closed (skin covering intact) or open (compound). An open fracture, in which a break in the skin allows a communication between the fracture and the external environment, may be caused by a fracture fragment penetrating the skin from within or by an external object penetrating or rupturing the skin from without (Fig. 1-4). These fractures carry the serious risk of infection. Treatment of open fractures is covered in Chapter 6.

Periosteum

Throughout most of childhood, the periosteum is thicker, more osteogenic, and more resistant to disruption than similar tissue in the adult. Because of its contiguity with the underlying bone, it is bound to be injured when the bone fractures. However, since the periosteum separates more easily from the bone in children, it is less likely to rupture completely, and a significant portion of the periosteum often remains intact, usually on the concave (compression) side. This intact periosteal hinge may lessen the degree of displacement, and may be used to assist in the reduction, as it imparts a certain degree of intrinsic stability (Fig. 1-5). Since the periosteum allows some degree of continuity, the subperiosteal new bone quickly bridges the fracture, leading to more rapid stability.

Joint disruption

Even though the ligaments exhibit a greater degree of laxity than they do in an adult, the capsule and ligaments are relatively more resistant to stress than the contiguous bone and cartilage. Consequently, ligament rupture and joint dislocations are infrequent in children. When major ligaments attach directly into an epiphysis, growth plate fractures are the most common failure mode. Joint dislocations in the child most commonly affect the elbow and hip. Knee and proximal tibio-fibular dislocations are less common. The other joints only rarely are dislocated prior to skeletal maturity.

Basics of Treatment

Since children can respond significantly differently than adults, they may require different and often specialized treatment. They have smaller respiratory and circulatory volumes, proportionately greater surface area, unique responses to drugs, surgery, and stress, and frequent difficulty in localizing and communicating symptoms. The margin for error in the pediatric age group is greater, and the response of the injured child is different quantitatively and qualitatively, physiologically, and psychologically from an adult. Abdominal distention and diaphragmatic elevation from post-traumatic ileus pose a much greater threat to a child's chest volume and ventilation than to an adult's. Similarly, the loss of a small amount of blood is proportionately more significant because of the child's lessened overall blood volume. The relatively large surface area (compared to body weight) allows rapid heat and water losses.

Factors requiring special consideration in the treatment of trauma in children include size, heat loss, respiratory reserve, fluid, electrolyte and caloric balance, drug therapy, congenital defects, and lability of a child's response to stress. Because small children have limited reserves, and because their conditions may deteriorate rapidly, speedy transport to an intensive care unit capable of managing seriously injured children assumes increased importance.

The problems requiring immediate attention in the management of the severely injured child are not different from those of the adult. Establishment and maintenance of an adequate airway, control of hemorrhage, detection and evaluation of head injury, replacement of blood loss, treatment of shock, recognition of serious skeletal injuries, and the pre-

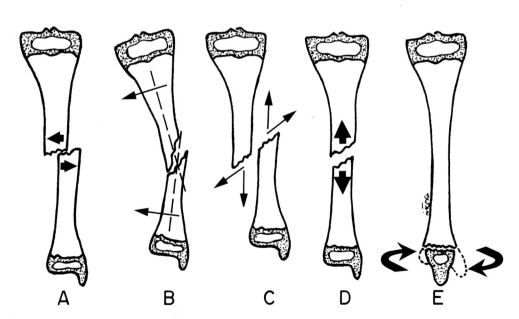

FIG. 1-3. Schematic of tibia from a six-year-old boy showing relationships of fracture fragments to each other. *A,* Translocation; *B,* angulation; *C,* overriding; *D,* distraction; and *E,* rotation in a distal epiphyseal fracture.

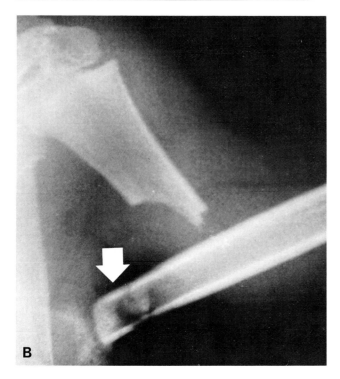

FIG. 1-4. *A,* Compound fracture of the proximal humeral metaphysis in a seven-year-old girl. *B,* Roentgenogram showing air in the soft tissues. The extracorporeal segment is indicated by the arrow.

vention of further injury through judicious and expeditious handling are of prime importance.

Head injury

Frequently, children injure their skull and brain, particularly if a vehicular accident is involved. The physician must be aware of some of the basic principles of treatment of head injuries. In children, fracture of the skull is generally less important than similar injury in an adult, unless the injury crosses a sinus or tears a nerve or blood vessel. The prime consideration is not the fracture, but damage to the brain. In the young infant with an elastic skull, much of the blow is absorbed by the osseous plates. Despite considerable depression of the bone, there may be little actual brain injury. Even the skull of a child with closing sutures and incomplete ossification absorbs a good deal of the blow in the osseous structure, transmitting less force to the brain itself. However, injuries to the tips of the frontal or temporal lobes may cause prolonged unconsciousness, extending for weeks or even months, but with complete recovery ultimately. Restlessness, agitation, and confusion may imply laceration and hemorrhage of the frontal and temporal lobes, whereas paralysis and deep shock suggest laceration of the brain itself. Extensor rigidity may be due to compression of portions of the temporal lobes, the cerebellum, or the brain stem. A child may fall and have momentary unconsciousness, followed by lucid intervals, then a second period of unconsciousness. This change in responsiveness suggests subdural or extradural hemorrhage. If the pupils are fixed, dilated, or contracted, or if the child cannot be aroused, serious brain damage must be suspected.

A child with head injury and multiple skeletal injuries should be permitted to assume a comfortable position in bed, unless he has a fracture of the cervical, dorsal, or lumbar spine, which would make such a posture inadvisable. Fractures of the extremities should be splinted for comfort, and treated more definitively several days later when the sensorium clears. Skeletal traction may be applied. Opiates, except codeine, should be avoided, and restlessness should be controlled by rectal aspirin or small doses of phenobarbitol. Lumbar puncture must be undertaken only after careful evaluation of the child, for elevation of pressure within the brain as a result of hemorrhage or soft tissue swelling may cause herniation through the tentorium, leading to further brain damage and death.

Sedation and anesthesia

Before satisfactory treatment can be provided, the fears and apprehensions of the child must be dispelled, and he must be given relief from pain. If reduction is necessary, proper levels of sedation and/or anesthesia are essential. In older, more cooperative children, one may infiltrate the fracture hematoma with a local anesthetic. Two points must be stressed in relation to this technique. First, unless the tip of the needle is in the fracture hematoma, as evidenced by aspiration of blood, anesthesia will be inadequate. Second, this must be done with rigidly sterile technique, after a thorough preparation of the skin with a bacteriocidal agent. Local infiltration may increase the risk of infection, with all its disastrous sequelae, because theoretically, local infiltration converts a closed fracture to an open fracture.

Intravenous regional block or even selective nerve blocks may be accomplished in the older child.[18] The use of intravenous diazepam must be undertaken with extreme caution. Appropriate anesthetic equipment must be available (mask, oxygen source, etc.). Further, one must remember that this latter drug is basically an amnesic, not an analgesic agent. The child will feel and react to pain, but will not remember doing so. The drug response may be delayed, and if the child must be sent to another area for postreduction films, he must be appropriately alert or a respiratory arrest may occur in an area where observation and resuscitation are difficult.

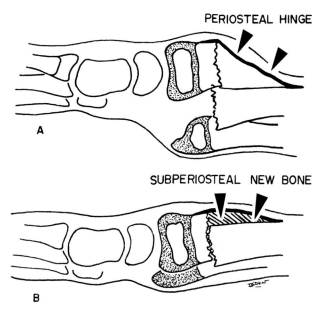

PERIOSTEAL HINGE

A

SUBPERIOSTEAL NEW BONE

B

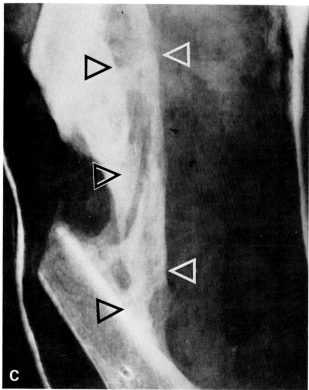

C

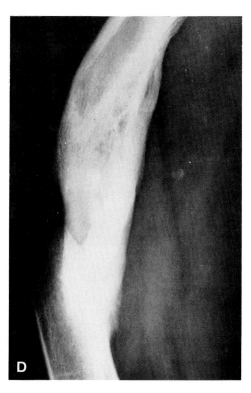

D

FIG. 1-5. Schematics of dorsally displaced, *A*, and reduced, *B*, distal radial metaphyseal fracture. The periosteum is connected to the proximal fragment by an intact dorsal periosteal hinge. When the fragment is reduced, this periosteal hinge prevents over-reduction. Fracture hematoma accumulates beneath the stripped periosteum and leads to extensive callus formation. *C*, Periosteal new bone (arrows) in the posteriorly displaced periosteal sleeve 11 weeks after multiple trauma to a 14-year-old boy. Following manipulation, the fragments were in better alignment, and a film taken a year later, *D*, shows extensive remodeling and incorporation of the subperiosteal new bone.

Basic guidelines

Since different treatment techniques can achieve similar desirable outcomes, making the appropriate decision becomes a focal step. An adequate approach should include: (1) a definition of the problem, particularly the complexity of the fracture and the extent of cartilaginous (i.e., radiologically invisible) involvement; (2) exploration of alternatives or options for treatment; and (3) choice of the best alternative for the given circumstances.

With few exceptions, fractures in children are due to relatively simple injuries, rather than the complex mechanical forces that usually cause adult skeletal injury. Accordingly, methods of treatment are generally simpler, with an appropriate emphasis on closed reduction.[1-3,10,12,15,17,19,20-43]

The basic principle of most fracture reductions, particularly in children, is reversal of the mechanism of injury. It is axiomatic that if a fracture is produced by an external force, it should be reduced by making the distal fragment retrace its steps. Reduction by this method, however, depends on the presence of the soft tissue linkage. Another axiom of fracture treatment is to align first the fragment you can con-

In any fracture requiring muscle relaxation for reduction, a general anesthetic is more useful. This is particularly true for supracondylar humeral and dorsally displaced distal radial fractures. If general anesthesia is used, the child often should be admitted to the hospital for overnight observation, not only of the recovery from anesthesia, but also of the peripheral neurovascular response to the injury, since displacement and manipulative reduction, which may be difficult, are certainly a further trauma to the already injured tissues.

trol more easily. Usually the distal fragment can be controlled more easily, and it should be aligned longitudinally with the displacing proximal fragment.[22] The proximal fragment adopts a position dictated by the pull of the muscles attached to it (e.g., the position of the proximal femur with a subtrochanteric fracture). Similarly, in considering fractures in the forearm, the key to reduction is the position of the proximal third. A proximal fragment may be strongly supinated by both the supinator and the biceps, and the forearm must be manipulated accordingly. A fracture at the lower levels adds the action of the pronator teres, placing the proximal fragment in a neutral position, between full supination and full pronation.

Closed reduction is adequate to maintain normal alignment of most fractures in children, because the plastic remodeling of their bones engenders good final anatomic and functional results. Certain fractures, especially those near the elbow, may require prompt open reduction. Much unnecessary surgery has been performed, sometimes resulting in permanent disability, because a physician failed to appreciate the recuperative powers of the child.

Rotational deformities *must* be corrected. Except in those fractures involving joints and epiphyses, absolute anatomic reduction of the bone fragments is not always necessary, and sometimes should be purposely avoided. Angulation in the middle third of long bones is unacceptable, and should be corrected, as close to normal as possible. In girls under 10 and boys under 12 years of age, angulation of fragments near the joints is more acceptable, if the angulation is less than 30°[36] and remains essentially within the plane of motion of the joint. Direct apposition of bone ends is less important. Bayonet or side-to-side apposition, especially in the midfemur, is desired, and leads to prompt, strong osseous union. After injury, the bones of children grow at an accelerated rate for six to eight months.[19] Overgrowth is a complication of the childhood fracture that may be avoided if general principles of treatment are understood well. The younger the child, the greater the amount of anticipated remodeling.

Open reduction

Fractures in growing bones are best treated by closed methods. However, there has been an increasing emphasis, particularly in the European literature, toward the use of open reduction techniques in children and adolescents.[7,44-67] Certainly, the trend in the treatment of skeletal injuries in adults is toward operative intervention, due in part to advances in the techniques of fixation and increases in understanding and control of wound infection. The drawbacks of conservative, closed treatment are the relatively long period of immobilization, the prolonged hospital stay, muscular atrophy, and joint stiffness,[67a] all of which may be lessened, if not eliminated, by active, aggressive, open treatment. In children, fractures usually unite more rapidly, restoration of function in muscles and joints is not as problematic, and even if perfect alignment cannot be achieved and maintained by external immobilization, remodeling and longitudinal growth certainly will correct lesser degrees of angular malunion.

Some authorities emphatically condemn internal fixation of almost all fractures in childhood, suggesting that all manners of dire consequences, such as nonunion, delayed union, altered growth, infection, and ugly scars, may arise.[19]

It is certainly correct that the thoughtless use of screws, plates, and pins should be strongly discouraged in treating fractures in children, but it is also certainly incorrect to deny their application altogether. A useful guide is that operative treatment of a child's fracture is indicated when conservative treatment cannot achieve an acceptable result. Open reduction and internal fixation are commonly indicated as an appropriate methodology in fracture-separations of the capitellum, trochlea, and the medial epicondylar regions.

Fractures of the shaft of the radius and ulna usually may be managed conservatively, but when there are exceptions, such as severely damaged bone and soft tissue, that may result in complete loss of intrinsic stability, open reduction should be considered, particularly for older children. Complete fractures of the shaft of the ulna with dislocation of the radial head provide a rare but important indication for surgery. Fractures of the neck of the femur are best treated by fixation with multiple pins.

At any age, complicating factors, such as burns, spasticity (developmental or due to head injury), or multiple osseous injuries, have an effect on treatment. For instance, fractures of the femoral shaft may be treated more satisfactorily by internal fixation in cases involving severe hypertonicity due to head trauma. The potential calamities of nonunion and infection should be avoidable through good surgical technique with, if necessary, prophylactic antibiotic treatment. Growth abnormalities should not occur if the vulnerability of the epiphyseal growth plates, both peripherally and centrally, is respected. Fixation plates should always be removed after satisfactory healing has occurred. External fixation devices, such as the Hoffman or Roger Anderson apparatuses, may also be applied effectively in children, as long as the growth regions are not violated by the pins.[68]

Many types of fractures of the physis and epiphysis are best treated by immediate open reduction and internal fixation. However, open reduction may be dangerous if performed several days or weeks after the epiphyseal injury, because the danger of damage to the growth plate increases. If displacement is still severe and open reduction is necessary, the surgeon can lessen, if not altogether avoid, these risks by handling the region around the growth plate with extreme care. The indications for surgical intervention in these injuries to the various chondro-osseous growth regions are discussed in detail in Chapter 4.

Immobilization

Because children devise ingenious methods for destroying immobilizing devices, casts or splints must be applied securely. As a general rule, one or more joints on either side of the fracture should be immobilized. Follow-up radiographs should be obtained at about five to ten days following reduction. During this time, the reactive swelling and pain are subsiding and the child's activity level is increasing, so the cast is somewhat likely to become loose and the reduction lost. This is also the period during which a loss of reduction or a less acceptable angulation is easiest to correct.

Rehabilitation

Physical therapy, in the otherwise normal child, has a negligible role in childhood fractures. Active use of the part by the child is almost constantly superior to the use of hand

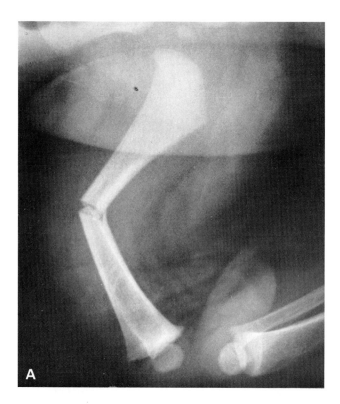

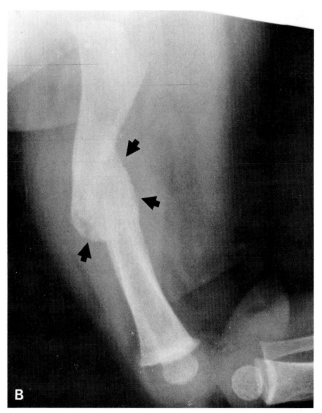

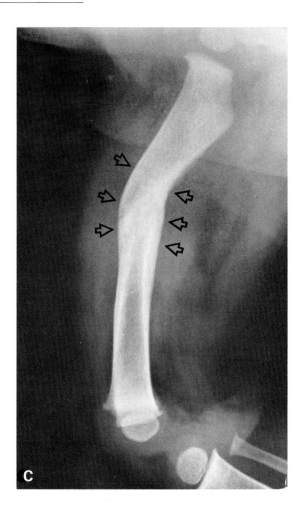

FIG. 1-6. *A,* Fracture of the midshaft of the femur in a seven-year-old girl. *B,* Callus formation (arrows) two months after the injury. This is limited by the relatively intact periosteal sleeve. *C,* Beginning remodeling and realignment (arrows) seven months after the original fracture.

massage and passive exercise by a therapist. Exaggerated limps gradually disappear and stiff elbows loosen, even if indifferent attention is paid to this phase of treatment. Normal use will invariably permit a return of motion. In the child, residual loss of motion probably is caused in part by anatomic malunion, and this will never be corrected by aggressive physical therapy. The therapist does play a major role, however, in rehabilitation of the child with a functional disability. In addition, children with neuromuscular disorders, such as cerebral palsy and myelomeningocele, sometimes require extensive physical therapy to attain pre-injury activity levels, since trauma may cause significant regression.

Remodeling

Children's fractures are easy to treat, but they do not always remodel, and results are sometimes bad. The remodeling capacity of a deformity caused by a fracture or epiphyseal injury is determined by three basic factors: (1) the age of the child; (2) the distance of the fracture from the end of the bone; and (3) the amount of angulation. The physiologic remodeling of a bone depends on periosteal appositional bone formation, resorption of some bone, and epiphyseal growth (Figs. 1-6, 1-7, and 1-8).

The criteria for an acceptable position of a fracture are based on the prediction of the remodeling in each case. For

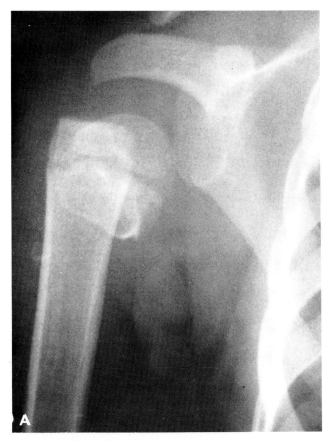

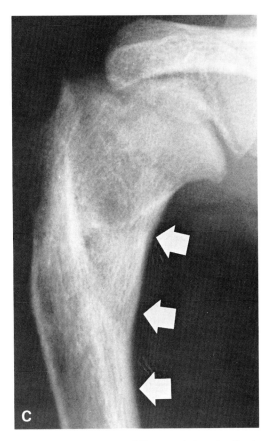

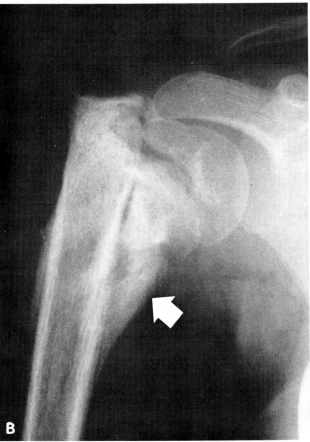

FIG. 1-7. Extensive remodeling and longitudinal overgrowth in a metaphyseal/epiphyseal fracture. *A,* Displaced fracture fragments in a three-year-old girl who fell two stories. She also sustained ipsilateral distal humeral and distal radial injuries. Repeated attempts at reduction under general anesthesia were unsuccessful. *B,* Four months after the injury, extensive subperiosteal new bone is evident, although it is still partially separated from the original cortex (arrow). *C,* Beginning realignment and correction of angular deformity nine months after the injury. The patient has full use of her glenohumeral joint. Extensive subperiosteal new bone has formed and is making a new medial cortex (arrows).

an axial deformity, remodeling capacity is better in the younger patient and for deformities nearer to the physis. For lateral displacement and shortening, remodeling capacity is good, but for rotational deformity, essentially *no* remodeling capacity exists. Additional factors that must be taken into account include: (1) skeletal age of the patient, which may differ from chronologic age; (2) the relative parts played by different epiphyseal plates in the longitudinal growth of a given bone; and (3) in some bones, stimulation of the longitudinal growth due to the fracture.

Remodeling is not something that can be totally or predictably relied upon, and every effort should be expended to attain as adequate an anatomic reduction as possible. Remodeling, in general, may be counted on in children with two or more years of growth ahead, in children with fractures near the ends of the bones, and in children with deformities in the plane of movement of the joint. Remodeling

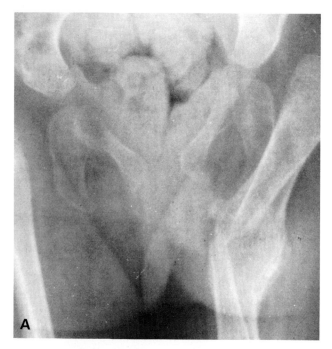

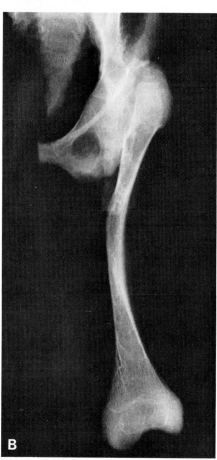

will not help with displaced intra-articular fractures, fractures toward the middle of the shaft of a bone (particularly when shortened, angulated, or rotated), displaced fractures where the axis of displacement is at a right angle to the normal plane of movement, and displaced fractures crossing the growth plate. Remodeling in the diaphysis is largely a process of rounding off of the bone, as evident in follow-up radiographs; it is *not* necessarily a true correction of longitudinal alignment. In fractures of the shaft, the periosteum drapes one side of the bone and this gradually fills in, whereas the other side is bare or denuded of normal periosteum and resorbs to some degree. This makes the fracture look less obvious when, in reality, there is minimal improvement in the alignment. Near an epiphysis, however, the growth plate can become realigned, and by realignment, assume a more normal growth pattern, by means of which metaphyseal remodeling will improve the overall appearance. In a supracondylar fracture that has healed with posterior displacement, the shaft acts as an anterior bone block and restricts movement until growth moves that portion away from the bone block. As the child grows, movement therefore increases. The wrist, one of the areas most commonly left to remodel, is an area in which malposition shows easily and readily, but also corrects relatively readily, although not necessarily rapidly.

Complications

The difference between complications in children and adults is mainly due to state of growth of the skeleton. Delayed union and nonunion are rare in children, because the healing capacity is better.[61,69] In Beekman's series of over 2000 fractures in children, there was not a single case of nonunion.[70] Post-traumatic joint stiffness is uncommon if the joint itself is not directly damaged. Mechanical hindrance due to malunion of the fracture rarely exists, sometimes being present in supracondylar fractures of the humerus. Refractures and myositis ossificans are less common in children than in adults, and there is a specific problem of injury to the growth area. All of these complications are discussed in detail in Chapters 4, 6, and 7.

References

1. Hanlon, C. R., and Estes, W. L.: Fractures in childhood—a statistical analysis. Am. J. Surg., *87:*312, 1954.
2. Surgical Staff of the Hospital for Sick Children: Care for the Injured Child. Baltimore, Williams & Wilkins, 1975.
3. Touloukian, R.: Pediatric Trauma. New York, John Wiley & Sons, 1978.
4. Giberson, R. G., and Ivins, J. C.: Fractures of the distal part of the forearm in childen: correction of deformity by growth. Minn. Med., *35:*744, 1952.
5. Stimson, B.: Growth correction of deformities resulting from fractures in childhood. Surg. Clin. North Am., *20:*589, 1940.
6. Bisgard, J. D.: Longitudinal overgrowth of long bones with special references to fractures. Surg. Gynecol. Obstet., *62:*823, 1936.
7. Iqbal, Q. M.: Long bone fractures among children in Malaysia. Int. Surg., *59:*410, 1974.
8. Dunn, P. M.: The Influence of the Intrauterine Environment in the Causation of Congenital Postural Deformities, with Special References to Congenital Dislocation of the Hip. M. D. Thesis, Cambridge University, 1969.

FIG. 1-8. *A,* Fracture of the left femur in a seven-month-old girl with arthrogryposis multiplex congenita. Note the bilateral hip dislocations. *B,* Postmortem roentgenogram at 15 months of age showing some remodeling and minimal remaining callus.

9. Dunn, P. M.: Perinatal observations on the etiology of congenital dislocation of the hip. Clin. Orthop., *119*:11, 1976.

10. Truesdell, E.: Birth Fractures and Epiphyseal Dislocations. New York, Paul Hoeber, 1917.

11. Reed, M. H.: Fractures and dislocations of the extremities in children. J. Trauma, *17*:351, 1977.

12. Ogden, J. A.: Injury to the Immature Skeleton. *In* Pediatric Trauma. Edited by R. Touloukian. New York, John Wiley & Sons, 1978.

13. Adams, J. G.: Bone injuries in very young athletes. Clin. Orthop., *58*:129, 1968.

14. Roser, L. A., and Clawson, D. K.: Football injuries in the very young athlete. Clin. Orthop., *69*:219, 1970.

15. Schenk, R. K.: Besonderheiten des Kindlichen Skelets im Hinblick auf die Frakturheilung. Langebecks Arch. Chir., *342*:269, 1976.

16. Alexander, C. J.: Effect of growth rate on the strength of the growth plate shaft junction. Skeletal Radiol., *1*:67, 1976.

17. Hartman, J. T.: Fracture Management: A Practical Approach. Philadelphia, Lea & Febiger, 1978.

18. Carrel, E. D., and Eyring, E. J.: Intravenous regional anesthesia for childhood fractures. J. Trauma, *11*:301, 1971.

19. Blount, W.: Fractures in Children. Baltimore, Williams & Wilkins, 1955.

20. Devas, M.: Stress Fractures. London, Churchill Livingstone, 1975.

21. Judet, R., Judet, J., and LaGrange, J.: Fractures des Membres chez l'Enfant. Paris, Libraire Maloine, 1958.

22. Ogden, J. A., and Southwick, W. O.: Adequate reduction of fractures and dislocations. Radiol. Clin. North Am., *11*:667, 1973.

23. Poland, J.: Traumatic Separation of the Epiphyses. London, Smith, Elder, and Co., 1898.

24. Pollen, A.: Fractures and Dislocations in Children. Baltimore, Williams & Wilkins, 1973.

25. Rang, M.: The Growth Plate and Its Disorders. Baltimore, Williams & Wilkins, 1969.

26. Rang, M.: Children's Fractures. Philadelphia, J. B. Lippincott, 1974.

27. Rettig, H.: Frakturen im Kindesalter. Munich, Verlag-Bergmann, 1957.

28. Rockwood, C. A., Jr., and Green, D. P.: Fractures. Philadelphia, J. B. Lippincott, 1975.

29. Schultz, R. J.: The Language of Fractures. Baltimore, Williams & Wilkins, 1972.

30. Sharrard, W. J. W.: Paediatric Orthopaedics and Fractures. Oxford, Blackwell, 1971.

31. Tachdjian, M.: Pediatric Orthopaedics. Philadelphia, W. B. Saunders, 1972.

32. Ecke, H.: Klinische und rontgenologische Diagnostik der Kindlichen Fraktur. Langenbecks Arch. Chir., *342*:277, 1976.

33. Ferguson, A. B., Jr.: Treatment of common childhood fractures. Am. J. Surg., *101*:684, 1961.

34. Godfrey, J. D.: Trauma in children. J. Bone Joint Surg., *46-A*:422, 1964.

35. Mays, J., and Neufeld, A. J.: Skeletal traction methods. Clin. Orthop., *102*:144, 1974.

36. Nonnemann, H. C.: Grenzen der Spontankorrektur fehlgeheilter Frakturen bei Jugendlichen. Langenbecks Arch. Chir., *324*:78, 1969.

37. Rang, M. C., and Willis, R. B.: Fractures and sprains. Pediatr. Clin. North Am., *24*:749, 1977.

38. Ryöppy, S.: Injuries of the growing skeleton. Ann. Chir. Gynaecol. Fenn., *61*:3, 1972.

39. Streicher, H. J.: Bericht uber 1500 kindliche und jugendliche frakturen. Hefte Unfallchir., *35*:129, 1956.

40. Wade, P. A.: Fractures in children. Am. J. Surg., *107*:531, 1964.

41. Weber, B. G.: Das Besondere bei der Behandlung der Frakturen im Kindesalter. Mschr. Unfallheilk., *78*:193, 1975.

42. Wilson, J. C., Jr.: Fractures and dislocations in childhood. Pediatr. Clin. North Am., *14*:659, 1967.

43. Zacher, D., Koob, E., and Schlegel, K. F.: Orthopadische Aspekte der Traumatologie im Kindesalter. Z. Kinderchir. Suppl. *11*:659, 1972.

44. Weber, B. G., Brunner, C., and Freuler, F.: Die Frakturenbehandlung bei Kindern und Jugendlichen. Berlin, Springer-Verlag, 1978.

45. Baijal, E.: Instances in which intramedullary nailing of a child's fracture is justifiable. Injury, *7*:181, 1976.

46. Debrunner, A.: Frakturen im Kindesalter. Konservative oder operative therapie. Zentralbl. Chir., *99*:641, 1974.

47. Ecke, H.: Traumatische Veranderungen an der Wachstumsfuge, Ihre Behandlung und Prognose. Z. Kinderchir., Suppl. *11*:699, 1972.

48. Editorial: Internal fixation for fractures in childhood. Br. Med. J., *1*:1301, 1976.

49. Ehalt, W.: Verletzungen bei Kindern und Jugendlichen. Stuttgart, Enke, 1961.

50. Eilenberger, S., and Feneis, J.: Der Versorgung der tibial spiral fraktur im Kindes—und Jugendalter durch Zugschraubenosteosynthese. Chir. Praxis, *17*:107, 1973.

51. Hackenbroch, M. H.: Die Indikation zur Osteosynthese bei der frischen Kindlichen Verletzung. Z. Kinderchir., Suppl. *11*:671, 1972.

52. Hamacher, O., and Pingel, P.: Die Verletzungen der Wachstumsfugen. Z. Allgemeinmed., *47*:176, 1971.

53. Hecker, W. C., and Daum, R.: Grundsatzliche Indikationsfehler bei Kindlichen Frakturen. Langenbecks Arch. Chir., *327*:864, 1970.

54. Hertel, P., and Klapp. F.: Epiphysenfugen verletzungen im Wachstumsalter. Mschr. Unfallheilk., *78*:206, 1975.

55. Jungbluth, K. H., Daum, R., and Metzger, E.: Schenkelhalsfrakturen im Kindesalter. Z. Kinderchir., *6*:392, 1968.

56. Kehr, H., and Hierholzer, G.: Technik der Osteosynthese bei Kindlichen Frakturen. Mschr. Unfallheilk., *78*:199, 1975.

57. Kumer, E. H., and Weyand, F.: Indikation zur operativen Behandlung Kindlicher Frakturen. Aktvel. Traumatol., *1*:63, 1971.

58. Muller, M. E., and Ganz, R.: Luxationen und Frakturen unterer Gliedmassen und Becken. In Unfallverletzungen bei Kindern. Edited by J. Rehn. Berlin, Springer-Verlag, 1974.

59. Probst, J.: Nachbehandlung und Begutachtung Kindlicher Frakturen. Langenbecks Arch. Chir., *342*:319, 1976.

60. Schweizer, P.: Indikationen zur operativen Knochenbruch behandlung in Kindesalter. Med. Welt, *27*:187, 1976.

61. Tscherne, H., and Suren, E. G.: Fehlstellungen, Wachstumsstorungen und Pseudarthrosen nach kindlichen frakturen. Langenbecks Arch. Chir., *342*:299, 1976.

62. Vinz, H.: Die Marknagelung kindlicher Oberschenkelsshaftfrakturen. Zentralbl. Chir., *97*:90, 1972.

63. Vinz, H.: Operative Behandlung von Knochenbruchen bei Kindern. Zentralbl. Chir., *97*:1377, 1972.

64. Vinz, H. and Grobler, B.: Osteosynthese in Kindesalter—biomechanische Aspekte und alter physiologische Osteosyntheseverfahren. Zentralbl. Chir., *100*:455, 1975.

65. Weber, B. G.: Indikationen zur operativen Frakturbehandlung bei Kindern. Chirurg., *38*:441, 1967.

66. Weller, S.: Spezielle Gesichtspunkte bei der Behandlung Kindlicher Frakturen. Z. Kinderchir., Suppl. *11*:655, 1972.

67. Witt, A. N., and Walcher, K.: Korrekturoperationen nach Kindlichen Verletzungen. Z. Kinderchir., Suppl. *11*:841, 1972.

67a. Odell, R. T., and Leydig, S. M.: The conservative treatment of fractures in children. Surg. Gynecol. Obstet., *92*:69, 1951.

68. Lehmann, L., and Gerbert, W. N.: Die Anwendung des Fixateur externe in der Behandlung Kindlicher schaft Frakturen. Mschr. Unfallheilk., *78*:401, 1975.

69. Kuntscher. G.: Die Behandlung der Pseudarthrose im Kindesalter. Langenbecks Arch. Chir., *304*:610, 1963.

70. Beekman, F., and Sullivan, J.: Some observations of fractures of long bones in the child. Am. J. Surg., *51*:722, 1941.

2

Anatomy and Physiology of Skeletal Development

Compared to the relatively static mature bone of adults, there are major, variable, dynamic, structural and functional differences, both physiologic and biomechanical, in immature, developing bones that render them susceptible to different patterns of fracture. Further, the types of fracture patterns within a given bone also demonstrate temporal variations that can be correlated closely with the progressive anatomic changes that affect the epiphysis, physis, metaphysis, and diaphysis at macroscopic and microscopic levels. The key to understanding children's musculoskeletal injuries lies initially in an adequate appreciation of the anatomy and physiology of the multiple chondro-osseous components of the developing skeleton, and particularly, of how these components change with time as growth progresses from the extremely biologically resilient skeleton of the newborn to the much more rigid skeleton of the adult.

Bone Development

All skeletal structural elements initially form as mesenchymal cellular condensations during the embryonic period.[1-8] Some of these cellular groupings modulate to fibrocellular tissue and ossify directly, forming membrane-derived, or intramembranous, bone. This is characteristic of all cranial and most facial bones, as well as of the initial formation of the clavicle. In contrast, the appendicular and axial skeletal elements are derived from the initial transformation of the mesenchymal model to a cartilaginous model, and its subsequent transformation to an ossified structure by two discrete processes: (1) the formation of an osseous collar around the midshaft of the cartilaginous anlage, with associated vascular invasion to form the primary ossification center; and (2) a later, usually postnatal, vascular-mediated, osseous transformation of the chondroepiphysis to form the secondary epiphyseal ossification center at each end. This progressive, integrated replacement of the preexistent and continuously dynamic cartilage model by osseous tissue is termed endochondral ossification.

These two basic types of osseous tissue formation—intramembranous and endochondral—refer *only* to the primary pattern of development of each individual structural unit, whether femur or phalanx. Subsequent growth of any particular unit after this initial differentiation may involve discrete, juxtaposed, or interspersed areas of both basic patterns within the same bone. Endochondral-derived bones generally undergo intramembranous ossification by appositional bone growth from the periosteum. Similarly, membrane-derived bone may undergo subsequent growth and elongation by a modified endochondral process (e.g., the clavicle). These two processes—temporal changes and biologic response differences (whether normal or abnormal)—are essential to an adequate comprehension of general and specific skeletal development, and are presented in more detail in the ensuing sections.

Intramembranous bone formation

Primary intramembranous bone formation occurs in the cranial and facial bones, and in part, in the clavicle and mandible (which also subsequently develop epiphyses and physes), while the endochondrally-derived axial and appendicular bones become involved in membranous bone formation secondarily. The membrane-derived bones are formed from condensations of mesenchymal tissue that are structural analogues of the presumptive bone, similar to the cartilaginous precursor of endochondral bone. At a presumably genetically-determined site of presumptive primary ossification, small groups of cells differentiate and aggregate in short, randomly-directed strands. These cells elaborate a fibrous intercellular matrix that is quickly calcified and subsequently ossified to form the primary trabeculae. Ossification then rapidly spreads out from the primary ossification center so that relatively large areas are ossified. The trabecular orientation is a direct response to mechanical stresses, internal and external, to the developing fetus.

The clavicle is the first fetal bone to ossify (intramembranous), followed rapidly by the mandible. Both bones eventually form hyaline cartilage and convert, in part, to endochondral ossification, but only after primary intramembranous ossification is well under way. This subsequently-appearing cartilage is sometimes referred to as secondary cartilage.

Virtually all of the axial and appendicular skeletal elements are also involved in intramembranous ossification. The diaphyseal cortex of developing tubular bone is progressively modified by specialized mesenchyme which differentiates into the periosteum and perichondrium, and invests the chondro-osseous model. This peripheral periosteal process of membrane-derived bone is quite dramatic in disease states such as childhood osteomyelitis, in which the entire original diaphysis may become sequestrated, with the elevated periosteum forming a totally new shaft (involucrum) that is entirely membranous, rather than endochondral, in origin (Fig. 2-1). The replacement process also may be seen when portions of the diaphysis are removed for use as bone graft (Fig. 2-2). This membranous ossification process is an essential step in physiologic fracture healing, especially in children.

Endochondral ossification

Endochondral bone formation is the primary osseous formation process of axial and appendicular skeletal components, and may recur in selected areas of established bone in the normal process of fracture repair (i.e., formation and maturation of callus). Succinctly, this type of bone formation is the continuous replacement of preexistent cartilaginous tissue by osseous tissue. The overall process is a continuum, but it may be divided arbitrarily into a number of steps (Fig. 2-3):
—the formation of a highly cellular mesenchymal condensation, the basic anlage.
—increased extracellular matrix formation to create pre-cartilage.
—extensive ground substance elaboration to form the chondral anlage, with selective hypertrophy of the central chondrocytes.
—further intercellular, interstitial, and extracellular enlarge-

ment of the entire chondral anlage, with selective hypertrophy of the central chondrocytes.
—formation of a trabeculated primary bone collar, associated periosteum, and rudimentary vascular supply at the presumptive diaphysis.
—increased intracellular and extracellular biochemical activity, especially in the hypertrophied central chondrocytes, leading to calcification of the cartilage.
—penetration of the primary osseous collar by the fibrovascular irruption tissue, part of which will become the nutrient artery.
—central replacement of cartilage by bone, initially around the area of vascular invasion, followed by extension of the process (including the bone collar) longitudinally toward each end of the anlage. This forms the primary ossification center, which eventually will become the diaphysis and metaphyses.
—establishment of an orderly arrangement in the ossification/growth mechanism (physis), and an actively remodeling metaphysis.

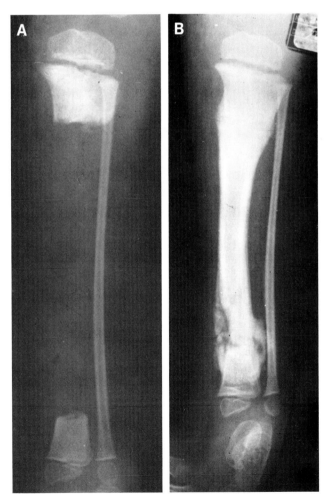

FIG. 2-2. *A,* The subperiosteal tibial diaphysis has been removed completely for use as a bone graft in a three-year-old child (intraoperative film). *B,* Six months later, extensive membranous new bone has filled in the periosteal sleeve.

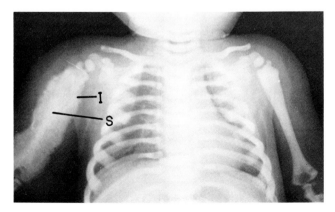

FIG. 2-1. Osteomyelitis involving the right humerus of a ten-month-old child. Extensive subperiosteal (membranous) reactive bone, the involucrum (I), surrounds the minimally visible endochondral shaft (S), comprising both metaphyses and diaphysis. This bone, if totally deprived of blood supply, may form a sequestrum.

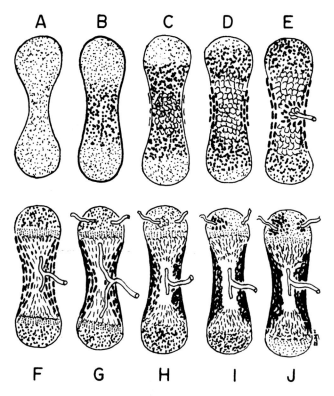

FIG. 2-3. Schematic of endochondral bone formation. *A,* Mesenchymal anlage; *B,* central chondrification; *C,* central cartilage hypertrophy; *D,* formation of primary bone collar; *E,* vascular irruption to form the primary ossification center; *F,* development of contiguous endochondral and membranous ossification, and well-established physeal cytoarchitecture; *G,* cartilage canal formation within the epiphysis; *H,* diaphyseal remodeling and cavitation, and formation of epiphyseal preossification center; *I,* formation of secondary ossification center; *J,* formation of accessory epiphyseal ossification centers (e.g., greater trochanter). See text for details.

—vascularization of the chondroepiphyses by the cartilage canal system.

—appearance of one or more secondary ossification centers within the chondroepiphysis. This is primarily a postnatal process.

On cursory examination, nontubular bones seem to have different patterns of endochondral ossification than the major and smaller tubular (longitudinal) bones. However, when schematically analyzed, it becomes evident that each of these bones is undergoing the same basic endochondral ossification process, albeit reorganized to conform to the specific contours of each particular bone. End-plate ossification of the vertebral centrum in adolescence closely resembles the process in a tubular bone, while the neural arch grows principally by periosteal appositional growth. However, there are selected areas at each end of the neural arch that function as growth regions. These are the spinous processes and the neurocentral synchondroses (Fig. 2-4). The scapula also can be conceived of as undergoing functionally and morphologically rearranged endochondral ossification along the vertebral border, the acromion, the coracoid, and

the glenoid. The calcaneus forms a posterior chondroepiphysis with a secondary ossification center, creating a situation similar to an end of a tubular bone.

Anatomic Regions

The major long bones of the child may be divided into several distinct anatomic areas—the diaphysis, metaphysis, epiphysis, and physis (Fig. 2-5). Each of these regions is prone to certain kinds of injuries, with this intrinsic susceptibility changing as the physiologic and biomechanical capacities of each region change in accord with postnatal developmental modifications at both the macroscopic and the microscopic levels.[9-12] These four regions originate, and subsequently become modified, as a result of the basic endochondral ossification process, but they are supplemented by intramembranous bone formation along the shaft, especially along the diaphysis.

Diaphysis

The diaphysis comprises the major portion of the cortical osseous tissue of each long bone. It is primarily a product of periosteal, intramembranous osseous tissue apposition on the original endochondral model, as well as of endosteal remodeling and bone formation (see Fig. 2-5). This leads to the progressive replacement of the primary ossification center and spongiosa, the latter first being replaced by secondary spongiosa in the metaphyseal region. These two processes also eventually replace most of the secondary spongiosa of the metaphysis.

At birth, the diaphysis is comprised principally of fetal, woven bone, which is characteristically lacking in Haversian systems. The neonatal femoral diaphysis is apparently the only area exhibiting any evidence of a prenatal change from this fetal osseous state to more mature (lamellar) bone with osteon systems. Periosteal-mediated, intramembranous, appositional bone formation with concomitant endosteal remodeling is characteristic of the postnatal period. This leads to enlargement of the overall diameter of the shaft, variably increased width of the diaphyseal cortices, and formation of the marrow cavity. Mature, lamellar bone with

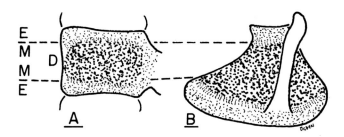

FIG. 2-4. Schematic of modified endochondral bone formation in nontubular bones. *A,* Vertebral body (sagittal section); *B,* scapular blade (spine and acromion are white). Note diaphyseal analogue (D), epiphyseal analogue (E), and metaphyseal analogue (M). Subperiosteal membranous bone plays a much less important role in the development of these bones.

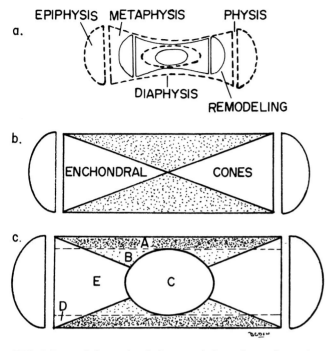

FIG. 2-5. *a,* Schematic of characteristic regions of growing tubular bone. *b,* The metaphyseal/diaphyseal unit of osseous tissue is derived from two basic patterns of bone formation. The endochondral bone may be thought of as two conical structures, apex-to-apex, capable of enlarging through physeal growth at the bases of the cones. Each cone may develop at a relatively independent rate, although both are integrated through the periosteal continuity. Membranous bone (stippled regions) progressively fills the "gap" between the conical, endochondral growth regions. *c,* As the shaft progressively enlarges longitudinally and latitudinally by the aforementioned basic bone formation patterns, remodeling will change both the macroscopic and the microscopic appearances. Note: (A) the formation of dense cortical (lamellar) bone by osteon maturation; (B) the formation of trabecular endosteal bone (of membranous derivation); (C) the formation of a fatty/erythropoietic marrow cavity essentially devoid of bone; (D) the peripheral metaphyseal cortex and remodeling; (E) the formation of trabecular endosteal bone (of endochondral derivation).

intrinsic, but constantly remodeling, osteonal patterns progressively becomes the dominant feature. This early bone is extremely vascular. When analyzed in cross section, it appears much less dense than the maturing bone of older children, adolescents, and adults (Fig. 2-6). Subsequent growth leads to increasingly complex Haversian (osteonal) systems and to the elaboration of increasing amounts of intercellular matrix, decreasing the relative porosity of the cross section, and increasing its hardness. In comparison to mature (adult) bone, the periosteum is much thicker, more vascular, more loosely attached to the underlying diaphysis, and capable of more rapid callus formation in response to similar injury (Fig. 2-7). The periosteum, rather than the bone per se, serves as the origin for most muscle fibers along the metaphysis and diaphysis. This allows growth of bone and muscle

units to be coordinated, a factor that would be impossible if all muscles attached directly into the developing bone. Exceptions include attachments of some adductor fibers into the medial distal femoral metaphysis. This attachment probably explains the irregularity of ossification often seen in this area, and often misdiagnosed as a neoplastic or traumatic response (see Chap. 17).

Metaphysis

The metaphyses are variably contoured flares at each end of the diaphysis. Their major characteristics are decreased thickness of the cortical bone and increased amounts of trabecular bone comprising both primary and secondary spongiosa. Extensive remodeling centrally and peripherally causes the primary spongiosa, which is a direct result of endochondral ossification, to be transformed into more mature secondary spongiosa, a process that involves osteolytic, osteoclastic, and osteoblastic activity. The metaphyses exhibit

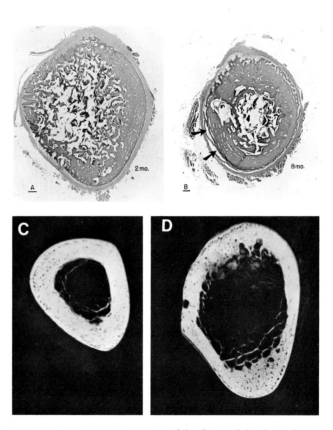

FIG. 2-6. Transverse sections of the femoral diaphyseal cortex at *A,* two months and *B,* eight months. The pattern of bone architecture varies considerably around the circumference, a factor that must be considered in doing biomechanical tests on developing bone. The initial cortical bone is extremely porous, but rapidly becomes less so as osteon formation commences. The laminar pattern of new bone formation is readily evident in *B* (arrows). *C,* Slab roentgenogram of midsection diaphysis. *D,* Slab roentgenogram of proximal shaft just below the tibial tuberosity. The tibial midshaft cortical bone exhibits a greater cross-sectional density (C). The tibial specimens are from a nine-year-old child.

considerable bone turnover compared to other regions of the bone. These active processes normally cause increased uptake of 99m-technetium-polyphosphate in a bone scan.

Like the diaphysis, the metaphyseal cortex also changes with time, although not as dramatically. Relative to the confluent diaphysis, the metaphyseal cortex is thinner and has greater porosity (trabecular fenestration). The metaphyseal cortical fenestration contrasts sharply with the thicker cortex of the diaphysis (Fig. 2-8). These cortical fenestrations contain fibrovascular soft tissue elements that connect the metaphyseal marrow spaces with the subperiosteal regions. The metaphyseal cortex exhibits greater fenestration near the physis than the diaphysis, with which it gradually blends as an increasingly thicker, denser type of bone. As temporal longitudinal growth continues, cortical fenestration becomes less frequent, and the overall width of the cortex increases, creating a greater morphologic transition between the juxtaphyseal and the juxtadiaphyseal cortices. The metaphyseal region does not develop significant Haversian systems until skeletal maturity approaches. These microscopic anatomic changes appear to be directly correlated with changing patterns of fracture occurrence, and they undoubtedly influence the possibility of torus (buckle) fractures, as opposed to complete metaphyseal or epiphyseal/physeal fractures.

Another microscopic anatomic variation in the metaphysis may be seen at the juxtaposition of primary spongiosa with the hypertrophic region of the physis. In most rapidly growing bones, the trabeculae tend to be oriented longitudinally. However, in shorter growing bones, such as the metacarpals and phalanges, the trabecular origin is more predominantly horizontal (see Fig. 2-8). As growth decelerates in adolescence, a similar, more horizontal orientation may be seen even in the major long bones. Undoubtedly, these variations in trabecular orientation affect the responsiveness of various metaphyseal regions to abnormal stress, and favor certain fracture modes (see Chap. 4).

While the periosteum is attached relatively loosely to the diaphysis, it becomes increasingly more firmly fixed in the metaphysis. Undoubtedly, this is due to the continuity of fibrous tissue through the metaphyseal fenestrations (Fig. 2-9). Since most experimenters have found it necessary to sever, completely and circumferentially, the metaphyseal periosteum to duplicate epiphyseal fractures, the implication is that this intermingling of endosteal and interosseous fibrous tissues with the periosteal tissue imparts considerable, additional biomechanical strength to the region. The periosteum subsequently attaches densely into the peripheral physis, blending into the zone of Ranvier, as well as the epiphyseal perichondrium. The metaphyseal cortex extends to the physis, and continues as the osseous ring of Lacroix (see Fig. 2-9).

As in the diaphysis, there are no significant direct muscle attachments into the metaphyseal bone. Instead, muscle fibers blend primarily into the periosteum.

Epiphysis

At birth, with the exception of the distal femur, each epiphysis is a completely cartilaginous structure at both ends of each long bone. This includes the small longitudinal bones of the hands and feet. This cartilaginous structure will be referred to as the chondroepiphysis, while the corresponding ossifying structure will be termed the chondro-osseous epiphysis, or simply, epiphysis. At a time characteristic for each of these chondroepiphyses, a secondary center of ossification gradually enlarges until virtually the entire cartilage model has been replaced by bone at skeletal maturity; only articular cartilage remains. As the ossification center expands, it undergoes structural modifications. Particularly, the region adjacent to the physis begins to form a distinct subchondral plate parallel to the metaphysis, creating the roentgenographically characteristic physeal line (Fig. 2-10). Certain chondroepiphyses exhibit variations in the appearance of the ossification centers, a factor that must be considered to appropriately diagnose fractures of these regions. In particular, the distal humerus shows an extremely variable pattern of ossification, beginning with a small, solitary center of ossification within the capitellum during the first year, subsequently developing multiple ossification foci in the trochlea at approximately seven to eight years, and eventually developing a focus in the lateral epicondyle during adolescence. The appearance and progressive development of the secondary center of ossification within the chondroepiphysis undoubtedly plays a role in the susceptibility of this region, as well as adjacent physeal and metaphyseal regions, to certain fracture patterns. As the osseous tissue expands, the ossification center imparts increasing rigidity to the more resilient epiphyseal cartilage.

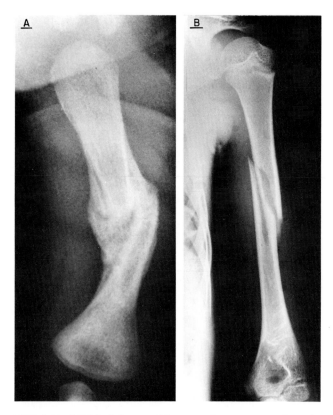

FIG. 2-7. Midshaft humeral fractures in a neonate, *A*, and a nine-year-old child, *B*, showing a significant difference in the rates of subperiosteal and callus ossification four weeks following fracture. The injury is almost completely healed in the neonate, whereas little roentgenographically-evident reparative bone appears in the older child.

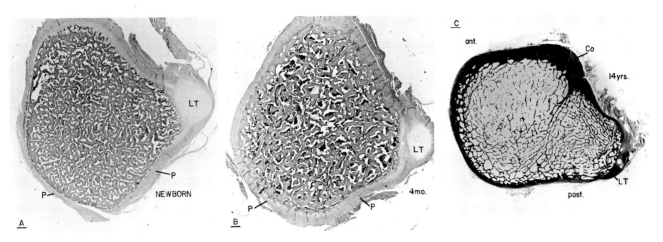

FIG. 2-8. Transverse sections of the proximal femur at the level of the lesser trochanter (LT) in, *A*, a newborn, *B*, a 4-month-old child, and, *C*, a 14-year-old child. The thick periosteum (P) is quite evident in *A* and *B*. Even in the 4-month-old child, there has been considerable thickening and remodeling of the central trabeculae, and the peripheral trabecular density has increased to create a more mature cortex. Near skeletal maturation, dense cortical (Co) bone with established osteons is present, although this varies considerably from anterior (ant.) to posterior (post.) surfaces.

When the hyaline cartilage of the chondroepiphysis first forms, there are no demonstrable differences between the cells of the joint surface and the remainder of the hyaline cartilage. However, at some point, a finite cell population becomes stabilized and functionally different from the remaining epiphyseal cartilage. McKibbin has described an interesting experiment which established that these two cartilage types are different physiologically and, by implication, biochemically.[13] If a core of articular and hyaline cartilage is removed, turned 180°, and reinserted, the transposed hyaline cartilage eventually forms bone at the joint surface, whereas the transposed articular cartilage remains completely cartilaginous and becomes surrounded by the enlarging secondary ossification center. Under normal circumstances, articular cartilage does not appear to be capable of ossification. As skeletal maturity is reached, a tidemark develops as a demarcation between the articular and epiphyseal hyaline cartilages.

An important aspect of the aforementioned experiment is an explanation of nonunion of certain fractures, such as those of the lateral condyle of the distal humerus, in which the fragment may be rotated up to 180°, causing the articular surface to lie against metaphyseal and epiphyseal bone. Union will not occur in such a situation, because the articular surface is incapable of osteogenic response, a most essential component of bone healing. This type of nonunion has been attributed incorrectly to the fragment being surrounded by synovial fluid, which alledgedly prevents union chemically. However, this same fluid does not seem to prevent spontaneous union of osteochondral defects and other types of epiphyseal fractures in which no significant displacement occurs. In these instances, both apposed surfaces are capable of an appropriate conjoint osteogenic and/or chondrogenic healing response.

Physis

The growth plate, or physis, is the essential mechanism of endochondral ossification prenatally and postnatally.[14-17] For most physes, the basic structural contour remains similar throughout development. For a few, there are major changes in contour. This is particularly true in the proximal humerus and proximal femur (Fig. 2-11), the physes of which change from initially transverse to highly contoured structures as they grow. The contour of the distal femur also changes from transverse to binodal (see Chap. 17). Because the contours are undergoing constant change, fracture pattern susceptibilities also change.

Since the physeal cartilage always remains radiolucent, except in the final stages of physiologic epiphysiodesis, the roentgenographic appearance of the physis can only be inferred from the metaphyseal contour, which follows the physeal contour closely. The changing size of the epiphyseal ossification center more effectively demarcates the physeal contour on the epiphyseal (germinal layer) side. As the secondary center of ossification enlarges and approaches the physis, the originally spherical shape of the ossification center begins to flatten and gradually develops a contour that parallels the metaphyseal contour. Similar contouring also occurs as the ossification center approaches the lateral and subarticular regions of the epiphysis. The region of the ossification center juxtaposed to the physis forms a discrete subchondral bone plate through which the epiphyseal vessels penetrate to reach the physis.

From a macroscopic viewpoint, there are two basic types of growth plates—discoid and spherical. Most primary growth plates of the major long bones are discoid. They are characterized by a relatively planar area of rapidly differentiating and maturing cartilage that grades imperceptibly from the epiphyseal hyaline cartilage. The primary function of the physis is to cause rapid longitudinal growth. Initially, most discoid physes are transversely planar, but as they respond to subsequent growth and biomechanical stresses, they assume characteristic contouring, while retaining their basic planar nature. Additionally, small interdigitations of cartilage extend into the metaphyseal bone; these are termed mammillary processes (Fig. 2-12). Contouring and mammillary processes appear to contribute to the intrinsic stability the physis has against shearing forces. Discoid (planar) growth plates also may be found between the metaphysis and an apophysis, which may be defined as an epiphyseal/physeal extension subjected primarily to tensile, rather than to compressive forces. The tibial tuberosity is such a structure. Instead of the normal columnar cytoarchitecture (Fig. 2-13), tension-responsive structures are characterized by variable amounts of fibrocartilage (Fig. 2-14) that apparently represent a microscopic structural adaptation of the physis to the high tensile forces imparted by the quadriceps mechanism.[18]

In the short, tubular bones (metacarpals, metatarsals, phalanges), two discoid physes and contiguous chondroepiphyses initially form, but with subsequent skeletal growth, only one end maintains a true chondroepiphysis and physis, and these become the primary mechanism for longitudinal

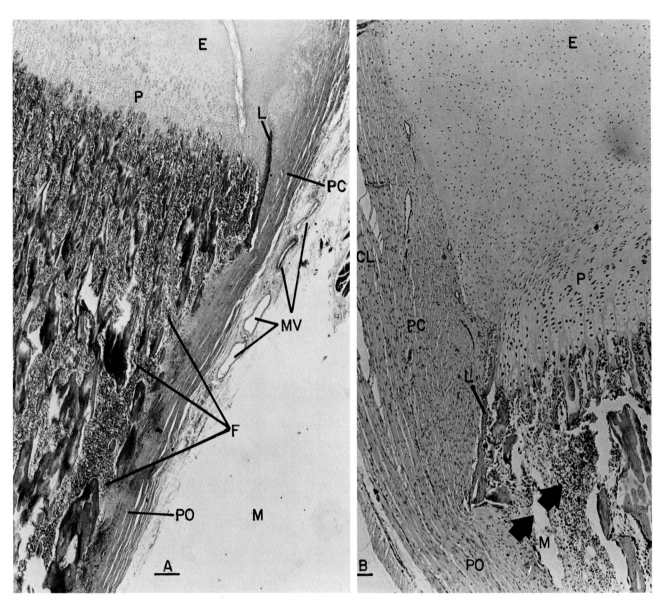

FIG. 2-9. *A,* Sagittal section of lateral proximal femur from six-month-old boy showing epiphysis (E), physis (P), and metaphysis (M). Multiple peripheral metaphyseal vessels (MV) are just outside the periosteum. The cortical bone of the metaphysis is fenestrated (F), allowing continuity of the intertrabecular soft tissue with the periosteum, which makes this region of periosteum more firmly fixed to the underlying bone than it is along the diaphysis. The metaphyseal cortex ends as the osseous ring of Lacroix (L), which surrounds the physis. The periosteum (PO) of the metaphysis is continuous with the perichondrium (PC) of the epiphysis. *B,* Sagittal section of distal femur from two-month-old girl. A large gap (arrows) exists between the trabecular cortex and the peripheral trabeculae associated with the ring of Lacroix. Note the continuity of the periosteum (PO) and perichondrium (PC). The perichondrium blends densely into the hyaline cartilage of the epiphysis (E). Collateral ligaments (CL) of the knee joint insert into the perichondrium. Note the physis (P), the metaphysis (M), and the ring of Lacroix (L).

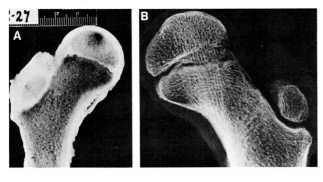

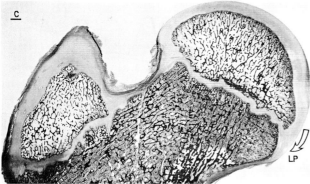

FIG. 2-10. Proximal femur from a ten-year-old boy. *A,* Slab section of specimen; *B,* roentgenograph of specimen; *C,* histologic section. The epiphyseal (secondary) ossification center has expanded out to the margins of the metaphyseal bone. However, physeal and epiphyseal cartilage extends latitudinally beyond this osseous margin, creating a lappet formation (LP, arrow) that contributes to fracture-resistance. Note the thickening of the subchondral plate above the center of the capital femoral physis.

growth of each bone (Fig. 2-15). The metaphyseal bone tends to have more transverse septa than comparable regions of major long bones in addition to the usual longitudinal pattern of the primary spongiosa. While this difference may impart a greater degree of resistance to shear fractures, it is primarily a reflection of relative rates of longitudinal growth and metaphyseal remodeling (see Chap. 4). In contrast, the epiphyseal hyaline cartilage of the opposite end is replaced relatively rapidly, until only a small amount remains between the articular surface and metaphysis. The associated physis assumes a spherical contour with decreased cell column length underneath the articular cartilage. This spherical physis contributes minimally to longitudinal growth, but it does allow contoured expansion of the metacarpal head. An epiphyseal ossification center rarely appears in the epiphysis associated with such a spherical growth plate, although a structural variation, the pseudo-epiphysis, is sometimes encountered (Fig. 2-16). This occurs most commonly in the distal end of the thumb metacarpal, where it should be considered a normal variant. The pseudo-epiphysis is not a true ossification center, but rather an upward, and subsequently expansile, enlargement of metaphyseal ossification.[19] It does not appear to be subject to

fracture, as true physes are, but it may radiologically mimic a fracture in an acutely injured child.

The spherical growth plate, which is the major growth mechanism of the epiphyseal ossification center, is also found in the small bones of the carpus and tarsus (Fig. 2-17). By progressive centrifugal expansion, each spherical growth plate gradually assumes the contours of the particular bone or epiphysis. In the epiphysis, this enlargement of the secondary ossification center leads to juxtaposition of part of the spherical growth plate against the primary discoid physis, creating a bipolar growth zone (Fig. 2-18). A bipolar growth zone also may be found in the arms of the acetabular triradiate cartilage and between the proximal tibial and the tuberosity ossification centers.

The physis has a characteristic and essentially unchanging basic cytoarchitecture from early fetal life until skeletal maturation.[1,20,21] Differences among the physes, which are reflections of growth rates and biomechanical stresses, can be found in the relative amounts of cells in each zone, the overall height of the physis, and any specific cellular modification, such as replacement of the zone of hypertrophic cartilage by a zone of fibrocartilage. These basic patterns may be analyzed upon either functional or morphologic criteria (see Fig. 2-13).

The zone of growth is directly involved in both longitudinal and latitudinal (diametric) expansion of the bone. It is the area of most concern in any fracture involving the growth plate, for damage to cells in this zone, in contradistinction to other zones of the physis, may have serious, long term consequences for normal growth patterns. It is in this cellular zone that mitosis and new cell formation occur. The resting and dividing cells are intimately associated with blood vessels of the epiphysis (a factor that is discussed in detail later in this chapter). Additional cells also may be added peripherally through a specialized region surrounding the physis—the zone of Ranvier. This zone contains fibrovascular tissue, undifferentiated mesenchymal tissue, differentiated epiphyseal and physeal cartilage, and the osseous ring of Lacroix (see Fig. 2-13). Adjacent to the resting cell layer is the layer of active cell division. Mitoses appear to occur in both longitudinal and transverse directions, although principally the former, leading to the earliest evidence of cell column formation. In an active growth plate, such as the distal femur, these cell columns may comprise half of the overall height of the physis. The randomly dispersed collagen of the resting and dividing regions gradually becomes longitudinally oriented between the columnar cells.[22]

The next functional area is the zone of cartilage maturation. In this zone, increased intercellular matrix is formed, principally between cell columns, rather than between successive cells in a given column (which remain separated by a thin transverse septum). This matrix is comprised of a distinct type of collagen that appears specifically related to endochondral ossification.[22] The intercellular matrix then exhibits cell-mediated biochemical changes, becoming metachromatic and then calcifying, a necessary prelude to ossification. The chondrocytes become hypertrophic, and eventually degenerate. While some authors feel that all chondrocytes are replaced by osteoblasts, others feel that the cells may modulate into osteoblasts under the influence of vascularization.[23]

The final functional zone is that of cartilage transforma-

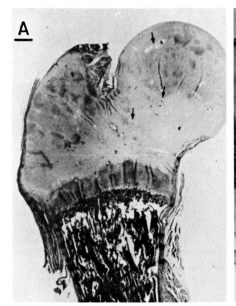

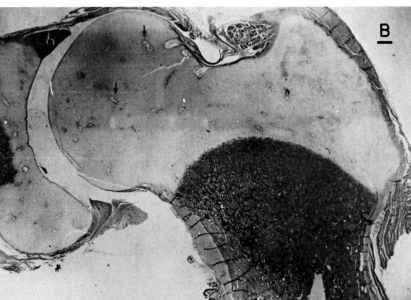

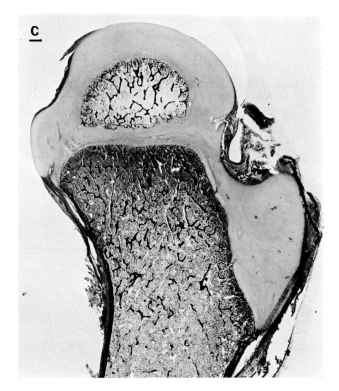

FIG. 2-11. Development of the physeal contour at, *A*, 4 months prenatal, *B*, full-term, and, *C*, 14 months postnatal. Initially, the physis is transverse, but by full-term, it is developing a curvilinear contour. By one year of age, the contour emphasizes the dominance of capital femoral growth over greater trochanteric growth. The small arrows in *A* and *B* indicate intraepiphyseal vasculature (cartilage canals).

be greatly widened because the matrix fails to calcify. This prevents capillary invasion from the metaphysis, so the hypertrophic zone cannot be replaced by osseous tissue. Addition to the hypertrophic cartilage zone continues, resulting in a progressively wider region which becomes more mechanically unstable and eventually results in epiphyseal displacement (see Chap. 8).

Patterns of physeal growth

Characteristically, the growth of the tubular bones is considered a longitudinal phenomenon.[24] However, expansion can, and must, occur in other significant ways. Certainly, appositional growth has been described for the diaphysis through the combined mechanisms of periosteal osteogenesis and endosteal remodeling. The physis also may expand in a diametric, or latitudinal fashion (Fig. 2-19).[25] This occurs by cell division and matrix expansion within the physis (interstitial growth), and by cellular addition peripherally at the zone of Ranvier (appositional growth).[26] Interstitial growth of the discoid physis appears to be related directly to enlargement of the secondary center of ossification. When the epiphysis is completely cartilaginous, or when it contains only a small, spherical ossification center, the biologically plastic cartilage does not present a total mechanical barrier to interstitial expansion of the juxtaposed physis. Both regions appear to undergo integrated interstitial expansion. But with increasing development of the epiphyseal ossification center, a discrete subchondral bone plate forms. Further interstitial expansion of the physis is effectively precluded in those areas directly apposed to the subchondral plate. Lat-

tion. The cartilage matrix must be sufficiently calcified to allow vascular invasion by the metaphyseal vessels, which break down the transverse cartilaginous septa to invade the cell columns, laying down primary spongiosa along the preformed intercolumnar matrix. This cartilage/bone composite will be remodeled, removed, and replaced by a more mature, secondary spongiosa, which contains no remnants of the cartilaginous precursor.

The regions of cellular hypertrophy and transformation appear to be structurally weak and also the regions most likely to be involved in a physeal fracture (see Chap. 4). In certain diseases, such as rickets, the hypertrophic zone may

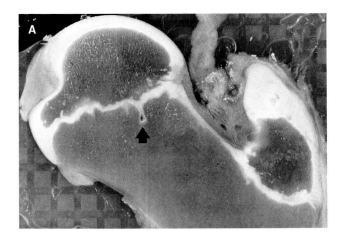

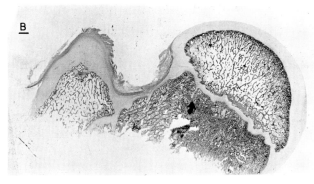

FIG. 2-12. *A,* Sagittal cut of proximal femur from a nine-year-old boy. The physis has an irregular, convoluted pattern, with a mammillary process extending into the metaphysis (arrow). *B,* Histologic section from an eight-year old girl with similar convolutions and mammillary process (arrow).

itudinal expansion thus becomes progressively limited to appositional growth from the peripheral zone of Ranvier as the subchondral bone plate enlarges. Once the ossification center has expanded to the epiphyseal margin, relatively minor damage to the peripheral zone of Ranvier may lead to rapid formation of an osseous bridge, severely limiting growth potential both latitudinally and longitudinally.

Control of growth

The factors affecting growth of the physis are not completely understood.[27] The physis appears to respond to various hormones, with cartilage growth being stimulated by thyroxin, growth hormone, sulfation factor, and testosterone. Estrogen appears to have a greater effect on stimulating the growth of already differentiated osseous tissue, and it actually may slow down cartilage growth, either primarily or secondarily, by affecting the subchondral plates on either side of the physis (see section on physiologic epiphyseodesis). Simmons[28] has shown a definite circadian pattern to longitudinal growth. This may reflect diurnal variations of different hormones. Mechanical factors, such as the intrinsic tension within the periosteal sleeve, also may control growth rates.[2] Disruption of this periosteal sleeve, as well as increased vascularity, may be important factors in the longitudinal overgrowth that often accompanies fractures.[29-36]

Metaphyseal changes

The metaphysis is the site of extensive osseous remodeling, both peripherally and centrally. The metaphyseal cortex consists of fenestrated, modified, trabecular bone on which the periosteum elaborates new membranous bone to thicken the cortex progressively. Similar but less extensive endosteal bone formation occurs. As this region thickens, the trabecular bone is invaded progressively by the osteon systems, a process not unlike osteons traversing the fracture site in primary bone healing (see Chap. 5). This converts peripheral trabecular bone (woven or fiber) to lamellar bone (osteonal), which has different biomechanical properties. A torus (buckle) fracture will occur only in a metaphyseal region with a trabecular cortex. Centrally, a considerable amount of trabecular reorientation and remodeling occurs. This is an area of intense osteoblastic activity, a factor readily evident on a bone scan in a child. This osteoblastic activity also explains the rapid healing of fractures through the metaphysis. This transitional area of bone formation and re-

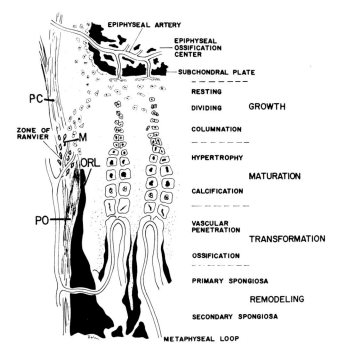

FIG. 2-13. Schematic of the major patterns of endochondral growth. Longitudinal growth occurs in the cell columns, which may be divided on the basis of physiologic function (growth, maturation, transformation, and remodeling), or histologic structure and appearance. Two relatively independent vascular systems supply the two sides of the physis. Additional branches supply a specialized region, the zone of Ranvier, where undifferentiated mesenchymal cells (M) give rise to chondroblasts. The periosteum (PO) and perichondrium (PC) are continuous in this region. The metaphyseal cortex also extends into this region, becoming the osseous ring of Lacroix (ORL), which acts as a peripheral restraint to the cell columns, but does not impede latitudinal growth of the adjacent zone of Ranvier or the more external periosteum and perichondrium.

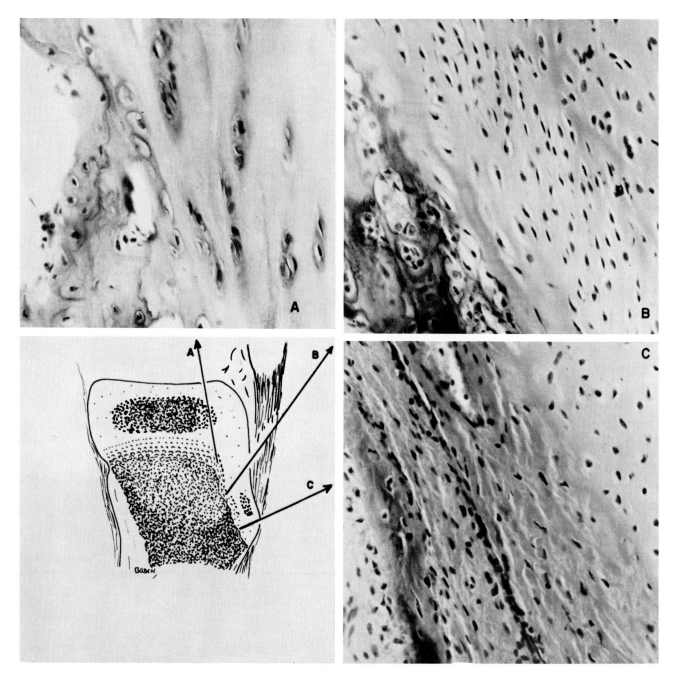

FIG. 2-14. Schematic and histologic sections showing the development of the various cellular zones underlying the tibial tuberosity (tubercle) of a four-year-old child. *A,* Region adjacent to the proximal tibial physis, showing increased intercellular matrix among irregular cell columns. *B,* Middle of tuberosity physis showing regularly aligned fibrocartilage with membranous bone formation. *C,* Distal region of tuberosity physis showing fibrous tissue between cartilage and bone.

modeling, which is continuously changing and responding to biologic stresses, is one of the most susceptible regions of the developing skeleton to fracture. The distal humeral and distal radial metaphyses are certainly the most commonly involved areas.

Many bones exhibit transversely oriented, dense trabecular patterns in the metaphysis. These patterns usually duplicate the appropriate physeal contour (Fig. 2-20). They often appear after generalized illnesses or even after localized processes within the bone (e.g., osteomyelitis). Apparently, they represent a temporary slowdown of normal longitudinal growth rates during the illness, and are often referred to as Harris "growth arrest" lines. Because of the slowdown, as the trabeculae of the primary spongiosa form, they become more transversely than longitudinally oriented, creating a temporary subchondral thickening in the primary spongiosa. Once the illness is over, normal longitudinal growth rates resume, and the primarily longitudinal trabecular orienta-

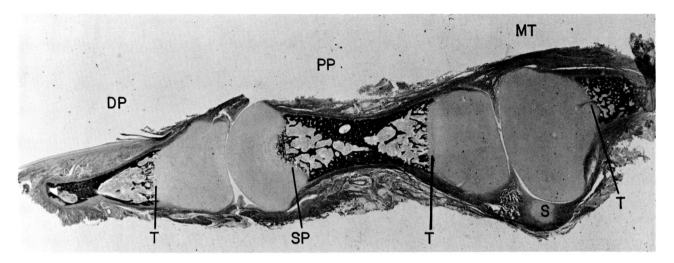

FIG. 2-15. Histologic section of first toe from a three-month-old girl showing distal phalanx (DP), proximal phalanx (PP), and metatarsal head (MT). The distal phalanx exhibits only one epiphysis and has a transversely oriented physis (T). The proximal phalanx also has a transversely oriented physis (T) at its proximal end. The transverse physis (T) of the metatarsal is also evident. Both structures eventually will develop secondary ossification centers. At the distal end of the proximal phalanx, a spherical (curvilinear) physis (SP) is beginning to develop. Much of the epiphyseal cartilage will be replaced by bone, without concomitant longitudinal growth of the shaft. Contributions to the growth of the overall length of a phalanx or metatarsal (metacarpal) from such a physis are less than those from the transversely oriented physis at the other end. A sesamoid (S) is evident beneath the metatarsal head.

tion is restored. The thickened, transverse plate is "left behind" to be gradually remodeled, as primary spongiosa becomes secondary spongiosa and medullary cavity. These particular metaphyseal changes will be discussed in more detail in Chapter 3.

Physiologic epiphysiodesis

Physiologic epiphysiodesis refers to the normal, gradual replacement of the physis during adolescence. The process commences with the formation of small osseous bridges between the epiphyseal ossification center and the metaphysis, and it ends with the complete replacement of the cartilaginous physis by osseous tissue.[5,37] This transversely oriented replacement may be evident radiographically at any age during adulthood, although it is usually progressively remodeled until no longer evident. Each physis appears to have its own pattern of closure, a factor which predisposes different physes to certain types of fractures (e.g., Tillaux fracture of the distal tibia).

Histologically, several significant changes occur during normal epiphysiodesis. Similar changes also must occur in damaged physes, although usually in more localized regions of the physis. The juxtaphyseal subchondral bone plate thickens (Fig. 2-21). A similar thickening of the metaphyseal bone also occurs, with formation of the transverse osseous septa instead of the more characteristic longitudinal trabeculae. The basic cellular arrangement of the physis does not change significantly while these osseous plates initially are forming. However, there is a distinct cessation of cellular proliferation and biochemistry is altered, with progressive calcification and mineralization extending into the germinal and resting zones to form multiple tide lines. The cell columns are rapidly replaced as they are progressively calcified.

The extension of ossification from both sides leads to eventual perforation of the physis in several areas by small osseous bridges. Ossification then progresses outward from these perforations, replacing the cartilage and leaving a thick, osseous, physeal "ghost," which is comprised of coalesced,

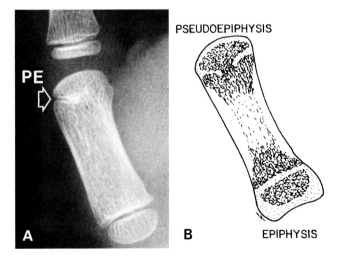

FIG. 2-16. *A*, Thumb of a normal seven-year-old boy being evaluated for hand trauma. A pseudoepiphysis (PE) is present at the distal end of the metacarpal. *B*, Schematic of development of a pseudoepiphysis, based on the work of Haines. Ossification extends directly into the epiphyseal cartilage from the metaphysis, which is the normal mode of epiphyseal ossification in primitive mammals, some marsupials (e.g., a kangaroo), and monotremes (e.g., a platypus).

thickened, subchondral plates of the metaphysis and epiphysis, and is evident on roentgenograms. Usually, the process starts centrally and proceeds centrifugally, so that small remnants of the physis may be found peripherally. However, certain physes show altered patterns. In particular, the distal tibial physis closes first over the middle and medial regions, and subsequently over the lateral region, a factor which leads to certain types of fractures (see Chap. 19).

Physiologic epiphysiodesis begins earlier in the female than in the male, and like the appearance of primary and secondary ossification centers, it follows a reasonably predictable sequence from bone to bone. The earlier closure in the female appears to be the direct effect of estrogenic compounds, which accelerate cartilage replacement and osseous

maturation, versus the effect of androgenic compounds, which stimulate cartilage growth and matrix elaboration. The times of both the onset and the completion of fusion are influenced significantly by sex hormones, and girls undergo the process much earlier than boys, but the sequence in which bones undergo closure is the same in both sexes (see Chap. 3 for closure patterns).

Vasculature

Developing bone, both osseous and cartilaginous, is extremely vascular.[5,38-43] The periosteum contains multiple, small vessels that play a role in osteogenesis and contribute to the increasingly complex Haversian systems of the maturing diaphyseal cortex. The endosteal surface of the diaphysis receives blood through the nutrient artery, a major vessel which sends branches to each metaphysis as well as throughout the diaphysis. The epiphysis receives its blood supply from vessels that penetrate and ramify through the cartilage. These two major circulatory patterns—epiphyseal vessels and metaphyseal vessels—appear to be functionally and anatomically separate. The physis derives a blood supply from three regions—epiphyseal vessels, metaphyseal vessels, and perichondral vessels of the zone of Ranvier.

Epiphyseal circulation varies significantly in conjunction with development and enlargement of the secondary ossification center. Vessels distribute through the chondroepiphysis as specialized structures termed cartilage canals (Fig. 2-22).[5,44] These canals course throughout the chondroepiphysis and send branches to the resting/germinal zones of the physis. Infrequently, these small vessels also may communicate across the physis, anastomosing with the metaphyseal circulation. These particular transphyseal vessels may be found in the larger epiphyses; they are usually more frequent near the peripheral than the central regions; and they become less frequent as the secondary ossification center enlarges. By the time the subchondral plate forms, these vessels are no longer present centrally.

The cartilage canals contain a central artery, one or more accompanying veins, and a capillary complex that surrounds the larger, central vessels (see Fig. 2-22). The capillary network forms a "glomerular" tuft which serves as the end-arterial termination of each canal system. These canals have several important functional and morphologic characteristics: (1) they supply discrete regions of the epiphysis and physis, where there are no significant intraepiphyseal anastomoses; (2) the mesenchymal tissue within the canals may serve as a source of chondroblastic cells for continued interstitial enlargement of the chondroepiphysis; (3) the canals are surrounded by differentiating hyaline cartilage that contains hypertrophic cells, and which may form an internal structural network prior to ossification; and (4) the canals play an integral role in the formation of the secondary center of ossification (Fig. 2-23).

Once the secondary center of ossification forms and begins to enlarge, changes commence within the epiphyseal circulation. Several cartilage canal systems may contribute to enlargement of the ossification center, thus creating anastomoses between canal systems that were initially end-arterial. Once the secondary center enlarges to form a subchondral plate, small vessels penetrate the plate to supply the physis. This circulatory pattern retains a territorial (end-arterial) pattern.

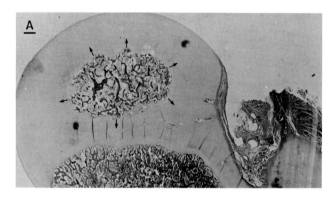

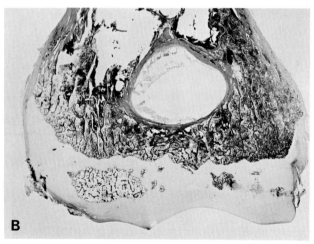

FIG. 2-17. *A,* Spherical ossification developing in the capital femoral epiphysis. Cells around the periphery of the ossific nucleus have the histologic appearance of foreshortened cell columns from a longitudinal growth physis. This type of growth plate (i.e., spherical) does *not* contribute to an increase in the size of the epiphysis. Instead, it represents a mechanism for replacement of the epiphyseal cartilage, which contributes to the overall increase in size through both interstitial and peripheral (perichondral) growth. The arrows indicate the centrifugal direction of ossification expansion. *B,* Multifocal ossification centers in the trochlear region of the distal humerus of a nine-year-old boy. Contrast these with the more mature ossification center in the capitellum.

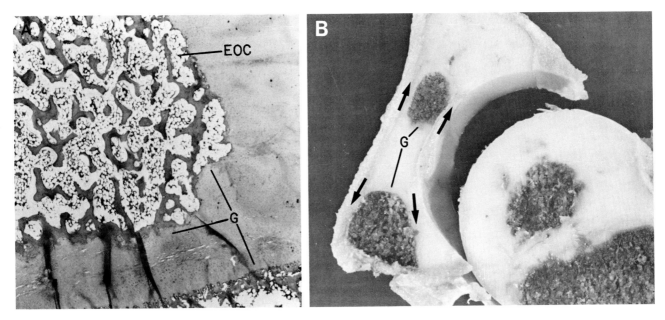

FIG. 2-18. *A,* Bipolar growth zone that develops between the epiphyseal ossification center (EOC) and the metaphysis. Germinal cells (G) are present on both sides of this plate, but significant longitudinal growth will occur only on the metaphyseal side. *B,* In other areas, such as the triradiate cartilage of the acetabulum, longitudinal growth may occur from both sides (arrows). Note the germinal cells (G).

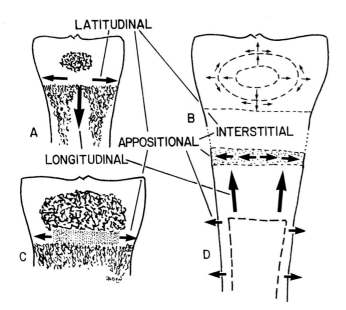

FIG. 2-19. Schematic of growth patterns of endochondral bones. *A,* The two primary patterns for physeal growth are longitudinal (elongation of cell columns) and latitudinal (diametric). *B,* The developing ossification center enlarges by interstitial growth between rudimentary columnar cartilage. *C,* Such interstitial growth (elaboration of extracellular matrix) also occurs in the physis. In addition, there are peripheral areas of appositional growth. *D,* Once a relatively mature epiphyseal ossification center is present, latitudinal development of the physis is limited essentially to appositional growth, which occurs primarily from the zone of Ranvier.

If a segment of the epiphyseal vasculature is compromised, either temporarily or permanently, then the zones of growth associated with those vessels cannot undergo appropriate cell division. Unaffected regions of the physis continue longitudinal and latitudinal growth, thus leaving behind the affected region (Fig. 2-24). The growth rates of the cells directly adjacent to the infarcted area are more mechanically compromised than cellular areas further away, resulting in an angular growth deformity.

Metaphyseal circulation is derived from two sources—the nutrient artery, which supplies the central region, and the perichondral vessels, which supply the peripheral regions (Fig. 2-24C). The terminal portions of both systems form a series of loops that penetrate between trabeculae to reach the margin of the hypertrophic zone of the physis (see Fig. 2-13). The venular side of the loop enlarges to form a sinusoid.

Interruption of metaphyseal circulation has no effect upon initial chondrogenesis and subsequent cartilage maturation within the physis. However, the subsequent transformation of cartilage to bone is blocked. This causes widening of the affected area as more cartilage is added to the cell columns (in a hypertrophic mode), but none is replaced by bone (Fig. 2-24D). Once metaphyseal circulation is reestablished, the widened, provisionally calcified region is penetrated rapidly, and ossified, returning the physis to normal width. This is the mechanism seen in fractures of the growth plate, and less frequently in fractures of the metaphysis. The metaphyseal blood supply is blocked temporarily by fracture-caused separation or impaction, and three to four weeks are required for its restoration. If the circulatory compromise has been caused by a metaphyseal fracture, bone formation in the ischemic portion of the metaphysis may increase temporarily once revascularization occurs, leading to a transient

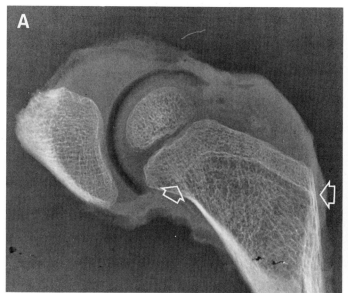

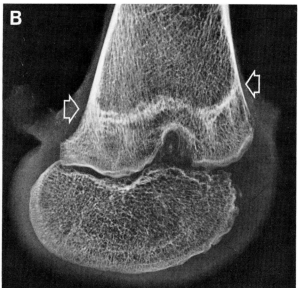

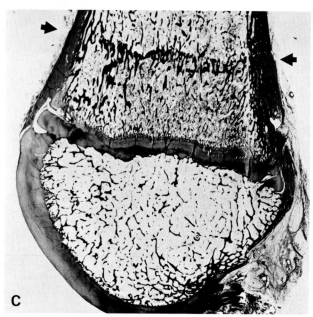

FIG. 2-20. Harris "growth arrest" lines. *A,* Three-year-old child suffering from malnutrition (kwashiorkor) and, possibly, mild rickets. At the time of the first onset of disease a transverse line was laid down (arrows). The child was treated in a hospital, provided with dietary supplements and grew more rapidly. He died a year later from Salmonella enteritis. Note the relative growth contributions of the trochanteric, neck, and capital femoral regions. *B,* Harris growth arrest line in the distal femur of a ten-year-old boy (arrows). This line occurred with the onset of leukemia. Subsequent growth occurred over the next 14 months while the boy was on chemotherapy. The disease recurred shortly before death, and a second line of growth slowdown is occurring at the physis. *C,* Distal femur from a nine-year-old child who had a severe septicemic episode approximately a year before death. Black arrows indicate the transverse trabeculae of the Harris line. Note the longitudinal orientation of the trabeculae between the Harris and physeal lines.

osseous overgrowth and apparent sclerosis (Fig. 2-25). Compromise of the metaphyseal circulation has a minimal effect on longitudinal and latitudinal physeal development, particularly as compared to the effects of epiphyseal circulatory compromise.

The perichondrial vascular network courses circumferentially around each physis. However, this circulatory pattern is quite variable, as dictated by individual epiphyseal anatomy. The small vessels of this system may provide peripheral circulation to the epiphysis, physis, and metaphysis. The most important branches supply the zone of Ranvier. The functional integrity of these vessels is essential to continued appositional growth at the periphery of the physis. Disruption of the perichondrial circulation, which can occur in certain kinds of growth plate injuries (fracture, burn, radiation, etc.), may lead to isolated areas of ischemia along the periphery of the physis, and subsequent eccentric growth with premature, localized epiphysiodesis.

Remodeling

On a developmental basis, cortical bone, which becomes the dominant skeletal tissue by the time chondro-osseous maturation is completed, may be categorized as either primary or secondary bone. As described previously, primary bone may be formed by either endochondral ossification or subperiosteal membranous deposition, and such bone is always the first bone formed in any region. During subsequent growth, and even beyond skeletal maturation (as defined by closure of the growth plates), there is a continuous process of osteoclastic (and possibly osteocytic) resorption of existing primary bone followed by osteoblastic deposition of new bone. These remodeling processes may involve several generations of bone absorption and accretion. All bone formed by the process of bone resorption and subsequent bone deposition is called secondary bone.

Three basic types of primary bone may be found in most large mammals: (1) circumferential lamellar bone, (2) woven-fibered bone, and (3) primary osteons. At birth, the differentiated metaphyseal and diaphyseal cortical bone

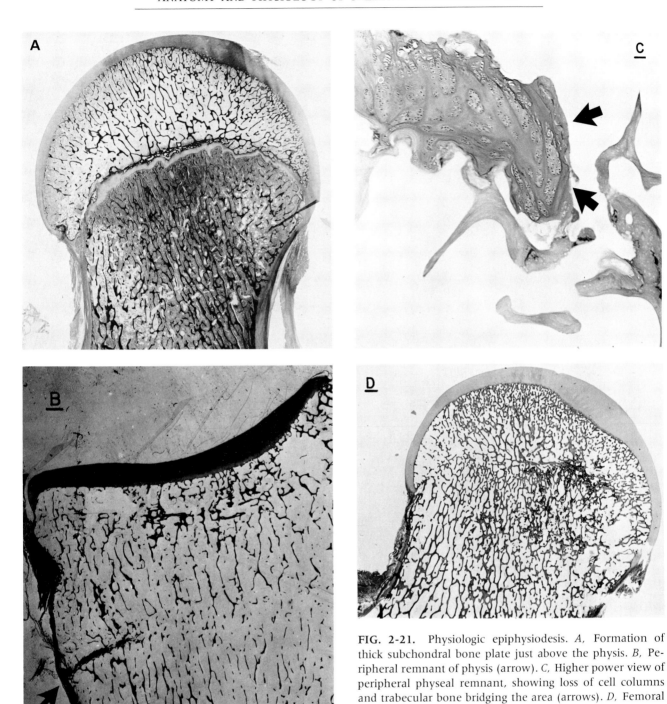

FIG. 2-21. Physiologic epiphysiodesis. *A,* Formation of thick subchondral bone plate just above the physis. *B,* Peripheral remnant of physis (arrow). *C,* Higher power view of peripheral physeal remnant, showing loss of cell columns and trabecular bone bridging the area (arrows). *D,* Femoral head from a 16-year-old showing remnant of thickened subchondral bone, the physeal "ghost" that is sometimes seen radiographically.

consists principally of woven-fibered bone, with a few areas such as the femur also having primary osteons. The girth of mammalian long bone is increased during growth by the deposition of primary bone along the subperiosteal surface. The structure of this new bone varies considerably in different species and also at different stages of development. In the human, this new bone normally consists of circumferential, laminar bone comprised of orderly collagen bundles, while in more rapidly growing quadripedal species (which

usually reach skeletal maturity in one to five years) the more common pattern consists of woven-fibered bone with randomly arranged collagen bundles.[6]

Woven-fibered bone generally contains large, irregularly shaped vascular spaces with osteoblasts on the surrounding bone surface. These osteoblasts deposit successive layers (lamellae) of new bone, progressively diminishing the caliber of each original vascular space. The resulting anastomosing, convoluted areas of bone, occupying what were previously

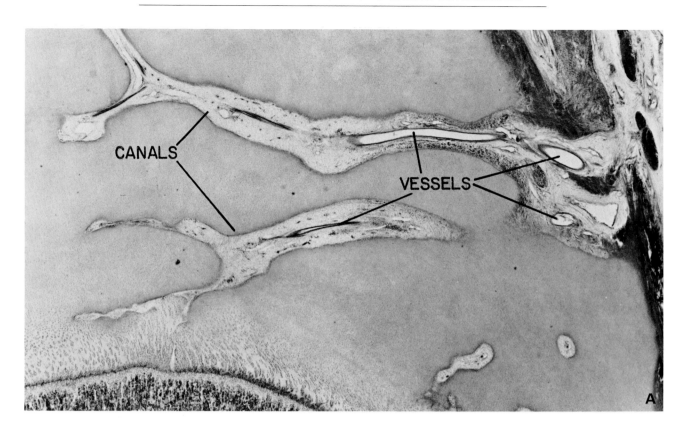

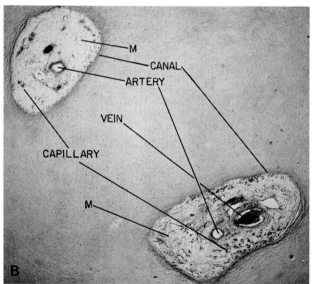

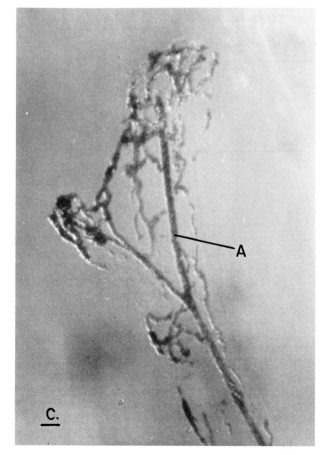

FIG. 2-22. *A,* Penetration of cartilage canals into capital femoral epiphysis. The vessels distribute throughout the epiphyseal cartilage and also send selected branches to the germinal zone of the physis (arrow). *B,* Higher power view (20×) of two adjacent cartilage canal systems. They are both reasonably well demarcated from the surrounding cartilage. Much of the canal is occupied by undifferentiated, perivascular mesenchyme (M). Each canal generally has a central artery (artery), one or more veins (vein), and a peripheral capillary network (capillary). *C,* India ink injection of terminal cartilage canal unit. Note the "glomerular" structure of the capillaries peripheral to the central artery (A).

vascular spaces, are called primary Haversian systems, or primary osteons. Primary osteons are usually, but not always, parallel to the long axis of a bone; they may contain from one to several vascular canals, and they are always surrounded initially by woven-fibered bone.[45,46]

The continuous process of remodeling that occurs throughout chondro-osseous development constantly and dynamically changes the internal architecture of each bone (see Fig. 2-6). The remodeling process is initiated by the osteoclastic resorption of bone and results in longitudinally oriented, anastomotic tubular cavities. Osteoblasts on the surfaces of these cavities then deposit successive layers of new bone with an orderly fiber orientation. The caliber of each cavity is thereby gradually reduced until only a small, single, vascular canal remains. The newly formed cylinders of bone are called secondary Haversian systems or secondary osteons.[45,46] Secondary osteons consist of concentric sheets of lamellar bone. Unlike primary osteons, secondary osteons are always bounded by cement lines that are formed when osteoclastic activity is superseded by osteoblastic bone formation. The irregular areas of bone between secondary osteons are called interstitial bone, and consist of remnants of both the primary and the remodeled bone previously deposited in the area. Interstitial bone may consist of woven-fibered bone, circumferential lamellar bone, portions of primary osteons, or portions of secondary osteons.

The two principal bone types, woven-fibered and lamellar, are in part a reflection of skeletogenic response to various biologic demands. As such, the fourth dimension, time, becomes an integral factor in the progressive development of three-dimensional bone structure. Woven-fibered bone, with or without primary osteons, is formed during rapid bone development and accretion. It is the normal bone of skeletal growth and the initial responsive bone in fracture callus formation. In contrast, lamellar bone, which may be found in primary osteons, secondary osteons, and circumferential lamellar bone, is formed when the rate of bone deposition is moderate or slow.

Biomechanics

During normal childhood activity and growth, the developing chondro-osseous skeleton is subjected to a complex pattern of forces that may cause microdeformations of the bone and is usually followed by appropriate biologic response patterns, such as replacement of epiphyseal and physeal cartilage by osseous tissues, increased amounts of osseous tissue, changing trabecular orientation, and varying amounts of different histologic types of bone. These local microdeformations are referred to as strains, and the local force concentrations at these points are termed stresses. The biologic relationships between stresses and strains at a particular point in the developing skeletal unit are governed by the material properties of the local chondro-osseous and fibrous/fibro-osseous tissues, the direction and magnitude of imposed loads, and the geometric configuration of the region being loaded.

The effects of normal biologic forces on the physis, epiphysis, and metaphysis are minimally understood. The development of the epiphyseal ossification center appears to be controlled both genetically and biomechanically. At a certain point in time, summated joint reaction forces reach a maximum within a given region of the chondroepiphysis, stimulating osteogenesis in an area with appropriate vascular supply. If forces are abnormal, as in congenital hip dysplasia or

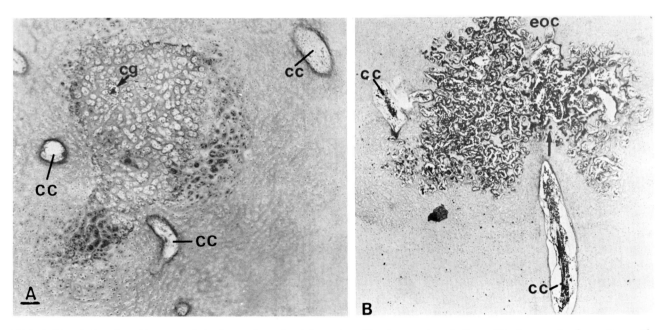

FIG. 2-23. Role of cartilage canals in formation of epiphyseal ossification center. *A,* Preossification center formation with hypertrophy of a zone of epiphyseal cartilage within several canals (cc). A portion of the capillary glomerulus (cg) is present within the hypertrophied cartilage. This vessel is analogous to the irruption artery that initiates primary ossification in the embryo or fetus. If this vessel is not functional, secondary (epiphyseal) ossification may be delayed. *B,* Early formation of bone in epiphyseal ossification center (eoc). Portions of cartilage canals (cc) are sending small vessels into this structure.

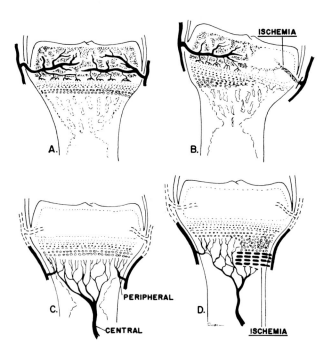

FIG. 2-24. Schematic of epiphyseal and metaphyseal circulatory patterns. *A,* The epiphyseal circulation vessel (E-vessel) enters the epiphysis and distributes to the enlarging epiphyseal ossification center. It also either directly supplies the germinal cells of the physis or crosses the subchondral plate to reach the physis. *B,* If the E-vessel is cut off, the germinal cells are deprived of nutrition and either decrease or cease the cell division necessary for longitudinal growth. Then, the part of the physis with good vascularity continues to grow, leading to eccentric growth. *C,* The metaphyseal circulation (M-vessels) is derived from both central (nutrient artery) and peripheral sources, and is essential to vascular invasion of the hypertrophic regions of the physis. *D,* If the M-vessels are disrupted, as in a metaphyseal fracture, the physis continues to grow, and the height of the cell columns increases, while adjacent regions maintain normal structure. This leads to remnants of cartilage that extend into the metaphysis (see Fig. 2-20*B*). Since the germinal cells are normally supplied, there is no growth angularity, but the physis is abnormally thick in the involved regions. Normal physeal thickness in such areas is replaced rapidly once metaphyseal circulation is reestablished.

congenital dislocation of the head of the radius, this ossification process may be delayed, irregular, or eccentrically located. Physiologic stress appears necessary for the continued, orderly development of both the physis and the secondary ossification center.

Stress is basically the internal resistance of bone and cartilage to deformation. It is not a directly measurable physical phenomenon, but may be considered as force applied per unit area. Rate of application of the force is also important. Three types of stress are seen in developing bones under normal conditions: tension, compression, and shear. If these are increased beyond the physiologic response capacities of a given portion of the developing bone or cartilage, failure

(fracture) may result. Compression and tension forces normally tend to act on bone at various angles. The growth plate develops undulations and mammillary processes, apparently as a means of aligning the physis either reasonably parallel or reasonably perpendicular to major force patterns, whether compression or tension. Similarly, developing trabecular patterns within the metaphysis and epiphysis also seem to be a direct alignment response to normal weight-bearing or functional stresses. Shear stress acts at any angle other than 90°. Again, the undulations in the physis and the appearance of fibrocartilage rather than columnar cartilage appear to be biologic adaptations to minimize shear stresses. Extrinsic forces acting on developing cartilage and bone may therefore evoke a normal response (i.e., stimulation of growth and remodeling) or an abnormal response (i.e., fracture/failure), contingent upon the magnitude, duration, and direction of the evocative forces, as well as upon the rate at which the responsive tissue is loaded.

It is important to realize that there is a normal biologic range of compression/tension response within each physis, and that a given physis is responsive to more than one type of stress.[47-49] Within this physiologic limit, increased tension or compression accelerates growth. Compression appears to elicit a more rapid rate of growth than tension. Beyond the

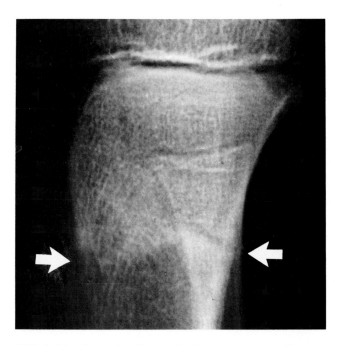

FIG. 2-25. Sclerosis of metaphysis consequent to fracture (arrows). Because of temporary deprivation of vascularity, the metaphysis did not continue normal remodeling. With remodeling of the still vascularized area, as well as some osteoporosis resulting from disuse of this segment, which is distal to the fracture, a contrast is obvious between involved and uninvolved sections of the metaphysis on either side of the fracture. This roentgenogram was taken three weeks after the fracture and immobilization in a non-weightbearing, long leg cast. By six weeks after injury, the metaphysis was the same throughout because vascularity had been reestablished.

physiologic limits of either stress, growth may be significantly decreased or even stopped.[50-53] This may occur in certain types of physeal fractures (see Chap. 4).[54] These principles are often referred to as the Heuter-Volkmann law of cartilage growth response.[55]

Ruysce was one of the earliest experimentalists (1713) to demonstrate that a massive force was required to separate the epiphysis from the metaphysis, because each epiphysis was firmly connected externally by the periosteum and internally by the undulations and mammillary processes existing between the metaphysis and physis.[56] In 1820, James Wilson showed that a longitudinal force of 550 lbs was required to detach the epiphysis from the metaphysis, but if the periosteum was divided first, the force required was only 119 lbs.[56] Bright and Elmore showed that both the age of the animal and the direction in which the force was applied were significant factors.[57] The growth plate is most resistant to traction and least resistant to torsion. Furthermore, the epiphysis can probably be displaced at least $\frac{1}{2}$ mm before any gross separation begins. A more detailed description of physeal and epiphyseal responses to injurious forces is in Chapter 4.

Besides the effects of extrinsic biomechanical forces on growth plates, there is an intrinsic anatomic control factor—the periosteum. The periosteum attaches directly and firmly into the zone of Ranvier at each end of the developing bone; however, it is attached more loosely to the diaphysis and metaphysis. Experimental circumferential resection of a portion of the periosteum may cause accelerated longitudinal growth.[58] It thus appears that the stimulus to longitudinal growth caused by joint reaction forces may be tempered by the intrinsic tensile restraint imposed by the periosteal sleeve (cylinder). When this restraint is temporarily released, as in a fracture, overgrowth may occur.

Besides the effect of factors extrinsic to bone, four major intrinsic factors also affect the response of developing bone and cartilage to potentially injurious forces: (1) energy absorbing capacity; (2) the modulus of elasticity; (3) fatigue strength; and (4) density. Each of these factors is influenced by the changes that occur in developing bone over the period of progressive maturation. The increasing size of the secondary center of ossification affects the energy absorbing capacity of the physis, and contributes to the greater incidence of physeal injuries in older children. Increasing diaphyseal (and less so, metaphyseal) cortical width and the development of primary and secondary osteons affect the modulus of elasticity and relative density and, thereby, cause different fracture patterns (e.g., greenstick versus complete). Much experimental work still has to be accomplished with developing bone, rather than mature bone, in order to answer many of these unknowns.

In order to understand specific biomechanical changes that take place during postnatal development, it is absolutely necessary to relate changing function to changing morphology. To date, there are only three brief studies on the mechanical properties of children's bones. Hirsch[59] showed that the tensile strength and the modulus of elasticity of bone tissue from 9 children (all under 2 months of age) were less than those from similar bone tissue from a 14-year-old. Vinz[60] conducted a more comprehensive study showing that tensile strength and modulus of elasticity increased progressively throughout growth, but that strain and fracture pattern decreased slightly. Currey,[61,62] using specimens of femoral cortical bone from 18 subjects between 2 and 48 years of age, conducted three-point bending tests. Compared to adult bone, he found that children's bone had a lower modulus of elasticity, lower bending strength, and lower ash (mineral) content; and children's bone also reflected more absorbed energy before breaking and tended to absorb more energy after fracture propagation had started. The typical greenstick fracture surface required more energy for its production than the relatively smooth surfaces of adult fractures.

It is reasonable to suggest that progressive maturation of porous cortical bone causes a gradual shift in the distribution of bone strength and stiffness in the various regions of the bone, especially the metaphysis and diaphysis. In younger persons, bone in the cortical center is probably the strongest and stiffest, although with aging (after physiologic epiphysiodesis) there is gradual shift of strength and stiffness toward the periosteal surface. In addition to the varying porosity distribution, a definite, progressive change also takes place in the osseous microstructure from the endosteal to the periosteal surface as the child matures. Bone near the endosteal surface undergoes more remodeling and thus contains more osteons and osteon fragments. However, inherent to such osteonal structure are numerous cement lines that have been shown to be sites of weakness in cortical bone.[45] In contrast, bone near the periosteal surface has undergone less remodeling and is often surrounded by a layer of circumferential laminar bone containing few, if any, cement lines.

Mechanical properties are determined by microstructure. The dynamic variations in microstructure throughout cortical bone undoubtedly reinforce the mechanical property distributions created by the porosity gradients. The strongest type of bone is circumferential lamellar bone, followed in order of decreasing strength by primary laminar, secondary Haversian, and woven-fibered bone.

The effects of varying histology on bone mechanics have also been studied.[45,46,63-65] Maj[66] investigated the correlation between breaking load and collagen fiber orientation, finding that bone cut longitudinally took three to six times more applied force to break then similar bone cut tangentially, transversely, or radially; and he concluded that breaking strength of bone was proportional to the number of collagen fibers in the plane of the applied force, and that the mechanical anisotropy of bone depended upon the distribution and direction of collagen fibers. Maj also found, with the exception of the distal metacarpals, that the variation in porosity was not specifically responsible for the variations in breakability between different parts of the skeletal system. Toajari[67] concluded that the modulus of elasticity and the breaking strength of bone were directly proportional and attributable to the orientations and quantity of collagen fibers. While these studies were directed specifically at bone, they present concepts that seem applicable to failure of the growth plate, since there are significant differences in collagen fiber orientation among the different regions of the physis. Ascenzi[68,69] found that the ultimate tensile strength of a single osteon system was found in the osteon in which the majority of the collagen fibers were oriented parallel to the longitudinal axis of the test specimens. Evans and Vincentelli[70] also felt that their experimental results showed tensile strength was related to the predominant direction of the collagen fibers in the osteon. These studies gain further import in the child, considering the fact that Haversian (osteon) systems must develop postnatally. Osteons with longitudinally oriented collagen fibers are stronger in tension than osteons with transversely oriented fibers, which are stronger in compression.

Therefore, children's bone is susceptible to fracture in different modes than adult's bone and it will fail differently because of the fact that they are in the process of forming these various osteon systems. Young bone certainly appears more porous on cross section, with the cortex having a greater relative number of open osteon systems compared to the adult (see Fig. 2-6). These pores may have further effects on the extension of a fraction line. Compact adult bone principally fails in tension,[71] whereas the more porous nature of the child's bone, particularly in the metaphysis, probably allows failure in compression as well (especially in those bones that go into greenstick failure or simple plastic deformation).

Smith and Walmsley[72] studied the factors affecting the elasticity of bone and found that the relationship between the modulus of elasticity in tension and in bending was extremely dependent upon the vascular pattern within the bone, and that an adequate, functioning vascular supply was necessary to effect a normal stress-pattern response. The usual equations expressing the reactions of materials to tensile and bending stresses are founded on the assumption that the experimental material is homogenous. However, an obvious tissue discontinuity exists in the multiple, small, vascular canals in the cortical, mature lamellar bone and in the fenestrated cortical bone of the metaphysis. The vascular pattern of bone varies considerably, not only among species, but among age groups and throughout regions of a single bone. It is evident that when a vascular gradient exists, the value of Young's modulus of elasticity must vary progressively from the periosteal to the endosteal aspect of bone, and from the diaphysis to the metaphysis. In some bone, the vascular pattern is such that it causes a partial lamination of the tissues, since solid bone alternates with relatively porous layers. This is more characteristic of developing bone, particularly in the metaphysis. The orientation of the irregular intertrabecular spaces shows a distinct preferential orientation in which the intervening bone is in the form of thin sheets that lie parallel to the bone surface and have infrequent radial interconnections. Subsequently, primary osteons form within this vascular labyrinth. The longitudinal vascular canals of these osteons lie within the sites occupied by the original vascular spaces and are consequently seen, in transverse section, to lie in rows parallel to the bone surface. Areas of solid bone intervene between adjacent vascular rows. In other regions, however, the vascular canals of the primary osteons undergo local enlargement to form erosion cavities, and these cavities are subsequently occupied by secondary osteons. Because this erosion phase of the reconstruction and remodeling process usually proceeds eccentrically from the primary osteons, the canals of the secondary osteons are not always aligned with the original vascular planes. Consequently, as the remodeling process becomes more extensive, the subdivision of the bone into vascular/nonvascular laminae becomes progressively less distinct until, in many skeletally mature bones, it is no longer discernible. This alternation of strong and weak layers particularly characterizes bone at the junction of the metaphysis and diaphysis, and possibly renders this area more susceptible to injury.

Cortical bone is stronger in compression than tension. The shear strength for torsional loading about the longitudinal axis is less than the tensile strength. Because secondary Haversian bone is an anisotropic material that is transversely isotropic, it is stronger and stiffer in the longitudinal direction than it is in the transverse direction.[45] Furthermore, bone has poor fatigue resistance.

Classically, bone was considered a brittle material when loaded in tension. But over the past few years it has become evident that bone initially exhibits a type of ductile behavior; that is, elongation of bone tissue under tensile or elongating loads may continue beyond 1% elongation, depending on the age of the individual and the area of the bone.[73,74] This may result in an elongation between 2 and 7% of the overall length of the bone. However, after elongation reaches about ¾%, continued elongation in the 2 to 7% level results in permanent, plastic elongation (Fig. 2-26). Plastic deformation is essentially an irreversible deformation. If a plastically deformed bone is subsequently cyclically loaded, the total deformation will increase to a point at which the next load applied will result in failure. The clinical importance of this behavior of bone tissue is that bone as a structure can sustain permanent damage, even though no gross fracture or decrease in load carrying capacity is noted. Furthermore, such damaged bone tissue is capable of sustaining a load virtually identical to that of the previous cycle. When it has been loaded a sufficient number of times at that level or slightly above that level, a fracture may result. The only detectable damage during plastic deformation appears to be the production of microvoids within the osseous tissue.

Tensile behavior of bone tissue varies within an individual from bone to bone, and also with age. The most dramatic change is a decrease in the amount of total strain that bone

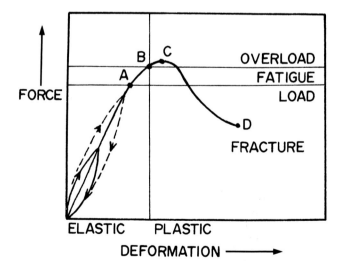

FIG. 2-26. Graphic relationship of osseous deformation (bowing) and force (longitudinal compression). In the zone of elastic deformation, bone deforms but springs back to its original contour (loop). Eventually, the bone is overloaded (C) and develops acute permanent deformation (bowing). If force increases beyond this point, fracture results. In the child, remodeling will bring a plastically deformed bone back into the normal response zone of elastic deformation (modified from Chamay[73]).

tissue can undergo. This amount decreases from almost 4% strain capacity to slightly more than 2%, and the decrease occurs gradually throughout adult life. It is possible that children have a capacity for total strain even greater than 4% although this has not been measured because of the minimal number of available specimens.

Another significant change in the mechanical properties of femoral bone tissue during deformation is the increase in slope in the second region of loading, or the region of fatigue. This increase probably reflects an increase in the stiffness of the bone collagen, again a factor that gradually increases with age.[45,63-65] Different bones exhibit different capacities for plastic deformation and strength, even in the same individual. For instance, between the third and eighth decades of life, femoral bone exhibits less plastic deformation and is somewhat weaker than tibial bone.

Bending stress in developing tubular bone often causes an incomplete fracture through only a portion of the cortical circumference. The remaining cortex is grossly intact, but in actuality probably has microfractures. This "intact" cortex is invariably plastically deformed, whereas the fractured area has gone through the phase of plastic deformation to complete failure. Since plastic failure, by definition, means permanent deformation, this will have an effect on reducibility and ability to maintain longitudinal alignment. Such greenstick fractures usually must be completed, which is relatively easy to do since the bone has already undergone a certain degree of failure. Clinically, some bones may undergo only plastic deformation, causing an increased bowing. This is most likely in the ulna and the fibula.[75,76]

In experimental work with puppies, bone subjected to bending stress showed increased stiffness or initial slope of the curve as the animal aged.[57] This is a reflection not only of the increasing amount of material in the cross section of the bone, but also of the increasing strength of the bone tissue as well. The amount of plastic deformation which a bone can undergo decreases with increasing age. Bone with thin cortices will plastically deform to a greater extent than bone with thick cortices, which invariably has a better developed osteon structure (Fig. 2-27).

Bending is not the only load situation that may cause permanent damage to bones without causing concomitant fracture. Axial or compressive loads may cause permanent injury even though no fracture is noticeable, even by roentgenography. Since the predominant mode of loading of a long bone is axial compression, it is not surprising that

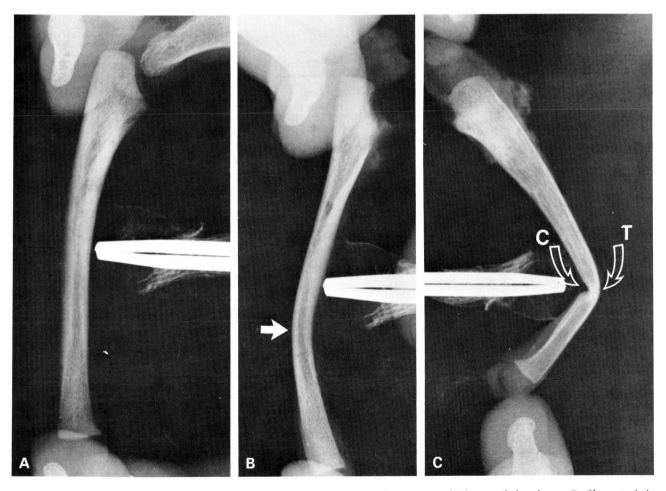

FIG. 2-27. Deformation capacity of neonatal ulnae (human). *A,* Bending was applied toward the clamp. *B,* Characteristic degree of deformation in most of the bones, with bowing beginning (arrow). These bones characteristically spring back to their original shape, but not always instantly. *C,* Most extreme deformation capacity in one specimen. Note the buckling (compression deformation—C) which is occurring opposite the tensile (T) deformation.

overload conditions exist in which the compressive yield strength of bone tissue is exceeded, and upon further increasing the load, the tissue plastically deforms. Plastic deformation of cortical bone under a compressive load is really a microfracture mechanism. These microfractures, due to the large shear stresses in oblique planes, may or may not coalesce into larger shear cracks or buckling as is characteristic of the torus fracture of the distal radius. Occurrence of a compression overload does not appreciably reduce the load strength of a bone in axial loading. However, it may weaken the bone's response to a subsequent bending load, which may help to explain the phenomenon of refracture sometimes complicating distal radial fractures.

The compressive behavior of bone tissue is quite different from tensile behavior. The application of a load again results in a linear, reversible range, and then a second, nonlinear, irreversible range. Failure occurs by a microfracture mechanism within the tissue, with most of the microfracture characteristically appearing at approximately 35° angles to the loading direction.[14] Although the bone has undergone microfracture in the compressive mode, it may still sustain continued load application. In fact, it is possible to continue foreshortening the bone tissue by as much as 10 to 12% of its total length and still have the tissue remain grossly intact.

Tendons and ligaments

As previously alluded to, the periosteum is attached relatively loosely to the diaphysis, and its external surface serves as the attachment (origin) of muscle units (both muscle fibers and encircling mysial sheaths). The muscle tissues usually do not originate directly from the developing osseous surface, and with the exception of a few areas such as the medial distal femur, they never develop a direct relationship with mature osseous tissue, although soft tissue components contiguous with the muscle fibers may have fairly rigid relationships. The most obvious example is the linea aspera. Even in a child, the periosteum is densely attached along this structure, and must be elevated by sharp dissection in contrast to the ease with which the majority of the periosteum can be elevated.

In the metaphyseal region, the periosteum is more densely attached to the underlying bone, and also blends continuously into the epiphyseal perichondrium and physeal zone of Ranvier. These latter regions are densely contiguous with the underlying physeal and epiphyseal cartilage. Ligaments and tendons insert, for the most part, into these fibrous and fibrocartilaginous regions, and not directly into the osseous tissue of the metaphysis or secondary ossification center (Fig. 2-28). Such attachment mechanisms not only allow active, integrated growth of muscular and chondro-osseous structures, but also permit a tensile-responsive unit, such as a ligament or tendon, to insert into a similarly tensile-responsive component of the developing skeleton, rather than directly into bone, which is characteristically more susceptible to failure in tension. Such an arrangement allows progressive, rather than abrupt, gradations of moduli of elasticity.

Only with progressive skeletal maturation, especially in the epiphyses, do the characteristic Sharpey's fibers develop. These are collagen continuities between tendon or ligament and cortical bone. These differing and developing interrelationships between soft tissue and chondro-osseous compo-

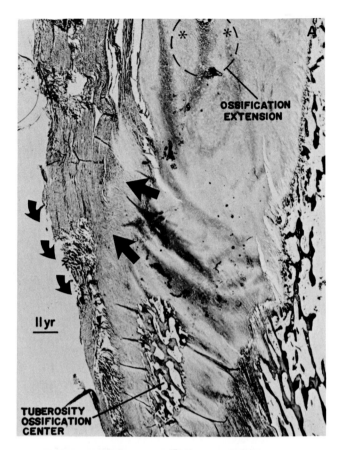

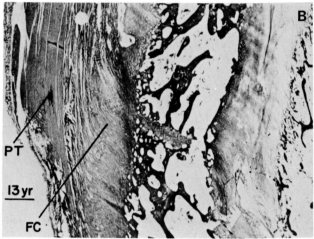

FIG. 2-28. Insertion of patellar tendon (PT) into chondro-osseous epiphysis of the tibial tuberosity. *A,* Section from an 11-year-old with early ossification center formation in the distal end of the tuberosity. *B,* More mature ossification in a 13-year-old. Note the blending of tendon fibers into the hyaline cartilage in *A* (large arrows) and the continuity of the tendon with the perichondrium/periosteum complex (small arrows). As the epiphyseal ossification center matures further, the tendon fibers blend into fibrocartilage (FC), which then blends into the ossification center. This is the initial step in the formation of the Sharpey's fibers of an adult. Ligament insertion into a chondrous or chondro-osseous epiphysis is similar to tendon insertion.

nents are major factors in the tendency toward soft tissue/bone interface avulsion in the adult and intra-osseous failure in a child. For example, a child will avulse the tibial spine, whereas an adult will avulse the cruciate ligament, either at the insertion or within the ligament proper. If skeletal chondro-osseous transformation progresses more rapidly than the normal adaptive response patterns, failure may result, as in Osgood-Schlatter's disease (see Chaps. 4 and 19).

References

1. Gardner, E.: Osteogenesis in the human embryo and fetus. *In* The Biochemistry and Physiology of Bone. Edited by G. Bourne. New York, Academic Press, 1971.

2. Jaffe, H. L.: Metabolic, Degenerative and Inflammatory Diseases of Bones and Joints. Philadelphia, Lea & Febiger, 1972.

3. Lacroix, P.: The Organization of Bone. London, J. & A. Churchill, 1951.

4. Ogden, J. A.: Development of the epiphyses. *In* Orthopaedic Surgery in Infancy and Childhood. Edited by A. B. Ferguson. Baltimore, Williams & Wilkins, 1975.

5. Ogden, J. A.: The development and growth of the musculoskeletal system. *In* The Scientific Basis of Orthopaedics. Edited by J. A. Albright, and R. A. Brand. New York, Appleton-Century-Crofts, 1979.

6. Ogden, J. A.: Chondro-osseous development and growth. *In* Fundamental and Clinical Bone Physiology. Edited by M. R. Urist. Philadelphia, J. B. Lippincott, 1980.

7. O'Rahilly, R., and Gardner, E.: The timing and sequence of events in the development of the limbs in the human embryo. Anat. Embryol., *148:*1, 1975.

8. O'Rahilly, R., and Gardner, E.: The embryology of movable joints. *In* The Joints and Synovial Fluid. Edited by L. Sokoloff. Vol. 10. New York, Academic Press, 1978.

9. Ogden, J. A.: Injury to the immature skeleton. *In* Pediatric Trauma. Edited by R. Touloukian. New York, John Wiley & Sons, 1978.

10. Alexander, C. J.: Effect of growth rate on the strength of the growth plate shaft junction. Skeletal Radiol., *1:*67, 1976.

11. Siffert, R. S.: The growth plate and its affections. J. Bone Joint Surg., *48-A:*546, 1966.

12. Siffert, R. S.: The effect of trauma to the epiphysis and growth plate. Skeletal Radiol., *2:*21, 1977.

13. McKibbin, B., and Holdsworth, F.: The dual nature of epiphyseal cartilage. J. Bone Joint Surg., *49-B:*351, 1967.

14. Rang, M.: The Growth Plate and Its Disorders. Baltimore, Williams & Wilkins, 1969.

15. Hall-Craggs, E.: Influence of epiphyses on the regulation of bone growth. Nature, *221:*1245, 1969.

16. Hall-Craggs, E.: The effect of experimental epiphyseodesis on growth in length of the rabbit tibia. J. Bone Joint Surg., *50-B:*392, 1968.

17. Lufti, A. M.: The role of cartilage in long bone growth: a reappraisal. J. Anat., *117:*413, 1974.

18. Ogden, J. A., Hempton, R., and Southwick, W.: Development of the tibial tuberosity. Anat. Rec., *182:*431, 1975.

19. Haines, R. W.: The pseudoepiphysis of the first metacarpal in man. J. Anat., *117:*145, 1974.

20. Dodds, G.: Row formation and other types of arrangements of cartilage cells in endochondral ossification. Anat. Rec., *46:*385, 1930.

21. Gardner, E., and Gray, D.: The prenatal development of the human femur. Am. J. Anat., *129:*121, 1970.

22. Von der Mark, K., and Von der Mark, H.: The role of three genetically distinct collagen types in endochondral ossification and calcification of cartilage. J. Bone Joint Surg., *59-B:*458, 1977.

23. Crelin, E., and Koch, W.: An autoradiographic study of chondrocyte transformation into chondroblasts and osteocytes during bone formation in vitro. Anat. Rec., *158:*473, 1967.

24. Digby, K.: The measurement of diaphyseal growth in proximal and distal directions. J. Anat. Physiol., *50:*187, 1915.

25. Hert, J.: Growth of the epiphyseal plate in circumference. Acta Anat. (Basel), *82:*420, 1972.

26. Shapiro, F., Holtrop, M., and Glimcher, M.: Organization and cellular biology of the perichondrial ossification groove of Ranvier. J. Bone Joint Surg., *59-A:*703, 1977.

27. Rose, S., Bradley, T. R., and Nelson, J. F.: Factors influencing the growth of epiphyseal cartilage. Aust. J. Exp. Biol. Med. Sci., *44:*57, 1966.

28. Simmons, D. J.: Chronobiology of endochondral ossification. Chronobiologia, *1:*97, 1974.

29. Edvardson, P., and Syversen, S. M.: Overgrowth of the femur after fractures of the shaft in childhood. J. Bone Joint Surg., *58-B:*339, 1976.

30. Jenkins, D. H., Cheng, D. H., and Hodgson, A. R.: Stimulation of bone growth by periosteal stripping. J. Bone Joint Surg., *57-B:*482, 1975.

31. Keck, S. W., and Kelly, P. J.: The effect of venous stasis on intra-osseous pressure and longitudinal bone growth in the dog. J. Bone Joint Surg., *47-A:*539, 1965.

32. Reidy, J. A., Lingley, J. R., Gall, E. A., and Barr, J. S.: The effect of roentgen irradiation on epiphyseal growth. J. Bone Joint Surg., *29:*853, 1947.

33. Ring, P. A.: The influence of the nervous system upon the growth of bones. J. Bone Joint Surg., *43-B:*121, 1961.

34. Rohlig, H.: Periost und Langenwachstum. Beitr. Orthop. Traumatol., *13:*604, 1966.

35. Sola, C. K., Silberman, F. S., and Cabrini, R. L.: Stimulation of the longitudinal growth of long bones by periosteal stripping. J. Bone Joint Surg., *45-A:*1679, 1963.

36. Weinman, D. T., Kelly, P. J., and Owen, C. A.: Blood flow in bone distal to a femoral arteriovenous fistula in dogs. J. Bone Joint Surg., *46-A:*1676, 1964.

37. Haines, R. W.: The histology of epiphyseal union in mammals. J. Anat., *120:*1, 1975.

38. Brodin, H.: Longitudinal bone growth. The nutrition of the epiphyseal cartilages and the local blood supply. Acta Orthop. Scand., Suppl. 29, 1955.

39. Brookes, M.: The Blood Supply of Bone. New York, Appleton-Century-Crofts, 1971.

40. Trueta, J., and Morgan, J. D.: The vascular contribution to osteogenesis. J. Bone Joint Surg., *42-B:*97, 1960.

41. Trueta, J., and Cavadias, A. X.: A study of the blood supply of the long bones. Surg. Gynecol. Obstet., *118:*485, 1964.

42. Trueta, J.: Studies of the Development and Decay of the Human Frame. Philadelphia, W. B. Saunders, 1968.

43. Trueta, J.: Bone growth. Mod. Trends Orthop., *5:*196, 1972.

44. Haines, R. W.: Cartilage canals. J. Anat., *68:*45, 1933.

45. Carter, D. R., and Spengler, D. M.: Mechanical properties and composition of cortical bone. Clin. Orthop., *135:*192, 1978.

46. Enlow, D. H.: The functional significance of the secondary osteon. Anat. Rec., *142:*230, 1962.

47. Pauwels, F.: Eine klinische Beobachtung als Beispiel und Beweis fur funktionelle Anpassung des Knochens durch Langenwachstum. Z. Orthop., *113:*1, 1975.

48. Porter, R. W.: The effect of tension across a growing epiphysis. J. Bone Joint Surg., *60-B:*252, 1978.

49. Strobino, L. J., French, G. O., and Colonna, P. C.: The effect of increasing tensions on the growth of epiphyseal bone. Surg. Gynecol. Obstet., *95:*694, 1952.

50. Haas, S. L.: Retardation of bone growth by a wire loop. J. Bone Joint Surg., *27:*25, 1945.

51. Hert, J.: Acceleration of the growth after decrease of load on epiphyseal plates by means of spring distractors. Folia Morphol. (Praha), *17:*194, 1969.

52. Kessel, L.: Annotations on the etiology and treatment of tibia vara. J. Bone Joint Surg., *52-B:*93, 1970.
53. Sijbrandij, S.: De invloed van mechanische factoren op de groei van de epifysaire schijf, in het bijzonder bij genua valga en genua vara. Ned. Tijdschr. Geneeskd., *116:*1363, 1972.
54. Warrell, E., and Taylor, J. F.: The effect of trauma on tibial growth. J. Bone Joint Surg., *58-B:*375, 1976.
55. Thompson, D. W.: On Growth and Form. Cambridge, University Press, 1942.
56. Poland, J.: Traumatic Separation of the Epiphyses. London, Smith, Elder, and Co., 1898.
57. Bright, R. W., and Elmore, S. M.: Physical properties of epiphyseal plate cartilage. Surg. Forum, *19:*463, 1968.
58. Crilly, R. G.: Longitudinal overgrowth of chicken radius. J. Anat., *112:*11, 1972.
59. Hirsch, C., and Evans, F.: Studies on some physical properties of infant compact bone. Acta Orthop. Scand., *35:*300, 1965.
60. Vinz, H.: Die Festigheit der reinen Knochensubstanz. Naherungsverfahren zur Bestimmung der auf den hohlraumfreien Querschnitt bezogenen Festigkeit von Knochengewebe. Gegenbaurs Morphol. Jahrb., *117:*453, 1972.
61. Currey, J. B.: Differences in tensile strength of bone of different histology types. J. Anat., *93:*87, 1959.
62. Currey, J. B., and Butler, G.: The mechanical properties of bone tissues in children. J. Bone Joint Surg., *57-A:*810, 1975.
63. Black, J., Mattson, R., and Korotsoff, E.: Haversian osteons: size, distribution, internal structure, and orientation. J. Biomed. Mater. Res., *8:*299, 1974.
64. Hert, J., Kucera, P., Vavra, M., and Volenik, V.: Comparison of the mechanical properties of both primary and Haversian bone tissue. Acta Anat. (Basel), *61:*412, 1965.
65. Simkin, A., and Robin, G.: Fracture formation in differing collagen fiber pattern of compact bone. J. Biomech., *7:*183, 1974.
66. Maj, F.: Osservazioni sulla differeze topographiche della resistenze meccanica del tessuto osseo di uno stesso segmento schletrico. Monitore Zool. Ital., *49:*139, 1938.
67. Toajari, E.: Resistenze meccanica et elastica del tessuto oddeo studiata in rapporto alla meniche struttura. Monitore Zool. Ital., *48:*178, 1938.
68. Ascenzi, A., and Bonucci, E.: The tensile properties of single osteons. Anat. Rec., *158:*375, 1967.
69. Ascenzi, A., and Bonucci, E.: The compressive properties of single osteons. Anat. Rec., *161:*377, 1968.
70. Evans, F. G., and Vincentelli, R.: Relation of the compressive properties of human cortical bone to histological structure and calcification. J. Biomech., *7:*1, 1974.
71. Panjabi, M. M., White, A. A., and Southwick, W. O.: Mechanical properties of bone as a function of rate of deformation. J. Bone Joint Surg., *55-A:*322, 1973.
72. Smith, J. W., and Walmsley, R.: Factors affecting the elasticity of bone. J. Anat., *93:*503, 1959.
73. Chamay, A.: Mechanical and morphological aspects of experimental overload and fatigue in bone. J. Biomech., *3:*263, 1970.
74. Chamay, A., and Tschantz, P.: Mechanical influences in bone remodeling. Experimental research on Wolff's law. J. Biomech., *5:*173, 1972.
75. Borden, S.: Roentgen recognition of acute plastic bowing of the forearm in children. A. J. R., *125:*524, 1975.
76. Manoli, A., II: Traumatic fibular bowing with tibial fracture: report of two cases. Orthopedics, *1:*145, 1978.

3

Radiologic Aspects

Radiology is extremely important in the evaluation of chondro-osseous trauma involving the developing skeleton. However, fractures in children are not always easy to visualize radiographically. Roentgenograms must be of sufficiently good technical quality to adequately elucidate not only the grossly evident skeletal trauma, but also the normal and distorted soft tissue contours, the fascial planes, and the intra-articular fat-fluid levels in appropriate cases.[1-3] Technically poor films should never be accepted. Standard positional radiographs (anteroposterior and lateral) must be supplemented, as indicated, with appropriate oblique views and special procedures.

Ultimately, the diagnostic proof of a fracture is roentgenographic demonstration. During the entire process of skeletal maturation, there are many pitfalls to avoid when evaluating radiograms. Fractures will be missed if proper views are not requested, particularly in children. It is imperative to get as many views as necessary to absolutely rule out a fracture, as well as to define differences in the anatomy. Efforts must be made to appreciate the wide variety of fractures that may occur in children as a result of various biologic responses to trauma at different ages.

Roentgenographic Evaluation

The roentgenographic evaluation of chondro-osseous injury must be based on a thorough knowledge of changing anatomy and response patterns in the developing skeleton. The importance of an orderly approach to the differential diagnosis of childhood skeletal trauma cannot be overemphasized. Even in the case of a simple fracture, care must be taken to thoroughly evaluate other areas, such as the joints above and below the injury, the soft tissue (for possible complications), and the extent of the injury to the opposite of two paired bones when one is not obviously fractured. In particular, it is easy to overlook plastic deformation of the ulna or fibula, or dislocation of the radial or fibular head, any of which injuries may cause major difficulties in anatomic

reduction, healing, and subsequent rehabilitation, and lead to significant growth deformity.

Unfortunately, when the skeletal elements are incompletely shown, as when the epiphysis is still partially or completely cartilaginous, or when a specific injury is seen infrequently, as is the case with less common types of fractures of the developing skeleton, few individuals will have sufficient diagnostic experience, and a systematized, correlative examination and review of clinical and radiographic findings will be absolutely essential.

Adequate films

In general, any bone *must* be visualized in at least two views, these ideally being true anteroposterior and lateral projections 90° apart. Nonstandard projections, while sometimes unavoidable because of pain, displacement, or limitation of motion, are treacherous, because the variable radiographic appearances of normal structures, especially the epiphyseal ossification patterns, may confuse even an experienced person. Improperly positioned films may place the physis in an unusual projection, making it appear fractured to the inexperienced eye.[4]

Not all injuries to the developing skeleton are readily evident in standard views. Minimally displaced areas of the lateral or medial condyles of the distal humerus, as well as the tibial and fibular malleoli, may be obscured by overlapping bone and thus not easily visualized by routine radiographs. Oblique radiographs often will show fractures not readily evident on standard views. They are particularly helpful in interpreting degrees of displacement in phalangeal fractures of the finger.

It is imperative that the joints above and below a fracture be radiographed so that the complete chondro-osseous unit(s) can be seen, since dislocations, especially those of the hip or radial head, are not uncommon in association with diaphyseal fractures.

The extremity must be adequately splinted and protected *prior* to sending the child for roentgenographic evaluation. While it may seem axiomatic, the physician must state that the *entire* arm be rotated to assess a forearm fracture. Otherwise, the technician may simply turn the unprotected distal region 90°, leaving the rest of the arm in the original position. This problem is encountered in supracondylar humeral fractures as well.

Comparison views

Radiographs may demonstrate the injury adequately, but since the appearance of displaced epiphyses may be quite subtle, the inexperienced observer may not recognize the injury initially. Sometimes a comparison view is necessary. In many hospitals it has become common practice to obtain comparison views of the contralateral extremity as a way of differentiating fractures from growth variants. *This generally is unnecessary*, particularly when the films are interpreted by someone with sufficient experience. In most cases, this practice only exposes the child to unnecessary additional radiation. Furthermore, there may be asymmetric epiphyseal ossification, which might confuse, rather than clarify. When an inexperienced observer must make the immediate interpretation of the film, or when sufficient doubt exists, comparison films are warranted, if only to avoid excessive confusion, multiple re-examinations, and inappropriate treatment.

Soft tissues

All of the normal soft tissues of the extremities, except adipose tissue, absorb x-rays to a similar degree and cast shadows of approximately equal radiodensity.[2] The nonfatty soft tissues, including epiphyseal cartilage, appear roentgenographically as a uniform, composite shadow with a density intermediate between the heavier density of the underlying bone, and the lighter density of the overlying subcutaneous fat. Adipose tissue has a specific gravity of 0.92, and is more radiolucent than the other soft tissues.[5] The shadows of fatty tissues may serve as a contrast density, partially outlining the margins of other, more dense soft tissues. The external margins of muscular masses often are clearly delineated by the overlying and intervening envelopes of more radiolucent fat. The large fat pads near the elbows, knees, and ankles may outline contiguous epiphyses, tendons, bursae, and muscular bundles. Injury to such soft tissues is frequently concomitant to fractures, and should be assessed as accurately as possible as part of the roentgenographic evaluation of the injury.[1,3]

Interstitial and intra-articular gas shadows

Gas in the soft tissues casts shadows of variable radiolucency. Air may be introduced through a wound (Fig. 3-1) or gas may be generated subsequently by various types of opportunistic bacteria. After traumatic lacerations, the presence of gas in the contiguous soft tissues always raises the question of gas gangrene. Gas shadows *may* develop in subcutaneous planes of many traumatized patients without any clinical or bacteriologic evidence of infection. The gas that enters the soft tissues from local lacerations is primarily subcutaneous, while the gas generated in clostridial infections tends to be within the muscular masses, and is usually accompanied by considerable edema of the skin and the superficial soft tissues. Wounds penetrating a joint may introduce

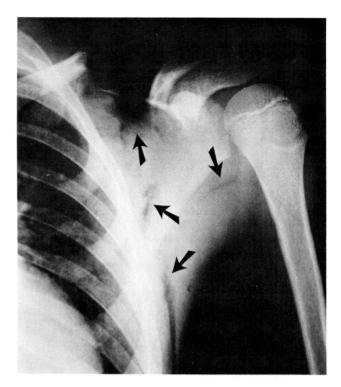

FIG. 3-1. Subcutaneous gas shadows throughout clavicular and subscapular tissues (arrows) secondary to severe open injury with fracture of clavicle and avulsion of brachial plexus at root level. The thoracic cavity was not injured.

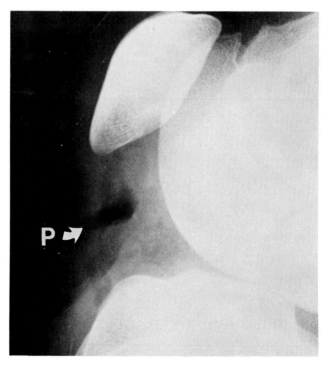

FIG. 3-2. Injury to knee of a 12-year-old boy. A small puncture wound was present (P). The penetration tract has introduced air into the knee (arrow). Arthrotomy also revealed damage to the articular surface.

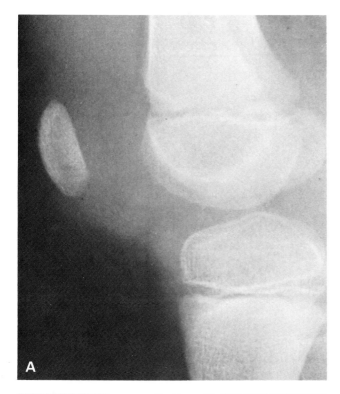

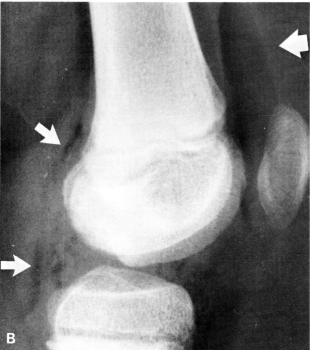

FIG. 3-3. Elevation of patella from hemarthrosis and joint effusion. *A,* Cartilage from the medial femoral condyle was floating in the joint. Since the subchondral plate was intact, no significant fat and marrow elements were present in the reactive fluid. *B,* Fat and marrow elements (large arrow) create a more lucent appearance than the reactive effusion in this boy, who had a relatively undisplaced type 1 fracture of the distal femoral physis. Similar radiolucencies are present in the posterior joint (small arrows).

air (Fig. 3-2), a factor that definitely confirms the diagnosis of an open joint injury, especially when the overlying skin lesion appears innocuous.

Intracapsular fat-fluid level

A fat-fluid level sometimes occurs in the knee if a fracture involves the articular surface of the femur or tibia, thus allowing the passage of fat and blood from the bone marrow into the joint. Although the fracture itself may be difficult or impossible to demonstrate radiographically, a definite diagnosis of fracture is possible because of the presence of liquid fat and fat-fluid interface in the suprapatellar region. The liquid intracapsular fat may be observed floating on the blood and joint fluid, which has the density of water (Fig. 3-3).

Fat pads

Minimally displaced fractures of the supracondylar region, the condyles, the epicondyles, and the radial head may be difficult to detect in the routine radiographic studies of the elbow. However, periarticular soft tissues may show swelling, thus allowing an accurate diagnosis.

Fairly large extracapsular pads of fat are present over the olecranon fossa, the coronoid fossa, and the radial fossa (Fig. 3-4). From the normal anatomic position, the dorsal (posterior) fat pad cannot be visualized in a roentgenogram. It is lodged in the olecranon fossa and overshadowed by bone, even in the lateral view. This does not apply as much to the pads of fat in the coronoid (anterior) and radial fossae, which are more shallow. Due to the differences in absorption of fat, muscular tissue, and bone, some of this fat is readily recognizable in routine radiographs. The anterior fat pads, which fit into the coronoid-radial fossae, are seen in a single triangular area of radiolucency in the lateral flexion view of the normal elbow.

Displacement of these fat pads appears to be related to the extent of bleeding, both intracapsularly as well as subperiosteally. This latter process in particular pushes the dorsal fat pad further posteriorly, so that it becomes more easily evident radiographically. Norell[6] erroneously described the dorsal fat as extracapsular. Bledsoe[7] showed that the pads of fat are, in actuality, extrasynovial, but intracapsular.

Norell[6] studied over 300 normal children with and without elbow trauma, and found that invariably the roentgenographic fat pad on the dorsal aspect of the humerus was diagnostic of injury, whereas a fairly thin, elongated layer of fat was consistently observed along the antecubital aspect in both injured and uninjured children.

When displaced, the posterior fat pad may be seen as a radiolucent area posterior to the humerus at the upper border of the olecranon fossa (Fig. 3-5). Traumatic rupture of the synovial membrane and articular capsule may permit intra-articular fluid to escape into the surrounding soft tissues, so that there is no synovial distension, and consequently, no roentgenographically evident displacement of the posterior fat pad. A fracture involving portions of the bone outside the limits of the synovial membrane does not necessarily produce synovial effusions, since the fracture may not communicate with the joint. Displacement of the fat pad is not necessarily concomitant to all fractures in the elbow region.

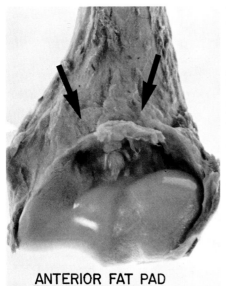

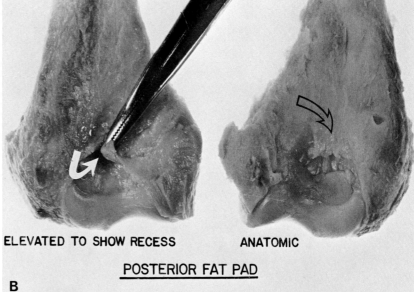

ELEVATED TO SHOW RECESS   ANATOMIC

ANTERIOR FAT PAD   POSTERIOR FAT PAD

A   B

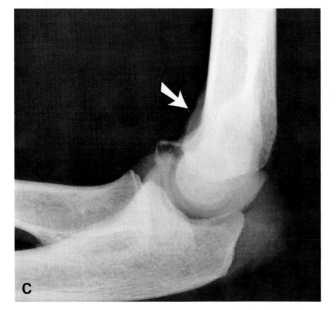

C

FIG. 3-4. Specimens of distal humerus from a six-year-old boy showing, *A,* anterior and, *B,* posterior fat pads. *C,* Roentgenogram of dissected specimen (fat left intact) showing normal location of anterior fat extending beyond fossa (arrow), while large posterior fat pad is not evident in the normal anatomic position.

Foreign bodies

Opaque foreign bodies of sufficient size to be readily detected radiographically frequently are found following seemingly insignificant trauma in children (Fig. 3-6). Fragments of lead-containing glass may be visible in the more radiolucent areas of skin, muscle, and joints (Fig. 3-7). Small, minimally radiopaque, foreign bodies may be invisible in the standard, heavily penetrated film made for the demonstration of bone detail, and they will become visible only on special, soft tissue exposures made with lower voltage. Many non-radiopaque foreign bodies are invisible because they have water density similar to the surrounding tissues.

Metallic foreign bodies in soft tissue, whether introduced accidentally or surgically, may remain at the original site of introduction, or may move considerable distances away with little or no disability to the patient. It is likely that the localized resorption of bone around the foreign body allows the movement to start, and then muscular forces probably propagate the migration. Migrating foreign bodies that are sharp should be removed as soon as their movement is detected, although it is not always imperative to remove them at the time of injury, especially if extensive dissection is necessary. Fluoroscopy is useful when attempting to remove these objects.

Roentgenographic response to trauma

Even in bone, the initial fracture lines may be difficult to demonstrate radiographically in children. Since the bones of children are relatively pliable, they do not sustain the same fracture patterns, especially in comminution, as they do later in life. Incomplete cortical disruptions are common in children, and may not be visualized well on initial roentgenograms (Fig. 3-8). The first roentgenographic sign of a fracture may be callus formation. The actual fracture line may never be discerned. Stress or ''march'' fractures may be manifested by pain with or without periosteal reaction; again, the fracture line itself may never be visible.

Whether the inciting injury is located in the metaphyseal, diaphyseal, or even juxtaphyseal regions, the new bone that forms at the cortical periphery in response to fracture takes the form of two basic patterns.[7a,7b] These may be described radiographically as either solid or interrupted (Fig. 3-9). Solid periosteal reaction is of uniform density, and the entire sheet of old periosteal and new subperiosteal bone looks the same on routine radiologic examination. The newly formed

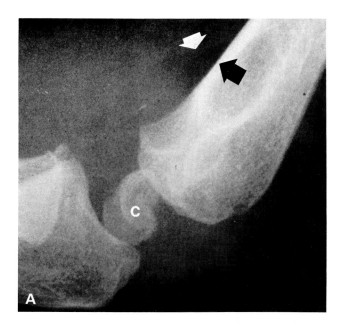

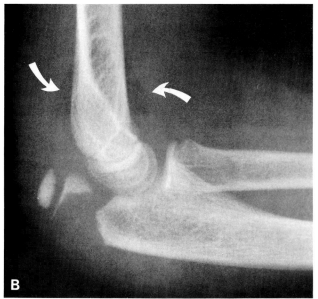

FIG. 3-5. *A*, Positive sign of anterior fat pad (arrows) in a boy with a type 3 capitellar fracture (C). No posterior fat pad was evident. *B*, Anterior and posterior fat pad signs (arrows) in a 10-year-old with a fracture of the olecranon.

bone is deposited as the result of periosteal reaction to trauma and has an even, uniform appearance. After several weeks, the subperiosteal new bone gradually becomes indistinguishable from the antecedent cortical bone. Thickness seems to be related to: the degree of trauma, the amount of periosteal stripping due to displacement of the bone relative to the periosteum, and the possible presence of factors promoting increased subperiosteal hemorrhage (e.g., hemophilia).

In contrast, interrupted periosteal reactions are pleomorphic, with varying roentgenographic patterns. Lamellar (onion-skin) or perpendicular (sunburst) periosteal reac-

tions are classic examples (Fig. 3-10), and are often encountered in neoplastic or infectious disorders, from which they must be diagnostically differentiated. They may occur consequent to fracture-induced hemorrhage, particularly in the neonate or in the metaphyseal regions of older children, in whom the normal as well as the trauma-responsive bone formation occurring in the thin metaphyseal cortex tends to be more irregular than that occurring in the diaphyseal fracture response. This response is also caused by repeated hemorrhage, which can easily occur with the repetitive trauma of child abuse or sensory neuropathy (e.g., myelodysplasia or congenital insensitivity to pain).

Roentgenographic Appearance of the Developing Skeleton

The ossified portions of the growing bone cast radiopaque shadows of variable density, whereas the noncalcified skeletal components (i.e., chondroepiphyses) cast shadows that are virtually impossible to distinguish from the contiguous soft tissues of comparable water density.[5,8,9,9a-c] Depending upon the degree of skeletal maturation, cortical bone varies considerably in thickness, especially at the metaphyseal/diaphyseal junction. The central diaphyseal spongiosa and the primary and secondary metaphyseal spongiosa appear as tightly meshed networks of linear shadows that always are partially obscured by heavier, superimposed shadows of cortical bone. The peripheral spongiosa and the cortices of the metaphysis fuse with the central spongiosa at the ends of the bones. Along the borders of the medullary canal, the peripheral spongiosa may give rise to a roughening of the endosteal surface of the cortex, or it may be invisible (Fig. 3-11).

The uncalcified, unossified portions of the growing bone (epiphyses and physes) cast shadows similar to those of the surrounding soft tissues and usually are difficult to visualize, except when there is a fluid or gas of different density adja-

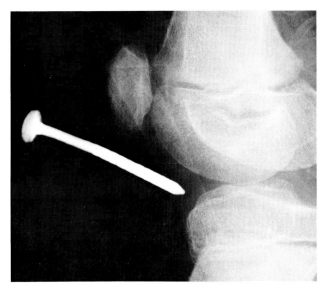

FIG. 3-6. Roentgenogram of an 11-year-old boy who fell on a piece of wood with a protruding nail (the wood is not evident). No air has entered the joint.

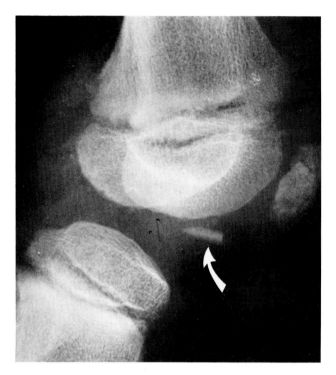

FIG. 3-7. Lateral roentgenogram of an eight-year-old girl who fell on a piece of glass, which she claimed did not enter her knee. The film showed that a small piece of the glass, sufficiently radiopaque (arrow), had entered the joint.

cent to the cartilage (e.g., blood, fatty marrow, or air in a joint consequent to trauma). Infrequently the cartilage may be outlined in a routine film (Fig. 3-12).

Radiographic demonstration of epiphyseal cartilage

Part of the diagnostic problem is our present inability to obtain radiographs of the cartilaginous portions of the skeleton (Fig. 3-13).[10] There have been repeated attempts, such as those by Gordon,[11] to use experimental methods to delineate the cartilage by taking advantage of potential contrast between cartilage, bone, and joint fluid. However, these have proved neither technically feasible nor clinically applicable.

Placing the joint under angular or longitudinal stress may cause a "vacuum" phenomenon, with a radiolucent line following the cartilage contours (see Fig. 3-12). This is due to cavitation of dissolved gases within the joint fluid. Arthrography, which will be discussed later in this chapter, is not always feasible in the acute injury, since hemarthrosis may interfere.

Radiography of growth plate

As previously emphasized, the radiographic evaluation of any skeletal injury requires, at the minimum, two views. Epiphyseal injuries occasionally may be seen in only one, not necessarily standard, projection. Rogers[12] reported 15 to 20% of such injuries being evident only in an oblique view, rather than the standard anteroposterior and lateral views. The majority of epiphyseal injuries are manifested by dis-

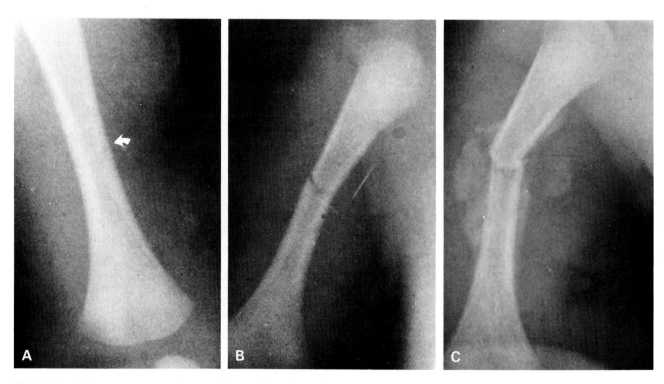

FIG. 3-8. *A,* Roentgenogram taken two hours after traumatic birth. The nutrient foramen is evident (arrow), but no fracture is obvious. *B,* Two days later, a lateral cortical lucency is noted. The angle of the lucency duplicates the nutrient foramen. However, the nutrient foramen, while almost at the same level, is a medial structure. *C,* Ten days later, angulation and completion of the transverse fracture are evident, and massive amounts of callus are forming.

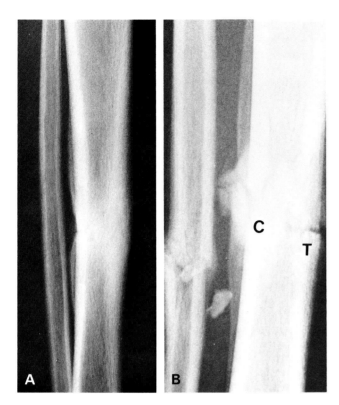

FIG. 3-9. *A,* Early subperiosteal new bone formation three weeks after a fracture. Note that no bone formation is evident at the fracture site where the periosteum presumably was disrupted. *B,* Similar patient five weeks after combined tibiofibular fracture. A solid sheet of bone is traversing the fracture sites on the compression (C) side, but is not yet complete on the tension (T) side.

placement of the shaft relative to the secondary ossification center, as well as by widening of the growth plate. However, widening of the physis may be extremely difficult to interpret, depending upon the size of the secondary ossification center relative to the entire epiphysis (i.e., the secondary ossification center has not yet formed a definitive subchondral plate). The greater the displacement, the more evident the injury. However, at times, both displacement or widening of the plate are minimal, necessitating comparative views of the opposite extremity. A detailed discussion of injuries to the various growth regions is in Chapter 4.

Teates[4] described an 18-year-old man in whom a remnant of the growth plate was misinterpreted as an acute fracture. This can be done easily, particularly if true lateral and anteroposterior views are not obtained. Oblique views, such as semi-supination, may result in growth plate remnant appearing much closer to the joint than it actually is. The growth plate tends to persist laterally (peripherally) in the major epiphyses during the last stages of physiologic epiphysiodesis (Fig. 3-14). If the position of the plate is unusual, or if the plate persists an unusually long time after closure, an erroneous diagnosis of fracture may be made.

In the type 2 injury, a triangular fragment of the metaphysis (Thurston Holland sign) accompanies a displaced

epiphysis, and aids in the demonstration of the injury. Werenskiöld[13] emphasized the presence of a thin flake or lamella of bone accompanying the epiphysis. The flake is detached from the metaphysis and lies within or near the epiphyseal line. This lamellar sign differs from the corner sign of Thurston-Holland in its size and position. The corner sign (triangular metaphyseal fragment) is created, in part, by a compressive failure on the side of the fulcrum. In contrast, the lamellar sign, formed more by an avulsive force, is found on the tension failure side opposite the fulcrum (Fig. 3-15). In general, the greater the epiphyseal displacement, the larger the metaphyseal fragment. If the fragment is small, the displacement tends to be less. If the only evidence is widening of the growth plate, a transverse lamella may exist.

Nutrient canals

Nutrient canals enter the bones in reasonably predictable anatomic regions (Fig. 3-16). Usually there is one canal per diaphysis. However, the humerus and femur may have two canals. Nutrient canals appear as roentgenographic "de-

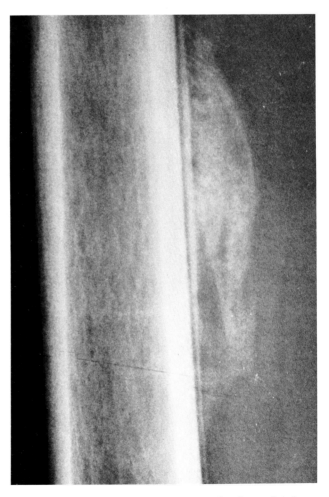

FIG. 3-10. The response to trauma in this femur has been the formation of an initial layer of layered, solid bone, followed by formation of a more irregular area of bone. This eventually formed myositis ossificans.

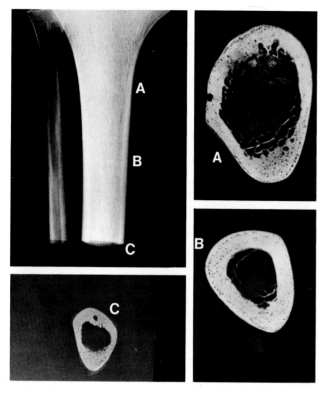

FIG. 3-11. Anteroposterior and cross-sectional (slab) roentgenographs showing the difficulty in visualizing endosteal bone when the cortical bone is increasingly dense.

fects" in the cortical bone. When a nutrient canal is projected in profile, its oblique channel through the cortex can be demonstrated clearly. However, in other projections, the nutrient canals are partially or completely obscured by the heavy shadow of the cortex surrounding them. These canals may be extremely misleading and highly suggestive of fracture, particularly if visualized in nonstandard views.

Plastic deformation

If a longitudinal compression force is applied to each end of a naturally curved, tubular bone, the curvature is increased and the ends of the bone are approximated slightly. Up to a certain point, the bone responds (deforms) in an elastic manner, and loses all such deformation once the force is removed (see Chap. 2).

Laboratory investigations have confirmed these elastic and plastic responses in the normal dog ulna, both in vitro and in vivo.[14,15] Skeletally immature canine bones stressed at forces within the range of elastic deformation were histologically normal. With progressive stresses, microscopic fatigue lines (microfractures) were documented in increasing numbers. These prefracture lines were oblique, found only in areas of maximum compression of cortical and heavy trabecular bone, and oriented at approximately 30° to the longitudinal axis of the bone. These shear lines varied in length and were independent of the lamellar structure, often traversing the entire periosteum to the medullary cavity. They were found to parallel zones of fragmentations within the bone architecture and to represent areas of incomplete bone shearing. Broad, plastic curvatures of 15 to 30° were produced routinely in these otherwise normal dog ulnae. In

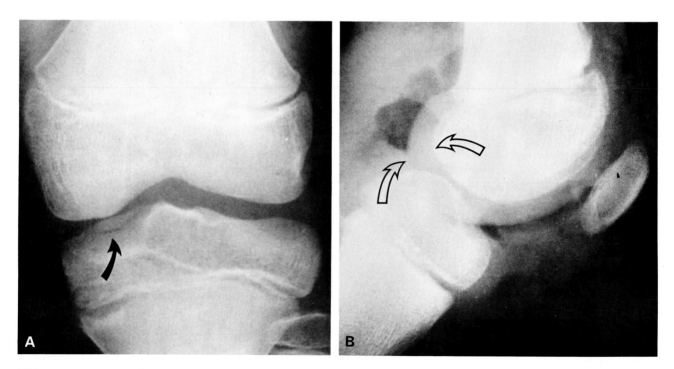

FIG. 3-12. *A*, Stress film of an adolescent with an injured knee reveals a "vacuum arthrogram" phenomenon (arrow) delineating the articular surface and contour of the medial femoral condylar cartilage. Initially, this was mistaken for a fracture. *B*, Delineation of femoral epiphyseal cartilage (arrows) in a patient with an open knee injury.

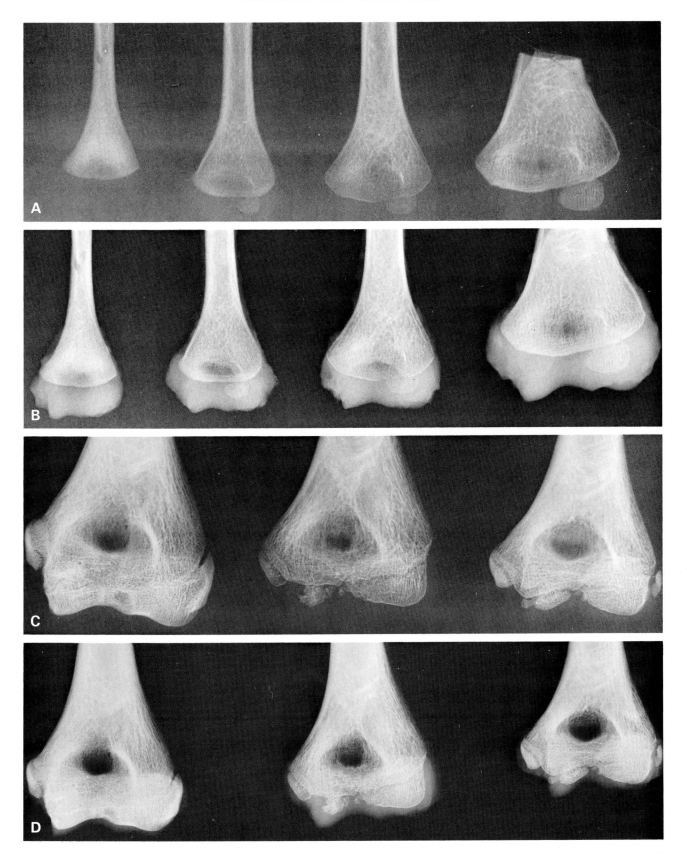

FIG. 3-13. Roentgenograms taken, *A,* under water and, *B,* with air interfacing in specimens from children aged newborn, 15 months, 24 months, and 36 months. The water immersion films duplicate the clinical situation of radiolucent cartilage. *C-D,* Similar films taken of children aged 14, 11, and 10 years (left to right).

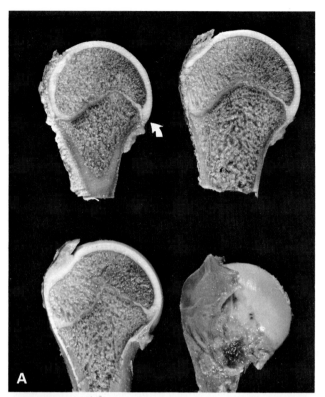

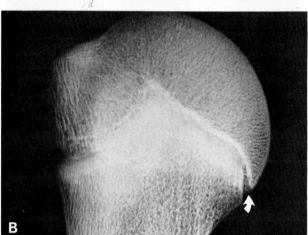

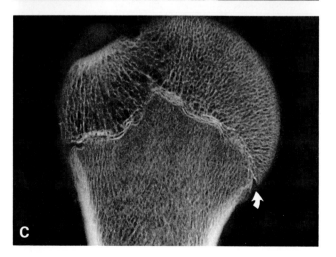

FIG. 3-14. *A,* Slab sections of proximal humerus from a 14-year-old girl. Notice the different contours of the physis at different depths. The physis is closing centrally, but remains open peripherally (arrow). *B,* Roentgenogram of entire specimen. Again, note central closure with the peripheral area still open (arrow). *C,* Roentgenogram of central slab. Again, note the closure of the physis centrally, with some peripheral function. Also note the differences among the trabecular patterns of the greater tuberosity, the capital tuberosity, and the capital humerus.

those bones with plastic curvatures, microscopic sections showed prefracture lines in the concave cortex, hemorrhaging in the periosteum, and less than 5% enlargement of the diaphyseal shaft diameter. No roentgenographic periosteal reaction was found up to two months after plastic deformation.

Traumatic bowing of forearm bones (Fig. 3-17) or the fibulae in children, while not generally recognized as a significant clinical problem until recently, is a definite manifestation of trauma that may occur because of the plastic deformation capacity of developing bones.[16] Borden[17] felt that the biomechanics of plastic deformation explained traumatic bowing. He described eight children with traumatic bowing of the forearm bones. None of these patients had evidence of subsequent, responsive subperiosteal new bone formation, although this certainly may occur. Traumatic bowing also may occur in the fibula when the tibia fractures.[16]

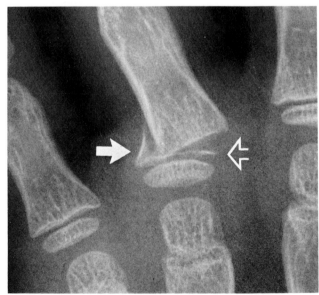

FIG. 3-15. Fracture of the distal phalanx of the finger in a 12-year-old child showing the avulsion fragment (open arrow) on the tension failure side and the triangular fragment (solid arrow) on the compression failure side. This linear fragment (open arrow) was described by Werenskiöld[13] and contrasts with the more frequent triangular metaphyseal fragment (solid arrow) known as the Thurston Holland sign.

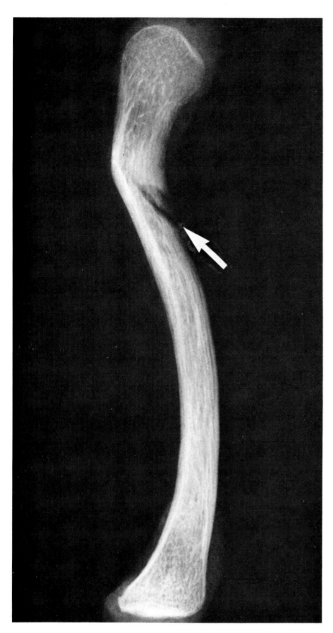

FIG. 3-16. Roentgenogram of clavicle from a three-year-old boy. The nutrient foramen (arrow) causes a significant radiolucency, which easily could be confused with a fracture if there were injury to the pectoral girdle. This particular nutrient foramen is frequently misinterpreted as a fracture in persons of any age.

Transverse lines of Park (Harris lines)

Radiopaque, transverse lines across the entire width of the metaphysis in growing long bones may be found in both healthy and sick children.[5,18-21] The lines may form during late childhood and persist into adult life. However, they do not occur de novo in adult bone.

Usually, transverse lines are distributed relatively symmetrically through the skeleton and occupy identical sites in the corresponding bones on either side of the body. The lines

are thickest in the metaphyses that grow most rapidly, such as those of the distal femur and proximal tibia (Fig. 3-18). In the metaphyses of slowest growth, lines may either not form at all or be exceedingly thin and lie at the very end of the shaft, directly under the provisional zone of calcification. These transverse lines are juxtaposed and parallel to the contours of the physeal provisional zones of calcification. When several transverse lines are present at the end of a shaft, they tend to parallel one another, each duplicating the contours of the others. The lines nearest the end of the shaft are ordinarily the thickest and widest. Lines farther away from the physis tend to be thinner, less distinct, and usually broken and irregular. Eventually, as they approach the diaphysis, they disappear completely with endosteal remodeling.

The exact cause of formation of transverse lines is not known, but they appear to develop whenever the growing

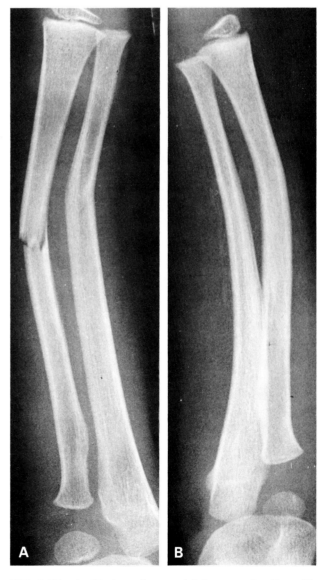

FIG. 3-17. A, AP view of greenstick fracture of radius with accompanying plastic deformation of the ulna. B, Plastic deformation of both radius and ulna.

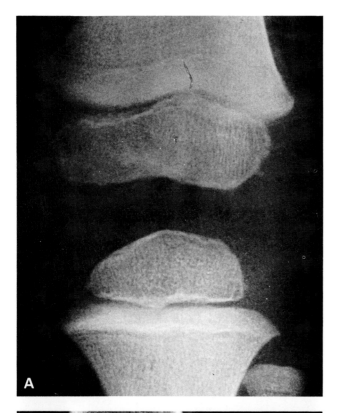

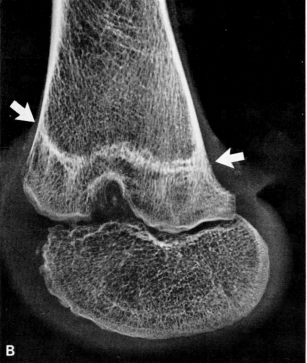

FIG. 3-18. *A,* Patient with Harris growth arrest lines in distal femur and proximal tibia following nine weeks of immobilization in a long leg cast for a femoral fracture. *B,* Section of the distal femur in a child dying from complications of leukemia. Notice that the contour of the Harris line (arrows) reflects the contour of the adjacent physis. The radiolucent area in the middle is ischemic physeal cartilage.

skeleton is subjected to a biologic stress of sufficient severity over a sufficient period of time, especially such stresses as starvation and fever.[22] Harris produced transverse lines experimentally in growing animals by starving them,[19] while Park induced transverse lines in rats by feeding them diets deficient in protein and fat, but high in carbohydrate.[21]

According to Park, a reasonable hypothesis for the cause of the lines was persistence of excessive cartilage due to transitory oligemia of the metaphyseal arteries.[21] However, the anatomic changes consist of transversely directed bony trabeculae that extend entirely across the medullary cavity, parallel the juxtaposed provisional zone of calcification, and run perpendicular to the normally longitudinally directed trabeculae.

These transverse lines have been called "growth arrest" lines in the belief that they develop during periods of decreased growth rates. However, in some cases, radiographic findings indicated that these lines were formed during periods of accelerated growth, because in cases in which the velocity of growth on the two sides of the body was different, the transverse lines were formed only in the more rapidly growing bone.[5] Park's studies indicated that longitudinal growth arrest of a growing bone was a prerequisite to the formation of a transverse line. During this initial phase of growth stoppage or slowing, a thin, transverse, osseous template on the underside of the zone of proliferative cartilage was formed. When longitudinal growth in the proliferative cartilage resumed, a period which Park termed the recovery phase, a transverse line became visible radiographically.

If one observes the normal, constantly changing morphology of the different bones, the more rapidly growing ones are associated with longitudinally oriented trabeculae in the juxtaphyseal region, whereas the slower growing bones, particularly the proximal radius, the metacarpals, metatarsals, and phalanges, normally have a greater amount of transversely oriented, juxtaphyseal primary spongiosa. Because this is the standard pattern of orientation in many smaller bones, transverse septae and their slower rates of growth are normal findings. The orientation of trabeculae in these particular bones will not become sufficiently different to be radiographically evident.

However, if growth slows down in the areas that grow more rapidly and are normally characterized by longitudinal orientation of trabeculae, then more primary spongiosa is formed in a transverse orientation. This bone can be quite thick, a factor probably related to the duration of the biologic stress. Once normal rates of longitudinal growth and trabecular orientation have been reestablished, the transversely oriented septal subchondral plate contrasts to the pre- and postdisease longitudinally oriented trabeculae and appears as a specific transverse line radiographically. As remodeling occurs, the epiphysis migrates away from this region, the primary spongiosa is converted to the secondary spongiosa, the secondary spongiosa is converted to the medullary cavity, and the transverse trabecular orientation is gradually broken up.

Special Techniques

Because of difficulty visualizing epiphyseal contours and microscopic fractures, an absolute diagnosis of skeletal injury in children sometimes requires the use of techniques other than routine roentgenography. Among the special procedures are: (1) stress films; (2) arthrography; (3) computerized tomography (e.g., CAT scan); (4) scintigraphy; and (5) arteriography and venography.

Stress Films. Because of the elastic capacity of developing bone and contiguous soft tissues, the injured part often "springs" back into anatomic position after the deforming force is removed. This is particularly common in epiphyseal fractures around the knee. These fractures are the childhood and adolescent analogue of ligamentous injuries in the adult, and one can test for them using similar diagnostic methods. Stress application, utilizing fluoroscopy or routine radiography, may "open" a fracture sufficiently to document the injury (Fig. 3-19).

Arthrography. This technique probably is more useful in chronic problems than in acute injuries, although it certainly can be used in the latter circumstance. In infants and young children with suspected epiphyseal fractures of a radiolucent distal humerus or proximal femur, arthrographic evaluation often may allow a correct diagnosis (Fig. 3-20) and proper treatment. In the case of chronic problems, arthrographic techniques may make unusual injuries visible (Fig. 3-21).

Computerized Tomography. This new technique is particularly useful in the evaluation of spinal trauma (Fig. 3-22). It allows an accurate assessment of narrowing of the spinal canal due to fracture of the posterior or anterior elements, or translation of one vertebra onto the next.[10] It also is the most useful diagnostic method for evaluating fractures of the C1 vertebra, a difficult area to assess with routine radiography or standard AP/lateral tomographic techniques, especially in children.

Scintigraphy (Radionuclide Imaging). Systemic application of nuclear medicine procedures probably has been underutilized in children's trauma.[23] The simple, noninvasive nature of isotope studies makes them attractive as a screening procedure. The reduced radiation dosage permits repeat and follow-up studies to be done with relative safety.

Applications of bone scans currently of clinical use include: (1) evaluation of fractures; (2) discovering osteomyelitis or a tumor as the cause of acute bone pain following an injury; (3) evaluation of aseptic (ischemic) necrosis of the capital femoral ossification center following hip dislocation or fracture of the femoral neck; and (4) evaluation of radiographically normal-appearing bone to detect stress fractures, thus allowing early diagnosis of these lesions (see Chap. 8).

Vascular Radiography. Trauma to blood vessels is an infrequent accompaniment to fractures but it represents a potential catastrophe when present. Because of the difficulty of visualization on routine radiography, arteriography is especially helpful in adequately delineating vascular injury (Fig. 3-23). Fortunately, the increasing awareness of soft tissue injury and vascular compromise has led to a significant decrease in Volkmann's contracture, whether involving the upper or lower extremity. A more detailed description of concomitant vascular injuries, diagnosis, and treatment may be found in Chapters 7, 10, and 18. Venography has less use in childhood and adolescence because phlebitis and thrombosis are rare complications of chondro-osseous injury prior to skeletal maturation (see Chap. 7).

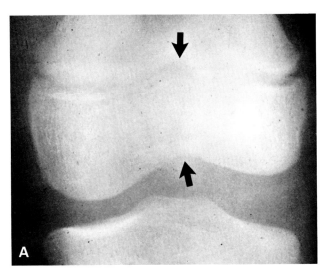

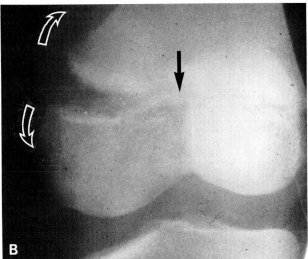

FIG. 3-19. *A,* Injured knee in adolescent with a lucency apparent through the intercondylar notch (arrows) that is suggestive of fracture. *B,* Application of a valgus stress separated the type 3 epiphyseal fracture of the medial condyle (epiphyseal ossification center) away from the metaphysis (open arrows). The solid arrow indicates the fracture involvement through the ossification center.

Skeletal Growth

Orthoroentgenographic methods have been employed increasingly for accurate measurement of normal and abnormal upper and lower extremity osseous length.[23a,23b] Bertelsen introduced the term "anisomelia" to replace the much longer term "inequality of leg length."[24] Green, Wyatt, and Anderson[9] were the first to use roentgenographic measurement extensively. Goldstein and Dreisinger[25] described a spot-orthoroentgenographic method in which each joint was exposed separately. The error due to distortion was computed to a maximum of 1.3%. Nordentoft's studies showed that movements of the legs between single exposures and inaccuracy of positioning at separate exami-

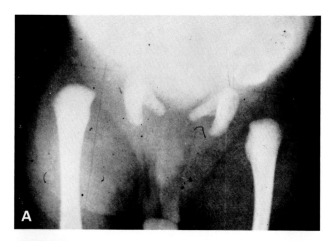

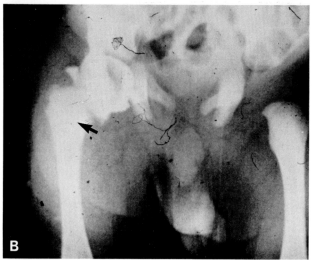

FIG. 3-20. *A,* Neonatal film of child with symptoms suggestive of congenital hip dysplasia (CDH), but with pain on examination of the hip. *B,* Arthrogram shows location of capital femur and lateral displacement (arrow) of shaft (see Chapters 8 and 17 for discussion of this injury). Follow-up examination 20 years later showed an unremarkable hip.

nations were the major sources of error.[24] He felt that ortho-roentgenographic measurement was sufficiently exact for clinical use, but that the errors might influence the accuracy of scientific results.

The technique that I currently use is to take spot roentgenograms centered directly over the hips, knees, and ankles, using a moveable 14″ × 17″ cassette. A steel ruler with radiopaque measurements is placed next to each extremity (Fig. 3-24). Direct measurements may then be made from the films and recorded on growth charts.

Development of ossification centers

Development of the primary ossification centers of major longitudinal bones occurs prenatally. In contrast, the only long bone with a secondary ossification center present at birth is the distal femur, and this is a reliable indicator of a full-term pregnancy. The carpal and tarsal bones develop

primary ossification centers to some degree prenatally, but extensively postnatally, a factor of consequence in the estimation of skeletal age. However, of all human carpal and tarsal bones, only the calcaneus develops a secondary ossification center.

Roentgenologic studies of skeletal development consist essentially of determining the rate and time of appearance of ossification centers of epiphyses and small bones (Fig. 3-25). The age at which union of the epiphyses occurs is also important (Fig. 3-26).

Skeletal maturation is affected variably by the multitude of skeletal dysplasias. A complete description of these is certainly beyond the scope of this book. Caffey[5] and Edeiken,[8] as well as many other authors, have adequately presented the highly variable radiologic appearances of bones affected by these disorders. The ossification patterns may be affected in any region—diaphyseal, metaphyseal, physeal, or epiphyseal—and major distortion of the bone can result. The orthopaedist should have some familiarity with these disorders, since the milder forms may not be diagnosed until observed fortuitously during the evaluation of trauma.

Postnatal growth of human limbs

An understanding of the growth of the individual human long bones is of primary importance to any physician concerned with the potential problem of unequal limb length consequent to trauma. Whether the result of shortening, overgrowth, incomplete or complete premature epiphysiodesis, or traumatic amputation, the correct estimation of anticipated growth enhances the results of any elective corrective surgery. Unfortunately, appropriate decisions are fre-

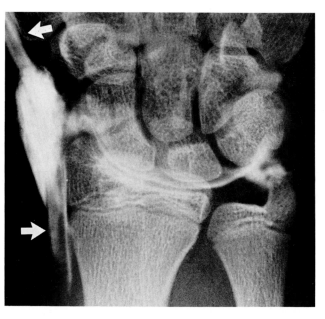

FIG. 3-21. Normal views of the wrist in a boy who complained of chronic pain following a fall but whose hand showed no abnormalities. An arthrogram of wrist, however, showed communication with the thumb tendon sheath (arrows). Closure of the capsular tear produced relief of symptoms.

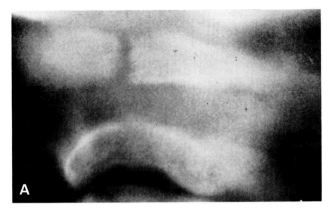

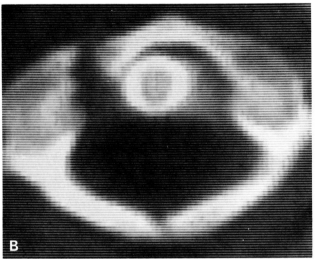

FIG. 3-22. Fracture of C1 vertebra in a six-year-old boy. *A,* Routine radiography does not reveal the fracture. Multiple tomographic cuts were required to diagnose one fracture of the ring of C1. *B,* CAT scan illustrated fractures of both the anterior and posterior rings. This method was used subsequently for follow-up examinations.

quently impossible owing to the lack of practical information and the difficulty in adapting the findings of academic interest to the immediate needs of the patient.

Figure 3-27 shows the contributions of the various growth plates of the upper and lower extremities to growth both of individual bones as well as to the overall length of each extremity. The contributions of the various epiphyseal plates to linear growth of the long bones were studied initially by Digby,[26] using the nutrient canal as a point of reference. These studies must be considered rough estimates, because the two major bones, the humerus and the femur, often have two or more nutrient canals. In dealing with these particular figures, it must be emphasized that they represent the percentage of *relative* growth derived from each physis (the ratio of growth expected from a given physis relative to the overall length of the respective bone).[26a] Specific charts must be used for anticipated *actual* length of growth (see Appendix II). It must be remembered that these are based on selective population samples and are not necessarily accurate for the given individual, although the *ratio* values appear to be

relatively constant in either boys or girls and whether dealing with short or tall children.

When such graphs are used to predict growth and time of surgery properly, the role of relative maturity and various other clinical factors must be taken into account. Maximal length of the long bones in girls is attained in earlier skeletal and chronologic ages than it is in boys.[27,28] The relative physical maturity, which includes skeletal maturity, of a child is of primary importance in predicting the growth patterns of the long bones. The growth potential following an injury in two 10-year-old boys obviously differs if one has a skeletal age of 8 and the other 12 years. Because the 10-year-old with the higher skeletal age has fewer years remaining before the normal closure of his epiphyseal growth plates, his long bones will grow less than those of the skeletally more immature 10-year-old. He will have less time in which deformity due to growth arrest could occur, but he also will have less time in which malunion could be corrected.

Estimation of skeletal age

The skeleton does not develop at a constant rate from fetus to adult.[29,30] Initially there is a relative acceleration during early childhood, followed later by another acceleration during the adolescent growth spurt. Few individuals follow the idealized developmental curve exactly. Most stay within the boundaries of a normal range throughout, but some entirely healthy children show sufficient variations to be judged at least temporarily advanced or retarded.[31]

Because it can be studied with relative ease, the skeleton is referred to most frequently in maturation studies. It has long been realized that skeletal development is divisible into two components: increase in size, and increase in maturity. Although closely integrated in a healthy child, each basically follows its own pattern and rate. Increase in size is relatively

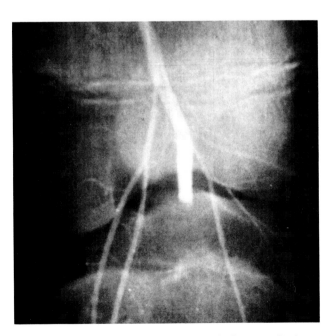

FIG. 3-23. Arteriogram in patient with fracture-displacement of the proximal tibial epiphysis, showing complete block of popliteal artery.

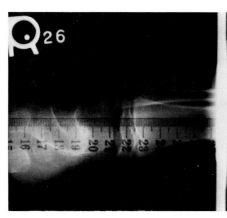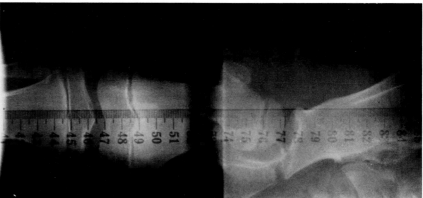

FIG. 3-24. Routine method of orthoroentgenography utilizing steel ruler with radiopaque numbers under the extremity of the patient.

easy to assess. Skeletal maturation, however, is not only elusive of measurement, but also difficult to define.[9,27,28,32-38]

The hand, including the wrist, has received most attention because it radiographs easily and includes a wide range of bone development suitable for study.[39-43] The most popular method of assessing maturity, therefore, has been to base comparison on a series of films typical of the various age groups.[40-46] However, these inspectional methods involve considerable subjective error. To eliminate such errors, efforts were made to assess maturity by measuring the actual size of various bones on the radiographs.[47] However, these techniques were seldom used outside of the centers in which they were derived, because they were slow, cumbersome, and inaccurate.

A third method entails radiographing all the joints on one side of the body and counting the number of centers that have fused.[48,49] This system involves many radiographic films and ignores the structural changes that occur in the epiphyses between initial ossification and fusion. Acheson[50] presented a new method, called the "Oxford Method," in which each bone is awarded a unit designation depending upon its stage of development. This system is similar to the Tanner-Whitehouse[51] technique for the hand and wrist. Both are rather time consuming and not ordinarily utilized in clinical situations.

There may be some mild asymmetry within the body. Dreizen[52] and colleagues, in a radiographic study of the hands of 450 children, found identical bilateral symmetry of bone maturation in only 117 children, a factor that must be considered when relying upon comparison films to evaluate either injury or skeletal age. The same side always should be radiographed on subsequent examinations. According to others, significant skeletal developmental asymmetry, with the exception of a few specific abnormal conditions (e.g., dysplasia hemimelia), does not, for all practical purposes, occur.[47] The left center is the side of the skeleton sampled by convention.

In the small bones of the wrist and ankle, there is a great variation in the time of appearance and the order of appearance of the primary ossification centers. Robinow[53] found that in the same individual, the appearance of the secondary centers in the epiphyses of the tubular bones of the hands and feet often shows wide discrepancies in comparison to

the appearance of the primary centers in the tarsals and carpals. These discrepancies between round bones and epiphyseal centers sometimes make it difficult to appraise the skeletal age according to the standards of Vogt and Vickers, Todd, or Flory.[40,43,46] Robinow[53] made the interesting sugges-

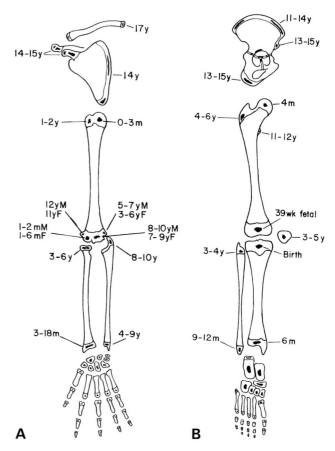

FIG. 3-25. Schematic of ages of onset of secondary ossification of major long bones in, *A,* the arm and, *B,* the leg. Specific patterns in the hand and foot may be obtained from Caffey.[5]

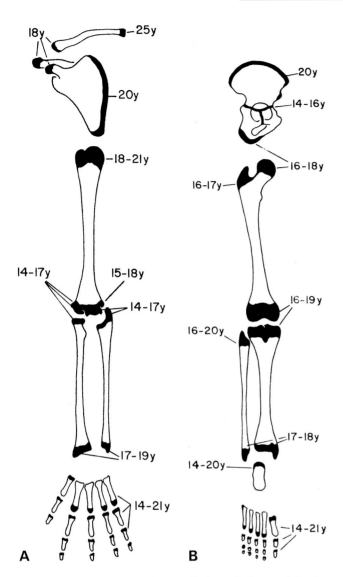

FIG. 3-26. Schematic of ages of physeal closure (physiologic epiphysiodesis) in the major long bones of, *A,* the arm and, *B,* the leg.

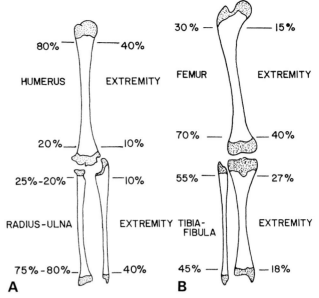

FIG. 3-27. Schematic of relative contributions of individual growth regions to overall length of an individual bone and composite extremity in, *A,* the arm and, *B,* the leg.

End of skeletal growth

To establish skeletal criteria for onset of adolescence, it appears that ossification is present in the crest of the ilium within six months of menarche (12.9 years) in ⅔ of a number of studies.[54] The age of inception of crest ilial ossification in the male probably represents a maturational level analogous to the female maturational level at the menarcheal date. In males, iliac ossification appears on the average at 14.5 years, or 1.6 years later than in females. In the proximal phalanx of the second digit of the hand, fusion of the epiphysis with the shaft begins near the menarcheal date. Completion of ossification along the iliac crest generally coincides with the cessation of longitudinal growth in the arms and legs. However, additional overall body height may still be added by continued longitudinal development of the thoracolumbar vertebral bodies, which may not stop growth until the third decade.

tion that two categories of skeletal age be established; namely "round bone skeletal age" and "epiphyseal skeletal age." Further findings suggest that the radial epiphyseal center is even more variable than the epiphyseal centers in the small, tubular bones of the hands.

Errors in determination of skeletal age by the Greulich and Pyle atlas methods have been particularly well elucidated by Roche.[42] It is noteworthy that experienced radiologists show a mean replicability of three to four months with the standard deviation in most cases being approximately the same on repeated evaluations of sample radiographs, and this can be improved by averaged dual reading only in about 30% of all cases. The accuracy obtained in assessing interval changes in serial studies was even less encouraging.[53] Interestingly, exclusion of the carpal centers has no real effect on replicability.[47] In fact, evaluation of the carpals may decrease the overall accuracy of the hand and wrist assessments.

References

1. Drey, L.: A roentgenographic study of transitory synovitis of the hip joint. Radiology, *60:*588, 1963.
2. Frantzell, A.: Soft tissue radiography: technical aspects and clinical applications in the examination of limbs. Acta Radiol. [Suppl.] (Stockh.), *85:*1951.
3. Hermel, M., and Sklaroff, D.: Roentgen changes in transient synovitis of the hip. Arch. Surg., *68:*364, 1954.
4. Teates, C. D.: Distal radial growth plate remnant simulating fracture. A. J. R., *110:*578, 1970.
5. Caffey, J.: Pediatric X-ray Diagnosis. 6th Ed. Chicago, Yearbook Medical Publishers, 1972.
6. Norell, H. G.: Roentgenologic visualization of the extracapsular fat. Acta Radiol. [Diagn.] (Stockh.), *42:*205, 1954.
7. Bledsoe, R. C., and Izenstark, J. L.: Displacement of fat pads in disease and injury of the elbow. Radiology, *73:*717, 1959.

7a. Lodwick, G. S.: Reactive response to local injury in bone. Radiol. Clin. North Am., 2:209, 1964.

7b. Lodwick, G. S.: The Bones and Joints: An Atlas of Tumor Radiology. Chicago, Yearbook Medical Publishers, 1971.

8. Edeiken, J., and Hodes, P. J.: Roentgen Diagnosis of Diseases of Bone. Baltimore, Williams & Wilkins, 1967.

9. Green, W. T., Wyatt, G. M., and Anderson, M.: Orthoroentgenography as a method of measuring the bones of the lower extremities. J. Bone Joint Surg., 28:60, 1946.

9a. Keats, T. G., and Smith, T. H.: An Atlas of Normal Developmental Roentgen Anatomy. Chicago, Yearbook Medical Publishers, 1977.

9b. Ogden, J. A., Conlogue, G. J., and Jensen, P.: Radiology of postnatal skeletal development: I. The proximal humerus. Skeletal Radiol., 2:153, 1978.

9c. Schmid, F.: Epiphysenkern-entwicklung. Fortschr. Med., 90:4, 1972.

10. O'Connor, J. F., and Cohen, J.: Computerized tomography (CAT Scan, CT Scan) in orthopaedic surgery. J. Bone Joint Surg., 60-A:1096, 1978.

11. Gordon, A. E.: The experimental x-ray demonstration of epiphyseal cartilages: a technique of freezing and high contrast. A. J. R., 83:674, 1964.

12. Rogers, L. F.: The radiography of epiphyseal injuries. A. J. R., 96:289, 1970.

13. Werenskiöld, B.: A contribution to the roentgendiagnosis of epiphyseal separations. Acta Radiol. [Diagn.] (Stockh.), 8:419, 1927.

14. Chamay, A.: Mechanical and morphological aspects of experimental overload and fatigue in bone. J. Biomech., 3:263, 1970.

15. Chamay, A., and Tschantz, P.: Mechanical influences in bone remodeling. Experimental research on Wolff's law. J. Biomech., 5:173, 1972.

16. Manoli, M.: Traumatic fibular bowing with tibial fracture: report of two cases. Orthopedics, 1:145, 1978.

17. Borden, S., IV: Roentgen recognition of acute plastic bowing of the forearm in children. A. J. R., 123:524, 1975.

18. Garn, S. M., Silverman, F. N., Hertzog, K. P., and Rohmann, C. G.: Lines and bands of increased density. Their implication to growth and development. Med. Radiogr. Photogr., 44:58, 1968.

19. Harris, H. A.: The growth of the long bones in childhood with special reference to certain bony striations of the metaphysis and to the role of vitamins. Arch. Int. Med., 38:785, 1926.

20. Park, E. A.: Bone growth in health and disease. Arch. Dis. Child., 29:269, 1954.

21. Park, E. A.: The imprinting of nutritional disturbances on growing bone. Pediatrics, 33 (Suppl):815, 1964.

22. Acheson, R. M.: Effects of starvation, septicaemia and chronic illness on the growth cartilage plate and metaphysis of the immature rat. J. Anat., 93:123, 1959.

23. Khan, R. A., Hughes, S., Lavender, P., Leon, M., and Spyrou, N.: Autoradiography of technetium-labelled disphosphonate in rat bone. J. Bone Joint Surg., 61-B:221, 1979.

23a. Maresh, M. M.: Growth of the major long bones in healthy children: a preliminary report on successive roentgenograms of the extremities from early infancy to 12 years of age. Am. J. Dis. Child., 66:227, 1943.

23b. Maresh, M. M.: Linear growth of long bones of extremities from infancy through adolescence. Am. J. Dis. Child., 89:725, 1955.

24. Nordentoft, E. L.: The accuracy of orthoroentgenographic measurements. Acta Orthop. Scand., 34:283, 1964.

25. Goldstein, L. A., and Dreisinger, F.: Spot orthoroentgenography. Methods for measuring length of bones of the lower extremity. J. Bone Joint Surg., 32-A:449, 1950.

26. Digby, K.: The measurement of diaphyseal growth in proximal and distal directions. J. Anat. Physiol., 50:187, 1915.

26a. Swinyard, C. A.: Limb Development and Deformity: Problems of Evaluation and Rehabilitation. Springfield, Charles C Thomas, 1969.

27. Hansman, C. F., and Maresh, M. M.: A longitudinal study of skeletal maturation. Am. J. Dis. Child., 101:305, 1961.

28. Harding, V. S. V.: A method of evaluating osseous development from birth to 14 years. Child. Dev., 23:247, 1952.

29. Christie, A.: Prevalence and distribution of ossification centers in the newborn infants. Am. J. Dis. Child., 77:355, 1949.

30. Fischgold, H., Bernard, J., and Bandey, J.: Les cartilages epiphysaires de l'enfant. J. Radiol., 40:429, 1959.

31. Anderson, M., Green, W. T., and Messner, M. B.: Growth and predictions of growth in the lower extremities. J. Bone Joint Surg., 45-A:1, 1963.

32. Bayley, N., and Pinneau, S. R.: Tables for predicting adult height from skeletal age. J. Pediatr., 40:423, 1952.

33. Eklof, O., and Ringertz, H.: A method for assessment of skeletal maturity. Ann. Radiol., 10:330, 1967.

34. Falkner, F.: The physical development of children: a guide to growth charts and development assessments, and a commentary on contemporary and future problems. Pediatrics, 29:441, 1962.

35. Garn, S. M., and Rohmann, C. G.: Variability in the order of ossification of the bony centers of the hand and wrist. Am. J. Phys. Develop., 18:219, 1960.

36. Liliequist, B., and Lundberg, M.: Skeletal and tooth development: a methodologic investigation. Acta Radiol. [Diagn.] (Stockh.), 11:97, 1971.

37. Pyle, S., and Hoerr, N.: A Radiographic Standard of Reference for the Growing Knee. Springfield, Charles C Thomas, 1969.

38. Seyss, R.: Zu den Grund prinzipen der Verknocherring des menschlichen Skelettes. Paediatr. Grenzgeb., 9:315, 1970.

39. DeRoo, R., and Schroder, J. J.: Pocket Atlas of Skeletal Age. Baltimore, Williams & Wilkins, 1977.

40. Flory, C. D.: Osseous development in the hand as an index of skeletal development. Monogr. Soc. Res. Child Develop., 1:3, 1936.

41. Greulich, W. W., and Pyle, S. I.: Radiographic Atlas of Skeletal Development of the Hand and Wrist. Stanford, University Press, 1959.

42. Roche, A. F., Wainer, H., and Thissen, D.: Skeletal Maturity. The Knee Joint as a Biological Indicator. New York, Plenum Publishing, 1975.

43. Todd, T. W.: Atlas of Skeletal Maturation. St. Louis, C. V. Mosby, 1937.

44. Elgenmark, O.: Normal development of the ossific centers during infancy and childhood: clinical, roentgenologic and statistical study. Acta Paediatr. Scand. [Suppl.], 33, Suppl. 1, 1946.

45. MacKay, D. H.: Skeletal maturation in the hand: a study of development in East African children. Trans. R. Soc. Trop. Med. Hyg., 46:135, 1952.

46. Vogt, E. C., and Vickers, V. S.: Osseous growth and development. Radiology, 31:441, 1938.

47. Graham, C. B.: Assessment of bone maturation—methods and pitfalls. Radiol. Clin. North Am., 10:185, 1972.

48. Sontag, L. W., Snell, D., and Anderson, M.: Rate of appearance of ossification centers from birth to the age of five years. Am. J. Dis. Child., 58:949, 1939.

49. Sontag, L. W., and Lipford, J.: The effect of illness and other factors on appearance pattern of skeletal epiphyses. J. Pediatr., 23:391, 1943.

50. Acheson, R. M.: A method of assessing skeletal maturity from radiographs. J. Anat., 88:498, 1954.

51. Tanner, J. M. et al.: Assessment of Skeletal Maturity and Prediction of Adult Height (TW2 Method). New York, Academic Press, 1975.

52. Dreizen, S.: Bilateral symmetry of skeletal maturation in the human hand and wrist. Am. J. Dis. Child., 93:122, 1957.

53. Robinow, M.: Appearance of ossification centers: groupings obtained from factor analyses. Am. J. Dis. Child., 64:229, 1942.

54. Risser, J. C.: The iliac apophysis: an invaluable sign in the management of scoliosis. Clin. Orthop., 11:111, 1958.

4

Injury to the Growth Mechanisms

Approximately 15% of all fractures in children involve the physis.[1-24] Table 4-1 gives the relative incidence of specific areas of physeal injury from three series.[25,26] The series by Neer and Horwitz[25] covered 2500 consecutive physeal injuries. All series showed that males sustained physeal injuries more frequently than females. This is undoubtedly because of the greater exposure of boys to significant etiologic factors, especially uncontrolled and controlled trauma from athletic activities, and also because the physes of the male stay open longer than those of the female, extending the duration of possible exposure to injurious trauma.

TABLE 4-1. *Relative Incidence of Physeal Injuries*

	A*	B†	Author's Series
Proximal clavicle			3
Distal clavicle			1
Proximal humerus	72	22	27
Distal humerus (including epicondyles)	332	20	56
Proximal radius	124	1	5
Proximal ulna	21		3
Distal radius	1096	98	114
Distal ulna	136	12	11
Metacarpals		10	8
Phalanges (fingers)		39	41
Pelvis			23
Proximal femur		7	9
Trochanters			4
Distal femur	28	18	17
Proximal tibia	17	6	8
Proximal fibula	2		2
Tibial tuberosity			12
Distal tibia	238	59	60
Distal fibula	302	21	15
Metatarsals		6	3
Phalanges (toes)		11	21
TOTAL	2368	330	443

*Neer and Horwitz.[25]
†Peterson and Peterson.[26]

However, there may be intrinsic response differences, especially during the growth spurt. Morscher[27,28] has shown that there are hormone-mediated differences in the physeal response to experimentally applied stresses. Furthermore, as shown in Chapter 2, anatomic changes occurring in the metaphyseal cortex, primarily during the growth spurt, must affect injury response patterns.[29] Most studies have shown that in all long bones, the distal physes are injured more commonly than the proximal physes. This high incidence of injury to certain physes, such as the distal radius, distal tibia, and phalanges, may result from increased exposure of these more distal regions to trauma, rather than from any unique physiologic susceptibility of these particular physes. Peterson's series revealed more phalangeal physeal injuries than did all the previous series combined,[26] a factor which the authors felt drew attention to the need for more accurate and complete recording of meaningful statistics.

The ages at which most physeal fractures occur, excluding those of the distal humerus, are from 9 to 12 in girls and from 12 to 13 in boys, suggesting that, from the standpoint of a physiologic chronology, most physes are comparably vulnerable to injury.

Classification

While epiphyseal fractures have been recognized with increasing frequency since the early nineteenth century, the first classification scheme was espoused by Foucher.[30] He described: (1) pure separation of the epiphysis from the diaphysis, with no osseous tissue adhering to it ("divulsion epiphysaire"); (2) separation of the epiphysis with a thin, finely granular layer of osseous material attached to it ("fracture epiphysaire"); and (3) solution of continuity of the diaphysis in the osseous spongy tissue near the epiphysis, at a time when the epiphyseal growth plate is closing ("fracture preepiphysaire").

Over the next 40 years, increasing attention was given to these injuries,[31] and in 1898, based upon a comprehensive review of cases described throughout London (including specimens from various anatomic museums), as well as upon some experimental work on child cadavers, Poland[32] advanced a classification system which divides fractures into four types. Aitken[4] subsequently presented a classification scheme designating only three types of fractures. He was the first to emphasize that deformity consequent to initial malunion or potential growth disturbance was probably rare, although displacement was often significant. Aitken emphasized that the third type of fracture, a compression injury, was extremely difficult to diagnose, was frequently thought to be of little clinical significance, and could easily lead to major growth deformities.

The most complete classification scheme was proposed by Salter and Harris.[33] This scheme was based on a combination of: (1) mechanism of injury; (2) relationship of the fracture line to the various cellular layers of the physis; and (3) prognosis concerning subsequent disturbance of growth. Salter and Harris recognized five, radiologically definable types of injury. Type 1 was a complete separation of the epiphysis and physis from the metaphysis, with the fracture occurring through the zone of the hypertrophic cells. In type 2 a similar fracture occurred, except that a metaphyseal fragment was included on the compression side of the fracture. Types 1 and 2 were supposedly virtually free of long term complications, such as premature growth arrest. Type 3 involved a fracture along part of the growth plate, with propagation through the epiphyseal ossification center into the joint. Type 4 involved a fracture through the epiphyseal ossification center and a juxtaposed portion of the metaphysis. Type 5 was a crushing injury to the growth plate. These latter three types of injury were associated with a greater risk of premature growth arrest.

While the classification scheme of Salter and Harris is concise, and certainly has proved to be of major diagnostic and clinical importance, certain types of epiphyseal and physeal injuries cannot be readily classified by it, and complicated combinations of injuries obviously occur. Furthermore, injury to other growth mechanisms such as the metaphysis, diaphysis, periosteum, zone of Ranvier, and epiphyseal perichondrium are not included in the scheme. Accordingly, an enlarged and more inclusive scheme has been devised. Types 1 and 2 are given subtypes in this system to explain the probable cause of the infrequently encountered, premature, localized growth plate closure and osseous bridging, a complication that is being described more frequently.

Type 1 (Fig. 4-1)

The epiphyses and most of the cellular regions of the contiguous growth plate separate from the metaphysis with no roentgenographically evident osseous fragments (type 1A). The plane of cleavage essentially undulates through the zones of hypertrophic and degenerating cartilage cell columns, leaving the resting and dividing cell layers of the germinal region of the physis undamaged and still connected to the epiphysis. While the basic defect appears to be a separation through the hypertrophic zone, the propagation plane is not always a smooth, transverse plane. Undulation of the normal physis as well as of the fracture line may cause propagation into regions of the germinal/resting zones of the physis or metaphysis, such that microscopic pieces of primary spongiosa may be included on the "epiphyseal" side of the fracture. This variable failure pattern occurs more frequently in those growth plates that are beginning to develop

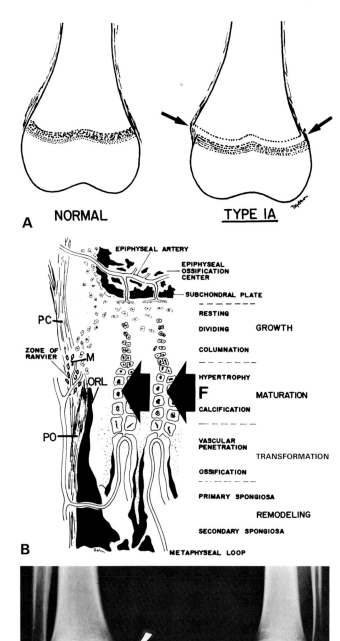

FIG. 4-1. *A,* Schematic of the usual type 1A growth plate injury. The majority of the physis remains with the epiphyseal fragment. Only the calcifying and terminal hypertrophic regions remain with the metaphysis. *B,* Schematic showing region of fracture propagation (F-arrows) at the histologic level. This same pattern exists in type 2 and 3 injuries in which the fracture propagates transversely across the physis. Note the perichondrium (PC); periosteum (PO); mesenchymal cells (M); and ossification ring of Lacroix (ORL). *C,* AP view of type 1A distal tibial injury with mild widening of the physis (arrow) compared to the uninvolved side.

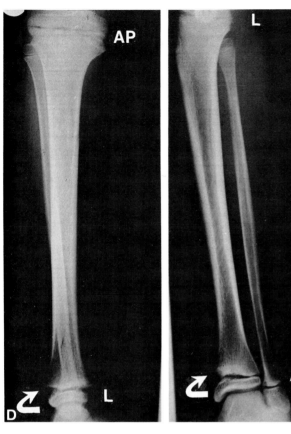

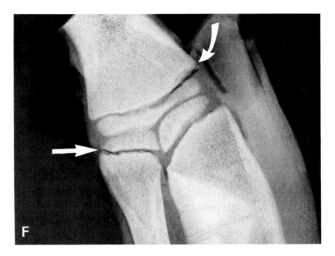

FIG. 4-1 (Continued). *F,* Roentgenogram of specimen shown in *E.* Lucencies indicate the fracture planes across the physeal/metaphyseal junction.

contour changes in response to dynamic biomechanical forces. The changes in contour may include small mammillary processes extending into the metaphysis, or larger curves such as the binodal contour of the distal femoral physis. In infants and young children, such extensive remodeling and contouring (undulation) of the growth plate with formation of mammillary processes usually has not commenced, so the fracture line tends to be relatively smooth and transverse.

Displacement of the epiphyseal fragment from the metaphysis is generally much less in type 1 than in other types of growth plate injuries, because most of the thick periosteal attachment into the zone of Ranvier remains intact and mechanically prevents significant displacement. This lack of displacement frequently makes radiologic diagnosis difficult, if not impossible. Slight widening of the physis may be the only sign, but if the secondary ossification center is small, this is difficult to assess. In such a situation, clinical diagnosis assumes greater import. However, complete displacement of the epiphysis and physis may occur (Fig. 4-2), usually as a result of a shearing or tensile (avulsion) force.

Type 1A injuries are more commonly encountered in neonates and infants with limited development of the secondary ossification center. The size of the secondary ossification center, relative to the overall size of the epiphysis, probably plays a major role in dissipation of fracture forces during propagation of the acute injury across the physis, particularly on the compression side of the fracture. The larger the ossification center, the greater the tendency of a fracture to propagate into the metaphysis and create a type 2 injury. Type 1 injuries also may occur as pathologic fractures complicating underlying diseases such as rickets and osteomyelitis (Fig. 4-3).

A subclassification of these fractures, type 1B, may occur in children with systemic disorders affecting the ossification patterns in the metaphysis (Fig. 4-4). These disorders may occur in children with myeloproliferative disorders such as leukemia (in which a fracture is often the initial presentation of the disease), or neuromuscular sensory disorders such as congenital insensitivity to pain and myelomeningocele.

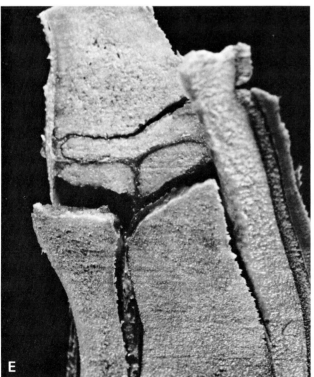

FIG. 4-1 (Continued). *D,* AP view and lateral views of type 1A injury of distal tibia with 90° rotation of fragment (arrow). *E,* Displaced type 1 injuries of distal humerus and proximal radius and ulna in a skeletally immature whale.

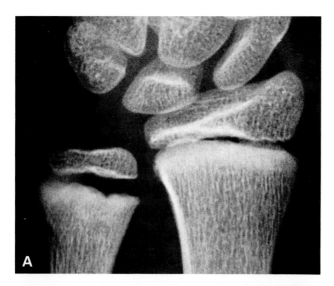

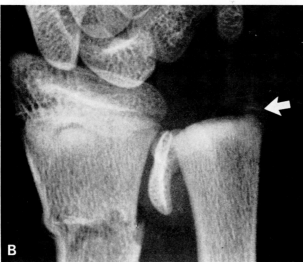

FIG. 4-2. *A,* Undisplaced type 1A injury of distal ulna. *B,* Type 1A injury with complete displacement of the distal ulnar epiphysis. Note that a small segment of the epiphysis remains (arrow). This is the Werenskiöld fragment, as discussed in Chapter 3, which represents tension failure through the ossification center just above the subchondral plate.

In contrast to type 1A fractures, which propagate primarily through the zone of hypertrophic cartilage, type 1B fractures occur in the zone of cartilage degeneration and primary spongiosa formation. If the fracture complicates a cellular proliferative disorder such as leukemia, the initial fracture tends to be a microscopic trabecular injury consequent to cellular hyperplasia, cystic expansion, and displacement of the primary spongiosa. These are probably compression injuries. If the primary disease can be controlled, the microfractures improve. Major displacements and long term complications are uncommon in these situations. However, in other types of cellular proliferative disorders such as thalassemia, the microscopic fractures and mild hyperplasia may lead to destruction of portions of the growth plate and for-

mation of osseous bridges (Fig. 4-5). If these fractures occur in cases of myelodysplasia, they are often unrecognized and inadvertently subjected to frequent motion as the child is moved in and out of bed, or in and out of braces, and considerable amounts of new bone may form in the subperiosteal metaphyseal region (see Fig. 4-4). A more detailed presentation of these disorders is given in Chapter 8.

Generally, subsequent growth is normal in type 1A and 1B fractures, since the essential germinal elements, the resting and dividing cellular layers of the growth plate, and the attendant epiphyseal and peripheral metaphyseal blood supplies are usually undisturbed. There may be a temporary cutoff of the central metaphyseal circulation such that the invasive arcades of the metaphyseal vessels cannot reach the hypertrophic, degenerating cartilage, and this causes a temporary widening of the growth plate in the hypertrophic zone. But once central metaphyseal revascularization occurs, the thickened cellular layer is rapidly re-invaded and restored to its normal thickness. In some situations, such as injury to the proximal femur, the major blood supply to the epiphysis may be damaged (Fig. 4-6). The ischemic condition may lead to osseous necrosis and deformity within the developing ossification center and growth irregularities in the physis. These changes may be localized and cause asymmetric growth, or they may involve the complete growth plate and result in an overall slowdown of the rate of growth of the capital femoral physis. In either instance, premature closure of some or all of the growth plate may occur. Depending upon the remaining growth potential, partial closure is a significant complication, leading to severe angular growth deformities as well as to decreased longitudinal growth.

While type 1 injuries seem relatively straightforward as indicated by types 1A and 1B, a further subclassification, type 1C, defines those infrequent fractures in which an associated injury occurs to a germinal portion of the physis (Fig. 4-7). Birth or early infancy are the most likely times for such injuries to occur. The major part of the growth region of the physis is uninvolved, but a localized region is subjected to a crushing injury of *all* layers of the physis. An osseous bridge eventually forms after the secondary ossification center has developed and expanded to reach the damaged region. Attempts to duplicate the mechanism of injury using stillborn cadavers resulted in disruption of the epiphysis from the metaphyseal shaft and localized crushing and fragmentation in the medial portion of the epiphysis and metaphysis (Fig. 4-8). In these type 1C cases, the initial injury occurred either before the secondary ossification center had formed, or just after it had appeared. Yet once the secondary center had grown sufficiently to reach the originally damaged area, an osseous bridge eventually formed across the physis, a complication comparable to that of a type 3 or type 4 injury. The type 1C injury is less likely to occur in children older than two years of age, after which time the failure pattern is more likely to create a metaphyseal fragment (type 2 injury).

Due to the immense growth potential of the longitudinal bones in young children, and the possible multiple-year delay between injury and eventual roentgenologic evidence of any complications, adequate long term follow-up care is essential to ascertain whether such physeal injury and complication may have occurred. Furthermore, as more detailed studies of growth following type 1 and type 2 injuries to such

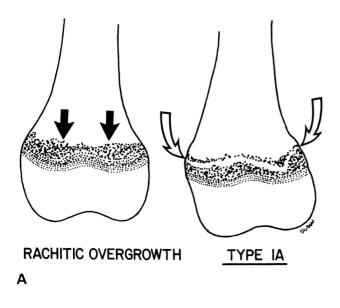

RACHITIC OVERGROWTH   TYPE IA

A

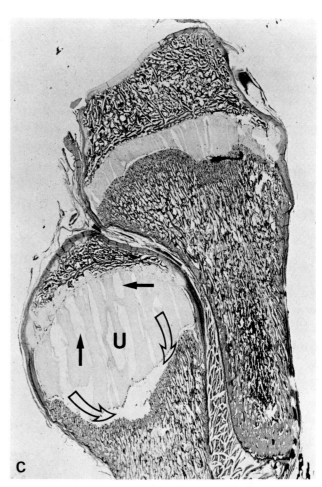

C

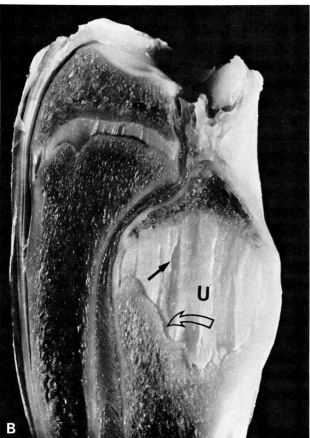

B

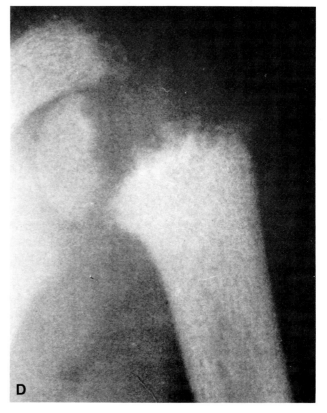

D

FIG. 4-3. *A,* Schematic of a pathologic type 1A injury occurring as a result of rickets. The hypertrophic zone widens considerably and fails through this region. *B-C,* Gross and histologic sections from a juvenile arctic fox (Alopex lagopus). Note the massive widening of the distal ulnar physis (U). Clefts with fluid developed between cell columns (closed arrows) and between the cartilage and metaphyseal bone (open arrows). *D,* Apparent epiphysiolysis in three-year-old boy with renal rickets.

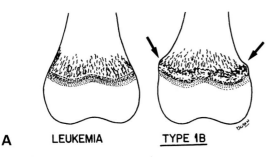

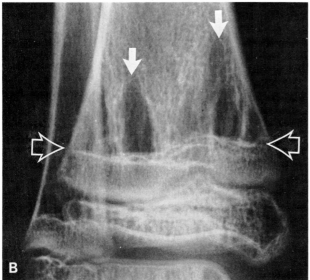

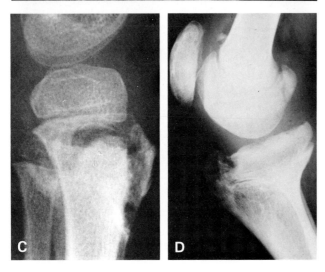

regions as the proximal humerus and distal femur are undertaken, it is becoming evident that decreased longitudinal growth may occur *without* premature epiphysiodesis or angular deformation. The decreased growth may be only a few millimeters, but it does represent subtle, permanent injury to the entire growth plate.

Type 2 (Fig. 4-9)

The type 2A injury is the most common of all growth plate injuries. Similar to type 1, it is generally caused by a shearing or avulsion force. It occurs frequently in young children who have undergone the first major growth spurt (from three to seven years), and it is certainly the most frequent type of physeal separation in children over the age of ten. Like type 1, some of these injuries may be extremely difficult to diagnose, although the presence of a very small fragment of metaphysis makes the diagnosis certain. Any child who presents a history of trauma and swelling around a joint or epiphysis must be suspected of having this type of injury, and should be treated as having a fracture, even if the diagnosis cannot be absolutely confirmed by routine radiography.

Similar to type 1 injuries, the line of fracture propagates along the hypertrophic and provisionally calcified zones of the physis. However, in contrast to type 1, propagation along the physeal/metaphyseal junction is quite variable, with a point being reached at which the fracture line turns and propagates through a variably-sized portion of the metaphysis. The metaphyseal fragment, which is generally triangular and may be extremely small, is diagnostic of this pattern of injury (Fig. 4-10). This radiologically evident metaphyseal

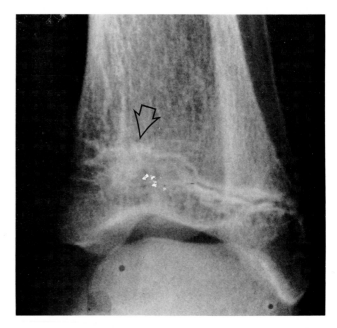

FIG. 4-4. *A,* Schematic of type 1B injury. The fracture is in the primary spongiosa rather than the hypertrophic cartilage. *B,* One year after chemotherapy for leukemia, residuals of the fractures are visible as metaphyseal lucencies (closed arrows), with subsequent normal metaphyseal bone and a Harris growth line (open arrows). *C,* Myelodysplastic patient with chronic type 1B epiphysiolysis of the proximal tibia. The metaphysis is widened (open arrow), and new metaphyseal bone is forming (closed arrow). This child's presenting symptoms were a fever and a swollen knee. *D,* The long term consequences are destruction of overall growth potential and premature epiphysiodesis.

FIG. 4-5. Premature epiphysiodesis (arrow) in 11-year-old girl with severe thalassemia. This girl had similar osseous bridges in both proximal humeri and one distal radius. The contiguous metaphysis is more radiolucent, probably from marrow hyperplasia.

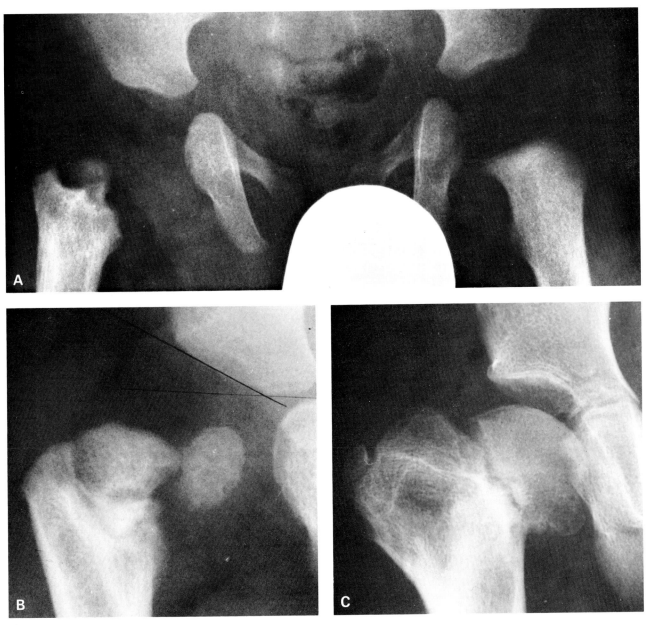

FIG. 4-6. Birth injury to right proximal femur. *A,* Appearance at three months. *B,* At one year, just prior to performance of a valgus osteotomy. *C,* At six years, after several operative procedures.

fragment is frequently referred to as the Thurston-Holland sign.[34] It represents compression phase redirection of fracture stresses into the metaphysis, which, in the individual shown in Figure 4-10, is structurally (biomechanically) less able to withstand these propagating fracture-failure forces than are the adjacent portions of the physis and epiphysis.

Although it may be separated from the metaphyseal cortex, the periosteum usually remains intact on the "compression" side with the metaphyseal fragment, whereas on the opposite side, where initial separation occurred under tension, the periosteum is often stripped and torn from the metaphysis (although it usually remains attached to the epiphysis and peripheral physis). In fact, the periosteum may invaginate into the gap between epiphysis and metaphysis, a

phenomenon that has been described often in proximal humeral fractures (Fig. 4-11). The tendency of segments of the periosteum to remain attached to the epiphysis and physis while shearing away from the metaphysis is due to the thick attachment of the periosteum into the growth plate at the zone of Ranvier and the blending of the more superficial fibers of the periosteum into the contiguous perichondrium of the epiphysis. In sharp contrast, the periosteum is attached relatively loosely to the metaphysis and diaphysis, particularly in the age-range susceptible to physeal injuries.

Displacement is quite variable and may be extreme, to the point of total displacement of the epiphysis from the metaphysis (Fig. 4-12). These injuries certainly should be reduced as closely as possible to their original anatomic state.

However, when attempting reduction, great care must be taken to have the musculature as relaxed as possible (this may require general anesthesia), so that the physis is not "grated" over the metaphyseal fragments, a potential cause of further microscopic physeal damage, and an event more likely to occur if the child is experiencing pain and resisting the reduction. In general, closed reduction is relatively easy and may be maintained without difficulty. As previously mentioned, the periosteum is attached on the compression side and may be used as a hinge to help in reduction. Further, the metaphyseal bone fragments, especially if large, will usually prevent over-reduction.

As with type 1 injuries, subsequent physeal growth is infrequently disturbed significantly since the germinal layers of the physis remain attached to the epiphysis and the epiphyseal circulation is usually uninterrupted. However, normal undulations of the physis, especially in the distal femur, may cause selective regions of more severe injury.

A subclassification, type 2B, involves further propagation of the fracture forces on the tensile side to create a free metaphyseal fragment (Fig. 4-13). The free metaphyseal fragment makes reduction more difficult and may necessitate open reduction to stabilize the comminuted fragments.

Another subclassification, type 2C, is the inclusion of a thin layer of metaphysis along with, or instead of, the larger triangular fragment. This osseous layer traverses most of the metaphysis (Fig. 4-14). This subtype is more common in slowly growing regions, such as the phalanges, which normally have increased transverse trabeculation in the juxtaphyseal metaphysis (primary spongiosa).

Again, as in type 1 injuries, these injuries may not be "pure" type 2. When the fracture force turns to propagate through the metaphysis, an angular moment change is produced at this site. Because of the forces of injury, this area of metaphysis may be driven into a segment of the growth plate, causing compression damage (type 5 injury) to a localized area (Fig. 4-15). This complication occurs particularly in injuries to the distal femur and distal tibia, and certainly is of sufficient potential risk to warrant follow-up care for many years after the injury.[35,36] This type 2D injury may occur even before an ossification center is present in the distal tibia, as in the aforementioned complication of type 1B. However, as the ossification center appears with skeletal growth, an osseous bridge to the metaphysis may progressively form.

Since type 2D is generally a localized injury, rather than complete growth plate compression, subsequent growth abnormality is eccentric and leads to angular deformation. If a growth plate has significant normal contour variations, rather than a relatively smooth, transverse structure, there is an increased risk of type 2D localized damage consequent to the shearing forces causing fracture propagation between the various regions of the growth plate and the metaphysis (Fig. 4-16). This may be a mechanism of growth slowdown, complete premature closure, or localized angular deformity in epiphyseal fractures of the distal femur.

The anatomy of the epiphysis and physis shown in Figure 4-16 is one of progressive development of binodal curves in both the coronal and sagittal planes. A central region extends farther into the metaphysis than it does into the midregions associated with either condyle. This central region is probably particularly susceptible to more extensive damage when the fracture propagates across it during varus

or valgus displacement. This anatomic contouring is not unique to the distal femur, but it certainly may explain its greater predisposition to growth injuries, particularly premature epiphysiodesis, than most other physeal regions have. Physeal contour variations in other regions, such as the proximal humerus or proximal tibia, also may predispose those regions to more severe cellular damage.

Type 3 (Fig. 4-17)

This is an intra-articular fracture primarily involving the epiphysis, with the plane of fracture extending from the articular surface through the epiphysis, epiphyseal ossification center (if present), and physis to the aforementioned zone of

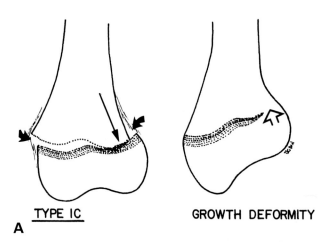

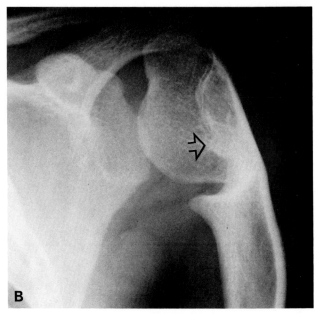

FIG. 4-7. *A,* Schematic of type 1C injury. On the compression side, there is a crushing injury (type 5) to a localized segment of the physis. Eventually, an osseous bridge will form. *B,* Humerus varus in an 11-year-old boy who had sustained a birth injury to his shoulder. An osseous bridge has impeded the growth of the medial physis (arrow), causing progressive angular deformity by differential growth.

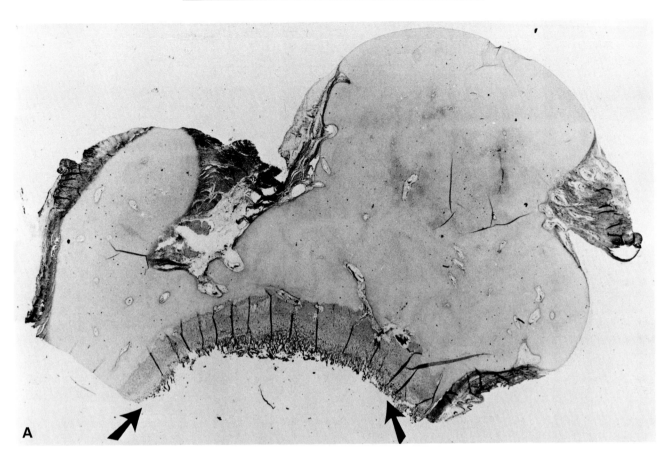

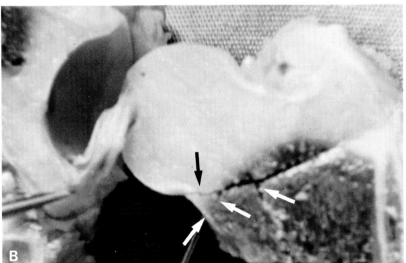

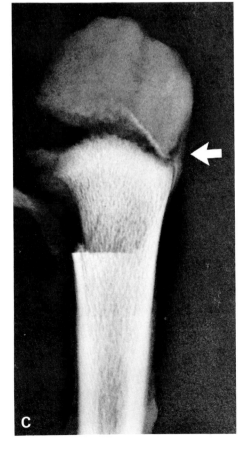

FIG. 4-8. *A,* Characteristic fracture in the proximal femur propagated through various layers of the hypertrophic and calcified cartilage (arrows). The medial physis is undamaged. *B,* In two specimens the fracture comminuted, and the failure extended into the epiphyseal cartilage (arrows), creating a crushing injury which could explain a deformity like the one seen in Figure 4-6. *C,* Failure patterns in neonatal proximal humerus. Notice how the capital humerus has been medially compressed (arrow). Such an injury may have been responsible for the type of deformity shown in Figure 4-7B.

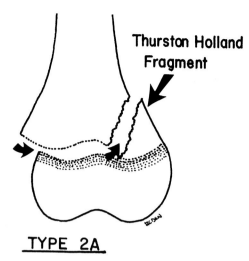

TYPE 2A

FIG. 4-9. Schematic of usual type 2A injury. The fracture propagates across the physis, as in type 1A injuries, but then it turns to enter the metaphysis, creating a piece of metaphyseal bone still attached to, and displacing with, the physis and the epiphysis. This fragment, which is diagnostic of the injury, is termed the Thurston-Holland sign.

weak hypertrophic columnar cells, and then turning approximately 90° to extend along this layer of the growth plate toward the peripheral margins (type 3A). In some instances, transverse fracture propagation may be through the primary spongiosa, leaving a thin layer of metaphyseal bone with the epiphyseal fragment (type 3B). This may occur in the lateral humeral condyle (Fig. 4-18). These type 3 fragments also may undergo significant rotational deformation.

There is a tendency for this fracture to occur as the growth plate is undergoing the final phases of physiologic epiphysiodesis. Such an injury is common in the distal tibial epiphysis (Tillaux fracture).

Restoration of congruency of both the articular surface and the physis is essential, particularly in younger children. Open reduction frequently is indicated to obtain accurate anatomic restoration. Prognosis for future growth is reasonably good, provided that circulation to the separated fragment of the epiphysis and physis is not impaired. Futhermore, since many of these fractures occur when skeletal maturity is approaching, the chances for eventual growth disturbance are minimized by the lesser amount of anticipated longitudinal growth.

The type 3C subclassification includes injuries involving epiphyses that have developed major contour changes, such as the ischial tuberosity, in which epiphyseal fracture propagation may not necessarily involve a joint surface (Fig. 4-19). These seemingly isolated epiphyses have radiolucent cartilaginous and fibrocartilaginous attachments to contiguous regions, such as the symphysis pubis. The epiphysis is avulsed from the metaphysis and attentuates or fractures the cartilaginous/fibrocartilaginous growth region intervening between the injured portion of the epiphysis and the remaining, functionally separate portion of the originally contiguous epiphysis. In some instances, this connecting region may be injured significantly and lead to growth disturbance.

Type 4 (Fig. 4-20)

Like type 3 injuries the type 4A fracture line involves the articular surface, extending through the epiphysis (and ossification center, if present), across the full thickness of the physis, and subsequently through a significant segment of the metaphysis, causing a complete vertical (longitudinal)

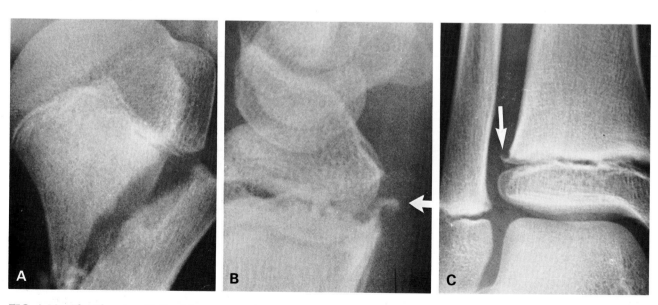

FIG. 4-10. The Thurston-Holland fragment varies significantly in size among the various regions, although it tends to be of comparable size in a given epiphysis. *A,* The conical nature of the proximal humerus is associated with a large medial fragment. *B,* The distal radius often has an extremely small fragment on the dorsal surface (arrow). Oblique views may be necessary to visualize such an injury. *C,* Undisplaced distal tibial type 2 fracture. A mortise view enabled visualization of the small metaphyseal fragment (arrow).

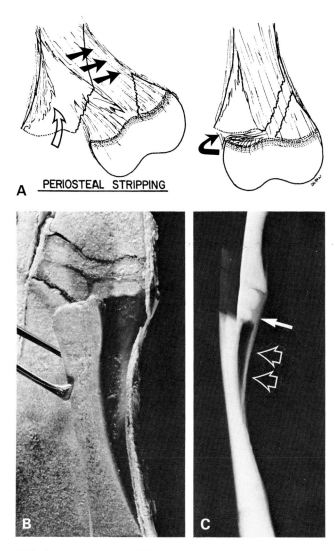

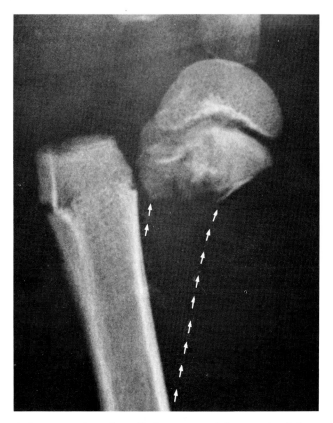

FIG. 4-11. *A,* In most of these injuries, the periosteum tends to strip away from the metaphysis while remaining attached to the epiphysis and physis. Portions of this may invaginate into the fracture defect, impeding normal repair processes or preventing reduction. *B,* Specimen from an immature narwhale showing how the metaphysis and diaphysis may displace from the periosteal sleeve. *C,* Roentgenogram showing how the periosteal sleeve (open arrows) remains attached to the epiphysis (solid arrow).

split of all zones of the physis, including the germinal layer. This injury commonly involves the medial and lateral condyles and epicondyles of the distal humerus. It may also involve the medial malleolar region of the distal tibia. The fracture fragments may be displaced to a highly variable extent, as a result of the original injury as well as the subsequent pull of specific attached muscles (such as the extensor mass of the forearm). If the secondary ossification center is small, the type 4 pattern may not be easily recognized (Fig. 4-21). However, the presence of a small metaphyseal fragment without evidence of other physeal separation (clinically or radiographically) should make one suspect a type 4 rather than a type 2 injury.

Anatomic reduction is imperative for restoration of both a smooth articular surface and normal cytoarchitectural relationships of the growth plate, which, in turn, minimize the risk of subsequent osseous bridging and localized premature growth arrest. Only fine, smooth Kirschner pins should be used for internal fixation if they must cross the growth plate. If possible, pins or screws should be placed transversely through the epiphyseal ossification center fragments and through the metaphyseal fragments, rather than across the growth plate (Fig. 4-22). If they must be directed across the growth plate, the pins should be placed as nearly perpendicular to the physis as possible, and they should be removed within four to six weeks. They should also be placed as centrally as possible to avoid the more active peripheral physeal regions.

Despite accurate reduction, growth damage and premature, localized epiphysiodesis still may occur, most likely as a result of microscopic, compression-type injury to regions of the growth plate. When attempting open reduction, care must be taken not to excessively strip periosteum in order to visualize the fracture completely, since this may damage the peripheral cellular activity of the zone of Ranvier and thereby contribute to the possibility of premature growth arrest.

The subclassification type 4B involves the aforementioned epiphyseal/metaphyseal unit, plus additional propagation of the fracture through remaining portions of the physis to create an additional free fragment comparable to an accom-

FIG. 4-12. Complete displacement of the proximal fragment toward the side of the Thurston-Holland fragment. The arrows show the periosteal course.

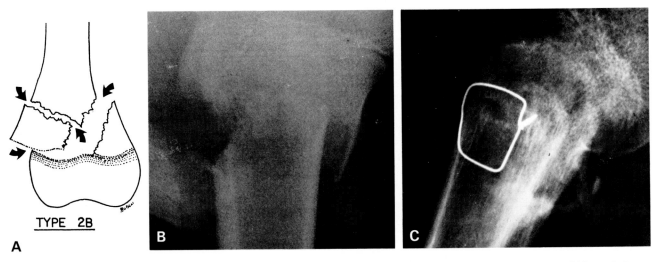

FIG. 4-13. *A,* Schematic of type 2B injury with a free metaphyseal fragment. *B,* Type 2B injury in a 12-year-old boy. *C,* Open reduction was necessary to stabilize the fracture.

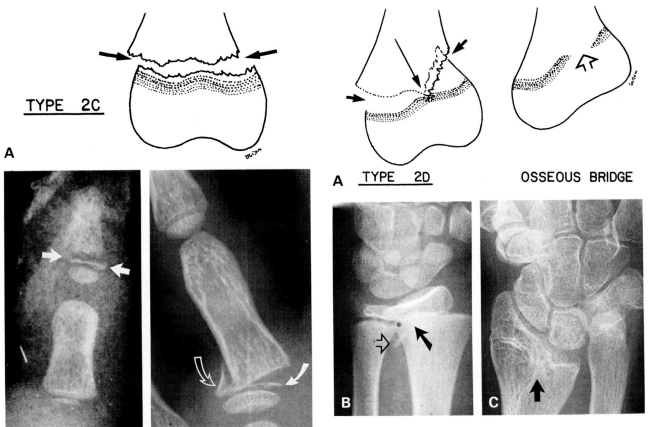

FIG. 4-14. *A,* Schematic of type 2C injury, in which the more transversely oriented primary spongiosa remains on the physeal side of the fracture. *B,* Type 2C injury (arrows) in the distal phalanx of the thumb. This injury pattern is fairly typical of phalangeal physeal injuries. *C,* Type 2C injury of proximal phalanx of digit with concomitant metaphyseal Thurston-Holland (open arrow) and Werenskiöld (closed arrow) signs.

FIG. 4-15. *A,* Schematic of type 2D injury in which there is compression of metaphysis into the physis, leading to permanently arrested growth and formation of an osseous bridge. *B,* At the age of eight, this patient sustained this typical type 2 distal radial injury with a metaphyseal fragment (open arrow). The angulation of the ossification center on the edge of the metaphysis (closed arrow) should make one suspect a 2D rather than a 2A injury. *C,* Four years later, growth arrest and osseous bridging (arrow) have occurred, confirming a type 2D injury.

panying type 3 injury (Fig. 4-23). This tendency for multiple fragmentation is again more common in people approaching skeletal maturity, a time when the growth plate is susceptible to different fracture propagation modes than it is in younger children.

As in type 3C, the type 4C fracture may propagate through radiolucent cartilaginous regions. Figure 4-24 shows a proximal femur, with the fracture propagating from the

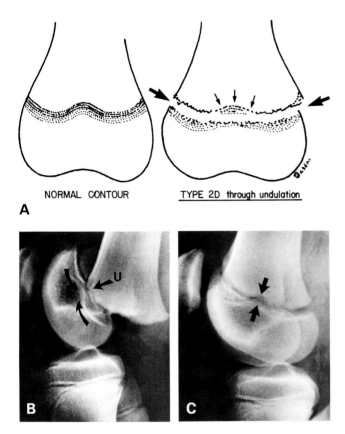

FIG. 4-16. *A,* Schematic showing effect of physeal undulation on fracture propagation. The binodal contour in the more central regions of the distal femur probably predisposes it to type 2D injuries with growth slowdown or arrest. *B-C,* Injury to distal femur showing effect of undulation. Note the undulation (U) in *B,* and its central peak (arrows) in *C.* This is the probable area of maximum damage.

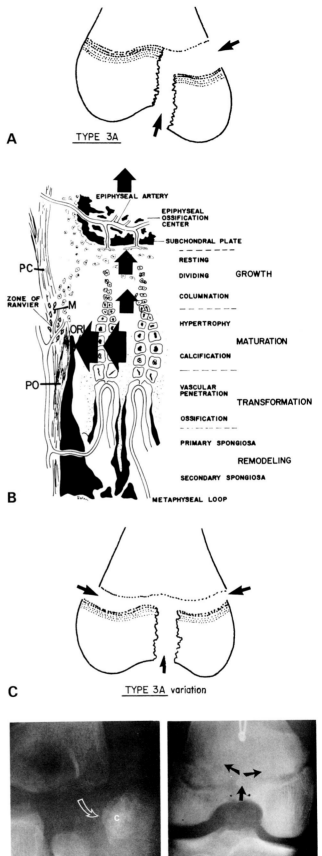

FIG. 4-17. *A,* Schematic of type 3A injury. *B,* Histologic schematic showing how the involvement of the growth plate in this fracture is bidirectional. The larger arrows show transverse propagation and the smaller arrows show longitudinal propagation across epiphyseal components. *C,* Schematic of variation of type 3A, with production of at least two separate epiphyseal fragments. *D,* Type 3A injury of lateral condyle (capitellum = c) of distal humerus (arrow). *E,* Type 3A injury involving both condyles (arrows) showing fracture propagation. Initially, it was felt that only the lateral condyle was involved. However, after an arthrotomy was performed, the less severely displaced medial condyle was also discovered.

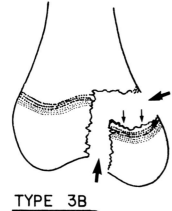

A TYPE 3B

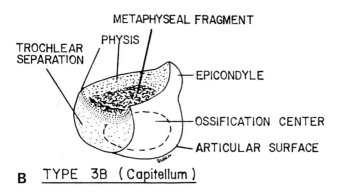

B TYPE 3B (Capitellum)

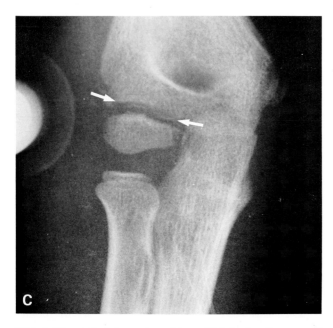

FIG. 4-18. *A-B*, Schematics of type 3B injuries. Because of the extensive lappet formation anterior to the physis, posteriorly and laterally, the fracture is through the physis, but centrally it tends to propagate across the primary spongiosa. This defect of bone is not the same as either the Werenskiöld or the Thurston-Holland sign. *C*, Type 3B injury involving the distal humerus (capitellum). The arrows show the thin layer of metaphyseal bone.

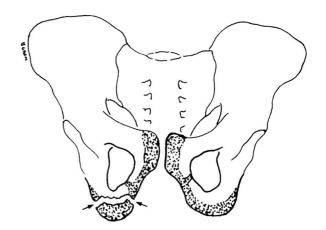

A TYPE 3C - Ischial tuberosity

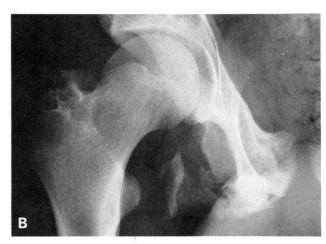

FIG. 4-19. *A*, Schematic of type 3C injury involving non-articular epiphyseal cartilage. These injuries particularly involve the pelvis. *B*, Type 3C injury of avulsion of ischial tuberosity.

metaphysis through the contiguous physis into the epiphyseal region between the trochanter and the capital femur. Such a type 4C injury involves metaphysis, physis, and epiphysis.

The frequent accidents involving rotary lawn mowers may result in multiple metaphyseal-physeal-epiphyseal fragments (type 4D). This only increases the risk of traumatically induced, localized epiphysiodesis (Fig. 4-25).

Type 5 (Fig. 4-26)

This injury occurs infrequently, is difficult to diagnose and usually involves weightbearing epiphyses around the knee or ankle—those articulations that normally move significantly in only one plane (flexion-extension). The application of a significant abduction or adduction (valgus or varus) strain to such regions causes transmission of a compression force through certain segments of the epiphysis and physis, which crushes germinal regions of the chondrocytes as well as adjacent hypertrophic, columnar regions. Displacement of the epiphysis is minimal, and virtually unrecognizable by

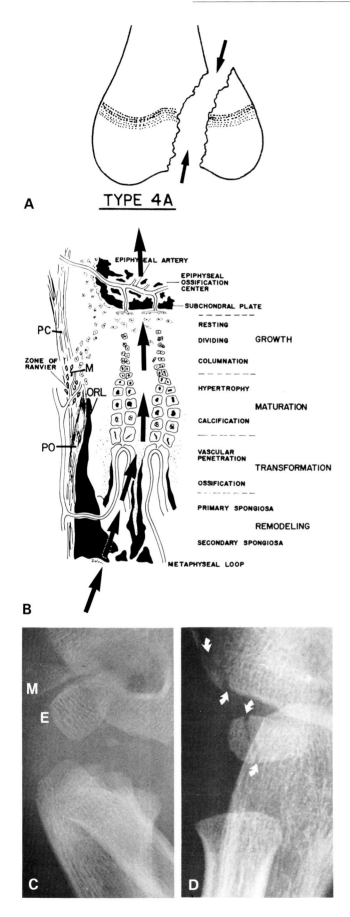

A **TYPE 4A**

standard diagnostic techniques. Often, the serious nature of the condition is unsuspected, and the injury may be diagnosed as a simple sprain. Diagnosis frequently must be empirical, with treatment directed at non-weightbearing (lower extremity) and cast immobilization for three to four weeks.

The prognosis in type 5 injuries is poor, since premature growth arrest almost always occurs. However, this premature growth arrest may not occur for several years after the initial injury, at which time the child may present with an angular deformity and minimal memory of the original injury (Fig. 4-27). Infrequently, the metaphysis may be driven completely through the growth plate into the epiphysis (Fig. 4-28).

While indirect crushing trauma is presumably the major cause of this type of injury, additional mechanisms may lead to the same type of localized growth arrest. One such mechanism is electrical injury due to high voltage wires, or to being struck by lightning.[4,37-39] The unique aspects of propagation of electrical forces through the extremities cause highly variable, localized injuries to the growth plates which result in premature slowdown of growth and eventual arrest in certain areas of the physis (Fig. 4-29). Another cause of generalized or localized growth slowdown or arrest is radiation. Innumerable reports document the deleterious effects of radiation delivered for "therapeutic" reasons, as well as the experimentally produced effects of roentgen rays on the physis.[40-59] Frostbite also may lead to growth retardation, possibly due to ischemia rather than the direct thermal effect on the physeal cartilage.[60-69] Decreased arterial supply to the physis, whether due to extraosseous or intraepiphyseal disruption, certainly may lead to irregular growth (Fig. 4-30). The physis and epiphysis seem to assume a characteristic "cone-shape" in such circumstances.[70-72] These various "noncompression" factors are discussed in more detail in subsequent sections of this Chapter.

Type 6 (Fig. 4-31)

This type of injury involves the peripheral region of the growth plate, particularly the zone of Ranvier. Such an injury may not always be associated with a major fracture. More frequently, it results from a localized contusion or avulsion of the portion of the growth mechanism concerned specifically with latitudinal or appositional cartilaginous growth. The injury may even result from a glancing type of trauma primarily involving avulsion of overlying skin and subcutaneous tissues, such as might occur from a lawn mower (Fig. 4-32), or from extension of a traumatically induced infection or severe burn (Fig. 4-33). Because of the

FIG. 4-20. *A-B,* Schematics of type 4A injury, in which the fracture propagates across both the epiphysis and the metaphysis. The arrows show the direction of fracture propagation through the metaphysis, physis, and epiphysis. *C,* Type 4D injury of the distal humerus (capitellum), with the entire chondro-osseous unit separating from the trochlea. Note the metaphyseal fragment (M) and the epiphyseal ossification center (E). *D,* Similar type 4A injury, but with the fracture propagating (arrows) through the capitellar ossification center and metaphysis.

highly selective and localized nature of these lesions, peripheral osseous bridge formation frequently occurs, and leads to peripherally localized epiphysiodesis and subsequent progressive angular deformity.

While the exact mechanism is not clear, trauma to this peripheral region may also cause solitary osteochondroma formation. Rang[73] suggested that particular types of experimentally produced injury to the periphery of the growth plate and periosteum could lead to osteochondroma formation, and certainly, many children with solitary exostoses do have significant history of specific trauma to the area (Fig. 4-34).

Involvement of the zone of Ranvier undoubtedly occurs in types 3 and 4 physeal injuries in which the fracture propagates to the periphery of the bone. At such points, localized type 6 damage may occur, leading to osseous bridge formation. When type 3, 4, or 6 injuries are treated, care must be taken not to strip the zone of Ranvier away from the underlying epiphysis when elevating periosteum. This may disrupt the blood supply, as well as directly traumatizing these important peripheral germinal cells.

Type 7 (Fig. 4-35)

These fractures are completely intraepiphyseal and represent propagation of the fracture from the articular surface through the epiphyseal cartilage into the secondary ossification center or preossification center, depending upon the stage of maturation. They do not involve the primary physis at all, although they may affect the smaller, spherical physis around the secondary center of ossification. This type of injury is common at the malleoli, and within the distal humerus (capitellum) or distal femur as an osteochondral fracture.

There are two basic subtypes. The first type (7A) involves propagation of the fracture through both the epiphyseal and the articular cartilage, as well as the bone of the secondary ossification center. The second type (7B) is more difficult to diagnose and represents a propagation of the fracture primarily through the cartilaginous portions, with involvement of some of the pre-ossifying regions of the expanding secondary ossification center, which are analogous to the hypertrophic, fracture-susceptible zone of the main physis. This type of fracture is likely to occur in the distal tibia, and it also may involve non-articular regions such as the tibial tuberosity, the greater trochanter, and the fifth metatarsal at its proximal base (Fig. 4-36).

Osgood-Schlatter's disease, and perhaps other lesions classified as osteochondroses, possibly represent stress-type fractures involving regions of the chondro-osseous tissue that are beginning to undergo the normal transition from cartilage to bone. During this transition phase, if subjected to high tensile forces (a phenomenon particularly evident in the tibial tuberosity), the pre-ossification region may be avulsed partially away from the main portion of the tuberosity. This may occur prior to the appearance of the ossification center, creating a type 7B injury, or after its appearance, creating a type 7A lesion. The fingers and toes may have small type 7 intraepiphyseal fractures which are comparable to the mallet finger injury. In the case of avulsion of portions of the phalangeal physes and epiphyses concomitant with tendon ''ruptures,'' the failure to adequately reduce the injury may result in formation of a region of overgrown cartilage in the epiphysis and the creation of a structure analogous to an osteochondroma (see Fig. 4-34).

Osteochondral fractures involve a fragment containing both bone and cartilage. If the fragment is replaced by closed or open reduction, the bone may heal, permitting the cartilage laceration to heal with fibrocartilage. The cartilage attached to the stabilized fragment may retain normal viability through nutritional diffusion from the synovial fluid. If the bone fragment does not heal promptly, the fragment may be unstable and the normal diffusion process disturbed. Both bone and cartilage may become necrotic, frequently being extruded into the joint as a loose body.

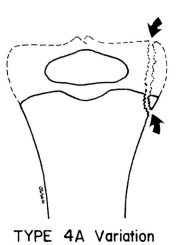

TYPE 4A Variation

A

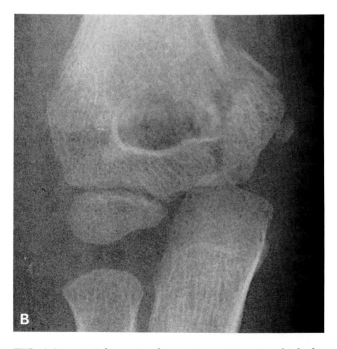

FIG. 4-21. *A*, Schematic of type 4A variation in which the epiphyseal fracture propagates through radiolucent cartilage. *B*, Fracture of medial portion of distal humeral metaphysis. This resembles the Thurston-Holland sign. However, the capitellum is obviously uninjured, indicating a diagnosis of a type 4, not a type 2 injury.

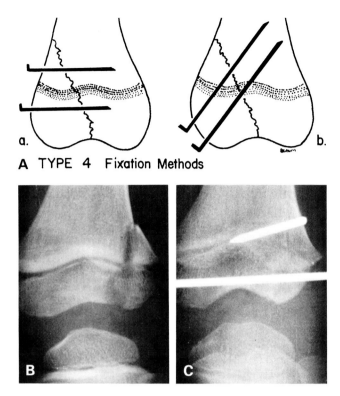

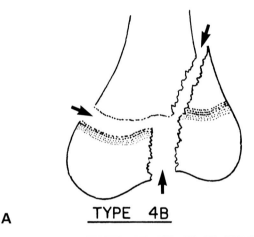

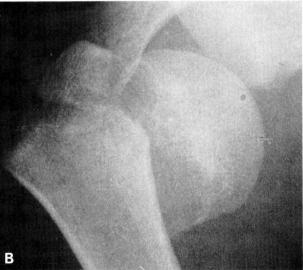

FIG. 4-22. *A,* Schematic of proper fixation for type 4 injuries. The method shown in (a) is preferred to that shown in (b). *B,* Type 4A injury of lateral distal femur. *C,* Fixation pins placed through epiphyseal fragments, and through metaphyseal fragments, with neither pin crossing the physis.

Osteochondritis dissecans probably is produced as a result of a sharp impact of one joint surface against another in a rotatory or angular fashion. The cartilage, being resilient, may remain intact and a fragment of subchondral bone may fracture.[74-77] The more common sites of occurrence for this fracture type are the inner aspect of the medial femoral condyle, the capitellum, and the talus. These lesions are discussed in more detail in Chapters 11, 18, and 20.

Type 8 (Fig. 4-37)

These are injuries that occur to the metaphyseal growth and remodeling mechanisms and represent transient phenomena primarily related to vascularity. If a significant fracture occurs through the normal, central or peripheral vascular supply patterns (which may occur in normal bone as well as pathologic situations), the metaphyseal circulation involved in formation of primary spongiosa from the cartilage cell columns is temporarily disrupted, leading to failure of normal osseous remodeling and subsequent, transiently increased osseous density as the area is revascularized (Fig. 4-38). Experimentally, Spira and Farin[78] showed that in the rabbit, blood vessels (E-vessels) could penetrate from the epiphysis through the physis to substitute temporarily for the primary spongiosa M-vessels. As the latter circulation was restored, these transphyseal vessels regressed. Whether a similar phenomenon can occur in the skeletally immature human is open to conjecture.

Following rapid revascularization, the junction of primary spongiosa and hypertrophic cartilage may become biomechanically weaker, not unlike the revascularization phase of Legg-Perthes disease, and as a result, epiphysiolysis may be a complication of temporary metaphyseal ischemia (Fig. 4-39).

Type 9 (Fig. 4-40)

Type 9 injuries are selective injuries to the diaphyseal growth mechanisms that are controlled by appositional, membranous new bone formation from the periosteum. Any direct injury causing permanent damage to the periosteum may affect the ability of the bone to remodel and to increase cortical volume circumferentially. This may be associated with severe compounding and fragmentation of portions of the diaphysis (Fig. 4-41), which is a significant problem if the damaged bone requires a thick diaphyseal cortex

FIG. 4-23. *A,* Schematic of type 4B injury, in which the type 4 fragment is accompanied by a type 3 fragment. This is a pattern encountered in the distal tibia. *B,* Type 4B injury of the proximal humerus. The epiphyseal/metaphyseal fragment involves the capital humerus, while the epiphyseal fragment involves the tuberosity.

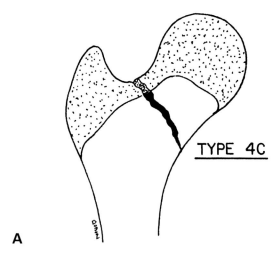

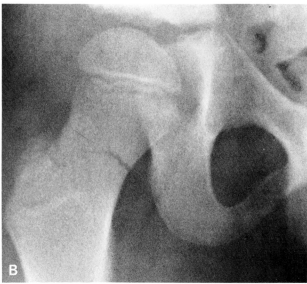

FIG. 4-24. *A,* Schematic of type 4C injury involving non-articular epiphyseal cartilage. *B,* Clinical roentgenogram of such an injury does not show cartilaginous involvement.

for normal biomechanical function, as the tibia does. The periosteum may be damaged in a localized area, and this may lead to unusual patterns of extra-periosteal bone formation (Fig. 4-42).[79] Wringer injuries may be associated with significant avulsion damage to the periosteum.[80,81] Damage to the interosseous area, particularly in paired bones, also may cause contiguity of damaged periosteal elements between tibia and fibula or radius and ulna, leading to synostosis formation (Fig. 4-43).

While these injuries may not be conceived of as typical to a growth mechanism, it must be remembered that one of the major mechanisms for longitudinal as well as appositional bone growth is the control imparted by the highly osteogenic periosteal sleeve. Damage to this soft tissue "skeletal" component by compound injury, burn, or infection must affect localized areas of diaphyseal bone growth, either transiently or permanently. Furthermore, significant loss of periosteal growth mechanisms may also affect intrinsic periosteal control of longitudinal (physeal) growth (see Chap. 2).

Specific Injuries

Athletic injuries

Athletics play an especially important role in the lives of children and adolescents; and more and more children of both sexes are participating, in increasing numbers, in contact and noncontact sports. Collins[82] reviewd 2137 cases of athletic injuries in children, but found only 58 epiphyseal injuries, the majority of which were acutely symptomatic cases of Osgood-Schlatter disease. He felt that the incidence of epiphyseal injuries was no higher than might be expected in other, nonstructured activities of youth. Larson[83] also found a similar low incidence of epiphyseal injuries in adolescent athletes. It appears that there is *not* a greater risk of epiphyseal and physeal injury during competitive athletics. However, specific types of epiphyseal injury, such as the "little league elbow," do occur frequently in certain competitive situations. A more detailed discussion of athletic injuries is presented in Chapter 8.

Electrical injuries

Brinn[37] noted that many factors determine the effects of electrical current on chondro-osseous tissue. The principal factors are: (1) type of current, with alternating current being three to four times as dangerous as direct current; (2) voltage; (3) amperage; (4) duration of contact with the electrical current; (5) path taken by current through the body; (6) resistance at the points of contact and exit and elsewhere in the body; and (7) individual's general state of health. Death from low voltage electrical injury, especially below 220 volts, is usually due to inhibition of the central nervous system, especially the respiratory center. During electrical accidents, tissue temperature may reach several thousand degrees centigrade momentarily, and cause heat-induced liquefaction and necrosis of bone. The changes in the bone that is liquefied and transformed into a gel may be attributed to the pathway of the electricity (Fig. 4-44). In general, the tissues offering the greatest resistance to current flow suffer the greatest damage. Electrical injury may result in cell death or may alter cellular activity either temporarily or permanently. After electrical accidents, tissue repair, including callus formation, is poor.

Much more basic research is needed before the modifications occurring in developing chondro-osseous structure and physiology as a result of electrical trauma are intelligently understood. Granberry and Janes[38] attempted to influence bone growth by stimulating the epiphyseal plates of bones in dogs with implanted electrodes. In their study, no acceleration of growth occurred with such electrical stimulation. However, the doses were deliberately small, so this experiment did not allow observation of the detrimental effects of high voltage electricity.

Children may show osseous changes similar to those shown by adults, but they may also have additional abnormalities secondary to the effect of the current on the epiphyseal cartilage.[84] The epiphyseal center and the epiphyseal cartilage may be affected by the current, and the metaphyseal region will undergo little remodeling. Ahstrom[85] described electrical burns caused by treatment of a scrotal swelling by a chiropractor who used "electrical treatment." The patient sustained a severe burn to the lateral aspect of

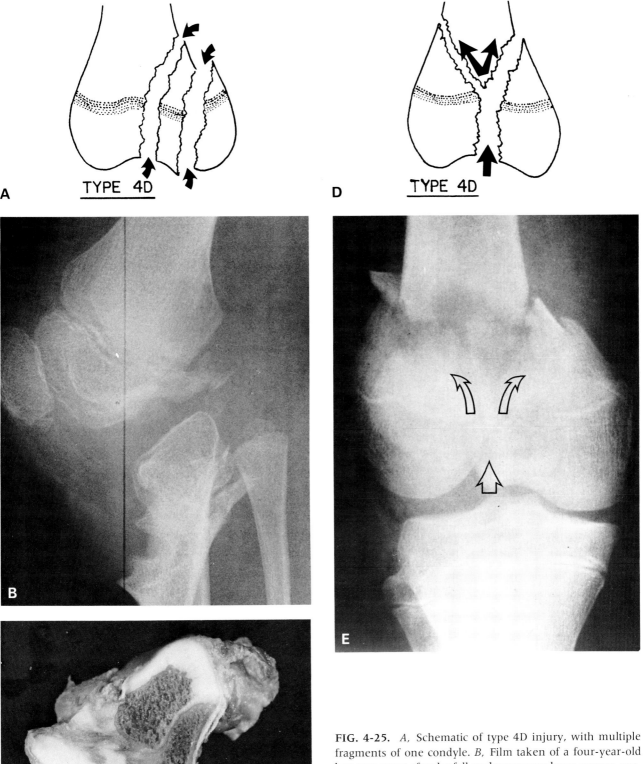

FIG. 4-25. *A,* Schematic of type 4D injury, with multiple fragments of one condyle. *B,* Film taken of a four-year-old boy two years after he fell under a power lawn mower, sustaining type 4D injuries of the distal femur and proximal tibia. *C,* Sagittal section showing severe long term damage to articular surface and epiphysis consequent to this injury (see Fig. 4-55). *D,* Schematic of type 4D injury involving the entire epiphysis, with a splitting of the fragments. *E,* Type 4D injury of the distal femur, with arrows indicating directions of fracture propagation.

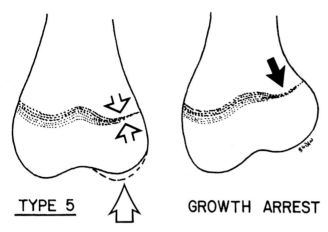

TYPE 5   GROWTH ARREST

FIG. 4-26. Schematic of type 5 injury. This is a direct compression injury of all layers of the physis and eventually leads to growth arrest. Unfortunately it is difficult, if not impossible, to diagnose at the time of initial injury.

the left knee and thigh, and eventually developed premature lateral growth arrest of the distal femur. Kolar[39] reported three cases in which electrical accidents resulted in extensive tissue burns requiring amputation of phalanges. In these cases, several of the remaining phalanges showed an abnormal elongation. This overgrowth could be secondary to chronic hyperemia resulting from the extensive soft tissue injuries, with infection contributing to the hyperemia as well. None of these studies described the actual histologic changes, illustrated in Figure 4-44, that affected the bone and the growth plate.

Frostbite

Cold thermal injury to the physes has been described infrequently. Epiphyseal changes from frostbite were reported in a 16-year-old boy who had lost the distal phalangeal epiphyses of the four fingers of the right hand.[86] Bennett and Blount[61] reported an 8-year-old girl who had frozen her left hand three years before, and as a result, lost the epiphyses of the middle phalanges of the index, middle, and ring fingers and all the distal phalangeal epiphyses. Thelander[68] described a 9-year-old boy who had sustained a severe frostbite injury of the hand two and one-half years previously. Thelander thought that the overexposure to cold temperatures might have caused vascular damage. The subsequent radiographic changes included absence of the distal phalangeal epiphyses, thinning of the joint space and cartilage, and diaphyseal roughening of the second digits. The phalanges were shortened, and it was presumed that the epiphyses had been destroyed, and the growth arrested. Dreyfuss and Glimcher[62] presented an excellent study of the clinical course of a child two and one-half years after frostbite. Thiemann[87] reported a peculiar case, in which the epiphyseal ossification centers of the phalanges disappeared during puberty, only to reappear a few years later. Bigelow[6] reported on 13 patients who experienced frostbite of the hands during childhood, all of whom had lost one or more physes when evaluted 4 to 50 years after exposure. Several authors have contributed further case experiences, with most feeling that vascular injury was the main effect of frostbite.[63-65,67,89] Epiphysiolysis was found after Volkmann's ischemic contracture[54] and after severe arm injuries.[61]

In Bigelow's study, the index and little fingers were involved in every frostbitten hand, the ring finger slightly less, while the middle finger was the least often involved. In each digit, the distal phalanx and distal interphalangeal joint were involved most often. The proximal phalanx and proximal interphalangeal joint were never involved if the distal phalanx of that same digit was not also involved.

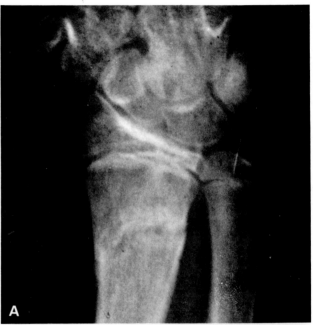

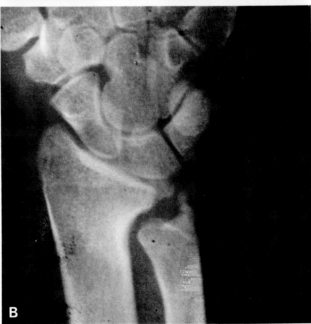

FIG. 4-27. *A*, Nine-year-old girl with seemingly innocuous injury to distal radial metaphysis. *B*, Four years later there has been a type 5 injury to the distal ulna and a secondary impairment of distal radial growth.

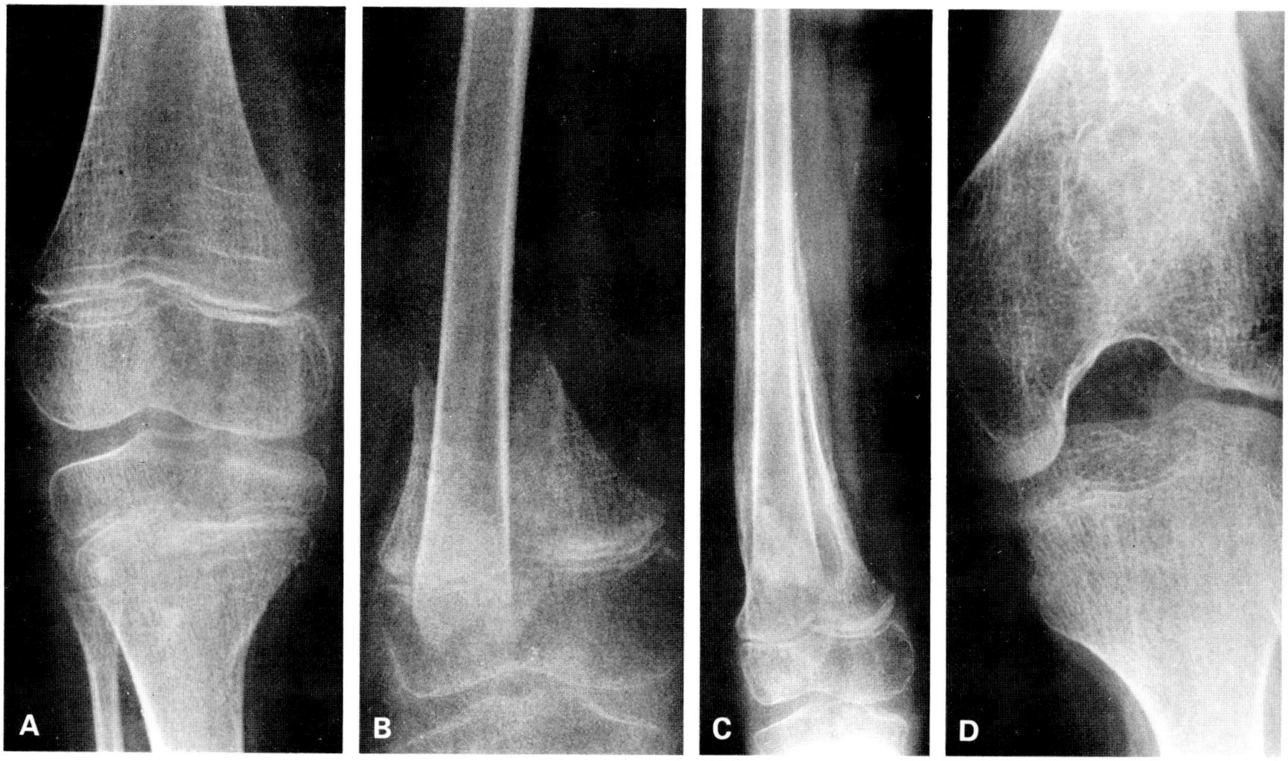

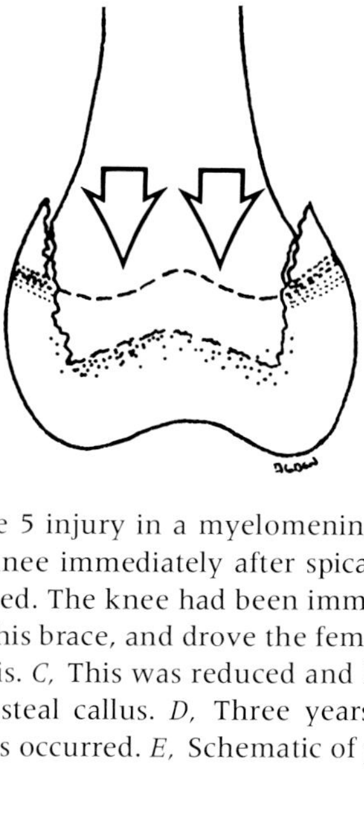

FIG. 4-28. Type 5 injury in a myelomeningocele child. *A,* Appearance of knee immediately after spica cast (spine fusion) was removed. The knee had been immobilized. *B,* The patient stood in his brace, and drove the femoral metaphysis into the epiphysis. *C,* This was reduced and healed with extensive subperiosteal callus. *D,* Three years later, obvious growth arrest has occurred. *E,* Schematic of probable mechanism.

In children, frostbite causes a characteristic radiographic appearance, particularly at the articular ends of the bones on both sides of the joint (Fig. 4-45). The affected phalanges are shorter and smaller than normal, the juxta-articular bone is expanded and irregular with the spongiosa altered to show a coarse cancellous pattern. The same expanded and irregular appearance is seen on the contiguous surface of the more proximal phalanx, where there is no epiphysis. The joint surfaces are irregular and uneven, but the width of the joint space does not appear to be altered. Usually the epiphysis

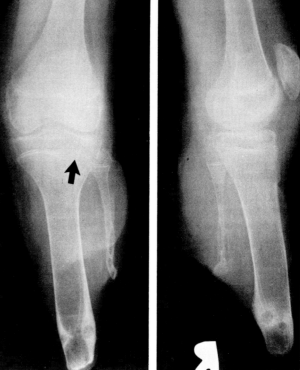

FIG. 4-29. Twelve-year-old boy who sustained a high voltage electrical injury and required a below-knee amputation. Premature epiphysiodesis occurred in the lateral tibial physis (arrow), along the probable line of electrical impulse propagation.

disappears completely, but it may be only partially destroyed, with the undestroyed portion taking part in the joint disfiguration. Not uncommonly, the base of an involved phalanx has a pronounced V-shape, presumably due to ischemic damage.[72,90] There may be no obvious acute destruction of the epiphysis, but eventual premature fusion of a part of the epiphyseal line may lead to varus or valgus angulation.

Shumacker and Lempke[91] confirmed that vascular channels were closed while the extremity was frozen and that the capillaries became contracted just before freezing. This constriction contributed to tissue anoxia. Within a few minutes of the return of blood flow on thawing, there was perivascular edema of the subcutaneous tissues, a precapillary cuffing of the eosinophils, and swelling and engorgement of the capillary endothelium.[92-94] The edema resulted from increased permeability of the capillary walls. The edema continued, and extracapillary pressure increased, further augmenting capillary stasis.[95] Agglutination of blood cells in the small vessels obstructed the circulation.[91,96] Thrombi occurred in the veins and venules. After a few hours, there was dissolution of the endothelium of the small arterioles, with further vascular occlusion, tissue edema, transudation of fluid, and perivascular hemorrhage. Tissue necrosis resulted because the sudden demands of the increased metabolism could not be met. Using angiography, Hurley[97] showed that the vascular supply in the surviving tissue was abundant because of the opening of side branches and the development of new capillary outgrowths in both the arterial and the venous sides of the vascular tree. The budding and revascularization were prolific, especially in the borderland zones between necrotic and viable tissue.

The freezing of articular cartilage produces changes immediately after thawing.[60] The articular surface becomes darker, and the nuclei of the cartilage cells lose their normal staining properties. Cartilage degeneration begins, and eventually the cartilage may be completely absorbed. Lohr[86] said that epiphyseal and physeal cartilage also goes through a

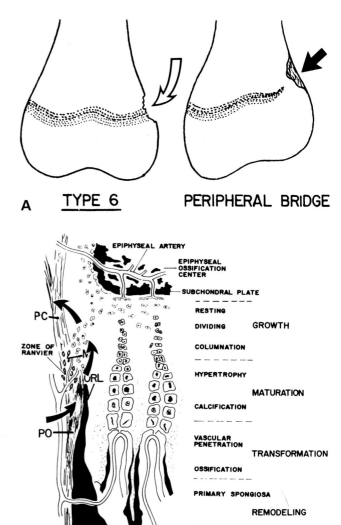

A   TYPE 6   PERIPHERAL BRIDGE

B

FIG. 4-31. *A,* Schematic of a type 6 injury, which involves the peripheral region. Damage may lead to osseous bridging. *B,* Histologic schematic showing area of involvement in this injury. Arrows show area of fracture involvement.

series of degenerative stages, and the destruction may be such that the cartilaginous tissue is replaced by connective scar tissue. Scow[66] showed that growth arrest was evident as early as three or four days following freezing of the tail vertebrae of newborn rats.

Irradiation

Therapeutic irradiation has been used for a number of neoplastic problems involving the skeleton and contiguous soft tissues. Unfortunately, it is injurious and may result in physeal growth impairment (Fig. 4-46). Desjardins[46] reported a nine-year-old girl irradiated for tumor of the upper humerus; five years later there was marked shortening of the humerus with atrophy of the shoulder musculature. Stevens[98] described a child who had been irradiated for a cutaneous tumor in the groin, with subsequent retardation

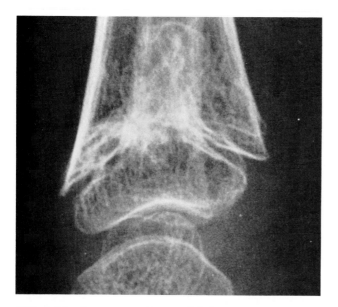

FIG. 4-30. Severe type 5 central defect resulting from ischemia. There is some retention of peripheral growth.

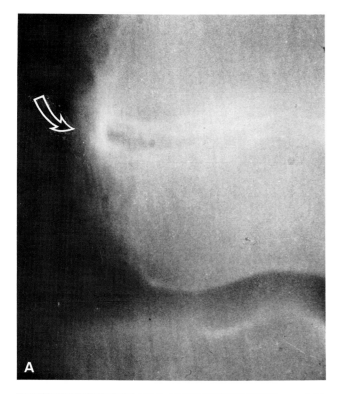

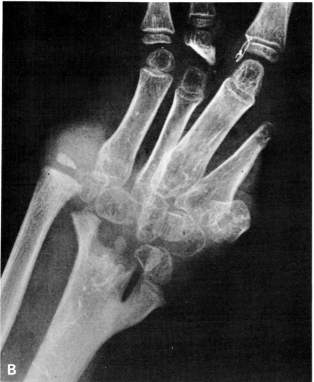

of proximal femoral growth. Langenskiöld[53] described a child who had received radiation for telangiectasia; the growth plate did not spontaneously close completely, but there was a slowdown of growth, creating a varus deformity affecting both the distal femoral as well as the proximal tibial growth plates. Judy[51] described changes affecting growth regions in three children submitted to irradiation to correct asymmetry in the length of lower extremities. Spangler[58] tried to use irradiation to cause epiphysiodesis in children with leg length inequality.

The effects of radiation on growth have been demonstrated in man as well as in experimental animals.[99] Nevertheless, some aspects of the effect on the growth plate have not been shown clearly; significantly, whether the apparent histologic lesions in the growth plate and the consequent retardation of growth are caused by direct radiation effect on the chondrocytes or are secondary to damage of neighboring tissues such as blood cells, osteoblasts, and marrow cells. It appears that a number of factors influence the histologic changes found in the growth plate after irradiation. The changes are proportional to the radiation delivered and inversely proportional to the age of the animal at the time of irradiation.

The dosage and type of rays are undoubtedly the most important factors. Experimentally, up to 800 rads produced a retardation of bone growth that was temporary and reversible. With 800 to 1800 rads cellular survival was less, bone growth was held back for a longer time, and if the germinal cells were damaged irreparably, growth would cease prematurely. With doses of more than 1800 rads, complete arrest of growth occurred, although evidence of later regeneration has been reported.[40]

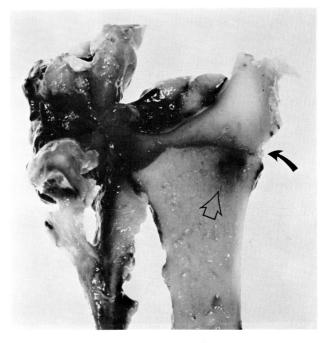

FIG. 4-32. *A,* Tomogram showing (arrow) bridge formation in a child struck in the knee by an automobile bumper. The injury led to full thickness avulsion down to and including the periosteum, but no obvious osseous damage occurred. *B,* Erratic post-traumatic ossification after compound trauma (blast injury from fireworks) to hand and periphery of distal radius.

FIG. 4-33. Peripheral burn injury (closed arrow) with concomitant deeper involvement of the metaphysis (open arrow).

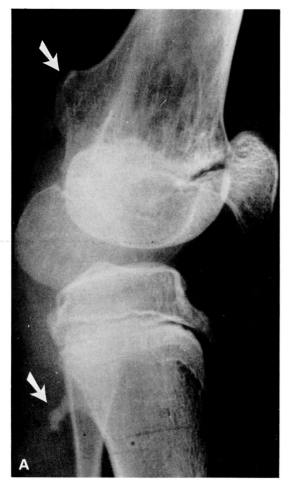

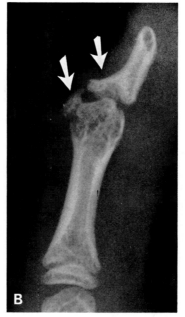

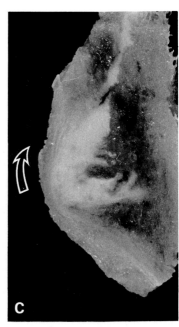

FIG. 4-34. *A,* Formation of osteochondroma (arrows) of the posterior femur and tibia in a child who sustained a severe hyperextension injury 17 months earlier. *B,* Formation of osteochondroma (arrows) following displaced fracture of the distal phalangeal epiphysis. *C,* Osteochondroma formation complicating combined type 4 and type 6 injury. The physeal cartilage is extending proximally along the femoral metaphysis (arrow).

Burns (Type 6 injury)

Bone and joint changes occurring as a result of severe burns are of clinical interest both from the standpoint of pathogenesis and because of the significance of the rehabilitation phase. Burns may extend down to the zone of Ranvier and the peripheral growth plate, and cause impairment of growth and subsequent angular deformity, if not complete disruption (Fig. 4-47; also see Fig. 4-33).

Multiple osseous changes occur consequent to burns, including osteoporosis, ectopic bone, periosteal new bone formation, pericapsular calcification and ossification, osteophyte formation, and progressive joint destruction with ankylosis (Fig. 4-48). Many of these changes have been reported in young children as well as in adults. Evans[100] felt that skeletal alterations fell logically into three groups: (1) alterations limited to bone, which included osteoporosis and periosteal new bone formation; (2) alterations involving para-articular structures, including pericapsular calcification, osteophytes, and hetertopic, para-articular ossification; and (3) alterations involving the joint proper, which included progressive articular destruction and ankylosis.

If an area of bone is denuded by a burn, eventual sequestration of the avascular portion may occur. This necrotic bone may remain exposed until adequate granulation tissue has developed. This represents damage to the periosteal and

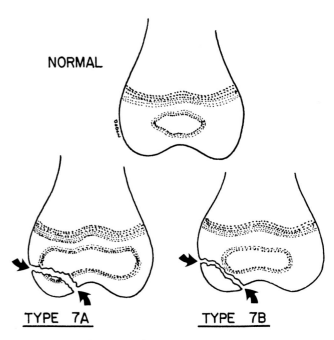

FIG. 4-35. Schematic of type 7 injuries.

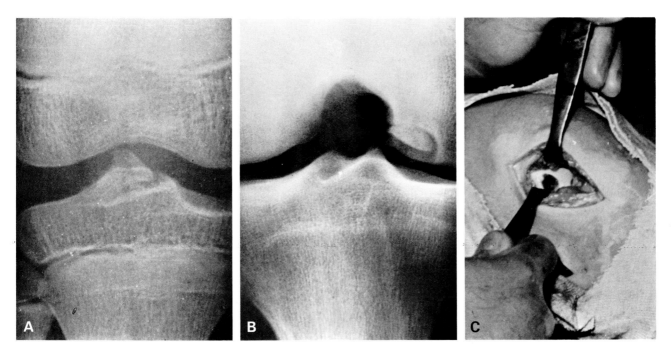

FIG. 4-36. *A,* Type 7 injury involving avulsion of the attachments of the anterior cruciate ligaments. *B-C,* Type 7 injuries of the femoral condyles.

physeal growth mechanisms in several areas, potentially creating type 5, 6, or 9 injuries. Cartilage dessicates, and becomes necrotic. Direct involvement of the joints frequently results in septic arthritis, articular destruction, and ankylosis. The wrist and hand joints are most frequently involved.

Skeletal alterations after burns seem to occur more often and to a greater degree in children than in adults, a factor that Evans ascribed to the exuberant granulation tissue response that is characteristic of youth.[100] Growth spurts in children after severe burns have been described, and it may be that skeletal growth is stimulated by stasis, passive hyperemia, or chronic inflammatory processes.

The precise mechanisms causing growth retardation in severely burned lower limbs are not well understood.[101] Evans and Smith[100] suggested that retardation could result from the restrictive or strangling effect of thick scar about the distal tibial metaphyseal and ankle joint areas, with inhi-

bition of epiphyseal growth. Their amputation specimens clearly demonstrated the destructive processes existing in and around the ankle joint. In addition to alterations visible in the bone and in the periarticular and interarticular structures, there probably is initial thermal damage to the margins of the epiphyseal plate, particularly the zone of Ranvier, as demonstrated in Figure 4-46. This damage to the appositional chondro-osseous growth mechanisms may be the most significant factor leading to eventual growth deformity.

Osteochondroma formation (Type 6 injury)

Ford and Key[102] showed that an osteocartilaginous exostosis might result when a patch of epiphyseal cartilage cells was displaced outside the shaft of the bone. This was an incidental finding during their efforts to experimentally traumatize the distal femur in rabbits. Rang[73] and D'Ambrosia and Ferguson[103] produced osteochondromata by damaging and redirecting the peripheral periosteal/zone of Ranvier complex. Many cases of solitary osteochondromata possibly result from such damage to the periphery of the growth plate, although it is extremely difficult to document this problem with any degree of causal certainty (see Fig. 4-34).

Osteochondral fractures (Type 7 injury)

Olsson[76,77] reviewed the problems of osteochondrosis in a number of animals. It appeared that the common denominator was a disturbance of endochondral ossification in animals exhibiting rapid musculoskeletal maturation. The most important manifestation of the osteochondrosis was osteochondritis dissecans, which began as a thickening of the articular and underlying epiphyseal cartilage, with necrosis of the deepest layer. Cracks and fissures then occurred, sponta-

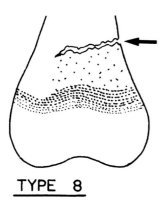

TYPE 8

FIG. 4-37. Schematic of type 8 injury.

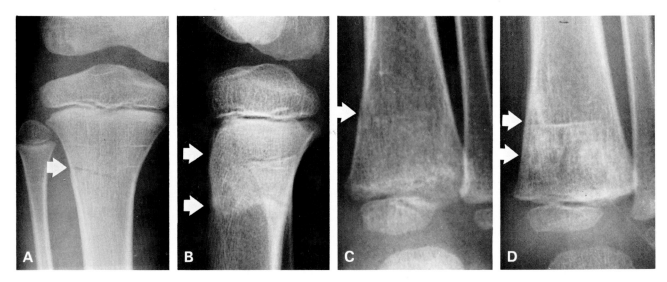

FIG. 4-38. *A,* Undisplaced proximal metaphyseal fracture (arrow). *B,* Two weeks later, the metaphyseal bone is sclerotic between the fracture and the physis (arrows). *C,* Almost invisible compression fracture of distal tibial metaphysis (arrow). *D,* Mottled sclerosis and transverse fracture line evident three weeks after injury (arrows).

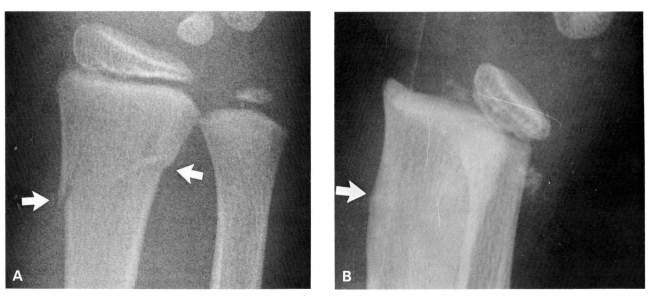

FIG. 4-39. *A,* Metaphyseal fracture of distal radius (arrows). *B,* Three weeks later the cast was removed. Two days later, the patient reinjured the arm, but had an epiphyseal injury instead. The metaphyseal fracture (arrow) is well healed.

neously dissecting a piece of cartilage to eventually form a flap or loose body. The initial crack occurred between the hypertrophic cartilage and the underlying bone, which appeared not to be forming a typical subchondral plate. Subsequently, the cracks propagated toward the articular surface (Fig. 4-49).

Meachim[104] took skeletally immature rabbits and created para-articular defects of the cartilage with injury to the subchondral bone plate. Bone healing of the defects in the osseous plate took place in both the articular and the para-articular drill holes. This was a fibrous reparative tissue. There was also a nonspecific osteochondrogenic reaction that occurred only in those animals in which the overlying

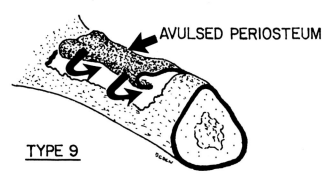

FIG. 4-40. Schematic of type 9 injury.

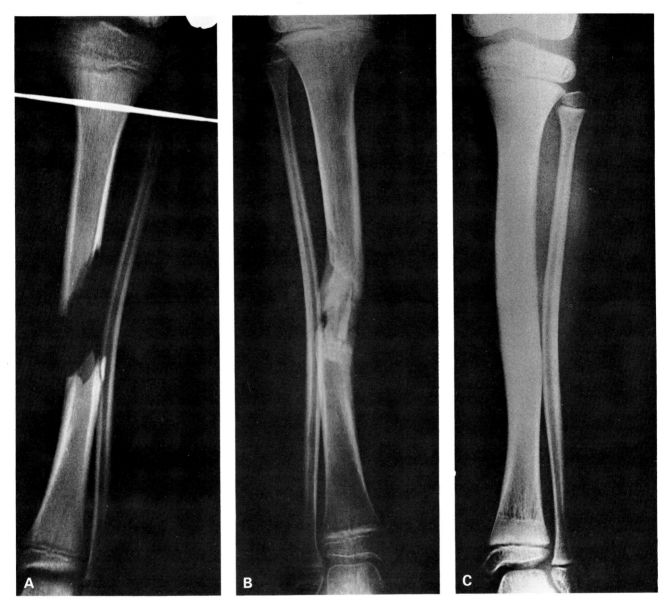

FIG. 4-41. *A,* Compound (open) injury to lower leg in which a diaphyseal fragment was extruded. Unfortunately, the periosteum was also moderately damaged. *B,* Subperiosteal bone formation and bone graft allowed reconstitution of the shaft. *C,* Extent of graft incorporation one year later.

cartilage had been removed and the subchondral plate drilled.

In contrast, nondrilled surfaces of the subarticular bone exposed by removal of the overlying cartilage showed virtually no response following the operation. Meachim concluded that chondrogenesis during the initial stages of healing of a full thickness defect of articular cartilage was a phenomenon in no way peculiar to the articular surface and was, in fact, an integral part of the osteogenic response of the subarticular plate to a fracture. However, in the later stages of the repair process, a difference became apparent between the articular and para-articular responses. The tissue that had repaired the articular drill holes usually showed cartilaginous plaques where it abutted the synovial cavity. The new articular cartilage contained rounded clusters of chondrocytes.

Wringer injury (Type 9 injury)

These injuries usually involve the upper limb, being sustained by a child whose hand has been drawn into the power-driven rollers of a washing machine. Maximum damage to the soft tissues generally is sustained in the antecubital fossa, although maximum trauma may occur in the axilla if the elbow is extended and allows the arm to go farther. The extent of the injury is increased by applying countertraction to the extremity or by reversing the direction of the roller, thus subjecting the arm to a second crushing. Other factors determining severity of damage are length of time during which the limb is caught between the rollers, size of the limb, tension of the rollers, and rapidity of the revolution. The crushing injury is primarily to soft tissues such as skin, subcutaneous tissue, muscles, tendons, and nerves. The bones are rarely fractured. However, periosteal damage (crushing, tearing) may be significant. This is primarily a type 9 injury.

Akbarnia and Campbell[80] reported a case of wringer injury in a 29-month-old child on whom they did a 24-year follow-up study. Initially, there was extensive loss of the diaphysis and periosteum of both the radius and the ulna, thus limiting the capacity for spontaneous restoration of the diaphyseal shaft. The child was subjected to repeated on-lay grafts to fill in the defects and had a rather dramatic restoration of a functional radius and ulna. Akbarnia and Campbell felt that the circulatory disturbances were a major factor in the distal shortening of the bone.

Comparable compression/avulsion injuries may occur when the ankle is caught in bicycle spokes. The ankle is severely twisted and massive swelling of the soft tissues may occur. Roentgenographic evidence of injury may be extremely subtle. Shearing damage consequent to a limb being run over by an automobile tire also produces an injury similar to a ''wringer injury'' (see Fig. 4-43).

Physiology of Epiphyseal/Physeal Injury

Biomechanics of the physis

The specific three-dimensional configuration of epiphyseal plates in growing mammals is extremely variable and probably develops primarily in response to the principal stresses applied to each specific epiphysis,[88,105-107] although a genetically programmed, basic developmental pattern (contour) also contributes to control of development. The overall complexity of the large undulations of the growth plate, as well as of the many smaller mammillary processes, cannot be fully appreciated in standard, two-dimensional radiographs. Because the human is not as highly specialized for rapid, twisting locomotion, the configurations of the epiphyseal plates of the lower extremity in humans are not as geometrically complex as they are in animals specialized for rapid running (e.g., the artiodactyls). In such animals, the attachments of ligaments to the epiphysis and the patterns of gait are such that a considerable rotatory force is applied, especially during an abrupt directional change.

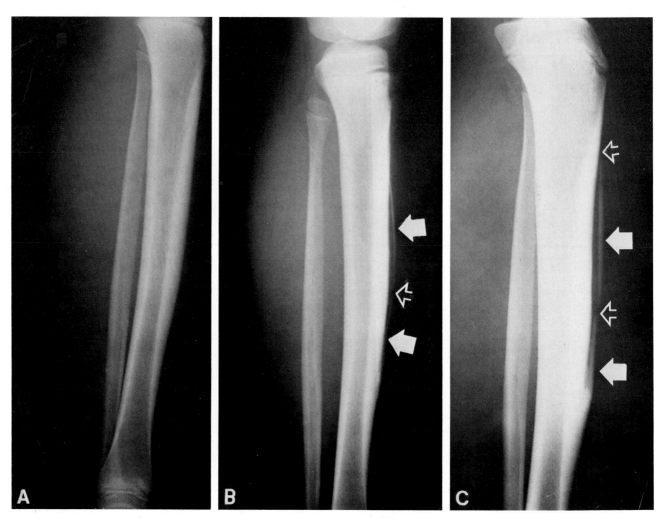

FIG. 4-42. Type 9 injury to the tibia of a young girl whose leg was run over by a bus wheel. *A,* Initial appearance. *B-C,* Progressive development of apparent heterotopic bone (solid arrows). Open arrows indicate pseudarthroses in the new bone. These were painful.

shearing transversely across only the hypertrophic cellular zone.

The strength of the physis probably is provided by both the cytoarchitectural types and arrangements as well as the intercellular cartilaginous matrix. In the first two zones of the physis, the cartilage matrix is abundant, and the growth plate is intrinsically strong. In contrast, in the third zone, the hypertrophic chondrocytes enlarge, making this zone potentially the weakest portion of the epiphyseal plate. This weakness is to shearing, bending, and tension stresses, but not to compression. The fourth zone is reinforced by the addition of calcification, but it still is weaker than the first and second zones. Fractures generally involve the third and fourth zones, propagating a variable distance into each one, and not cleaving neatly between the two zones.

The weakest part of the physis appears to be the third layer, the zone of hypertrophic cartilage cells. This was demonstrated by Haas,[108,109] who found that if the periosteum around the periphery of an epiphyseal plate was incised, the epiphysis could be detached relatively easily from the metaphysis by gentle pressure. He felt that the plate of cleavage was constant and that it went through the layer of hyper-

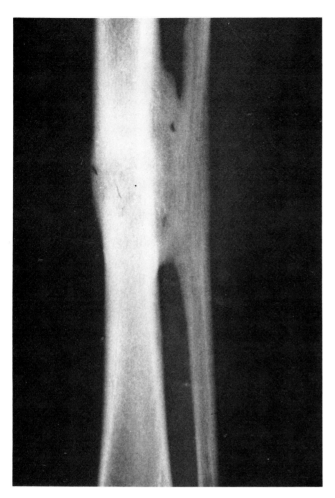

FIG. 4-43. Transverse fracture of the tibia and greenstick fracture of the fibula apparently led to sufficient periosteal and interosseous disruption sufficient for formation of a synostosis.

The distal femur in these animals represents a portion of a joint that is essentially a hinge joint; the epiphysis contains four cone-shaped projections from the metaphyseal side which fit into appropriate, concave-shaped areas of the epiphysis and physis. These effectively prevent displacement in anterior-posterior, medial, and lateral directions, as well as specifically preventing epiphyseal rotation. There is also a lappet formation around the periphery of the epiphysis to further anatomically resist varus-valgus and anterior-posterior displacements (Fig. 4-50). This particular configuration of the epiphysis is seen only moderately in the human (Fig. 4-50). The major import is that the epiphysis and growth plate are reasonably protected from major rotatory and shearing forces, but when the epiphysis is traumatically translocated in any direction from its normal position, the degree of potential deformity to the cone-shaped projections will depend on their degree of development. In the adolescent, these cone-shaped projections are more significantly developed, and a lateral or medial transverse fracture and displacement may shear through these projections and induce fractures in multiple regions of the growth plate, metaphysis, and epiphyseal ossification center, rather than

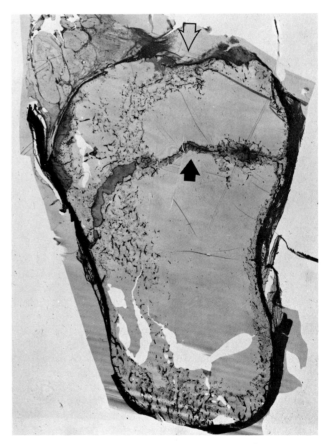

FIG. 4-44. Sagittal section showing severe involvement of proximal tibia in a patient who sustained a high voltage electrical injury. Liquefaction of trabecular bone is evident. The articular surface was destroyed (open arrow) and had undergone fibrous ankylosis to the femur. The physis (solid arrow) was destroyed except for the region under the tibial tuberosity.

trophic cartilage. Harris[110,111] designed an apparatus to determine shearing strength of the upper tibial epiphysis in the rat and confirmed that when the epiphysis separated from the metaphysis, the plane of cleavage consistently passed through the third layer. The clinical significance of these early experimental findings was that the growing cartilage cells in the physis remained with the epiphyseal fragment.

The region of trabecular formation in the metaphysis also contributes to the strength of the physis, though the thinness and fenestration of the metaphyseal cortex makes it susceptible to certain kinds of injuries (e.g., compression or torus failure) that are not seen in adults.

The epiphysis renders a certain shock-absorptive effect as long as it is primarily cartilaginous. In this situation, the fracture-producing forces are transmitted more directly into the metaphysis, resulting in torus fractures. However, as the epiphyseal ossification center enlarges, this resiliency and ability to absorb stress probably are lessened, and the deforming forces tend to be transmitted more directly into the growth plate, which, as a potentially weaker region, may be sheared through the third and fourth cellular zones.

The dense periosteal attachments around the physeal periphery seem to increase the resistance of the physis to shear and tensile failure. The physeal periosteum also blends into the epiphyseal perichondrium and joint capsule/ligament complex, further increasing its strength. In contrast, the periosteum is attached relatively loosely to the underlying, fenestrated metaphysis, although there is continuity of fibrous tissue from the intertrabecular spaces. In the child, the diaphyseal periosteum is attached even more loosely than the continuous metaphyseal and physeal periosteal regions. The diaphyseal periosteum seems not to contribute significantly to the strength of the bone in adults,[112] and since it is attached even more loosely in children, it is unlikely that it plays any major role in mechanically protecting the developing diaphysis from fracture/failure. However, it certainly contributes to stability if incompletely disrupted, and it is extremely osteogenic, leading to rapid subperiosteal new bone formation and fracture stabilization in the child.

Bright[113] showed that viscoelasticity of physeal cartilage was dependent on rate of loading. The total load before failure was substantially higher when rapid loading rates were used. Morscher[27,28] showed that the load-to-failure of epiphyseal cartilage with intact periosteum is almost twice that of epiphyseal cartilage with the periosteum removed. However, the fibrous periosteal membrane is much softer than cartilage and has a lower elastic modulus. Therefore, it can only play a secondary role in load distribution. The periosteum should be considered a checkrein on the epiphysis, once the cartilage plate has failed. It may prevent marked displacement if the load is insufficient to rupture its fibers, but its ultimate tensile properties probably are not tested until the cartilage has failed. This concept is in keeping with the clinical finding that epiphyseal injury often occurs without roentgenographic evidence of significant epiphyseal displacement (i.e., a type 1 injury).

Morscher[27,28] showed that the quality of the physeal cartilage, in terms of ultimate tensile strength, was physiologically reduced during sexual maturation, particularly in male animals (rats). Male and female animals differed with regard to the morphology and strength of their epiphyseal cartilage during this phase of sexual maturation (corresponding to the growth spurt of human adolescence). The

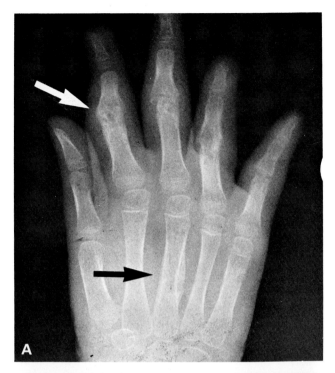

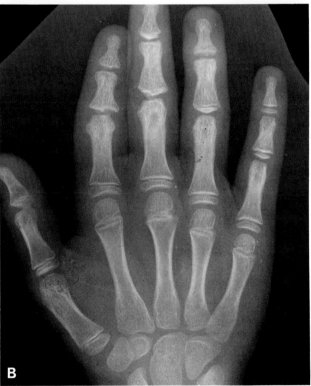

FIG. 4-45. *A,* This child sustained frostbite of the hand seven months before this roentgenogram was taken. Note the extensive damage to the proximal interphalangeal joints (white arrow) and contiguous bone, and the closure of the physes of the middle phalanges. There is also reactive subperiosteal bone around the third metacarpal (black arrow). *B,* This similar case shows involvement of index and long finger PIP joints.

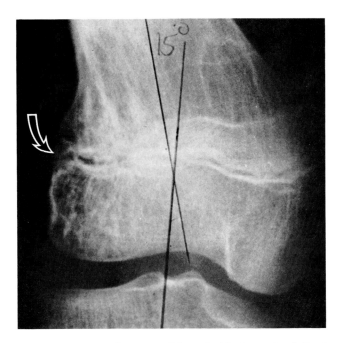

FIG. 4-46. Growth arrest of lateral side (arrow) of distal femur secondary to irradiation of vascular malformation during first year of life.

decrease in the quality of cartilage during sexual maturation, and the difference between the sexes with regard to morphology and strength were due to the influence of the various hormones, which generally included sex hormones and somatotrophic hormone.

These results suggested that both androgens and somatotrophic hormone (STH) reduced the overall (total) strength of the growth cartilage, or at least delayed its age-conditioned increase, whereas female sex hormone(s) increased the tensile strength of the cartilage. Both STH and androgens possessed a positive action on nitrogen balance. STH and androgens also promoted physeal and epiphyseal cartilage cell proliferation, whereas estrogens had insignificant, if any, effects.

On the other hand, osseous maturation was not affected by STH, and reacted to androgens only if they were administered in high doses for a reasonably long time; but osseous maturation was markedly accelerated by estrogens, which may effect their function by several methods, one of which is increasing the rigidity (decreasing the elasticity) of the collagen and the tensile nature of the periosteal sleeve, and thereby secondarily controlling the rate of longitudinal (and perhaps diametric) growth.

In essence, the effect of hormonal changes during adolescence appears to be a slight physiologic decrease in the overall tensile strength of the cartilage in the male in response to STH and androgens, and greater mechanical strength of the epiphyseal plate in females in response to the estrogen compounds, with the former hormones tending to increase physeal column height (which is a reflection of growth rates) and the latter tending to slow down growth, decrease cell column height, and precipitate physiologic epiphysiodesis. Subsequently, Bright[113,114] showed a definite sex difference in failure-response modes.

Physeal Responses to Trauma

Experimental trauma to the physis

Experimental investigations of the effects of injury to the physis are numerous. In 1867, Ollier[115] made linear incisions across the epiphyseal plate in skeletally immature rabbits and cats; superficial cuts did not affect growth, but deep incisions led to growth arrest. Vogt[116] was unable to disturb growth in goats and sheep by separating the epiphysis through the natural line of cleavage. Brashear[117] produced fractures through the distal femoral epiphysis of rats by a varus angulation force. This resulted in tensile disruption. On the distraction side, the cleavage plane passed through the aforementioned plane of hypertrophic cells, whereas the compression side fracture line usually propagated into the metaphyseal trabeculae. A combination of shearing and compression stresses pushed the metaphyseal bone into the epiphyseal plate, damaging *all* layers of cells, rather than just the hypertrophic layer.

Friedenberg[118] showed that resection of portions of the epiphysis in rabbits often resulted in premature growth arrest. Probably the major factor preventing regeneration of the cartilage was the fact that the ossification ring of Lacroix and zone of Ranvier, which were regarded as the areas of greatest regenerative capacity, were part of the resected segment.[119,120] Friedenberg found that he could not fully control the reactive osteogenesis secondary to the trauma with various interposition substances. The greater the degree of resection or the more extensive the overall length of the growth plate damage, the worse the response to interposition of tissue. He did note small peripheral bony bridges histologically in animals with minor deformities and felt that these regions were capable of continued growth because they constantly induced microfractures of the osseous bridge.

How significant this might be to human injury, and whether it might be possible for the human to avoid such injury by similarly breaking these small osseous bridges, is difficult to say, but it is likely that, with the elongated period of bony growth, a bridge of significant size will eventually form and lead to a radiologically evident bridge and growth arrest.

Ford and co-workers perforated the epiphyseal cartilage of young rabbits with a $\frac{1}{8}$-inch drill.[102,121,122] This did not cause any major shortening in spite of osseous or fibrous bridging between the epiphysis and the metaphysis. When larger drill sizes were used, shortening became more marked. Campbell and others resected minor areas of the peripheral growth cartilage and surrounding bone without observing major deformities.[123,124] They seldom saw retardation of growth, provided that the fragments were reduced immediately. But if the fragments were deprived of blood supply, as is often done in clinical situations by periosteal stripping to better visualize the edges of the fracture and effect anatomic reduction, or if the fragment was fixed in alcohol, growth was permanently inhibited. Again, they also observed epiphysiodesis if the growth plate was damaged by larger bone drills.

Harris and Hobson[111] studied displaced proximal femoral epiphyses in rabbits, finding a line of cleavage in the zone of hypertrophic cartilage cells. In monkeys, Dale and Harris[13] described experimental fractures with a cleft through the junction of hypertrophic cartilage cells and the calcified portion of the growth plate.

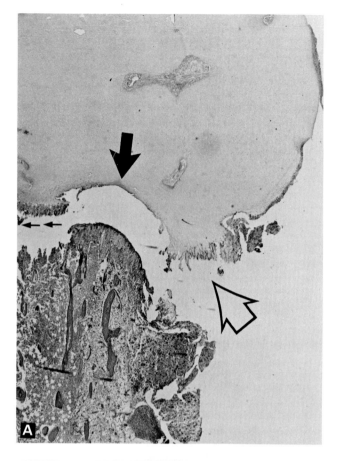

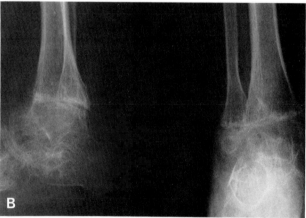

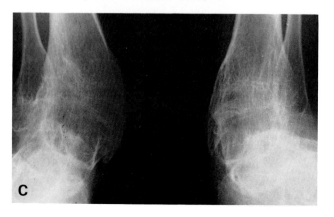

In other experiments, short linear cracks developed within the physis after partial failure.[113] The repeated presence of these cracks deep within the germinal physeal cartilage, rather than just in the hypertrophic zone, before the rupture of the fibers in maximum tension, lends support to the concept that these internal changes are the first evidence of cartilage failure that results from subcritical loading. Many of these cracks were also planes of expected high shear stress.

The final failure of the plate occurred after the structure that was being subjected to the increasing load had absorbed about 50% of its expected failure energy, at which time shear cracks began to occur within various levels of the growth plate along those planes of high shear stress. If the load was released, the shear cracks remained, and their presence weakened the plate to further applications of similar transverse loads. If the deforming force continued to increase, a secondary crack occurred, and the outermost fibers that were in maximum tension ruptured. The secondary crack then became the propagating crack and passed through the plate to cause cartilage failure.

Such a failure crack may or may not coalesce with the smaller, primary shear cracks in other levels of the physis. In older animals, it appeared to do so more frequently than in younger ones. Finally, no matter which species was studied, if the load application continued, the periosteum also reached its ultimate tensile strength and ruptured, allowing epiphyseal displacement in the direction of the applied force.[113]

Whether the human epiphysis and physis fail in a similar fashion is yet to be determined. Complete extrapolation from these animal models must be questioned because of differences in the biomechanics of the bone, the histologic patterns in the growth plates, and the fact that the physes remain open and functional throughout the life of some experimental animals (e.g., rat).

Transphyseal pins

Johnson and Southwick,[125] in animal experiments, showed that when drill holes were made across the central portion of the distal femoral growth plate and a fibular graft inserted through the defect, the epiphysis and physis sometimes fused microscopically to the fibular graft. Despite this, a microscopic cleft developed between the bone graft and the epiphysis/metaphysis such that physeal growth continued in the majority of cases. These bony defects or stretch factors were accompanied by an intense cellular reaction, and it was felt that, at least in central defects, premature

FIG. 4-47. *A,* Section of distal ulna from case also shown in Figure 4-33. Thermal damage and secondary osteomyelitis have caused an epiphysiolysis. The infection and burn destroyed a portion of the physis (solid arrow) and the zone of Ranvier (open arrow), but then the fracture line propagated in a more anticipated manner through the zones of cellular hypertrophy and calcification (small arrows). *B,* Severe bilateral burns of the feet and lower legs. Early closure of the distal tibial and fibular physes. *C,* Complete closure of the physes and ankylosis of the ankle joint. On the right, eccentric closure of the physis has caused valgus deformation.

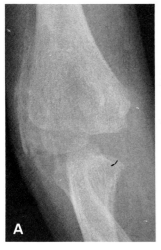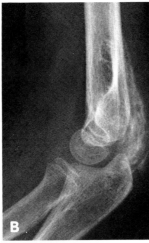

FIG. 4-48. *A-B*, Elbow of ten-year-old sustaining extensive burns around the elbow joint, which led to extensive periarticular calcification and ossification along the posterior and medial aspects of the joint.

epiphysiodesis and permanent growth arrest were not necessary sequelae. However, the longer period of skeletal growth in humans may decrease the likelihood for formation of these clefts and increase the chances for osseous bridge formation.

In the past, surgeons operating for fusion for tuberculosis of the knee have driven bone grafts across the center of the epiphyses of both the distal femur and the proximal tibia without necessarily causing deformity or clinical shortening.[125] However, damage to the periphery of the growth plate at the metaphyseal margin definitely will cause prompt ossification at the site of injury with resultant growth disturbance.

Great care should be taken in the type and manner of insertion of any internal fixation devices in the region of the physes. These devices should be sufficiently smooth to avoid damage to the plate and, whenever possible, should be inserted so they traverse the center of the epiphysis and physis without concerning the physeal plate at its peripheral margins.

Certainly, large central bridges will halt growth completely, while small central ones may have little effect. In contrast, peripheral injury seems to have a more dramatic effect on growth potential. Therefore, wires that traverse from metaphyseal to epiphyseal bone to fix displaced, unstable, slipped epiphyses or fragments in type 3 and type 4 injuries do not generally result in epiphysiodesis.

Thin, unthreaded wires across the central growth plate occupy such a small volume of the plate that even a local tether that occurs from metaphyseal to epiphyseal bone when the wires are removed or overgrown probably has little or no clinical effect on the growth potential of the plate as a whole. Threaded wires, which have a firmer hold in the epiphysis and metaphysis and prevent longitudinal growth plate expansion, eventually cause compression of the germinal cells and produce subsequent premature epiphysiodesis. However, even smooth pins placed across the physis, epiphysis, or articular surface may lead to significant histologic

changes that may predispose the physis to osseous bridge formation during subsequent skeletal maturation (Fig. 4-51).

Hemiepiphyses

Barash and Siffert[126,127] showed that a longitudinal, bifurcation osteotomy extending through the epiphysis, growth plate, and metaphysis of experimental animals subsequently produced variable deformities. The degree of deformity produced was apparently directly proportional to the volume of the epiphyseal ossification center present at the time of surgery. If the secondary ossification center had a large volume, early epiphysiodesis and deformity occurred as a consequence of new bone formation, and a bridge quickly formed between the epiphysis and the metaphysis.

If the epiphyseal ossification center was small at the time of surgery and a larger portion of epiphyseal cartilage separated the osteogenic sites, (that is, the ossification center and the metaphysis), relatively normal growth continued until the centrum came to rest against the growth plate, at which time premature epiphysiodesis and deformity occurred. If the bifurcation procedure was performed prior to the appearance of the osseous centrum, relatively normal, undeformed growth of the divided halves occurred. This latter observation is in contradistinction to the situation in humans, in whom an injury to a totally cartilaginous epiphysis appears to lead to subsequent growth deformity which is often manifested during the adolescent growth spurt (see Fig. 4-7).

Intraepiphyseal osteotomy

Transverse intraepiphyseal osteotomy performed on the proximal end of the rabbit tibia and subsequently packed with fragments of homogenous iliac cortical bone, polyethylene plastic films, or stainless steel showed no untoward effects on the intraepiphyseal vascularity, and normal endochondral ossification continued at the growth plate as well as within the epiphysis.[127] This represents a possible way of correcting growth plate angular deformities by performing the osteotomy in the epiphyseal ossification center, rather than within the metaphysis. Such an approach has been tried in Blount's disease.[128]

Circulation/ischemia

The effects ischemia has on the physis have been studied extensively by Trueta and co-workers.[130-131] Cutting off the epiphyseal circulation leads to either temporary or complete cessation of growth. The central region seems more sensitive to ischemia than the periphery, which may have a capacity to continue growth.[116] This leads to differential rates of growth and significant changes in physeal contour. Immunosuppressive drugs may affect growth in a similar fashion by differentially decreasing rates of cellular multiplication in the physis.[132] Metaphyseal circulatory compromise appears less sensitive to permanent change (see Fig. 2-24).

Morscher[72] described the development of a cone-shaped epiphysis after injury to the distal tibia in a two-year-old boy. This apparently occurred as a result of the temporary inhibition of growth of a central, rather than peripheral, part of the epiphyseal cartilage plate. This inhibition appeared to occur without the formation of a significant osseous bridge,

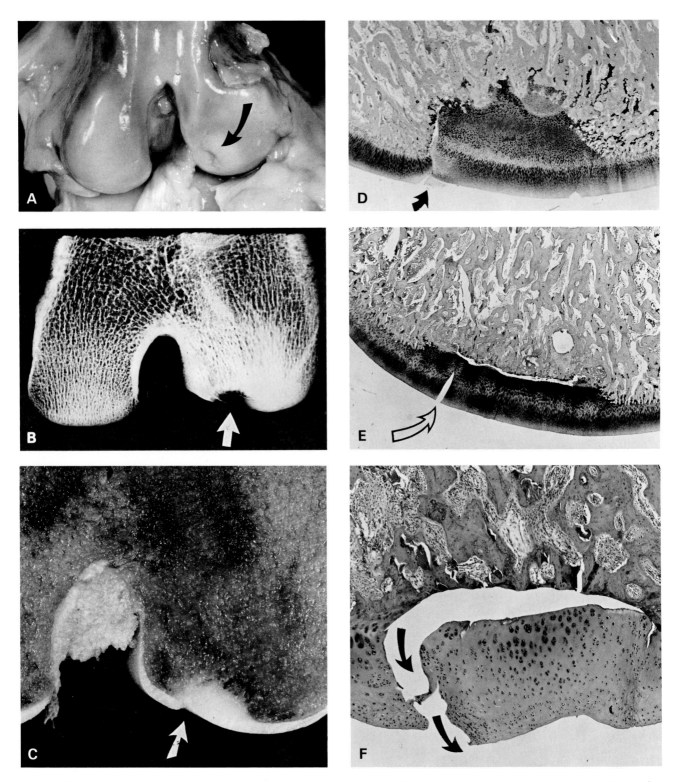

FIG. 4-49. Osteochondritis dissecans in a dog (case courtesy of Dr. S. Olsson). *A,* Cross view showing defect of articular surface (arrow). *B,* Slab roentgenogram showing defect (arrow) and irregular ossification of trabecular bone compared to other condyle. *C,* Slab shown in radiograph. The defect is actually cartilage extending into the trabecular bone. Note the defect in the articular surface (arrow). *D,* Histologic section showing that the lesion is incomplete ossification of a segment of the epiphyseal cartilage. A small crack extends inward from the articular surface (arrow). *E,* Incomplete crack in articular surface (arrow) associated with an extensive subchondral crack separating the cartilage from bone. *F,* Final stage in development of dissecans lesion, with fragment beginning to separate to become a loose body (arrows). Again, note that no bone is attached to this fragment.

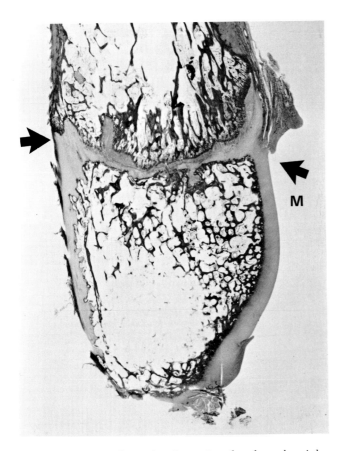

FIG. 4-50. Lappet formation (arrow) at the physeal periphery of the distal fibula. This is prominent on the medial side (M). This is a further mechanical/cytologic adaptation to minimize shear and tension stresses. Also, notice that a definite subchondral plate has formed under the medial fibular articular surface, while laterally the endochondral ossification is more irregular.

at least in the early stage of development, although it seemed possible that a bridge would occur by the time the patient reached skeletal maturity. Also, the cessation of growth appeared to be of the cartilage cells situated in the center of the growth cartilage, and it appeared to be caused by an interruption of the epiphyseal circulation, possibly followed by revascularization. A similar case, shown in Figure 4-30, has a permanent deformity. In contrast, the peripheral cells in the area of Ranvier's ossification groove, which are supplied by the relatively separate perichondrial vascular system, continue to be active, and thus, support further growth in width and length of the epiphyseal cartilage plate. The development of these cone-shaped epiphyses is further proof that significant growth of the epiphysis and physis may take place peripherally.

Trueta and Trias,[131] on the basis of rabbit experiments, concluded that persistent compression affected the growth plate by interfering with the blood flow on one or both sides of the physis. Despite exertion of the same pressure upon both sides of the growth plate, only the metaphyseal side is readily affected in the early stages. As long as no damage is caused to the epiphyseal side of the growth plate, the lesions appear fully reversible. Interference with growth is directly

proportional to the damage caused by compression of the epiphyseal side of the growth plate; and in general, the duration of severity of compression of the epiphyseal plate will affect its growth primarily by interrupting the microvascular blood supply.

Healing patterns

The physis heals primarily by temporarily increased endochondral bone and cartilage formation and gradual reinvasion by the disrupted metaphyseal vessels which eventually replace the widened growth plate. Very little experimental work has been directed at post-traumatic normal cellular response patterns, with most work having been done in the rat.[117]

Contingent upon the level(s) of cellular injury within the epiphyseal plate, three types of chondro-osseous healing may be observed:

1. If the fracture-separation occurs through the more recently formed regions of cell columns (before significant cellular hypertrophy has occurred), healing takes place primarily by continued, relatively rapid increases in the cells within the columns, which causes moderate widening of the physis. Since there are some small epiphyseal vessels in this region, some resorption of fracture debris may occur early in the healing process. These vessels also exhibit a hyperemic response, increasing cellular proliferation rates, especially peripherally in the zone of Ranvier.

The healing response of the metaphysis is continued, perhaps rate-increased, replacement of the hypertrophic cell

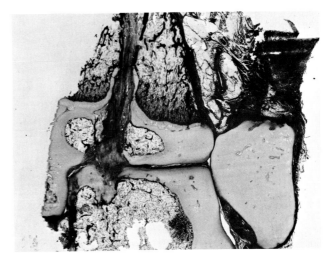

FIG. 4-51. Effect of a transphyseal pin. This patient underwent attempted reconstruction for pseudarthrosis of the tibia seven months prior to a below knee amputation. The pin had been in place for eleven weeks. Note how the physeal cartilage extends along the fibrous tissue filling the pin tract into the metaphysis. The secondary ossification center has been split and has not replaced the fibrous tissue. Further, a fibrous ankylosis is developing between the tibia and the talus. Pins across the physis and articular surface should be used with great caution in children, as similar changes may complicate subsequent growth and rehabilitation.

columns by endochondral bone. Once the level of fibrosis and debris within the physis is encountered, the vessels rapidly invade this damaged area to reach the maturing, newer cell columns on the other side. These cellular response patterns lead to restoration of normal anatomy and strength within three to four weeks.

2. If the fracture-separation occurs through the transition of hypertrophic cells to primary spongiosa (probably the most commonly involved cellular level), there may be marked separation, with the gap being filled by hemorrhage and fibroblastic tissue. This region may then progressively form disorganized cartilaginous tissue, not unlike the initial cartilaginous callus in a diaphyseal fracture (see Chap. 5). Meanwhile, cellular proliferation, cell column formation, hypertrophy and calcification continue on the ''epiphyseal'' side of the disorganized callus, leading to widening of the physis, while vascular invasion of the remnants of hypertrophic, calcified cartilage rapidly occurs on the ''metaphyseal'' side of the fracture.

However, once invading metaphyseal vessels reach the disorganized cartilaginous callus, vascular-mediated bone replacement is temporarily slowed down, since there is no pattern of cell columns to invade in an organized fashion. As the callus cartilage matures, the metaphyseal vessels begin to invade irregularly and replace the cartilage with bone. The thickness of this callus varies, depending upon the degree of longitudinal and lateral displacement and periosteal continuity with the physeal periphery. The callus will be replaced at different rates, and the invading metaphyseal vessels will reach the normal cell columns, which have been maturing in a normal sequence, but osseous replacement will not take place. The widened physis is rapidly invaded by the vessels, replaced by primary spongiosa, and progressively restored to normal physeal width (Fig. 4-52).

The callus in the subperiosteal region contributes to early stability. This region heals by vascular invasion of the callus, through which process trabecular bone forms between the original metaphyseal cortex and the subperiosteal membranous bone that is forming continuously, external to the metaphyseal cartilaginous callus. These three microscopic bone regions progressively merge and remodel, making the region biomechanically strong. With further growth and remodeling this coalescent bone will be completely replaced. These initial cellular replacement processes in both metaphyseal and physeal regions probably take four to six weeks. However, remodeling may continue for months.

3. If the injury extends through all cell layers of the physis, as it would in type 3, 4, and 7 injuries, the repair processes differ slightly. Fibrous tissue initially fills the gap between

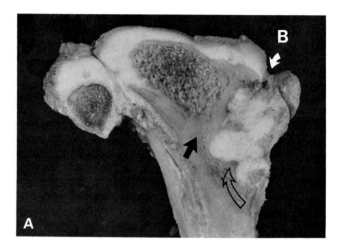

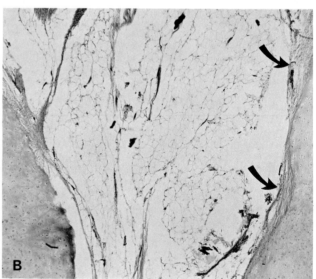

FIG. 4-53. *A,* Result of a type 4 injury to the proximal tibia leading to a varus deformity and formation of an osseous bridge (solid black arrow) between the epiphyseal ossification center and the metaphysis. The physis lateral to the bridge is relatively normal, whereas the epiphysis medial to the bridge has failed to ossify or form normal physeal cytoarchitecture (open black arrow). The white arrow indicates a region shown in *B* at a higher power. *B,* Higher power view showing fatty tissue in cartilaginous gap. Fibrocartilage is developing at the margins (arrows).

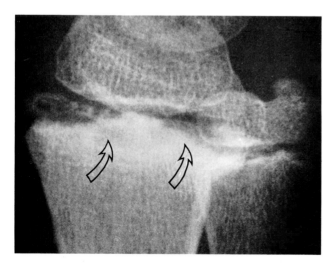

FIG. 4-52. Healing of type 1 or type 2 fractures leads to excessive bone formation in the metaphysis (arrows). This increases the stability of the region. With remodeling and further longitudinal growth this will gradually be restored to normal roentgenographic density.

separated physeal components, while typical callus formation occurs in the contiguous metaphyseal spongiosa and/or epiphyseal ossification center. If large surfaces of non-ossified epiphyseal cartilage also are involved, fibrous tissue initially forms in the intervening region. The reparative response shows irregular healing of the epiphyseal and physeal cartilage, with loss of normal cellular architecture (Fig. 4-53).

Within the central physeal regions diametric expansion of cell columns is minimal, so closure of a large defect by physeal cartilage is unlikely. The gap remains fibrous, but has the potential to ossify. Toward the physeal periphery, diametric expansion is more likely, but still may not lead to closure of large gaps by progressive replacement of fibrous tissue. This replacement process consists essentially of diametric expansion of the germinal and hypertrophic cell regions by cell division, maturation, and matrix expansion. The intervening fibrous tissue disappears through growth, but only if the cell gap closes. Since blood supply to this region is minimal, the fibrous tissue, similarly, is not well vascularized, and significant cell modulation, especially to osteoblastic tissue, is less likely over a short term.

However, the larger the gap filled with fibrous tissue, and the longer the time remaining from fracture to skeletal maturity, the greater the likelihood of developing sufficient neovascularity to commence an osteoblastic response and form an osseous bridge (Fig. 4-54). Furthermore, in the young child with minimal epiphyseal ossification, the blood supply to the physeal germinal region is not defined as well, whereas once the ossification center expands and forms a subchondral plate over the germinal region, microvascularity probably increases, and the chances for vascularization and ossification of the fibrous region increase, thus explaining the delayed appearance of the osseous bridge.

If accurate anatomic reduction is carried out, then a very thin gap should be present, which would fill in with minimal fibrous tissue and allow progressive replacement of the tissue by diametric expansion of the physis. However, if the fragment has been partially or completely devascularized by either the initial trauma or subsequent dissection to effect an open reduction, cellular growth and diametric and longitudinal expansion may not occur, increasing the chances of cellular disorganization, fibrosis, and eventual osteoblastic response (Fig. 4-55). Failure to correct anatomic displacement, especially in type 4 injuries, increases the possibility of apposition of epiphyseal ossification center and metaphysis, thereby enhancing the risk of osseous bridge formation between the two regions.

Angular deformity

Angular deformity of growing long bones, whether acquired as a growth variation, a consequence of a pathologic process (e.g., rickets) or a secondary result of trauma has long been recognized in clinical practice.[19,133-138] However, the basic mechanism of the process of correction and the

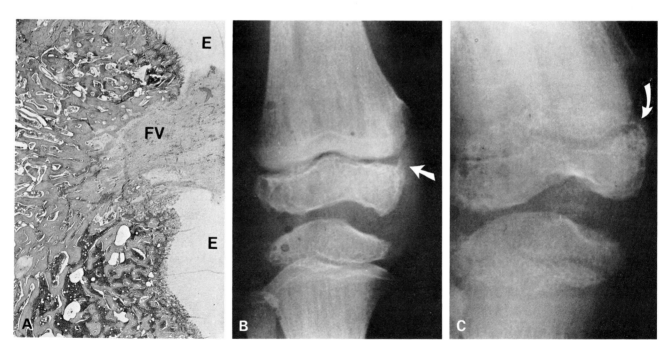

FIG. 4-54. *A,* Early fibrovascular (FV) response bridging region between metaphyseal bone and epiphyseal (E) cartilage. This region is filled with small vessels that cross a region of the physis normally not traversed by blood vessels. As the child grows, this communication may gradually ossify and create an osseous bridge between the epiphyseal ossification center and the metaphyseal bone. *B,* Nine-year-old boy with thalassemia who sustained a type 6 power lawn mower injury to the medial femur two years before this film. The epiphyseal ossification center is beginning to extend toward the metaphysis (arrow), which is also deformed and suggestive of early osteochondroma formation. *C,* A year later a distinct bridge has formed (arrow). Presumably, fibrovascular tissue formed as the initial reparative response, and subsequently, this ossified to lead finally to a solid bridge between the epiphysis and the metaphysis.

factors that influence it are not well known. It is generally accepted that the straightening of a deformity caused by a malunited fracture is due mainly to variable apposition and resorption at the fracture site (Wolff's law).[139]

Normally, chondro-osseous tissues are exposed to the action of muscles that attach into the periosteum along the diaphysis and metaphysis, and may, thereby, affect the intrinsic tension of the periosteal sleeve, which, in turn, may affect the physes. In the growing organism, these combined muscular periosteal forces seem capable of modifying the growth pattern.[140-143] Further, changes in the tension in different regions of the periosteum also may contribute to increased growth in one portion of the physis.[144] Extremely mild forces may inhibit or modify epiphyseal

growth.[119,145,146] Experimentally increased pressure on the end of the bone modifies the direction of growth of an epiphysis and physis. The experiments of Arkin and Katz[145] suggested that pressure acting obliquely on the epiphysis and physis will deflect the direction of growth.

Ryoppy[147] showed that a number of factors contribute to the remodeling process of a long bone (Fig. 4-56). A major factor seems to be local remodeling by asymmetric epiphyseal growth as well as by changes in the process of resorption and apposition in the metaphysis. Interestingly, Ryoppy failed to demonstrate stimulation of longitudinal growth in accord with the generally accepted view that a diaphyseal fracture stimulates growth of the affected bone.[148,149]

However, this may relate to the method by which he pro-

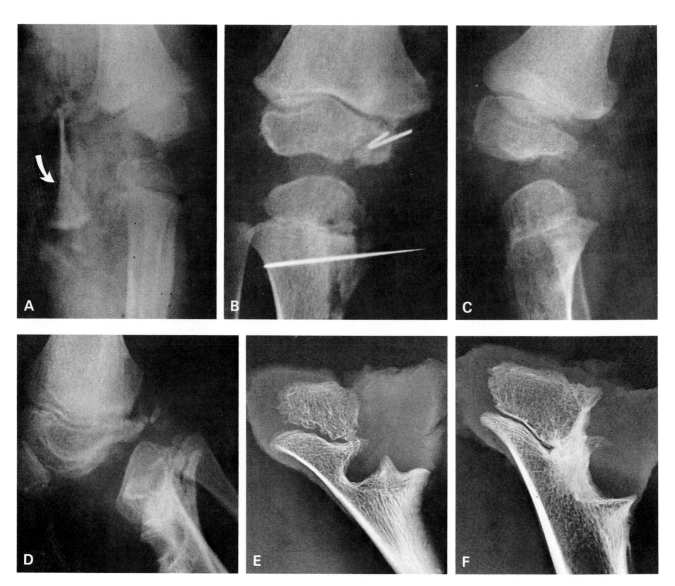

FIG. 4-55. Six-year-old boy who fell under a power lawn mower. *A*, Initial injury, showing one of several type 4 fragments (arrow) of the distal femoral and proximal tibial epiphyses. *B*, Post-reduction film showing apparent anatomic reductions. *C*, Eight months later, mild growth deformities are evident, although no osseous bridges have formed. *D*, Thirty months later, severe deformities of both the distal femur and the proximal tibia are evident. The boy underwent a knee disarticulation at this point. *E-F*, Serial slab roentgenograms of the proximal tibia showing lack of growth medially and the formation of a significant osseous bridge in the more posterior region.

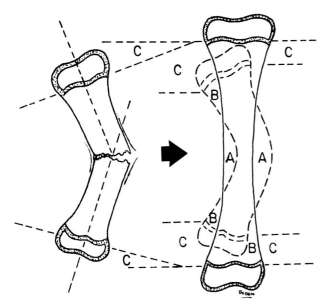

FIG. 4-56. Corrective mechanisms proposed by Ryoppy[147] for restoration after malunion of a metaphyseal or diaphyseal fracture. Local remodeling takes place at the fracture site by both apposition and resorption (A). As remodeling takes place in the metaphysis, resorption is more extensive on the concave side (B). Growth across the physis is asymmetric (C).

duced the fracture, which was by closed means, and may not have led to complete, circumferential disruption of the periosteum, which has been described as one of the possible mechanisms for controlling longitudinal growth and, presumably, overgrowth.[150,151] Ryoppy's experimental animal, the rabbit, reaches skeletal maturity in three to four months, and since the rabbits were several weeks old at time of fracture, time for significant overgrowth to develop may have been insufficient.

Ryoppy et al. also showed that asymmetric growth at the epiphyses was independent of the stimulation of longitudinal growth. The generally accepted view has been that increased pressure on the concave side results in retardation of growth.[140,141,143] However, in experimentally induced scoliosis it has been found that the number of cells on the concave side in the epiphyseal plate may be increased and that growth may also take place in the direction of the concavity.[51] Ryoppy's finding of asymmetric epiphyseal growth was not in complete accord with the law of Heuter-Volkmann.[141,143]

Pauwels[136,137] demonstrated that the growth plate responds eccentrically to changes in pressure and will, through selective growth in different regions, attempt to reorient itself perpendicular to the major joint reaction forces going across the physis (Fig. 4-57). This explains the gradual correction of some deformities, both in the plane of motion of the joint axis as well as in those at right angles to it, such as varus or valgus. Certainly in fractures around the knee and particularly with fractures in the tibia, there is some mild correction of varus and valgus deformation, which is not seen in fractures around the elbow. In part, this may reflect the relative rates of growth, as well as the relatively small contribution to longitudinal growth made by the upper extremities, in the region of the elbow, compared to the significant portion of longitudinal growth of the lower extremity that occurs around the knee.

The distal and proximal fragments must be accurately aligned, whether dealing with diaphyseal, metaphyseal, or epiphyseal injuries. While 30° are generally the acceptable maximum for acute deformity,[152] correction depends on anticipated, and often unpredictable, subsequent growth. Epiphyseal-physeal fractures should be reduced as accurately as possible, including correction of both angular and rotational malalignments (Fig. 4-58). Rotation, in contrast to angulation, does *not* correct (see Fig. 4-1E).

Epiphyseal regeneration

Experimentally, cellular epiphyseal components in small mammals (i.e., rat) will partially regenerate following incomplete and complete physeal/epiphyseal resection.[153-155] However, the extent of regeneration is unpredictable and never equal to the amount of growth that takes place in the original epiphyseal/physeal unit. In larger-boned animals, including humans, regeneration of the physis, for practical purposes, does not exist. The physeal cartilage adjacent to an injury cleft tends to lose columnar orientation and form rounded, clone-like structures, which introduce randomness to growth (Fig. 4-59).

Approach to Epiphyseal Injuries and Complications

General principles of management

All reductions, whether closed or open, should be performed with utmost gentleness in order to prevent further damage to the physis. Forceful, painful manipulations are to be condemned and avoided. During open reduction, direct pressure on the physis by blunt instruments also must be avoided.

Type 1, 2, 3, 4, and 7 injuries consolidate very rapidly, usually in about half the time required for a fracture through the diaphysis of the same bone. If significant amounts of cartilage are present in type 3, 4, and 7 injuries, healing may be delayed. The child should be immobilized for at least three to four weeks, as fracture callus is biologically plastic and may deform if early activity is allowed. Children usually become asymptomatic and willing to use the injured part vigorously long before sufficient healing has occurred.

Due to rapidity of repair, epiphyseal separations should be reduced as soon as possible, each day of delay making reduction progressively more difficult. In fact, after ten days, type 1 and 2 physeal injuries probably cannot be manipulated without exerting undue force, which may damage the cartilaginous growth plate and disrupt early callus. When a type 1 or 2 injury is seen late, (that is, after seven to ten days), it probably is best to accept the malunion rather than cause significant growth arrest by forceful manipulation or open surgery. Any residual malunion may be corrected subsequently by appropriate osteotomy. In type 3 or 4 physeal injuries, restoration of articular surfaces is essential. Delayed reduction should be performed, if only to restore joint congruity.

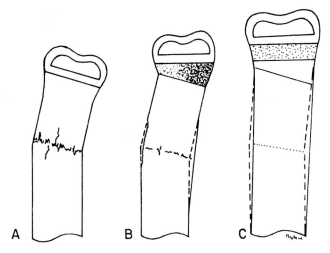

FIG. 4-57. Concept for correction of angular malunion proposed by Pauwels.[136] He emphasized eccentric growth across the physis, with minimal correction at the fracture site itself.

Type 3, 4, and 7 injuries require anatomic reduction. In types 1 and 2, anatomically perfect reduction, while desirable, is not absolutely essential, as chondro-osseous remodeling will correct mild to moderate residual angular deformities (but not rotational deformities, which must be corrected accurately). In general, one can accept a greater degree of deformity in multiplane joints, such as the shoulder, than in single plane joints, such as the knee and ankle.

Reduction of type 1 and 2 fractures usually can be attained and maintained readily by closed means. However, some fractures require open reduction. In type 3 fractures, open reduction may be indicated to restore congruous articular surfaces and good apposition of the ends of the physis. Open reduction is required in almost all type 4 fractures of the epiphyseal plate. Caution must be exercised in order to prevent injury to the circulation of the epiphysis. Excessive stripping of the already damaged periosteum must also be avoided. Only smooth Kirschner wires should be used for internal fixation if they must cross the growth plate. **Threaded screws or wires should not be inserted across the physis.** Internal fixation devices should be removed as soon as the fracture is adequately healed.

Fractures involving the physis must be followed closely for possible development of growth disturbance during the first 12 to 18 months after the injury, and then they should be examined annually or biannually until skeletal maturity is reached, since many growth disturbances do not manifest themselves until the adolescent growth spurt, not unlike the "rapid" onset of scoliosis. Parents must be warned of potential complications, and the importance of long term follow-up must be stressed.

Premature closure of the physis

Many authors have recognized that acute injuries to the growth mechanisms may lead to chronic, later-appearing, growth discrepancies.[8,33,156-178] Ecke[179] stipulated that growth arrest could only follow type 3 and 4 injuries, and that type 1 and 2 injuries were without consequence; however, a con-

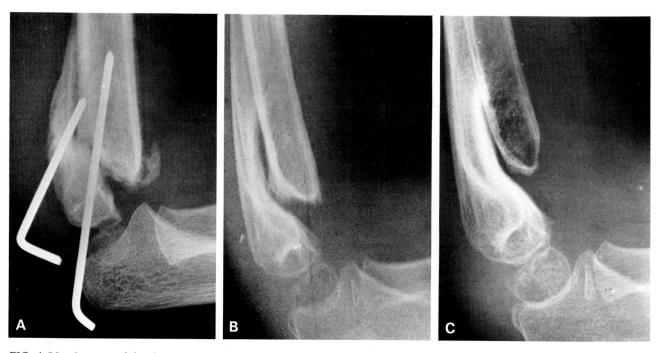

FIG. 4-58. Supracondylar fracture of the distal humerus. *A*, The posterior angulation of the fragment was not completely corrected at the time of percutaneous pinning. *B*, Eight months later, some correction has occurred. Note the gap between the original metaphysis and the subperiosteal new bone. *C*, Two years later, the epiphysis exhibits normal anterior angulation. If malunion is in the plane of joint motion in a growing child, correction is quite likely. However, malunion not in the plane of motion (e.g., varus or valgus) usually will not correct, nor will a rotational deformity.

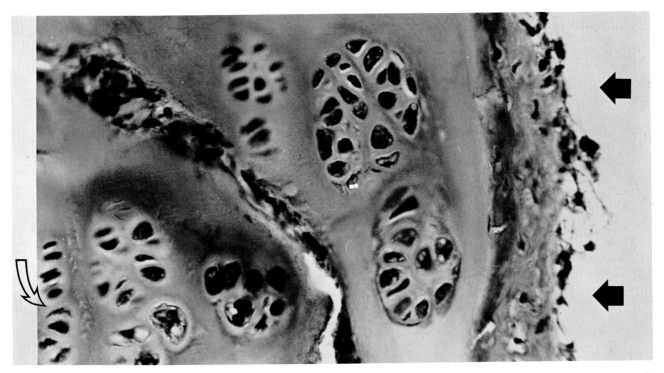

FIG. 4-59.   Resected specimen in a child with osseous bridging following a physeal fracture. The osseous bridge is indicated by the arrows. The cells have lost normal columnar orientation and formed clones surrounded by increased amounts of matrix. A rudimentary cell column is evident at the left (open arrow).

trasting study by Oh of 162 epiphyseal fractures indicated that the type 2 injury, which has long been considered a "safe" injury, also may be responsible for significant discrepancy and distortion in bone growth.[170] Recognizing that type 2 injuries involving the distal femur have led to significant problems, Oh went on to emphasize that more common sites of injury such as the ankle and wrist may also lead to this particular problem.[170] Interestingly, in his series there were no type 5 injuries. My experience with type 1 and 2 injuries is similar, and many examples are shown in the chapters that follow.

Nordentoft[180,181] found that drilling through the growth cartilage with small bone drills did not result in permanent arrest of growth, and similar curettage of approximately 10% of the growth cartilage seldom arrested growth. On the other hand, epiphysiolysis, as well as epiphysiolysis plus curettage of the cartilage, did cause permanent osseous bridging in almost ¾ of the cases in which the procedure was combined with drilling through the basement subchondral plate of the epiphyseal ossification center. Excision of the periosteum and perichondrium combined with epiphysiolysis and curettage did not alter the course of growth significantly. Further, resection of minor bone bridges aggravated the growth disturbance. Resection of the metaphysis below experimentally produced injuries to the growth plate resulted in somewhat, but not significantly, improved growth, as compared to the control leg, which was subjected to the same injury, but without subsequent metaphyseal resection. Nordentoft felt that metaphyseal resection was unjustified on the basis of the experiments, in contradistinction to the work of Langenskiöld.[162]

Several other experimental studies of the pathophysiology of osseous bridge formation after growth plate injury have been reported.[102,108,121,122,124,182,183] Siffert[127,184] and Campbell et al.[124] demonstrated effects of longitudinal, transepiphyseal types of injury. All documented the fact that extensive injuries are more likely to develop substantial bridging. Johnson and Southwick[125] demonstrated that growth may occur after bridging of the epiphysis by bone graft, if the osseous bridge is central rather than peripheral. The tension of growth may cause continuing microfracture of such osseous bridges and thereby permit longitudinal advancement.

Other investigators[13,108,181,185] have suggested that the epiphyseal blood supply is probably the most important determinate in the development of the bone bridges. Nordentoft[181] showed experimentally that the tendency for the development of an epiphyseal bone bridge is increased if the blood supply from the metaphysis also is disrupted by partial transverse section of the metaphysis.

Premature arrest of longitudinal growth may occur either due to destruction of the germinal cells of the growth cartilage, which may be traumatic and/or ischemic, or due to the establishment of a bone bridge between the epiphysis and the metaphysis (Fig. 4-60; also see Fig. 4-55). It also seems accepted that minor bone bridges, especially those located centrally, may be fractured by the continuation of growth, and that growth will definitely be arrested if the bridge is so strong that the growth pressure is unable to break it.

Most of the early work on traumatically induced epiphysiodesis and subsequent release was done by Langenskiöld,[161-163] and this work evolved into a clinical method of treatment that involved resection of the osseous

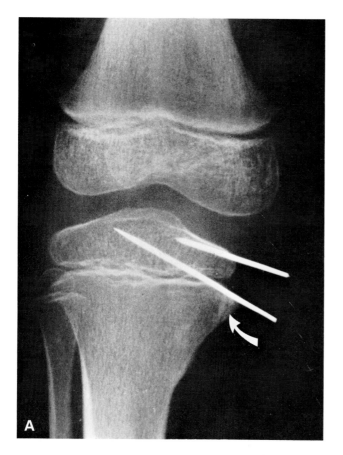

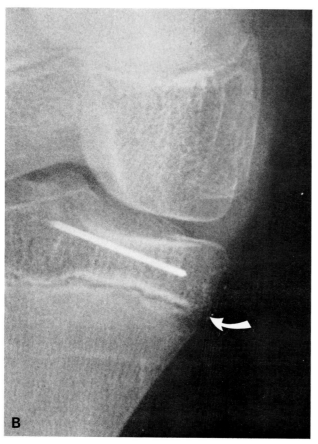

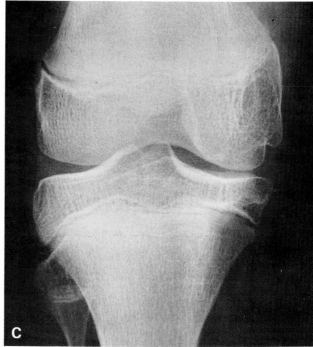

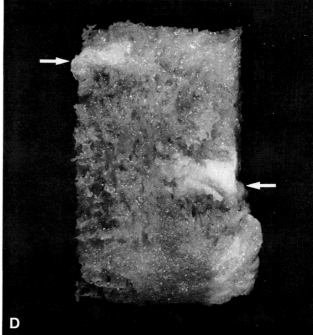

FIG. 4-60. Seven-year-old girl sustaining extensive injury to both legs following power lawn mower injury. *A,* A small metaphyseal fragment (arrow) did not indicate the true extent of the type 4 injury, which did not involve the epiphyseal ossification center (only epiphyseal cartilage was damaged). Open reduction and pin fixation were undertaken. *B,* Six years later, an osseous bridge had formed (arrow) and was causing a varus angulation deformity. *C,* This bridge was resected, leading to improved growth and spontaneous correction of the varus deformation. *D,* Specimen showing osseous bridge between segments of physis (arrows).

bridge and interposition of autogenous fat. Langenskiöld[161] reported that following correction of an angular deformity, a bony bridge spontaneously disappeared. He also reported a case in which a bridge was resected from the proximal tibia under the tuberosity and replaced with fat.

Mallet and Rey[186] reported five cases of post-traumatic partial epiphysiodesis that were treated by surgical epiphyseal release. One case was treated also with corrective osteotomy. Another case had a rapid recurrence of the deformity and the three other cases were not felt to be illustrative, because they were operated on toward the end of skeletal growth.

More recently, Österman[187] has experimentally created osseous bridging, and attempted resection and implantation of various materials to prevent rebridging. Cartilage worked quite well, especially epiphyseal (physis included), but such material is not readily available for grafting in humans (rib cartilage possibly could be used).

Bright[156] created a model epiphysiodesis in which partial closure of the distal femoral plate caused a secondary varus deformity. The resultant osseous bridges were then resected and covered with various types of silicone/silastic rubber implants that consistently prevented osseous bridge reformation and further angular deformities. Absolute contact of implant against the growth plate seemed to be necessary, but it may be essential only for peripheral lesions, and lesions in children who will attain skeletal maturity within one year or less. It may not be necessary in those who have different rates of growth and maturation.

Elimination of partial premature epiphyseal closure

Prior to 1967, the only reported successful treatment for angular deformities in long bones was corrective osteotomy or completion of epiphysiodesis. Depending upon the patient's age, osteotomy might have to be performed repeatedly during the course of growth. Investigators have attempted to prevent the reformation of osseous bridges by implanting a variety of substances such as gelfoam,[102,188] bone wax,[122] methylmethacrylate,[155] beeswax,[118,189] cartilage[187] and muscle flaps.[189] Unfortunately, each of these implant materials provided only limited protection, although materials such as allograft cartilage and autogenous fat were notably better than others. However, none of these materials provided completely and consistently satisfactory results.

The advantage of fat tissue transplant is that under experimental and clinical conditions it is readily available and easy to implant.

However, because fat tissue may become partially necrotic, a phenomenon described by Österman,[187] the rapidly growing bone may displace the necrotic fat tissue. The postoperative hematoma may also provide a bony bridge by intruding between the transplant and the bone. Some of the failures in treatment probably can be explained on the basis of these disadvantages. The best end-results in Österman's study, with regard to both the correction and final results, were achieved with a heterogenous cartilage transplant. Increased metabolism caused by reaction against foreign tissue possibly stimulated growth in this group. The use of bone wax had a significant hemostatic effect, and exposed areas perhaps should be coated with this material prior to the application of fat.

Evaluation of an osseous bridge should include uniplane or biplane tomography to define the extent of bridging. If the bridge is peripheral, then it should be removed, along with overlying periosteum. The growth plate should be exposed by careful curetting or burring with a dental drill until a white line is evident throughout the defect (Fig. 4-61). The defect then is packed with autologous fat.

If the osseous bridge is centrally located, and completely surrounded by normal physeal tissue, a different approach is recommended. Only a metaphyseal defect is made (Fig. 4-62). The metaphyseal side of the physis is exposed to make the bridging bone evident and it then can be curetted carefully until the epiphyseal bone is exposed. The defect is then packed at the site of the bridge, and more fat is placed in the metaphyseal defect. Figure 4-63 shows a representative case on which such a technique was used. While the opportunity may be rare, interposition of fat during open reduction of an acute growth plate injury is also possible, especially if the evident or suspected risk of damage to the growth plate is high (Fig. 4-64).

Epiphyseal transplantation

The only other reported procedure used to correct significant physeal/epiphyseal injury is transplantation of an epiphyseal plate.[153,163,190-208] This technique has provided only limited success when autografts were used, and it failed completely when allografts were attempted. Since an injured child has no expendable source of growth plate cartilage for transplantation, this technique has minimal clinical application. Few indications for transplanting an entire bone in a child are sufficiently compelling to attempt the operation (Fig. 4-65).

In 1966, Wilson[208] reviewed the subject and reported 11 cases in which an epiphysis had been transplanted. Early evidence of longitudinal growth was present in only two patients, and full longitudinal growth was present in only one. Whitesides[209] reported a case in which transplantation was followed by normal growth; the particular patient was first seen because of osteomyelitis which had obviously destroyed the periosteum (type 9 injury). The patient was followed to skeletal maturity at the age of 15. The transplanted phalanx grew and functioned. The transplanted phalanx was approximately the same length as the corresponding phalanx in the normal hand.

Eades and Peacock[193] transplanted the proximal interphalangeal joint and epiphysis of the middle phalanx from the long finger to the metacarpophalangeal areas of the adjacent ring finger, reversing it 180° so that the epiphysis became a metacarpal. The functional result was reasonably good. However, the transplanted epiphysis failed to remain functional or to produce longitudinal growth in the metacarpal area. This result was also observed by others.

Allografting

Certainly, techniques for transplantation preclude large epiphyseal transplants. However, microsurgical anastomosis may increase the potential for survival of growth areas. In a patient approaching skeletal maturity, allografting, with replacement of deformed articular surfaces and correction of angular deformity, offers an additional means of dealing with major structural changes consequent to physeal/epiphyseal damage (Fig. 4-66).

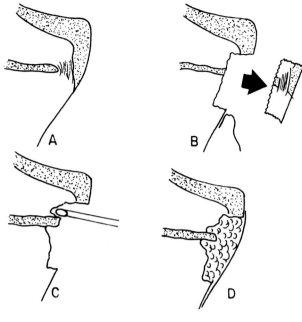

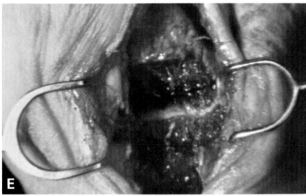

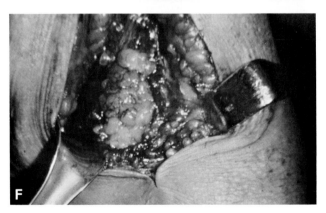

FIG. 4-61. Schematic of correction of peripheral bridge. *A,* Location of bridge at margin of epiphyseal ossification center. *B,* A block is removed. This includes epiphysis, metaphysis and osseous bridge. Bone should be removed until the physis is well visualized. *C,* The area on either side of the physis is undermined with a currette. *D,* The area is packed with fat. *E,* Surgical exposure, with block removed, and normal physis (white line) evident across surgical site. *F,* Surgical exposure showing the defect packed with fat (in this case, removed from the margins of the surgical incision).

Growth estimation

The difficulty of estimating the expected remaining growth of a long bone is highlighted more and more by the increased interest in the problem of equalization of length of traumatically shortened lower extremities, particularly when the shortening is due to epiphysiodesis.[7,210,211] Menelaus[212] based calculations for the correction of leg length discrepancy on chronologic rather than skeletal age. The calculations he used were based on the observation that the lower femoral epiphysis provides $\frac{3}{8}$ of an inch, and the upper tibial epiphysis $\frac{1}{4}$ of an inch, of growth per year.[212] His original calculations show that growth stops at the age of 17 in boys and 16 in girls, but this was later modified to 16 and 14, respectively.

More recently, Moseley[213,214] discussed a new method for recording and interpreting data in cases of leg length discrepancy. This method provides a mechanism for predicting future growth and automatically takes into account the child's growth percentile and the degree of growth inhibition in the short leg. It can be used to predict the effects of corrective surgical procedures and to choose a surgical timetable. The computation methods are discussed in Appendix II.

Whatever method of calculation is employed, good results depend on accurate records. These should be kept on a standard chart included in the history of all children with leg length discrepancy. Measurements should be recorded at regular intervals. These should include measurements from the anterior/superior iliac spine to the medial malleolus and to the heel, as discrepancies may exist between the malleolus and the heel due to concomitant foot injury.

Epiphysiodesis

The most commonly employed procedure for equalizing leg lengths is an appropriately timed surgical epiphysiodesis of the contralateral, normal leg.[210,212-223] Timing is based on accurate computation of the anticipated discrepancy. The major drawback to this approach is that both legs end up shorter than they normally would have been.

Several experimenters have performed epiphysiodesis to study the effect of the procedure on bone growth.[144,224] One of the significant findings was a greater growth contribution from the remaining functional physis.[144] There may be a limit for the combined rates of growth of the two physes of a long bone, and either one may increase the respective rate of growth if, because of trauma or surgery, it becomes the only active growth region. Whether such a phenomenon may occur in the skeletally immature human is unknown, but it certainly is a factor to be considered.

Phemister's method of epiphysiodesis should be used.[223] The epiphysis is exposed through oblique incisions on the medial and lateral aspects. A rectangle of cortex is removed. The growth plate may be isolated readily by raising a flap on the metaphysis and extending it gradually down to the growth plate, where it will be firmly adhered. This will allow adequate placement of the transverse cuts so that $\frac{1}{3}$ of the piece removed will consist of epiphysis and $\frac{2}{3}$ of metaphysis. This block, which should be at least a centimeter deep and a centimeter wide, is removed and the physeal line is curretted as much as possible. The rectangle of bone is then reversed and replaced (Fig. 4-67).

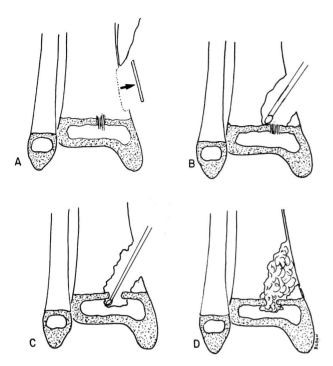

FIG. 4-62. Schematic of correction of central osseous bridge. *A,* A window is made in the metaphyseal cortex. The physis (especially the zone of Ranvier) is left intact. *B,* A metaphyseal "cyst" is carefully made, exposing the metaphyseal side of the physis and the osseous bridge. *C,* The bridge is selectively removed and the physis is undermined. *D,* The defect is packed with fat, the fat impacted through the former site of the bridge.

Stapling

Another method for equalizing length is temporary slowing of growth by inserting staples around the physis.[111,135] When equal length is attained, these staples theoretically can be removed. However, the results are not dependable, and the stapled physis may cease to function.

Christensen[225] found that a significant number of animals did not resume growth even if the staples were removed three to four weeks after original placement. The growth plate could still be recognized, but it was functionless as far as longitudinal growth was concerned. In a few cases, unilateral epiphysiodesis was seen as a result of a massive bony union within half of the growth region. Variable degrees of bridging across the growth plate were seen even where growth was resumed. Christensen's study points out the significantly high probability that staples will cause permanent growth impairment and it questions the standard technique of using them to slow growth temporarily with the intent of removing them at a subsequent phase.

Leg shortening

Segments of diaphyseal bone may be removed from the femur or the tibia of the longer leg.[226,227] However, this technique should not be used until skeletal maturity is reached, and it is a more difficult method than epiphysiodesis. It is also possible to remove a section of femur from the longer leg and insert it into the shorter femur.

Physeal stimulation

Attempts to stimulate the physis to increase the rate of growth, such as increasing rates of blood flow, implantation of ivory chips, etc., have been unsuccessful.[228,229] At present, there is no applicable method of stimulating bone growth.

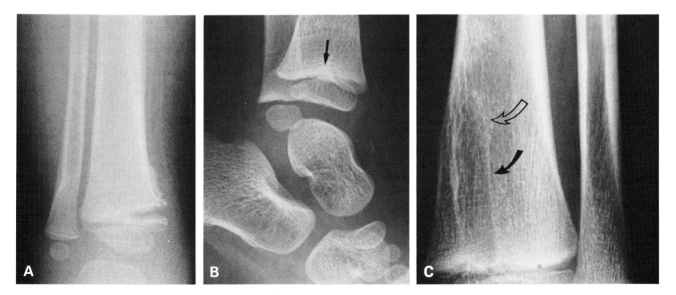

FIG. 4-63. *A,* Eighteen-month-old child sustaining a seemingly innocuous fracture (type 2) of the distal tibia. *B,* Six months later, an osseous bridge has formed (arrow). This was resected utilizing the technique shown in Figure 4-62. *C,* Three years later, the physis has grown normally without any recurrence of the bridge. The open arrow indicates the upper limit of the metaphyseal surgical opening, while the solid arrow indicates the level of the physis at the time of surgery.

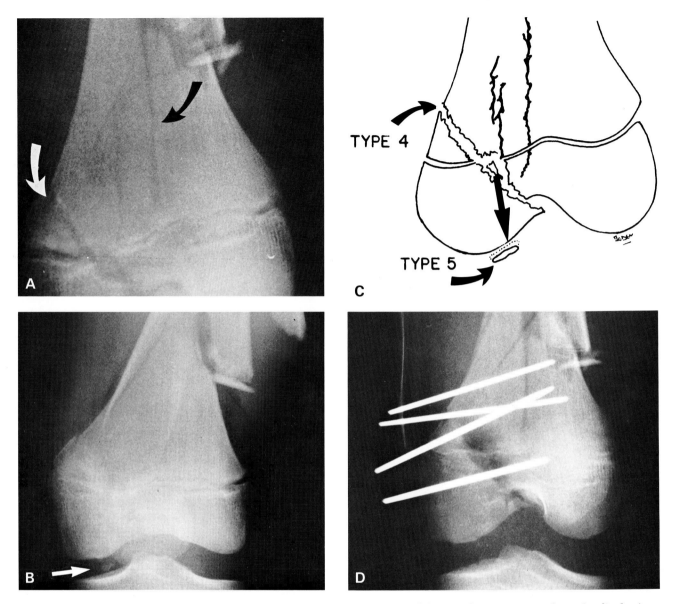

FIG. 4-64. *A,* Extensive comminution of femur in an 11-year-old girl. Several fracture lines propagate from the diaphysis to the physis (black arrow), and at least one type 4 fracture is evident (white arrow). *B,* An apparent osseous body was present in the joint (arrow). This proved to be a segment of physis (radiolucent) and the epiphyseal ossification center which had been impacted into the joint when the condyle was acutely separated. *C,* Schematic of injury. *D,* At the time of anatomic reduction (three days post-injury), the defect created by the fragment impacted into the joint was packed with fat in a manner similar to resection of a large osseous bridge.

Porter[230] inserted stainless steel distraction springs across the upper tibial epiphyseal growth, but did not find a sufficient increase in longitudinal growth. Crilly,[150] using chickens, and Warrel,[231] using rats, showed that reduction of pressure on the epiphyseal cartilage through resection of the periosteum permitted increased longitudinal growth. It has been recognized for some time that compression retards epiphyseal growth.[232]

Increased epiphyseal growth has been observed experimentally in dogs with arteriovenous fistulae, and in association with venous stasis.[233-236] Edvardsen[237] suggested that increased skeletal growth after femoral fracture was a vascu-

lar-mediated phenomenon. Kessel[238] recognized increased growth after metaphyseal forage. Sola[239] recorded experimental overgrowth consequent to periosteal stripping and Jenkins[233] applied this to reduce minor limb inequality in children with poliomyelitis. Sola[239] suggested that increased epiphyseal activity after periosteal stripping was the result of a relative increase in blood to the epiphysis, although this was never adequately substantiated.

Crilly[150] postulated that release of periosteal tension and decompression of the growth plate might explain considerable overgrowth from complete transverse sectioning of the periosteum in domestic fowl. This effect of circumferential

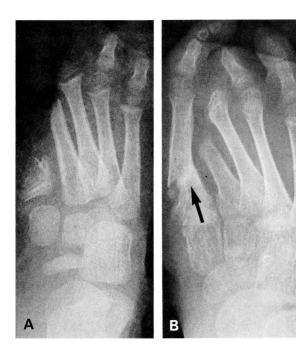

FIG. 4-65. Child sustaining bilateral partial foot amputations secondary to power lawn mower injury. *A,* Left foot after debridement. The right foot had only the great toe remaining. The feet were joined in a "cross-leg" pedicle and the right great toe grafted to the left foot. *B,* Six months later the grafted toe has formed an osseous union (arrow).

division of the periosteum was confirmed by Warrell[231] in rats. He concluded that overgrowth could have resulted either from diminution of pressure on the growth plate or from increased vascularity following trauma.

Any experiment to determine the effect of tension across the growing epiphysis must recognize that surgical insult

alone may affect bone growth, and the control limb must be subjected to an identical operative procedure, excluding tension. Overgrowth did occur in Porter's studies but with angulation which was attributed to the design of the distraction spring. Ring[240] has shown that genetic factors and, possibly, neurologic factors have a considerable effect on bone shape. It is not known if an epiphysis stimulated by increased tension (as by tension springs) will fuse permanently, nor is it known what effect distraction of one epiphysis has on the other epiphyses in the same limb. In fact, there are some indications that premature physiologic epiphysiodesis may accompany this type of distraction.[119]

Distraction epiphysiolysis

Several authors have suggested that the epiphysis could be detached and pulled away from the metaphysis, stimulating a greater rate of longitudinal growth.[241-246] Ray produced partial physeal closure in the distal femurs of dogs and subsequently corrected the angular/length deformity by controlled physeal distraction.[173] This distraction method produced a "pull out fracture" which occurred primarily at the junction of the physis and the primary spongiosa. Interestingly, the fracture line was not confined to a single histologic layer, but in no area was the epiphyseal subchondral plate involved. Resection of the osseous bridge was essential prior to distraction. Elongation of cell columns, not unlike that seen in rickets, occurred in the early distraction phase. Up to 2.6 cm of lengthening was achieved.

Distraction epiphysiolysis has been used experimentally by Connolly (unpublished) and Monticelli (unpublished) in large animals with considerable success. Monticelli found that closure occurred shortly after lengthening was accomplished, and recommended that the procedure not be used until the final phases of the growth spurt. Monticelli has now performed the procedure in several patients. This procedure is still in the phase of a clinical trial and should not be used routinely.

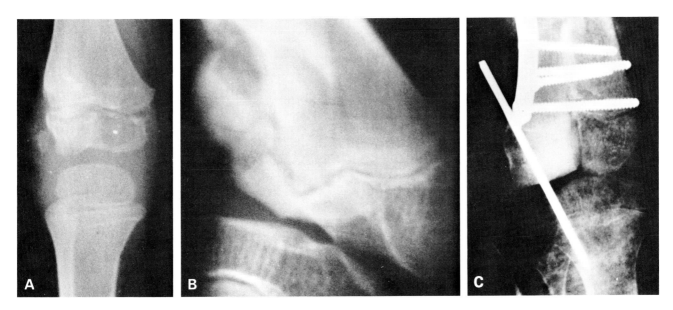

FIG. 4-66. *A,* Type 4 injury to the lateral epicondyle. *B,* Several years later, major structural deformity of physis, epiphysis, and articular regions is evident. *C,* This was treated by resection and allograft replacement (case courtesy of D. MacEwen).

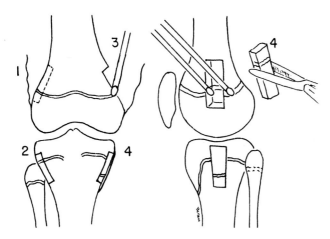

FIG. 4-67. Schematic of technique of epiphysiodesis. The periosteum is elevated as a flap toward the physis (1). This requires sharp dissection at the zone of Ranvier and the contiguous perichondrium. A block including ⅔ metaphysis and ⅓ epiphysis is removed (2). The physis is ablated with a currette (3). The block is turned 180° and reinserted into the defect, with periosteal flap being reattached (4).

Leg lengthening

In an effort to maintain length of the unaffected leg, efforts have been made to surgically lengthen a damaged femur or tibia.[190,211,247-253] Timing of such a procedure is important, and it may be combined with epiphysiodesis, depending upon the anticipated length of the inequality. Wagner has the most extensive experience, and his work should be consulted for operative details.[253]

References

1. Ogden, J. A.: Injury to the immature skeleton. *In* Pediatric Trauma. Edited by R. Touloukian. New York, John Wiley & Sons, 1978.
2. Rang, M.: Children's Fractures. Philadelphia, J. B. Lippincott, 1974.
3. Tachdjian, M.: Pediatric Orthopaedics. Philadelphia, W. B. Saunders, 1972.
4. Aitken, A. P.: Fractures of the epiphyses. Clin. Orthop., *41:*19, 1965.
5. Bergenfeldt, E.: Beitrage zur Kenntnis der traumatischen Epiphysenlosung an den langen Rohrenknochen der Extremitaten. Acta Chir. Scand. [Suppl.], *28,* 1933.
6. Bigelow, D. R., and Ritchie, G. W.: The effects of frostbite in childhood. J. Bone Joint Surg., *45-B:*122, 1963.
7. Bisgard, J. D., and Bisgard, M. E.: Longitudinal growth of long bones. Arch. Surg., *31:*508, 1935.
8. Bouyala, J. M., and Rigault, P.: Les traumatismes du cartilage de conjugaison. Rev. Chir. Orthop., *65:*259, 1979.
9. Bowen, D. R.: Epiphyseal separation-fracture. Interstate Med. J., *17:*607, 1915.
10. Brashear, H. R., Jr.: Epiphyseal fractures of the lower extremity. South. Med. J., *51:*845, 1958.
11. Budig, H.: Ergebnisse bei Epiphysenlosungen und Oberarmbruchen am proximalen Ende von Kindern und Jugendlichen. Arch. Orthop. Trauma. Surg., *49:*521, 1958.
12. Cassidy, R. H.: Epiphyseal injuries of the lower extremities. Surg. Clin. North Am., *38:*1125, 1958.
13. Dale, G. G., and Harris, W. R.: Prognosis of epiphyseal separation. J. Bone Joint Surg., *40-B:*116, 1958.
14. Eliason, E. L., and Ferguson, L. K.: Epiphyseal separation of the long bones. Surg. Gynecol. Obstet., *58:*85, 1934.
15. Harris, W. R.: Epiphyseal injuries. AAOS Instr. Course Lectures, *15:*206, 1958.
16. Harsha, W. N.: Effects of trauma upon epiphyses. Clin. Orthop., *10:*140, 1957.
17. Lovell, W. W., and Winter, R. B.: Pediatric Orthopaedics. Philadelphia, J. B. Lippincott, 1978.
18. O'Brien, T. R., Morgan, J. P., and Suter, P. F.: Epiphyseal plate injury in the dog: a radiographic study of growth disturbance in the forelimb. J. Small Anim. Pract., *12:*19, 1971.
19. Roberts, J. M., et al.: Symposium update on epiphyseal injuries. AAOS 47th Annual Meeting, Atlanta, Ga., Feb. 12, 1980.
20. Ruckensteiner, E.: Erwargungen zum Rontgenbild ortlicher Erfrierungen. Zentralbl. Chir., *72:*163, 1947.
21. Sakadida, K.: Clinical observations on the epiphyseal separation of long bones. Clin. Orthop., *34:*119, 1964.
22. Steinert, V.: Epiphysenlosung und Epiphysenfrakturen. Arch. Orthop. Unfallchir., *58:*200, 1965.
23. Sussenbach, F.: Anatomie, Prognose und Behandlung von Epiphysenfugenverletzungen. Chir. Praxis, *16:*117, 1972.
24. Witt, A. N., and Mittelmeier, H.: Epiphysenverletzungen des Unterschenkels. Handb. f. Orthop., *IV:*1174, 1961.
25. Neer, C. S., II, and Horwitz, B. S.: Fractures of the epiphyseal plate. Clin. Orthop., *41:*24, 1965.
26. Peterson, C. A., and Peterson, H. A.: Analysis of the incidence of injuries to the epiphyseal growth plate. J. Trauma, *12:*275, 1972.
27. Morscher, E., Desaulles, P. A., and Schenk, R.: Experimental studies on tensile strength and morphology of the epiphyseal cartilage at puberty. Ann. Paediatr., *205:*112, 1965.
28. Morscher, E.: Strength and morphology of growth cartilage under hormonal influence of puberty. Animal experiments and clinical study on the etiology of local growth disorders during puberty. Reconstr. Surg. Traumatol., *10:*3, 1968.
29. Adams, J. G.: Bone injuries in very young athletes. Clin. Orthop., *58:*129, 1968.
30. Foucher, M.: De la divulsion des epiphyses. Cong. Med. France, Paris, *I:*63, 1863.
31. Hutchinson, J.: Lectures on injuries to the epiphysis and their results. Br. Med. J., *69:*669, 1894.
32. Poland, J.: Traumatic Separation of the Epiphyses. London, Smith, Elder, and Co., 1898.
33. Salter, R. B., and Harris, W. R.: Injuries involving the epiphyseal plate. J. Bone Joint Surg., *45-A:*587, 1963.
34. Holland, C. T.: Radiographical note on injuries to the distal epiphyses of radius and ulna. Proc. R. Soc. Med., *22:*695, 1929.
35. Tanner, J. M., et al.: Assessment of Skeletal Maturity and Prediction of Adult Height (TW2 Method). New York, Academic Press, 1975.
36. Teates, C. D.: Distal radial growth plate remnant simulating fracture. A. J. R., *110:*578, 1970.
37. Brinn, L. B., and Moseley, J. E.: Bone changes following electrical injury. A. J. R., *97:*682, 1966.
38. Granberry, W. M., and Janes, J. M.: Effect of electrical current on epiphyseal cartilage. A preliminary experimental study. Proc. Staff Meet. Mayo Clin., *38:*87, 1963.
39. Kolar, J., and Vrabec, R.: Roentgenological bone findings after high voltage injury. Fortschr. Roentgen., *92:*385, 1960.
40. Arguelles, F., Gomar, F., Garcia, A., and Esquerdo, J.: Irradiation lesions of the growth plate in rabbits. J. Bone Joint Surg., *59-B:*85, 1977.
41. Barnhard, H. J., and Geyer, R. W.: Effects of x-radiation on growing bone. Radiology, *78:*207, 1962.
42. Barr, J. S., Lingley, J. R., and Gall, E. A.: The effect of roentgen irradiation on epiphyseal growth. I. Experimental studies upon the albino rat. A. J. R., *49:*104, 1943.

43. Bisgard, J. D., and Hunt, H. B.: Influence of roentgen rays and radium on epiphyseal growth of long bones. Radiology, 26:56, 1936.

44. Brooks, B., and Hillstrom, H. T.: Effect of roentgen rays on bone growth and bone regeneration. Am. J. Surg., 20:599, 1933.

45. Dahl, B.: Effects des rayons-x sur les os longs en developpement. J. Radiol. Electr., 18:131, 1934.

46. Desjardins, A. U.: Osteogenic tumor: growth injury of bone and muscular atrophy following therapeutic irradiation. Radiology, 14:296, 1930.

47. Frantz, C. H.: Extreme retardation of epiphyseal growth from roentgen irradiation. A case study. Radiology, 55:720, 1950.

48. Gall, E. A., Lingley, J. R., and Hilcken, J. A.: Comparative experimental studies of 100 kilovolt and 1000 kilovolt roentgen rays. I. The biological effects on epiphysis of the albino rat. Am. J. Pathol., 16:605, 1940.

49. Hinkel, C. L.: The effect of roentgen rays upon the growing long bones of albino rats. I. Quantitative studies on the growth limitation following irradiation. A. J. R., 47:439, 1942.

50. Hinkel, C. L.: The effect of roentgen rays upon the growing long bones of albino rats. II. Histopathological changes involving endochondral growth centers. A. J. R., 49:321, 1943.

51. Judy, W. S.: An attempt to correct asymmetry in leg length by roentgen irradiation. A. J. R., 46:237, 1941.

52. Kember, N. F.: Cell survival and radiation damage in growth cartilage. Br. J. Radiol., 40:496, 1967.

53. Langenskiöld, A.: Growth disturbance appearing 10 years after roentgen ray injury. Acta Chir. Scand., 105:350, 1953.

54. Redell, G.: Retardation of growth after traumatic epiphyseal separation. Acta Orthop. Scand., 25:97, 1955.

55. Regen, E. M., and Wilkins, W. C.: The effect of large doses of x-rays on growth of young bone. J. Bone Joint Surg., 18:61, 1936.

56. Ring, P. A.: Experimental bone lengthening by epiphyseal distraction. Br. J. Surg., 196:169, 1958.

57. Segale, G. C.: Sull azione biologica dei raggi Roentgen e del radium sulle cartilagini apofisarie. Radiol. Med., 7:234, 1920.

58. Spangler, D.: The effect of x-ray therapy for closure of epiphyses. Radiology, 37:310, 1941.

59. Stevens, R. H.: Retardation of bone growth following roentgen irradiation of an extensive nevocarcinoma of the skin in an infant four months of age. Radiology, 25:538, 1935.

60. Ariev, T. J.: Monograph on Frostbite. Translated by J. Steiman. Narkomzdrov, U.S.S.R. State Health Committee, 1940.

61. Bennett, R. B., and Blount, W. P.: Destruction of epiphyses by freezing. J.A.M.A., 105:661, 1935.

62. Dreyfuss, J. R., and Glimcher, M. J.: Epiphyseal injury following frostbite. N. Engl. J. Med., 253:1065, 1955.

63. Florkiewicz, L., and Kozlowski, K.: Symmetrical epiphyseal destruction by frostbite. Arch. Dis. Child., 37:51, 1962.

64. Hakstian, R. W.: Cold-induced digital epiphyseal necrosis in childhood (symmetric focal ischemic necrosis). Can. J. Surg., 15:168, 1972.

65. Lindholm, A., Nilsson, O., and Svartholm, F.: Epiphyseal destruction following frostbite. Acta Chir. Scand., 134:37, 1968.

66. Scow, R.: Destruction of cartilage cells in the newborn rat by brief refrigeration, with consequent skeletal deformities. Am. J. Pathol., 25:143, 1948.

67. Tempsky, A.: Gelenkschadigung durch Erfrierung. Zentralbl. Chir., 58:339, 1931.

68. Thelander, H. E.: Epiphyseal destruction by frostbite. Pediatrics, 36:105, 1950.

69. Wenzl, J. E., Burke, E. C., and Bianco, A. J.: Epiphyseal destruction following frostbite in hands. Am. J. Dis. Child., 114:668, 1967.

70. Brashear, H. R., Jr.: Epiphyseal avascular necrosis and its relation to longitudinal bone growth. J. Bone Joint Surg., 45-A:1423, 1963.

71. Giedion, A.: Cone-shaped epiphyses (SCE). Ann. Radiol., 8:135, 1965.

72. Morscher, E.: Posttraumatische Zapfenepiphyse. Arch. Orthop. Unfallchir., 61:128, 1967.

73. Rang, M.: The Growth Plate and Its Disorders. Baltimore, Williams & Wilkins, 1969.

74. Landells, J. W.: The reactions of injured human articular cartilage. J. Bone Joint Surg., 39-B:548, 1957.

75. Langenskiöld, A.: Can osteochondritis dissecans arise as a sequal of cartilage fracture in early childhood? Acta Chir. Scand., 109:204, 1955.

76. Olsson, S. E.: En ny typ av armbagsledsdyplasi hos hund? Sv. Vet., 26:152, 1974.

77. Olsson, S. E.: Osteochondros hos hund. Patologi, rontgendiagnostik och klinik. Sv. Vet., 29:577, 1977.

78. Spira, E., and Farin, I.: The vascular supply to the epiphyseal plate under normal and pathologic conditions. Acta Orthop. Scand., 38:1, 1967.

79. Ogden, J. A., et al.: Ectopic bone secondary to avulsion of periosteum. Skeletal Radiol., 4:124, 1979.

80. Akbarnia, B. A., Campbell, C. J., and Bowen, J. R.: Management of massive defects in radius and ulna wringer injury. Clin. Orthop., 116:167, 1976.

81. Allen, J. E., Beck, R., and Jewett, T. C.: Wringer injuries in children. Arch. Surg., 97:194, 1968.

82. Collins, H. R.: Epiphyseal injuries in athletes. Clev. Clin. Q., 42:285, 1975.

83. Larson, R.: Epiphyseal injuries in the adolescent athlete. Orthop. Clin. North Am., 4:839, 1973.

84. Ogden, J. A., and Southwick, W. O.: Electrical injury involving the immature skeleton. Skeletal Radiol., 6:187, 1981.

85. Ahstrom, J. P., Jr.: Epiphyseal injuries of the lower extremity. Surg. Clin. North Am., 1:119, 1965.

86. Lohr, W.: Die Verschiedenheit der Auswirkung gleichartiger bekannter Schaden auf den Knochen Jugendlicher und Erwachsener, gezeigt und Epiphysenstorungen nach Erfrierlangen und bei der Hamophile. Zentralbl. Chir., 57:898, 1930.

87. Thiemann, H.: Juvenile Epiphysenstorungen. Fortschr. Roentgen., 14:79, 1909.

88. Bectol, C. O.: The biomechanics of the epiphyseal lines as a guide to design considerations for the attachment of prothesis to the musculoskeletal system. J. Biomed. Mater. Res., 4:343, 1973.

89. Selke, A. C.: Destruction of phalangeal epiphyses by frostbite. Radiology, 93:859, 1969.

90. Straub, G. F.: Anatomic survival, growth and physiological function of an epiphyseal bone transplant. Surg. Gynecol. Obstet., 48:687, 1929.

91. Shumacker, H. B., Jr., and Lempke, R. E.: Recent advances in frostbite with particular reference to experienced studies concerning functional pathology and treatment. Surgery, 30:873, 1951.

92. Blaustein, A., and Siegler, R.: Pathology of experimental frostbite. NY State J. Med., 54:2968, 1954.

93. Pirozynski, W. J., and Webster, D. R.: Redistribution of K and Na in experimental frostbite. Surg. Forum, 3:665, 1953.

94. Pirozynski, W. J., and Webster, D. R.: Experimental investigation of changes in axis cylinders of peripheral nerves following local cold injury. Am. J. Pathol., 29:547, 1953.

95. Crimson, J. M., and Fuhrman, F. A.: Studies on gangrene following cold injury. J. Clin. Invest., 26:486, 1947.

96. Greene, R.: The immediate vascular changes in true frostbite. J. Pathol. Bact., 55:259, 1943.

97. Hurley, L. A.: Angioarchitectural changes associated with rapid rewarming subsequent to freezing injury. Angiology, 8:19, 1957.

98. Stephens, D. C., Herrick, W., and MacEwen, G. D.: Epiphysiodesis for limb length inequality: results and indications. Clin. Orthop., 136:41, 1978.

99. Baserga, R., Lisco, H., and Cater, D. B.: The delayed effects of external gamma irradiation on the bones of rats. Am. J. Pathol., 39:455, 1961.

100. Evans, E. B., and Smith, J. R.: Bone and joint changes following burns. J. Bone Joint Surg., *41-A:*785, 1959.

101. Frantz, C. H., and Delgado, S.: Limb-length discrepancy after third-degree burns about the foot and ankle. J. Bone Joint Surg., *48-A:*443, 1966.

102. Ford, L. T., and Key, J. A.: A study of experimental trauma to the distal femoral epiphysis in rabbits. J. Bone Joint Surg., *38-A:*84, 1956.

103. D'Ambrosia, R., and Ferguson, A. B., Jr.: The formation of osteochondroma by epiphyseal cartilage transplantation. Clin. Orthop., *61:*103, 1968.

104. Meachim, G.: Repair of the para-articular bone plate in the rabbit knee. J. Anat., *113:*359, 1972.

105. Ogden, J. A.: The development and growth of the musculo-skeletal system. *In* The Scientific Basis of Orthopaedics. Edited by J. A. Albright, and R. A. Brand. New York, Appleton-Century-Crofts, 1979.

106. Ogden, J. A.: Chondro-osseous development and growth. *In* Fundamental and Clinical Bone Physiology. Edited by M. R. Urist. Philadelphia, J. B. Lippincott, 1981.

107. Karaharju, E. O.: Deformation of vertebrae in experimental scoliosis. Acta Orthop. Scand. [Suppl.], *105,* 1967.

108. Haas, S. L.: The changes produced in growing bones after injury to the epiphyseal cartilage. J. Orthop. Surg., *1:*67;166;226, 1919.

109. Haas, S. L.: Further observations on the transplantation of the epiphyseal cartilage plate. Surg. Gynecol. Obstet., *52:*958, 1931.

110. Harris, W. R.: Endocrine basis for slipping of upper femoral epiphysis. J. Bone Joint Surg., *32-B:*5, 1950.

111. Harris, W. R., and Hobson, K. W.: Histological changes in experimentally displaced upper femoral epiphyses in rabbits. J. Bone Joint Surg., *38-B:*914, 1956.

112. Huller, T., and Nathan, H.: Does the periosteum contribute to bone strength? Isr. J. Med. Sci., *6:*630, 1970.

113. Bright, R. W., and Elmore, S. M.: Physical properties of epiphyseal plate cartilage. Surg. Forum, *19:*463, 1968.

114. Bright, R. W., Burstein, A. H., and Elmore, S. M.: Epiphyseal-plate cartilage. A biomechanical and histological analysis of failure modes. J. Bone Joint Surg., *56-A:*688, 1974.

115. Ollier, L.: Traite Experimental et Clinique de la Regeneration des Os et de la Production Artificielle du Tissu Osseux, Vol. 1. Paris, Masson et Fils, 1867.

116. Vogt, P.: Die traumatische Epiphysenntrennung und deren Einfluss auf des Langenwachstum der Rohrenknochen. Arch. Klin. Chir., *22:*343, 1978.

117. Brashear, H. R., Jr.: Epiphyseal fractures. A microscopic study of the healing process in rats. J. Bone Joint Surg., *41-A:*1055, 1959.

118. Friedenberg, Z. B.: Reaction of the apophysis to partial surgical resection. J. Bone Joint Surg., *39-A:*332, 1957.

119. Hindrichsen, G. J., and Storey, E.: The effects of force on bone and bones. Angle Orthod., *38:*155, 1968.

120. Solomon, L.: Diametric growth of the epiphyseal plate. J. Bone Joint Surg., *48-B:*170, 1966.

121. Ford, L. T., and Canales, G. M.: A study of experimental trauma and attempts to stimulate growth of the lower femoral epiphysis in rabbits. III. J. Bone Joint Surg., *42-A:*439, 1960.

122. Key, J. A., and Ford, L. T.: Study of experimental trauma to the distal femoral epiphysis in rabbits, II. J. Bone Joint Surg., *40-A:*887, 1958.

123. Campbell, C. J.: The healing of cartilage defects. Clin. Orthop., *64:*45, 1969.

124. Campbell, C. J., Grisolia, A., and Zanconato, G.: The effects produced in the cartilaginous epiphyseal plate of immature dogs by experimental surgical trauma. J. Bone Joint Surg., *41-A:*1221, 1959.

125. Johnson, J. T. H., and Southwick, W. O.: Growth following trans-epiphyseal bone grafts. J. Bone Joint Surg., *42-A:*1381, 1960.

126. Barash, E. S., and Siffert, R. S.: The potential for growth of experimentally produced hemiepiphyses. J. Bone Joint Surg., *48-A:*1548, 1966.

127. Siffert, R. S., and Katz, J. F.: Experimental intra-epiphyseal osteotomy. Clin. Orthop., *82:*234, 1972.

128. Storen, H.: Operative elevation of the medial tibial joint surface in Blount's disease. Acta Orthop. Scand., *40:*788, 1969.

129. Troup, H.: Nervous and vascular influence on longitudinal growth of bone. Acta Orthop. Scand. [Suppl.], *51,* 1961.

130. Trueta, J., and Amato, V. P.: The vascular contribution to osteogenesis. J. Bone Joint Surg., *42-B:*571, 1960.

131. Trueta, J., and Trias, A.: The vascular contribution to osteogenesis, IV. The effect of pressure upon the epiphyseal cartilage of the rabbit. J. Bone Joint Surg., *43-B:*800, 1961.

132. Bright, R. W., and Elmore, S. M.: Some effects of immunosuppressive drugs of the epiphyseal plates of rats. Surg. Forum, *18:*485, 1967.

133. Sharrard, W. J. W.: Paediatric Orthopaedics and Fractures. Oxford, Blackwell, 1971.

134. Abbott, L. C., and Gill, G. G.: Valgus deformity of the knee resulting from injury to the lower femoral epiphysis. J. Bone Joint Surg., *24:*97, 1942.

135. Blount, W. P., and Clarke, R. G.: Control of bone growth by epiphyseal stapling. J. Bone Joint Surg., *31-A:*464, 1949.

136. Pauwels, F.: Grundniss einer Biomechanik der Frakturheilung Verhandlungen. Deutsch. Orthop. Gesellschaft, *34:*62, 1940.

137. Pauwels, F.: Uber die mechanische Bedeutung der groberan Kortikalisstruktur beim normal und patologisch verbogenen Rohrenknochen. Anat. Nachr., *1:*53, 1950.

138. Ruter, A., and Burri, C.: Fehlwachstum nach Epiphysenverletzungen der unteren Extremitat. Aktuel. Traumatol., *5:*157, 1975.

139. Wolff, J.: Das Gesetz der Transformation der Knochen. Berlin: Hirschwald, 1892.

140. Delpech, J. M.: De l'orthomorphie, par rapport a l'espice humaine. Paris, Gabon, 1829.

141. Heuter, C.: Anatomische Studien an der Extremitatengelenken Neugeborner und Erwachsener. Virchows Arch., *25:*572, 1862.

142. Siegling, J. A.: Growth of the epiphysis. J. Bone Joint Surg., *23:*39, 1941.

143. Volkmann, R.: Chirurgische Erfahrungen uber Knochenverbiegungen und Knochenwachstum. Arch. Pathol. Anat., *24:*512, 1862.

144. Hall-Craggs, E.: Influence of epiphyses on the regulation of bone growth. Nature, *221:*1245, 1969.

145. Arkin, A. M., and Katz, J. F.: The effects of pressure on epiphyseal growth. J. Bone Joint Surg., *38-A:*1056, 1956.

146. Tschantz, P., and Rutishauser, E.: La surcharge mecanique de l'os vivant. Ann. Anat. Pathol., *12:*223, 1967.

147. Ryoppy, S., and Karaharju, E. O.: Alteration of epiphyseal growth by an experimentally produced angular deformity. Acta Orthop. Scand., *45:*490, 1974.

148. Blount, W.: Fractures in Children. Baltimore, Williams & Wilkins, 1955.

149. Sunden, G.: Some aspects of longitudinal growth. Acta Orthop. Scand. [Suppl.], *103,* 1967.

150. Crilly, R. G.: Longitudinal overgrowth of chicken radius. J. Anat., *112:*11, 1972.

151. Lufti, A. M.: The role of cartilage in long bone growth: a reappraisal. J. Anat., *117:*413, 1974.

152. Nönnemann, H. C.: Grenzen der Spontankorrektur fehlgeheilter Frakturen bei Jugendlichen. Langenbecks Arch. Chir., *324:*78, 1969.

153. Banks, S., and Compere, E.: Regeneration of epiphyseal cartilage. An experimental study. Ann. Surg., *114:*1076, 1941.

154. Hellstadius, A.: An investigation by experiments in animals of the role played by the epiphyseal cartilage in longitudinal growth. Acta Chir. Scand., *95:*156, 1947.

155. Ring, P. A.: The effects of partial or complete excision of the epiphyseal cartilage of the rabbit. J. Anat., 89:79, 1955.

156. Bright, R. W.: Operative correction of partial epiphyseal plate closure by osseous-bridge resection and silicone-rubber implant. J. Bone Joint Surg., 56-A:655, 1974.

157. Compere, E. L.: Growth arrest in long bones as a result of fractures that include the epiphysis. J.A.M.A., 105:2140, 1935.

158. Hessels, G. J., Dereymaeker, G., and Fabry, G.: Epiphyseal arrest following prolonged immobilization. Acta Orthop. Belg., 39:752, 1973.

159. Iwahara, T.: Fracture observed from the standpoint of longitudinal growth of bone. Jpn. Med., 5:429, 1959.

160. Kobayaski, S.: A study of the effect caused by repeated movement of the displaced fragment on longitudinal growth of bone. J. Jpn. Orthop. Assoc., 32:718, 1958.

161. Langenskiöld, A., and Edgren, W.: The growth mechanism of the epiphyseal cartilage in the light of experimental observations. Acta Orthop. Scand., 19:19, 1950.

162. Langenskiöld, A.: The possibilities of eliminating premature closure of an epiphyseal plate caused by trauma or disease. Acta Orthop. Scand., 38:267, 1967.

163. Langenskiöld, A.: An operation for partial closure of the epiphyseal plate in children and its experimental basis. J. Bone Joint Surg., 57-B:325, 1975.

164. Langenskiöld, A., and Österman, K.: Surgical treatment of partial closure of the epiphyseal plate. Reconstr. Surg. Traumatol., 17:48, 1979.

165. Lehner, A., and Dubas, J.: Sekundare Deformierungen nach Epiphysenlosungen und epiphysenliniennahen Frakturen. Helv. Chir. Acta, 20:388, 1954.

166. Lipshultz, O.: The end results of injuries to the epiphyses. Radiology, 28:223, 1937.

167. Lutken, P.: Two cases of abnormal skeletal growth following trauma. Acta Orthop. Scand., 33:358, 1963.

168. Mallet, J.: Les epiphysiodeses partielles traumatiques de l'extremite inferieure du tibia chez l'enfant un traitement avec disepiphysiodese. Rev. Chir. Orthop., 61:5, 1975.

169. Milch, H.: Epiphyseal pseudarthrosis. J. Bone Joint Surg., 24:653, 1942.

170. Oh, W. T.: Type II epiphyseal fractures may also be responsible for bone growth distortions. Orthop. Rev., 6:95, 1977.

171. Ohyoshi, K., and Miura, T.: Five cases of the epiphyseal detachment of long bone. Hokkaido Igaku Zasshi, 5:37, 1959.

172. Rampoldi, A., and Boni, M.: I distacchi epifisari traumatici. Proc. 42nd Congr. Soc. Ital. Orthop. Traumatol., 1957.

173. Ray, S. K., Connolly, J. F., and Huurman, W. W., Jr.: Distraction treatment of deformities due to physeal fractures. Surg. Forum, 29:543, 1978.

174. Sarnat, B. G., and Creeley, P. W.: Effect of injury upon growth and some comments on surgical treatment. Plast. Reconstr. Surg., 11:39, 1963.

175. Sledge, C. B., and Noble, J.: Experimental limb lengthening by epiphyseal distraction. Clin. Orthop., 136:111, 1978.

176. Smith, M. K.: Premature ossification after separation of lower radial epiphysis. Ann. Surg., 75:501, 1922.

177. Smith, M. K.: The prognosis in epiphyseal line fractures. Ann. Surg., 79:273, 1924.

178. Snyder, C. H.: Deformities resulting from unilateral surgical trauma to the epiphyses. Ann. Surg., 100:335, 1934.

179. Ecke, H.: Diagnose und Prognose von Epiphysenfugen verletzungen. Aktuel. Traumatol., 5:97, 1975.

180. Nordentoft, E. L.: Den Operative Epifyseodese. Copenhagen, Munksgaard, 1964.

181. Nordentoft, E. L.: Experimental epiphyseal injuries. Acta Orthop. Scand., 40:176, 1969.

182. Simmons, D. J., and Nunnemacher, R. F.: Growth of the rat epiphyseal cartilage plate following partial amputation. Am. J. Anat., 117:221, 1965.

183. Yoshida, H.: Experimental studies on the repair of injured epiphyseal cartilage plate. J. Jpn. Orthop. Assoc., 33:993, 1959.

184. Siffert, R. S.: The effect of staples and longitudinal wires on epiphyseal growth. J. Bone Joint Surg., 38-A:1077, 1956.

185. Silverskiöld, N.: Uber Langen Wachstum der Knochen und Transplantation von Epiphysen schieben. Acta Chir. Scand., 75:77, 1934.

186. Mallet, J., and Rey, J. C.: Traitement des epiphysiodeses partielles traumatiques chez l'enfant par desepiphysiodese. Int. Orthop., 1:309, 1978.

187. Österman, K.: Operative elimination of partial premature epiphyseal closure. An experimental study. Acta Orthop. Scand. [Suppl.], 147, 1972.

188. Reynolds, F. C., and Ford, L. T.: An experimental study of the use of gelfoam to fill defects in bone. J. Bone Joint Surg., 35-A:980, 1953.

189. Serafin, J.: Effect of longitudinal transection of the epiphysis and metaphysis on cartilaginous growth. Am. Dig. Orthop. Lit., 1:17, 1970.

190. Anderson, W. V.: Lengthening of the lower limb: its place in the problem of limb length discrepancies. Mod. Trends. Orthop., 5:1, 1972.

191. Barr, J. S.: Autogenous epiphyseal transplant. J. Bone Joint Surg., 36-A:688, 1954.

192. Benum, P.: Autogenous transplantation of apophyses. Acta Orthop. Scand. [Suppl.], 156, 1974.

193. Eades, J. W., and Peacock, E. E.: Autogenous transplantation of an interphalangeal joint and proximal phalangeal epiphysis. J. Bone Joint Surg., 48-A:775, 1966.

194. Ecke, H.: Die Transplantation der Epiphysenfuge. Stuttgart, Enke, 1967.

195. Freeman, B. S.: Growth studies of epiphyseal transplant by flap and by free graft: a brief survey. Plast. Reconstr. Surg., 36:227, 1965.

196. Haas, S. L.: Transplantation of the articular end of bone, including the epiphyseal cartilage line. Surg. Gynecol. Obstet., 23:301, 1916.

197. Harris, W. R., Martin, R., and Tile, M.: Transplantation of epiphyseal plates. An experimental study. J. Bone Joint Surg., 47-A:897, 1965.

198. Hoffman, S., Siffert, R. S., and Simon, B. E.: Experimental and clinical experiences in epiphyseal transplantation. Plast. Reconstr. Surg., 50:58, 1972.

199. Key, J. A.: Survival and growth of an epiphysis after removal and replacement. J. Bone Joint Surg., 31-A:150, 1949.

200. MacDonald, W. F., Barnett, R. J., and Bray, E. A.: The viability of transplanted epiphyseal cartilage. U.S. Armed Forces Med. J., 7:59, 1956.

201. Obata, K.: Uber Transplantation von Gelenken bei jungeren Tieren, mit besonderer Berucksichtigung des Verhaltens des Intermediarknorpels. Beitr. Pathol. Anat., 59:1, 1914.

202. Ring, P. A.: Transplantation of epiphyseal cartilage. J. Bone Joint Surg., 37-B:642, 1955.

203. Ring, P. A.: Excision and reimplantation of the epiphyseal cartilage of the rabbit. J. Anat., 89:231, 1955.

204. Sarrias, M.: The vulnerability of the growth cartilage to survive after transposition. J. Anat., 101:113, 1967.

205. Spira, E., and Farin, I.: Epiphyseal transplantation. J. Bone Joint Surg., 46-A:1278, 1964.

206. Volkow, M., and Bizer, V.: Homotransplantation of Bone Tissue in Children. Moscow, Mir Publishers, 1972.

207. Wenger, H. L.: Transplantation of epiphyseal cartilage. Arch. Surg., 50:148, 1945.

208. Wilson, J. N.: Epiphyseal transplantation. A clinical study. J. Bone Joint Surg., 48-A:245, 1966.

209. Whitesides, E. S.: Normal growth in a transplanted epiphysis. J. Bone Joint Surg., 59-A:546, 1977.

210. Hendryson, I. C.: An evaluation of the estimated percentage of growth from the distal epiphyseal line. J. Bone Joint Surg., 27:208, 1945.

211. Wilson, P. D., and Thompson, T. C.: A clinical consideration of the methods of equalizing leg length. Ann. Surg., *110*:992, 1939.

212. Menelaus, M. B.: Correction of leg length discrepancy by epiphyseal arrest. J. Bone Joint Surg., *48-B*:336, 1966.

213. Moseley, C. F.: A straight-line graph for leg-length discrepancies. J. Bone Joint Surg., *59-A*:174, 1977.

214. Moseley, C. F.: A straight-line graph for leg-length discrepancies. Clin. Orthop., *136*:33, 1978.

215. Fries, I. B.: Growth following epiphyseal arrest. A simple method of calculation. Clin. Orthop., *114*:216, 1976.

216. Gill, G. G., and Abbott, L. C.: Practical method of predicting growth of the femur and tibia in a child. Arch. Surg., *45*:286, 1942.

217. Green, W. T., and Anderson, M.: The problem of unequal leg lengths. Pediatr. Clin. North Am., *2*:1137, 1955.

218. Green, W. T., and Anderson, M.: Epiphyseal arrest for the correction of discrepancies in length of the lower extremities. J. Bone Joint Surg., *39-A*:853, 1957.

219. Green, W. T., Wyatt, G. M., and Anderson, M.: Orthoroentgenography as a method of measuring the bones of the lower extremities. Clin. Orthop., *61*:10, 1968.

220. Gross, R. H.: Leg length discrepancy: how much is too much? Orthopedics, *1*:307, 1978.

221. Masse, P., and Taussig, G.: Inegalites de Longeur des Membres Inferieurs chez l'Enfant. Paris, Bailliere, 1978.

222. Morein, G., Gassner, S., and Kaplan, I.: Bone growth alterations resulting from application of CO_2 laser beam to the epiphyseal growth plates. Acta Orthop. Scand., *49*:244, 1978.

223. Phemister, D. B.: Operative assessment of longitudinal growth of bones in the treatment of deformities. J. Bone Joint Surg., *15*:1, 1933.

224. Younge, D., and Colliou, L.: Fermeture experimentale d'une plaque par epiphysiodese. Union Med. Can., *105*:866, 1976.

225. Christensen, N. O.: Growth arrest by stapling. Acta Orthop. Scand. [Suppl.], *151*, 1973.

226. Bianco, A. J., Jr.: Femoral shortening. Clin. Orthop., *136*:49, 1978.

227. Winquist, R. A., Hansen, S. T., Jr., and Pearson, R. E.: Closed intramedullary shortening of the femur. Clin. Orthop., *136*:54, 1978.

228. Wilson, C., and Percy, E. C.: Experimental studies on epiphyseal stimulation. J. Bone Joint Surg., *38-A*:1096, 1956.

229. Yabsley, R. H., and Harris, W. R.: The effect of shaft fractures and periosteal stripping on the vascular supply to epiphyseal plates. J. Bone Joint Surg., *47-A*:551, 1965.

230. Porter, R. W.: The effect of tension across a growing epiphysis. J. Bone Joint Surg., *60-B*:252, 1978.

231. Warrell, E., and Taylor, J. F.: The effect of trauma on tibial growth. J. Bone Joint Surg., *58-B*:375, 1976.

232. Hert, J.: Acceleration of the growth after decrease of load on epiphyseal plates by means of spring distractors. Folia Morphol. (Praha), *17*:194, 1969.

233. Jenkins, D. H., Cheng, D. H., and Hodgson, A. R.: Stimulation of bone growth by periosteal stripping. J. Bone Joint Surg., *57-B*:482, 1975.

234. Keck, S. W., and Kelly, P. J.: The effect of venous stasis on intra-osseous pressure and longitudinal bone growth in the dog. J. Bone Joint Surg., *47-A*:539, 1965.

235. Trueta, J., and Morgan, J. D.: The vascular contribution to osteogenesis. J. Bone Joint Surg., *42-B*:97, 1960.

236. Weinman, D. T., Kelly, P. J., and Owen, C. A.: Blood flow in bones distal to a femoral arteriovenous fistula in dogs. J. Bone Joint Surg., *46-A*:1676, 1964.

237. Digby, K.: The measurement of diaphyseal growth in proximal and distal directions. J. Anat. Physiol., *50*:187, 1915.

238. Kessel, L.: Annotations on the etiology and treatment of tibia vara. J. Bone Joint Surg., *52-B*:93, 1970.

239. Sola, C. K., Silberman, F. S., and Cabrini, R. L.: Stimulation of the longitudinal growth of long bones by periosteal stripping. J. Bone Joint Surg., *45-A*:1679, 1963.

240. Ring, P. A.: The influence of the nervous system upon the growth of bones. J. Bone Joint Surg., *43-B*:121, 1961.

241. Eydelstehyn, B. M., Udalova, N. F., and Bochkarov, G. F.: Dynamics of reparative regeneration after lengthening by the method of distraction epiphyseolysis. Acta Chir. Plast. (Prague), *15*:149, 1973.

242. Fishbane, B. M., and Riley, L. H.: Continuous transphyseal traction: experimental observations. Clin. Orthop., *136*:120, 1978.

243. Jani, L.: Tierexperimentelle Studie uber Tibiaverlangerung durch Distraktionepiphyseolyse. Z. Orthop., *111*:627, 1973.

244. Jani, L.: Die Distraktionepiphyseolyse: Tierexperimenter Studie zum Problem der Beinverlagergung. Z. Orthop., *113*:189, 1975.

245. Letts, R. M., and Meadows, L.: Epiphyseolysis as a method of limb lengthening. Clin. Orthop., *133*:230, 1978.

246. Marsh, H. O., Adas, E., and Laroia, K.: An experimental attempt to stimulate growth by a distracting force across the lower femoral epiphysis. Ann. Surg., *27*:615, 1961.

247. Cauchoix, J., and Morel, G.: One stage femoral lengthening. Clin. Orthop., *136*:66, 1978.

248. Coleman, S. S., and Stevens, P. M.: Tibial lengthening. Clin. Orthop., *136*:92, 1978.

249. D'Aubigne, R. N., and Dubousset, J.: Surgical correction of large length discrepancies in the lower extremities of children and adults. J. Bone Joint Surg., *53-A*:411, 1971.

250. Eyring, E. J.: Staged femoral lengthening. Clin. Orthop., *136*:83, 1978.

251. Hungerford, D. S., ed.: Leg Length Discrepancy: The Injured Knee. New York, Springer-Verlag, 1977.

252. Ilizdrov, G. A., and Soybelman, L. M.: Some clinical and experimental data on the bloodless lengthening of lower limbs. Expr. Khir. Anestez., *4*:27, 1969.

253. Wagner, H.: Operative lengthening of the femur. Clin. Orthop., *136*:125, 1978.

5

Biology of Chondro-Osseous Repair

The progressive changes that make up the normal process of osseous fracture healing, whether in the diaphysis, metaphysis, or epiphyseal ossification center, may be grouped conveniently into a reasonably chronologic series of phases. There are a number of factors influencing bone healing that may be identified from clinical observation as well as from experimental work, and these must be considered in order to place treatment of childhood fractures on a rational basis. Much experimentation has been undertaken on animals which, because of differences in macroscopic and microscopic bone structure and skeletal homeostatic mechanisms, may respond differently than the skeletally immature human.[1-3] Much of this work has been done in skeletally mature animals, and the particular relevance of such data to fracture healing in the developing skeleton of the child is not always clear. Furthermore, as shown in Chapter 4, certain areas of the developing skeleton, particularly the physis and epiphyseal hyaline cartilage, probably do not heal by classic callus formation at all. In fact, if this type of osseous (callus) repair does occur in these cartilaginous regions, an osseous bridge may form and lead to significant growth deformities.

As in the adult, fracture healing in the immature skeleton may be divided into three integrated, sequential phases: (1) the inflammatory phase; (2) the reparative phase, and (3) the remodeling phase. In a child, the remodeling phase is temporally more extensive and physiologically more active, depending on the age of the child, than the comparable phase in an adult. The phase is further complicated by the responses of the growth plate to changing joint reaction forces and biologic stresses that alter angular growth dynamics.[4-6] These complications occur even when the fracture is mid-diaphyseal, and significantly distant from the active longitudinal growth regions.

Inflammatory phase

Immediately following a fracture through any of the osseous portions of the developing skeleton (diaphysis, metaphysis, or epiphyseal ossification center), a number of cellular processes commence. The damaged periosteum, contiguous bone, and soft tissues begin to bleed. If the fracture is localized in the maturing diaphysis, there is bleeding from the Haversian systems, as well as from the multiple small blood vessels of the microcirculatory systems of the endosteal and periosteal surfaces and the contiguous soft tissue anastomoses. In the metaphysis, bleeding may be extensive because of the anastomotic ramifications of the peripheral and central metaphyseal vascular systems. This hemorrhaging leads to the accumulation of a hematoma within the medullary canal at the fracture site, beneath the elevated periosteum, or extra-periosteally if the fracture has disrupted the periosteum.

In contrast to the adult, the periosteum strips easily away from the underlying bone in the child, allowing the fracture hematoma to dissect along the diaphysis and the metaphysis, a factor evident in the amount of subsequent new bone formation along the shaft (Fig. 5-1). However, the dense attachments of the periosteum into the zone of Ranvier limit formation of subperiosteal hematoma to the metaphysis and diaphysis (Fig. 5-2). Since the perichondrium of the epiphysis is densely attached, a hemorrhagic response in the epiphyseal ossification center is uncharacteristic; thus, formation of subperichondrial callus, and its subsequent stabilization effect, are limited. Furthermore, because of the partial or completely intra-articular nature of some epiphyses, propagation of the fracture into the joint allows decompression of the hematoma into the joint, and, again, limits the volume available for callus formation.

The multiple small vessels of the Haversian and Volkmann systems are fractured and disrupted, leading to internal bleeding. The periosteal vessels and the endosteal medullary vessels become involved, bleed, and form a larger, more inclusive clot. This may lead to temporary cessation of blood supply to the osteocytes for a distance of a few millimeters on either side of the cortical fracture site, creating juxtaposed, avascular trabecular and cortical bone.

In the metaphysis, this can lead to a complete (although temporary) cutoff of the blood supply of a segment 2 to 3 cm in length within the endosteal region (see Fig. 4-38). Because of the nuances of the periosteal circulation, particularly the peripheral metaphyseal circulation, there is some blood flow to the more peripheral regions of the metaphysis, especially the cortex. The segments of ischemic bone eventually will be replaced by viable bone through a process of

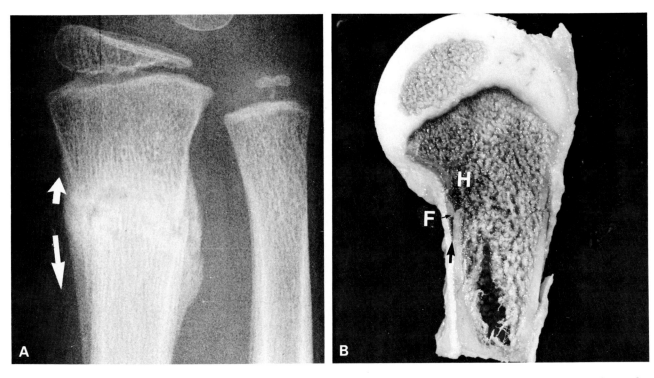

FIG. 5-1. *A*, Normal subperiosteal new bone formation. In a torus (compression) fracture of the distal radial metaphysis, the periosteum is usually intact, limiting the spread of the acute hemorrhage. Dissection of this specimen was more extensive proximally (arrows) as the periosteum in this region is attached more loosely and can be elevated by fluid under pressure more easily than in the opposite region over the metaphysis. *B*, Early subperiosteal hemorrhage (arrow) in a proximal humeral metaphyseal fracture (F). Hemorrhage is also present within the trabecular bone of the metaphysis (H).

simultaneous bone resorption and new bone deposition, the latter leading to an initial appearance of sclerosis, while the former makes the fracture line more obvious two or three weeks after an injury than it is during the initial stages of healing.

In a relatively undisplaced fracture, most of the internal bleeding in and around the fracture site comes from the disrupted nutrient artery or the branches of it in the periosteal sleeve; therefore, the resultant fracture hematoma is localized around the bone ends. If the fracture is more severely displaced, the periosteal sleeve may be disrupted, leading to decompression of the hematoma into the surrounding soft tissues. Whether this has any significant effect on the rate of the inflammatory and reparative phases is unknown. In children, the periosteal sleeve is more likely to remain intact and able to effect a coordinated osteogenic response.

Areas temporarily deprived of vascular supply develop microscopic areas of damage and necrosis in bone, cartilage, and soft tissue. In this ischemic material, as well as in the fracture itself, an inflammatory response is a normal biologic process. In general, children's bones are much more vascular and capable of a greater hyperemic response than adult's bones. Accompanying the vasodilation is a cellular response in which inflammatory cells, including polymorphonuclear leukocytes and macrophages migrate into the region of injury (Fig. 5-3).[7,8] Macrophages appear to be a major factor in any type of wound healing, and they may be a significant producer of collagen, an important component for eventual organization and maturation of the fracture callus.

The cellular response apparently begins shortly after injury and reaches a maximum within 24 hours. Tonna and Cronkite[3] showed that activity is seen first in the subperiosteal region, but may extend the whole length of the injured

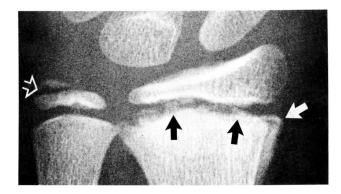

FIG. 5-2. Pattern of subperiosteal callus response in an epiphyseal fracture. New bone is limited by the dense attachment of the periosteum into the physis (closed white arrow). The physis continues to widen and is irregularly invaded to create random ossification (black arrows). The ulnar styloid has also fractured and may heal by cartilaginous and fibrous tissue to lead to a nonunion (open white arrow). This is an underemphasized problem of fracture healing in children.

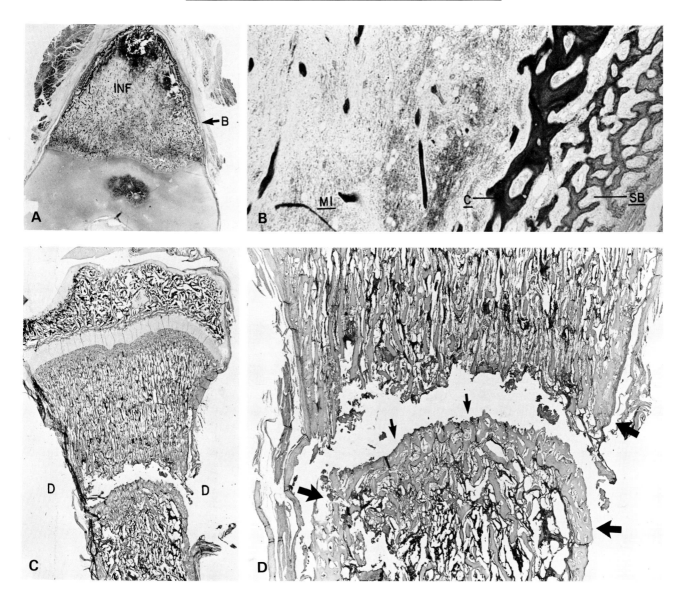

FIG. 5-3. *A,* Diffuse inflammation (INF) through the metaphysis of a neonate with osteogenesis imperfecta. Fracture through the metaphysis has stimulated subperiosteal new bone. (Arrow points to area shown in *B.*) *B,* High-power view of metaphyseal inflammation (MI), cortical bone (C), and new subperiosteal bone (SB). *C,* Low-power view of a metaphyseal fracture in the tibia of an arctic fox (Alopex lagopus). (D marks area shown in *D.*) *D,* Higher power view of part *C* showing necrotic tissue and inflammation on the proximal side, and inflammation and trabecular thickening (small arrows) forming the early callus. Subperiosteal callus is present in various stages (large arrows).

bone (Fig. 5-4). Within a few days, this generalized cellular activity becomes confined to the area juxtaposed to the fracture (Fig. 5-5).

At this early stage, the ends of the broken bone, at least in the diaphysis, are not participating in the proliferative activity of cellular division. Instead, they are undergoing localized cellular necrosis, as evidenced by the presence of empty osteocyte lacunae, which extend for a variable distance away from the fracture. Cell division appears to occur primarily in the endosteal and subperiosteal regions. It occurs in the former region particularly in the metaphysis, and in the latter in both the metaphysis and the diaphysis. This phenomenon occurs because of anatomic arrangements and microanastomotic connections of blood vessels in the diaphysis as well as in the metaphysis. Therefore, it is best to conceptualize the ends of the broken bone as playing a passive role in bridging the macroscopic fracture gap, particularly in incomplete fractures in children, and as rendering a certain intrinsic stability to the more complicated bridging process that occurs between the separated regions of viable bone (Fig. 5-6).

If one appreciates that the basic repair process of an injured, immature skeletal element is the progressive circumvention of localized, juxtaposed dead bone, with new, initially peripheral connections between the separated regions of viable bone, it is easier to understand why metaphyseal

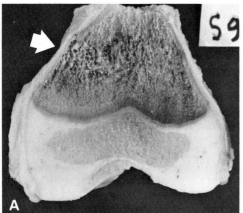
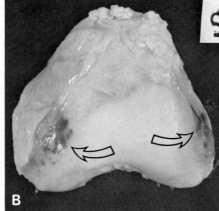
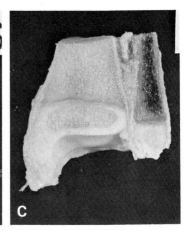

FIG. 5-4. Hemorrhagic response in a three-year-old boy who was struck by a car and died shortly thereafter. *A*, Distal femur showing torus fracture (arrow) with mild trabecular bleeding. *B*, However, the same specimen had obvious dissection of subperiosteal and extraperiosteal hematoma (arrows). *C*, The fibula was fractured in the midshaft, but hemorrhage extended down to the distal metaphysis.

fractures heal more readily than diaphyseal fractures, and why diaphyseal fractures in children heal more readily than those in adults. In both situations, we are dealing with tissues that normally undergo extensive remodeling, particularly in the metaphysis; thus, the normal, extremely active processes of bone replacement and remodeling participate in fracture healing.

When the fracture involves the growth plate through the region of new endochondral bone formation, it becomes necessary to unite the region of continuing post-fracture endochondral bone formation with the fractured region of the metaphyseal bone. This causes minimal disruption of the vascular pattern and allows rapid reconstitution of solid, structurally functional bone. This can come about because the hypertrophic zone of cartilage through which the fracture passes is not as dependent on blood supply as is the adjacent bone; therefore, only one side of the fracture is temporarily devascularized.

MacEwen[9] stated that the periosteum was nothing more than a limiting membrane, and that the cells responsible for production of new appositional bone belonged properly to the surface of the bone. Ham[10,11] pointed out that this was largely a matter of definition and that the periosteum should be regarded as consisting of at least two layers: an outer fibrous layer and an inner cambial layer. This latter layer consisted of cells termed osteoprogenitor cells, in order to distinguish them from osteoblasts, which have modulated to become functional, rather than dividing, cells.[12,13]

If the periosteum is stripped away traumatically, the bone is not totally deprived of osteogenic potential (Fig. 5-7). When periosteum is stripped away from bone, it does carry along some of these osteoprogenitor (osteogenic) cells. If a segment of bone is excised, the remaining periosteal tube sometimes will regenerate a new bone (see Fig. 2-2).[14-16] However, if the periosteum is significantly damaged or destroyed during the fracture, the potential for repair may be irrevocably lost, necessitating bone graft (Fig. 5-8), although this is extremely unusual in children's fractures.

The initial cellular repair process is organization of the fracture hematoma. Fibrovascular tissue replaces the clot

with collagen fibers and matricial elements, which will eventually become mineralized and form the woven bone of the provisional (primary) callus.[17,18] Initial invasion and cell division occur around the damaged bone ends, but proceed centrifugally away from the actual fracture site, thus allowing the most mature tissues of the repair process to be closest to the actual fracture site. In some areas, particularly at the periphery of the callus, an early type of cartilage forms that eventually will be converted to bone by endochondral ossification.

However, endochondral ossification can occur only in the presence of a microvascular supply. If vascular supply is defi-

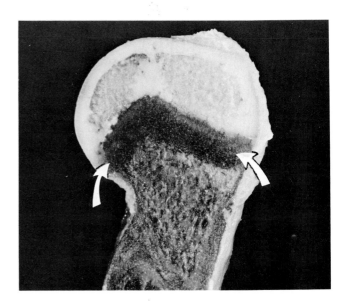

FIG. 5-5. Localization of the hemorrhagic-inflammatory response to juxtaphyseal metaphysis (arrows) after epiphyseal fracture of the proximal humerus in an eight-year-old child.

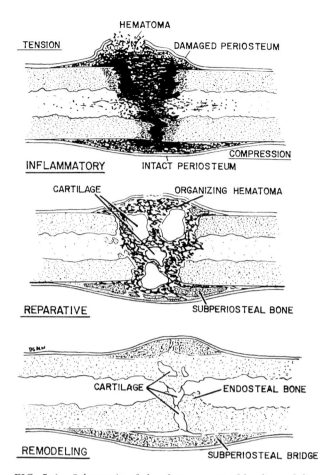

FIG. 5-6. Schematic of the three stages of healing of diaphyseal and metaphyseal bone—inflammatory, reparative, and remodeling. Subperiosteal new bone dominates in undisplaced diaphyseal fractures, whereas endosteal healing tends to dominate metaphyseal healing. In the child, the periosteum tends to be intact on the compression side of the fracture, and disrupted on the tension side. The subperiosteal callus is more extensive and mature on the compression side at any given stage of fracture healing.

cient, this modulation of cartilaginous to osseous tissue cannot occur readily. This is unlikely in children, but does occur in adults and may be one reason for the greater incidence of nonunion in adults.

The amount of cartilage that forms is variable. It appears to be a more prominent feature of fracture healing in lower animals,[2] and in cases in which excessive movement is permitted. A common factor here is probably low oxygen tension, a hypothesis that is compatible with some of the studies of chondro-osseous metabolism.[10,19-22] Theoretically, cartilage provides a suitable material with decreased oxygen demands that will temporarily bridge the fracture gap until a microvascular system can be adequately established to begin the gradual transformation to bone.

Concomitantly, similar cellular activity begins in the medullary region, although vascular response is much slower there than it is on the periosteal side.[5] Again, this factor may be highly variable in children, inasmuch as their trabecular bone is more vascular than that of adults. If the fracture involves the metaphysis, the vascular response is extremely rapid. The more mature the cortex, and the greater the amount of osteon bone involved, the more likely it is that the vascular response will be slow. This readily explains the rate-response differences between the fenestrated, woven bone of the metaphyseal cortex and the mature, lamellar bone of the diaphyseal cortex.

The amount of new endosteal bone is variable and depends on the nature of the bone involved. It is, of course, the principal method of union in cancellous (trabecular) bone of the metaphysis and epiphysis, but it can also form in predominantly cortical bone such as the diaphysis. While there is considerable cortical, lamellar bone in the diaphysis, the demands of growth and appositional increase in diameter necessitate the presence of some trabecular bone along the surfaces of the diaphyseal shaft (periosteal and endosteal) in children.

The process of new bone formation is enhanced when the fracture surfaces are offset, in which case the responsive, new endosteal bone from one side of the fracture may unite with the responsive subperiosteal bone of the opposite fragment (Fig. 5-9). In such situations, as in overriding fractures, this tends to be a dominant fracture healing pattern, and

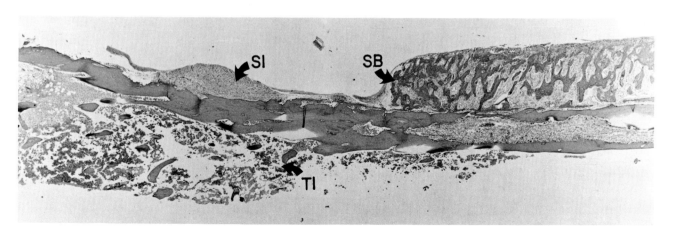

FIG. 5-7. Subperiosteal new bone formation (SB) and subperiosteal inflammation (SI) adjacent to normal cortex. Trabecular inflammation (TI) is also present.

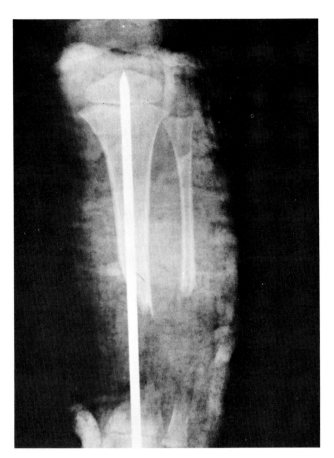

FIG. 5-8. Loss of extensive amounts of periosteum severely limits reparative response capacity, even in the young child. Eventually, amputation was necessary in this case.

leads to acceptable fracture stability with relatively rapid union. Remodeling eventually corrects contour changes.

Opinions differ regarding the relative importance of these basic cellular processes, although, as mentioned previously, some of the differences may be due to an effort to impute a simple, common mechanism to repair of all types of bone injury in all animal species (including the human), no matter what the degree of skeletal maturity. As described by McKibbin,[23] many of the differences in emphasis that appear in various accounts of fracture healing probably can be explained by differences between particular types of bones, the species studied, and even the experimental mode by which the fracture was produced.

Ham[10] has questioned the role of the hematoma. He described a zone of intense cellular activity in the subperiosteal region that resulted in the formation of two encircling collars of callus, appearing as wedge-shaped areas on a longitudinal section, which gradually approach each other until they meet and unite. This process may take place external to the hematoma, which is thereby bypassed and resorbed later.

Pritchard,[2] in contrast, has drawn a distinction between the reparative tissue, or blastema, that arises from the outer fibrous layer of the periosteum and the reparative tissue that emanates from the cambial layer of the medullary cavity, which he terms the osteogenic blastema. Normally, the oste-ogenic blastema, being more centrally placed, invades the hematoma, produces new bone, and bridges the fragments, while the more peripheral zones, which are fibrous in character, restore the continuity of the periosteum. Pritchard further feels that if the peripheral fibrous tissue invades the fracture gap before the osteogenic blastema, then conditions are set up for the development of nonunion.[2]

Because of the extreme osteogenic blastemal activity in the child, whether dealing with metaphyseal or diaphyseal osseous response, predominance of the fibrous response is unlikely, a factor that may be important in explaining the rarity of nonunion in children's bone. However, in fractures within the epiphyseal or physeal cartilage, particularly if the secondary ossification center has not developed or is quite small, the fibrous response seems to be more prone to develop (Fig. 5-10).

A more fundamental argument concerning these cellular processes is the differing concept of the source of the osteo-genic tissue. There are two basic, somewhat diametrically opposed, theories regarding these cells. According to one theory, the repair tissue arises from specialized cells with a predetermined commitment to bone formation. These specialized cells are the osteoprogenitor cells, which occur only in close association with the surface of the periosteal bone or the endosteal bone marrow.[24-26] As the osseous cells proliferate, the fibrous periosteum is pushed away from the bone to produce the apposed collars of callus that eventually fuse with each other (see Fig. 5-6).

The alternative theory is that repair tissue does not arise, per se, from these specialized cells, but rather that it arises from the activity of previously uncommitted fibroblasts that are capable of developing osteogenic potential if given the appropriate microenvironmental stimulus. This school of opinion feels that reparative tissue arises not from the bone itself, but from the surrounding soft tissues. However, these two theories may not be totally opposed, as the uncommitted fibroblasts may also be considered potential osteoprogenitor cells. This phenomenon, by which unassociated soft tissues are recruited in the osseous repair response, is known as osteogenic induction.[25,27-29]

Normally, the cortex is supplied largely through the medullary vascular system, the flow of which is centrifugal; and the periosteum makes only a small arterial contribution to the outer cortex (although in situations of trauma this may become a more dominant blood supply).[30] Following a fracture, an extensive, extra-osseous blood supply derived from the surrounding soft tissue develops.[31,32] While it assists in revascularizing any peripheral, necrotic tissue of the cortex, its main purpose appears to be participation in the formation of the external callus.

Reparative phase

The next step within the enveloping hematoma is cellular organization. During this stage, the circumferential tissues play only a small role in mechanical stabilization of the fracture. Instead, they serve primarily as a fibrous scaffold over which subsequently appearing cells may migrate and orient to induce a more stable type of repair. The cells that migrate are pluripotential mesenchymal cells theoretically capable of modulation into cartilage, bone, or fibrous tissue. Seemingly common stem cells migrate into the area and modulate, probably in response to variations in the microenvironment

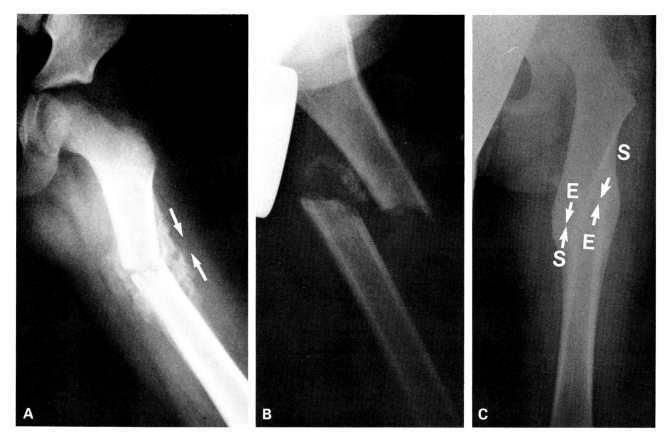

FIG. 5-9. *A,* Subperiosteal repair response with end-to-end apposition. Note that the subperiosteal callus of each segment is growing toward the other (arrows). *B,* Early response in side-to-side apposition. There is a combination of subperiosteal and endosteal callus. *C,* Later stage of repair showing maturation of endosteal (E) to subperiosteal callus (S). A new medullary communication will develop.

(e.g., changes in pH and the mechanical stresses of tension and/or compression).[19]

In the child, because of the osteoblastic activity of the inner layer, the periosteum contributes immensely to new bone formation by accentuating the normal process of membranous ossification to supplement the increasingly cellular organization within the hematoma. The region directly around the fracture site thus repeats the process of endochondral ossification in juxtaposition to membranous ossification from the elevated periosteum. Similar processes occur within the medullary cavity, where endosteal new bone and cartilage cells are forming. An integral part of the reparative process at this stage is microvascular invasion, a process that occurs rapidly and readily in children because of the state of vascularity within and without their bone and the surrounding soft tissues. Vessels come from the periosteal region, as well as from the nutrient artery and endosteal vessels.

The progressive organization of the hematoma by vascular invasion leads to the production of varying amounts of fibrous and cartilaginous cells that go through cellular and extracellular maturation processes in the presence of vascular supply to create immature, fibrous bone. As more and more of this cartilage and bone (callus) forms, the stability of the fragments gradually increases. However, until this bone goes through the final stages of maturation, it is still biologically plastic and, if not protected, may deform inexorably.

The microenvironment plays a significant role in this stress-responsive process.[29,33-36] Compression, or at least the absence of tension, discourages the formation of fibrous tissue.[25,37] Variations in oxygen tension probably modulate cellular formation of bone or cartilage, with cartilage being formed in lower oxygen tensions and bone in higher oxygen tensions. The cartilage that is formed eventually is replaced by bone through a process indistinguishable from prenatal and postnatal endochondral bone formation, with two exceptions: the cell columns are minimally formed, and there is nothing remotely resembling the modified spherical growth plate in the epiphyseal ossification center. The ossification transformation process appears randomly directed.

The fracture hematoma is the medium in which the early stages of healing take place. Osteogenic cells proliferate from the internal layer of the periosteum to form the external callus, and to a lesser extent, they also proliferate from the endosteum to form an internal callus. However, when the periosteum is severely disrupted, healing cells must differentiate from the ingrowth of undifferentiated mesenchymal cells within the hematoma. A few weeks after the fracture, the fracture callus consists of a thick enveloping mass of osteogenic tissue around the periphery. The callus itself does not contain any bone, and therefore is radiolucent and not apparent radiographically. The callus becomes progressively firmer and changes from undifferentiated tissue into a cartilaginous state. The cartilage is progressively invaded by new blood vessels and ossifies. This new bone is primarily woven bone.

Therefore, two types of healing are occurring: accelerated membranous bone formation in the child, and endochondral ossification within the fracture callus as cells modulate from fibroblasts to chondroblasts to osteoblasts. Clinical union is reached when the fracture site no longer appears to move and attempts at manipulation do not cause pain.

However, by no means is the bone restored to its original strength at this time. As time progresses, the primary callus gradually is replaced. This is enhanced in the child, because appositional growth and increasing diameter simply envelop the original fracture region. When the cartilage and woven bone have been replaced by mature, lamellar bone, the fracture is said to be consolidated, and essentially, has returned to its normal biologic standards and stress responsivity.

The cancellous bone of the metaphyses of long bones, the epiphyseal ossification center, the short bones of the hands and feet, and even flat bones such as the pelvis and ribs have a much more delicate, interconnected trabecular network with a much thinner cortex. Fracture healing in this cancellous bone occurs principally through the formation of an internal, endosteal callus, but also is accompanied by a periosteal or external callus. Minimal "cortical" callus is formed. Because of the rich blood supply to the trabecular region, much less necrosis of bone occurs at the fracture surfaces, and there is a larger area of osseous contact to consolidate.

Union proceeds more rapidly than it does in the dense cortical bone of the diaphysis. The osteogenic cells brought in by neovascularity and the existing vascularity proliferate to form primary woven bone throughout the hematoma and fracture area, resulting in a rapid and widely formed internal callus that readily fills the open spaces of the spongy, cancellous fracture surfaces. There is accompanying subperiosteal bleeding to create the external, membranous type of callus. Woven bone gradually is replaced by more mature bone, although there is not a great deal of conversion to osteonal or lamellar bone, since such bone is not characteristic of this region except at the periphery, and only as skeletal maturation approaches.

The initial stages of medullary callus formation in diaphyseal regions probably are not much different from those of periosteal callus formation, but it seems that a second stage of medullary callus formation exists that is different and appears later in the healing process. The obvious difference of this type of healing is on mechanical stability. Although motion appears to inhibit the development of external callus, medullary callus appears unaffected and may even flourish under motion (see Fig. 5-9). It appears to form without any intermediary stage of cartilage. One of its important functions is apparently as the tissue that initially replaces fracture gaps. New, immature, woven bone is preparatory for the subsequent development of lamellar, osteon bone. This type of fracture healing occurs in displaced (overriding) fracture fragments uniting subperiosteal and medullary callus. In the developing skeleton, there is often a significant amount of trabecular endosteal bone adjacent to more dense cortical bone. This medullary bone may respond more rapidly than the lamellar bone, thereby improving the rate of fracture healing in the child.

During the reparative phase, the ends of the bone gradually become enveloped in this confluent, fusiform mass of callus containing fibrous and cartilaginous tissue with increasing amounts of bone. The fragments become more rigid because of internal (fracture site) and external (periosteal) callus formation, and eventually, clinical union occurs. However, it must be stressed that "rigid" union, as a specific endpoint, does not exist yet. At some point during the reparative phase, the last phase of healing (remodeling) begins, with resorption of mechanically and physiologically unnecessary, inefficient portions of the callus, and the subsequent orientation of trabecular bone along the lines of stress. Thus, the reparative phase is characterized by relatively rapid formation of a randomly oriented bone collar composed primarily of immature fibrous bone and capable of imparting reasonable stability to the fracture site, although the bone is still capable of some plastic deformation if inappropriate stress is applied.

Since the two (or more) fracture fragments remain connected by the periosteum or related material in a child, it is easy to see how reparative activity could be conducted from one side to the other relatively easily and rapidly. Phillips and McKibbin[23] showed that well-developed callus formed rapidly, but after two weeks, if the collars of the opposing fragments did not make any cellular contact, they began to undergo involution, and even if interposed soft tissue was subsequently removed, the periosteum never became reactivated. The time period within which the fragments must make contact may be longer in the more osteogenic skeleton of a child.

Remodeling phase

The remodeling phase is the longest of the three phases, and in the child it is theoretically possible for this phase to continue unabated until skeletal maturation, and even beyond, in response to constantly changing stress patterns imposed by continued skeletal growth. The new bone that initially is laid down by both the fracture callus and the more extensive, but confluent, subperiosteal tissue is randomly oriented and certainly not capable of withstanding all biologic stresses imposed on it.[37,38] However, as the bone grows diametrically in the diaphyseal or metaphyseal regions, the new bone is gradually and increasingly incorporated into the already existent cortical bone, aligned in accord with predominant stress patterns, and to a great extent, inexorably replaced by physiologic remodeling processes. The younger the child, the greater the degree of remodeling and progressive replacement.

The end result of fracture remodeling in the presence of the continuing normal processes of growth of the immature skeleton is that the bone almost invariably returns to its original form, or at least is altered in a way that enables it to perform the functions demanded of it during subsequent growth and stress.

There is some suggestion that the control mechanism modulating much of this cell behavior is electrical (piezoelectrical), such that when a bone is subjected to compressive, tensile, and shearing stresses, electropositivity occurs along the more convex surfaces, and electronegativity along the more concave.

Using tissue culture, Bassett[19,39] and Brighton[20] have shown that differentiation of the fibroblast may be influenced by mechanical factors which may be acting through bioelectric phenomena. The piezoelectric effect appears to be more a function of collagen than of the mineral crystals of bone. It appears that electronegativity favors bone formation, and electropositivity favors bone dissolution. Such an observation suggests a hypothesis whereby Wolff's law is explained as a self-regulating feedback mechanism in which stresses and strains in the bone modify the bioelectrical environment in such a way as to direct cellular behavior. This is a complex and interesting new field, and the reader is referred to the references for further information.[20,23,28,39-42]

A number of factors influence the rates of fracture healing. Factors promoting bone healing appear to be growth hormone, the various thyroid hormones, calcitonin, insulin, vitamins A and B in physiologic doses, anabolic steroids, chondroitin sulfate and hyaluronidase (which certainly are present in variable concentrations in the developing skeletal system), certain types of electrical current, low dosages of hyperbaric oxygenation, and exercise.[43-47]

Factors that appear to retard bone healing are corticosteroids, diabetes, endocrinopathies, high doses of certain vitamins (e.g., A and D), anemia, unusual chemicals such as aminoacetonitrile or beta-aminopropionitrile, denervation, irradiation, high doses of hyperbaric oxygenation, some antibiotics and anticoagulants.[6,44,48-50]

A local factor affecting the rate of healing is the degree of trauma. The more extensive the soft tissue damage, the more delayed the normal reparative responses, especially if the highly osteoblastic periosteum is involved. The degree of bone loss is of import. But in view of the decreased incidence of compound injuries in children, there is rarely any significant bone loss. The type of bone involved is also a factor. Cortical and cancellous bone, the major components of the metaphyses and the epiphyseal ossification centers, unite rapidly, while osteon bone, the major component of the diaphyses, takes much longer. However, compared to the external, cortical bone of adults, the Haversian bone of children is more porous and capable of greater osteoblastic responses.

The degree of immobilization also affects the rate of healing. While the emphasis in adult orthopaedics is increasingly on absolutely rigid immobilization, often coupled with internal fixation, this is rarely necessary in children. Nonunion is essentially nonexistent, implying that a certain amount of biologic (muscular) stress, or motion, applied in a reasonably appropriate and anatomic fashion will lead to fracture healing. Infections will delay healing, but will not necessarily prevent it. Pathologic conditions such as malignancy may retard or preclude healing.

The critical step between the reparative and remodeling phases is the establishment of an intact bony bridge between the fragments, and since this involves the joining of separated segments of hard tissue, it follows that the whole system must become immobile, at least momentarily.[51] Once the bridge has been established, and provided that adequate mechanical protection is given, subsequent biologic failure is unlikely.

Once the fracture has been satisfactorily bridged by the external callus, it is necessary for this new bone to adapt to normal function. Again, this is an easier circumstance in children, in whom the skeleton is actively and continually remodeling in response to stress, as opposed to the more static skeleton of an adult.

There are two important points to stress. First, the processes of replacement and repair are going on continuously and concomitantly in the normal developing skeleton, and the mechanisms involved in fracture healing are essentially the same (again, these processes are more active in the child, and more active in the metaphysis than in the diaphysis). Second, there are differences in the process depending on whether it is occurring in compact or cancellous bone. Both essentially involve a process of simultaneous bone removal and replacement through the respective agencies of osteoclast and osteoblast. In the case of the cancellous bone of the metaphysis or the endosteal surface of the diaphysis, the cells are never far away from blood vessels, and the whole process of bone apposition and replacement can take place on the surface of the trabeculae.

However, in compact bone, the more deeply placed cells require the presence of an adequately functioning perfusion system that must be restored after the injury-related disruption.[52] This is a much longer sequence of events, and is not a common method of bone repair in the child, except when the fracture involves a densely cortical region such as the femoral shaft. The reader is referred to McKibbin's article for a more extensive discussion of this process, which is sometimes referred to as "primary bone union," since no intermediate cells are involved.[8,23]

Cartilage Repair

Unlike bone, the differentiated hyaline cartilage comprising the joint surfaces, and probably, the relatively undifferentiated hyaline cartilage of the epiphyses, appear to have a limited ability to repair or regenerate.[53] In fractures involving the articular surface in skeletally mature individuals, the hyaline articular cartilage apparently cannot be healed by the same tissue (i.e., proliferating articular chondrocytes), but is healed instead by fibrous granulation tissue and fibrocartilage, which is certainly inferior as a weightbearing joint surface.

If fracture surfaces of the cartilage are reduced perfectly, the thin scar of fibrocartilage is probably of little significance to normal joint function, even in a major weightbearing joint. However, if there is a gap, the fibrocartilage may be unable to withstand normal wear and tear and may contribute to early degenerative changes, particularly in weightbearing joints. Such degenerative changes may occur even before the end of skeletal maturation (see Fig. 5-10).

It was first pointed out by Strangeways,[54] and is a commonplace observation in joint pathology, that articular cartilage even in the skeletally immature, may live, grow, and calcify, but not ossify, when completely detached from the subchondral bone, provided that it has free access to the synovial fluid. Because of this capacity and the absence, or minimal presence, of blood vessels, articular cartilage nutrition is mainly synovial, although there is evidence of some diffusion from underlying (subchondral) bone.

In intra-articular fractures, an additional problem is imposed. Synovial fluid apparently contains fibrinolysins.[48] These fibrinolysins have the capacity to lyse initial clot formation and retard the aforementioned first stage (inflammatory phase) of fracture healing. However, to attribute this as the cause of total nonunion in fractures such as those involving the lateral condyle of the distal humerus is inappropriate, since the real problem in many of these fractures is rotation of the fragments and apposition of non-

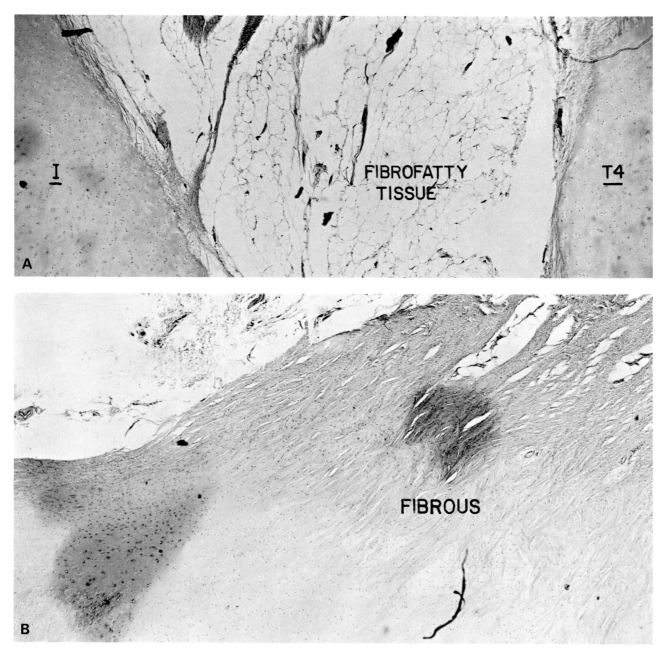

FIG. 5-10.   *A,* Fibrous tissue filling defect between intact (I) and type 4 fragment (T4). *B,* Similar fibrous tissue covered the joint surface.

ossifying articular cartilage to the normal reparative osseous regions. McKibbin[55] has adequately demonstrated that articular cartilage will not ossify under normal circumstances, and therefore, cannot participate effectively in the normal biologic repair process of a fracture of the ossification center.

The physical and chemical structure of normal hyaline articular cartilage has been studied extensively, but little has been published regarding reactions to injury and repair, particularly in the skeletally immature human.[47] Animal observations have been described.[56-58] The slow metabolism and physiologic inactivity of joint cartilage, emphasized by Bywaters,[59] were established mainly from animal material,

and the general view is that if cartilage has any reactions at all, they are so slow that they can be neglected. While this may be true for articular cartilage in the skeletally mature individual, the growing chondro-osseous skeleton is quite active biologically, and capable of considerable change, even when injured. Undoubtedly, this applies to cartilaginous as well as osseous components.

Along with the rearrangement of cartilage cells and the appearance of subchondral bone that takes place with increasing age, there are conspicuous changes in the cartilage matrix. In the fetus and young child, there is little collagen but more glycosaminoglycans than there are in more mature humans. The developing matrix progresses through biochemical changes characterized as metachromasia. From a histochemical standpoint, this phenomenon consists of a strong reaction with toluidine blue, but a weak or absent periodic acid-Schiff (PAS) reaction.[60] With increasing skeletal maturation, the PAS reaction becomes stronger, and the metachromasia less intense, although never completely lost. The collagen component becomes increasingly obvious and prominent.

It is reasonable to suggest that during growth, cartilage cells first form an excessive amount of highly polymerized, sulfated acid-glycosaminoglycans. The cartilage first loses its metachromasia, then part, but not all, of the epiphysis or articular region becomes PAS positive. The considerable variations in the shape of the cartilage cell and the extent and shape of the metachromasia around it are evidence of the variable physiologic state of the cell, which is by no means inert.

The repair of immature cartilage originates from several sources. Proliferation of cells from the intact cartilage and perichondrium may play a significant role in repair of defects within the epiphyseal cartilage, particularly along the nonarticular margins. However, such cellular responses are not as dominant in the repair of defects in the articular cartilage. Extension of tissue from the synovial margins may result in fibrous ankylosis and surface necrosis and does not contribute to healing (Fig. 5-11). The two principal methods of repair of linear defects in articular and epiphyseal cartilage are: (1) by extension of granulation tissue from the subchondral tissue and ossification center; and (2) by granulation tissue originating in the transected cartilage canals.

Calandruccio[56] found that the articular and epiphyseal cartilages of the femoral condyles of skeletally immature dogs were capable of proliferation, regeneration, and even complete repair with true hyaline cartilage, although the conditions leading to this desirable type of repair were not well elucidated. The observed differences in the repair of incomplete and complete defects suggested that granulation tissue from the subchondral bone of the epiphyseal ossification center inhibited cartilage formation, and that if this initial cellular inflammatory response could be prevented or minimized (i.e., by accurate anatomic reduction), the full potential of cartilage repair might be realized.

Calandruccio noted that cartilage proliferation was indicated by the presence of *chondrons,* which were cartilage lacunae with multiple nuclei. However, chondron formation was a slow process, and could occur only in the absence of granulation tissue. Such granulation tissue is neither primarily chondrogenic nor disposed to form cartilage secondarily, except perhaps by gradual fibrocartilaginous metaplasia. These workers were the first to suggest a possible role for the cartilage canal vessels in chondro-osseous healing.[56]

Marshall[58] studied cartilage repair in Holstein calves (distal femur) and firmly established the primary roles played by the subchondral region and cartilage canals in the formation of reparative granulation tissue. Whenever cartilage canal systems were present at or near the fracture site, capillary proliferation was evident (Fig. 5-12).

Tendon and Ligament Repair

Traumatic injury to developing tendons and ligaments is rare prior to complete skeletal maturation. Biomechanically immature chondro-osseous tissue is usually the weakest component of attached musculotendinous or ligamentous units. Tendons and ligaments do not always attach directly into the developing skeleton by Sharpey's fibers as they do

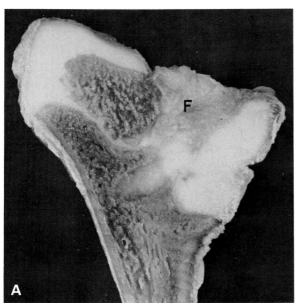
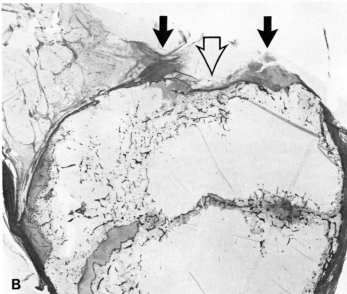

FIG. 5-11. *A,* Much of the medial tibial plateau of this type 4 injury (which occurred two years before this specimen was taken) has been replaced by fibrous tissue (F) which created a fibrous ankylosis to the distal femur. *B,* Sagittal section of proximal tibia from a 14-year-old who sustained a high voltage electrical injury. Extensive fibrosis (solid arrows) and loss of the articular cartilage (open arrow) led to a fibrous ankylosis.

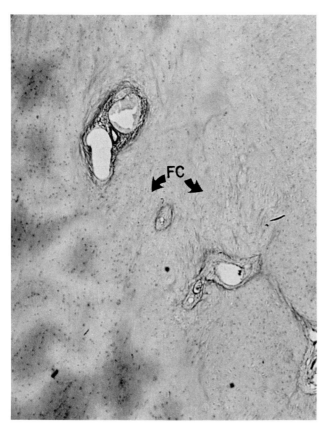

FIG. 5-12. Cartilage canals in type 4 fragment of case shown in Figure 5-11A. The cartilage forming around some of these appears more like fibrocartilage (FC) than the anticipated hyaline cartilage.

The principal blood supply of a tendon is not from the chondro-osseous insertion nor from the muscle origin, but rather from the mesotenon. The best known examples are the vincula of the digital tendons. Anastomoses are minimal between mesotendon supply areas. Any tendon deprived of its blood supply will degenerate and die.

The ends of a damaged tendon, as compared to osseous fracture surfaces, do not contribute significantly to the initial healing process. Instead, the essential source of reparative tissue is fibroblastic infiltration from the surrounding soft tissues. If the tendon ends retract, they may not reapproximate each other. However, in the child, such spontaneous reattachment may occur, especially if the disruption is near the cartilaginous insertion. This region has a cellular structure not unlike the physis,[61] and may facilitate repair without surgical intervention.

The joint ligaments and capsules generally attach directly and densely into the epiphyseal perichondrium. Under polarized light, continuity of the collagen elements between ligament and cartilage is evident. With time, the epiphyseal ossification center expands and gradually reaches the epiphyseal margins, forming a subchondral plate of bone into which the Sharpey's fibers will attach. The closer the ossification center is to the ligament attachment, the more likely it is to be avulsed (Fig. 5-14). This osseous region is certainly most susceptible to failure. The laxity of the developing ligaments allows a much greater degree of distortion without failure. However, this laxity decreases with increasing age, and the ligament becomes increasingly susceptible to disruption within its substance.

If the ligament fails at the osseous level, healing is by "fracture healing," and is usually quite rapid. However, if

in the adult skeleton. Instead, the tendons may attach into the cartilage of modified growth regions (e.g., the lesser trochanter or the tibial tuberosity) through a fibrocartilaginous intermediary tissue,[61-64] or into regions of the perichondrium or periosteum more densely associated with the underlying bone (i.e., near the physis and metaphysis).

Such methods of soft tissue/chondro-osseous continuity allow the attachments to "grow" as the bone undergoes elongation. The intrinsic capacity for elastic and plastic deformation without failure is much greater in the ligaments and tendons than it is in bones, and only when the child is nearing the end of the adolescent growth spurt do these structures exhibit decreasing laxity and increasing tendency to failure.

Experimental work has demonstrated that in an intact, mature musculotendinous-osseous system, the muscle belly itself is the weakest point, and will rupture under idealized circumstances.[65] However, in children, muscle ruptures are rare, and failure in these systems, at least in vivo, appears to be through the nearest bone, which invariably fails in tension (Fig. 5-13). The collagen orientation flows smoothly from tendon into perichondrium and subsequently into the epiphyseal cartilage. Ossification introduces a "disruption" in a unit that is specifically adapted to tensile stress. This certainly appears to be the failure mode in Osgood-Schlatter disease,[61] which is discussed in detail in Chapter 19.

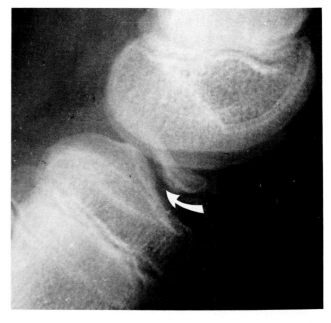

FIG. 5-13. Cruciate failure pattern in an adolescent. The chondro-osseous spine is more likely to fail, and may not heal by callus response, as in this case in which the fragment has developed a fibrous nonunion (arrow). This was reattached surgically.

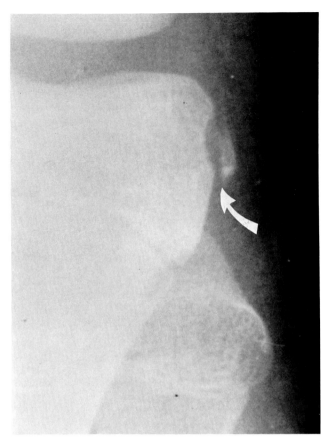

FIG. 5-14. Pattern of "ligament failure" in an adolescent. As in the previous figure of the cruciate, the collateral ligaments are stronger than the developing ossification center, and they cause a fracture (arrow), rather than soft tissue disruption.

the ligament itself is damaged, it will heal best if reapproximated.[57] Sutured ligaments subsequently tested under tension are stronger than nonsutured ones, which frequently fail through the area of scar tissue.

Both tendinous and ligamentous healing are based upon sufficient anatomic reapproximation to allow bridging with collagen and fibroblastic tissue (analogous to callus formation), and the subsequent reorientation of the collagen to re-establish the tensile strength. Again, because these tissues normally are growing and undergoing considerable remodeling, the capacity for repair, even spontaneous repair, is much greater in the musculoskeletally immature child than in the adult.

References

1. Panjabi, M. M., White, A. A., and Southwick, W. O.: Mechanical properties of bone as a function of rate of deformation. J. Bone Joint Surg., 55-A:322, 1973.
2. Pritchard, J. J., and Ruzicka, A. J.: Comparison of fracture repair in the frog, lizard, and the rat. J. Anat., 84:236, 1950.
3. Tonna, E. A., and Cronkite, E. P.: Cellular response to fracture studied with tritiated thymidine. J. Bone Joint Surg., 43-A:352, 1961.
4. Nonnemann, H. C.: Grenzen der Spontankorrektur fehlgeheilter Frakturen bei Jugendlichen. Langenbecks Arch. Chir., 324:78, 1969.
5. Gothman, L.: Vascular reactions in experimental fractures: microangiographic and radioisotope studies. Acta Chir. Scand. [Suppl.], 284, 1961.
6. Gudmundson, C.: Oxytetracycline-induced disturbance of fracture healing. J. Trauma, 11:511, 1971.
7. Lindholm, R., et al.: The mast cell as a component of callus in healing fractures. J. Bone Joint Surg., 51-B:148, 1969.
8. Wray, J. B.: Acute changes in femoral arterial blood flow after closed tibial fracture in dogs. J. Bone Joint Surg., 46-A:1262, 1964.
9. MacEwen, W.: The Growth of Bone. Glasgow, Maclehose, 1912.
10. Ham, A. W.: A histological study of the early phase of bone repair. J. Bone Joint Surg., 12:825, 1930.
11. Ham, A. W.: Histology. 6th Ed. Philadelphia, J. B. Lippincott, 1969.
12. Hall, B. K.: Developmental and Cellular Skeletal Biology. New York, Academic Press, 1978.
13. Young, R. W.: Cell proliferation and specialization during endochondral osteogenesis in young rats. J. Cell Biol., 14:357, 1962.
14. McClements, P., Templeton, R. W., and Pritchard, J. J.: Repair of a bone gap. J. Anat., 95:616, 1961.
15. Mulholland, M. C., and Pritchard, J. J.: The fracture gap. J. Anat., 93:590, 1959.
16. Zucman, J., and Piatier-Piketty, D.: Le role du perioste dans la cicatrisation des fractures. Acta Chir. Belg., 69:649, 1970.
17. Duthie, R. B., and Barker, A. N.: The histochemistry of the preosseous stage of bone repair studied by autoradiography. J. Bone Joint Surg., 37-B:691, 1955.
18. Potts, W. J.: The role of hematoma in fracture healing. Surg. Gynecol. Obstet., 57:318, 1933.
19. Bassett, C. A. L., and Herrman, I.: Influence of oxygen concentration and mechanical factors on differentiation of connective tissue in vitro. Nature, 190:460, 1961.
20. Brighton, C. T., Cronkey, J. E., and Osterman, A. L.: In vitro epiphyseal plate growth in various constant electrical fields. J. Bone Joint Surg., 58-A:971, 1976.
21. Brighton, C. T., and Heppenstall, R. B.: Oxygen tension in zones of the epiphyseal plate, the metaphysis and diaphysis. An in vitro and in vivo study in rats and rabbits. J. Bone Joint Surg., 53-A:719, 1971.
22. Girgis, F. G., and Pritchard, J. J.: Experimental production of cartilage during the repair of fractures of the skull vault in rats. J. Bone Joint Surg., 40-B:274, 1958.
23. McKibbin, B.: The biology of fracture healing in long bones. J. Bone Joint Surg., 60-B:150, 1978.
24. Crelin, E., and Koch, W.: An autoradiographic study of chondrocyte transformation into chondroblasts and osteocytes during bone formation in vitro. Anat. Rec., 158:473, 1967.
25. Crelin, E. S., White, A. A., III, Panjabi M. M., and Southwick, W. O.: Microscopic changes in fractured rabbit tibias. Conn. Med., 42:561, 1978.
26. Owen, M.: The origin of bone cells. Q. Rev. Cytology, 28:213, 1970.
27. Hall, B. K.: Cellular differentiation in connective tissue. Biol. Rev., 45:455, 1970.
28. Lokietek, W., Pawluk, R. J., and Bassett, C. A. L.: Muscle injury potentials: a source of voltage in the undeformed rabbit tibia. J. Bone Joint Surg., 56:361, 1974.
29. Urist, M. R., and McLean, F. C.: Osteogenetic potency and new bone formation by induction in transplants to the anterior chamber of the eye. J. Bone Joint Surg., 34-A:443, 1952.
30. Brookes, M.: The Blood Supply of Bone. New York, Appleton-Century-Crofts, 1971.
31. Rhinelander, F. W.: Tibial blood supply in relation to healing. Clin. Orthop., 105:34, 1974.

32. Rhinelander, F. W., et al.: Microangiography and bone healing. II. Displaced closed fractures. J. Bone Joint Surg., 50-A:643, 1968.

33. Bier, H.: Experimentelle Erfahrungen uber Pseudarthrosenbildung. M. M. W., 67:22, 1920.

34. Chalmers, J., Gray, D. H., and Rush, J.: Observations on the induction of bone in soft tissues. J. Bone Joint Surg., 57-B:36, 1975.

35. Friedenstein, A. Y.: Induction of bone tissue by transitional epithelium. Clin. Orthop., 59:21, 1968.

36. Goldhaber, P.: Osteogenic induction across millipore filters in vivo. Science, 133:2065, 1961.

37. Yamagishi, M., and Yoshimura, Y.: The biomechanics of fracture healing. J. Bone Joint Surg., 37-A:1035, 1955.

38. Tonino, A. J., et al.: Protection from stress in bone and its effects. J. Bone Joint Surg., 58-B:107, 1976.

39. Bassett, C. A. L., and Becker, R. O.: Generation of electric potentials by bone in response to mechanical stress. Science, 137:1063, 1962.

40. Becker, R. O., and Murray, D. G.: The electrical control system regulating fracture healing in amphibians. Clin. Orthop., 73:169, 1970.

41. Friendenberg, Z. B., Harlow, M. C., and Brighton, C. T.: Healing of nonunion of the medial malleolus by means of direct current. J. Trauma, 11:883, 1971.

42. Fukada, E., and Yasuda, I.: On the piezoelectric effect of bone. Nippon Seirigaku Zasshi, 12:1158, 1957.

43. Burger, M., Sherman, B. S., and Sobel, A. E.: Observations on the influence of chondroitin sulphate on the rate of bone repair. J. Bone Joint Surg., 44-B:675, 1962.

44. Herbsman, H., et al.: The influence of systemic factors on fracture healing. J. Trauma, 6:75, 1966.

45. Herold, H. Z., and Tadmor, A.: Chondroitin sulphate in treatment of experimental bone defects. Isr. J. Med. Sci., 5:425, 1969.

46. Herold, H. Z., Mobel, T. A., and Tadmor, A.: Cartilage extract in treatment of fractures in rabbits. Acta Orthop. Scand., 40:317, 1969.

47. Lack, C. H.: Proteolytic activity and connective tissue. Br. Med. Bull., 20:217, 1964.

48. Hsu, J. D., and Robinson, R. A.: Studies on the healing of long bone fractures in hereditary pituitary insufficient mice. J. Surg. Res., 9:535, 1969.

49. Rokhanen, P., and Slatis, P.: The repair of experimental fractures during long-term anticoagulant treatment. Acta Orthop. Scand., 35:21, 1964.

50. Rothman, R. H.: Effect of anemia on fracture healing. Surg. Forum, 19:452, 1968.

51. Charnley, J.: The Closed Treatment of Common Fractures. London, E. & S. Livingstone, 1970.

52. Schenk, R., and Willenegger, H.: Morphological findings in primary fracture healing. Symposia, Biologica Hungarica, 8:75, 1967.

53. Bennett, G. A., Baur, W., and Maddock, S. J.: A study of the repair of articular cartilage. Am. J. Pathol., 8:499, 1932.

54. Strangeways, T. S. P.: Observations on the nutrition of articular cartilage. Br. Med. J., 1:661, 1920.

55. McKibbin, B., and Holdsworth, F.: The dual nature of epiphyseal cartilage. J. Bone Joint Surg., 49-B:351, 1967.

56. Calandruccio, R. A., and Gilmer, W. S.: Proliferation, regeneration and repair of articular cartilage of immature animals. J. Bone Joint Surg., 44-A:431, 1962.

57. Clayton, M. L., and Weir, G. L., Jr.: Experimental investigations of ligamentous healing. Am. J. Surg., 98:373, 1959.

58. Marshall, J. L., and Bullough, P. G.: Repair of full thickness defects in the articular cartilage. Rev. Hosp. Special Surgery, 1:60, 1971.

59. Bywaters, E. G. L.: The metabolism of joint tissues. J. Pathol. Bact., 44:247, 1937.

60. Rosenberg, L.: Chemical basis for the histological use of safranin 0 in the study of articular cartilage. J. Bone Joint Surg., 53-A:69, 1971.

61. Ogden, J. A., Hempton, R., and Southwick, W.: Development of the tibial tuberosity. Anat. Rec., 182:431, 1975.

62. Ogden, J. A.: Development of the epiphyses. In Orthopaedic Surgery in Infancy and Childhood. Edited by A. B. Ferguson. Baltimore, Williams & Wilkins, 1975.

63. Ogden, J. A.: The development and growth of the musculoskeletal system. In The Scientific Basis of Orthopaedics. Edited by J. A. Albright, and R. A. Brand. New York, Appleton-Century-Crofts, 1979.

64. Ogden, J. A.: Chondro-osseous development and growth. In Fundamental and Clinical Bone Physiology. Edited by M. R. Urist. Philadelphia, J. B. Lippincott, 1980.

6

Open Injuries and
Traumatic Amputations

Open (compound) injuries involving the musculoskeletal system of children have received little attention (Fig. 6-1). Although such injuries represent only a small portion of all fractures and associated musculoskeletal injuries in children, they must be treated carefully and aggressively, as they are in the adult, to avoid devastating, possibly unnecessary, growth deformities and chronic diseases.[1-3] Childhood and adolescent injuries are increasingly being caused by more violent mechanisms, such as rotary lawn mowers, trail bikes, go-karts, and skateboards, as these devices become more common in the developing individual's milieu.[4] Figure 6-2 shows an injury sustained by a four-year-old child who fell under a tractor-type rotary lawn mower.

An open fracture involves a skeletal injury associated with a break in the skin, underlying subcutaneous tissue, and muscle, which usually leads to the fracture site and contiguous hematoma. While emphasis usually is placed on direct continuity between skeletal and cutaneous injuries, a fracture in the vicinity of any laceration should be treated as open, even if a definite communication cannot be established. Once the deforming, injurious force has been removed, the osseous fragments may snap back underneath muscle, so that the original communication is not always easy to find. Conversely, a laceration down to the periosteum, but not resulting in or associated with a fracture, should still be considered an open skeletal injury and treated as such. Such injuries frequently are encountered in children who catch their ankle in a spoked bicycle wheel, avulsing skin and subcutaneous tissue over a malleolus, and exposing the periosteum and perichondrium.

The specific consequence of open injury is the potential for direct inoculation with bacteria from either the skin or

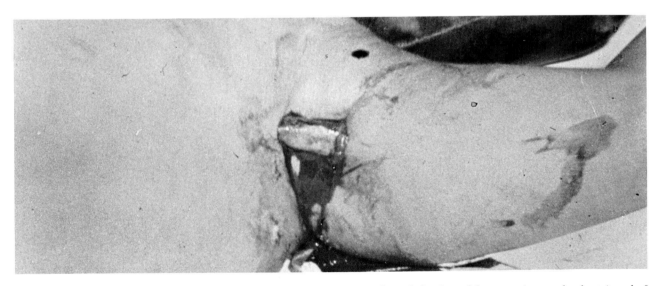

FIG. 6-1. Compound fracture of the left proximal humerus. The metaphyseal-diaphyseal fragment is completely stripped of its periosteum. The wound was treated with debridement, then left open after the fracture was reduced back within the periosteal sleeve. The wound closed secondarily over a period of two weeks while the girl was kept on parenteral antibiotics. No soft tissue or osseous infections developed.

the external environment. Traumatized tissue has a greater propensity for developing infection and may be infected by a much lower quantity of bacteria than would be required for a clinically significant infection to be established in otherwise normal tissue.[5-10]

The stripping of soft tissues that takes place to variable degrees consequent to the original injury renders both the soft tissues and the bone they cover more susceptible to active infection by creating dead spaces as well as potentially and actually less vascularized regions. The destruction or loss of soft tissue, especially the highly vascular and osteogenic periosteum that normally ensheaths developing bone, may affect the normal physiologic methods of bone repair.

For example, stripping of the periosteum, particularly in the child in whom it is of extreme osteogenic potential, may seriously impair the ability to unite the fracture rapidly and continue subsequent, normal, appositional bone growth in that portion of the metaphysis or diaphysis. These consequences vary with the extent of soft tissue damage. A major compounding injury may even indicate a need for immediate or delayed amputation, although this is highly unusual in children, and should be avoided.

The primary problem of any open fracture is associated soft tissue injury, because the degree to which this facet of the injury can be managed effectively ultimately determines the outcome of the bone or joint injury. When bone is not debrided and covered adequately, osteomyelitis or septic arthritis may be a sequela,[11-13] usually involving the diaphysis, which is less common than the metaphysis as a site of infection in children,[14-17] and also more difficult to treat because of the increased amounts of dense cortical bone in the diaphysis. Whether open or closed, soft tissue injury associated with a fracture necessitates adequate treatment of the soft tissue injury as well as the specific osseous problem.

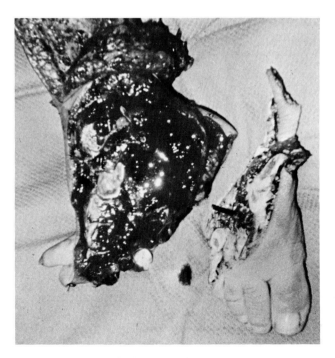

FIG. 6-2. Severe degloving and amputation in an eight-year-old girl who fell under a power lawn mower.

Wound examination

After the patient's general condition has been stabilized, the obviously injured extremity may be approached more deliberately. In evaluating the severity of any extremity with an open wound, one must note the state of the blood supply distal to the injury. It is also extremely important to assess the general condition of the skin about the actual wound. Is there an associated burn? Is it contaminated with dirt, clothing, or organic material? Are any fragments of foreign material superficially evident, implying that they may have been dragged deeper into the wound? What are the dimensions of the wound? Is the surrounding tissue abraded, contused, or flayed from its fascial bed? Is the bone protruding from the wound, or has it retracted into the ensheathing muscles? Manual exploration of the depth of the wound is contraindicated at this time, because these wounds should be treated in an operating room, where careful debridement and inspection are possible. Furthermore, there may be considerable clot formation within the wound, and manual exploration may renew venous or arterial bleeding that has spontaneously tamponaded.

Even a small wound, or one that does not seem to communicate with the underlying bone, should be adequately debrided if it goes down to the muscle area overlying a fracture. It is possible for the bone to penetrate the muscle, be involved in the laceration, then retract, leaving no obvious communication or grossly evident muscle damage. Furthermore, devitalized soft tissue can create a hazard to infection just as easily at the superficial surface as it can further down at the level of the bone, so it is still imperative to treat this as a potentially significant complication.

Use of antibiotics is discussed later, but assuming that they will be used, broad-spectrum coverage should be started at the time of initial evaluation, before the patient is taken to the operating room. However, it is essential that swabs for culture and sensitivity be taken from the wound in the emergency room *prior* to the administration of any antibiotics.

Debridement

The basic objective of the treatment of open wounds is the conversion of a contaminated wound to a clean, eventually closed wound. Debridement is undertaken to accomplish the removal of pieces of foreign material, necrotic tissue, and wound detritus. In a borderline case, particularly one in which a decision must be made about whether to proceed with an amputation of a severely traumatized limb, adequate debridement allows a more effective means of evaluating the overall extent of tissue damage and whether it might be feasible to salvage some or all of the extremity. As is discussed later in this chapter, techniques of amputation in children require different approaches to levels of amputation and handling of soft tissue injuries than similar injuries in skeletally mature adults (Fig. 6-3).

A constantly asked question is whether a small, minor wound, perhaps even an apparent puncture wound made outward from within by displaced, slightly protruding bone should be treated similarly to an obviously major compounding injury with a large laceration. *No wound is minor*

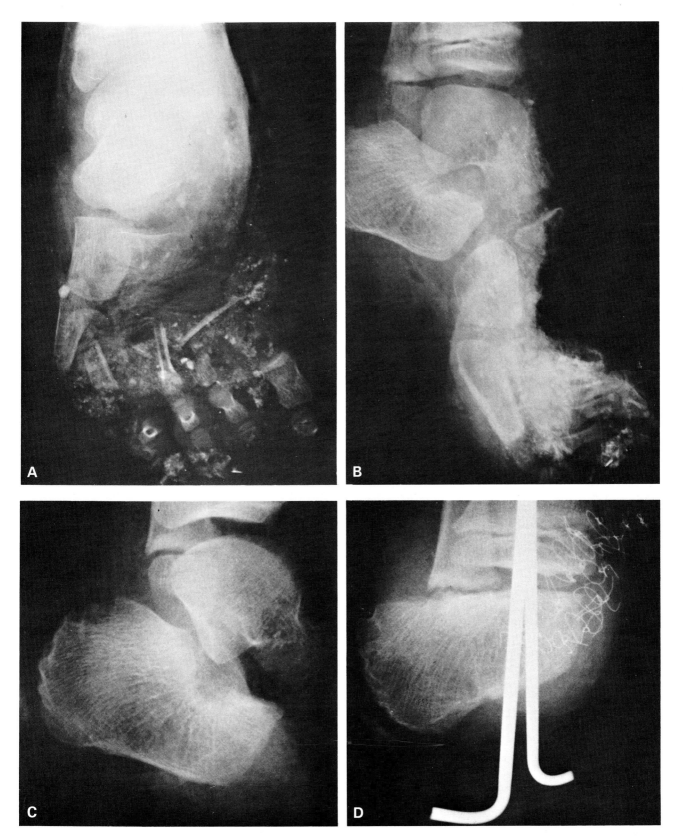

FIG. 6-3. *A-B,* Roentgenograms of the foot of a boy who fell under a power lawn mower. There are multiple metatarsal fractures and extensive debris in the soft tissue. *C,* Initial extensive debridement was carried back to the talus and calcaneus. *D,* Ten days later, after healing of the wounds without any evidence of infection, the talus was resected and the calcaneus fused to the distal tibial and fibular ossification centers (modified Syme).

when it is directly associated with a fracture. The presence of any wound makes the fracture a potentially open fracture because of the greater propensity to both hematogenous and direct spread of infection.

Any wound is enough of a break in the continuity of the skin to allow the introduction of bacteria that may cause extensive soft tissue infection in the subcutaneous region and proceed down to the muscle where more serious damage may eventually be caused. It may be argued that the conservative approach to such a wound is exploration and debridement, while the radical approach is to simply clean and dress the wound in the emergency room. The actual size of a wound often belies the maximum skin opening at the time of impact or injury. Since skin is quite distensible, the wound may have been four to five times its apparent size, but retracted quickly to a small size once the deforming force was removed.

The general objectives of debridement are: (1) the detection and removal of nonvital tissues; (2) the detection and removal of foreign materials, especially organic foreign material; (3) the reduction of bacterial contamination (it is becoming increasingly apparent that certain, quantitative amounts of bacteria are necessary to start clinical infections, and that microorganism populations lower than these levels usually can be adequately handled by the normal body defense mechanisms;[8] however, the amount of bacteria that devitalized musculoskeletal tissue can handle may be significantly different); and (4) the creation of a wound whose viable tissue surfaces help render it capable of coping with the residual bacterial contamination.

Incisions play an important role. Small puncture wounds may be elliptically excised and subsequently closed (however, this is *not* recommended except as a secondary procedure), or they may close spontaneously, leaving a relatively simple scar that may be revised later. It is always advisable to convert a puncture-type wound into an elliptical incision to make closure by normal means easier, rather than to simply trim the wound edges irregularly.

In planning incisions for debridement, one should consider: (1) the initial amount of skin and subcutaneous tissue loss; (2) the extent to which remaining, seemingly viable skin is separated from underlying subcutaneous or muscular regions; (3) the need to extend existing wounds for adequate inspection of deeper tissues, and the best direction in which to do so; (4) the usefulness of connecting adjacent, but separate, wounds; (5) the prospect for survival of flaps created by initial injury or planned, exploratory incision; (6) the amount of skin that may be sacrificed (if any) to effect the most appropriate subsequent closure; (7) the usefulness of counter-incisions to facilitate adequate debridement and arrange coverage of tissue or bone to provide adequate wound drainage; and (8) the likelihood that a planned incision will transect a major superficial venous drainage system and compromise distal tissue physiology.

Debridement should proceed layer by layer from the skin to the complete depths of the wound. Evident, deeper hemorrhage usually can be controlled by packing or a tourniquet, thus allowing an orderly, sequential approach. Damaged, contaminated subcutaneous tissue must be excised, but clean, intact tissue planes usually need not, and should not, be opened, since the supporting circulation of skin often is transmitted across such planes. Undermining subcutaneous tissue flaps as the wound is debrided is contraindicated.

Muscle

Muscle tends to respond differently than skin to direct trauma and may develop localized areas of nonvital tissue that are easily overlooked. This devitalized tissue offers an excellent culture medium for subsequent bacterial growth, especially infections caused by anaerobic and facultatively anaerobic microorganisms. If there has been significant damage to a major arterial supply of the severely damaged muscle, then it may be necessary to resect the entire muscle.

Several factors may be used to assess viability of muscle. Color may be misleading. What presents as dark tissue on the surface may be only a thin layer of blood beneath the epimysium. When the epimysium is incised and this seemingly necrotic tissue removed, the underlying muscle generally is found to be quite normal.

Consistency is a subjective qualification and basically relates to the firmness of the tissue. The less firm the tissue, the greater the probability of damage, and need for resection. Contractility most readily defines muscle viability. Muscle tissue that retracts from the incising edge of the scalpel is obviously alive and active.

The capacity to bleed must be qualified. The presence of an active arterial bleeder may simply mean that a conduit through the muscle has been transected. This conduit may be conveying blood to another area, and is not necessarily providing capillary perfusion to the area under treatment. Persistent bleeding from capillaries indicates the muscle is probably viable.

Scully[18] concluded that consistency and capacity to bleed were the most significant criteria for judging viability of the muscle, with color being the least useful indicator of potential viability.

Periosteum

When debriding in the region of the actual fracture, care must be taken not to remove any more periosteum than is absolutely necessary. This tissue is necessary to the ability of the diaphysis or metaphysis to heal the fracture, as well as to "regenerate" any cortical fragments that may have been missing. Loss of both bone and overlying periosteum may cause a permanent defect that subsequently may require use of bone graft. As shown in Chapters 2, 4, and 5, the periosteum is an extremely osteogenic tissue that not only has a dominant role in membranous, appositional bone formation along the shaft, but also significantly controls longitudinal growth by imparting tension to regions of the growth plate. Extensive dissection and removal of portions of the periosteum, particularly in a circumferential manner, may affect longitudinal growth as well.

Infection

Role of antibiotics

One of the most important aspects of an open fracture is whether to treat it prophylactically with a broad-spectrum antibiotic.[19] Patzakis[20] reviewed 310 patients with open fractures, many of whom were children. These patients were divided into three groups: those receiving penicillin and streptomycin, cephalothin, or no antibiotics. The incidence of infection was 14% in the untreated group, while in the group receiving a combination of penicillin and streptomycin it was 10%. This difference is statistically insignificant.

However, the group receiving cephalothin did have a significantly lower infection rate of 2%. This data would seem to substantiate the value of prophylactic antibiotic administration. The incidence of staphylococcal infection was high, and many, though not all, of the presently used cephalosporins have some degree of efficacy against staphylococcus, particularly when used prophylactically. However, once a staphylococcal infection is clinically established, the most effective antibiotics are undoubtedly cloxacillin and dicloxacillin.

The fact that several days of bacteriologic culturing must elapse before a wound can be considered sterile should support the use of a regimen of antibiotic prophylaxis that may be applied to all skeletally immature patients with open fractures, then discontinued when and if cultures are truly negative, or if the microorganism is more sensitive to a different antibiotic.

Clinical and experimental studies have shown that early administration of either a bacteriocidal or a bacteriostatic antibiotic prolonged the period between initial wounding and the development of localized infection, and decreased the incidence of systemic toxicity, bacteremia, and death, provided that the wounds were primarily contaminated with bacteria sensitive in vitro to the specific antibiotic administered.[21-25] The early administration of antibiotic exerted little, if any, beneficial effect if the wounds were contaminated with bacteria insensitive to the antibiotic. Burke[26] showed that the optimum period for effective administration

of prophylactic antibiotics in contaminated wounds was approximately three hours after wounding. The ability of different antibiotics to penetrate normal and damaged chondro-osseous tissue and joints varies significantly.[27-31]

Adequate debridement enhances neovascularity, even within bone, and thereby increases perfusion of blood and antibiotics. *The use of antibiotics should not be misconstrued as a substitute for the extremely important principle of adequate surgical debridement.*

Osteomyelitis

Compared to adults, direct osseous infection occurs infrequently in children, probably because of the lower overall incidence of open wounds. However, since children get osteomyelitis most commonly by the hematogenous route (Fig. 6-4), such spread in children with localized trauma from a source of infection elsewhere must be considered.[32-35]

Direct inoculation with bacteria may cause osteomyelitis at the fracture site. Adequate debridement, as discussed earlier, is essential to the prevention of such infection. Leaving the wound open to allow continued drainage and observation certainly will lessen the risk of an undiagnosed infection. Many open injuries occur on the street, in playgrounds, and in other areas where the risk of bacteria other than staphylococcus (the most common cause of hematogenous osteomyelitis) may be present. In such cases, broad-spectrum antibiotic prophylaxis is essential. Left untreated or inadequately treated, a severe osteomyelitis may supervene, with loss of cortical bone, destruction of periosteum, sequestration, and chronic disease.

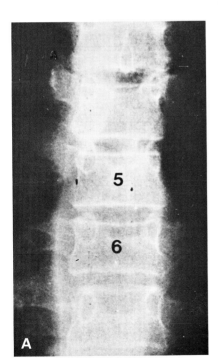 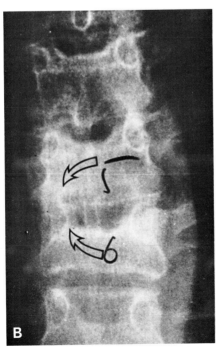 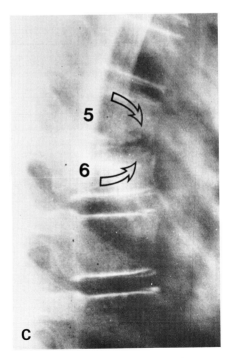

FIG. 6-4. Girl, 14 years old, who fell backwards and struck her midback against a bus bumper. *A*, Two weeks after the accident, because of recurrent pain, this roentgenogram, which appears normal, was obtained. *B-C*, Two months later pain persisted. Repeat roentgenography showed lytic collapse of T4 and T5. A decompressive costotransversectomy revealed osteomyelitis due to anaerobic microorganisms.

Hematogenous osteomyelitis secondary to soft tissue injury has been reported as a rare complication.[36-40] In a study by Waldvogel,[10] one third of the cases of osteomyelitis had an association between the infection and a seemingly trivial, blunt trauma, though not necessarily a fracture. Farr[33] found no evidence of related trauma in 98 cases of hematogenous osteomyelitis.

Canale described three children with post-traumatic osteomyelitis.[32] One had a wrist fracture and epiphyseal injury that subsequently went on to sequestration of a considerable portion of the metaphysis and diaphysis, but without any major evidence of growth deformity. The child, however, had not completed skeletal growth, and a future deformity could not be totally ruled out. The other two were femoral fractures. The first developed osteomyelitis seven weeks after the skeletal injury, following onset of acute tonsillitis. The other had a documented urinary tract infection with pyelonephritis and developed his infection ten days after the injury. In both, the microorganism causing the primary infection also caused the secondary, distant osteomyelitis at the fracture site.

A delay in recognizing the acute, complicating osteomyelitis was the rule in these three patients, and it was not until fluctuance developed that infection of the fracture site was seriously considered as the cause of toxicity. Several clues should have been noted. First, after the initial pain and swelling had subsided, pain of a different character became a complaint, and this pain was constant, progressive, and unrelieved by immobilization. A definite decrease in the local signs of the skeletal injury should have been present. All the patients had an obvious primary focus of infection and exhibited a persistent febrile course much out of proportion to that seen with an uncomplicated fracture or with an uncomplicated urinary or respiratory infection.

If hematogenous osteomyelitis complicates a fracture, particularly in a child, open debridement and evacuation of the infected area is indicated. At the time of initial injury, a dead space is created that is filled with hematoma, and this may be transformed rapidly into a cavity filled with purulent material. Many of the enzymes released by bacteria, as well as the reactive granulocytes, may be extremely destructive to developing chondro-osseous tissue.[41] Penetration of an abscess by systemic antibiotics invariably will be slow, if achieved at all.[31] There also is a variable amount of devitalized bone that may sequestrate. Drainage should be through a reasonable incision with adequate irrigation and debridement, and the wound must be left open.

Few papers are directed toward the specific problem of extensive open fractures in children. Anderson and Argammaso[11] approached the problem in adolescents by using percutaneous, transosseous pin fixation stabilization, skin grafts, and debridement to treat fractures with complicating, post-traumatic osteomyelitis, as well as fractures that were difficult to close by routine methods. For many years, surgeons have suggested that large compound defects of the lower extremity should be covered with pedicle flaps, yet most have advised against using these flaps, especially cross-leg flaps, in children. It has been felt that children could not adjust to the temporary postural restrictions that are necessary for the success of such pedicle flaps.

However, children adapt amazingly well, and pedicle flaps can be used (Fig. 6-5). The main indication for pedicle flaps, even in children, is that they provide a better-padded cover-age to bone and tendon than the split thickness skin graft does, and are more resistant to infection.[42] Further, an abundant blood supply, which is potentially beneficial to fracture healing, is brought into the affected, devitalized area. Newer techniques of microvascular anastomosis also raise the possibility of using free grafts based on arterial distribution patterns (e.g., groin flap).

Late infection

Late appearing osteomyelitis also may complicate fractures in children.[43-47] Usually, these cases are due to low-virulence microorganisms. Figure 6-6 shows a boy who sustained an open distal radial fracture that was successfully treated with no evidence of infection. However, several years later he presented with a swollen, tender forearm and biopsy-proven osteomyelitis (Serratia marcescens). It is likely that he had harbored the infection from the time of the initial injury. Such delay is not uncommon in osteomyelitis caused by Serratia.[45]

Figure 6-7 shows a similar problem. This boy cut himself in the thumb web space. Purulent drainage persisted for several days, but the boy never was treated with antibiotics. Three years later, because of a fall on the wrist, a roentgenogram was taken. During the subsequent operation, a membranous cavity was found, and cultures grew Staphylococcus aureus. This boy had been asymptomatic for almost three years and symbiotic with a microorganism that is normally extremely virulent when invading the developing skeleton.

Puncture wounds and osteomyelitis

Brand and Black[48] demonstrated that seemingly innocuous puncture wounds may lead to osteomyelitis. Further, infection with nonstaphylococcal microorganisms, especially Pseudomonas, are more prevalent. This particular problem is discussed in detail in Chapter 20.

Joint involvement

Open joint injuries accompanying musculoskeletal trauma are relatively infrequent in children. However, if intra-articular involvement is not recognized, or inadequately treated, serious damage to the articular surfaces, loss of normal joint function, fibrous ankylosis, or septic arthritis may occur. Since articular cartilage may have some regenerative capacity in a child, appropriate debridement and joint lavage may allow full restoration of the articular surface.

Many of the open injuries occurring in children are to the joints of the lower extremity, with the knee being the most commonly involved major joint. Power lawn mowers are a common cause, and may introduce significant amounts of foreign material into the joint. More frequently, the child falls on a sharp object (see Fig. 3-6). Many times the only objective evidence of injury is air or air-fluid levels within the joint. A less common cause is inflicted trauma, as in a stab wound of the knee (Fig. 6-8). When a sharp object penetrates a joint, the articular surface may be damaged directly. Adequate inspection of the joint surface and removal of the foreign body to prevent further damage are two major indications for immediate arthrotomy. In the event of accompanying type 3, 4, or 7 fractures, arthrotomy also allows anatomic reduction of the fracture.

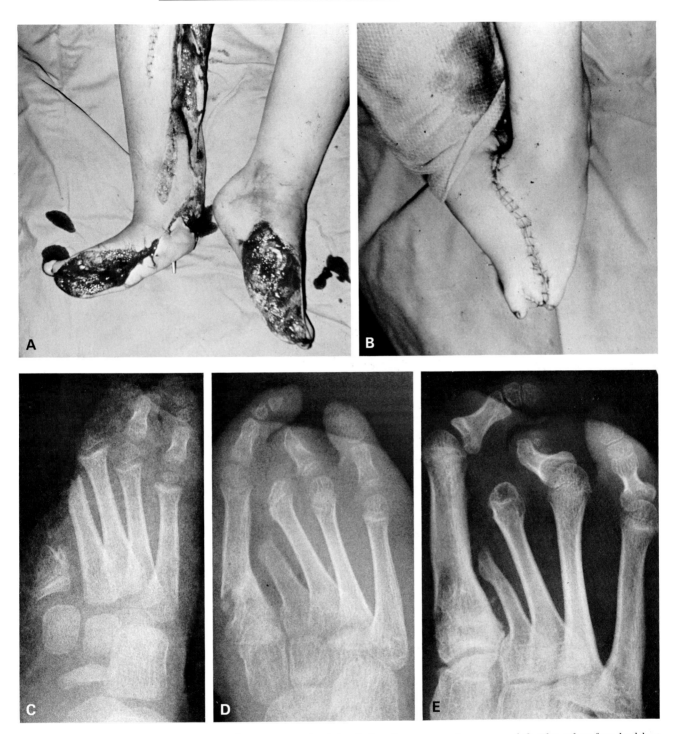

FIG. 6-5.   *A,* Following debridement, only one toe and minimal chondro-osseous tissue were left. The other foot had lost several toes. *B,* A cross foot pedicle flap procedure transferred the remaining metatarsal-phalangeal unit. *C,* Roentgenogram of remaining foot (left) after debridement. *D,* Three months after graft. *E,* Seven years later, at skeletal maturation.

However, the most important reason for arthrotomy is the prevention of subsequent septic arthritis. Curtis[28] has demonstrated experimentally that articular infection with various types of microorganisms, especially staphylococci, causes enzymatic destruction of the joint cartilage. The joint must be approached with an incision that includes the pene-tration wound, the margins of which should be adequately debrided. The joint should be irrigated profusely with saline and/or antibiotic solutions, and drains left in place. The surgeon should not hesitate to repeat this procedure two or three days later. An alternative is continuous lavage for two to three days, although this technique is not easy and should be used only if the support services, such as nursing, are familiar with it. Figure 6-8 illustrates the sequential osseous changes in a young boy stabbed in the knee.

Clostridia

Clostridial infections (such as gas gangrene) or similar infections due to other facultatively or completely anaerobic bacteria easily can become significant, even in the more superficial tissue planes. Clostridial infections frequently are dismissed as insignificant problems in civilian populations. However, Brown[49] described the occurrence of this type of infection in a major urban community. Figures 6-9 and 6-10 demonstrate classic forms of clostridial infection following trauma to an extremity (open injuries). In fact, it is possible for children to develop rare types of clostridial infection without an open wound injury,[50] inasmuch as they are more susceptible to hematogenous osteomyelitis (Fig. 6-11).

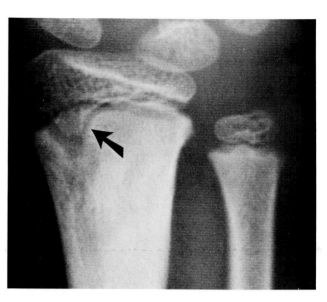

FIG. 6-7. Osteomyelitis of distal radial metaphysis. This probably occurred three years before, following an infected hand injury. The growth plate has been damaged, leading to retarded longitudinal growth (arrow). This proved to be chronic, minimally suppurative osteomyelitis, even though caused by coagulase-positive Staphylococcus.

Gas gangrene

Fractures of both bones of the forearm are frequently compounded by small lacerations or puncture wounds, particularly on the palmar aspect of the extremity. Severe clostridial infection and myonecrosis, while decreasingly common, may complicate these injuries.[49,51-53] Fee[54] described five cases, four of which were in children. Three of these cases, all caused by Clostridium perfringens, eventually required amputation, two at the elbow and one at the junction of the proximal and middle thirds of the humerus. This apparently was because of the particular demarcation. In one case, subperiosteal resection of large portions of the diaphysis of each bone was necessary. The ulna completely regenerated, and the radius later required an en bloc bone graft. Such regeneration may occur as long as reasonable longitudinal and circumferential amounts of the periosteum remain intact.

Common to these injuries is protrusion of the proximal fragment through the skin and into soil contaminated by clostridial microorganisms. The wounds may be relatively small and deceptively innocuous in appearance. These cases point out the need for aggressive initial management, with adequate debridement of the skin and underlying tissues. Under no circumstances should the wound be closed. Debridement is best performed in the operating room where an adequate amount of irrigation and complete exploration may be accomplished.

The symptoms of these infections evolve insidiously, and the serious nature of the complication usually is not noted until two to three days after the injury. Once it begins, the course of the disease is rapid. The earliest symptom is usually pain in the affected area, followed by chills, tachycardia, confusion, and other evidence of toxemia. In the early

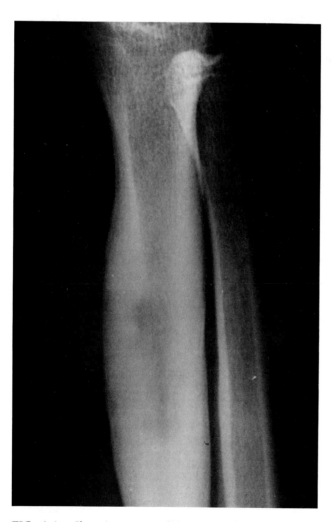

FIG. 6-6. Chronic osteomyelitis at site of an open distal radial (metaphyseal) fracture that was sustained several years before this roentgenogram. The distal radius and ulna have grown normally, but the chronic osteomyelitis has caused diaphyseal widening and sclerosis. Serratia marcescens was cultured from the marrow cavity.

stages, the skin around the wound is cool and quite edematous, but it is seldom crepitant. Later, it becomes brawny, discolored and crepitant, with exudation of a serous, brown fluid from the wound. The gram stain of the fluid usually will show the gram positive rods, confirming the diagnosis.

While local cleansing of a wound is advocated for pinhole openings, consideration must be given to a more aggressive form of treatment when soil contamination is suspected. Any injury occurring outdoors may be contaminated by soil microorganisms, so treatment should include an exploratory extension of the wound sufficient to provide adequate visualization of the bone ends to ensure that all foreign material has been removed. Meticulous debridement and thorough irrigation should be part of the procedure, and the wound should never be closed primarily. Removal of damaged and necrotic tissue is essential to lessen the local environment the bacteria have in which to grow.[9]

Once the diagnosis is suspected, treatment must be instituted immediately to avoid serious complications. The most important aspects of treatment consist of immediately opening the wound and adequately debriding it, even if debridement was part of the initial treatment. Decompression must be wide and extensive in order to get all areas that might be involved. Usually the degree of involvement is much greater than is first apparent. All involved muscle must be excised. Early surgical treatment may avert the need for amputation. General supportive measures also are essential.

Prophylaxis with antibiotics is of proven value in gas gangrene.[40] The role of antibiotics in well-established cases is to prevent recrudescence of the clostridial infection in traumatized tissue and to prevent secondary infection with other opportunistic microorganisms. Penicillin has demonstrated superiority in both prophylaxis and treatment of gas gangrene microorganisms. Certainly, any compound wound already should have been placed on an appropriate antibiotic, but the addition of penicillin in high doses may prevent the progression of gas gangrene.

The use of passive immunization with polyvalent gas gangrene serum for prophylaxis and treatment of gas gangrene is controversial, with some people believing that there is considerable evidence that the serum is useful in both the prevention and the treatment of gas gangrene, and that it should be used in all cases. However, most people feel that the value of the serum is uncertain, that it subjects the patient to the risk of a sensitivity reaction, and that it should not be in general use. In the series reported by Fee,[55] it was used in all cases without any side effects, but no beneficial effects on the disease process were evident.

The use of hyperbaric oxygenation, introduced by Brummelkamp[56,57] allows oxygen to gain access to anaerobic areas and has been shown, experimentally, to decrease the effect of clostridial endotoxins, as well as to affect the metabolic activity and release of further toxins.[13,40,58,59] Hyperbaric oxygen therapy leads to a higher concentration of dissolved oxygen, and allows increased diffusion of oxygen through the tissues. Most authors recommend a pressure of three times atmospheric pressure for an optimum effect. The arterial oxygen tension should be in the range of 1200 to 1700 mm Hg, with an exposure period of 60 to 90 minutes. The treatment should be repeated for 3 to 5 minutes every 8 to 12 hours. However, aggressive early debridement may obviate the need for hyperbaric oxygenation, which should

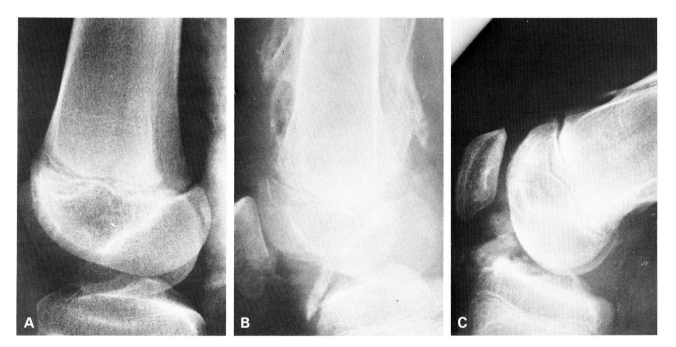

FIG. 6-8. *A*, Roentgenogram of boy stabbed in knee, with penetration to the articular surface. The injury occurred 3 days previous to this roentgenogram, but the boy sought medical help only when the knee became hot and swollen. A pyarthrosis was drained, and the joint irrigated profusely several times over the next 10 days. *B*, Extensive reactive bone developed along the femur and within the joint. *C*, Six months later the osseous reaction was resolving and motion was returning to the knee. The knee functioned normally 18 months after the injury.

be reserved for the more critical cases not well controlled by other means.

Clostridial cellulitis

A less common and less severe clostridial infection is that of anaerobic cellulitis (see Fig. 6-10). This usually occurs several days after an injury, in an inadequately debrided wound. The onset is more gradual and toxemia may be slight. It is easy to confuse with gas gangrene because of the foul smelling and abundant formation of gas, as well as the comparable brown and seropurulent exudate. Treatment should consist of adequate debridement and antibiotics.

Tetanus

This is an extremely rare complication in our urban, immunized society. It is to be feared in seemingly innocuous wounds, such as puncture wounds of the feet. The organism produces both tetanospasmin, a neurotoxin, and tetanolysin, a cardiotoxin.[58] These are exotoxins that have severe affects on human tissue, causing massive muscle spasm. It is important to treat this disease prophylactically, since antitoxin is unable to neutralize the toxin once it is tissue-bound in the nervous system. Most children in this country have been actively immunized and merely need a booster. The patient who has not, or may not have, been put through this type of normal prophylaxis should be treated with high doses of penicillin and streptomycin as well as tetanus immunoglobulin (250 to 500 U).

If tetanic spasm develops, anesthesia, muscle relaxants, respiratory assistance, and tracheostomy should be part of the treatment.[60,61] Excessive spasticity during treatment may cause vertebral compression fractures; extremity fractures are much less likely. Myositis ossificans and extension of ossification along tendons are significant complications.[62]

Atypical clostridial infections

It is becoming increasingly evident that many other types of clostridia may be part of the normal anaerobic flora of the human colon.[13,40] Following blunt trauma to various portions of an extremity, local tissue damage may create sufficient anaerobiasis to allow establishment of an infection by the hematogenous route. Figure 6-11 shows a case of a C. sphenoides osteomyelitis following a fall and direct blow to the lateral thigh. The laminated subperiosteal layering in this and other cases may lead to an erroneous diagnosis of a primary bone malignancy such as Ewing's sarcoma.[13]

Botulism

Botulism may be caused in open wounds infected by C. botulinum.[55,63,64] The microorganisms may cause a variable wound infection, and release a neurotoxin. The neural symptoms include a descending, progressive, symmetrical cranial-nerve paralysis with motor weakness, but no changes in sensory or mental status. Botulin affects cholinergic nerve endings, blocking the release of acetylcholine and producing pharmacologic denervation.[64,65] Symptoms may not begin for 4 to 14 days following injury.

Treatment should include extensive debridement and supportive care, especially adequate ventilatory support. Death in this disease usually results from respiratory failure. Neural symptoms usually resolve in time. High dose parenteral penicillin is essential. The effectiveness of botulinum antitoxin is not clear. Trivalent antitoxin effective against type A, B, and E toxins usually is given.

Crushing and Avulsion Injuries

These injuries are among the most unpredictable and difficult to manage of all musculoskeletal trauma. The skin wound initially may appear quite innocuous. But in the ensuing 24 to 48 hours, demarcation and skin slough may involve areas that looked viable. Furthermore, tissue necrosis may extend progressively to the underlying skeletal components, especially to those that are superficial (e.g., the malleoli). Common to all the wounds discussed in this section is a combined injury mechanism of crushing and avulsion. As the extremity is rolled over by the deforming object, whether bicycle spokes, washing machine wringer, or automobile tire, tissue may be subjected to shearing, compression, burning, and bursting forces. Primary wound healing without supervening infection is the goal of treatment. Adequate debridement and skin grafting, as necessary, usually will suffice. More extensive reconstruction and pedicle grafts may be utilized on an elective basis.

The simplest type of injury, and one likely if the child catches a leg in bicycle spokes, is a crush-burn. This results from a shearing, abrading mechanism, may be patchy in distribution, and linear in orientation, with streaks of dermal injury and more diffuse surrounding changes similar to a second degree burn. These wounds must be treated as burns, with daily observation for localized, deeper, tissue necrosis. The wound should be washed with sterile fluid and dressed

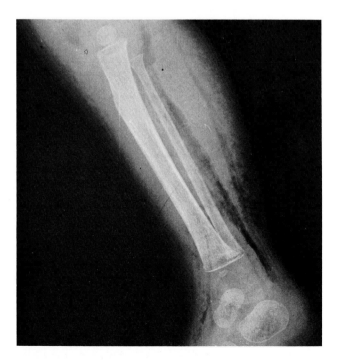

FIG. 6-9. Gas gangrene in a young child following a deep laceration.

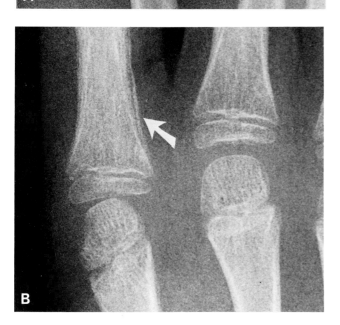
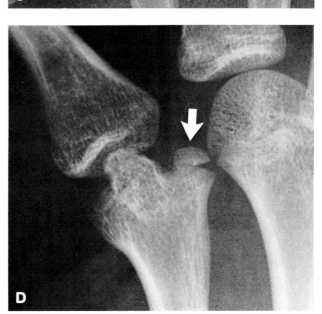

FIG. 6-10. *A*, Compound dislocation of the index metacarpophalangeal joint. This was "debrided" in an emergency room and closed primarily (i.e., the dislocation was not reduced). The next day, presenting symptoms were a fever of 105° and a frothy fluid exuding from the wound. The child developed clostridial cellulitis which responded to extensive debridement. The dislocation also was reduced. *B*, A few weeks later, some reactive bone is still evident along the metacarpal (arrow), and the metacarpal metaphysis and epiphysis are developing some lucent areas. *C*, A few months later, the physis appears to have closed, and the epiphyseal ossification center is damaged. *D*, When the patient appeared for follow-up examination four years later, he had 60° of motion, and an unusual attempt had been made to reform the ossification center (arrow).

with mafenide acetate cream (Sulfamylon), silver sulfadiazine cream (Silvadene), and fine mesh gauze, with daily dressing changes under sterile conditions. Within 7 to 10 days, the wound should be re-epithelializing, unless there is a deeper injury. If foreign material (e.g., macadam from a driveway surface) has been abraded into the initial wound, it may become permanently embedded in the dermis, resulting in a traumatic tattoo after the wound heals and re-epithelializes. Rigorous scrubbing during the initial treatment often will completely prevent this complication.

When more trauma is involved, tissue loss may be more extensive. A common pattern is a central zone of maximum destruction (which may take several days to demarcate) and a larger, peripheral zone of less severe injury. These central injuries are analogous to third degree burns and should be treated accordingly, with excision of the severely involved tissue, daily dressing with sulfadiazine, and subsequent secondary closure or a split-thickness skin graft when the condition of the wound permits.

Frictional abrasion of the soft tissue may extend down to

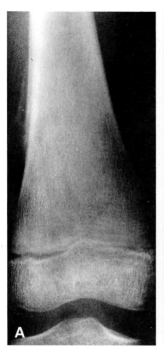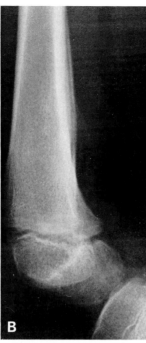

FIG. 6-11. *A*, AP, and *B*, lateral, roentgenograms of an eight-year-old boy who had struck the side of the femur three weeks before. The laminated appearance suggests Ewing's sarcoma as one diagnostic possibility. An open biopsy was done. A small amount of fluid grew Clostridium sphenoides, and the boy was treated only with oral penicillin.

fascia, periosteum, and perichondrium, especially at the ankle, where the malleoli are readily exposed to injury. Disruption of normal peripheral chondro-osseous development (type 6 injury) may occur with no roentgenographic evidence of physeal injury. Long term follow-up is necessary to rule out subsequent osseous bridge formation. Damage extending to and involving the peroneal tendons and sheaths also may occur. Adequate coverage by fascial-fat flaps is necessary if either chondro-osseous or tendinous elements are exposed. If tissue conditions do not permit flap rotation, free split-thickness skin grafts are accepted well, especially by children, and they have a great survival capacity, even when placed on perichondrium or periosteum, both of which are more vascular in children than in adults.

Avulsion of soft tissue flaps may occur without a major crushing component, since tissue response to shearing force is failure through the subcutaneous/fascial interface. Most flaps are viable structures. Potential for flap survival is dictated by several factors: (1) general vascular supply to the injured area, and specific supply to the flap (i.e., is there an arterial supply that will maintain perfusion, and sufficient venous outflow so as not to impede capillary dynamics); (2) whether the flap is proximally or distally based; (3) dimensions of the flap (length-to-base ratio); (4) depth of the cleavage-separation planes; (5) condition of the skin edges; and (6) extent of crush-contusion of the flap before cleavage failure.

If chances are good that the flap will survive, it should be debrided, irrigated, replaced, and sutured primarily, unless there is significant chondro-osseous injury. In the latter case, loose approximation of the flap edges to prevent contracture will allow observation for infection and subsequent secondary closure. Occasionally, flaps that seem to satisfy all criteria for viability will become necrotic over the ensuing days. This usually is due to microscopic crush injury that is not grossly evident in the acute stage. Such a flap can be excised and replaced with a split-thickness skin graft. Larger areas of avulsion, or exposure of significant neurovascular structures, often are better treated by local or distal pedicle flaps.[67] Complex avulsions, such as degloving, are beyond the scope of this book. Appropriate consultation with a plastic surgeon is beneficial in such injuries.

Wringer injuries

While becoming less frequent, these complex injuries still occur occasionally. These injuries damage the soft tissue extensively, but rarely cause fractures. However, they are extensive, often comminuted, and frequently difficult to manage. Larger roller devices (presses, etc.) increase the extent of soft tissue and chondro-osseous injury. Occasionally, amputation may occur.[68-71]

Osseous injuries tend to involve the more distal regions, especially the distal radius and ulna. Because of the direct crushing mechanism, greenstick fractures are more common. Furthermore, the periosteal tube is usually intact, and may act as an internal splint. The thumb may follow the rest of the hand through the rollers in an abducted, hyperextended position, leading to separation of the first interosseous web space, and the possibility of significant soft tissue injury. The metacarpophalangeal joint may be disrupted acutely, but spontaneously reduced on removal from the wringer. An epiphyseal Bennett's fracture also may occur (Fig. 6-12).

Akbarnia and Campbell[72] reported a case of wringer injury in a 29-month-old child on whom a 24-year follow-up study was done. Initially, there was extensive loss of the diaphysis and periosteum of both the radius and the ulna, thus limiting the capacity to otherwise restore the diaphyseal shaft. The child was subjected to repeated on-lay grafts to fill in the defects and the restoration of function to the radius and ulna was rather dramatic. The circulatory disturbances were felt to be a major factor in the shortening of the bone by disturbing distal radioulnar physeal growth.

Maximum damage to the soft tissues generally is sustained in the forearm and antecubital fossa, although, if the elbow is extended and allows the arm to go further, maximum trauma may occur in the axilla. The extent of injury may be increased if countertraction is applied to the extremity by reversing the direction of the limb or increasing the tension of the rollers or the rapidity of revolution.

Various degrees of superficial abrasion/burning occur, as well as an equally variable, and often changing, amount of deep shearing and muscular damage. Both these types of injuries may initially look benign. The skin should be treated as a burn; dressed (with a well-padded compression dressing), and elevated accordingly. If an extensive hematoma develops, it may be evacuated by proximal and distal fascial incisions. If there is an increase in compartment pressures, which can be measured with wick-catheter techniques, partial or complete fasciotomy also may be indicated.

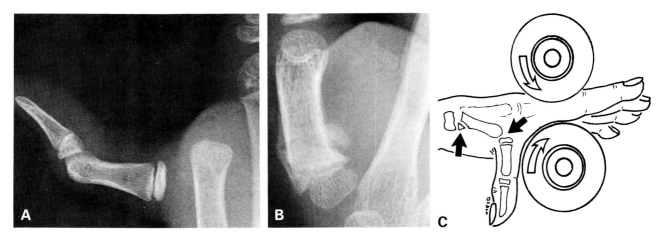

FIG. 6-12. *A*, Dislocation of thumb metacarpophalangeal joint. *B*, Bennett's epiphyseal fracture of metacarpal. Both injuries occurred when the hand was pulled through rollers, probably by the mechanism schematized in *C*.

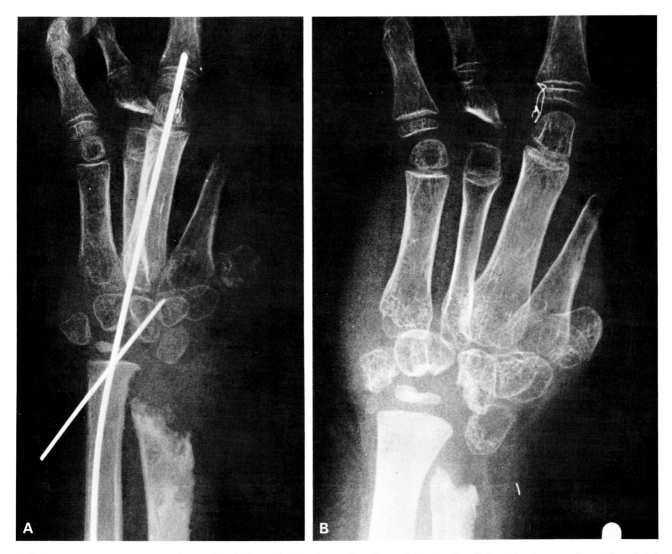

FIG. 6-13. *A*, Lawn mower injury of a child resulted in immediate loss of the distal radial epiphysis, as well as other distal injuries. After soft tissue wound care, the hand was centralized on the ulna. *B*, A year later, the ulna has grown and widened considerably to compensate for the radial loss.

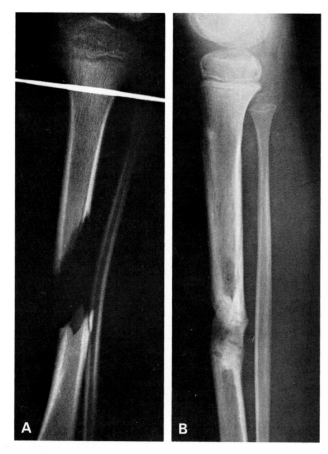

FIG. 6-14. *A*, Total loss of a segment of diaphysis in a child with compound tibial wound. The fibula was intact. The wound was debrided. The periosteum was extensively damaged. The tibial fragments were kept apart by external fixation pins placed away from the grossly injured tissues. *B*, When soft tissue conditions were deemed satisfactory, a graft was inserted in the defect.

One of the most significant problems is edema and venous congestion resulting from disruption of normal superficial venous and lymphatic drainage patterns. A pedicle flap may be of benefit in allaying this increased tissue perfusion pressure, which may lead to additional tissue infarction. The efficacy of sympathetic blocking agents, anticoagulants, and antisludging parenteral therapy (e.g., dextran 40 [Rheomacrodex]) is unclear.

Bone Loss

Complete extrusion of developing skeletal elements from an open wound is extremely unusual in childhood injuries, primarily because comminution of the fracture is infrequent. However, those cases in which significant bone loss occurs present major problems in management.[73,96] Most are associated with violent injury, especially power lawn mower or farm machinery accidents. As such, extensive, soft tissue injury is usually concomitant. Primary management must be directed at adequate debridement of devitalized tissue with

an attempt to save as much of the periosteal and skeletal components as possible.

Debridement should be repeated as indicated, until the tissue components, both soft and skeletal, are unquestionably viable and there is no further risk of infection. Foreign material is often embedded in tissue interstices, and must be completely removed. All wounds should be left widely open, and *never* closed primarily. Cultures should be taken initially to assess contaminants. Quantitative bacteriology allows an effective means of following the potential for subsequent infection and may be used to assess optimum timing for wound closure and reconstruction of the skeleton.

Replacement of devitalized, contaminated chondro-osseous fragments is usually contraindicated (Fig. 6-13). If a segment of bone has been extruded (Fig. 6-14), the remaining skeletal elements need to be stabilized. An intact fibula renders some intrinsic stability, and may be augmented by an external fixation device with the skeletal fixation pins placed in normal tissue above and below the injured area. This allows daily wound care without jeopardizing overall stability. Metallic stabilization should not be placed within the actual area of acute injury (Fig. 6-15), as the presence of a foreign body increases the risk of infection.

If segments of the periosteal tube can be salvaged, every attempt should be made to do so. As shown in Chapter 2, the periosteum is extremely osteogenic and capable of considerable new bone formation (see Fig. 2-2). However, damage to this structure, a type 9 injury, may necessitate placement of bone graft (see Fig. 6-14), which should not be attempted until there is absolutely no evidence of infection and the wound is well granulated. Quantitative bacteriology again is helpful in timing grafting. If the remaining skeleton has been stabilized, several weeks can elapse before grafting. If possible, the graft should be placed by a separate incision through nontraumatized tissue.

When soft tissue and osseous damage have been extensive, external fixation and primary wound management allow time to devise a more appropriate long term scheme of treatment. In the case shown in Figure 6-15, a possible scheme would have been initial control of the soft tissue injury and infection, subsequent shortening by grafting the remaining tibial ends together to create an intact longitudinal unit, and a Syme ankle disarticulation. This would have created a "below-knee" lever arm capable of some longitudinal growth without diaphyseal stump overgrowth. Unfortunately, the wound was closed primarily, became infected, and required diaphyseal amputation, with subsequent stump overgrowth. Methods of treating this particular complication are discussed in the following section on amputations.

Amputation

Since traumatic amputation during childhood has received minimal attention, management guidelines for confronting these problems are difficult to find; and yet, the extent to which optimal function may be provided, both initially and in the long term until skeletal maturity is attained, frequently is determined by appropriate or inappropriate initial management. The major factors to consider must be infection, vascular status, and the effect the amputation will have on anticipated skeletal growth and development.

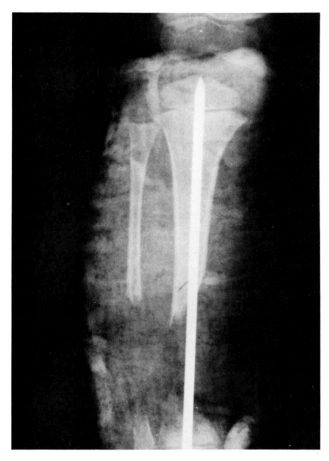

FIG. 6-15. Extensive osseous loss treated initially with intramedullary rod. Soft tissue complications necessitated amputation. More aggressive soft tissue care, and use of external fixation devices might have allowed further tissue to be saved, and perhaps even have allowed bone grafting.

Trauma is not a frequent cause of childhood amputation.[70,71,74-76] Only 17% of patients (21 out of 120) under active treatment at the Newington Children's Hospital Juvenile Amputee Clinic sustained traumatic amputations.[76] Spring and Epps[70] described 19 traumatic amputations out of 39 acquired amputations. The mechanisms of injury included thermal and electrical burns, washing machine wringer injury, automobile accidents, shotgun injury, and power mower and farm machinery accidents.

Unfortunately, relative to other forms of amputation, children with traumatic amputations have an extremely high incidence of infections, wound healing complications, and chronic prosthetic problems. In the severely traumatized and contaminated wound, avoidance of further infection and increased vascular compromise are essential. Constructive, long term planning and particular consideration of the effects of growth, and optimal stump condition throughout growth may dictate the need for considerable staging in the management of the child's amputation. Most problems encountered in the management of traumatic childhood amputation may be attributed to complications in the primary management, which have precluded construction of an optimal amputation stump.

The most common patterns of trauma leading to amputation are those in which the limb is crushed or partially or totally avulsed. Often, both mechanisms occur concomitantly. In some cases, major arterial injury may occur in the presence of less severe musculoskeletal trauma, endangering the part of the limb distal to the actual injury. Causes other than direct musculoskeletal trauma that may eventuate in childhood amputation include burns, gas gangrene, meningococcal septicemia, and electrical injury.

If the traumatic amputation is complete, but the amputated part is available, one should consider the possibilities of limb reimplantation. Most hospitals are not equipped to undertake such an extensive procedure. If possible, the child should be referred to a reimplantation unit where a multidisciplinary team is available to attempt such a procedure. Reimplantation is discussed in more detail in a subsequent section. If the amputation is incomplete, surgical care of the residual tissue is the major problem, with control of the vascular pedicle being a primary consideration.

Every effort should be made to save a limb, even if it means delaying eventual amputation. However, one of the most difficult problems is that of a delayed amputation in which the surgeon finds he is tempted to retain a limb that will only serve as an eventual burden to the child. This problem occurs not only in cases of traumatic injury, but also with many types of congenital deformities in children for whom function with a prosthesis is infinitely superior to that of a braced, deformed extremity.[77]

Principles of amputation for children differ from those for adults in three major respects: (1) preservation of functional epiphyseal/physeal units must assume a major priority, particularly when the distal femoral epiphysis is involved. An above-knee stump in a baby eventually becomes an extremely high thigh amputation in the adult, since 70% of the growth of the femur is eventually contributed by the distal femoral physis. Similarly, an ankle disarticulation with preservation of the lower tibial epiphysis leads to a much better stump than a short below-knee amputation. (2) The excellent healing potential of the young child makes possible the use of flaps that might be precarious in an adult.[42,67,78] Skin grafts may be very useful; it is sometimes possible to preserve a knee joint with a below-knee stump covered by a split-thickness skin graft, which, with continued growth, suitable modification, and eventual conversion to a knee disarticulation, will withstand the use of a prosthetic. (3) Stump overgrowth is the major problem with amputations in the child. In children, disarticulation through the joint will always be preferable to more proximal metaphyseal or diaphyseal amputation.

In dealing with a child's traumatic amputation, a great deal of constructive planning is required to salvage the best possible initial and long term functions. Planning for optimal amputee function and prosthetic use must take a secondary role to initial treatment of the injury, but the surgeon must keep in mind the types of prosthetic devices the patient may use, as well as the problems that may occur consequent to skeletal growth, whether normal or abnormal. Good amputee function requires an optimal conversion site, pliable skin cover with sensation, uncomplicated healing, freedom from infection, good vascular stump nutrition, and if possible, a well-muscled stump. In order to provide these objectives safely and with assurance, staging of treatment may be necessary.

Guidelines for the management of traumatic wound amputations, which are often caused by the mutilating forces of lawn mowers, firecracker blasts, propellers, etc., must take into consideration the extensive soft tissue damage as well as the chondro-osseous injury and the introduction of significant amounts of contaminating material (see Fig. 6-3). In order to effect optimum results, several guidelines should and must be recognized; these are:

(1) The amputation should be at the most distal, viable level. In the child, this must include ablation at the most distal, viable joint whenever possible.

(2) Viable skin should be preserved.

(3) Primary closure of the wound should *not* be attempted.

(4) Following debridement, skin traction should be used.

(5) The proximal joint should be immobilized in a functional position.

(6) The plaster should be longitudinal splints, not circumferential, to avoid constriction.

Any wound that can be closed at the time of initial debridement can be repaired *with equal facility and far greater safety* 7 to 10 days after the original injury, particularly if considerable contaminating material has been introduced. Increasing vascular embarrassment due to closed space edema cannot occur in a completely debrided, fasciotomized, open wound. Because many of these injuries are caused by blunt trauma, it is not always easy to estimate tissue viability and wound contamination at the time of injury, and a secondary debridement of residual necrotic tissue is necessary at the time of delayed closure or at some intervening time prior to closure. In any severely traumatized, potentially contaminated limb wound with bone exposure, infection usually does not occur in the completely debrided, open wound with viable tissue. This is particularly true for the introduction of the anaerobic bacteria, including clostridia.

Once wounds are healing satisfactorily, major revisions and grafting may be considered. If both feet are extensively involved, cross-leg pedicle transplants may allow reconstruction of at least one good, functional foot and a Syme amputation of the other (see Fig. 6-15).

Above and below knee amputations should be avoided in children whenever possible and knee disarticulations in which the distal femoral epiphysis is left should be performed instead. The presence of the distal femoral epiphysis with a tough prepatellar skin cover may provide good end-bearing control for a prosthesis. Knee disarticulation also allows later (if necessary), muscular, above-knee stump revision.

Diaphyseal amputations are sometimes necessary, but in young children, the cause of trauma is often the power rotary mower, and the majority of the resulting injuries involve the foot. The skin over the heel, though traumatized, may be salvaged. In severe foot injuries in the growing child, the Syme ankle disarticulation level is the site at which to amputate. The Chopart or Lisfranc levels can be fitted and tolerated in the child, but give a less functional prosthetic result after skeletal maturity is reached. The Syme amputation is almost mandatory in children if optimal function is to be achieved; so possible complications of the procedure should be considered during primary wound management to see how they best may be avoided.

If the tissues about the heel and plantar surface are trau-

matized, a well-drained, debrided wound is essential. Most of these injuries are contaminated by dirt or grass. If the tissues are traumatized but still viable, as is the case with most severe foot injuries, it is unwise to subject the heel pad to the trauma of major surgical dissection beyond adequate debridement. After open-flap treatment and subsequent delayed closure, these heel pads are often scarred, tender, and poorly adapted for end-bearing function.

There is another reason for rejection of the open-flap Syme technique in young children. The operation is not performed as it is in adults with resection of the cartilage surfaces of the ankle, but it is a disarticulation, which leaves the distal epiphysis of the tibia and fibula undisturbed. Open disarticulations may be troublesome. Articular cartilage deprived of nutrition may undergo necrosis and desquamation, and the recesses of the joint may invite persistent bacterial invasion. Therefore, in a child with a severe foot injury in which the heel pad is thought to be viable, an open, more distal forefoot amputation may be performed initially. All surface cartilage and bone is debrided. After the edema has resolved and nutrition of the tissues is established, a delayed, formal revision to a Syme ankle disarticulation may be performed with relative safety. In cases in which the edema or surface infection persists, or restoration of tissue nutrition is delayed, the application of a very thin, split-thickness skin graft as a temporary wound cover will usually result in a clean, closed wound that may subsequently be revised to a Syme ankle disarticulation with safety.

Overgrowth

In younger children, in whom significant longitudinal growth remains, any type of diaphyseal amputation leaves much to be desired in terms of ultimate adult function. Not only may there be a small, flabby, poorly-muscled stump, but loss of the distal epiphysis results in progressive, relative shortening of the amputated extremity compared to the uninvolved extremity. Overgrowth stemming from terminal, appositional, endosteal proliferation (rather than physeal growth) is a frequent complication, often requiring multiple revisions which result in further shortening.[79-82] This overgrowth results from a combined process of both periosteal and endosteal new bone formation, as well as from terminal remodeling. There is also a phenomenon of traction, with the remaining periosteum becoming fixed to the bone at the distal site and having no remaining control over diametric or latitudinal expansion. The end progressively becomes tapered because it fails to grow adequately in a diametric fashion compared to the more proximal portions, although longitudinal growth (appositional-membranous, not endochondral) does occur (Fig. 6-16).

Osseous overgrowth presents itself clinically as an increasing inequality in length between the stump skeleton and its soft tissue covering. As this inequality increases, the end of the stump becomes tented over the sharp bone and becomes tender. Sometimes an adventitious bursa develops between the skin and the bone, and this may or may not be acutely tender. In neglected cases, the sharp end of the bone may perforate the soft tissue covering. Ulceration develops about the area of perforation. There is generally an abundant local production of granulation tissue, and the possibility of osteomyelitis becomes significant.

This ability to produce bone in such an additive manner is

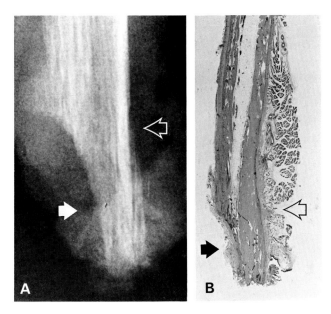

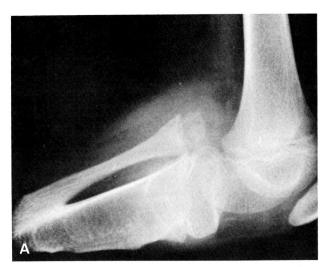

FIG. 6-16. Distal tibia of childhood below knee amputation, showing overgrowth of bone (solid arrow) beyond original amputation level (open arrow). There is subperiosteal and endosteal new bone. *A,* Radiologic section. *B,* Histologic section.

a characteristic of long bones in which the epiphyses are open. Certainly the phenomenon does not occur in adult amputees. Hellstadius[83] demonstrated that if he resected long bones at the midportion in rats with open epiphyses, regeneration would be consistent. It is possible that in juvenile amputees we observe the clinical counterpart of that experiment.

Radiologically, bony overgrowth has a characteristic appearance (see Fig. 6-16). The distal end of the stump skeleton seems to elongate; the medullary canal in the area of overgrowth is diminished or absent; the normal parallelism of the cortical surfaces is lost; the involved bone becomes sharply pointed; and the trabecular details of the area of overgrowth are poorly differentiated.

In cases in which the amount of overgrowth does not require treatment and the new bone has an opportunity to mature, the trabecular pattern becomes better defined. Radiologically, one can liken early overgrowth to immature, undirected callus formation. Over a period of several years, Aitken has been revising these stumps, and has placed metal clips in the revised bone ends.[81] Subsequent roentgenograms have shown conclusively that the overgrowing bone is added *distal* to the implanted metal marker, presumably by the periosteal remnants (i.e., by membranous ossification).

The treatment for the condition is revision of the overgrowing stump. There is *no* use for proximal epiphysiodesis in the management of this complication. Metallic implants in the overgrowing stumps have shown conclusively that this is a distal additive process. The ablation of the next proximal physis will not destroy distal additive bone formation. Appositional (distal additive) bone growth probably is an inherent characteristic of growing bone. It does not appear in patients whose epiphyses are physiologically closed, and who also have much less osteogenic periosteum.

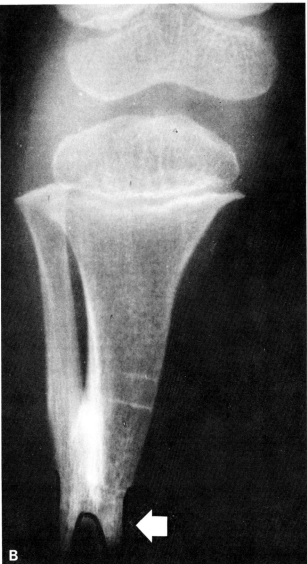

FIG. 6-17. *A,* A synostosis was created between the tibia and fibula. *B,* Overgrowth of both bones occurred despite this (arrow).

Recurrence of overgrowth is more likely than is the development of it in a patient who has never had the problem. Because this is a recognized clinical fact, efforts to prevent recurrence have been made following the first revision. These efforts have been basically to develop a synostosis[84] between the tibia and the fibula (Fig. 6-17). Often the synostosis fails to develop. Aitken[81] believed that continuing overgrowth of the fibula produced tibia vara.

Epiphyseal grafting

As an alternative to tibiofibular synostosis, the possibility of grafting epiphyseal/physeal composites onto the diaphyseal end has been suggested on the basis of clinical and animal experiments.[2,24,85-87] While the majority of the transplant may not survive unless microvascular anastomoses are undertaken, peripheral (appositional) physeal growth may be sufficient to prevent the bone from tapering (Figs. 6-18 and 6-19). It is important to realize and accept that longitudinal growth potential is limited in such a procedure. However, if latitudinal growth occurs, it will prevent tapering and conical tension in the distal periosteum.

Prosthesis

Guidelines for selection and use of prosthetics are readily available.[50,88] A stump should be fitted with a prosthesis as soon as it will tolerate pressure. In most traumatic amputations this requires three to four weeks after the completion of surgical treatment. While immediate postoperative prosthetic fitting has been advocated for adults, this is usually after an elective, nontraumatic amputation. Wound management, which is essential to the care of the traumatic amputation, precludes the immediate fitting of a prosthesis. If a significant amount of time elapses before the child is fitted with a prosthesis, he may become dependent on the contralateral extremity and reject the substitute device.

Delayed amputation

As stated earlier, adequate initial care for soft tissues and bone may prevent the immediate need for amputation, even in extremely damaged regions. Figure 6-20 shows the sequence of events in a young boy who had severe distal femoral and proximal tibial injuries as a result of a power lawn mower accident. The various injuries were treated initially without a major complication. However, over the next few years, angular growth deformity at the physes and restriction of joint motion became major factors. Eventually, a knee disarticulation was performed. This amputation would have been difficult if done initially, when there were severe, open chondro-osseous and intra-articular injuries. The child now functions extremely well in his prosthesis. In his case, because of severe soft tissue damage, earlier amputation probably would have necessitated the distal femoral diaphyseal level. Instead, the boy has a good, end-bearing stump, which will eventually become a good "above-knee" level because of impaired longitudinal growth in the distal femur.

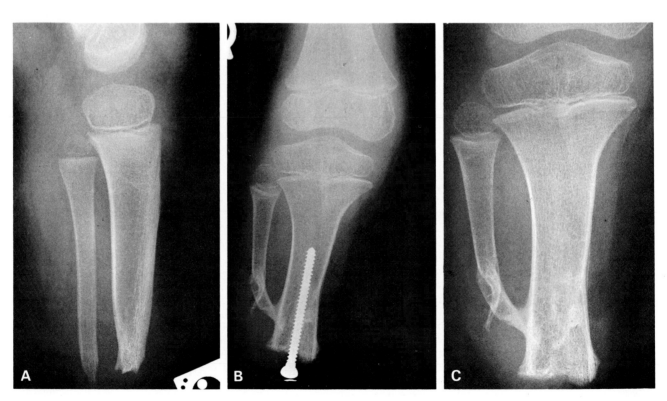

FIG. 6-18. Result of amputation in patient shown in Figure 6-15. *A,* Irregular stump overgrowth is evident. *B,* The fibula was synostosed to the tibia, and a graft of iliac crest, including epiphyseal cartilage, was attached to the tibia. *C,* Several months later there is no evidence of tibial overgrowth.

Reimplantation

A major question in partial or complete traumatic amputation in a child is whether to reimplant the arm, leg, or portion thereof (Fig. 6-21). This should be contingent upon the availability, and technical ability of, a team of orthopaedic, plastic, vascular and neurologic surgeons, as well as: the overall extent of soft tissue injury, the mechanism of injury, the time elapsed since injury, the presence or absence of other serious injuries, the condition of the severed limb, and a warm ischemic time of less than 10 hours or a cold ischemic time of less than 20 hours. Adequate discussion of what is involved must be held with the parents, and they must be informed that partial or complete amputation still may be necessary.

Clean, sharp, guillotine-type injuries are those for which reimplantation is most feasible. Avulsion mechanisms causing long, linear stretch injuries are least suitable, as are crushing injuries. Major soft tissue injury may seriously compromise attempted reimplantation. Anastomosis of nerves has a better chance of reasonably functional recovery in a child than in an adult. To facilitate vascular and neural anastomosis, it is generally easier to shorten the major involved bone at the site of the amputation by a centimeter or two. If possible, this should be done in the diaphyseal region. If the involved bone is a femur or a humerus, the normal capacity for overgrowth cannot be relied upon, particularly since very few long term studies have been done to show whether overgrowth really can occur due to the particular type of trauma.

Specific operative techniques may be obtained from the literature.[41,89-93,95] At one time, major limb reimplantation was not indicated in young children because of the problems of shock due to fluid loss in the limb and the technical problems of small vessel anastomosis. These concerns are less real now that microvascular surgery and use of the operating microscope have become more readily available, allowing successful anastomosis of small vessels and recognition of the need to repair enough veins to provide adequate drain-

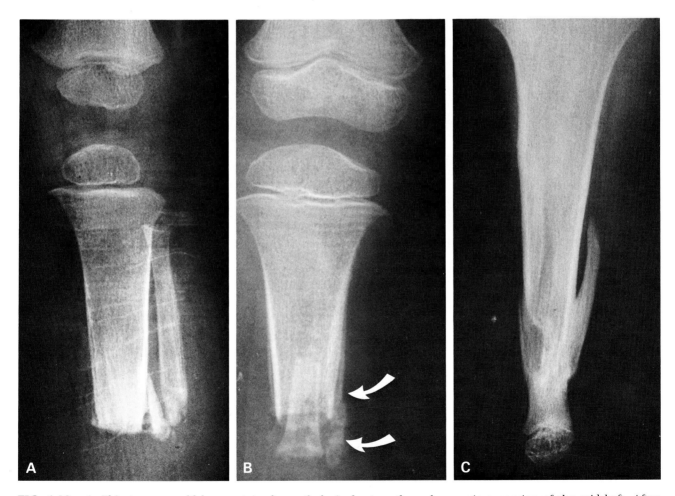

FIG. 6-19. *A,* This two-year-old boy sustained a pathologic fracture through a cystic expansion of the midshaft. After repeated grafts a below knee amputation was done, with an attempt to create a synostosis. Because of irregular distal bone formation, the fibula was removed 16 months later, reversed and implanted into the tibial endosteal cavity, with the periosteal sleeves being sutured together. *B,* Two months after this procedure, reactive subperiosteal bone is forming (arrows). The boy was placed back in his prosthesis at this time. *C,* One year later, the graft is fully incorporated and shows no osseous overgrowth.

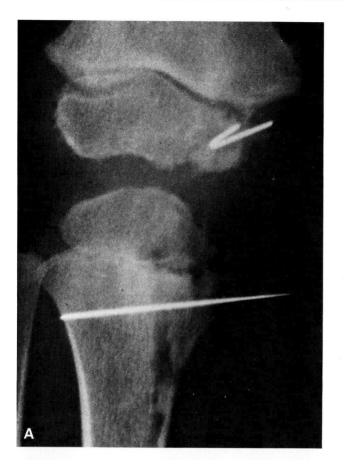

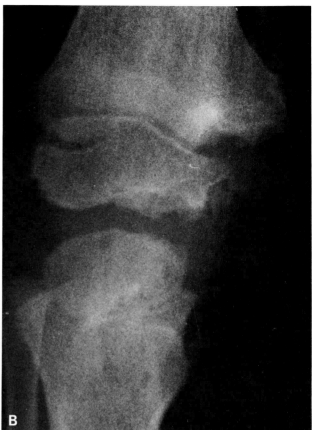

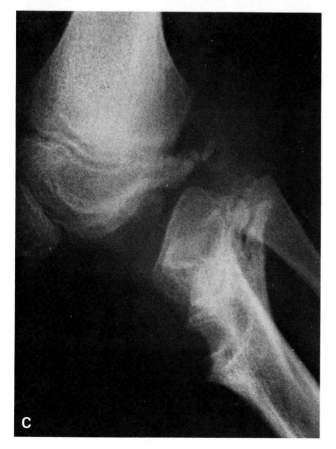

FIG. 6-20. *A,* Young child who sustained a severe, compound injury of the distal femur and proximal tibia as a result of a power lawn mower accident. Multiple type 4 fragments were separated by the lawn mower blades, *B,* One year later, beginning growth irregularities are evident. *C,* Three years later, severe deformity has developed (also see Figs. 2-55 and 4-25).

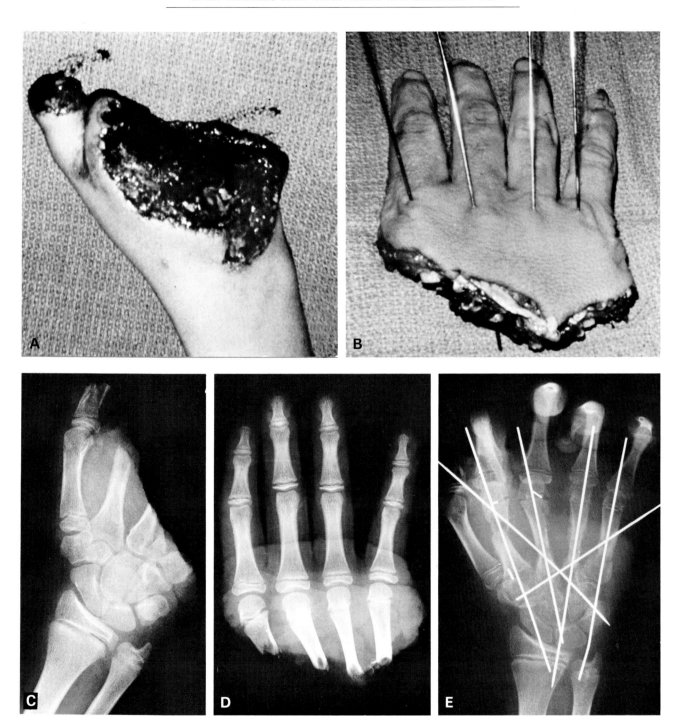

FIG. 6-21. *A-B,* Gross specimens of hand amputation in a 14-year-old boy. *C-D,* Roentgenograms of the two specimens. *E,* Roentgenogram of reconstructed hand.

age of the part and reduce blood loss. Even with reanastomosis of the circulation, the long term viability of the physis is not certain. It appears that premature growth arrest is likely (Fig. 6-22).

Sehayik[16] presented the results of upper extremity reimplantation in children. Results were good for the hand, good to excellent for the digits, and best for the thumb. Digits amputated distal to the flexor digitorum sublimis usually had excellent recovery of neurovascular function. However,

the overall success rate was lower for the child than for the adult, primarily because of microvascular problems. The vessels are smaller in the child, and there is more vasospasm. Because of the latter, Sehayik recommended waiting 7 to 10 days for the first dressing change. No comment was made regarding epiphyseal/physeal growth, although others have indicated it may be impaired,[94] as in the case shown in Figure 6-22.

Many authors feel there is no place for reimplantation of

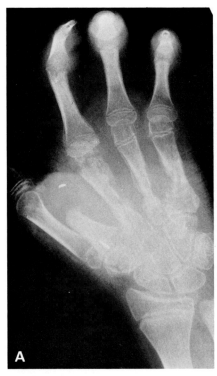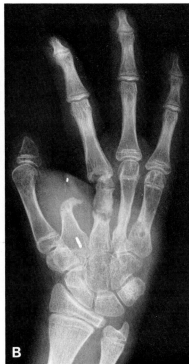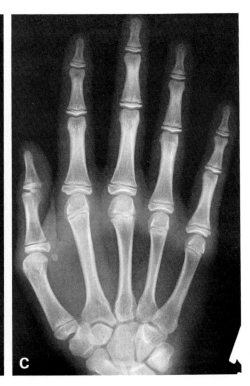

FIG. 6-22. Unfortunately, the index finger in the case shown in Figure 6-21 did not survive the immediate postoperative period. *A*, Film taken eight weeks after surgery. *B*, Film taken three months after surgery. Note premature closure of the third metacarpal physis. *C*, Normal contralateral hand, for comparison.

severed, lower limbs, although recent success has been described.[92] Weightbearing and locomotive function probably are better served by a prosthesis. Exceptions to this are severance of the limb above the knee in a young child when successful reimplantation may mean retention of the lower femoral epiphysis, which contributes much to the lower limb length, or reimplantation of a distal amputation (ankle or foot levels), which is comparable to wrist/hand procedures. Even if a true knee disarticulation is required later, a great service will have been done to the patient in terms of function. In the upper limb, however, sensation and manipulation are all-important, and even a reimplanted hand that has little of either is superior to a prosthesis.

References

1. Brav, E. A.: Open fractures: fundamentals of management. Postgrad. Med., *39:*11, 1966.
2. Heikel, H. V. A.: Experimental epiphyseal transplantation. III. The influence of age. Acta Orthop. Scand., *36:*371, 1965.
3. Lindseth, R., and DeRosa, G.: Fractures in children. General considerations and treatment of open fractures. Pediatr. Clin. North Am., *22:*465, 1975.
4. Barry, T. P., and Linton, P. C.: Biophysics of rotary mower and snowblower injuries of the hand: high vs. low velocity "missile" injury. J. Trauma, *17:*211, 1977.
5. Cluff, L. E., et al.: Staphylococcal bacteremia and altered host resistance. Ann. Intern. Med., *69:*859, 1968.
6. Gordon, S. L., Greer, R. B., and Craig, C. P.: Recurrent osteomyelitis. Report of four cases culturing L-form variants of staphylococci. J. Bone Joint Surg., *53-A:*1150, 1971.
7. Hamblen, D. L.: Hyperbaric oxygenation: its effects on experimental Staphylococcal osteomyelitis in rats. J. Bone Joint Surg., *50-A:*1129, 1968.
8. Krizek, T. J., and Robson, M. C.: Biology of surgical infection. Surg. Clin. North Am., *55:*1261, 1975.
9. Loesch, W. J.: Oxygen sensitivity of various anaerobic bacteria. Appl. Microbiol., *81:*723, 1969.
10. Waldvogel, F. A., Medoff, G., and Swartz, M. N.: Osteomyelitis: a review of clinical features, therapeutic considerations, and unusual aspects. N. Engl. J. Med., *282:*198;260;316, 1970.
11. Anderson, R. S., and Argamaso, R.: Management of extensive open fractures in children and teenage patients. J. Natl. Med. Assoc., *68:*20, 1976.
12. Curtiss, P. H., Jr.: Some uncommon forms of osteomyelitis. Clin. Orthop., *96:*84, 1973.
13. Ogden, J. A., and Light, T. R.: Pediatric osteomyelitis. III. Anaerobic microorganisms. Clin. Orthop., *145:*230, 1979.
14. Ogden, J. A.: Pediatric osteomyelitis. Orthop. Trans., *3:*95, 1979.
15. Ogden, J. A., and Lister, G.: The pathology of neonatal osteomyelitis. Pediatrics, *55:*474, 1975.
16. Sehayik, R.: Reimplantation in children. Orthop. Trans., *3:*84, 1979.
17. Trueta, J.: The three types of acute hematogenous osteomyelitis. A clinical and vascular study. J. Bone Joint Surg., *41-A:*671, 1959.
18. Scully, R. E., Artz, C. P., and Sako, Y.: An evaluation of the surgeon's criteria for determining muscle viability during debridement. Arch. Surg., *73:*1031, 1956.
19. Waterman, N. A., Howell, R. S., and Babich, N.: The effect of a prophylactic antibiotic (cephalothin) on the incidence of wound infection. Arch. Surg., *98:*365, 1968.
20. Patzakis, M., Harvey, J., and Ivler, D.: The role of antibiotics in the management of open fractures. J. Bone Joint Surg., *56-A:*532, 1974.

21. Alexander, J. W., et al.: Concentration of selected intravenously administered antibiotics in experimental surgical wounds. J. Trauma, *13:*423, 1973.

22. Fogelberg, E. U., Zitzmann, E. K., and Stinchfield, F. E.: Prophylactic penicillin in orthopaedic surgery. J. Bone Joint Surg., *52-A:*95, 1970.

23. Sanford, J. P., et al.: An experimental evaluation of the usefulness of antibiotic agents in the early management of contaminated soft tissue wounds. Surg. Gynecol. Obstet., *105:*5, 1957.

24. Wang, G. J., Baugher, W. H., and Stamp, W. G.: Epiphyseal transplant in amputations. Clin. Orthop., *130:*285, 1978.

25. Winters, J. L., and Cahen, I.: Acute hematogenous osteomyelitis. A review of sixty-six cases. J. Bone Joint Surg., *42-A:*691, 1960.

26. Burke, J. R.: The effective period of preventive antibiotic action in experimental incisions and dermal lesions. Surgery, *50:*161, 1961.

27. Bowers, W. H., Wilson, F. C., and Greene, W. B.: Antibiotic prophylaxis in experimental bone infections. J. Bone Joint Surg., *55-A:*795, 1973.

28. Curtiss, P. H., Jr.: The pathophysiology of joint infections. Clin. Orthop., *96:*129, 1973.

29. Evaskus, D. S., Laskin, D. M., and Kroeger, A. V.: Penetration of lincomycin, penicillin and tetracycline into serum and bone. Proc. Soc. Exp. Biol. Med., *130:*89, 1969.

30. Kanyuck, D. O., et al.: The penetration of cephalosporin antibiotics into bone. Proc. Soc. Exp. Biol. Med., *136:*997, 1971.

31. Wilson, F. C., et al.: Antibiotic penetration of experimental bone hematomas. J. Bone Joint Surg., *53-A:*1622, 1971.

32. Canale, S. T., et al.: Acute osteomyelitis following closed fractures. J. Bone Joint Surg., *57-A:*415, 1975.

33. Farr, C. E.: Acute osteomyelitis in children. Ann. Surg., *83:*686, 1926.

34. Ogden, J. A.: Pediatric osteomyelitis and septic arthritis: the pathology of neonatal disease. Yale J. Biol. Med., *52:*423, 1979.

35. Watson, F. M., and Whitesides, T. E.: Acute hematogenous osteomyelitis complicating closed fractures. Clin. Orthop., *117:*296, 1976.

36. Gerszten, E., Allison, M. J., and Dalton, H. P.: An epidemiologic study of 100 consecutive cases of osteomyelitis. South. Med. J., *63:*365, 1970.

37. Gilmour, W. N.: Acute hematogenous osteomyelitis. J. Bone Joint Surg., *44-B:*841, 1962.

38. Gledhill, R. B., and McIntyre, J. M.: Various phases of pediatric osteomyelitis. In AAOS Instructional Course Lectures, *22:*245, St. Louis, C. V. Mosby, 1973.

39. Shandling, B.: Acute hematogenous osteomyelitis: a review of 300 cases treated during 1953–1959. S. Afr. Med. J., *34:*520, 1960.

40. Youmans, G. P., Paterson, P. Y., and Sommers, H. M.: The Biologic and Clinical Basis of Infectious Diseases. Philadelphia, W. B. Saunders, 1975.

41. Lazarus, G. S., et al.: Human granulocyte collagenase. Science, *159:*1483, 1968.

42. Argamaso, R., et al.: Cross-leg flaps in children. Plast. Reconstr. Surg., *51:*662, 1972.

43. Burton, D. S., and Nagel, D. A.: *Serratia marcescens* infections in orthopaedic surgery. Clin. Orthop., *89:*145, 1972.

44. Derian, P. S., Fisher, L. C., and Adkins, J.: Acute osteomyelitis from *Serratia marcescens*. Am. J. Orthop., *8:*96, 1966.

45. Kelly, P. J., Wilkowske, C. J., and Washington, J. A.: Musculoskeletal infections due to *Serratia marcescens*. Clin. Orthop., *96:*76, 1973.

46. Khanna, S., and Sharma, S. U.: Fungal bone cyst developed at the site of a healed compound fracture. Int. Orthop., *2:*343, 1979.

47. Nelms, D. K., et al.: *Serratia marcescens* osteomyelitis in an infant. J. Pediatr., *72:*222, 1968.

48. Brand, R. A., and Black, H.: Pseudomonas osteomyelitis following puncture wounds in children. J. Bone Joint Surg., *56-A:*1637, 1974.

49. Brown, P. W., and Kinman, P. B.: Gas gangrene in a metropolitan community. J. Bone Joint Surg., *56-A:*1445, 1974.

50. Ogden, J. A., and Light, T. R.: Pediatric osteomyelitis. II. *Arizona hinshawii* osteomyelitis. Clin. Orthop., *139:*110, 1979.

51. Filler, R. M., Griscom, N. T., and Pappas, A.: Post-traumatic crepitation falsely suggesting gas gangrene. N. Engl. J. Med., *278:*758, 1968.

52. MacLennan, J. D.: The histotoxic Clostridial infections of man. Bacteriol. Rev., *26:*177, 1962.

53. Pappas, A. M., et al.: Clostridial infections (gas gangrene). Diagnosis and early treatment. Clin. Orthop., *76:*177, 1971.

54. Fee, N. F., Dobranski, A., and Bisla, R. S.: Gas gangrene complicating open forearm fractures. J. Bone Joint Surg., *59-A:*135, 1977.

55. Cherington, M., and Ginsburg, S.: Wound botulism. Arch. Surg., *110:*436, 1975.

56. Brummelkamp, W. H., Boerema, I., and Hoogendyk, L.: Treatment of Clostridial infections with hyperbaric oxygen drenching. A report of 26 cases. Lancet, *1:*235, 1963.

57. Brummelkamp, W. H., Hogendijk, J., and Boerema, I.: Treatment of anaerobic infections (clostridial myositis) by drenching the tissue with oxygen under high atmospheric pressure. Surgery, *49:*299, 1961.

58. Brooks, V. B., Curtis, D. R., and Eccles, J. C.: The action of tetanus toxin on the inhibition of motorneurones. J. Physiol., *135:*655, 1957.

59. McCord, J. M., Kaele, B. B., and Fridovich, I.: An enzyme-based theory of obligate anaerobiasis; the physiologic function of superoxide dismutase. Proc. Nat. Acad. Sci. USA, *68:*1024, 1971.

60. Smythe, P. M.: Studies on neonatal tetanus and on pulmonary compliance of the totally relaxed infant. Br. Med. J., *1:*565, 1963.

61. Smythe, P. M.: The problem of detubating an infant with a tracheostomy. J. Pediatr., *65:*446, 1964.

62. Jajic, J., and Rulnjevic, J.: Myositis ossificans localisata as a complication of tetanus. Acta Orthop. Scand., *50:*547, 1979.

63. Hansen, N., and Tolo, V.: Wound botulism complicating an open fracture. J. Bone Joint Surg., *61-A:*312, 1979.

64. Kennedy, T. L., and Merson, M. H.: An infected wound as a cause of botulism in a 12-year-old boy. Clin. Pediatr., *16:*151, 1977.

65. DeJesus, P. V., Jr., et al.: Neuromuscular physiology of wound botulism. Arch. Neurol., *29:*425, 1973.

66. Gutman, L., and Pratt, L.: Pathophysiologic effects of human botulism. Arch. Neurol., *33:*175, 1976.

67. Braithwaite, F., and Moore, T. F.: Skin grafting by cross-leg flaps. J. Bone Joint Surg., *31-B:*228, 1949.

68. Golden, G. T., Fisher, J. C., and Edgerton, M. T.: Wringer arm reevaluated. A survey of current surgical management of upper extremity compression injuries. Ann. Surg., *177:*362, 1973.

69. MacCollum, D. W., Bernhard, W. F., and Banner, R. L.: The treatment of wringer arm injuries. N. Engl. J. Med., *247:*750, 1952.

70. Spring, J. M., and Epps, C. H.: The juvenile amputee. Some observations and considerations. Clin. Pediatr., *7:*76, 1968.

71. White, A. A., III: Instantaneous washday amputation. A plea for prevention. J.A.M.A., *220:*123, 1972.

72. Akbarnia, B. A., Campbell, C. J., and Bowen, J. R.: Management of massive defects in radius and ulna wringer injury. Clin. Orthop., *116:*167, 1976.

73. Borgi, R., Butel, J., and Finidori, G.: La regenerescence diaphysaire d'un os long chez l'enfant. Rev. Chir. Orthop., *65:*413, 1979.

73a. Varma, B. P., and Srivastava, T. P.: Successful regeneration of large extruded diaphyseal segments of the radius. J. Bone Joint Surg., *61-A:*290, 1979.

74. Baumgartner, R. F.: Amputation und Prosthesenversorgung beim kind. Stuttgart, Ferdinand Enke, 1977.

75. Baumgartner, R. F.: Above knee amputation in children. Prosthet. Orthot. Int., *3:*26, 1979.

76. Cary, J. M.: Traumatic amputation in childhood—primary management. Interclinic Inform. Bull., *14:*1, 1975.

77. McKenzie, D. S.: The prosthetic management of congenital deformities of the extremities. J. Bone Joint Surg., *39-B:*233, 1957.

78. Dederich, R.: Plastic treatment of the muscles and bone in amputation surgery. J. Bone Joint Surg., *45-B:*60, 1963.

79. Aitken, G. T.: The lower extremity juvenile amputee. In AAOS Instructional Course Lectures, *14:*329, St. Louis, C. V. Mosby, 1957.

80. Aitken, G. T.: Surgical amputation in children. J. Bone Joint Surg., *45-A:*1735, 1963.

81. Aitken, G. T.: Osseous overgrowth in amputations in children. *In* Limb Development and Deformity. Edited by C. A. Swinyard. Springfield, Charles C Thomas, 1969.

82. Frantz, C. H., and Aitken, G. T.: Management of the juvenile amputee. Clin. Orthop., *14:*30, 1959.

83. Hellstadius, A.: An investigation by experiments in animals of the role played by the epiphyseal cartilage in longitudinal growth. Acta Chir. Scand., *95:*156, 1947.

84. Barber, C. G.: Amputation of the lower leg with induced synostosis of the distal ends of the tibia and fibula. J. Bone Joint Surg., *26:*356, 1944.

85. Heikel, H. V. A.: Experimental epiphyseal transplantation. I. Roentgenological observations on survival and growth of epiphyseal transplantations. Acta Orthop. Scand., *29:*257, 1960.

86. Heikel, H. V. A.: Experimental epiphyseal transplantation. Acta Orthop. Scand., *30:*1, 1961.

87. Knoeler, A., and Matzen, P. F.: Experimentelles zur Epiphysentransplantation. Beitr. Orthop. Traumatol., *7:*1, 1960.

88. McCullough, N. C., Fryer, M. A., and Glancy, J.: A new approach to patient analysis for orthotic prescription—part I: the lower extremity. Artif. Limbs, *14:*68, 1970.

89. Malt, R. A., and McKhann, C. F.: Replantation of severed arms. J.A.M.A., *189:*114, 1964.

90. Malt, R. A., Remensnyder, J. P., and Harris, W. H.: Long-term utility or replanted arms. Ann. Surg., *176:*334, 1972.

91. O'Brien, B. M.: Replantation surgery. Clin. Plast. Surg., *1:*3, 1974.

92. Usui, M., et al.: Experience in reimplantation of the totally severed lower limb in a child. Shujutsu, *28:*1349, 1974.

93. White, S. C.: Nerve regeneration after replantation of severed arm. Ann. Surg., *170:*715, 1969.

93a. Rosenkrantz, J. G., et al.: Replantation of an infant's arm. N. Engl. J. Med., *276:*609, 1967.

94. Curtis, R. M.: Personal communication.

7

Complications

While children develop fewer complications than adults from comparable musculoskeletal injuries, as shown in Chapters 4 and 6, certain types of chondro-osseous injuries result in complications relatively unique to the developing skeleton. In this chapter, a variety of more generalized complications are discussed, with emphasis on how they differ if a child is involved. Fortunately, most of these complications are rare in children. However, this minimizes each orthopaedist's familiarity and experience with the nuances the complications have in children, even though he might be quite familiar with the problem in an adult.[1] Approaches to treatment that might be applied in an adult often must be modified for use in a child. The ability to effectively diagnose and treat complications rests on a thorough knowledge of what to look for and where to look.

A small child often responds differently than an adolescent or an adult to major injuries. Following blunt abdominal trauma, paralytic ileus may be of greater consequence in children, because abdominal distension may elevate the diaphragm and interfere with the relatively limited pulmonary function. Similarly, small blood losses assume greater consequence in infants and children, because infants and children have a more limited circulating blood volume. A closed fracture of the femur may be associated with a 300 to 400 ml loss of blood into the contiguous soft tissues. In a six-year-old, this may represent 15 to 25% of the total circulating blood volume and may contribute to hypovolemic shock. In contrast, the adolescent or adult suffers less consequences from a similar volume depletion.

Major heat losses may occur quite rapidly in children. A drop in core temperature of only a few degrees may interfere with normal enzyme function and other metabolic processes, adding further insult to the child's response to traumatic stress.[2] The rapidity with which metabolic and cardiovascular responses can occur serves to emphasize the importance of good monitoring systems. Minor changes in response to treatment must be detected early to prevent serious sequelae.

Congenital abnormalities rarely complicate the management of traumatized adults. However, they may cause serious complications in young children, particularly if previously undetected. Trauma may precipitate cardiogenic shock in a child with a previously asymptomatic ventricular septal defect.[2]

Shock

In contrast to adult skeletal injuries, shock is an uncommon accompaniment to most children's fractures, although it does occur in a small number of multiple-system injuries, particularly those resulting from vehicular accidents. Varieties of shock encountered in children include: (1) hypovolemic shock, (2) septic (endotoxic) shock, and (3) cardiogenic shock. In children, shock following injury nearly always is due to blood loss. In the pediatric age group, cardiogenic shock will be seen almost exclusively in patients with a congenital cardiomyopathy. Trauma to the central nervous system practically never causes shock, and circulatory collapse due to autonomic response to fear or pain is usually of such brief duration that it is no longer present when the child arrives in the emergency room. Shock resulting from infection is a late and infrequent complication, due in part to the low incidence of compound (open) injuries in children (see Chap. 6).

When any type of shock is encountered, treatment must be specific and prompt. While children have a much greater capacity for eventual recovery, their initial "downward" response to blood or fluid volume loss may be unexpectedly rapid.

Hemorrhagic shock is characterized by hypotension, tachycardia, cool, pale or slightly cyanotic extremities, restlessness or obtunded sensorium, and oliguria. Hypotension is caused directly by the decreased blood volume, with tachycardia and peripheral vasoconstriction being the compensatory mechanisms. The hypotension, in turn, causes inadequate cerebral and renal perfusion, leading to hypoxia as a result of the former, and hypoxia and decreased filtration as a result of the latter.

Compared to adults, children can tolerate a greater degree of blood loss as a percentage of total fluid volume, and take a longer time to manifest an overt response to blood loss; therefore, it is extremely rare, with the exception of injuries involving a major vascular or organ laceration, for a child to lose sufficient blood from a skeletal injury to manifest a shock response. Any child presenting with or developing shock should undergo complete evaluation to rule out intrathoracic, intra-abdominal or retroperitoneal injury.

The specific effect that shock has upon the kidney is decreased renal function, mediated, in part, by decreased blood flow. Excessively decreased flow to the kidneys initially may lead to progressive renal ischemia and eventually to renal tubular necrosis. Proper management and attention to fluid and electrolyte administration early in the course of the shock state will aid in the prevention of renal insufficiency. Again, children have a better capacity than adults for complete recovery of renal function, even if they are temporarily anuric.

Management of shock should be directed at general, supportive measures as well as at the actual, causative mechanism, which should be specifically rectified. Immediate steps include: (1) maintenance of an airway; (2) insertion of a sufficiently large intravenous line to allow rapid transfusion; (3) maintenance of arterial blood pressure (early infusion of Ringer's lactate followed by properly matched blood); (4) insertion of a nasogastric tube; and (5) cardiac monitoring. The use of adequate monitoring equipment (e.g., central venous pressure and arterial pressure lines) is also helpful in following these problems through their acute phases.

Familiarity with normal values is fundamental to rational management of shock. A child's blood volume relates directly to body weight and is approximately 40 ml/lb, regardless of age or size. Pulse rates gradually decrease with age, the upper limits of normal being 160 per minute in infants, 140 in preschool children, and 120 for all other children. The normal systolic blood pressure, in mm Hg, is 80 plus twice the age (in years), while the normal diastolic pressure is $\frac{2}{3}$ of the systolic. Normal urine outputs average 1 ml/lb/hr in small children and 0.5 ml/lb/hr in older children.

Most children suffering from hemorrhagic shock have a blood loss of approximately 10 to 20 ml/lb (25 to 50% of circulating volume). Initial treatment should consist of rapidly infused Ringer's lactate solution (10 ml/lb of body weight). Blood should be given as necessary, and particularly in younger children, it should be warmed to body temperature before infusion.

Respiratory distress

A discrete type of acute respiratory insufficiency following trauma and shock is called the post-traumatic respiratory insufficiency syndrome (shock-lung, traumatic wet lung, or respiratory distress syndrome). The insufficiency is manifested initially by tachypnea and increased respiratory effort. A progressive decrease in pulmonary compliance takes place, along with an increase in airway resistance, and a decrease in arterial oxygen tension and pulmonary arteriovenous shunting. While the lungs may sound dry to auscultation, the chest roentgenogram may reveal a few infiltrates. The management of post-traumatic pulmonary insufficiency is well outlined by Shires.[3] The major treatment is ventilatory support in conjunction with correction and management of the underlying disorders responsible for the shock, which are direct pulmonary injury, fat embolism, multiple blood transfusions, embolic phenomenon, and fluid overload.

Vascular Injury

Arterial injury

Blunt trauma severe enough to fracture the long bones of a limb may seriously damage adjacent arteries by either direct or indirect force.[4] Disruption or thrombosis of the traumatized artery may ensue, and the viability of the extremity may be jeopardized. Delay in diagnosis lessens the opportunity to salvage the extremity. Often, temporizing measures are utilized in the false hope that the vascular impairment does not represent damage requiring prompt operative treatment. Guidelines for the management of this complex problem in children are not readily available, since the incidence of fracture and concomitant arterial injury involving the immature skeleton is extremely uncommon (Fig. 7-1). Effective management of these concomitant injuries requires the avoidance of two principle mistakes. One, the delay in recognition of the arterial injury, and two, inappropriate or-

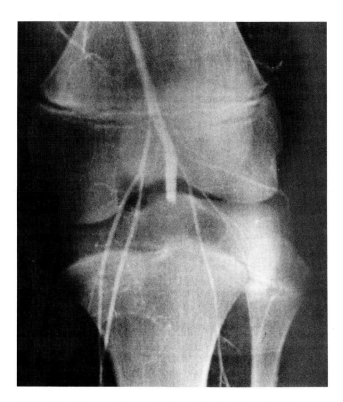

FIG. 7-1. Transection and thrombosis of popliteal artery complicating a proximal tibial epiphyseal fracture in a 14-year-old boy tackled in a football game. Arteriogram shows a complete block of the popliteal artery with some collateral flow. However, retrograde filling did not occur because of extensive thrombosis within the artery. "Poor" retrograde circulation through collaterals may be normal and should not be relied upon to sustain functional muscle demands.

thopaedic management. The successful management of a child who has sustained an arterial injury in association with fracture of a long bone requires the rapid recognition that there is significant circulatory compromise due to vascular damage.[5]

Arterial injury must be suspected in any patient who has been injured by direct or indirect trauma of sufficient magnitude to fracture a long bone, particularly if the fracture is displaced. Both the appearance of the extremity and the presence or absence of the pulses must be scrutinized carefully. The color, temperature, state of sensation, and motion of the limb may suggest diminished arterial inflow. Relative diminution of the pulses in comparison to the contralateral extremity may be significant.

However, the presence of a distal pulse does not positively exclude damage to a proximal artery. If doubt remains regarding the intactness of the peripheral artery after critical evaluation of the circulatory status of the involved limb, angiographic studies must be undertaken promptly. As a diagnostic tool, arteriography is not always necessary, since in at least half of the cases, the diagnosis can be made firmly on clinical grounds alone. This is particularly true in cases of compound fractures. However, arteriography is useful in ways independent of diagnostic assistance, for it supplies valuable details of confirmation about the exact location and extent of arterial damage and the status of collateral circulation.

There are several anatomic types of vascular injury: (1) lesions in discontinuity, in which the vessel is completely transected; (2) lesions in continuity, including intimal lesions; and (3) contusions causing either partial or complete occlusion of the vessel. Spasm also may cause a lesion in continuity. Traction on the vessel, particularly that which occurs during acute injury, is well recognized as capable of producing vasospasm. Compression, either from the cast externally or from a fracture fragment internally, may cause variable occlusion of a vessel. Prolonged occlusion may lead to thrombosis and permanent occlusion.

Relative to the anatomic injury patterns, different alterations in vascular pathophysiology may occur. In complete occlusion, the pulse is generally absent and the venous system relatively empty. The limb gradually will become white and cold. It may take more time for anesthesia and paralysis to develop. Pain is extreme until nerve loss begins to occur.

Incomplete occlusion or compartment ischemia, sometimes known as Volkmann's ischemia, is quite compatible with an intact pulse and seemingly adequate peripheral circulation. There may be resting pain in specific muscle groups and increased pain on stretching the involved muscles. If the flow in the main artery is reduced, the flow through collaterals may be sufficient to maintain a pulse in the distal circulation, but insufficient to maintain perfusion through specific muscle groups, especially during activity. These muscles become hypoxic and swell within the closed fascial compartments. Arterial inflow, capillary throughflow, and venous outflow become occluded, leading finally to ischemic necrosis of the muscle with ischemic contraction.

Further, in areas that are commonly problematic in children, such as the forearm in supracondylar humeral fractures, selective occlusion of a smaller vessel, such as the anterior interosseous artery, may also lead to this syndrome. Since the main vessel is intact, major signs of vascular problems are not as obvious.

In compensated occlusion, the extremity may be cool, but there are no signs of nerve or muscle ischemia. The collaterals are maintaining adequate resting circulation. Usually the pulse will return. However, in this situation and in the previous one of incomplete occlusion, consultation with a vascular surgeon should be sought in the event there is concern over the patency or adequacy of the circulation, as a feeble pulse that remains feeble may create a painful subsequent deformity as a result of ischemia occurring during function, even though the child has no symptoms apparent while resting.

Prevention requires the application of adequate casts, without excessive flexion, in areas such as the elbow or knee. Bivalving the cast may be sufficient to relieve temporary vascular insufficiency. True ischemia, particularly around the elbow and forearm, that does not improve after a short period of time (which should be well within 30 minutes) should be evaluated rapidly and completely to ascertain the diagnosis. Fasciotomy may be indicated when there is no doubt that the artery is intact and that the symptoms primarily represent a compartment syndrome. This requires preoperative establishment of normal distal circulation. If more than three to four hours have elapsed since injury and the vessel must be explored and repaired, a fasciotomy should be included in the composite surgical procedure. Repair of lesions should be done in conjunction with a vascular surgeon, if available.

The damaged arterial segment often must be excised, and the remaining portions sufficiently mobilized and debrided to ensure normal arterial structures for reconstruction. The exact pattern of reconstruction varies according to the demands of the injury. If the extent of injury requires so much sacrifice of vascular tissue that primary reanastomosis is not possible, the use of an autogenous vein graft is the next most desirable form. Prosthetic vascular grafts probably should be avoided in children.

If it is necessary to excise a portion of the vessel and reanastomose it, then it is imperative that the fracture be treated with internal fixation at the same time. An unstable fracture, particularly a supracondylar humeral fracture, will only jeopardize the vascular suture line. This is probably one of the infrequent situations in which open reduction and fixation are indicated in the child. The open reduction should be carried out first, followed by the vascular repair. Firm stabilization of the fracture site is essential for the protection of the subsequent vascular reconstruction.

While vascular (arterial) injuries are most often associated with neuromuscular involvement, one must not forget the potential long term consequences of ischemia on longitudinal and latitudinal physeal growth. Circulatory compromise may cause central physeal growth arrest and the development of conical physes.[6-9] Such growth slowdown or arrest may not be evident clinically for many years after the vascular injury.

Compartment syndrome

A compartment syndrome is caused by increased tissue pressure in a closed fascial space or compartment, which compromises the circulation to the nerves and muscles within the involved compartment. The syndrome may be caused by fracture, severe contusion, drug overdose with limb compression (which is increasingly becoming a problem in adolescence), a burn, or vigorous exercise. The initial insult causes hemorrhage, edema, or both in the closed fascial compartments of the extremities. An increase in intra-compartmental fluid pressure causes ischemia. Damage to the contents of the compartment, if permanent, may result in Volkmann's contracture. To prevent such complications, a prompt diagnosis must be made. Decompression of the involved compartments must be done quickly if the pressure is high.[10,11]

Swelling and palpable tension over a muscle compartment are the first signs of compartment syndrome, and are manifestations of increased pressure within the compartment. However, these signs are only crude indications of increased pressure, and other physical findings must be sought. Pain with stretching of the muscles is a common finding, but it is subjective and unreliable because the sign may be enhanced by the chondro-osseous trauma, rather than the ischemia. Furthermore, pain on stretching may be absent later because of anesthesia secondary to ischemia of the nerve. Paresis also is a difficult sign to interpret, because it may arise secondary to either neural involvement or primary ischemia of muscle, and there may be a guarding secondary to the pain that stimulates paresis.

The most reliable physical finding is a sensory deficit. Although it may appear early in the compartment syndrome, it may manifest only as a paresthesia rather than anesthesia. Each compartment of the leg and forearm has at least one nerve coursing through it that has sensory fibers, and with careful physical examination, selective confirmation of the involved compartment will be possible because of the sensory deficit in the area appropriate to the involved nerve.

The common denominator of compartment syndromes is an elevated interstitial fluid pressure which causes vascular occlusions in the compartments containing muscle. Although it may be high enough to cause ischemia of muscle and nerve, elevation of intracompartmental pressure only rarely is sufficiently high to occlude a major artery (even though venous occlusion and capillary occlusion are feasible). Failure to appreciate that arterial circulation may be maintained in the face of small vessel and venous occlusion may lead to a false sense of security. Several investigators have demonstrated the relationship between increased tissue pressure and ischemia of muscle.[12-14] Analysis suggests that when tissue fluid pressure exceeds 30 mm Hg, the capillary pressure is not sufficient to maintain blood flow through the muscles.[15-16]

Intracompartmental pressures may be measured by the wick catheter technique in patients suspected of having acute compartment syndromes.[14,17,18] By such methods, the range of normal pressure is 0 to 8 mm Hg. A pressure of 30 mm Hg or more lasting for six to eight hours is an indication for decompressive fasciotomy. Using intraoperative wick catheter measurements, fasciotomy should restore pressures to normal, except in buttock and deltoid compartments where epimysiotomy may be required to supplement the fasciotomy. Continuous intraoperative monitoring of pressure may allow selection of a few cases in which primary closure of the wounds is appropriate.

Fasciotomy in the leg should be done by an open method and not through percutaneous and subcutaneous incisions. It is necessary, particularly with the lower leg, to decompress all compartments through anterior and posterior incisions, particularly in violent trauma or major vascular injury. Fas-

ciotomy-fibulectomy, which has been described for adults,[19] should not be used for children because it may lead to major growth impairment, especially at the ankle.[20]

Volkmann's contracture/ischemia

Decreased arterial perfusion appears to be the primary initiating factor of Volkmann's ischemia, although other factors also may be involved.[5] Lesions caused by temporary arterial occlusion are different from the lesions caused by venous occlusion. Venous obstruction does not appear to be significant in the pathogenesis of experimental or clinical ischemic necrosis of skeletal muscle.[12,21] However, the extension of ischemic muscle necrosis, once initiated by arterial occlusion, may proceed by other pathways.

Several types of intramuscular vascular patterns have been demonstrated in adults, and it is reasonable to assume further variations in the developing muscle of skeletally immature patients. There are peculiarities of the vascularity to specific muscle groups, and anastomotic pathways are such that whole muscles, or segments thereof, may be affected by vascular occlusion despite no signs of distal ischemia. Certain muscle groups, such as the forearm flexors, appear more susceptible.

The vulnerability of a muscle to vascular injury is determined by the specific pattern of intramuscular anastomoses and the relationship between volume of muscle and size of the main nutrient vessels. For example, the sole blood supply to the flexor digitorum profundus and flexor pollicis longus muscles is the anterior interosseous artery (Fig. 7-2). Since the circulatory pathways are still developing in a child,

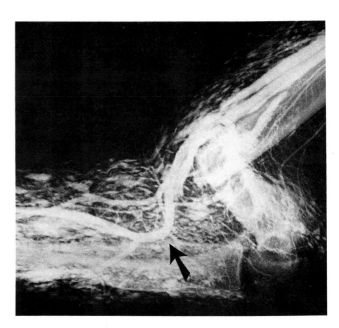

FIG. 7-2. Injection of cadaver arm of a 14-year-old. A supracondylar fracture has been duplicated by osteotomy. The lacertus fibrosis anchors the artery distal to the joint, and causes a retrograde kinking (arrow) as the fracture displaces posteriorly. Note that in this instance, acute angulation occurred near the origin of the anterior interosseous artery, rather than at the fracture site.

some vessels may subsequently enlarge to bring in sufficient flow. However, ischemic muscle damage, per se, is irreversible.

Direct damage to the blood supply of the median nerve may be a cause of some of the problems encountered in this syndrome. The median nerve deficit is consistent in all cases, and the ulnar deficit may be found in most instances. The median nerve is vulnerable to compression, as it lies actually on the undersurface and within the investing facia of the flexor sublimus muscle. As the muscle expands because of ischemic changes, it may compress the median nerve directly and cut off the arterial supply.

Specific involvement of the forearm and lower leg in these vascular complications will be discussed in Chapters 10, 11, and 18.

Venous Disorders

Thromboembolic disease

Thrombosis of the deep veins, particularly those of the lower extremity, has been well described in adults. Its incidence in childhood and adolescence is believed low, even in the presence of such predisposing factors as trauma, immobilization, surgery, pregnancy, malignancy or estrogen medication.[22-25]

Horwitz described ten adolescent patients who were admitted with diagnoses of primary or secondary deep vein thrombosis.[26] In three, the venous thrombosis occurred in the iliofemoral vein, while in five others the popliteal-deep saphenous system was involved. One patient had a primary occlusion of the right axial area and subclavian vein following weight-lifting. This condition, known as "effort" thrombosis of the axillary vein or Paget-Schroetter syndrome, occurs in healthy individuals after a forceful event produces direct or indirect injury to a vein.[27,28] One patient, a 16-year-old white male, developed sudden dyspnea, sharp central chest pains, tachycardia, fever, and pleural effusion, but was not resuscitated after the massive embolism. The site of thrombosis was not apparent. Three additional patients developed pulmonary embolism. One of the patients sustained thrombosis of the left calf after trauma, while two patients sustained thromboses postoperatively, one after a craniotomy for a fractured skull and the other after the pinning of a slipped epiphysis.

Clyne reported a five-year-old boy who sustained thrombosis and required thrombectomy of the iliofemoral vein for occlusion.[29] Marks and Sussman described a case of superficial thrombophlebitis in an eight-year-old girl and commented that only one other case of phlebitis in children had been reported in the English literature in the previous ten years.[30]

Deep vein thrombosis seen in children, adolescents, and adults has many common features. In a study of 13 adolescents and 14 children, deep vein thrombosis in 8 of the 13 adolescent patients occurred postoperatively or following trauma, whereas this predisposing factor was present in only 3 of 14 children.[25] In contrast, 7 of 14 children had a predisposing infective process, whereas only 3 of the 13 adolescents did. Horwitz noted that an obesity factor was known to increase the risk of thrombosis following surgery and immobilization, but had not been implicated in spontaneous venous thrombosis in healthy, non-obese, young individuals.[26] The patient shown in Figure 7-3 was an overweight 14-year-old suffering bilateral thromboembolic disease.

Children appear relatively immune to venous thrombosis, possibly because of their short veins and their continual, almost constant movement in bed when ill or in skeletal traction.

Dehydration may be important in vessel wall injury and may have played a part in many reported cases. There are a number of reports on the deleterious effects of cannulation of the deeper limb veins.[31-33]

These experiences suggest that deep vein thrombosis may be more frequent in children than is generally believed. Dif-

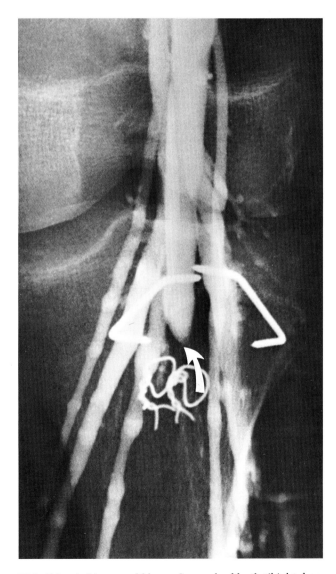

FIG. 7-3. A 14-year-old boy who avulsed both tibial tuberosities while running. Five weeks post-injury he had acute onset of shortness of breath, and a chest film showed opacification of the left lower lung field. A venogram of the right leg showed small vessel thrombosis. The left leg was more severely involved, with thrombosis of much of the deep system (arrow).

ficulty in diagnosis may be one reason it is not thought to be more common. The specific detection of deep vein thrombosis is contingent upon several diagnostic tests. With phlebography (venography), the most useful test, the extent of thrombosis formation and its adherence to the vein wall can be shown.[34,35] I[125]-labeled fibrogen is a sensitive screening substance[36] which becomes concentrated in a forming clot, and is indicated by increased radioactivity over the clot site detected by a scintillation counter. The technique may not be useful if the thrombosis is more than a week old, and it is unreliable in the presence of excessive edema. The Doppler technique is a simple and inexpensive procedure that detects changes in velocity of flow in blood vessels.[37,38] Extensive experience with these techniques in children is not readily available.

Treatment should be directed at compression of the extremity, elevation, and appropriate anticoagulant therapy. Varicose veins represent a rare complication of deep vein thrombosis (Fig. 7-4).

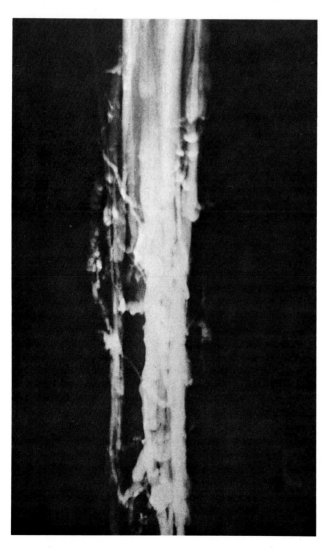

FIG. 7-4. Chronic multiple varicosities in a 14-year-old girl who sustained a tibial fracture at 3 years of age. Her major symptom was discomfort in the leg during strenuous athletic activity.

While thromboembolic disease is probably one of the most common and feared complications in adult orthopaedic patients, it is extremely unusual in children, especially in younger children who are otherwise normal.[39,40] It has been reported in a few adolescent children.[41] Certainly the risk rate is sufficiently low not to give prophylactic treatment for the disease, as one might in an adult. However, at least one-half of hospitalized adults develop venous thrombosis that cannot be diagnosed by current clinical means, so it also must be considered that thrombosis predisposing to embolic disease in children may be more common than we fully appreciate. A pulmonary embolic phenomenon is a rare complication of pediatric fractures in the lower extremity (see Fig. 7-3).

Hemorrhagic Complications

Hereditary coagulopathies

Certain hereditary hemorrhagic disorders may first manifest themselves in excessive bleeding following skeletal trauma. This may be the first indication of a disorder such as hemophilia, especially if the child has not had a previous injury that caused sufficient bleeding to make the diagnosis obvious, or if he has a mild clotting disorder.

A relatively common type of bleeding disorder is Von Willebrand's disease, which is a prolongation of normal bleeding time. This is probably the second most common inherited hemorrhagic disorder. The most common is hemophilia, which is a sex-linked disorder resulting in reduction of factor VIII. Christmas disease or hemophilia B (a deficiency of factor IX), can be differentiated from classic hemophilia. Many factors have been identified as necessary for proper coagulation. Interaction between these factors is probably best described by the "cascade" theory.

The goal of hematologic management in fracture treatment is to maintain sufficient levels of clotting factors for a sufficient period of time to forestall bleeding complications. This allows microhemostasis to occur. By this time, also, adequate treatment will have been rendered to minimize motion at the fracture site, which might cause further hemorrhage. Specific problems of fracture treatment in children with hemophilia will be covered in Chapter 8.

Acquired coagulopathies

Deficiencies of clotting factors may be acquired. Neonates may have excessive periosteal hemorrhage associated with birth injuries because of a relative deficiency of vitamin K. Children with malabsorption syndromes, liver disease, biliary atresia, and other similar conditions also may have deficient absorption of vitamins, so that they have an acute or chronic vitamin K deficiency.

Disseminated intravascular coagulation (DIC)

This term is given to a group of bleeding states of diverse etiology that usually present with accelerated, variable degrees of thrombosis and bleeding. They may accompany fat embolism syndrome, meningococcal sepsis (Fig. 7-5), mismatched blood, and massive blood transfusions. Their cen-

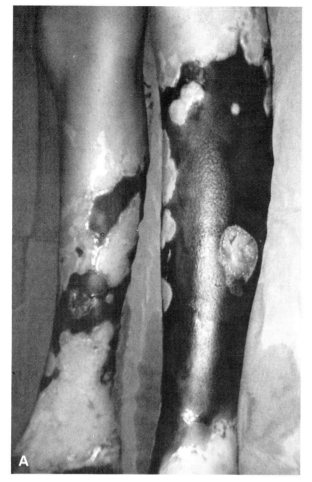

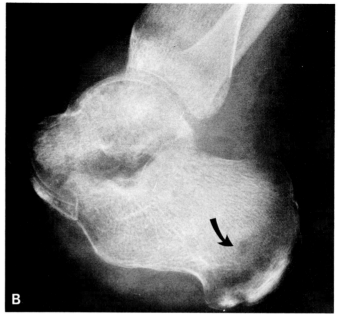

FIG. 7-5. A 13-year-old girl who sustained musculoskeletal complications of disseminated intravascular coagulopathy that was caused by meningococcal sepsis. *A*, Massive areas of cutaneous infarction required debridement and skin grafting. *B*, The feet were the most severely involved, with muscular infarction as well as cutaneous involvement. Amputations were done at the most distal levels possible, although revisions are anticipated depending on long term skin changes. Small areas of bone infarct (arrow) characterize the calcaneus, tibia, and fibula; these areas should not be misconstrued as osteomyelitic foci.

tral pathologic process appears to be a generalized activation or overactivation of the hemostatic mechanism beyond that expected for the local vascular response around a fracture. A notable feature of DIC is the reduced level of plasma fibrinogen, although this is variable because of the complex interaction of the many factors involved in DIC.

DIC usually causes bleeding at multiple sites, and occasionally it causes thrombotic episodes or acrocyanosis. Its diagnostic manifestations include a hemorrhagic-thrombotic diathesis, a specific coagulation test profile, the presence of fibrin thrombi, and a response to heparin therapy. Three abnormal screening tests that tend to be diagnostic are prothrombin time, fibrinogen level, and platelet function. If only two of the three are abnormal, a test for fibrinolysis (thrombin time, euglobulin clot lysis time, or fibrinogen degradation products) should be abnormal in order to establish the diagnosis.

The treatment of choice is heparin, which usually results in decreased bleeding.[42] The prothrombin time, fibrinogen level, and euglobulin lysis become normal within one to three days, although platelet levels do not respond uniformly to heparin therapy. Heparin should not be used if significant risk of intracranial bleeding is present. Epsilon aminocaproic acid (EACA) therapy aggravates DIC, and often results in thrombosis. There is no indication for its use in traumatized children.

Fat Embolism

This appears to be an infrequent complication in children, with adolescents being more likely to develop it than young children.[43] The greatest potential for developing fat embolism syndrome occurs in the presence of multiple fractures and multiple system injury.[44]

Onset may be immediate or in two to three days after the injury. Coma is the most severe presentation. There may be hemoptysis or pulmonary edema in the fulminant course. Early symptoms include shortness of breath, restlessness, and confusion. There may be progression to marked confusion, stupor, or coma. There may be urinary incontinence. Petechia may develop two to three days after injury. These are characteristically located across the chest, axilla, base of the neck, and under the conjunctiva. These lesions may be evanescent, and many milder cases can be overlooked. The diagnosis of "fracture fever" may be an unrecognized, mild variety of the fat embolism syndrome.

The most significant laboratory finding that characterizes the disease is decreased arterial oxygen tension. Arterial blood gases usually reveal hypoxemia and mild alkalosis. A sudden drop in hematocrit is also common. Urinary and sputum fat and serum lipase levels are probably of little value. The chest roentgenogram classically demonstrates interstitial infiltrates and obliterated peripheral vascular markings.

Scattered reports of fat embolism in children have occurred.[45,46] Limbird reported the complication in an 11-year-old boy with myelodysplasia.[47] He had been immobilized for anterior spine fusion, and sustained a fracture of the proximal tibial metaphysis. Shortly after the fracture he became tachypneic, febrile, mildly nauseated, and lethargic.

This syndrome is remarkably rare in normal children following major trauma. Drummond reported an incidence of 0.05% in 1800 children with pelvic and femoral fractures, compared to a 5.0% incidence in adults with similar injuries.[48] Carty found only six reports of fat embolism in children; however, he found a 90% incidence of fat embolism at autopsy in children dying from trauma, a statistic similar to that in the adult population.[49] It appears that children may sustain fat emboli relatively frequently, but do not develop the clinical syndrome as often as adults, due either to a difference in the type of embolized fat or to a decreased susceptibility to the toxic effects of the fat emboli. James noted that the fat content of the marrow in children, as compared with adults, is low, with relatively little of the more liquid fat, olein, and a higher proportion of palmitin and stearin.[50]

The pathogenesis of fat embolism syndrome is still controversial.[51] One possible source of embolic fat is the bone marrow (Fig. 7-6). Marrow and osseous fragments have been demonstrated in lung sections frequently enough to indicate that mechanical fat embolism probably does occur. However, more generalized blood lipid changes occur during stress, in combination with changes in blood coagulation systems, that may result in coalescence of chylomicrons into larger fat droplets. The physiochemical explanation of fat embolism postulates that changes occur in blood lipid stability after trauma, and the resultant altered microcirculatory flow patterns combine to result in inadequate tissue perfusion, subsequent tissue hypoxia, and the fat embolism syndrome. There certainly may be more than one source of fat in this syndrome.

Children with myelodysplasia, juvenile rheumatoid arthritis, collagen vascular disease, and various endocrine and metabolic disorders associated with osteoporosis are highly susceptible to the fat embolism syndrome.[48] All involved in the care of these children should be attuned to this potentially fatal complication.

Treatment should be directed at general respiratory support, as well as specific problems. The airways must be maintained, even if a tracheostomy must be performed. Blood volume should be restored and fluid and electrolyte balance maintained. The injured parts must be immobilized. Adequate oxygenation is the most important part of treatment, as respiratory failure is the most common cause of death from this syndrome. The use of steroids and heparin, while seemingly beneficial is still somewhat controversial. Albumin as an adjunct has also recently risen to popularity.

Neurologic Complications

Head injury

Head injuries occur much more commonly as a result of blunt trauma in children than in adults, and if present, they may complicate the overall evaluation of the child.[52] Possible reasons for the higher incidence in children are that the relatively larger head of a child may be more exposed to trauma, or that the child's head is less well supported on the neck and shoulder girdle. Whatever the exact explanation for the high incidence in children, the fact remains that head injuries are frequently associated with generalized blunt trauma in children. Aside from the errors in diagnosis that can result from evaluating an obtunded child, the lethal effects of subdural hematomas and progressive cerebral edema are a major cause of death in childhood.

Singer and Freeman provide an excellent review of approaches to handling the patient with mild head trauma and particularly address the issue of the importance of skull x-ray examinations.[53] They conclude with the following points: (1) patients with head trauma, especially if associated with loss of consciousness, should be examined and subsequently evaluated by reliable observers; (2) skull roentgenograms rarely provide information that affects medical management; (3) deterioration in the patient's clinical condition demands consultation and appropriate neuroradiologic studies; (4) the presence of a seizure or basilar skull fracture does not, in itself, necessitate therapy; and (5) continued evaluation of head trauma management is required to determine the optimal approach.

Head injury, particularly in children, presents a major problem in the treatment of fractures.[54] Many times, because of the severity of trauma necessary to create a head injury, there is a concomitant fracture of the postcranial skeleton. Problems then arise out of conflicting demands for treatment. The complications of one injury may interfere with the treatment of the other. An unconscious patient is frequently restless, whereas a fractured femur requires immobilization. A head injury requires cautious fluid replacement, whereas a femoral fracture may require copious fluid replacement. In the presence of a head injury, at least acutely, general anesthesia is better avoided, whereas the presence of

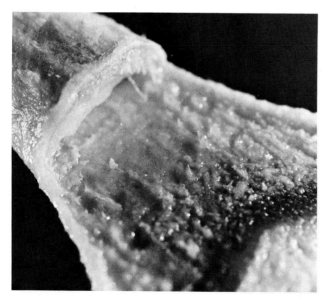

FIG. 7-6. Fatty marrow and trabecular replacement in an eight-year-old myelomeningocele child. This may explain the higher incidence of fat embolism in these children. However, this is not the normal appearance of a bone in a growing child with active hematopoietic marrow.

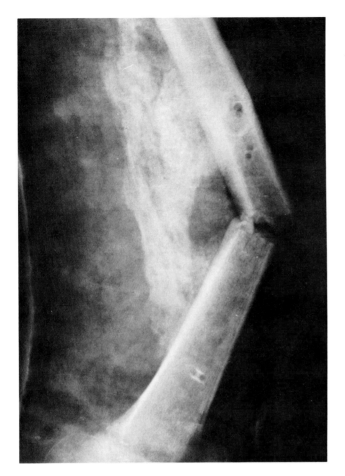

FIG. 7-7. Increased angulation in a 12-year-old with head injury. This occurred despite skeletal traction on the distal fragment. Notice the massive posterior callus, which probably indicates the extent of stripping and displacement of the periosteum that occurred due to hyperactivity and restlessness until the sensorium became more normal 5 weeks after injury.

a compound fracture necessitates adequate debridement under anesthesia. The patient may remain in a coma. Fat embolism from the femoral fracture may complicate assessment of the head injury. Deterioration in the level of consciousness usually is due to causes other than the head injury per se.

Fractures of the femur (Fig. 7-7) and humerus often are extremely difficult to manage in these restless, recumbent children.[55] If the head injury is minor and expected to clear in a day or two, the fracture should be immobilized by simple splinting and treated as indicated. When decerebration is likely to be prolonged beyond a few days, skeletal traction or internal fixation is recommended, depending upon the degree of restlessness and extent of other injuries. However, if the patient is a young child, classic intramedullary fixation could damage portions of the epiphysis and physis.

Herold reported accelerated fracture union, as determined radiographically, in fractured ulnae in brain-injured guinea pigs.[56] Massive heterotopic bone formation around joints may complicate severe head injuries (Fig. 7-8).[57]

Peripheral nerve injuries

Nerve injury associated with fracture or dislocation may be acute or delayed.[58-61] The diagnosis of primary nerve injury may be missed easily. The physican may discover the nerve complication several weeks after the injury, following removal of the splint or cast. In management, the *immediate* recognition of a primary nerve injury at the initial evaluation is important. Nerve involvement does not always occur at the time of trauma or during manipulation. Secondary nerve injuries may be attributed to scar and callus inclusion with pressure causing eventual dysfunction of the nerve.

In more chronic cases, there may be scarring about the nerve and adhesions to the bone. Such constriction of the nerve may cause neurotmetric degeneration at the site of the lesion. The nerve may even be caught between fracture fragments, with healing bone developing progressively around it. A third type of nerve involvement is the late (tardy) neuritis that frequently occurs many months or years after an injury, (particularly, progressive valgus deformity of the elbow with tardy ulnar palsy).[62]

During examinations, one should remember that a peripheral sensory nerve is manifest in the skin in three zones; autonomous, maximal, and intermediate.[63] The autonomous zone is supplied exclusively by a given nerve. After injury, whether contusion or transection, there is anesthesia in this isolated area. The maximal zone is the sensory area of a nerve that can be detected when function of adjacent sensory nerves is interrupted. This area is larger than the gross anatomic field of the nerve. Between these zones lies the intermediate zone where painful stimuli to pin pricks or extremes of hot and cold may be appreciated. This phenomenon is attributed to nerve overlap.

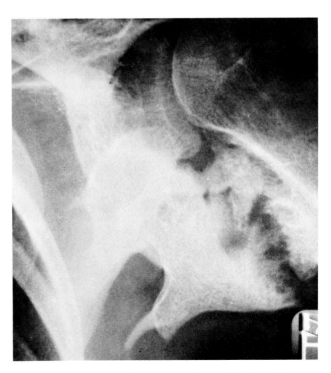

FIG. 7-8. Heterotopic bone around shoulder in a 16-year-old girl with severe head trauma.

Leonard felt that sensation in the digital nerve could return to skin "deprived" of nerve supply by proximal transection, even without nerve repair.[64] Probable mechanisms of this return of sensory function are fibers from adjacent nerves in the intermediate zone and budding from these adjacent nerves into the dermal plexus of the autonomous zone.[65,66] Adeymo demonstrated nerves running from the margins as well as from the bed into skin grafts.[67] This phenomenon seems to occur primarily in pure peripheral sensory nerves. Local extension could replace regeneration in nerve recovery in large sensory fields.[68]

In children, this recovery is sometimes surprisingly complete.[69] Further, return of sensation in transplanted skin in children is more complete than in adults.[70] Almquist, based on sensory nerve conduction velocity studies, concluded that better results of nerve repair in children were due to the adaptability of the sensory cortex rather than to increased maturation of the nerves.[71]

Experimentally, growth of nerve fibers into denervated areas in tadpoles has been demonstrated by Speidel.[72] Weddell suggests that the rapid recovery of sensation observed in baby rabbits after nerve section was due to local extension in the skin plexus of fibers from adjacent nerves.[73] Fitzgerald demonstrated reinnervation of the dermal plexus in young pigs.[74]

The parameters involved in recovery of sensation include the degree of neuronal regeneration and maturation, the maintenance of function in the end organs, the adaptability of the sensory cortex (relearning), and nerve overlap and budding. Nerve budding is probably more intense in children in whom the central nervous system is developing. In these children, overlap and budding may bring about a normal or almost normal return of sensation to the dermal plexuses. Even without repair of individual nerves the upper age limit at which sensation will return and whether the phenomenon is constant are unknown. This type of recovery of sensation appears to be most common in digital nerves.

The outcome of an injured peripheral nerve is contingent upon many factors, some of which are the age of the patient, the site of the lesion, the extent of the damage, the time interval before repair if the nerve has been severed, and accuracy of the repair.[75-78] Children seem to have a greater potential for neural repair and regeneration than adults.[79] It has been estimated that for every six days of delay before suturing, 1% of maximal performance is lost.[80] Therefore, early repair, at least by three months after injury, is encouraged. However, the time elapsed before repair does not seem to have as much effect on the recovery of sensory modalities. If repair has been delayed for more than a year, motor function rarely returns. However, sensation may return even if as many as two years have elapsed.

Altered fracture healing has been reported in many neurologic conditions, particularly peripheral nerve injury (Fig. 7-9). Many clinicians have observed more rapid union with exuberant callus in neurologically injured patients.[57,81-83] Others have noted decreased rates of healing. Despite clinical observations, little experimental investigation has been directed at this phenomenon, and most studies have been on skeletally mature animals.[56,84-87] Herold reported accelerated fracture healing in fractured ulnae of neurologically impaired guinea pigs.[56] Quilis showed a qualitative increase in callus formation in immature rats in which the primary rami of L3 through S1 had been sectioned.[86]

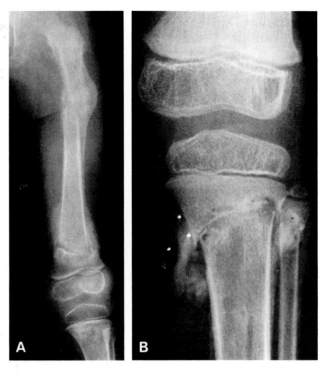

FIG. 7-9. Complications of sciatic nerve injury in a four-year-old girl sustaining sacroiliac and triradiate separations leading to a sciatic nerve-lumbosacral plexus injury. *A,* Healed femoral diaphyseal fracture complicated by fractures of proximal and distal femoral metaphyses through osteoporotic bone. *B,* One year later, following six weeks of immobilization after heel cord lengthening, the patient fractured her proximal tibia.

Post-traumatic reflex dystrophy

This syndrome has a number of descriptive terms, the most common of which is Sudeck's atrophy. This symptom complex is also known as causalgia, post-traumatic painful osteoporosis, minor causalgia, post-traumatic sympathetic dystrophy, shoulder-hand syndrome, and chronic traumatic edema.

The syndrome consists of continuous pain, hyperesthesia, and autonomic symptoms in an extremity, often following relatively minor trauma.[88,89] The precipitating insult occasionally may be infection, thrombosis, a burn, an animal bite, or frostbite. The signs and symptoms observed in the involved extremity are burning or aching pain, discoloration (cyanosis, plethora, or erythema), swelling, joint stiffness, hyperhydrosis, and altered sensation (hyperesthesia, hypesthesia, or parasthesia). These signs may occur in a glove or stocking distribution, or in a distinct sensory distribution.

Reflex sympathetic dystrophy is rare in children.[90-92] Fermaglich reported two cases.[93] In the first case, the patient was treated with a local block using triamcinolone acetonide and lidocaine. Treatment in the second case consisted simply of elevation and immobilization. Both cases resolved satisfactorily. Kozin described a three-year-old boy who developed this syndrome following an injection of pain medication in the buttock; this patient was treated successfully with prednisone.[94] While this syndrome appears to be uncommon in children, approximately 8% of the patients in a large study of post-traumatic reflex dystrophies were less than 19 years of age.[95]

Characteristically, the patchy osteopenia evident on radiographs may take five to seven weeks to develop, but it is infrequently seen in skeletally immature individuals (Fig. 7-10).

Although the progression of osteopenia can be reduced or halted in many patients, improvement in bone mineral content is not always seen.[89] Indeed, to Kozin's knowledge, the only prior case of this syndrome in which improvement of osteopenia occurred was in a child.[92] This may reflect an inability of adult bone to sufficiently remineralize and remodel when osteopenia has been present for a critical period.

Little is known about the pathophysiology of this syndrome, although increased local blood flow to the affected limb has been demonstrated. One popular hypothesis is that a reflex arc is established in the subcortical, internuncial neuronal pool, producing chronic and excessive activity in the autonomic nervous system.[96] A series of reflexes dependent upon cross-stimulation between sympathetic afferent fibers and damage to the myelin that sensory fibers depend upon may account for the underlying pathophysiology.

Another postulate is that chronic irritation of a peripheral sensory nerve leads to abnormal activity in the internuncial neuron center, which leads, in turn, to a continuum of increased stimulation of afferent motor and sympathetic neurons. As a consequence, normal vasoregulatory controls are disrupted, and local blood flow is increased, with secondary changes taking place in skin and subcutaneous tissue, and demineralization of bone.

Many therapeutic modalities have been advocated, including physical therapy, exercise, sympathectomy, and cor-

ticosteroids. Any or all of these measures may be effective when employed *early* in the disease, but the response rate progressively decreases the longer treatment is delayed. Recent studies have shown a predictable improvement in several objective clinical measurements with systemic corticosteroid therapy, even in patients who have had symptoms for several months or longer.[88]

Chondro-Osseous Complications

Hypercalcemia

Immobilization for the treatment of children's fractures normally does not produce significant changes in serum calcium levels. As part of the normal repair process, there is significant mobilization of calcium from the skeletal system during immobilization. This is reflected clinically as hypercalciuria, but a significant elevation of serum calcium levels generally does not occur in normal patients who are confined to bed rest or immobilized in body casts for treatment of fractures.

Cristofaro[97] reported that 7 of 20 patients admitted consecutively to the Rancho Los Amigos Hospital demonstrated hypercalcemia ranging from 10.7 to 13.2 mg% (upper range of normal is 10.5).[97,98] Return to normocalcemia coincided with mobilization in five of seven patients. Four patients developed heterotopic ossification; two of these had concurrent hypercalcemia. Cristofaro[97] concluded that hypercalcemia due to immobilization occurs more frequently than suggested by other authors. He also found that elevated alkaline phosphatase levels were associated with heterotopic ossification. However, the role of hypercalcemia in the development of heterotopic ossification must remain speculative.

Hypercalcemia complicating the treatment of pediatric fractures is encountered occasionally in immobilized patients with pre-existing metabolic or bone disease, and, although encountered less frequently, it may also accompany immobilization in patients with absolutely no predisposing factors.[99-104]

The classic description of hypercalcemia complicating the immobilization of a patient without pre-existing metabolic disease was by Albright, who named the condition "acute bone atrophy" and emphasized that it must be distinguished from hyperparathyroidism.[105] A review of previously reported cases showed that the complication is most common in adolescents, rather than younger children, in whom the normal rate of osseous metabolism prior to immobilization is already quite high because of the increase in growth rate.

All previously reported cases of immobilization hypercalcemia occurred in children between the ages of 9 and 14 years.[106] This occurrence is attributed to the fact that the rate of bone turnover during this particular growth period is more rapid. Normally there is a balance between bone formation and resorption in the active young individual. The balance is influenced by age, nutritional and hormonal factors, and degrees of activity. Bone formation decreases when immobilization eliminates these stimuli. The normal equilibrium is upset, resulting in bone demineralization that is excessive compared to bone formation, and release of calcium into the extracellular fluid. Ordinarily, this extra load is excreted by the kidney with resultant hypercalciuria and

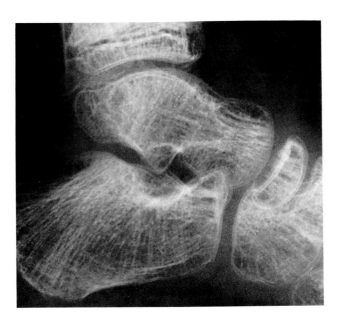

FIG. 7-10. Ten-year-old with reflex sympathetic dystrophy after an ankle sprain. Note the diffuse osteoporosis. The subchondral plate of the navicula has a double contour.

maintenance of a normal serum calcium level. Urinary excretion reaches a peak value approximately four weeks after immobilization begins.

It is important to recognize this syndrome, since its treatment is generally easy. The patient may complain of nausea and vomiting, abdominal pain and tenderness. There is anorexia. Dehydration is common. Lethargy, pain with movement, an apparent flaccid paralysis, and muscle hypotonia appear. Vision may be blurred. In cases such as this, immediate serum calcium levels should be drawn. The importance of this syndrome lies in the fact that it is readily treated if recognized early.

An elevation of serum calcium above 15 mg/100 ml should be considered an acute crisis. Levels between 10 and 15 mg/100 ml may be associated with milder symptoms. Usually the serum alkaline phosphatase level is normal, thus distinguishing the condition from hyperparathyroidism, in which this level is generally high. The differential diagnosis of immobilization hypercalcemia as distinct from primary hyperparathyroidism is probably best accomplished by parathormone essay.

Treatment is relatively easy and effective. A low calcium diet limits calcium ingestion. Mithramycin also effectively lowers serum calcium either by direct antagonism of bone resorption or by interference in metabolism of parathyroid hormone.[107] Dehydration usually is a factor, so fluid replacement assumes primary importance. Saline diuresis, with volumes of up to ten liters per day, appears effective. Phosphate ion, administered orally or intravenously, binds with calcium ion and is deposited in the bone. The most important therapeutic measure is immediate institution of as much movement and weightbearing as is practical and safe. If untreated, significant neurologic complications may occur, especially supratentorially, with residual convulsions and loss of hearing.

Institution of calcitonin therapy will relieve the symptoms rapidly.[108] Pezeshki described two adolescents in whom hypercalcemia was successfully treated by subcutaneous injections of salmon calcitonin.[109] The danger that an excessive drop in the calcium level will lead to tetany must be avoided.[110] Corticosteroid administration has also been effective in treating hypercalcemia.

Although profound hypercalcemia occurring as a result of immobilization is rare, it can progress to crisis levels. Henke reported a 13-year-old boy in whom failure to consider hypercalcemia as the source of progressive anorexia, nausea, vomiting, and irritability resulted in respiratory arrest and a nearly fatal outcome after a simple femoral fracture.[111] The case of Henke should be considered *immobilization hypercalcemic crisis.* The mortality rate from acute hypercalcemic crisis has been reported as high as 50%.[112]

Myositis ossificans

Traumatic myositis ossificans is a poorly understood condition in which heterotopic bone forms in injured muscle (Fig. 7-11) or around a joint (Fig. 7-12). Certain muscles are affected preferentially, and the condition seems to follow an orderly, predictable course. The condition is seen most frequently in teenagers, although occasionally in younger children.[113] Wilkes reported a case in a three-year-old boy; the lesion was removed seven months later.[114] Dickerson

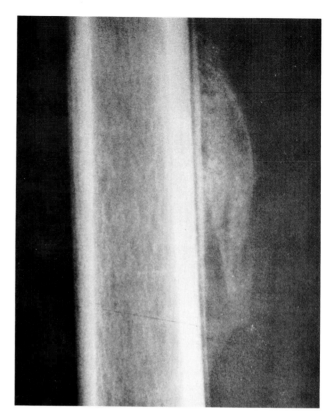

FIG. 7-11. Myositis ossificans in 11-year-old hockey player who was struck across the thigh. The thin, new bone formation is subperiosteal new bone, while the more superficial bone is probably forming extraperiosteally (intramuscularly).

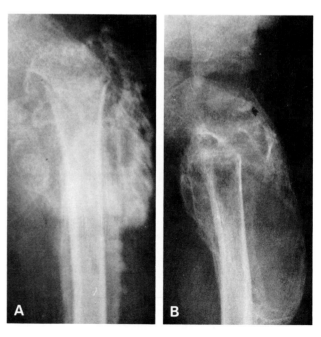

FIG. 7-12. *A,* Ectopic bone formation seven weeks after an intertrochanteric fracture. *B,* Four months later, maturation of the callus is evident.

described an occurrence of this condition in a five-year-old child.[115]

The relatively common incidence of myositis ossificans following dislocation of the elbow is even greater when there is an associated fracture. Incidence is also high if the elbow is treated by open reduction later than the first 24 to 48 hours after the injury (Fig. 7-13). Children are less prone to develop this complication after elbow injury. Even when ectopic calcification forms, there is a greater propensity to resorb it before it can become mature bone.[116]

Patients developing the complication generally have roentgenographic evidence within three to four weeks after their initial injury. This may gradually resorb with inception of joint motion (if periarticular). Resorption is less likely if the bone is adjacent or attached to the diaphysis. With no evidence of any osseous resorption for six to eight months post-injury, the condition is probably mature.

Attempts to excise the ectopic bone should be delayed until the process has completely matured, usually about one year after injury.

Pseudarthrosis

This complication is extremely rare in children (Fig. 7-14), undoubtedly because the periosteal/endosteal osteoblastic response in children is rapid and prolific, quickly bridging the fracture with primary callus. Compound injuries, which often are associated with pseudarthrosis, are infrequent in children. However, when they do occur, the child may lose sufficient periosteal tissue (type 9 injury) to predispose the fracture to pseudarthrosis (see Fig. 4-41). Underlying bone disorders (e.g., fibrous dysplasia) may create a predisposition to this pseudarthrosis, often after seemingly minimal trauma.

The cases tend to occur in older children, and show similar osseous involvement as adults.[117,118] The tibia is involved most often. Forearm fractures in adolescents who are nearing skeletal maturity may require operative treatment to prevent nonunion of at least one of the bones.

As in adults, the treatment of choice for pseudarthrosis is operative, with utilization of bone graft and, if necessary, some type of skeletal fixation. Complete (circumferential), subperiosteal stripping to expose the entire pseudarthrosis should be avoided. Leaving some of this tissue, which has mechanical integrity and the potential to modulate into osteoblastic tissue, may minimize or negate the need for metallic fixation. Once exposed sufficiently, the interposed fibrous tissue should be removed, although complete resection is generally not necessary in children. The exposed subchondral bone on either side of the pseudarthrosis impedes the normal endosteal response. It should be drilled so that the marrow cavity on each side is in communication with the pseudarthrosis. Iliac crest bone is easily obtained and fashioned into inlay/onlay grafts. If metallic fixation is used, the remaining growth potential of the bone must be respected when choosing the type of fixation.

Synostosis

Another complication, also due to type 9 periosteal injury, is the formation of a synostosis between the radius and the ulna or the tibia and the fibula (Fig. 7-15). Again, this complication is unusual in children, because severity of trauma is insufficient to disrupt interosseous tissues and lead to some type of continuity between paired bones. This complication may occur in the elbow region, although one must be careful not to attribute proximal radioulnar synostosis to trauma.

With diaphyseal lesions, careful resection may be successful after the lesion has matured. Since such an injury is comparable to myositis ossificans, early resection presumably enhances the possibility of recurrence. Since fibular rotation is essential for normal ankle function, resection of a synostosis is advisable in a young child, if only to redirect chondroosseous development along a more normal pathway.

Fracture recurrence

Arunachalam described 20 children with refractures, predominantly of the forearm.[119] He noted a significant increase of deformity occurring after refracture.

Refracture probably occurs either because the original fracture has not united soundly or because an identical mechanism of injury has occurred (Fig. 7-16). There is sufficient confidence in the certainty of rapid and effective union of injuries in children that delayed union is never seriously contemplated. Because of this, the tendency is to take children out of immobilization devices earlier than they probably should be, especially in view of their general hyperactivity. It was noted in the study of fracture recurrence that many of the children did not have roentgenograms taken at the time of discontinuation of immobilization, the decision that they were sufficiently healed being based on clinical examination. Children often deny pain. It is imperative that adequate fracture healing be documented roentgenographically before treatment is discontinued.

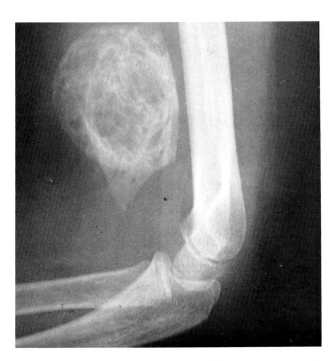

FIG. 7-13. Myositis ossificans is evident several months after elbow dislocation.

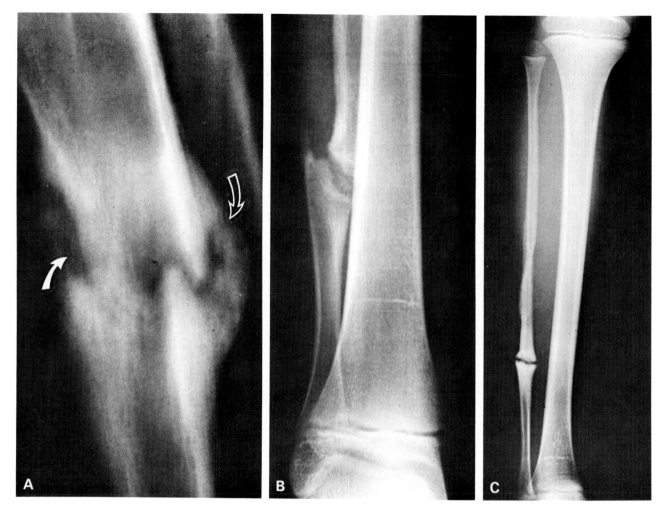

FIG. 7-14. *A*, Tomogram of painful tibial fracture 6 months after injury in a 13-year-old girl. There was mild subperiosteal callus posteriorly, and the cortical bone has almost fused to endosteal bone (solid arrow). Anteriorly, there is a better subperiosteal callus response, although the fracture line continues through it (open arrow). This girl was subsequently treated with bone grafting. *B*, Pseudarthrosis of the fibula. *C*, Pseudarthrosis of the fibula with overgrowth and flaring.

Epiphysiolysis

As shown in Chapter 4, a temporary type 8 growth mechanism impairment is caused by a blockage of the nutrient arterial circulation to the juxtaphyseal metaphysis. Since the epiphyseal side of the physis is unaffected, the physis continues to grow by deposition to the cell columns. Without concomitant replacement by the metaphyseal neovascularity, the physis widens and becomes slightly less mechanically stable. If a child treated for metaphyseal fracture inadvertently stresses the contiguous physis after removal of a cast, an epiphyseal fracture (type 1 or 2) may occur (Fig. 7-17). This should be treated by reduction and further immobilization.

Postfracture cyst

The pathogenesis of a variety of cystic bone lesions in children remains in doubt. Trauma has been implicated as the inciting factor in some cystic lesions, although the occurrence of bone cysts during fracture healing has not been well documented. Levine described a case of fracture of the tibia and fibula with development of a cystic lesion in the fibula during healing.[120] There seemed little doubt, in view of the exploration that was carried out, that vascular injury with hemorrhage into a closed space resulted in an encapsulated hematoma which produced the lesion. Presumably, the periosteum was stripped for several centimeters on each side of the fracture site, and it is possible that this lesion represented a false aneurysm. The lesion had an appearance quite similar to that of a pseudotumor complicating hemophilia.

Exostosis/osteochondroma

The possible role of trauma in causing the formation of exostoses or solitary osteochondromata is uncertain. Figure 7-18 shows a fracture of the distal radius and ulna that was left in side-to-side (bayonet) apposition after an unsuccessful closed reduction. While the ulna remodeled extensively in the ensuing 16 months, a small area of the proximal frag-

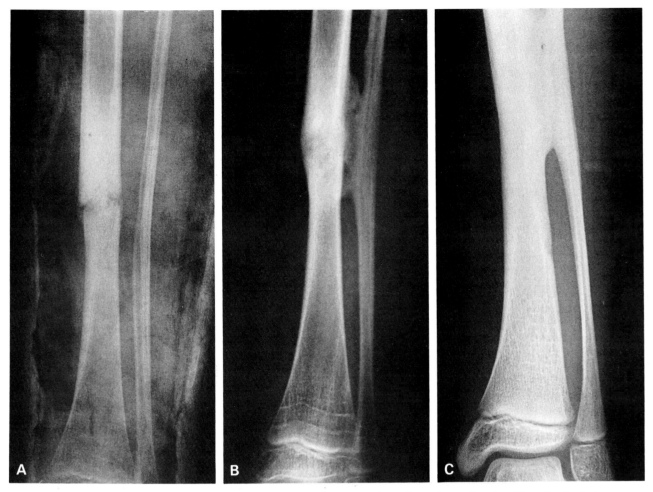

FIG. 7-15. *A*, Seemingly innocuous fracture of tibia. *B*, Four months later, bone formation is evident in the interosseous space. *C*, At one year, synostosis is present.

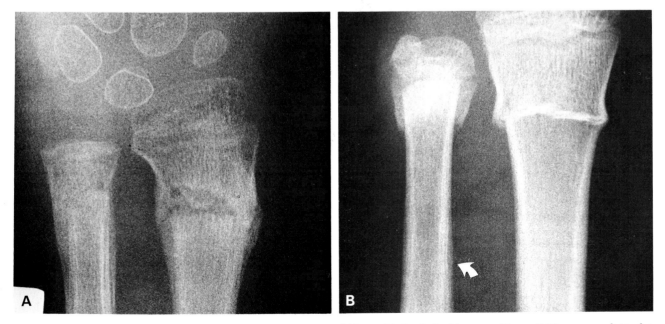

FIG. 7-16. *A*, Fracture of distal radius and ulna in a five-year-old boy. This healed without problems. *B*, Three years later, he fractured the region again. The arrow shows some residual subperiosteal bone from the first fracture.

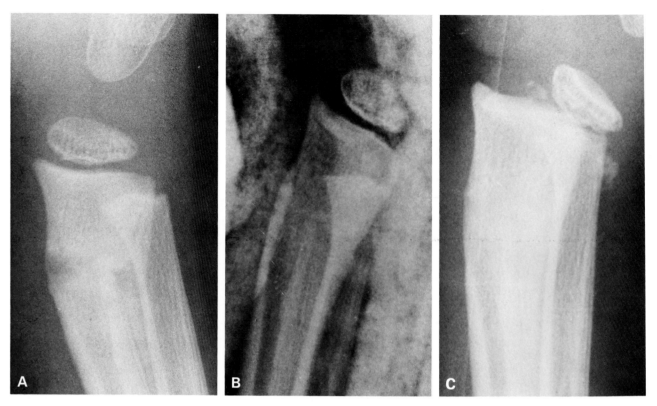

FIG. 7-17. *A*, Metaphyseal fracture in a five-year-old. *B*, This fracture was placed in a cast for four weeks. *C*, Three days after removal of the cast, the child fell and sustained an epiphyseal fracture (type 2). The metaphyseal fracture has healed.

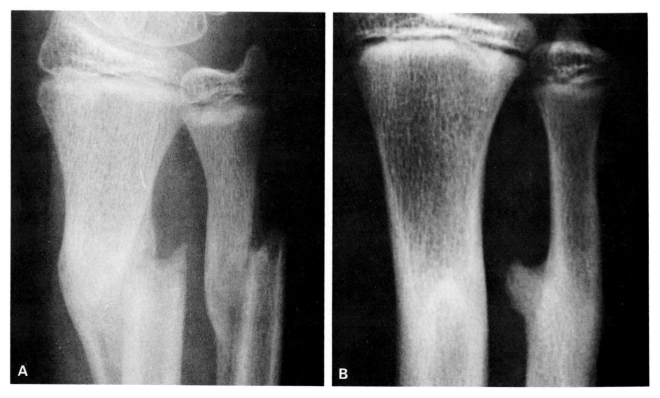

FIG. 7-18. *A*, Overriding distal radius and ulna fractures in an 11-year-old boy. *B*, The radius healed smoothly. However, a large exostosis developed in the ulna. This did not impair function.

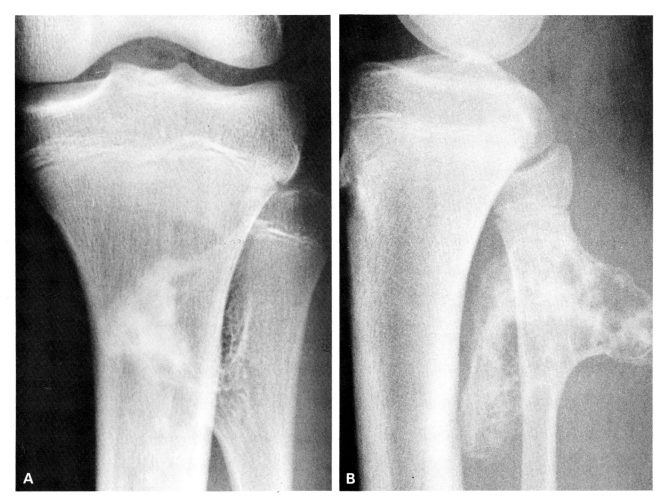

FIG. 7-19. Anterior, *A*, and lateral, *B*, views of large, proximal fibular osteochondroma. The boy had been kicked in the popliteal fossa, and a mass had developed within two years. However, roentgenograms were not taken until five years after the injury.

ment remained. Presumably this was herniated through the periosteal sleeve and was not subsequently surrounded by tissue capable of resorbing the fragment end. Another possible explanation is that heterotopic bone formed in the interosseous membrane.

If the peripheral growth plate (or epiphysis) is avulsed or otherwise damaged (type 6 or 7 injury), the normal restraints to appositional physeal cartilaginous growth may be disrupted and formation of an osteochondroma allowed. Figure 7-19 shows a teenager with a large, solitary fibular osteochondroma that developed progressively (based on clinical examination) over a five year period after he was kicked in the lateral popliteal fossa. Progressive peroneal neuropathy necessitated removal. Figure 7-20 shows a boy who sustained a type 3 distal femoral injury that was complicated primarily by an osseous bridge. However, at one margin, an osteochondroma is forming.

Malunion

Angular malunion is often encountered in pediatric fractures. In fact, it is commonly suggested that an angulation of up to 30° beyond normal longitudinal alignment will correct spontaneously. However, remodeling and physeal growth may not always realign the bone (Fig. 7-21), and every effort should be made to obtain longitudinal alignment of the fracture fragments (in both sagittal and coronal planes). Rotational malalignment never corrects itself (see Fig. 4-1). Therefore, it must be restored during fracture treatment. Some degree of rotational malunion (which often accompanies supracondylar fractures) may be compensated for in the upper extremity, primarily because of the nature of the scapulothoracic and glenohumeral joints. But in the lower extremity, rotational malunion can cause significant changes in the gait pattern.

Traction complications

Proper pin placement is essential in children (Fig. 7-22). Placement too close to the surface, because of the relative porosity of metaphyseal bone, may result in the pin pulling out of the bone. Placement too close to the surface may also result in the pin moving subperiosteally or extraperiosteally, so that there is no skeletal traction. The pin must not be placed near or through a physis, or long term growth complications may follow. The treating physician must be aware of the contours of the physes of the proximal ulna, distal femur, and proximal tibia, the areas used most often for placement of skeletal traction pins. While not often used in children, calcaneal traction must also be done carefully, as there is an epiphyseal/physeal growth mechanism in this region.

Miscellaneous Complications

Foreign bodies

Children frequently place objects beneath the cast. Neff reported a case in which a rubber band, placed around a plastic bag to protect the cast during bathing, had gotten under the cast and was constricting the common peroneal nerve and causing neuropraxia.[121]

Fat fractures

The most common cause of a fat fracture is a sharp, non-lacerating force, such as a dog bite. It may overlie an osseous injury. The phenomenon is fortunately rare, and usually late to appear, with an interval of several months between injury and initial observation. It is almost impossible to foresee this clinical entity because of the swelling accompanying the underlying skeletal injury. Fat fractures are probably caused by a shearing force through the subcutaneous fat, superficial fascia, and on occasion, deep fascia. This creates a diathesis in the fat compartment; and a degree of fat necrosis is present as a result of the original compression-contusion force. As resolution occurs, the proximal edge is elevated and the distal edge flattened. Attempts to restore normal planes by fat, fascial, and muscle rotation flaps are difficult and sometimes associated with major complications.

Cast syndrome

While this is an uncommon problem in the treatment of childhood fractures, the increased emphasis on immediate reduction and application of a spica cast for hip dislocations and femoral fractures as well as cast treatment of childhood spinal fractures increases the potential for its occurrence. The severity of the symptoms, the lethal potential, and need for prompt, effective treatment mandate recognition in the early stages. The term *cast syndrome* has been applied primarily to the association of arterio-mesenteric duodenal obstruction with immobilization. It has been reported relatively frequently in adolescents and young adults, with or without cast application, and particularly following spine surgery (e.g., scoliosis correction).[122,123]

Its signs and symptoms are typical of an upper gastrointestinal obstruction. They may develop acutely or insidiously. Initial symptoms include "fullness," nausea, vomiting, and progressive abdominal distension. Vomiting may lead to dehydration and metabolic alkalosis.

The pathogenesis appears to be localized to the junction of the third and fourth parts of the duodenum, where the duodenum is bound by the ligament of Treitz (Fig. 7-23). This is juxtaposed to the origin of the superior mesenteric artery. The duodenum may be compressed posteriorly by the lumbar spine and aorta, and anteriorly by the mesenteric artery. Recumbency further contributes to the compression as does increased lumbar lordosis. This leads to gastric outflow obstruction, gastric dilation, and a compounding of the problem.

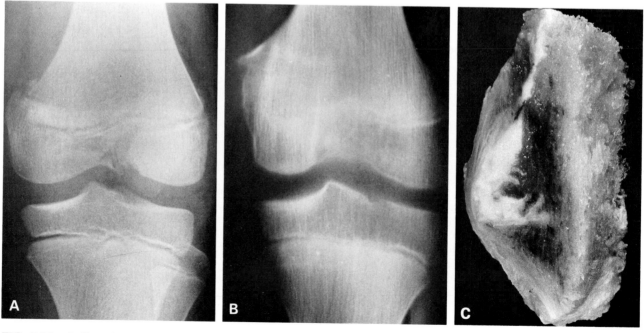

FIG. 7-20. *A,* Type 3 injury to distal femur. This was treated by open reduction and pin fixation. *B,* Premature osseous bridging and a peripheral osteochondroma developed. *C,* Pathologic specimen, showing remnant of physis, and larger portion of physeal cartilage along the metaphysis. The osseous bridge is adjacent to the physis.

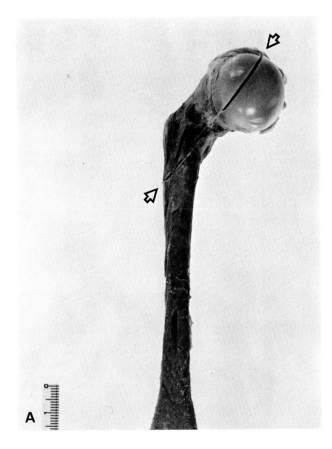

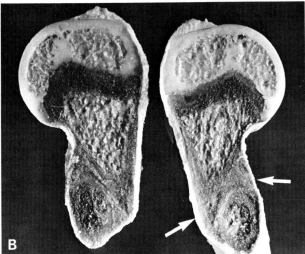

FIG. 7-21. *A*, Malunion of proximal humerus in seven-year-old child. This fracture was sustained five months prior to death from leukemia. The lateral view shows 40° of malunion from a proximal metaphyseal fracture. The plane of section used to create the "opened" fracture shown in *B* is indicated by the arrows. *B*, New bone and fibrous tissue fill the subperiosteal space and extensive remodeling has taken place in the five months, although the original cortex (arrows) is still evident. Juxtaphyseal metaphyseal changes (darkened trabeculae) are also grossly evident, reflecting the changes caused by decreased blood flow when the nutrient artery was disrupted.

Treatment is contingent upon the severity of the symptoms. Dietary restriction may be sufficient. Nasogastric intubation may be necessary to decompress gastric dilation. Intravenous hyperalimentation may be necessary. Electrolyte balance should be monitored closely, and corrected as indicated. Positioning the patient on the left side or prone may relieve the symptoms. Windowing the jacket over the abdomen rarely is successful. Very infrequently, surgery is necessary, with duodenojejunostomy being the most common relief procedure.

Infection

Infections certainly may complicate fracture treatment in children.[124] The infection may be introduced directly, as in an open fracture, or it may be caused by hematogenous seeding of the traumatized tissue from an extraosseous, often distant, source. Infection is discussed in detail in Chapter 6.

References

1. Epps, C. H., Jr., (ed.): Complications in Orthopaedic Surgery. Philadelphia, J. B. Lippincott, 1978.
2. Touloukian, R.: Pediatric Trauma. New York, John Wiley & Sons, 1978.
3. Shires, T., et al.: Fluid therapy in hemorrhage shock. Arch. Surg., *88:*688, 1964.
4. Smith, R. F., Szilagyi, E., and Elliot, J. P., Jr.: Fracture of long bones with arterial injury due to blunt trauma. Arch. Surg., *99:*315, 1969.
5. Shaker, I. J., White, J. J., and Signer, R. D.: Special problems of vascular injuries in children. J. Trauma, *16:*863, 1976.
6. Bloom, J. D., et al.: Defective limb growth as a complication of catheterization of the femoral artery. Surg. Gynecol. Obstet., *138:*524, 1974.
7. Boros, S. J., et al.: Leg growth following umbilical artery catheter-associated thrombus formation—a 4-year follow-up. J. Pediatr., *87:*973, 1975.
8. White, J. J., Talbert, J. L., and Haller, J. A.: Peripheral arterial injuries in infants and children. Ann. Surg., *167:*757, 1968.
9. Whitehouse, W. M., et al.: Pediatric vascular trauma. Arch. Surg., *111:*1269, 1976.
10. Holden, C. E. A.: Compartmental syndromes following trauma. Clin. Orthop., *113:*95, 1975.
11. Matsen, F. A., III: Compartmental syndrome: a unified concept. Clin. Orthop., *113:*8, 1975.
12. Rorabeck, C. H., and Clarke, K. M.: The pathophysiology of Volkmann's ischemia. Orthop. Trans., *2:*78, 1978.
13. Sheridan, G. W., and Matsen, F. A., III: An animal model of the compartment syndrome. Clin. Orthop., *113:*36, 1975.
14. Whitesides, T. E., Jr., et al.: Tissue pressure measurements as a determinant for the need of fasciotomy. Clin. Orthop., *113:*43, 1975.
15. Hargens, A. R., et al.: Fluid balance within the canine anterolateral compartment and its relationship to compartment syndromes. J. Bone Joint Surg., *60-A:*499, 1978.
16. Hargens, A. R., et al.: Peripheral nerve-conduction block by high muscle-compartment pressure. J. Bone Joint Surg., *61-A:*92, 1979.
17. Matsen, F. A., III, et al.: Monitoring of intramuscular pressure. Surgery, *79:*702, 1976.
18. Mubarak, S. J., et al.: Acute compartment syndromes: diagnosis and treatment with the aid of the wick catheter. J. Bone Joint Surg., *60-A:*1091, 1978.
19. Feagin, J. A., and White, A. A., III: Volkmann's ischemia treated by transfibular fasciotomy. Milit. Med., *38:*497, 1973.

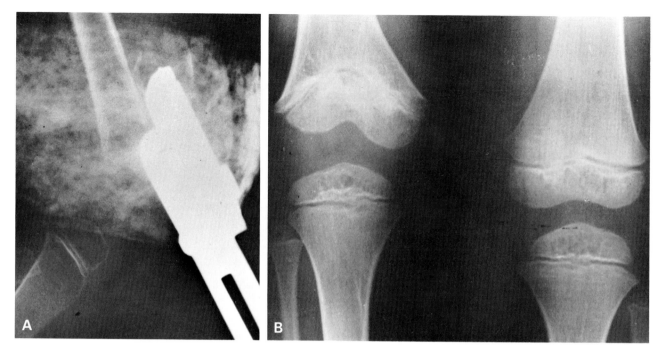

FIG. 7-22. *A,* Skeletal traction for a femoral fracture in a four-year-old. This was placed close to the distal femoral physis anteriorly. *B,* Five years later, significant disruption of physeal development and longitudinal growth is evident. A large central bridge formed, but peripherally, the physis has continued to grow.

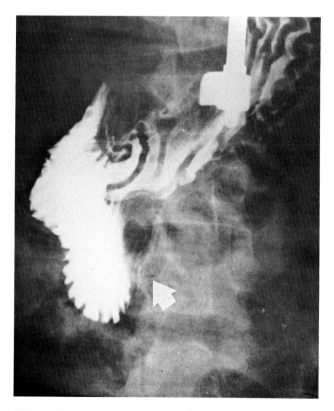

FIG. 7-23. Cast syndrome complicating a scoliosis fusion. There is obvious obstruction of the duodenum. This was relieved by changing the cast and placing the patient in less hyperextension with less molding over the pelvis.

20. Hsu, L. C. S., et al.: Valgus deformity of the ankle in children with fibular pseudarthrosis. J. Bone Joint Surg., *56-A:*503, 1974.
21. Volkmann, R.: Die ischamischen Muskellahmjungen und-kontrakturen. Zentralbl. Chir., *51:*801, 1881.
22. Jones, D. R. B., and McIntyre, I. M. C.: Venous thrombosis in infancy and childhood. Arch. Dis. Child., *50:*153, 1975.
23. Sobotka, M. R.: Postoperative deep venous thrombosis in a nine year old girl. Ned. Tijdschr. Geneeskd., *119:*916, 1975.
24. Tournay, R.: Venous thrombosis of the lower limbs in the child. Phlebologie, *21:*381, 1968.
25. Wise, R. C., and Todd, J. K.: Spontaneous lower-extremity venous thrombosis. Am. J. Dis. Child., *126:*766, 1973.
26. Horwitz, J., and Shenker, I. R.: Spontaneous deep vein thrombosis in adolescence. Clin. Pediatr., *16:*787, 1977.
27. Hughes, E.: Venous obstruction in the upper extremity. Br. J. Surg., *36:*155, 1948.
28. Kleincasser, L. J.: Effort thrombosis of the axillary and subclavian veins. Arch. Surg., *59:*258, 1949.
29. Clyne, C. A. C., et al.: Thrombectomy for ilio-femoral venous occlusion: the youngest reported case. J. Pediatr. Surg., *12:*703, 1977.
30. Marks, J. G., Jr., and Sussman, S. J.: Thrombophlebitis in an eight year old girl. J. Pediatr., *80:*336, 1972.
31. Fonkalsrud, E. W.: Post-infusion phlebitis in infants and children. Clin. Pediatr., *8:*135, 1969.
32. Fontaine, J. L., Lasfargues, G., N'ghiem-Minh-Dung: Les thromboses des veines profondes des membres chez l'enfant. Arch. Fr. Pediatr., *26:*249, 1969.
33. Joffe, S.: Postoperative deep vein thrombosis in children. J. Pediatr. Surg., *10:*539, 1975.
34. Kakkar, V. V.: The diagnosis of deep vein thrombosis using the I^{125} fibrinogen test. Arch. Surg., *104:*152, 1972.
35. Negas, D.: The diagnosis of deep-vein thrombosis. Br. J. Surg., *52:*830, 1972.
36. Flanc, C., Kakkar, V. V., and Clark, M. B.: The detection of

venous thrombosis of the legs using ^{125}I-labeled fibrinogen. Br. J. Surg., 55:742, 1967.

37. Evans, D. S.: The early diagnosis of thromboembolism by ultrasound. Ann. R. Coll. Surg. Engl., 49:255, 1971.

38. Strandness, D. E., and Summer, D. S.: Ultrasound velocity detector in the diagnosis of thrombophlebitis. Arch. Surg., 104:180, 1972.

39. Birzle, H., and Reinwein, H.: Beckenventhrombosen in Kindesalter. Beitr. Klin. Chir., 219:440, 1972.

40. MacIntyre, I. M., Jones, D. R., and Ruckley, C. V.: Venous thromboembolism in childhood. Thromb. Diath. Haemat., 34:563, 1975.

41. Greenwood, R. D., and Traisman, H. S.: Pediatric-pulmonary embolism: thromboembolism in a child. J. Kans. Med. Soc., 76:34, 1975.

42. Colman, R. W., Robboy, S. J., and Minna, J. D.: Disseminated intravascular coagulation (DIC): an approach. Am. J. Med., 52:679, 1972.

43. Shulman, S. T., and Grossman, B. J.: Fat embolism in children. Am. J. Dis. Child., 120:480, 1970.

44. Tedeschi, C. G., Walter, C. E., and Tedeschi, L. G.: Shock and fat embolism: an appraisal. Surg. Clin. North Am., 48:431, 1968.

45. Allred, A. J.: Fat embolism. Br. J. Surg., 41:82, 1953.

46. Richards, H. G.: A case of fat embolism in early childhood. Edinburgh Med. J., 57:252, 1950.

47. Limbird, T. J., and Ruderman, R. J.: Fat embolism in children. Clin. Orthop., 136:267, 1978.

48. Drummond, D. S., Salter, R. B., and Boone, J.: Fat embolism in children: its frequency and relationships to collagen disease. Can. Med. Assoc. J., 101:200, 1969.

49. Carty, J. B.: Fat embolism in children. Am. J. Surg., 94:970, 1957.

50. James, E. S.: Fat embolism. Can. Med. Assoc. J., 62:548, 1950.

51. Peltier, L. F.: Fat embolism: a current concept. Clin. Orthop., 66:241, 1969.

52. Knighton, R. S., Jackson, I. J., and Thompson, R. R.: Pediatric Neurosurgery. Springfield, Charles C Thomas, 1959.

53. Singer, H. S., and Freeman, J. M.: Head trauma for the pediatrician. Pediatrics, 62:819, 1978.

54. Hoffer, M., Garrett, A., and Brink, J.: The orthopaedic management of brain-injured children. J. Bone Joint Surg., 53-A:567, 1971.

55. Gibson, J. M. C.: Multiple injuries: the management of the patient with a fractured femur and a head injury. J. Bone Joint Surg., 42-B:425, 1960.

56. Herold, H. A., Tadmor, A., and Hurvitz, A.: Callus formation after acute brain damage. Isr. J. Med. Sci., 6:163, 1970.

57. Calandriello, B.: Callus formation in severe brain injuries. Bull. Hosp. Joint Dis., 25:170, 1964.

58. Collins, H. R.: Damage of peripheral nerve associated with orthopedic injuries. South Med. J., 60:355, 1967.

59. Gurdjian, E. S., and Smathers, H. M.: Peripheral nerve injury in fractures and dislocations of long bones. J. Neurosurg., 2:202, 1945.

60. Lewis, D., and Miller, G. M.: Peripheral nerve injuries associated with fractures. Ann. Surg., 76:528, 1922.

61. Seddon, H. J.: Nerve lesions complicating certain closed bone injuries. J.A.M.A., 135:691, 1947.

62. Simeone, F. A.: Acute and delayed traumatic peripheral entrapment neuropathies. Surg. Clin. North Am., 52:1324, 1972.

63. Moberg, E.: Criticism and study of methods for examining sensibility in the hand. Neurology (NY), 12:8, 1962.

64. Leonard, M. H.: Return of skin sensation in children without repair of nerves. Clin. Orthop., 95:273, 1973.

65. Guth, L.: Regeneration in the mammalian peripheral nervous system. Physiol. Rev., 36:441, 1956.

66. Gutmann, E., and Guttmann, L.: Factors affecting recovery of sensory function after nerve lesions. J. Neurol. Psychiatry, 5:117, 1942.

67. Adeymo, O., and Wyburn, G.: Innervation of skin grafts. Transplantation, 4:152, 1957.

68. McCarroll, H. R.: The regeneration of sensation in transplanted skin. Ann. Surg., 108:309, 1938.

69. Pollock, L. J.: Nerve overlap as related to the relatively early return of pain sense following injury to the peripheral nerves. Comp. Neurol., 32:357, 1920.

70. Thompson, H. G., and Sorokolit, W. T.: The cross-finger flap in children. A follow-up study. Plast. Reconstr. Surg., 39:487, 1967.

71. Almquist, E., and Erg-Olofsson, O.: Sensory-nerve-conduction velocity and 2-point discrimination in sutured nerves. J. Bone Joint Surg., 52-A:791, 1970.

72. Spiedel, C. E.: Studies of living nerves. Comp. Neurol., 61:1, 1935.

73. Weddell, G., Guttmann, L., and Gutmann, E.: The local extension of nerve fibers into denervated areas of skin. J. Neurol. Psychiatry, 4:206, 1941.

74. Fitzgerald, M. J. T., Martin, F., and Paletta, F. X.: Innervation of skin grafts. Surg. Gynecol. Obstet., 124:808, 1967.

75. Boswick, J. A., Jr., Schneewind, J., and Stromberg, W., Jr.: Evaluation of peripheral nerve repairs below the elbow. Arch. Surg., 90:50, 1965.

76. Clippinger, R. W., Goldner, J. L., and Roberts, J. M.: Use of the electromyogram in evaluating upper-extremity peripheral nerve lesions. J. Bone Joint Surg., 44-A:1047, 1962.

77. Howard, F. M., Jr.: Electromyography and conduction studies in peripheral nerve injuries. Surg. Clin. North Am., 52:1343, 1972.

78. Onne, L.: Recovery of sensibility and sudomotor activity in the hand after nerve suture. Acta Chir. Scand. [Suppl.] 300, 1962.

79. Lindsay, W. D., Walker, F. G., and Farmer, A. W.: Traumatic peripheral nerve injuries in children. Plast. Reconstr. Surg., 30:462, 1962.

80. Woodhall, B.: The surgical repair of acute peripheral nerve injury. Surg. Clin. North Am., 31:1369, 1951.

81. Benassy, J., Mazabraud, D., and Diveres, J.: L'osteogenese neurogene. Rev. Chir. Orthop., 49:95, 1963.

82. Freehafer, A. A., and Mast, W. A.: Lower extremity fractures in patients with spinal cord injury. J. Bone Joint Surg., 47-A:683, 1965.

83. Weisz, F. M., Fishman, J., and Steiner, E.: Callus formation in cases of cerebral fat embolism: a contribution of the theory of narcogenic influence on osteogenesis. Comp. Neurol., 31:362, 1969.

84. Cunningham, A. R., Marquez-Monter, H., and DeGuerrero, L. M.: Study of the bone callus in denervated extremities: experimental study in rats. Archives Invest. Med., 2:15, 1971.

85. Hulth, A., and Olerud, S.: Healing of fractures in denervated limbs: an experimental study using sensory and motor rhizotomy and peripheral denervation. J. Trauma, 5:571, 1965.

86. Quilis, A. N., and Gonzalez, A. P.: Healing in denervated bones. Acta Orthop. Scand., 45:820, 1974.

87. Rappaport, M. B.: Roentgen characteristics of reparative osteogenesis in long bones under conditions of disturbed denervation. Orthopedics Kiev Institute of Research, 14:153, 1967.

88. Kozin, F., et al.: The reflex sympathetic dystrophy syndromes. I. Clinical and histologic studies. Am. J. Med., 60:321, 1976.

89. Kozin, F., et al.: The reflex sympathetic dystrophy syndrome. II. Roentgenographic and scintigraphic evidence of bilaterality and periarticular accentuation. Am. J. Med., 60:332, 1976.

90. Carron, H., and McCue, F.: Reflex sympathetic dystrophy in a ten year old. South. Med. J., 65:631, 1972.

91. Guntheroth, W. G., et al.: Post-traumatic sympathetic dystrophy. Am. J. Dis. Child., 121:511, 1971.

92. Matles, A. L.: Reflex sympathetic dystrophy in a child: a case report. Bull. Hosp. Joint Dis., 32:193, 1971.

93. Fermaglich, D. R.: Reflex sympathetic dystrophy in children. Pediatrics, 60:881, 1977.

94. Kozin, F., Haughton, V., and Ryan, L.: The reflex sympathetic dystrophy syndrome in a child. J. Pediatr., *90:*417, 1977.

95. Patman, R. D., Thompson, J. E., and Peterson, A. V.: Management of post-traumatic pain syndromes: Report of 113 cases. Ann. Surg., *177:*780, 1973.

96. Steinbrocker, O., and Argyros, T. G.: The shoulder-hand syndrome: present status as a diagnosis and therapeutic entity. Med. Clin. North Am., *42:*1533, 1958.

97. Cristofaro, R. L., and Brink, J. D.: Hypercalcemia of immobilization in neurologically injured children: a prospective study. Orthopedics, *2:*485, 1979.

98. Heath, H., III, Earll, J. M., Schaaf, M., Piechocki, J. T., and Li, T-K: Serum ionized calcium during bedrest in fracture patients and normal men. Metabolism, *21:*633, 1972.

99. Claus-Walker, J., Carter, R. E., and Campos, R. J.: Hypercalcemia in early traumatic quadriplegia. J. Chronic Dis., *28:*81, 1975.

100. Dodd, K., Graubarth, H., and Rapoport, S.: Hypercalcemia, nephropathy and encephalopathy following immobilization. Pediatrics, *6:*124, 1950.

101. Halvorsen, S.: Osteoporosis, hypercalcemia and nephropathy following immobilization of children. Acta Med. Scand., *149:*401, 1954.

102. Hyman, L. R., Boner, G., and Thomas, J. C.: Immobilization hypercalcemia. Am. J. Dis. Child., *124:*723, 1972.

103. Lawrence, G. D., et al.: Immobilization hypercalcemia: some new aspects of diagnosis and treatment. J. Bone Joint Surg., *55-A:*87, 1973.

104. Scheller, A., and Crothers, O.: Immobilization hypercalcemia associated with multiple trauma. Orthopedics, *2:*19, 1979.

105. Albright, F., et al.: Acute atrophy of bone (osteoporosis) simulating hyperparathyroidism. Clin. Endocrinol., *1:*711, 1941.

106. Winters, J. L., et al.: Hypercalcemia complicating immobilization in the treatment of fractures. J. Bone Joint Surg., *48-A:*1182, 1966.

107. Ellas, E. G., Reynoso, G., and Mittleman, A.: Control of hypercalcemia with mithramycin. Ann. Surg., *175:*431, 1972.

108. Hantman, D. A., et al.: Attempts to prevent disuse osteoporosis by treatment with calcitonin, longitudinal compression and supplementary calcium and phosphate. J. Clin. Endocrinol. Metab., *36:*845, 1973.

109. Pezeshki, C., and Brooker, A. F., Jr.: Immobilization hypercalcemia. Report of two cases with calcitonin. J. Bone Joint Surg., *59-A:*971, 1977.

110. Schakney, S., and Hasson, J.: A precipitous fall in serum calcium, hypotension, and acute renal failure after intravenous phosphate therapy for hypercalcemia. Ann. Intern. Med., *66:*906, 1967.

111. Henke, J. A., Thompson, N. W., and Kaufer, H.: Immobilization hypercalcemic crisis. Arch. Surg., *110:*321, 1975.

112. Max, M.: Acute hypercalcemic crisis. Heart Lung, *5:*624, 1976.

113. Gold, R. H., et al.: Case report 68 (myositis ossificans circumscripta). Skel. Radiol., *3:*123, 1978.

114. Wilkes, L. L.: Myositis ossificans traumatica in a young child. Clin. Orthop., *118:*151, 1976.

115. Dickerson, R. D.: Myositis ossificans in early childhood. Report of an unusual case. Clin. Orthop., *79:*42, 1971.

116. Thompson, H. C., and Garcia, A.: Myositis ossificans: aftermath of elbow injuries. Clin. Orthop., *50:*129, 1967.

117. Rang, M.: Children's Fractures. Philadelphia, J. B. Lippincott, 1974.

118. Ter-Egiazarov, G. M., and Bolotzev, O. K.: Compression-distraction osteosynthesis in the management of sequelae of fractures of the long tubular bones in children. Orthop. Travmatol. Protez., *11:*19, 1971.

119. Arunachalam, V. S. P., and Griffiths, J. C.: Fracture recurrence in children. Injury, *7:*37, 1975.

120. Levine, B. S., Dorfman, H. D., and Matles, A. L.: Evolution of a post-fracture cyst of the fibula. J. Bone Joint Surg., *51-A:*1631, 1969.

121. Neff, R. S., Borwin, L. P., and Wissinger, A.: An unusual complication of a below-the-knee cast. J. Bone Joint Surg., *52-A:*165, 1970.

122. Berk, R. N., and Coulson, D. B.: The body cast syndrome. Radiology, *94:*303, 1970.

123. Warner, T. F., et al.: The cast syndrome. J. Bone Joint Surg., *56-A:*1263, 1974.

124. Robson, M. C., Krizek, T. J., and Heggers, J. P.: Biology of surgical infection. Curr. Probl. Surg., March 1973.

8

Special Fractures

General Injuries

Intrauterine fractures

Fractures of the fetal skeleton are infrequent and difficult to identify with certainty.[1-4] Intrauterine fractures may occur consequent to abdominal or uterine trauma during pregnancy, with indirect injury to the fetus (Fig. 8-1).[4a] The criteria for a true intrauterine fracture of normal bone are roentgenograms showing absence of generalized osseous disease and normal callus appearance. Films should be taken as soon after birth as possible, as callus forms so quickly in the newborn that roentgenograms taken even one week after delivery would not rule out birth trauma. Most intrauterine fractures are due to underlying, more generalized disease, including osteogenesis imperfecta, chondrodystrophies, congenital rubella, and syphilis.[5,6]

Experimentally produced fetal fractures have a less active inflammatory phase and smaller amounts of hematoma than experimental fractures in postnatal animals.[7] These characteristics have also been described in other fetal tissue wound responses. Proliferative activity in the periosteum and endosteum is more intense and appears earlier than in postnatal injury. Fetal callus is more abundant and differentiates into cartilage more rapidly. Chondro-osseous transformation is also rapid. Thus, it appears that the second phase of fracture healing predominates over the first. Possibly, the decreased inflammatory reaction in the first phase permits more rapid cellular differentiation in the callus. In general, these fractures heal uneventfully.

Fractures in the newborn

Since the advent of improved antenatal and perinatal care, birth trauma and skeletal injuries have been encountered less frequently.[8-11] Trauma to long bones in the newborn may be sustained during difficult delivery, particularly if the baby is large, the mother has a small pelvic outlet, or the presentation is breech (Fig. 8-2). When more than one fracture is present, one should suspect underlying metabolic bone disease, such as osteogenesis imperfecta.[12] Multiple birth fractures also may occur in babies with arthrogryposis, especially if there is rigid extension of a joint. Fetal anoxia

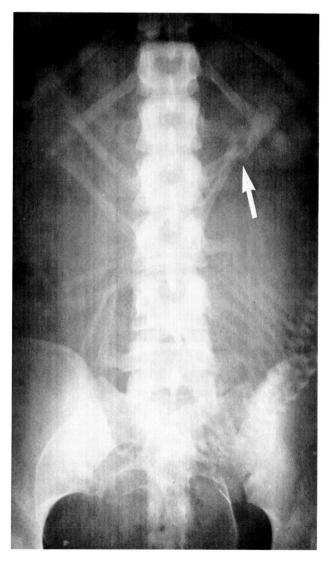

FIG. 8-1. Antenatal film following maternal abdominal trauma. A fracture of the fetal femur is evident (arrow).

171

and urgent delivery often necessitate unduly forceful extraction, increasing the likelihood of fractures.

Fractures of the diaphyses are usually easily recognized. Diaphyseal skeletal injuries, in order of decreasing frequency, usually involve the clavicle, humerus, and femur. Fractures distal to the elbow and the knee are unusual. Fracture of the tibia is often pathologic; congenital pseudarthrosis of the tibia should be considered.

Fractures of the epiphyseal regions are more difficult to recognize, and may require more definitive diagnostic techniques, such as arthrography. The most commonly involved epiphyses are those of the proximal and distal humerus and femur. Such epiphyseal separations are frequently misdiagnosed as acute, traumatic dislocations (Fig. 8-3). Dislocation, while often discussed as part of a differential diagnosis, is essentially nonexistent in the major joints of children younger than 12 to 18 months. Invariably, the suspected "dislocations" are epiphyseal/physeal separations (type 1 injuries).

Traumatic displacement of the proximal humeral physis may occur alone or, less frequently, in association with brachial plexus paralysis. The shoulder is markedly swollen and may be misdiagnosed as an acute dislocation or suppurative arthritis with secondary dislocation (Fig. 8-4).[13] The clinical symptoms of traumatic epiphysiolysis are pseudoparalysis, a functional disability, and internal rotation contracture of the arm. Initially, diagnosis is difficult because the cartilaginous head is ossified in only about 20% of full-term newborns. Arthrography may be undertaken, but it is rarely necessary. The diagnosis is established by the subsequent appearance of callus of the healing fracture. The arm should be bandaged across the chest. While prognosis generally is excellent, these children must be followed to skeletal maturity, because significant growth problems may occur.

Fracture of the humeral diaphysis usually occurs in the middle third. The fracture is either transverse or oblique and angulated laterally by the pull of the deltoid. Diagnosis generally is made by the obstetrician who feels the bone break. The infant will not use the arm (pseudoparalysis). Roentgenograms disclose the fracture, although care should be taken not to confuse a fracture line with the nutrient canal. Treatment consists of immobilizing the arm with the elbow flexed over the chest. The fracture will heal quickly, usually within two weeks, and angular deformities will be spontaneously corrected by the extensive growth that will occur. Transient radial nerve palsy may be associated with these fractures, but it usually resolves completely within six to eight weeks.

Fracture-displacement of the upper femoral epiphysis often is confused with congenital dislocation of the hip; the term "pseudodislocation" of the hip has sometimes been applied.[14,15] The diagnosis is primarily clinical, as radiologic signs only become evident after an interval of healing. The radiologic signs may, on the other hand, be misinterpreted as showing a congenital dislocation of the hip. Michail states that "so far as we are aware, the existence of an obstetrical (traumatic) dislocation of the hip has never been demonstrated," a statement with which I completely agree.[15]

The mechanism of injury is hyperextension, abduction, rotation, and forceful traction of the leg during delivery (breech presentations are common among those with this injury). The line of separation is distal to the combined proximal physis and extends in a crescentic line from the greater

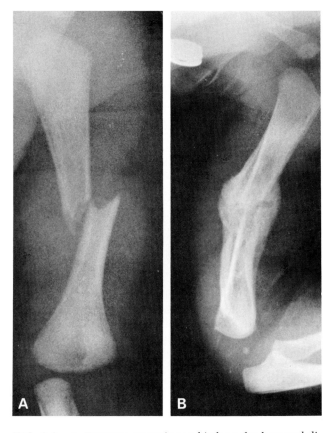

FIG. 8-2. *A*, Fracture occurring at birth to the humeral diaphysis. *B*, Appearance of callus three weeks later. Two types of new bone are evident. Extensive subperiosteal bone indicates the elevation of periosteum proximal and distal to the fracture. This is membranous bone. At the actual fracture site, a globular cluster of endochondral bone has formed within the fracture callus.

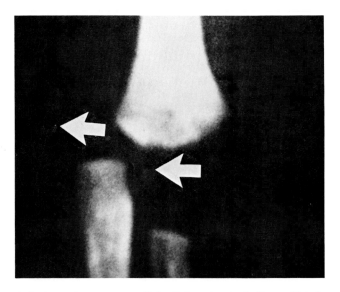

FIG. 8-3. Apparent medial "dislocation" of elbow. This is actually a fracture across the distal humeral physis, with a medial shift (arrows) of the entire elbow unit.

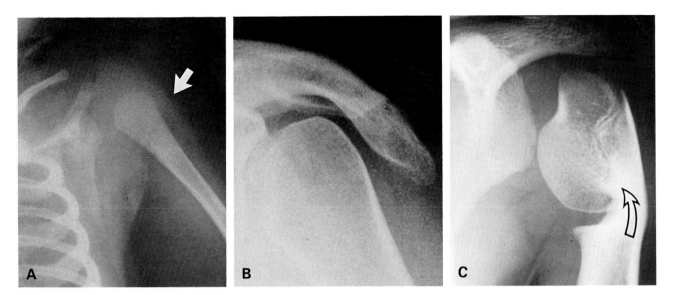

FIG. 8-4. *A,* Shoulder injury that occurred during birth. Soft-tissue swelling (arrow) is the only evidence of injury. *B,* No follow-up was done until this patient sought help for a painful shoulder during her third decade. The proximal humerus is deformed and the acromion has molded over it. In retrospect, the original injury may have been a proximal humeral fracture with progressive deformation and secondary remodeling of the acromion. *C,* Deformed left proximal humerus in a ten-year-old boy who sustained a "shoulder injury" at birth. Original roentgenograms are unavailable, but allegedly showed no injury. A medial osseous bridge (arrow) has led to a humerus varus.

to the lesser trochanter (Fig. 8-5). Acute injury is suggested by pseudoparalysis. At birth, the femoral head, neck, and greater trochanter are entirely cartilaginous, making roentgenographic diagnosis extremely difficult. The proximal femoral metaphysis is displaced upward and laterally. Because the femoral epiphysis has been in its normal position, the acetabula are developed symmetrically, which makes true congenital hip disease unlikely. Treatment should consist of immobilization of the hip in abduction, partial flexion, and

medial rotation in a spica cast for three to four weeks. However, diagnosis is frequently not made until the healing phase, when coxa vara may have developed. Although there is a high potential for remodeling and spontaneous correction in infants, coxa vara may persist or worsen (Fig. 8-6).

Traumatic separation of the distal femoral epiphysis presents less of a roentgenographic diagnostic problem, since the secondary ossification center of the distal femur is usually present at birth in the full-term child. However, the in-

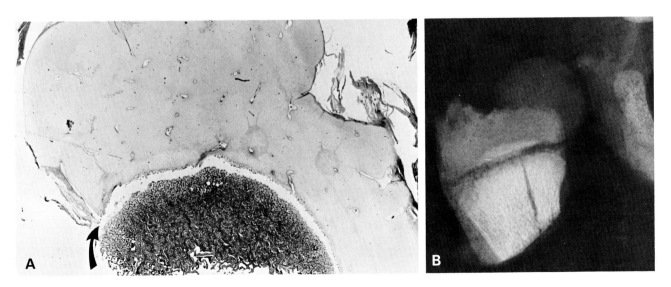

FIG. 8-5. Experimental fractures of the proximal femur caused during attempts to acutely dislocate the neonatal hip. *A,* Characteristic pattern of fracture (arrow) through primary spongiosa, with minimal involvement of any physeal cartilage layers. *B,* Roentgenogram showing comminuted fracture across and within the metaphysis and the physis.

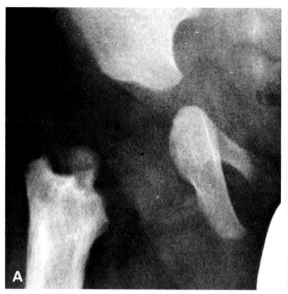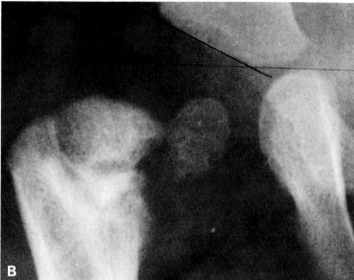

FIG. 8-6. *A*, Three-month-old child who sustained a fracture of right proximal femur during birth. The acetabulum is developing normally. The capital femur has ossified early (usually it appears from four to six months postnatally), probably because of the hyperemic fracture response. *B*, At one year a coxa vara is developing. The acetabulum is still developing normally.

jury frequently is unsuspected until the subperiosteal hematoma ossifies. The lower femoral epiphysis almost always is displaced posteriorly, with extensive stripping of the periosteum from the back of the lower femoral shaft. The fracture is a type 1 epiphyseal injury with an excellent prognosis for subsequent normal growth. Manipulative reduction must be undertaken carefully to minimize injury to popliteal vessels. A single leg hip spica cast with the knee in partial flexion, should be applied for three weeks. A residual angular deformity usually will correct spontaneously during the rapid growth the child undergoes in the first year of life.

Metaphyseal fractures in infancy

These fractures may occur in the neonatal period or in the first year of life,[16] and they must be differentiated from a number of predisposing factors such as syphilis, tuberculosis, scurvy, osteomyelitis, malignant tumors, and child-beating. Weston felt that many of these fractures were due to traumatic delivery, or child-beating.[17] A cause should be sought whenever metaphyseal fractures are found. Treatment is primarily symptomatic, as these usually are incomplete compression failures.

Diaphyseal injury

Most fractures of the shafts of long bones are readily recognizable. However, the appearance of subperiosteal new bone may cause some concern, especially regarding the possibility of child abuse. During infancy, the femur or the tibia commonly has a longitudinal layer of subperiosteal bone, often extending the entire length of the shaft (Fig. 8-7). Usually, this new bone is bilaterally symmetric, but it is less likely to be so in an abused child.[18]

Rickets

Vitamin D deficiency rickets is rarely encountered in this country. However, it remains a common problem for the large, malnourished, childhood populations in other parts of the world. Florid cases may be associated with progressive metaphyseal/epiphyseal deformation (Fig. 8-8), especially at the wrist or knee, which are areas of rapid growth in infancy and early childhood. Because of excessive widening of the physeal cell columns and irregular metaphyseal bone formation and remodeling, these areas become susceptible to gradual plastic deformation and failure. Most fractures are microscopic initially.

Rachitic changes in the physis result in the presence of excessive numbers of cells in the uncalcified hypertrophic zone. The metaphyseal vascular loops will not invade the cell columns unless they are calcified. With distortion of normal cell column integrity, cleavage planes may develop between the columnar clones, leading to further instability and failure (Fig. 8-9). Osteodystrophic changes in the metaphysis also increase susceptibility to fracture at this level, and may cause some delay in the repair of the fracture.

Treatment should be directed at the primary cause with injections of large doses of vitamin D, and the deformed or painful regions should be splinted until a drug response is seen. This may take several weeks or months. Permanent deformation may require subsequent osteotomy.

Rickets also may result from a variety of other causes. Vitamin D resistant rickets is relatively frequent in this country. Renal tubular abnormalities associated with phosphaturia and hypophosphatemia account for a large number of cases of rickets and may lead to proximal femoral failure and coxa vara (Figs. 8-10 and 8-11). Secondary hyperparathyroidism in association with the florid form of vitamin D

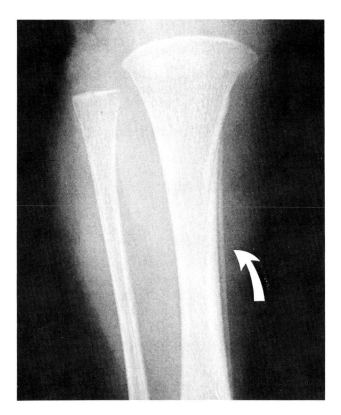

FIG. 8-7. One-month-old child with subperiosteal diaphyseal bone (arrow). This is a relatively normal finding and may be due to birth trauma to the lower leg. Rough handling of the neonate, as in child abuse, may cause a similar roentgenographic appearance (see Fig. 8-33).

deficiency, vitamin D resistant, or renal tubular rickets or with rare primary hyperparathyroidism also may occur.

Children under treatment for renal osteodystrophy, particularly those on dialysis, may show metaphyseal fractures or even slipping of the proximal femoral epiphysis. This may occur earlier than the classic slip and lead to coxa vara. Shea and Mankin reported three cases of slipped capital femoral epiphysis in patients with renal rickets.[19] Slipping appears to be associated primarily with renal or glomerular rickets.[20] Children with renal and glomerular rickets have not only calcium and phosphorus metabolic disorders, but also defects in protein synthesis, and this provides an additional possible explanation for slipping. Unlike the classic coxa vara, a slipped epiphysis will not occur until adolescence; and it is only in recent times that a significant number of children with these disorders have survived to this age.[19] The mechanics of coxa vara and a slipped epiphysis are probably not significantly different. They simply occur because of different degrees of chondro-osseous maturation along the developing femoral neck.

Endocrinopathy

Children with specific or generalized endocrinopathy may become increasingly susceptible to fractures as a result of the effect of hormonal alteration(s) on the chondro-osseous components. Hypothyroidism may have a profound effect

on protein metabolism and the production of chondroid and osteoid. Children with craniopharyngioma may have slipped capital femoral epiphyses. Comparably, a child with Schmidt's syndrome (diabetes, hypothyroidism) may develop a slipped epiphysis if placed on thyroid supplementation.

Osteogenesis imperfecta

These children appear to have a basic mesenchymal defect that is manifested primarily in the osseous tissue. In the developing skeleton, this causes generalized hyperosteocytosis, increased intertrabecular resorption, and immaturity of the

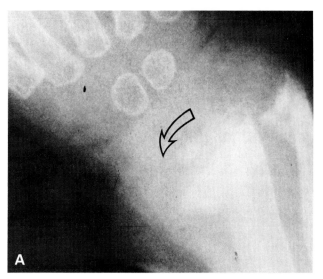

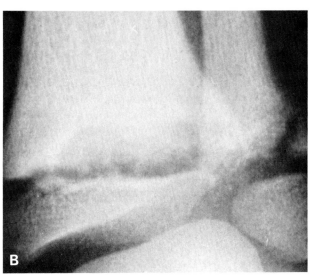

FIG. 8-8. *A*, Rachitic epiphysiolysis (arrow) in an infant suffering from kwashiorkor and dietary deficiency rickets. *B*, Four-year-old child with dietary deficiency rickets (decreased total body calcium). The distal tibial physis has widened. The fibular physis has widened similarly, and due to normal valgus forces at the ankle, it has developed a type 2 fracture. This did not heal until adequate calcium supplements were provided.

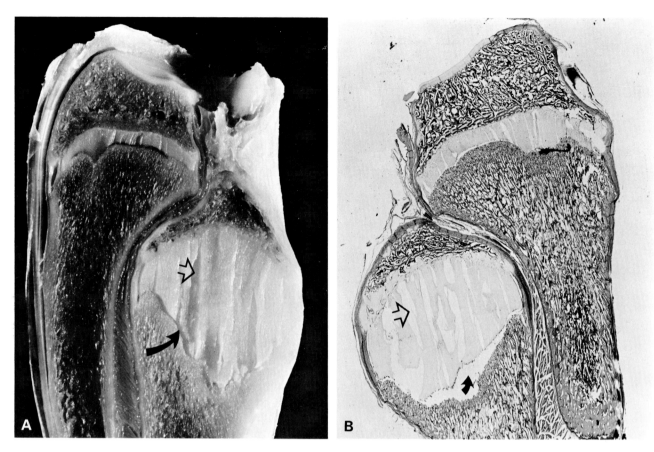

FIG. 8-9. Rachitic changes in distal radius and ulna of an arctic fox (Alopex lagopus). This fox had a deficient dietary intake of calcium. *A,* Slab section shows excessive widening of the distal ulnar physis, with the physis beginning to separate from the metaphysis (solid arrow) and cystic separations developing between the elongated cell columns (open arrow). *B,* Histologic section showing the same findings.

bony architecture (Fig. 8-12). Metabolism of some amino acids, particularly hydroxyproline, also may be defective. Infants with severe forms of the disease will have multiple fractures at birth (see Fig. 8-12). However, those with less severe involvement (e.g., tarda) may not be diagnosed until adolescence, when they may present with a fracture and short stature.

Basic principles of fracture treatment are the same as they are for normal children, except that angulation should be corrected as much as possible, since remodeling does not appear to be normal. Callus formation may be massive.[21] Mobilization and prevention of contractures assume major importance so that stresses predisposing the bones to subsequent fracture can be avoided.

Repeated fractures may lead to significant deformity (Fig. 8-13), and often require subsequent osteotomy at multiple levels. If possible, corrective surgery should be deferred until adolescence, when the bone has usually matured in strength and when the rate of fracture has decreased.

Multiple fractures of unresolved etiology

Fulkerson and Ozonoff reported a ten-year-old boy with multiple symmetric fractures.[22] The findings did not indicate osteogenesis imperfecta or osteomalacia, despite apparent

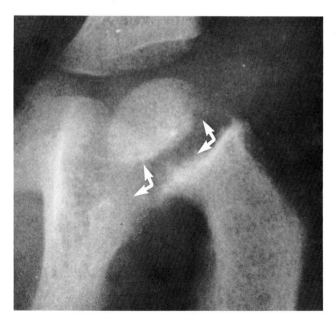

FIG. 8-10. Coxa vara in an infant with renal rickets. The physis has widened and the epiphysis has slipped medially (arrows).

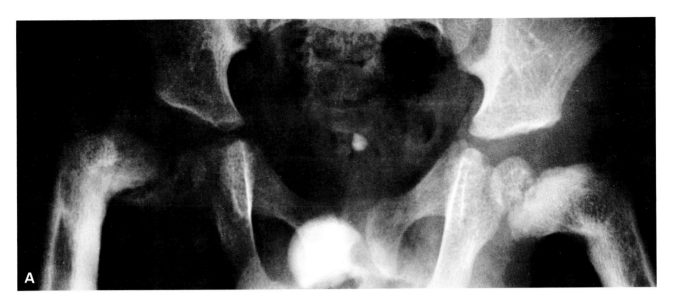

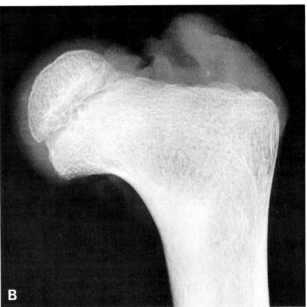

osseous fragility. Elevated serum pyrophosphate and low urine phosphate content suggested that abnormalities in phosphate metabolism contributed to the formation of bone that was biochemically and structurally deficient.

Osteopetrosis

Lack of remodeling in this disease leads to thickened trabeculae and cortical bone that is termed "brittle" (Fig. 8-14). Fractures are relatively common (Fig. 8-15) and must be protected for an adequate period of healing, which may be considerably longer than normal because of differences in remodeling of callus and patterns of bone formation. Recent studies of this disease have found isozymic changes in liver acid phosphatase, and comparable changes in the bone may explain the physiologic dysfunction.

Multiple dislocations

Multiple joint dislocations are unusual (Fig. 8-16). Bartsocas described familial multiple joint dislocation in a mother and child.[23] Larson's syndrome manifests itself in multiple congenital dislocations that are associated with osseous abnormalities and a characteristic flat facial pattern, with a depressed nasal bridge and prominent forehead. Other causes of hypermobility include Ehlers-Danlos syndrome and homocystinuria.

Loose joints

The cracking of joints is a common phenomenon that is even more common in children who have greater range of motion in the joints.[24] Translocation of the knee and hip tendons over chondro-osseous prominences can cause clicking, which may be palpable or audible. The tensor fascia lata is particularly prone to snap over the greater trochanter. Studies of cracking in the metacarpophalangeal joints suggested that bubbles of previously dissolved gases formed in the joints. Unsworth showed that the bubble was the effect, rather than the cause, of the crack, and that fluid cavitation was responsible for the cracking noise.[25]

FIG. 8-11. *A,* Older child with renal rickets in whom bilateral coxa vara is beginning to improve following renal transplant. One year later, the child died. *B,* Postmortem specimen of left hip showing coxa vara.

Studies of the geometry of metacarpophalangeal joints demonstrated that the joint surfaces were essentially spherical, and hydrodynamic equations for such configurations show that when the joint surfaces are close together, separation may produce large subatmospheric pressures. Under such pressures, the synovial fluid vaporizes, and dissolved gas is released from the solution (see Fig. 3-13*A*). The collapse of the vapor cavities gives rise to the noise.

Pathologic fractures

Due to the infrequent occurrence of benign and malignant tumors, the child's skeleton is not a frequent site of patho-

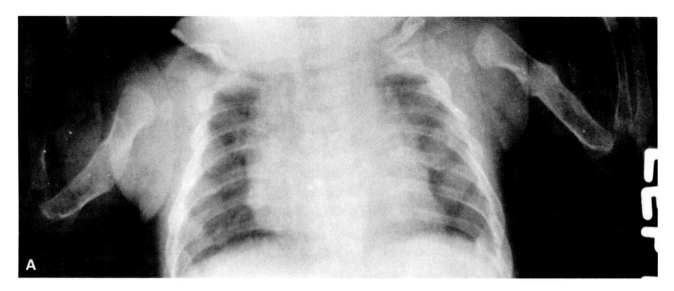

logic fracture compared to the adult's. However, fracture may be the initial presentation of many primary osseous malignancies, especially osteogenic sarcoma of the lower extremity in an active adolescent. The first presenting symptom of metastatic malignancies may also be an acute skeletal injury (Fig. 8-17). Treatment must be directed at the specific pathologic lesions. Fracture healing may be impaired by radiation or chemotherapy.

Simple bone cysts are most common in the proximal humerus, distal tibia, proximal tibia, and femoral neck. They are rarely symptomatic until developing into an acute, pathologic fracture (Fig. 8-18). Cysts that are fractured will infrequently heal spontaneously, but enlargement of the cyst and further fracture is more likely. These cysts may disappear slowly following skeletal maturation, but this is not an absolute. As long as they remain, they represent a weakness in the bone.

Cyst fractures usually are insignificantly displaced and exhibit only small, incomplete cortical fracture. The presence of a cyst does not interfere with the normal healing of the fracture, and certainly, if one is considering definitive treatment of a cyst with grafting, a sufficient period must elapse to allow adequate fracture healing. One should probably wait for a second pathologic fracture through the cyst before attempting curettage and grafting, unless a major weightbearing area is involved.

Neer found that 80% of all children had one to three refractures through a cyst (even after surgery), and 10% had some residual deformities; only 1 of 42 patients did not undergo surgery eventually.[26] Up to 30% required reoperation because of failure to totally incorporate the graft or because of complete dissolution of the graft.

Less commonly, cystic fractures occur in weightbearing bones, such as the femur or the tibia. Here, deformity is more likely to occur, and curettage and bone grafting are indicated once the diagnosis is made and the initial fracture has healed. Internal fixation may be a necessary adjunct, especially if the femoral neck is involved.

Recent evidence suggests that steroid injections may be beneficial.[27] However, this should not be done until a pathologic fracture has healed, as steroids may adversely affect the callus response necessary for fracture healing.

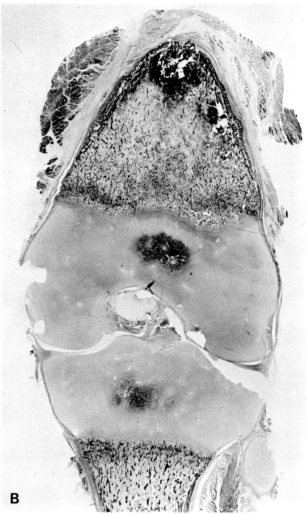

FIG. 8-12. *A*, Multiple fractures of humeri, clavicles, and ribs in neonate with osteogenesis imperfecta. *B*, Histologic appearance of distal femur and proximal tibia in a stillborn infant with severe osteogenesis imperfecta. Normal metaphyseal trabeculation is replaced by inflammatory tissue.

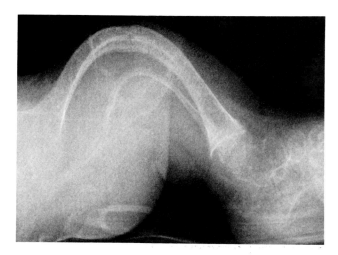

FIG. 8-13. Severe bowing resulting from osteogenesis imperfecta.

the round bones. This would not immediately damage the whole bone, but merely affect its chondro-osseous maturation processes.[30] The necrosis that follows is secondary to the original compression fractures in cancellous trabeculae.

Neurologic Disorders

The number of children with significant neurologic deficits is increasing because of the improved survival rate for myelodysplasia, the increased incidence of spinal cord injury, and the higher survival rate for patients with spinal tumors (e.g., neuroblastoma).[31] Fractures due to such disorders involve not only diaphyseal and metaphyseal bone, but also physes. Failure to recognize the latter may lead to significant growth deformity. Charcot-like fragmentation and destructive changes in the physis and metaphysis may lead to diagnostic errors and unnecessary diagnostic procedures (e.g., biopsy). Roentgenographic evidence of these injuries may resemble osteomyelitis, metabolic bone disease, or malignancy.

Nonossifying fibromas commonly involve the tibia and distal femur. These usually are located eccentrically in the cortex of the metaphysis, although they may involve the diaphysis. They are generally not large enough to cause a significant problem, but they may be quite painful if a small cortical fracture occurs. Nonosteogenic fibroma of bone seldom presents problems in diagnosis or treatment, but some lesions, by virtue of their size, may predispose the bone to fracture and lead to confusion in diagnosis.[28] The lesions may take two to six years to become obliterated, and they may not disappear until long after skeletal maturity has occurred. In those treated by bone graft, complete reossification occurs more rapidly.

Osteochondroses

Caffey[29] feels very strongly that most lesions called ischemic (avascular) necrosis and osteochondrosis are focal stress fractures and deformities of epiphyseal ossification centers. These lesions are characterized radiographically by focal compression of the provisional zones of ossification. Many of them pass through a series of progressive radiographic changes that include sclerosis, flattening, fibrous replacement of the sclerotic bone, and reossification of the fibrous tissue with complete healing, but sometimes with a severe crippling deformity (as in Legg-Perthes disease). Each of these cyclic changes may recur. The deformity and disability depend on the duration and degree of stress(es) to which the soft fibrous and cartilaginous parts of the bone were subjected. The exact cause and mechanisms are unknown, although excessive, repetitive mechanical stress appears to play an important role.

The traditional causal hypothesis suggests impairment of the local arterial blood supply as the primary cause, because it reduces the flow of essential nutrients and oxygen to the developing bone. Caffey feels that in coxa plana and in Blount's disease, the deformity and sclerosis follow a fracture.[29] Boznan proposed that the primary injury and causal mechanism might be direct mechanical compression of the convex edges of the epiphyseal ossification centers and of

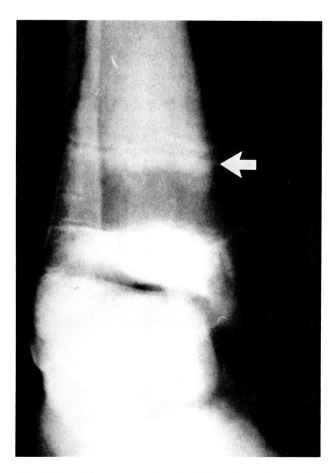

FIG. 8-14. Osteopetrosis. The distal tibia shows dense, sclerotic bone in the metaphysis, diaphysis, and epiphysis. A Harris line (arrow) shows new distal tibial growth occurring following an ipsilateral femoral fracture and prolonged immobilization in a cast (with relative osteoporosis of this newly formed bone).

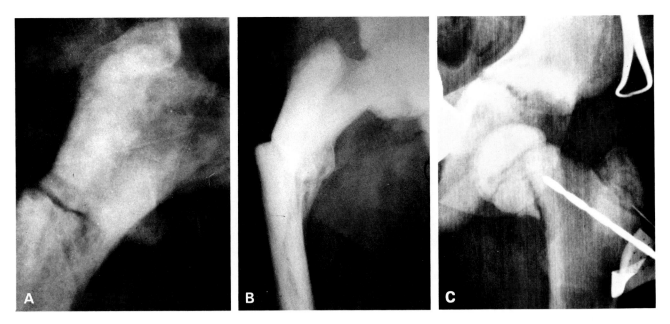

FIG. 8-15. Osteopetrosis. *A,* The dense proximal femoral bone predisposes to subtrochanteric fracture. *B,* Six months later, medial callus formation has been adequate but lateral callus formation has been minimal. *C,* Another characteristic fracture involves the femoral neck, creating coxa vara.

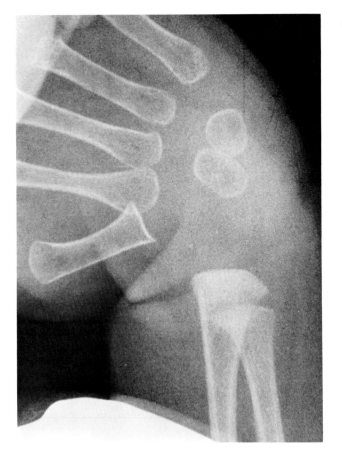

Myelodysplasia

The increased emphasis on mobility for children with myelodysplasia produces a greater incidence of injury to their poorly innervated lower extremities. Fractures in these children follow no definite pattern, occur in unusual sites, are of obscure etiology and are difficult to diagnose.[31-40] There is a predisposition toward metaphyseal and epiphyseal fractures, especially near the knee joint, in both the distal femur and the proximal tibia, although the latter area is not commonly involved in normal children (Fig. 8-19).

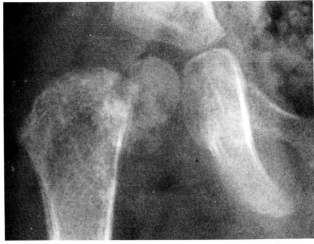

FIG. 8-16. Excessive laxity of wrist joint in one-year-old with generalized hyperlaxity. The wrist could be subluxated easily in virtually any direction.

FIG. 8-17. Pathologic fracture in three-year-old with metastatic neuroblastoma. This was the initial presentation of the disease.

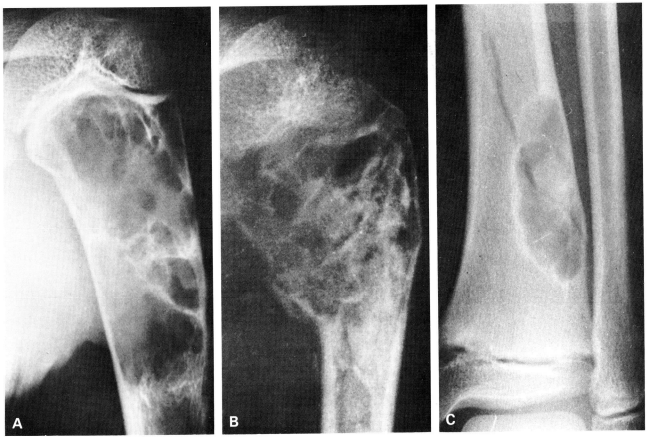

FIG. 8-18. *A*, Proximal humeral cyst in a boy with vague shoulder pain. *B*, Two weeks later the boy fell on the shoulder and sustained a fracture and varus collapse through the cyst. *C*, Spiral fracture complicating a non-ossifying fibroma of the distal tibia.

Because of the preponderance of fractures around the knee and ankle joints in young patients with impaired sensation, a great potential exists for the development of Charcot-type joints.[33] As advances in the care of these children allow more of them to live to adulthood, the development of significant joint deformity and dysfunction becomes a significant problem.

Norton and Foley described 43 fractures in 48 patients with spina bifida.[41] Quilis reviewed 130 children with myelodysplasia and found that 15 children had sustained a total of 55 fractures.[42] Only 3 of the children sustained one fracture; the remaining sustained multiple fractures, including one child who had 12 fractures. Of the injuries, 62% occurred around the knee joint. Callus formation was described as excessive in 19 (Figs. 8-20 and 8-21), moderate in 23, and minimal in 10. Interestingly, while 50% of the fractures occurred in children paralyzed below the L2 or L3 level, 16 of the 19 fractures that healed with excessive callus formation belonged to this group. Excessive callus formation has been reported by others,[42a] and may lead to significant complications such as further limitation of joint motion.

Thirty of the fractures occurred during limb manipulation, either during therapy, intraoperatively, or postoperatively following removal of the immobilization plasters; 4 were due to falls, 5 from an unknown cause, and 16 to walking. This contrasts with the feelings of other authors who have stated that walking protects the child. Only 3 cases involved a fracture-separation of the epiphysis, although in one case, this led to closure of the distal femoral growth plate (Fig. 8-22).

Drennan reported that 25 of 84 patients sustained at least one fracture of the lower extremity and a total of 58 fractures.[43] These fractures occurred in patients with levels of paralysis ranging from T8 to L3; 4 patients with a T8 level incurred a total of 24 fractures. Handlesman found that 11 of 77 children developed spontaneous fractures of the lower limbs, which were usually multiple and recurrent.[44] In 17 additional patients, plaster cast immobilization after surgery, particularly around the hip, was followed by juxtaepiphyseal fractures, usually at the level of the knee. Fractures of the shafts of long bones occurred in 9 patients with no apparent causal factor. Of the 34 fractures, 32 healed rapidly, usually with exuberant callus which was indicative of the excess motion allowed by the lack of painful response. Fractures involving the neck of the femur required subtrochanteric osteotomy for increasing coxa vara.

Similar susceptibility to fracture also occurs in children with paraplegia resulting from such causes as subdural hematoma, spinal injury, avulsion of lumbosacral roots, transverse myelitis, and cord tumors.[45-51] However, in children with atrophic limbs due to poliomyelitis, in whom sensation is intact, spontaneous fractures are much less frequent. Ab-

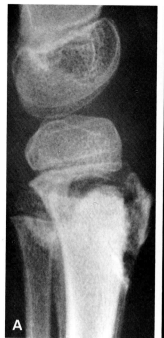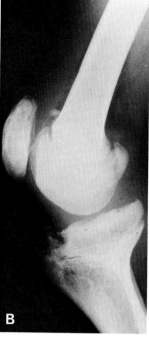

FIG. 8-19. *A,* Seven-year-old child with myelomeningocele whose presenting symptoms were a fever and a hot, swollen proximal tibia. A chronic fracture of the proximal tibia and tuberosity is evident. *B,* Such an injury may lead to premature epiphysiodesis. Charcot-type fractures of the posterior femoral physis and epiphysis are also evident.

sence of active movements in the limbs due to paralysis produces bone atrophy, and the prevention of passive movements caused by brace treatments enhances atrophy still further. Fractures occur in atrophic bone much more frequently when the limbs are also deprived of sensation, probably because strains applied to legs are not protectively restricted when normal sensation is absent.

Diagnosis is frequently delayed in these patients, particularly when the fracture is in an anesthetic part of the lower limb. The sensory deficit present in most patients with myelodysplasia makes the history of injury of doubtful value to the diagnosis. Many simply cannot specify the incident that may have caused the fracture. The symptoms, which are usually a fever and a swollen, red, hot limb, are similar to those usually seen in acute osteomyelitis. Often, decubiti are present in the area. In the abscence of pain, a fracture may be overlooked unless a roentgenogram is fortuitously obtained. Any child with myelodysplasia who has a fever should be evaluated for occult fracture as part of the diagnostic workup. The white blood count and sedimentation rate may be elevated, although the likelihood of concurrent urinary tract infection may make these findings of limited value.

Treatment of fractures in patients with sensory deficits is difficult. Eichenholtz condemned circular casts, skeletal and skin traction, and open reductions; he recommended simple, well-padded plaster shells.[52] Unfortunately, the immobilization itself may predispose the myelodysplastic patient to further spontaneous fractures elsewhere.

Treatment should be aimed at keeping the child as active as possible. Overriding and displacement are rarely problems because of the flaccid paralysis. However, the child who has contractures may accentuate them. Alignment and rotation must be maintained as nearly normal as possible. Because of the sensory neuropathy, it is wise to minimize motion in these children with bulky cotton dressings and plaster splints. This avoids the problem of cast pressure points. Since many of these children are in braces as part of their treatment program, they can be taken out of a relatively rigid, padded dressing early, and placed in their braces for the duration of fracture healing.

These fractures usually heal rapidly.[53] However, they are often associated with hyperplastic callus, undoubtedly because of repeated movement, an unspecified neurotrophic influence in bone formation, and hyperphosphatemia.[51,54]

Fractures occurring when plaster casts are removed after reconstructive surgery usually are incomplete and generally

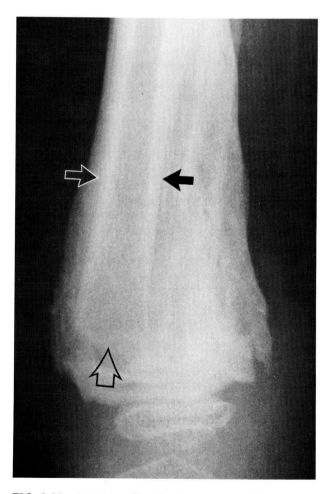

FIG. 8-20. Massive callus due to chronic epiphysiolysis in child with myelomeningocele. The solid arrows indicate the original limits of the cortical bone, while the open arrow demarcates the site of the original metaphyseal-physeal separation. Longitudinal growth has not yet been disrupted in this patient. However, she is only seven years old and must be followed closely to rule out eventual premature epiphysiodesis.

do not require manipulative reduction or major treatment. When braces are chosen as the method of treatment for fractures of the femur, tibia, and fibula in these children, the children are permitted to stand as soon as possible, because the fractures almost always are undisplaced and in good position. The use of braces is probably safe. Significant displacement, angulation, or rotation may preclude the use of these methods.

Fractures occurring in patients with myelodysplasia can lead to significant complications. Leg-length discrepancy, bowing, angulation, and rotational deformities have been described, but nonunion is quite rare. Skin necrosis can also result from the use of skin traction. Skeletal traction may be associated with a high incidence of pin tract infection and poor fixation in atrophic bone. Pressure sores may increase.

Edvardsen described damage to the growth plate of the lower extremities that resulted in a lesion characterized by broadening and loosening of the physis (see Fig. 8-19).[55] In one case, this proceeded to virtual pseudarthrosis. He described these epiphyseal lesions in 6 of 50 patients, and advocated annual examination of weightbearing epiphyses until the physes have fused. This is of major concern since both the growth rate and configuration of the affected bones are impaired beyond the usual shortening and deformity. These physeal injuries, if not properly recognized and treated, exhibit delayed healing. Treatment must be complete immobilization and avoidance of weightbearing until there is clinical and roentgenographic evidence of healing. Immobilization in a brace, as recommended for diaphyseal fractures, is not appropriate in physeal separations.

The prevention of conditions that predispose bones to fractures assumes paramount importance.[56] Vigorous passive stretching of contractures is quite applicable in these children. As dysfunctional as it may be, the continuous muscle activity of active exercise and ambulation may be the best prophylactic against disuse osteoporosis and consequent fractures. Muscle activity, not weightbearing, may be a major factor responsible for prevention of osteoporosis. Walton and Warwick relate bone atrophy in myopathies to the absence of stresses and strains by the muscles.[57] Katz found that fractures do not occur in myelodysplastic patients if they are actively ambulating in braces.[58]

Poliomyelitis

While acute poliomyelitis may be disappearing in certain areas, it is still quite prevalent in much of the world, and with patterns of migration, many of these children come under an orthopaedist's care. Robin reported 62 fractures in children under the age of 16 who had residual paralysis following polio.[59] Two-thirds of the fractures occurred while the children were inpatients, and one-third while they were outpatients. Only 5 fractures were in contralateral, normal limbs. The remaining 57 occurred in severely paralyzed limbs, and most commonly involved the femur (32 fractures; 29 in the supracondylar region), the tibia (18 fractures), and the humerus (7 fractures). Most were impaction types with little displacement. There were no epiphyseal fractures, and no cases of late deformation that could be attributed, in retrospect, to epiphyseal injury.

The most common causal pattern was antecedent plaster immobilization or some other corrective procedure such as an osteotomy. Of the 29 supracondylar femoral fractures, 17

involved patients with preexisting limitation of movement of the knee joint or contracture of the joint. Thirteen of the limbs had just been released from plaster cast immobilization for six weeks or less before the fracture occurred.

In view of the connection between joint stiffness and fracture, it is important that remobilization of the stiff joint be carried out as the first stage of rehabilitation following surgery, especially in the lower limb.[60] Until the knee joint is freely mobile, the patient should not be allowed complete freedom of activity.

Treatment of these fractures should be directed at rapid functional restoration, and early use of protective braces if they are already available. Manipulative reduction rarely is needed because of the compression nature of most of the fractures. There is no significant delay in rate of fracture healing.

Cerebral palsy

Fractures in children with spastic cerebral palsy are uncommon. The constant stimulation of hyperactive muscles probably results in strong bone that has minimal evidence of osteoporosis and little intrinsic susceptibility to fracture, unlike the previously discussed neuromuscular disorders.

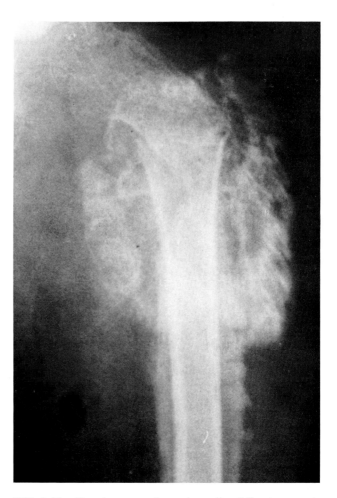

FIG. 8-21. Development of massive callus following proximal femoral fracture in child with myelomeningocele.

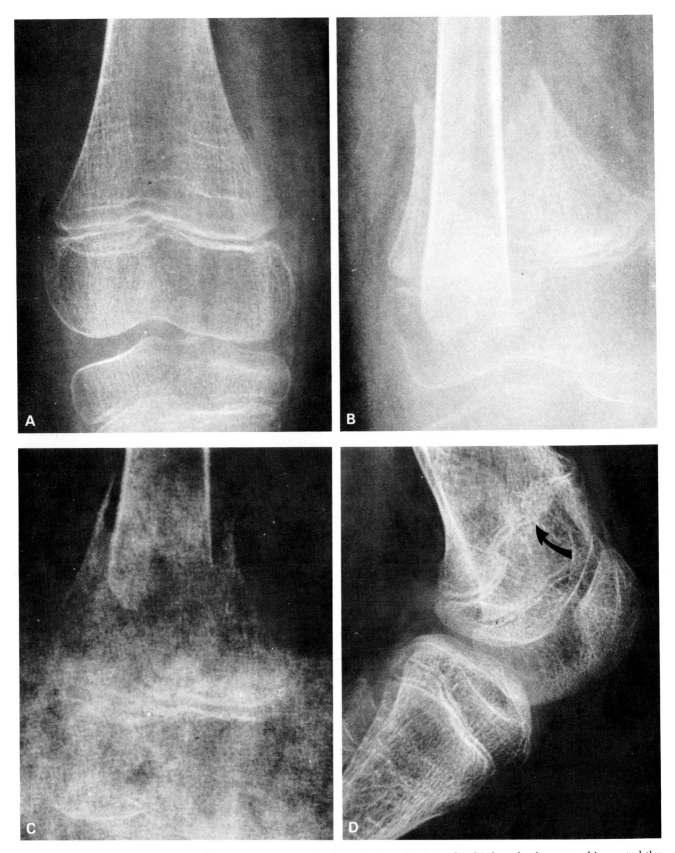

FIG. 8-22. *A,* Osteoporotic bone following removal of hip spica. *B,* The patient stood in his long leg braces and impacted the femur through the physis into the epiphysis. *C,* Roentgenogram taken after reduction. *D,* Growth arrest six months later, with osseous bridge (arrow).

Most fractures in cerebral palsied patients may be treated with casts. However, the type of plaster immobilization must be modified according to coexisting contractures of contiguous joints. Contiguous joints, whenever possible, should be included in the cast, although severe contractures of these joints may obviate more adequate immobilization.

Nonunion is rare. Malunion is infrequent, usually relating to a preexistent contracture, and usually occurring in severely spastic patients. Malunion is particularly a problem in femoral fractures, but it may also occur in the humerus (Fig. 8-23). The malunions never improve the situation by compensating for the joint contractures. Remodeling in children under ten usually is comparable to that in neurologically normal children. Significant growth disturbances are uncommon, and epiphyseal injuries are rare.

Refracture was encountered primarily in bedridden patients with severe deformities, and it was usually followed by malunion. Predisposing factors to refracture appear to be contractures, inadequate maintenance of reduction, and disuse osteopenia in bedridden patients.

Head injury

The partial maintenance of the position of a reduced fracture by the stabilizing action of the muscles with constant, normal tone is well recognized. If muscle tone is increased abnormally, a fracture may easily displace or angulate. Traction may increase muscle tone abnormally by overactivating the stretch reflexes, and displacement and angulation will increase. These factors must be considered in the conservative treatment of fractures of long bones associated with decerebrate rigidity due to brain stem or intracranial injury.[45,50] Decerebrate posturing results in full extension of the hips and knees and plantar flexion of the ankles. The arms may be extended or flexed, but they are held firmly in either position. The fluctuation in the level of consciousness determines the severity of the brain stem injury.

After a head injury, if consciousness is not lost or is regained rapidly, a serious injury to the brain stem probably has not occurred. The importance of this observation is that the original resistance present on testing joint movement in the patient will not be followed by permanent decerebrate rigidity, and the fractures may be treated temporarily by conservative methods, provided that the increased muscle tone is not displacing the fracture significantly.

Several factors must be considered in managing these patients: (1) The ultimate recovery potential of the head injury victim cannot be predicted accurately, particularly in the acute state and in children, who seem to have a greater capacity for recovery. The orthopaedist must proceed with effective treatment as if full neurologic recovery is going to occur. If the fractures of a head injured patient are only minimally treated, the child may recover almost completely and end up with severe, preventable deformities. (2) Anesthesia in head injured patients poses specific problems and may be delayed for a few hours or days to establish baseline neurologic levels before proceeding with treatment of severe or compound fractures. (3) Nursing and respiratory management in unconscious and/or uncooperative patients often are greatly improved by internal fixation of the fractures. If a patient exhibits either of these problems, appropriate fixation, using methods that will not affect longitudinal bone growth, may be indicated. A compression plate of a femoral

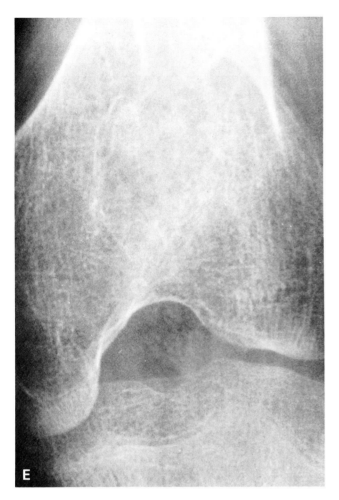

FIG. 8-22 (Continued). *E,* One year later, the physis is totally closed.

However, less common types of cerebral palsy, especially flaccid palsy, may have an increased incidence of functional osteoporosis. Further, if patients have been immobilized following surgery, particularly tendon-lengthening and transfer procedures, they may develop immobilization osteoporosis. More severe forms of cerebral palsy, particularly those associated with convulsions and severe spasticity, may include fractures. An overly aggressive therapy program may also cause fractures when trying to overcome joint contractures.

McIvor reviewed fractures in 57 cerebral palsied patients under 20 years of age.[61] Invariably they sustained closed fractures, with the exception of one open fracture. There was no definite correlation between the type of cerebral palsy and the incidence or location of fracture. The major causes of fractures appeared to be falls or direct blows (such as striking the side of the bed during a seizure). Only five fractures occurred following orthopaedic procedures. The more severe the disease involvement, the greater the number of fractures. A contracture or paralytic hip dislocation predisposed a patient to femoral fracture, and knee contractures predisposed patients to distal femoral and proximal tibial fractures.

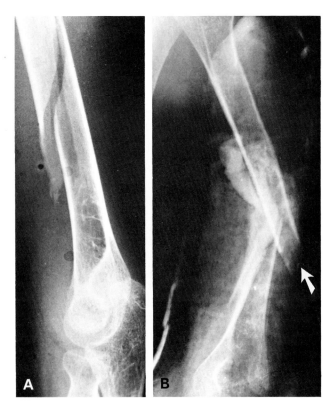

FIG. 8-23. *A*, Fracture of humerus in child with severe spastic cerebral palsy. *B*, This was placed in a long arm cast, but it angulated, and ten days later it became an open fracture due to ulceration (arrow).

fracture would be much preferred to a Küntscher rod that has to be placed through the proximal femoral growth plate (intraepiphyseal region).

Obstetric trauma to the spinal cord

Spinal cord injury resulting from obstetric trauma merits separate consideration. In a review of 15,000 infants delivered at the University of Pennsylvania Hospital, only one instance of spinal cord injury was recorded.[62,63] However, such injuries often escape diagnosis. There was a high incidence of vertebral artery damage and significant epidural hemorrhage in neonates in whom the spinal cord was examined during autopsy. Most reported cases of spinal injury have occurred during breech delivery with traction applied to the trunk while manipulating the aftercoming head. Caesarean section delivery has been suggested for infants shown radiographically to be in a hyperextended ("star-gazing") breech position.

Birth injuries of the spinal cord occur most commonly at the cervicothoracic junction. The spinal column of the infant consists of a series of elastic rings joined by relatively brittle discs and ligaments. The dura mater is attached to the vertebral canal by many strong fibrous bands in the cervical and lumbar region, but it is only loosely attached in the thoracic region. The cord itself is anchored firmly by the brachial plexus above, and the cauda equina and lumbar plexus below; and it is relatively inelastic.

Lateral traction on the head increases the tension on the cord at its junction with the brachial plexus and may result in avulsion of the cervical roots. Hyperextension with traction applied to the legs and the head held firmly by uterine contraction may result in actual rupture of the cords and meninges. The cartilaginous spine of the infant may be grossly distorted, but it usually does not disrupt completely because of its relative elasticity. Injuries occurring above the level of the phrenic nuclei are generally rapidly fatal. However, the neonate with a lower cervical or cervicothoracic injury may survive. Generally, the damage extends over several segments and the infant is noted at birth to be hypotonic with depressed respirations. Prompt resuscitative measures are followed by the appearance of reflex movement to stimulation, which sometimes leads to the diagnosis of primary muscle disease.

It should be noted that the spinal shock seen in adult patients following severe cord trauma generally is not present in the infant, and recovery of reflex function follows a time course similar to that of recovery of movement following any resuscitative procedure in the newborn. Continued flaccidity is probably due to destruction of the cord over many segments, either as a result of intramedullary hemorrhage or infarction. The demonstration of a sensory level is the key diagnostic criterion. The presence of an abnormal "wheal and flare" skin response and the lack of a cortical response to stimulation of the lower extremities may be helpful diagnostic signs.

Minor degrees of cord damage may account for some of the spastic diplegias now grouped with cerebral palsies. Secondary injuries to the cerebral cortex may result from hypoxia caused by the transient respiratory depression that is associated with reversible, undiagnosed neonatal cord injury. The true contribution of neonatal traumatic myelopathy to the broad group of neurologic diseases associated with birth injuries remains to be defined.

Treatment in these cases is generally supportive. Upper respiratory infections are common, and pneumonia is a frequent cause of death in infancy. Lack of vasomotor control below the level of the lesion may seriously impair temperature regulation in the infant.

Congenital sensory neuropathy

Several syndromes are associated with congenital insensitivity to pain in patients with otherwise normal muscle tone.[64] In particular, children with congenital sensory neuropathy have insensate joints. Progressive destruction of the articular surface is common (Fig. 8-24). Epiphyseal fractures also are relatively common and may lead to chronic epiphysiolysis, physeal damage, and premature physeal closure (Fig. 8-25).

Muscular dystrophy

Many of the progressive muscular dystrophies that commence in childhood, such as Duchenne muscular dystrophy, lead to excessive osteoporosis in the metaphyseal and diaphyseal cortices, and in the metaphyseal and epiphyseal trabecular bone.[64] This leads to increased tubulation of the bone and occurs primarily because growth stimulation from normal muscular tension is deficient.[57,65] Disease progression and weakness may be severe enough to cause frequent fall-

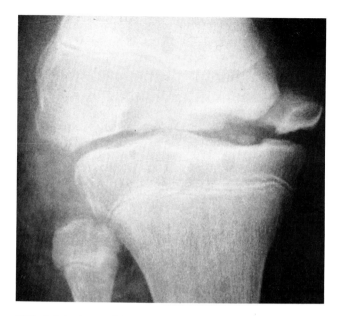

FIG. 8-24. Loss of joint space and fragmentation of distal femoral ossification center in a 13-year-old with a sensory neuropathy.

ing and worsening of contractures by the time the child is nine or ten years old, and wheelchair confinement in adolescence.[66] Fractures occur readily in porotic bones that lack protective muscle bulk and fat. Fractures are most common in the diaphyses, especially the femur and upper humerus. Fractures sustained falling out of wheelchairs are more common than those sustained from falling while in braces.[67] Usually, fracture fragments are minimally displaced and less painful than they are for the nondystrophic patient, because little muscle spasm accompanies the break. Healing appears to be unimpaired by muscular dystrophy. However, since these children lose strength rapidly when confined to bed, ambulatory treatment of fractures should be used whenever possible.[68]

Hematologic Disorders

Coagulation disorders

Hemophilia generally refers to deficiencies of factor VIII and IX. Other congenital coagulation disorders are described in Table 8-1. Patients with a severe deficiency of factor VIII or IX (less than 5% of the normal amount) have spontaneous bleeding episodes and usually come to medical attention in infancy. Patients with moderate deficiencies (10 to 20% of the normal amount) may come to medical attention because of unusual bleeding following relatively mild trauma. Mild deficiencies (20 to 50% of the normal amount) or deficiencies of another of the clotting factors shown in Table 8-1 are generally associated with few bleeding problems in daily life, but may cause bleeding complications following dental extractions, trauma, or surgery.

Fracture treatment of patients with congenital disorders of blood coagulation has become easier for three fundamental reasons:[69,70] (1) ease and specificity of diagnosis have been

TABLE 8-1. *Coagulation Disorders*

Factor VIII	Antihemophilic factor	Hemophilia A
—	von Willebrand's factor	von Willebrand's Disease
Factor IX	Christmas factor—plasma thromboplastic component	Hemophilia B
Factor X	Stuart-Prower	—
Factor XI	Plasma thromboplastin-antecedent	Hemophilia C

greatly facilitated by increased understanding of the coagulation mechanism and improved laboratory methods for making specific diagnosis of the disorders; (2) increased availability of concentrated clotting materials and experience in the medical management of patients with clotting disorders; and (3) a longer life expectancy which has led to increased probability of developing traumatic injuries prevalent in the general population as well as problems peculiar to bleeding disorders.

Many hemophiliacs, because of the current intensive replacement programs, do not suffer major musculoskeletal deformity. Children with moderate or severe hemophilia may be more susceptible to fracture because of limited joint movement, poor muscle function, and associated osteoporosis. Every effort should be made to maintain joint ranges of motion and promote isotonic and isometric exercises. Those who develop inhibitors, which lead to poorly controlled muscular and joint bleeds and contractures also may be predisposed to fracture. Recurrent bleeding in a child who has an inhibitor maximizes the immobilization necessary to treat bleeds, which will lead to osteoporosis. More significant in these children is bleeding into the forearm or lower leg compartment to create Volkmann's contracture.

Table 8-2 summarizes the requirements for ongoing treatment of fractures in patients with hematologic disorders. Inhibitor screening tests are mandatory. Presence of an inhibitor necessitates a modified approach to fracture treatment. When fracture treatment would be improved consid-

TABLE 8-2. *Requirements for Fracture Treatment (Closed and Open) in Patients with Coagulation Disorders*

1. Adequate, readily available replacement material (factors).
2. Survival studies of factor in patient.
3. Inhibitor screening.
4. Pretreatment hemoglobin, hematocrit, reticulocyte count, haptoglobins.
5. Capacity to do assays.
6. Blood bank facilities.

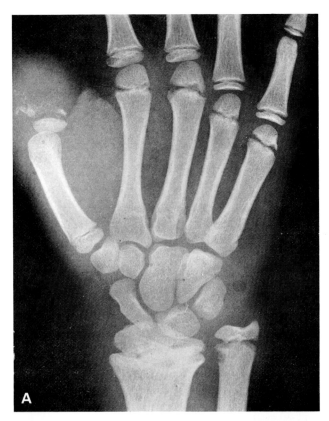

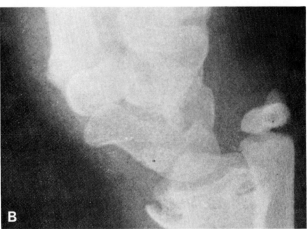

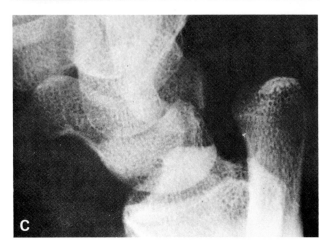

TABLE 8-3. *Therapeutic Guidelines for Patients with Coagulation Disorders*

1. Raise plasma level to 100% at time of fracture for 48 hours.

2. Maintain plasma level greater than 60% for one week.

3. Then maintain plasma level greater than 40% until subperiosteal new bone is evident (three to four weeks).

4. Increase level to 100% for three days during acute mobilization.

5. Decrease level to 40% for one week.

6. Monitor plasma levels with daily assays, when feasible, during the first seven to ten days, when the fracture is most unstable and more likely to bleed.

erably by the use of factor replacement and an inhibitor is present, several therapeutic options are available, including the use of high dose factor concentrates, exchange transfusion, or one of the experimental concentrates containing activated clotting factors.[71-73]

Use of the antifibrinolytic agent, epsilon-aminocaproic acid (EACA), has been recommended as an alternative to replacement material in patients undergoing active treatment for acute fractures. The use of EACA is contraindicated in patients for whom adequate replacement therapy is available.[73] The clots formed by EACA on the fibrinogen strands may not lyse for six months, and thus can cause considerable fibrosis, particularly in bleeds that complicate fractures around and within joints.

Proper dosage of specific replacement products must be based on a variety of factors, including the nature and severity of the bleeding defect, the patient's weight, and the biologic half-life of the infused factor. The orthopaedic surgeon should work closely with the hematologist in seeing that appropriate replacement product and levels are given. Careful monitoring of the patient is mandatory, particularly to detect the gradual build-up of an inhibitor that might affect the level of coagulation attained.

The goal of hematologic management of the fracture in the initial three to four week period, until the child has gotten into the remodeling phase, is to maintain sufficient clotting factor levels for a sufficient period of time to forestall bleeding complications. In general, the regimen outlined in Table 8-3 has proved efficacious. The distinction between major and minor fractures is fallacious in patients with a clotting disease, as a seemingly minor fracture (e.g., a meta-

FIG. 8-25. Chronic trauma leading to type 5 growth arrest of the distal radius in a child with sensory neuropathy. The ulna continued relatively normal growth. *A,* At 8 years of age. *B,* At 11 years of age, *C,* At 15 years of age. Also note the self-inflicted damage to the distal phalanx of the thumb.

carpal) may lead to severe bleeding and, potentially, to the loss of a hand or digit if too large a bleed occurs within a closed space. Hemostatic factors must be maintained at high levels for at least five days when the injured areas are immobilized. The degree of replacement can be tapered during subsequent healing until vigorous rehabilitation and mobilization is started, at which time sufficiently high factor levels must again be achieved.

When planning treatment, it is important to consider the lowest level to which the patient's clotting factor will fall between transfusions, because recurrence of bleeding is determined by this level. Certain damaged tissues may need higher clotting factor concentrations than others. In general, the more extensive the injury, the higher the required concentration. Second, transfusion should be continued at least for the shortest time necessary for the healing of a particular injury, because there is always considerable risk of recurrent bleeding during this period.

Finally, the importance of immobilization of the fracture must be emphasized, since even slight movement in children with clotting disorders can cause a recurrence of bleeding. Even maneuvers such as changing a cast may have to be accompanied by infusion of the appropriate replacement factor. Soft tissues may bleed enough to produce compression of nerves and vessels with consequent neuropraxia or ischemia.[74] Peripheral gangrene and Volkmann's ischemia have been observed in these patients.

No fracture or soft tissue injury in the limb of the hemophiliac should be immobilized in circumferential plaster unless hemostasis is absolute and swelling is subsiding. Any plaster applied during the first 24 hours should be adequately padded and completely split after application. Fracture healing, per se, in the hemophiliac is not delayed, even in patients who have not received treatment with coagulation factors.

Since most patients in major hemophiliac programs are on home transfusion programs, frequent treatment does not necessarily require hospitalization. However, if bleeding is excessive, it is wise to hospitalize the child for observation. This is particularly important if the patient has an inhibitor, in which case it is impossible to transfuse, and the patient must be kept in protected immobilization, elevation, and close observation for evidence of neurovascular compromise and the need to consider other methods of hemostasis.

An important observation is the relative lack of subperiosteal callus, which suggests that fracture healing in these cases is largely endosteal. Since healing does follow this pattern, great care should be taken in the post-fracture mobilization period. When fractures of certain bones, such as the femur, are treated by rigid compression, which emphasizes endosteal repair as opposed to periosteal repair, the incidence of refracture after removal of the hardware increases, implying that a longer period of immobilization may be necessary for remodeling adequate to support the weight and activity of the child.

Thalassemia

Thalassemia is a genetically determined hemoglobinopathy, classically transmitted in children whose ancestry can be traced to the Mediterranean area. The disease is inherited as a single, autosomal, incompletely dominant gene, and in the homozygous state, two defective alleles are present. The disease is characterized by a primary deficiency in the production of beta globin chains, which produces an abnormal hemoglobin that leads to a severe hemolytic anemia. The anemia and the secondary hemochromotosis then affect most organ systems, including the developing chondroosseous skeleton. Many patients have hypoparathyroidism and hypothyroidism with delayed sexual maturation. This also affects the developing skeleton and its biomechanical response to stress.

The skeletal changes basically reflect compensatory hyperactivity and hypertrophy of the bone marrow manifested by osteoporosis, widened medullary spaces, thinning of the intratrabecular cortices, and thinning of the diaphyseal and metaphyseal cortices with coarse reticulations.[75-77] In a rapidly growing skeleton, these changes can be particularly prominent in the metaphysis, especially in the juxtaphyseal area, where they may lead to small microfractures and damage to the zone of Ranvier, which can lead in turn to osseous bridging that may not manifest itself until the adolescent growth spurt (Fig. 8-26). These profound skeletal changes also may be caused by impaired ossification, a result of faulty protein metabolism.[78]

Other common roentgenographic findings are abnormal modeling of the bones. The reported skeletal manifestations include delayed skeletal maturation and premature fusion of the epiphyses of long bones. In one study, 11 of 79 patients, all of whom were older than 10 years, showed premature fusion, most often involving the proximal humerus and distal femur.[79] The presence of fusion did not relate to either the severity of the disease or the number of transfusions. Although the cause of the disturbance of growth is not yet understood, antecedent trauma, infection, or pathologic microfractures are obvious possibilities, with the last being most likely.

Dines, Canale, and Arnold made an extensive study of fractures in patients with homozygous beta thalassemia.[80] Of 75 patients, 25 had one or more fracture, and 7 had evidence of premature fusion of an epiphysis of one of the long bones. A total of 47 fractures were noted in these 25 patients. Ten patients had more than one fracture, and one patient had experienced nine separate fractures. Most of the fractures occurred in the long bones of the lower extremity. A permanent deformity had occurred by the time of diagnosis in all but two patients. These results indicate that these patients often sustain multiple fractures that frequently heal with deformities. These patients now can be expected to live longer because of the more adequate transfusion therapies; but these therapies, particularly when they are started early, allow growth plate damage to manifest itself as shortening or angular deformity.

Although actual data on healing time are lacking, the overall assumption is that healing is slow in most of these patients and that permanent deformities are common.[81] In addition, refractures were common and often resulted from minimal trauma. The high frequency of fracture undoubtedly is a consequence of the severe osteoporosis that commonly accompanies the marked erythroid hyperplasia of the marrow. Normal bone metabolism depends upon normal endocrine function and protein metabolism, and thalassemic patients often have demonstrated deficiencies in these areas. A possible abnormal thyroid function, impaired parathyroid and gonadotrophic hormone function as a result of pituitary dysfunction, and hemochromotosis of the affected end-

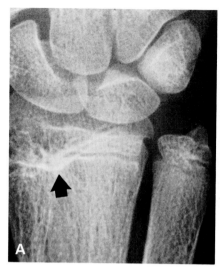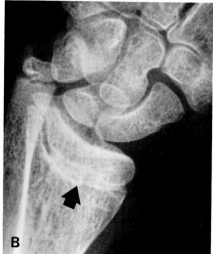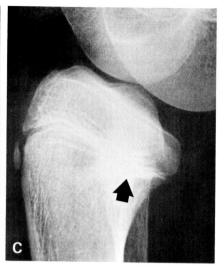

FIG. 8-26. Thalassemia. *A,* Mild osseous bridging (arrow) in left distal radius. *B,* More severe bridging (arrow) and relative growth retardation in right distal radius. *C,* Posterior bridge formation in the proximal tibia (arrow). None of these were associated with significant antecedent trauma.

organs secondary to the thalassemia have been reported as major causes of skeletal disorders. Protein hypermetabolism and increased catabolism, as evidenced by the increase in urinary excretion of hydroxyproline in these patients, interfere with normal chondro-osseous protein metabolism.[78] This may well contribute to the deficient ossification seen in the disease.

Treatment of pathologic fractures in these osteoporotic children has been limited to conventional techniques. Skeletal traction should be avoided in view of the extreme degrees of osteoporosis; although as these children are now being treated more effectively and from an earlier age, they do not have such severe chondro-osseous changes and probably can be treated safely and effectively with skeletal traction. However, if skeletal traction is chosen as treatment for a femoral fracture, the pin must be checked carefully to make sure that it does not migrate through mildly osteoporotic bone into the distal femoral physis or the proximal tibial tuberosity, if either of these is the site of pin placement.

Similarly, open reduction has rarely been contemplated in the past because of the relatively short life expectancy of the children. Again, because of improved treatment, these children are reaching skeletal maturation and young adult life with deformities that should be prevented. The changes causing premature fusion, particularly in the proximal humerus, seem to relate to small osseous bridges, and it is feasible that they might be resected. However, the primary consequence of the proximal humeral deformity is deficient length of the humerus. The deformity appears not to cause a major functional limitation, and it seems unlikely that an effort at bridge resection should be made in these cases. If the patient begins to exhibit functional limitation, then fusion of the more lateral portions under the greater tuberosity (epiphysiodesis) should be considered.

Maintenance of hemoglobin at greater than 12 g/100 ml may suppress both marrow hyperplasia and protein catabolism and significantly improve skeletal development. Further, Dines (unpublished data) reported that four children had clinical relief of bone and joint pain with vigorous transfusion regimens and replacement therapy with calcium and vitamin D_2.

Scott was one of the first to advocate the use of corrective osteotomies in children with thalassemia who had sustained either malalignment of fractures or premature closure of the epiphysis.[82] This approach was previously uncommon, because it had a poor prognosis in children, but as transfusion therapy in children improves, reconstructive surgery for skeletal abnormalities becomes a more realistic approach.

Leukemia

Pathologic fractures in the spine and lower extremities, or pain in the metaphyseal regions (possibly due to microscopic fractures) often are the presenting signs and symptoms of leukemia (Fig. 8-27). Multiple or even single vertebral compression fractures in an otherwise healthy child, especially in the absence of significant trauma, should make one highly suspicious. When pain in the joint region is the complaint, roentgenography of the metaphyses may show trabecular irregularities or collapse. Pain usually improves if the child is placed on effective chemotherapy, implying that many of the changes that occur are a skeletal response to expansile marrow hyperplasia caused by the disease.

Athletic Injuries

Injuries to the musculoskeletal system involving the young athlete appear to be much less prevalent than those involving the adolescent athlete, particularly when ligamentous injuries are considered.[83] Larsen reported a series of 4854 athletic injuries, of which only 933 occurred in children under 15 years of age, even though that group represented the greatest number of participants in organized athletic programs.[84] Selective examination of tackle football programs in this study showed the injury rate for the junior high school population to be 11%, whereas the injury rate in the high school population was 33%. Similar differences were seen in other sports activities such as baseball, basketball, track, gymnastics, wrestling, and cross-country. In these particular sports, junior high school students had an injury incidence of 2%, whereas the high school students had an injury rate of 12%.

Certain sports seem to have prevalent injury patterns.[85-87] Ice hockey is associated with a high incidence of cranial and facial trauma, a fact stressing the need to wear protective head gear including not only a helmet but also a face mask. Prior to skeletal maturation, injury to the lower back is relatively uncommon, but it becomes more frequent in the older (adolescent) age groups. Lower back injuries usually involve soft tissue inflammation and manifest themselves as a loss of lumbar lordosis due to paravertebral muscle spasm. An increase is apparent in discrete skeletal trauma to the low back in certain sports characterized by repetitive spinal stresses (Fig. 8-28). For example, spondylolysis and spondylolisthesis are being seen more frequently in young gymnasts and figure skaters.

Upon critical evaluation and comparison, the main difference between organized athletic programs and unorganized play appears to be adult supervision and participation. Without adult supervision, youngsters are not bound by rigid rules. They create their own rules, which conform to their physical abilities and enjoyment. Their activities are more varied, changing frequently from one game to another according to their moods. As a rule, they do not force themselves beyond their physical tolerance or ability and they stop playing when tired or slightly injured. If injured, medical attention is not complicated by pressures from parents and coaches, so healing progresses normally. In contrast, in organized sports the youngster's activities are completely dominated and regulated by adult supervision, both from the coach and the often overaggressive and demanding parents. This deprives the youngsters of much of the fun and enjoyment they should derive from sports. Although many rules of organized sports have been modified to conform to the age and size of the participants, basically most games are played the same no matter what the age level of the participants, and the tendency is to treat the youngsters as miniature adults. Instead of being varied, physical activity becomes repetitive, with persistent practice and the demand for maximum effort, and it is spurred on by the competitive pressures of winning at any cost, team spirit, and a spartan attitude toward injury.

The periods of increased athletic activity, particularly through the aegis of organized team sports, coincide with the times of developmental maturation of the male and female chondro-osseous skeletal systems. Any physician dealing with children who participate in organized sports must consider the variations in growth maturity and coordination of the musculoskeletal system (during both the preparticipation physical examination and the treatment of specific injuries); and he must have an appreciation for the development of the skeleton, particularly its response to stress and its normal and abnormal responses to injury. This should include not only an awareness of epiphyseal injuries, but an awareness of injuries to other areas of the metaphysis and diaphysis as well.

Any abnormalities of skeletal development, whether localized or generalized, as well as any chronic disorders must be evaluated on an individual basis that considers which ac-

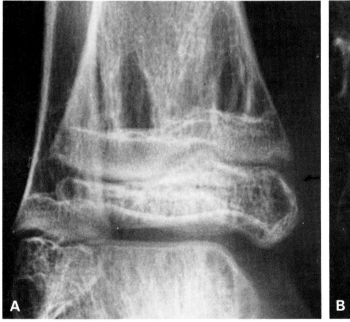 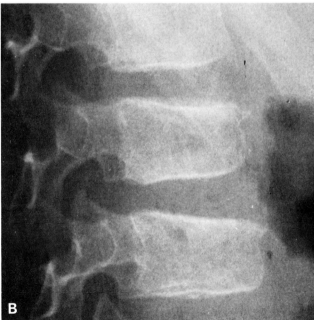

FIG. 8-27. *A*, Severe leukemic involvement in distal tibia and talus, with marrow hyperplasia and expansile destruction. The Harris growth arrest line demarcates the start of effective chemotherapy for the leukemia, after which the formation of more normal trabecular patterns is seen. *B*, Wedging of vertebral bodies due to leukemic involvement. Back pain is a relatively common initial presentation of children with leukemia.

tivities can be safely performed in view of the musculoskeletal problem or problems.[88] Certain injuries may effectively preclude participation in certain sports, but not others, thereby allowing the child an opportunity to participate in some degree of physical activity without risking further injury. As is discussed later, "little league elbow" is essentially a disorder affecting preadolescent pitchers. By changing to a fielding position or decreasing the amount of pitching, the youngster may continue to participate in the chosen athletic activity.

Athletic trauma, whether incurred during participation in organized or in recreational sports, usually has a recognizable cause. The most important factors leading to injury appear to be the following:

Conditioning. The young athlete must learn the fundamentals of both a specific sport and a generalized physical conditioning program. Injury most commonly occurs in novice participants in the early parts of the season or the early part of a game.[1,89] As a young athlete develops coordination, confidence, and experience, he lessens the risk of injury. It certainly is becoming recognized that ligament strength may increase with conditioning. This undoubtedly is important in the older adolescent, but may not be as crucial in the younger child, in whom ligamentous laxity is a normal musculoskeletal phenomenon.

Endurance. Continued physical conditioning and increased familiarity with the specific demands of a sport make an athlete less susceptible to injury. Fatigue is an important predisposing factor, but it becomes less consequential as the child learns to pace himself.

Antecedent Injury. Failure to diagnose and treat minor trauma can culminate in serious injury later. For example, repetitive unprotected ankle "sprains" in a young gymnast can lead to serious inversion injury with complete ligamentous disruption and a need for subsequent surgical reconstruction. Failure to recognize "back sprain" as being caused by traumatic spondylolysis, possibly in association with spondylolisthesis, can lead to serious impairment of the activity levels of a young gymnast.

Adherence to Rules. Many injuries are incurred during rule infractions. This includes failure to wear required protective equipment. It is the responsibility of the team physician to see that equipment rules are enforced strictly, and to discuss with officials any serious oversights regarding enforcement of rules that may affect the incidence of injury. It is extremely important that a physician on duty at a game identify himself to coaches as well as to officials, and that he establish a role for himself as final arbiter in any decision making process that affects the physical well-being of the participants.

Epiphyseal fractures, which are common in children, do not appear to occur more frequently as athletic injuries in organized or recreational sports during childhood.[84,90-92] Such fractures usually heal within three to four weeks, contingent upon the type of epiphyseal-physeal injury, and they are much stronger during the earlier phases of repair than healing fractures in the metaphysis or diaphysis. Return to athletic participation, however, must be individualized and include consideration of the patient's overall ability, assess-

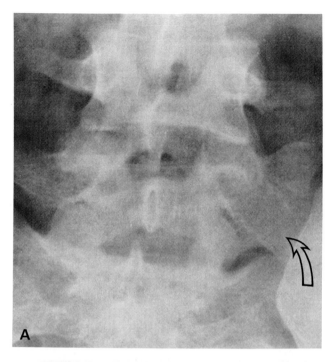

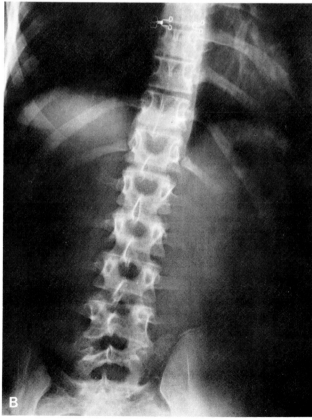

FIG. 8-28. *A,* Partial sacralization (arrow) of L5 in a 14-year-old who had acute onset of debilitating back pain following a gymnastic tournament. Tomograms suggested a stress fracture in this bone and a 99m-technetium scan was positive. *B,* Two months later, scoliosis was developing rapidly. She was treated with an L4-S1 fusion and has become completely asymptomatic.

ment of any damage to joint function (particularly when a type 3, 4, or 7 injury is involved) and appreciation of the particular musculoskeletal demands of the sport. When the epiphyseal fracture involves a joint, it is recommended that the child not participate in contact sports for at least a year, and that sports such as swimming, which allow joint exercise with lessened weightbearing stress, be encouraged.

One of the more common problems affecting the adolescent athlete has been termed "epiphysitis" or "apophysitis." These terms are used to describe "inflammatory" reactions involving the ligamentous or tendinous insertions into an epiphysis that is affected primarily by tensile forces (e.g., the ischial tuberosity, the tibial tuberosity, or the medial epicondyle of the distal humerus). Certainly the most publicized example is "little league elbow," a name applied to the mechanism that causes the clinical problem.[22,93-97a] Excessive duration of throwing, or of attempts to throw, a curve ball causes an immature elbow to change rapidly from acute flexion to forced extension or to severe hyperextension with a supinated forearm. This causes an excessive increase in muscular strain within the flexor-pronator muscle group and manifests itself in increased tensile force at the medial epicondyle of the distal humerus. Similarly, compressive stresses can damage the proximal radial epiphysis or capitellum, causing the development of an osteochondrosis in either region.[98-101]

Because of the hypervascularity associated with the normal repair response, these various areas may be the sites of excessive growth leading to localized overgrowth of the capitellum and radial head and, possibly, to a cubitus varus or valgus deformity. Furthermore, when the capitellum is involved, the articular surface may be fragmented and loose bodies may be created within the joint (see Chap. 11). Some degree of limitation of the amount of pitching would probably affect the incidence of this condition.

A similar sort of problem is now being recognized in young children playing intensely competitive tennis, in which the mechanism of the serve duplicates that of throwing a baseball. Torg described a nonunion of a stress fracture through the olecranon epiphyseal plate in an adolescent baseball pitcher. This represents another type of injury to the elbow that must be suspected in young adolescents who complain of persistent pain around the elbow.[102]

In the lower extremity, the insertion of the Achilles tendon into the epiphysis of the calcaneus sometimes leads to an entity known as Sever's disease (calcaneal apophysitis). This condition is best treated by rest and patients may benefit from the use of heel cups. The most frequently affected area in the lower limb is the tibial tuberosity, where Osgood-Schlatter's disease also becomes manifest. Recent anatomic and experimental studies suggest that this disease represents an avulsion of small portions of the patellar tendon and contiguous tibial tuberosity as the secondary ossification center is forming.[103] This leads to the formation of excessive osteocartilaginous tissue (callus) and a prominent deformity on the anterior tibia that may elevate the patellar tendon and patella enough to effect mechanical function along the patello-femoral axis.

Again, this disease is treated best by rest, and it may require immobilization in a cylinder cast for three to four weeks. Around the pelvis, the attachment of the rectus femoris to the anterior/inferior iliac spine, the psoas to the lesser trochanter, and the hamstrings to the ischial tuberosity are areas of potential apophysitis, as well as areas that can be completely avulsed as a result of excessively severe muscle contractures.[104]

Unless an obvious fracture, dislocation, or other musculoskeletal injury occurs, treatment often is recommended or instituted by coaches or parents. Their recommendations may be based on a minimal understanding of musculoskeletal disease, and knowledge and experience perhaps gained in training rooms during their own playing days in high school or college, usually at a much higher level of physical development than the young children whom they are "treating." Unfortunately, talented athletes, upon whom the coach and the team depend, often have their future and potential as "star" athletes jeopardized by either the lack of proper medical attention or the return to play before complete recovery from the injury.

Stress Fractures

A stress fracture results from the application of abnormal (muscular) stress or torque to a bone that has normal elastic resistance, a characteristic of most children's bone. Stress fractures often result from muscular activity on bone, rather than from direct impact. Most stress fractures share the following triad of causal factors: (1) the activity was new or different for the individual; (2) the activity was strenuous; and (3) the activity was repeated with a frequency ultimately producing the symptoms. Fractures also may occur when normal or physiologic stress is placed on a bone that has deficient elastic resistance. The fatigue type of stress fracture occurs in normal bone when abnormal muscular tension or torsion is placed upon it. The insufficiency type of stress fracture results when normal muscular stress is placed upon a bone in which elastic resistance is deficient. Most stress fractures are of the fatigue type and usually occur at reasonably predictable sites that relate to the activity that produced them.

One of the more common misconceptions regarding stress fractures is that they result from jarring injuries to the bones. Particularly with the fibula and calcaneus, there is antagonistic, forceful, muscle pull. When an individual jumps, an antagonistic pull of the Achilles tendon occurs in the calcaneus opposite the plantar tendons of the foot. The resulting action may overstress the calcaneus, producing the characteristic fracture parallel to the growth plate, but approximately a centimeter into the neck of the bone. The plantar fascia and much of the plantar musculature, as well as the Achilles tendon, attach into the inferior and superior regions of the calcaneal apophysis and certainly can stress it to create the condition known as Sever's disease, which may represent a mild stress fracture of the epiphyseal ossification center.[95]

When a bone-muscle system is stressed, changes take place that generally result in increased tone or strength of all components of the system. Bone will hypertrophy as a response to exercise. However, the rate of this response is much slower than it is for muscle. If an individual uses his increased muscle strength to perform an activity more vigorously, a stress fracture may result to bones that have not yet completely compensated for the new activity.

Stress fractures begin as small cortical cracks that progress as osseous strain increases or continues.[105] Crack propaga-

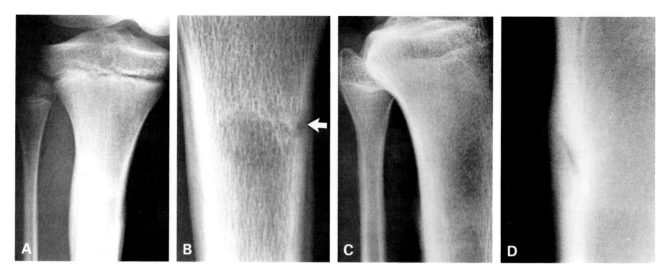

FIG. 8-29. *A*, Reactive bone around stress fracture in a 10-year-old child. *B*, Magnified view showing transverse fracture extending across the shaft (arrow). *C*, Early reactive bone in a 14-year-old complaining of "shin splints." *D*, Four weeks later, a small cortical fracture was evident.

tion is initiated by subcortical infractions ahead of the main crack. With increasing age, the elasticity of bone decreases and its predisposition to fracture increases. This particularly may occur in the adolescent going through major physiologic changes in the maturity of the bones during rapid longitudinal growth. In many instances, the patient may be unaware of the developing crack until it extends into a complete fracture. This is particularly common among young children, especially adolescents who often perform "with pain," attributing it to pulled muscles or "pointers" (Fig. 8-29).

The pattern of stress fractures in the child is different from that in the adult. In the child, the clinical course, radiographic features, and site of the lesion vary with age. Clinical and radiographic findings in children differ from those in adults, in part, because of the greater tendency of the young bone to undergo normal elastic and plastic deformation and remodeling, as well as because of the rich blood supply of the growing bone.

Stress fractures in children, particularly in the lower extremities may present diagnostic problems, because the child often also exhibits listlessness, slight irregular fever, swelling, and tenderness that must be distinguished from malignant tumors and osteomyelitis. A biopsy must be done if any uncertainty exists.

The most common sites of stress fractures in children are the upper third of the tibia (Fig. 8-30), the lower half of the fibula, and the metatarsal, rib, pelvis, femur, and humerus.[1,8,106-111] These become more common in the springtime when children increase their level of activity after a winter of relative inactivity.

In the tibia, it is nearly always the upper third of the bone that is affected by transverse fracture.[112] The child has a painful limp, usually of gradual onset but occasionally sudden. Younger children often refuse to bear weight on the affected leg. Sleep is usually unaffected. The pain improves with rest, but may not go away entirely. Tenderness may extend along the shaft, depending on the size of the subperiosteal reaction, and it certainly may be more marked on one

side than the other. Radiographically, there is a haze of internal callus across the shaft, subperiosteal new bone formation, and sometimes a slight disruption of the cortex. No linear fracture is radiographically evident because this is a compression stress fracture. The periosteum is elevated, presumably by hematoma formation, and as it calcifies, a long thin line of callus may be evident in the radiograph. The fibula may sustain a stress fracture at a younger age than most other bones. The youngest child in Devas' series was two.[113]

Routine radiography of suspected stress fractures should include repeat examinations in one to two weeks. Magnification studies with fine focal spot technique and tomography may prove helpful in making the diagnosis. Three major conditions should receive consideration in the differential diagnosis of stress fractures. These are osteoid osteoma, chronic sclerosing osteomyelitis, and Ewing's or osteogenic sarcoma.

The roentgenographic changes of stress fractures can be divided into three phases. Initially, there is a small area of radiolucency in the cortex on the posterior wall of the tibia. This is associated with some metaphyseal, endosteal increase in bone density and a fine haze of periosteal reaction. These findings usually are present two to three weeks after the onset of symptoms. This phase is often missed in children. Follow-up films reveal a gradual increase in the periosteal and endosteal new bone. This second phase is sometimes associated with the appearance of a definite, incomplete defect. If an actual fracture does occur, this periosteal and endosteal new bone matures and is partially resorbed. If a fracture line becomes apparent, the characteristic sequence of an undisplaced fracture follows.

Recently, radioisotope scanning with 99m-technetium compounds has proved useful in the evaluation of stress fractures.[114] This technique has allowed early diagnosis of suspected lesions, since the bone scan is usually positive before there are any radiographic findings (Fig. 8-31). However, the technique is not specific for stress fracture. Early osteomyelitis, which often has similar clinical signs and

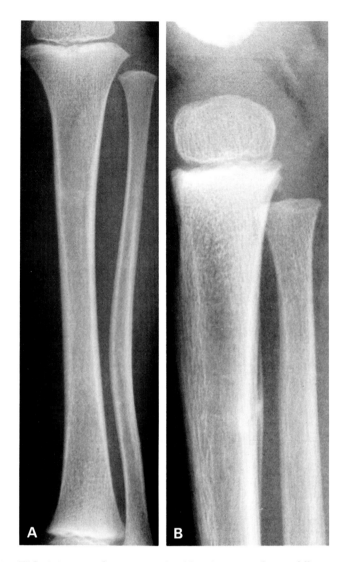

appears to be increased cortical resorption.[116] This resorption occurs by the formation of many hollow channels through the cortex. This process of osteoclastic tunneling normally occurs gradually throughout childhood, adolescence, and early adult life. The resorption spaces normally are filled with mature Haversian systems. In this fashion, the circumferential lamellar bone of childhood is converted gradually to osteonal bone, which is structurally more compatible with weightbearing stresses.

The most important stimulus to this conversion process is use. However, with excessive use, cortical resorption can be stimulated to an accelerated rate at which susceptibility to localized injury is increased. Relatively immature trabecular bone can be formed more rapidly than mature osteonal bone, and this is the normal healing response. If the temporary buttressing bone is not formed rapidly and if continued excessive stress is applied to the bone, microfracture or gross fracture may occur.

Resorption of cortical bone is a normal process taking place in childhood and adolescence. Osteoclastic activity results in many microscopic channels through the cortex, especially in the metaphyseal region. Eventually, these resorption cavities are filled by mature Haversian systems. The lamellar bone is gradually replaced by more structurally adapted osteonal bone.

The usual sites of stress fractures in children are areas of junction between metaphyseal and diaphyseal cortices in regions in which fenestration is less prominent (as compared to the juxtaepiphyseal region) and in which biomechanical stresses change between lamellar bone and osteonal bone.

FIG. 8-30. *A*, This 14-month-old girl sustained a "toddler's fracture" of the fibular diaphysis. *B*, One year later, she was limping again. The roentgenogram showed residual bowing of the fibula, but no acute injury. However, the area over the proximal tibia was tender. She was placed in a non-weightbearing cast. Three weeks later, reactive subperiosteal bone compatible with a tibial stress fracture was evident.

symptoms, may produce the same scintigraphic appearance. Prather reported the use of bone scanning in the evaluation of stress fractures.[115] In 15 patients roentgenographs were normal, while the bone scan was positive. The need to obtain total body scans, rather than focal spot films, should be emphasized, because four of the patients studied by Prather et al. had multiple areas of involvement (see Fig. 8-31). Bone scans offer a highly sensitive technique for the early diagnosis of stress fracture and abnormalities can be identified on scans long before there are roentgenographic changes.

Descriptions of the histologic appearance of stress fractures are limited (Fig. 8-32). The initial pathologic change

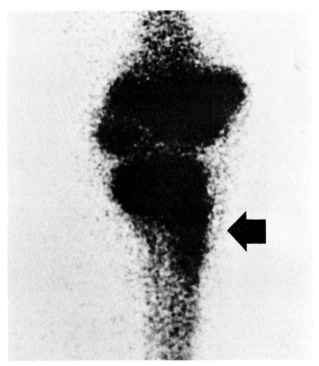

FIG. 8-31. Bone scan of patient shown in Figure 8-29*C* and *D*. There was positive uptake along the posteromedial region. Findings were similar in the other leg (symptomatic, but without any roentgenographic findings).

Bone responds to excessive stress and strain by acceleration of the normal process of cortical resorption and remodeling of the Haversian systems. The cortex may be weakened by formation of numerous resorption channels, but usually such structural changes are the consequence of normal anatomic variations.

If the child subjects himself to undue stress, particularly after a period of relative inactivity, the buttressing process that normally strengthens the bone at the metaphyseal/diaphyseal junction has not had a chance to occur, and excessive stress continuously applied to the bone may result in a subclinical fracture. In a stress fracture, cortical resorption is increased, periosteal and endosteal new bone forms, the resorption cavity in the cortex is filled in, and the periosteal and endosteal new bone matures. All this represents an excessive modification of the normal chondro-osseous developmental patterns.

Battered-Child Syndrome

A battered child is an unwitting victim of deliberate, physical trauma, usually inflicted by the person or persons responsible for the child's care. The radiographic and orthopaedic aspects of this syndrome were first elucidated by Caffey when he drew attention to the association of multiple fractures of the long bones with a significant number of cases of subdural hematoma.[116a] Initially, these fractures were thought to be pathologic. Silverman presented a report on multiple long bone fractures without subdural hematoma, and firmly established their deliberate basis.[117] Subdural hematoma is a common problem in the battered child, and possible brain damage due to repeated cranial trauma should receive prime consideration. The term "battered-child syndrome" was first used by Kempe.[118] Unfortunately, little information has appeared on this subject in the orthopaedic literature.[119]

Battered children tend to be young, with about ⅔ being under three years, and ⅓ under six months. Their general health is usually poor. They are underweight, malnourished, and retarded in development. Evaluation often reveals multiple fractures with evidence of repeated trauma. The fractures are usually in different stages of repair. There is a predilection for the metaphysis to fracture because of the poor nutrition (Fig. 8-33). It is possible that these areas are more susceptible to injury, because of "metabolic" bone disease. There is marked subperiosteal reaction and multiplicity of lesions in various stages of healing and repair. The trauma often is inflicted by vigorous pulling on the limbs, direct blows, or throwing the child. While one can be reasonably certain of the diagnosis, the differential must include osteogenesis imperfecta, congenital insensitivity to pain, scurvy, congenital lues, and infantile cortical hyperostosis.

Roentgenographic findings in the battered-child syndrome are well documented.[120] The classic picture in infants is multiple epiphyseal-metaphyseal fractures in various stages of healing. Spiral and transverse fractures of the long bones are also common, and one should not rely too heavily on the "classic" epiphyseal or metaphyseal fractures.[121] Multiple chondro-osseous injuries, especially if seen in various stages of healing must be considered highly suspicious, but not absolutely diagnostic of the battered-child syndrome. However, only 23% of the patients in Kogutt's paper showed this pattern of multiple, metachronous fractures; one should be suspicious of even solitary fractures with an incongruous clinical history.[120]

Fractures of the midshaft clavicle are fairly common, but it appears that fractures of the lateral margin of the clavicle are

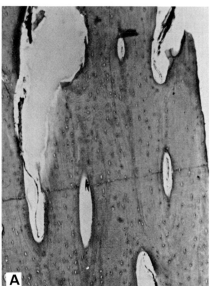 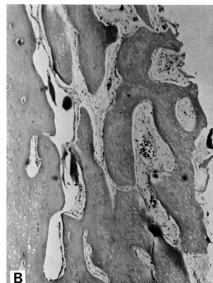 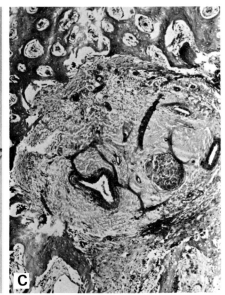

FIG. 8-32. Case shown in Figure 8-29C and D. A, Relatively normal cortical bone at periphery of biopsy margin (10×). B, Reactive subperiosteal new bone evident on roentgenogram shown in Figure 8-29C. The cortex is at the left side of the picture. C, Section through region of fracture shown in Figure 8-29D showing fibrovascular inflammatory tissue and reactive new bone adjacent to this tissue, which indicate a normal callus response. This should not be misinterpreted as osteogenic sarcoma.

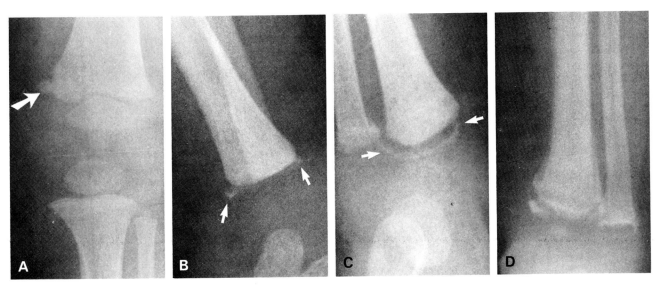

FIG. 8-33. Battered-child syndrome. *A*, Metaphyseal lipping of distal femur (arrow). *B*, Similar metaphyseal fractures involving the distal tibia (arrows). *C*, AP view in same patient shows that this fracture extends across the metaphyseal width (arrows). *D*, Chronic epiphyseal separation leads to avulsion of the entire periosteal sleeve, with formation of subperiosteal new bone along the entire shaft, not just the metaphysis. This must be differentiated from normal diaphyseal new bone in the neonate (see Fig. 8-7).

more common in cases of battered children. Sternal fractures are most unusual at any time and result from severe, direct blows to the chest. If such a fracture is present and there is no substantiating history, such as an automobile accident or crush injury, one should strongly consider the possibility of child abuse.

Rib fractures are also rather uncommon, particularly in the battered child age-range. The normal resilience of the young thorax, plus the need for a direct blow to have occurred, probably account for this fact. Healing rib fractures are sometimes seen shortly after birth, and may result from perinatal injury. If fractures are encountered later than this and a legitimate history of trauma is absent, the presence of the fractures should raise the possibility of intentional abuse (Fig. 8-34). In the battered-child syndrome, rib fractures are usually multiple and are seen most commonly in the posterior or lateral region of the ribs, but anterior costochondral separations also may occur.

Trauma to the spine and spinal cord in the battered-child syndrome have been reported, but are not common.[122-125] Generally, its appearance takes one of three configurations: (1) anterior notching of the vertebral body produced by hyperflexion injury with or without anterior herniation of the nucleus pulposus; (2) compression of the vertebral body; and (3) fracture-dislocation, which is certainly the most significant, since it is unlikely that such injury could have been sustained, in the abscence of significant vehicular or crushing trauma, other than from severe, purposeful, directed blows, violence, or shaking.

Akbarnia reviewed 231 patients with battered-child syndrome.[119] About $\frac{1}{3}$ of the patients required orthopaedic treatment. Among 74 children there were 265 fractures, with an average of 3.6 fractures per child and a range from 1 to 15. The distribution of the fractures was as follows: ribs, 72; humerus, 42; femur, 32; tibia, 31; skull, 25; hand, 15;

ulna, 12; radius, 11; and others, 24. Interestingly, only 1 of the 168 fractures of long bones in this study involved the growth plate.

Radiographic study of the bones will disclose the site, number, nature, and approximate age of the bone lesions. Since it is sometimes difficult to diagnose these lesions when

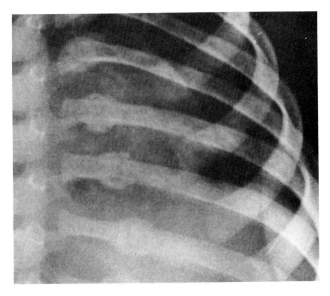

FIG. 8-34. Multiple posterior rib fractures in a child kicked repeatedly in the back. The child subsequently died from intra-abdominal injuries when sent back to the hostile home environment. (A second-degree manslaughter conviction was eventually obtained against the person who abused this child.)

radiographic signs of subperiosteal injury are minimal in the early stages, consideration should be given to a bone scan to detect areas of increased activity that might develop into fractures and warrant closer observation. The roentgen test of the skeleton for signs of trauma in parent-traumatized infants not only identifies the origin, but provides information that is valuable in several other ways. The presentation of positive roentgenographic evidence may persuade parents or other involved persons to tell the truth. In many cases, such evidence is a deterrent to further trauma.

The hypertrophic callus probably is caused by repeated abuse. Metaphyseal lesions are characterized by impactions, irregular metaphyseal deformity, and periosteal avulsion. Diaphyseal injuries are characterized by exuberant callus, multiple lesions in varying stages of healing, and gross deformity.

Most of the skeletal lesions in this syndrome result from traction or stretch stresses, rather than from impact or compression stresses. They are produced by stretching and shearing forces in the periosteum and in the tendinous and ligamentous attachments to the growing bones, rather than by direct compression from the hit of a hand or kick of a foot. The high frequency of these traction lesions indicates that the infant commonly is grabbed and held by the extremities while being shaken. In the extremities, the soft tissue stretching and squeezing are aggravated by the resistant counterforces of the infant as he twists and squirms.

Some battered children do not demonstrate the classic findings, but do demonstrate traumatic slipped epiphyses. These may be difficult to detect in initial studies, particularly if limited views are obtained. This injury is potentially harmful to the infant. If the injury is intracapsular, the periosteal pattern is not demonstrable along the shaft. If the displaced shaft is not realigned with its growth center, resorption of the primary shaft occurs and a new shaft forms in line with ossification centers. Sequential radiographs are sometimes strongly suggestive of osteomyelitis, and children have, on occasion, undergone unnecessary antimicrobial therapy. The prognosis in these injuries depends on the degree of cartilaginous physeal injury. Reconstitution may be almost complete, or if damage is severe, marked growth disturbances may occur (Fig. 8-35).

Whenever child abuse is suspected, a total skeletal survey must be done to rule out other fractures. It is impossible to say definitely that a given fracture, even the characteristic ones of infancy, is due to battering and not to other trauma such as a fall or vehicular accident. Most parents of a battered child are evasive about the mechanism of injury. They often simply state that the child fell out of the crib during a diaper change or fell down the stairs a few days before. Most concerned parents bring the child for examination immediately after an injury, and they are reasonably distraught about the circumstances. Therefore, lack of emotional interest in the injury should again arouse suspicion. Leven showed that of approximately 100 infants who had fallen (these were only the falls that had alarmed the mother), there was virtually no injury to the skeletal system.[119]

Statistics indicate that 10% of all injuries in children under the age of two years, and 25% of all fractures in children under the age of three years may be due to assault and battery. Fractures in these age groups always should be approached with a high index of suspicion. Whether or not the injury would normally demand admission to the hospital,

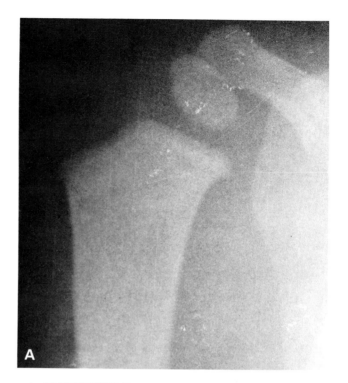

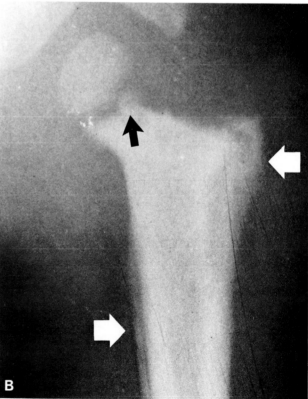

FIG. 8-35. *A,* Normal right proximal humerus. *B,* Damaged left proximal humerus with possible early osseous bridging (black arrow). Lateral metaphyseal and medial diaphyseal reactive bone has formed subperiosteally in response to the traumatic epiphysiolysis (white arrows). (The family abruptly moved out of the state when proceedings of child abuse were started.)

the child must be admitted for protection and to provide time for investigation. The child should also be examined to rule out generalized diseases of the skeleton such as scurvy, rickets, vitamin A toxicity of infantile cortical hyperostosis, pseudarthrosis, or osteogenesis imperfecta.

The orthopaedist can support the assertion that old as well as recent trauma is present, and that the changes are traumatic in nature, rather than due to other causes of periosteal new bone formation. A firm diagnosis such as that leads to the investigation of the home situation and the removal of the child from danger. When this has not been done, subsequent, repetitive, traumatic insults have caused permanent, crippling, deformities, and death has resulted from repeated brain, intrathoracic, and intra-abdominal damage.

It is the responsibility of the physician to report these cases of child abuse to the appropriate agency. In many states it is now legally mandatory for a physician to report a suspected case of child battering to allow the state the opportunity to prove or disprove the allegation. This type of legislation protects the physician from being sued for misrepresentation. Large medical centers have set up means of identifying suspicious cases and most pediatric emergency departments are attuned to recognizing these children and usually notice the injuries as part of their initial evaluation, so that the orthopaedist is rarely the first person involved.

References

1. Clement, D. B.: Tibial stress syndrome in athletes. J. Sports Med. Phys. Fitness, 2:81, 1974.
2. Dawson, G. R.: Intra-uterine fractures of the tibia and fibula. J. Bone Joint Surg., 31-A:406, 1949.
3. Smith, R. R.: Intra-uterine fracture. Report of a case and a review of the literature. Surg. Gynecol. Obstet., 17:346, 1913.
4. Snure, H.: Intrauterine fracture. Case report and review of roentgenologic findings. Radiology, 13:362, 1929.
4a. Bucholz, R., and Mauldin, D.: Prenatal diagnosis of intrauterine fetal fracture. J. Bone Joint Surg., 60-A:712, 1978.
5. Sacks, R., and Habermann, E. T.: Pathological fracture in congenital rubella. J. Bone Joint Surg., 59-A:557, 1977.
6. Sekeles, E., and Ornoy, A.: Osseous manifestations of gestational rubella in young human fetuses. Am. J. Obstet. Gynecol., 122:307, 1975.
7. Ris, P. M., and Wray, J. B.: A histological study of fracture healing within the uterus of the rabbit. Clin. Orthop., 87:318, 1972.
8. Bumbic, S., Lukac, R., and Najdanovic, Z.: Les epiphysiolyses obstetricales des nouveau-nes. Ann. Chir. Infant., 15:135, 1974.
9. Ekengren, K., Bergdahl, S., and Elstrom, G.: Birth injuries to the epiphyseal cartilage. Acta Radiol. [Diagn.] (Stockh.), 19:197, 1978.
10. Scott, W.: Epiphyseal dislocations in scurvy. J. Bone Joint Surg., 23:314, 1941.
11. Snedecor, S. T., and Wilson, H. B.: Some obstetrical injuries to the long bones. J. Bone Joint Surg., 31-A:378, 1949.
12. Hudson, R. T., Hutcherson, D. C., and Ortner, A. B.: Complete bilateral epiphyseal separation of the upper humeral epiphysis due to scurvy. J. Bone Joint Surg., 23:375, 1941.
13. Scaglietti, O.: The obstetrical shoulder trauma. Surg. Gynecol. Obstet., 66:868, 1938.
14. Kennedy, P. C.: Traumatic separation of the upper femoral epiphysis. A birth injury. A.J.R., 51:707, 1944.
15. Michail, J. P., Theodorou, S., Jouliaras, K., and Siatis, N.: Two cases of obstetrical separation (epiphysiolysis) of the upper femoral epiphysis. J. Bone Joint Surg., 40-B:477, 1958.
16. Singer, J., and Towbin, R.: Occult fracture in the production of gait disturbance in childhood. Pediatrics, 64:192, 1979.
17. Weston, W. J.: Metaphyseal fractures in infancy. J. Bone Joint Surg., 39-B:694, 1957.
18. Shopfner, C. E.: Periosteal bone growth in normal infants. A preliminary report. A.J.R., 97:154, 1966.
19. Shea, D., and Mankin, H. J.: Slipped capital femoral epiphysis in renal rickets. J. Bone Joint Surg., 48-A:349, 1966.
20. Mehls, O., Ritz, E., and Krempien, B.: Slipped epiphyses in renal osteodystrophy. Arch. Dis. Child., 50:545, 1975.
21. Schwarz, E.: Hypercallosis in osteogenesis imperfecta. A.J.R., 85:645, 1961.
22. Fulkerson, J. P., and Ozonoff, M. B.: Multiple symmetrical fractures of the bone of unresolved etiology. A.J.R., 129:313, 1977.
23. Bartsocas, C. S.: Multiple joint dislocation in mother and child. J. Pediatr., 80:299, 1972.
24. Roston, J. B., and Haines, R. W.: Cracking in the metacarpophalangeal joint. J. Anat., 81:165, 1947.
25. Unsworth, A., Dowson, D., and Wright, V.: 'Cracking joints.' A bioengineering study of cavitation in the metacarpophalangeal joint. Ann. Rheum. Dis., 30:348, 1971.
26. Neer, C. S., et al.: Current concepts on the treatment of solitary unicameral bone cyst. Clin. Orthop., 97:40, 1973.
27. Campanacci, M., Dessessa, L., and Bellando-Randone, P.: Bone cysts: review of 275 cases—results of surgical treatment and early results of treatment by methylprednisolone acetate injections. Chir. Organi. Mov., 62:471, 1976.
28. Butkin, W. J.: The avulsive cortical irregularity. A.J.R., 112:487, 1971.
29. Caffey, J.: Pediatric X-ray Diagnosis. 6th Ed. Chicago, Yearbook Medical Publishers, 1972.
30. Boznan, E. J.: Compression of cancellous bone. Am. J. Surg., 53:532, 1941.
31. Wenger, D. R., Jeffcoat, B. T., and Herring, J. A.: The guarded prognosis of physeal injury in paraplegic childen. J. Bone Joint Surg., 62-A:241, 1980.
32. Alliaume, A.: Fractures des os longs dans les myelo-meningoceles. Arch. Fr. Pediatr., 7:294, 1950.
33. Charcot, J. M.: Sur quelques arthropathies qui paraissant dependre d'une lesion du cervean ou de la moelle epiniere. Arch. Physiol. Norm. Pathol., 1:161, 1868.
34. Gillies, C. L., and Hartung, W.: Fractures of the tibia in spina bifida vera. Radiology, 31:621, 1938.
35. Golding, C.: Museum pages. III. Spina bifida and epiphyseal displacement. J. Bone Joint Surg., 42-B:387, 1960.
36. Gyepes, M. T., Newbern, D. H., and Neuhauser, E. B. D.: Metaphyseal and epiphyseal injuries in children with spina bifida and myelomeningocele. A.J.R., 95:168, 1965.
37. Johnson, J. T. H.: Neuropathic fractures and joint injuries. Pathogenesis and rationale of prevention and treatment. J. Bone Joint Surg., 49-A:1, 1967.
38. Korhonen, B. J.: Fractures in myelodysplasia. Clin. Orthop., 79:145, 1971.
39. Soutter, F. E.: Spina bifida and epiphyseal displacement. J. Bone Joint Surg., 44-B:106, 1962.
40. Zachary, R. B., and Sharrard, W. J. W.: Spinal dysraphism. Postgrad. Med. J., 43:731, 1967.
41. Norton, P. L., and Foley, J. J.: Paraplegia in children. J. Bone Joint Surg., 41-A:1291, 1959.
42. Quilis, A.: Fractures in children with myelomeningocele. Acta Orthop. Scand., 45:883, 1974.
42a. Ochme, J.: Periostale reaktionen bei myelomeningozele. Fortschr. Roentgen., 94:82, 1961.
43. Drennan, J. C., and Freehafer, A. A.: Fractures of the lower extremities in paraplegic children. Clin. Orthop., 77:211, 1971.
44. Handelsman, J. C.: Spontaneous fractures in spina bifida. J. Bone Joint Surg., 54-B:381, 1972.
45. Bellamy, R., and Brower, T. D.: Management of skeletal

trauma in the patient with head injury. J. Trauma, *14:*1021, 1974.

46. Caffey, J.: Multiple fractures in the long bones of infants suffering from chronic subdural hematoma. A.J.R., *56:*163, 1946.

47. Gillespie, G. A.: The nature of the bone changes associated with nerve injuries and disease. J. Bone Joint Surg., *36-B:*464, 1954.

48. Groher, W., and Heidensohn, P.: Ruchenschmerzen und roentgenologische Veranderungen bei Waysersspringer. Z. Orthop., *108:*51, 1970.

49. Jeannopoulos, C. L.: Bone changes in children with lesions of the spinal cord or roots. NY State J. Med., *54:*3219, 1954.

50. Merianos, P.: Treatment of fractures of the long bones in brain stem injury. Br. Med. J., *2:*316, 1975.

51. Robin, G. C.: Fractures in childhood paraplegia. Paraplegia, *3:*165, 1965.

52. Eichenholtz, S. N.: Management of long-bone fractures in paraplegic patients. J. Bone Joint Surg., *45-A:*299, 1963.

53. Navarro, A., and Peiro, A.: Healing in denervated bones. Acta Orthop. Scand., *45:*820, 1974.

54. Komprda, J.: Neurogenic osteogenesis following injuries of the lower extremities in children with myelomeningocoele. Acta Chir. Orthop. Traumatol. Cech., *31:*104, 1964.

55. Edvardsen, P.: Physeoepiphyseal injuries of lower extremities in myelomeningocoele. Acta. Orthop. Scand., *43:*550, 1972.

56. Corbin, K. B., and Hinsey, J. C.: Influence of the nervous system in bone and joint. Anat. Rec., *75:*307, 1939.

57. Walton, J. N., and Warrick, C. K.: Osseous changes in myopathy. Br. J. Radiol., *27:*1, 1954.

58. Katz, J. F.: Spontaneous fractures in paraplegic children. J. Bone Joint Surg., *35-A:*220, 1953.

59. Robin, G. C.: Fractures in poliomyelitis in childhood. J. Bone Joint Surg., *48-A:*1048, 1966.

60. Robin, G. C.: Prevention of fractures in the paralyzed child. Am. J. Orthop. Surg., *10:*16, 1968.

61. McIvor, W. C., and Samilson, R. L.: Fractures in patients with cerebral palsy. J. Bone Joint Surg., *48-A:*858, 1966.

62. Stern, W. E., and Rand, R. W.: Birth injuries to the spinal cord. Am. J. Obstet. Gynecol., *78:*498, 1959.

63. Yales, P. O.: Birth trauma to vertebral arteries. Arch. Dis. Child., *34:*436, 1959.

64. Siegel, I. M.: Fractures of long bones in Duchenne muscular dystrophy. J. Trauma, *17:*219, 1977.

65. Epstein, B. S., and Abramson, L.: Roentgenologic changes in the bones in cases of pseudohypertrophic muscular dystrophy. Arch. Neurol., *46:*868, 1941.

66. Taft, L. T.: The care and management of the child with muscular dystrophy. Dev. Med. Child Neurol., *15:*510, 1973.

67. Vignos, P. J., Jr., and Archibald, K. C.: Maintenance of ambulation in childhood muscular dystrophy. J. Chronic Dis., *12:*273, 1960.

68. Miller, J.: Management of muscular dystrophy. J. Bone Joint Surg., *49-A:*1205, 1967.

69. Feil, E., Bentley, G., and Rizza, C.: Fracture management in patients with haemophilia. J. Bone Joint Surg., *56-B:*643, 1974.

70. Kemp, H. S., and Matthews, J. M.: The management of fractures in haemophilia and Christmas disease. J. Bone Joint Surg., *50-B:*351, 1968.

71. Croom, R. D., III, Hutchin, P.: Surgical management of the patient with classical hemophilia. Surg. Gynecol. Obstet., *128:*793, 1969.

72. Dudley, N. E., Kernoff, P. B., and Gough, M. H.: Surgery in children with congenital disorders of blood coagulation. J. Pediatr. Surg., *6:*689, 1971.

73. Krieger, J. N., Hilgartner, M. W., and Redo, S. F.: Surgery in patients with congenital disorders of blood coagulation. Ann. Surg., *185:*290, 1977.

74. Jensen, P. S., and Putnam, C. E.: Hemophilic pseudotumor. Am. J. Dis. Child., *129:*717, 1975.

75. Baker, D. H.: Roentgen manifestations of Cooley's anemia. Ann. NY Acad. Sci., *119:*641, 1964.

76. Caffey, J.: Cooley's anemia: a review of the roentgenographic findings in the skeleton. A.J.R., *78:*381, 1957.

77. Choremis, C., Liakakos, D., and Tseghi, C.: Pathogenesis of osseous lesions in thalassemia. J. Pediatr., *66:*962, 1965.

78. Liakakos, D., Karpouzas, J., and Agathopoulos, A.: Hyperprolinemia and hyperprolinuria in thalassemia. J. Pediatr., *73:*419, 1968.

79. Currarino, G., and Erlandson, M. E.: Premature fusion of epiphysis in Cooley's anemia. Radiology, *83:*656, 1964.

80. Dines, D. M., Canale, V. C., and Arnold, W. D.: Fractures in thalassemia. J. Bone Joint Surg., *58-A:*662, 1976.

81. Herrick, R., and David, G.: Thalassemia major and non-union of pathological fractures. J. La. State Med. Soc., *127:*341, 1975.

82. Scott, W. N., Dines, D. M., and Insall, J. N.: Supracondylar osteotomy in Thalassemia. Clin. Orthop., *135:*42, 1978.

83. Rogers, L., et al.: "Clipping injury" fracture of the epiphysis in the adolescent football player: an occult lesion of the knee. A.J.R., *121:*69, 1974.

84. Larson, R.: Epiphyseal injuries in the adolescent athlete. Orthop. Clin. North Am., *4:*839, 1973.

85. Mack, R., et al.: The biomechanics of children's ski bindings. J. Sports Med. Phys. Fitness, *2:*154, 1974.

86. Quinby, W. C.: Athletic injuries in children. Clin. Pediatr., *3:*353, 1964.

87. Ryan, J. R., and Salciccioli, G. G.: Fractures of the distal radial epiphysis in adolescent weight lifters. Am. J. Sports Med., *4:*26, 1976.

88. Jokl, P.: Athletic injuries. Radiol. Clin. North Am., *11:*657, 1973.

89. McBryde, A.: Stress fractures in athletes. J. Sports Med. Phys. Fitness, *3:*212, 1975.

90. Collins, H. R.: Epiphyseal injuries in athletes. Clev. Clinic. Q., *42:*825, 1975.

91. Howard, F., and Piha, R.: Fractures of the apophyses in adolescent athletes. J.A.M.A., *192:*842, 1965.

92. Larson, R. L., and McMahon, R. O.: The epiphysis and the childhood athlete. J.A.M.A., *196:*607, 1966.

93. Adams, J. E.: Injury to the throwing arm: a study of traumatic changes in the elbow of boy baseball players. Calif. Med., *103:*127, 1965.

94. Adams, J. E.: Little league shoulder: osteochondrosis of the proximal humeral epiphysis in boy baseball pitchers. Calif. Med., *105:*22, 1966.

95. Cameron, H. U., and Fornasier, V. L.: Trabecular stress fractures. Clin. Orthop., *111:*266, 1975.

96. Lipscomb, A. B.: Baseball pitching injuries in growing athletes. J. Sports. Med. Phys. Fitness, *3:*25, 1975.

97. Torg, J. S., Pollack, H., and Sweterlitsch, P.: The effect of competitive pitching on the shoulders and elbows of pre-adolescent baseball players. Pediatrics, *49:*267, 1972.

97a. Brogdon, M. D.: Little leaguer's elbow. A.J.R., *83:*671, 1960.

98. Cahill, B. R., Tullos, H. S., and Fain, R. H.: Little league shoulder. J. Sports Med. Phys. Fitness, *2:*150, 1974.

99. Trias, A., and Ray, R. D.: Juvenile osteochondritis of the radial head. J. Bone Joint Surg., *45-A:*576, 1963.

100. Tullos, H. S., and King, J. W.: Lesions of the pitching arm in adolescents. J.A.M.A., *220:*264, 1972.

101. Tullos, H. S., et al.: Unusual lesions of the pitching arm. Clin. Orthop., *88:*169, 1972.

102. Torg, J. S., and Moyer, R. A.: Non-union of a stress fracture through the olecranon epiphyseal plate observed in an adolescent baseball pitcher. J. Bone Joint Surg., *59-A:*264, 1977.

103. Ogden, J. A., Hempton, R., and Southwick, W.: Development of the tibial tuberosity. Anat. Rec., *182:*431, 1975.

104. Lagier, R., and Jarret, G.: Apophysiolysis of the anterior inferior iliac spine. A histological, clinical and radiological study. Acta Orthop., *83:*81, 1975.

105. Daffner, R. H.: Stress fractures: current concepts. Skeletal Radiol., *2:*221, 1978.
106. Berkbile, R. D.: Stress fracture of the tibia in children. A.J.R., *91:*588, 1964.
107. Childress, H. M.: March foot in a seven-year-old child. J. Bone Joint Surg., *28:*877, 1946.
108. Griffiths, A. L.: Fatigue fracture of the fibula in childhood. Arch. Dis. Child., *27:*552, 1952.
109. Miller, F., and Wenger, D. R.: Femoral neck stress fracture in a hyperactive child. J. Bone Joint Surg., *61-A:*435, 1979.
110. Tullos, H., and Fain, R.: Little league shoulder: rotational stress fracture of the proximal epiphysis. J. Sports Med. Phys. Fitness, *2:*152, 1974.
111. Wilson, F. S., and Katz, F. N.: Stress fractures. An analysis of 250 consecutive cases. Radiology, *92:*481, 1969.
112. Spiedel, C. E.: Studies of living nerves. Comp. Neurol., *61:*1, 1935.
113. Devas, M. B.: Stress fractures in children. J. Bone Joint Surg., *45-B:*528, 1963.
114. Geslein, G. E., et al.: Early detection of stress fractures using 99m Tc-polyphosphate. Radiology, *121:*683, 1976.
115. Prather, J. L., et al.: Scintigraphic findings in stress fractures. J. Bone Joint Surg., *59-A:*869, 1977.
116. Engh, C. A., Robinson, R. A., and Milgram, J.: Stress fractures in children. J. Trauma, *10:*532, 1970.
116a. Caffey, J.: Traumatic cupping of the metaphyses of growing bones. A.J.R., *108:*451, 1970.
117. Silverman, F. N., and Gilden, J. J.: Congenital insensitivity to pain: neurologic syndrome with bizarre skeletal lesions. Radiology, *72:*176, 1959.
118. Kempe, C. H., Silverman, F. N., and Steele, B. F.: The battered child syndrome. J.A.M.A., *181:*17, 1962.
119. Akbarnia, B., et al.: Manifestations of the battered-child syndrome. J. Bone Joint Surg., *56-A:*1159, 1974.
120. Kogutt, M. S., Swischuk, L. E., and Fagan, C. J.: Patterns of injury and significance of uncommon fractures in the battered child syndrome. A.J.R., *121:*143, 1974.
121. Hiller, H. G.: Battered or not—a reappraisal of metaphyseal fragility. A.J.R., *114:*241, 1972.
122. Cullen, J. C.: Spinal lesions in battered babies. J. Bone Joint Surg., *57-B:*364, 1973.
123. Dickson, R. A., and Leatherman, K. D.: Spinal injuries in child abuse: case report. J. Trauma, *18:*811, 1978.
124. Swischuk, L. E.: Spina and spinal cord trauma in the battered child syndrome. Radiology, *92:*733, 1969.
125. Wenger, D. R., and Rokicki, R. R.: Spinal deformity secondary to scar formation in a battered child. J. Bone Joint Surg., *60-A:*847, 1978.

9

Chest and Pectoral Girdle

Except for the clavicle, which is probably the most frequently injured bone in the developing skeleton, the remainder of the components of the pectoral girdle are infrequently injured. The ribs and sternum are reasonably pliable and capable of much more elastic and plastic deformation than the major longitudinal bones. The scapula is also resilient, mobile, and well padded with muscles, all of which afford a great deal of protection except from a direct blow. In contrast, the clavicle is not as flexible as other elements of the pectoral girdle. It develops a thick cortex, anatomic curves, and relative fixation at the sternoclavicular and acromioclavicular joints, all of which function to increase susceptibility to fracture when the bone is loaded abruptly during a fall.

Anatomy

The clavicle extends from the acromial process of the scapula to the manubrium, serving as the only normal osseous connection between the arm and the trunk in the human. Consequently, it is constantly subjected to medially directed forces from the upper limb. The bone has a double curve, being convex forward in the medial two-thirds, and concave in the lateral third (Fig. 9-1). The pattern of the curve changes as the medial (sternal) segment elongates more rapidly than the lateral (acromial) segment (Fig. 9-2).[1] The double curve of the clavicle seems to be a poor mechanical shape, adequate in arboreal animals and some quadripeds, but definitely a point of weakness in the active child. Fur-

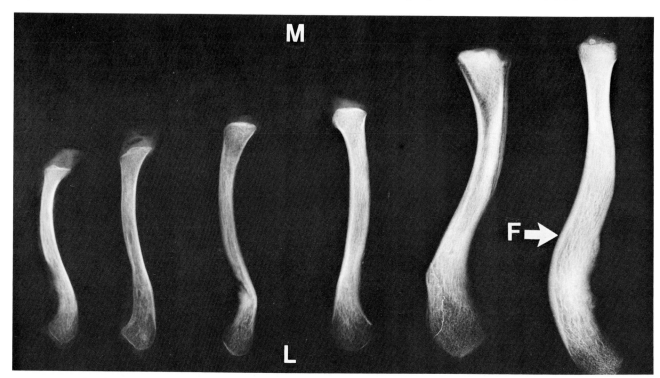

FIG. 9-1. Series of clavicles ranging from 3 months (postnatal) to 14 years. Note medial (sternal) ends (M); lateral (acromial) ends (L); and usual location of fractures (F).

202

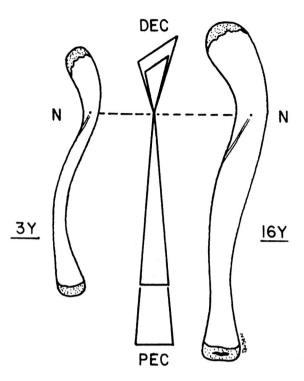

FIG. 9-2. Schematic of clavicular growth patterns between 3 and 16 years (relative sizes derived from specimen radiograms). The diagrammatic endochondral cones show relative increases in length and width from the proximal (sternal) and distal (acromial) ends, with the nutrient artery used as the base reference point. Note the nutrient foramen (N) and canal, the proximal endochondral cone (PEC), and the distal endochondral cone (DEC).

thermore, this double curve produces a good imitation of an undisplaced clavicular fracture on some radiographic projections, especially if the nutrient artery is visualized in an unusual position.

The lateral third of the clavicle provides attachment for the trapezius posterosuperiorly and for the deltoid anteriorly. In the medial two-thirds, the clavicular portion of the sternocleidomastoid muscle is inserted above and the pectoralis major muscle below. The subclavius muscle originates along the inferior clavicular groove. Knowledge of these various muscular insertions and origins is important for understanding directions of fragment displacement in complete clavicular fractures. There are strong costoclavicular ligaments proximally, while the conoid and trapezoid ligaments connect the distal clavicle to the coracoid process of the scapula.

The combination of various ligamentous and muscular insertions, the summation of forces acting on the clavicle, and the anatomic curves all combine to render the middle third of the clavicle the portion most vulnerable to injury. These injuries are generally greenstick fractures in the first decade of life, but are often complete or comminuted during adolescence. The superior surface of the clavicle is subcutaneous throughout the entire length. This subcutaneous location increases the risk of acute or subsequent penetration of the skin in a sharply angulated fracture, although this complication is still rare.

Normal primary ossification of the clavicle begins with two mesenchymal anlagen, each with its own center of ossification.[2] The clavicle is the first fetal bone to undergo ossification, doing so initially by membranous ossification with no prior endochondral staging. However, cartilaginous growth areas do develop at both ends. A secondary ossification center develops in the sternal end of the clavicle between the ages of 15 and 18 (Fig. 9-3), but it is rarely visible in routine radiographs, and is often difficult to visualize even in special sternoclavicular views taken to rule out anterior or posterior dislocation. The secondary center may not fuse

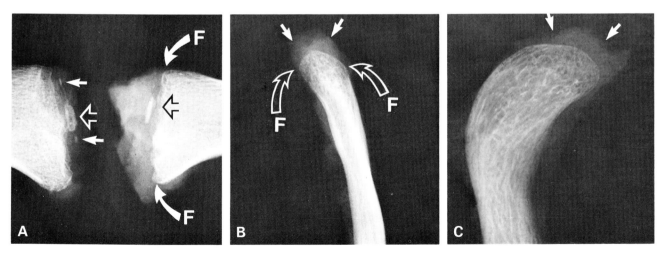

FIG. 9-3. *A,* Sternal clavicular ends from two adolescents show early development of proximal epiphyseal ossification centers (open arrows) and satellite ossification (small arrows). The usual location of a fracture of the medial clavicular epiphysis is shown (F). *B-C,* Lateral and anterior roentgenograms of distal clavicle show a radiolucent distal epiphysis (solid arrows). The level of distal "epiphyseal" fracture is indicated (F).

with the shaft until 25 years of age. This area may be the site of a true physeal fracture in children, rather than a sternoclavicular dislocation, as occurs in adults.[1] In some cases, an ossification center may develop at the acromial (distal) end, although it unites rapidly with the shaft. These centers must not be mistaken for fractures, and one must remember the propensity of the medial epiphysis to form a physeal fracture rather than a true sternoclavicular joint dislocation. The medial end of the clavicle is attached to the sternum and first rib by a heavy sheet of fibrous tissue that is difficult to disrupt in a child.[3] The attachments primarily involve the epiphysis rather than the clavicular shaft, further enhancing the likelihood of a physeal injury. This joint also has a meniscus that contributes to sternoclavicular stability (Fig. 9-4).

There are seven or more scapular ossification centers: one for the body, which is a prenatal ossification process; and two for the acromium, two for the coracoid process, one for the vertebral border, and one for the inferior angle, all of which are postnatal ossification centers (Fig. 9-5).

These postnatal ossification centers begin to form between 15 and 18 months of age, commencing with the middle of the coracoid process (Fig. 9-6). A separate coracoid ossification center forms in the base (at the glenoid) between 7 and 10 years of age and is sometimes called the subcoracoid bone. This bone rapidly fuses with the main bulk of the scapula, but it does not fuse with the earlier appearing midossification center until 14 to 16 years of age. A third coracoid ossification center at the tip appears around age 14 and fuses by age 18.[4,5]

Ossification of the acromial process (Figs. 9-6 and 9-7) originates from at least two centers, one at the base, and the other at the apex, which begin to ossify between the fourteenth and sixteenth years, and coalesce to form one epiphysis about the nineteenth year, finally fusing with the scapular spine from the twenty-second to the twenty-fifth year. Osseous union sometimes fails to take place between the acromium and the spine of the scapula, leaving a fibrous union that should not be mistaken for a fracture. The acromial metaphyseal ossification often has a crenated appearance (see Fig. 9-6E).

The ossification center for the inferior angle of the scapula appears at the fifteenth year and fuses by the twentieth year (Fig. 9-8). That of the vertebral margin of the scapula appears by the seventeenth year and fuses by the twenty-fifth year.

The sternum develops multiple ossification centers that reflect the original embryonic metamerism (Fig. 9-9). These sternebrae may appear separate on a lateral roentgenogram, and on an anteroposterior view they may show right/left segmentation as well. Such normal cartilaginous regions should not be misinterpreted as fractures.[6,7]

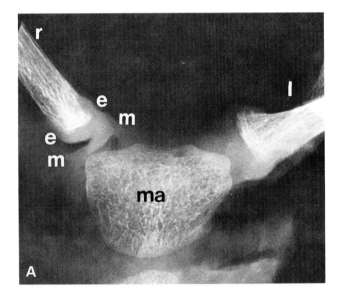

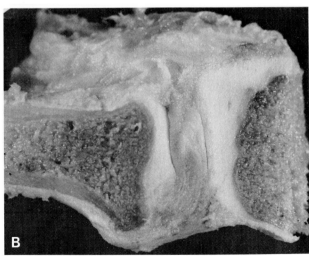

FIG. 9-4. *A,* Intact left (l) sternoclavicular joint, and exploded right (r) joint show actual anatomy. Note manubrium (ma), meniscus (m), and proximal clavicular epiphysis (e). *B,* Gross specimen of sternoclavicular joint.

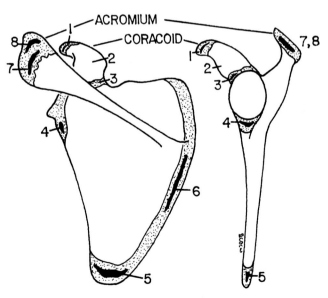

FIG. 9-5. Schematic of multiple areas of primary and secondary ossification in the scapula. 1,3—secondary coracoid centers; 2—primary coracoid center; 4—secondary infraglenoid center; 5—secondary center at tip of scapula; 6—secondary center of vertebral border; 7,8—secondary centers of acromion.

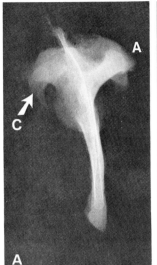
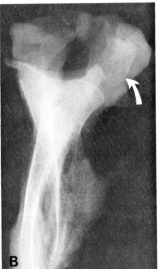
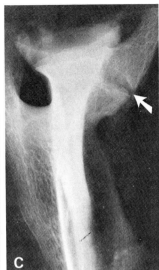
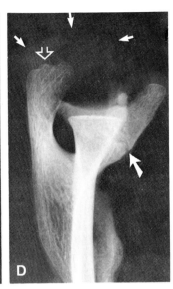

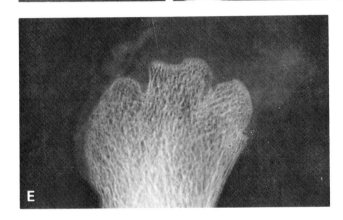

FIG. 9-6. *A,* "Y" view of scapula in 4-month-old child showing early development of primary ossification center (arrow) of (C), coracoid (number 2 in Fig. 9-5). Note the lighter appearing (normally radiolucent) cartilage in this and the remaining figures. Note acromion (A) and coracoid (C). *B,* Further development of coracoid ossification center by 1 year (arrow). *C,* Development of physis (arrow) at base of coracoid in 8-year-old. *D,* Beginning closure of physis at base of coracoid (closed arrow) in a 14-year-old. Compared to *C,* the acromion is developing an undulated appearance (open arrow). Also note the size of the unossified acromion, even at this age (small arrows). *E,* Magnified view of normal undulated appearance of acromial metaphysis.

Thoracic Cage

Injury to the sternum and ribs is extremely unusual in children.[8] The resiliency of individual ribs, as well as of the entire composite rib cage and sternum, allows significant elastic deformation without progression to plastic deformation or fracture. One need only observe an infant or young child with respiratory distress to fully appreciate the degree of elastic sternocostal deformation possible even without direct external pressure. Simple rib fractures comparable to those seen in adults are rare in children. The first rib may be involved with a stress fracture from seemingly inconsequential trauma. Most fractures involve several ribs and result from major trauma, especially as a consequence of child abuse or vehicular accidents (Fig. 9-10).

Healing of rib fractures is rapid, and usually requires only symptomatic treatment. The intrinsic resiliency of the ribs often causes spontaneous reduction after the immediate deforming force is removed. Further, the thick periosteum remains intact, at least on one surface, and contributes to the spontaneity of reduction and stability. This reducibility immediately after cessation of the injurious force, and the fact that in children, most of these fractures are greenstick deformations, makes roentgenographic diagnosis extremely difficult. Often the injury is not diagnosed until two to three weeks after it occurs, when the fracture callus becomes evident along the subperiosteal margins (Fig. 9-11).

Since the chest wall of a child is more resilient than that of an adult, the intrathoracic contents may be injured severely, even if the ribs are not fractured. In fact, the mortality rate for closed chest injuries may be higher in children without rib fractures than in those with fractures. Closed chest injuries vary significantly in severity and may be easily missed in the multiply-injured child with obvious severe trauma to the extremities or head. Closed chest wall injury produces few outward signs, but palpable crepitation from a rib fracture, changing level of consciousness due to hypoxia, and alteration of blood gases are the easiest to observe.

Lung contusion is the most common major complication of rib fracture in the child, but it usually presents itself insidiously. Because of greater pulmonary reserve, a child may be completely asymptomatic and the contusion may go unrecognized until there is blood-tinged sputum or obvious hemoptysis, or until a routine chest radiograph begins to demonstrate regions infiltrated by parenchymal hemorrhage. Most lung contusions resolve themselves within a week or two. General respiratory care is sufficient treatment.

Pneumothorax, with or without hemothorax, may accompany any lung contusion. In a simple pneumothorax, air enters the pleural cavity slowly through a laceration in the

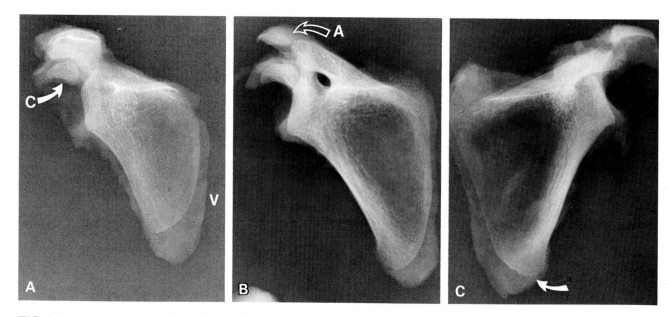

FIG. 9-7. Anteroposterior views of scapula. *A,* At 1 year, note the primary ossification of the coracoid (C, arrow), with overlying acromion. Also note the thick epiphyseal cartilage along the vertebral (V) border. *B,* Accessory ossification center in the acromion (A, arrow) in a 10-year-old. The vertebral cartilage border has thinned, except at the tip. *C,* Development of undulation of the physis at the scapular tip (arrow). This change precedes the appearance of the secondary ossification center shown in Figure 9-8.

pulmonary surface. A free exchange of air takes place between the pleural cavity and the exposed pulmonary air space. In contrast, the pulmonary or chest wall laceration may behave like a one-way valve, creating a tension pneumothorax when inspired air is continually pumped into the pleural cavity and maintained there under increasing pressure. Early detection of a tension pneumothorax is important, as immediate recognition and treatment with a chest tube will reverse the situation rapidly and markedly improve the respiratory distress, which can worsen rapidly and jeopardize the child's survival (Fig. 9-12). If the pulmonary laceration has been caused by a rib fracture, air may dissect into the soft tissues around the osseous injury, creating subcutaneous emphysema. The accumulated blood from a hemothorax must be removed with large intercostal tubes that are connected to underwater seal and suction. In children the

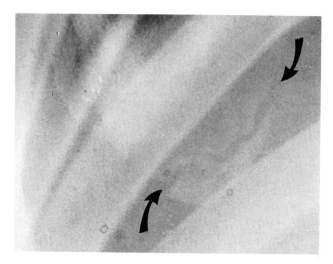

FIG. 9-8. A 16-year-old boy with chest trauma on the right side and pain over the scapula. The wavy line (arrows) is the normal physis separating the scapula from the secondary ossification center at the tip of the scapular epiphysis, rather than a fracture.

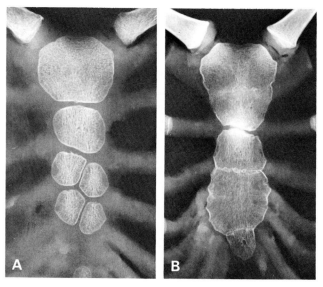

FIG. 9-9. Serial development of the sternum. *A,* Early development showing bifid sternal ossification. *B,* Beginning fusion of sternal units in an adolescent.

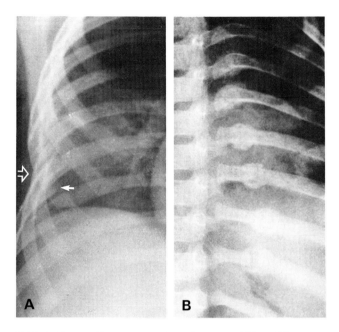

FIG. 9-10. *A,* Chest trauma in a six-year-old boy. The open arrow indicates a concavity suggestive of rib cage deformity, while the solid arrow points to a seemingly minimally displaced rib fracture (also see Figs. 9-12 and 9-13). *B,* Healing multiple rib fractures in a case of child abuse. (The child subsequently died.)

tube(s) should be inserted into the anterior axillary line in the fifth or sixth intercostal space.

Damage to major blood vessels may also occur with or without rib fracture. A widened or widening mediastinum should make one suspect an aortic injury. Aortography should be used to establish the diagnosis.

Injury to the lower rib cage may produce a ruptured diaphragm (Fig. 9-13) or intra-abdominal damage (to the liver or spleen). A ruptured diaphragm, which usually occurs on the left side, will produce immediate symptoms of respiratory distress. A chest film may demonstrate herniation of abdominal contents into the left pleural cavity. Thoracotomy is essential. The spleen is also frequently injured when the left side of the chest is traumatized. The overlying rib cage in this region is extremely resilient, and rarely fractures, but allows sufficient deformation to contuse, displace, or rupture the spleen. Blood loss may be immediate or delayed, especially if the splenic bleeding is intracapsular. In the past, immediate splenectomy has been advocated, although more recent clinical trials have suggested that complete removal may not be necessary.[9,10] Further, following splenectomy, many children exhibit regeneration of some splenic elements (the ''born-again spleen'').[11] Splenectomy is not without long term complications, the most severe being inappropriate function of the immune system.[12]

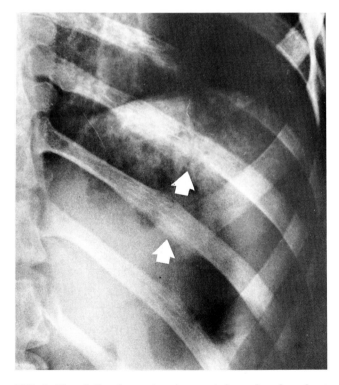

FIG. 9-11. Callus formation (arrows) 3 weeks after chest trauma in a 12-year-old girl. Actual fractures were never evident. Undoubtedly, incomplete fractures that sprang back into anatomic position were present.

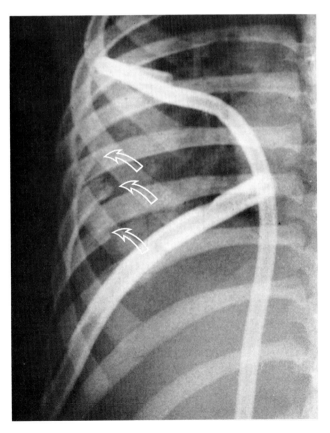

FIG. 9-12. Case shown in Figure 9-10*A*. This slightly more oblique film, taken six hours later, shows multiple, displaced rib fractures (arrows) which lacerated the right lung, creating a hemopneumothorax, and necessitating placement of chest tubes.

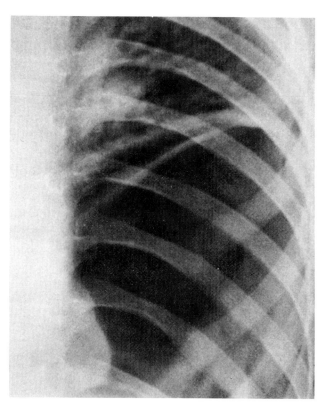

FIG. 9-13. Rupture of left side of diaphragm secondary to rib fractures. The stomach has herniated into the left thoracic cavity.

First rib fracture

When the first rib is fractured, it most often is a stress injury, especially in adolescents (Fig. 9-14), and particularly in those undergoing vigorous weight-training programs. Initial treatment should be symptomatic immobilization of the arm. Nonunion or delayed union are common complications.[13] If pain or neurologic symptoms supervene, bone grafting should be considered.

Several authors have described vascular complications of first rib fractures, especially arterial injuries.[14-16] Pseudoaneurysm formation is circumstantial evidence that injuries of the subclavian artery and brachial plexus may occur later, rather than concomitant with the initial trauma. Furthermore, destruction of a vein graft in one reported case constituted proof that fractures of the first rib, if left unstable, could produce delayed injuries.

Sternum

The sternum, like the ribs, is extremely resilient in a child. The manubrium and sternum have a cartilaginous junction that allows some motion. This manubriosternal joint may be displaced. The sternocostal cartilage is extensive. Fractures, which are extremely rare, invariably result from direct injury (Fig. 9-15). Most injuries occur in the older child approaching skeletal maturity, when the separate ossification centers have begun to coalesce and the capacity for elastic deformation has lessened considerably. The xiphoid may be depressed inward (see Fig. 9-15C) and may require removal or elevation if pain results.

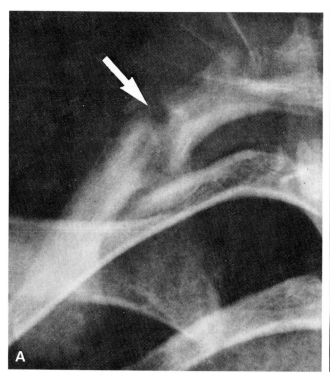
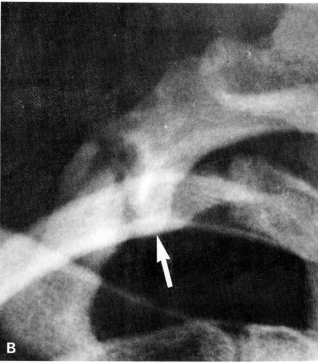

FIG. 9-14. *A,* Stress fracture (arrow) of first rib. *B,* Six months later, a characteristic pseudarthrosis is present, with hypertrophy of the ends (arrow). The roentgenographic appearance changed little after this time.

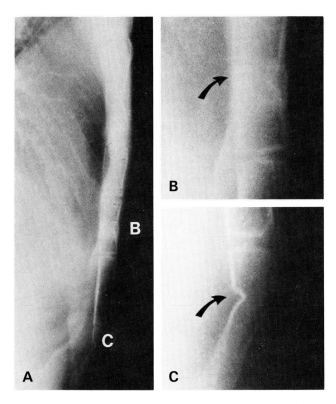

FIG. 9-15. *A,* Sternebral (B) and xiphoid (C) sternal fractures in a 15-year-old boy, sustained from a "bear hug" during a wrestling match. *B,* Magnification of the sternebral fracture (arrow). *C,* Magnification of the xiphoid fracture (arrow).

Clavicle

Over 60% of fractures of the clavicle occur in children under ten years of age. Furthermore, this is probably the most frequently injured bone in children during the first ten years. Fractures may occur at three regions: the diaphyseal shaft, the medial epiphyseal end, and the distal metaphyseal end (Fig. 9-16). Dislocation or subluxation of either proximal (sternoclavicular) or distal (acromioclavicular) joints is rare in children not yet approaching skeletal maturity.

Fractures of the midshaft are most common, and range from greenstick to complete, the latter being more common during adolescence. These fractures unite quickly, almost invariably with some degree of malunion. Remodeling is generally complete within a year, especially in young children (Fig. 9-17). This bone remodels adequately and quickly and may be left in a reasonable degree of angular deformity. In adolescents, anatomic realignment assumes more importance, since remodeling is less active and may not correct major malalignment. It is unwise to complete the greenstick fracture, as is taught with other bones, inasmuch as the subclavian vessels and brachial plexus lie directly beneath this, and rupture of the subclavian vessels has been described as a cause of death. Despite proximity of pleura, skin, brachial plexus, and brachial vessels, complications of this fracture are rare. Most often the deformation is anterior and away from major neuromuscular structures.

Mechanism of injury

The clavicle may be fractured in the neonatal period during a difficult delivery.[17-21] Such fractures are evident in most instances and may result in an apparent Erb's palsy (pseudoparalysis) because of reluctance of the neonate to use the arm. Once the child is ambulatory, the most common mechanism of injury is a fall. The patient may land on an outstretched hand or elbow, or directly on the shoulder.

Pathologic anatomy

The most frequent fracture site is the junction of the middle and distal third of the bone. In the infant and young child, the break usually is incomplete (greenstick), whereas older children and adolescents tend to have complete or comminuted fractures (Fig. 9-18), even though the fragments may not be displaced significantly, and some periosteal continuity is retained. Angulated, sharp fragments may penetrate the subcutaneous or cutaneous tissues (Fig. 9-19) and also may lacerate subclavian vessels, or the brachial plexus, although these complications do not generally occur in children. Anterior bowing, with or without fracture, also may occur, although this bone does not exhibit a great deal of capacity for plastic deformation.

When the fracture is complete, muscle forces maintain the deformation. The glenohumeral joint pulls the lateral fragment downward and inward. This displacement is a combination of the overall weight of the limb as well as the pull of the pectoralis muscles anteriorly and part of trapezius posteriorly, with their summated forces being directed in an inferior and medial fashion. In contrast, the medial half is pulled upward and backward by the sternocleidomastoid muscle (Fig. 9-20). The costoclavicular and sternoclavicular ligaments may act as checkreins.

Diagnosis

Birth fractures are not always easy to diagnose, since they often are asymptomatic. Fracture of the anteriorly positioned clavicle predominates over the more posterior clavicle. In a roentgenographic survey of 300 consecutively born living newborns, 5 had evidence of fractured clavicles (1.7%). In *none* of these cases was the fracture suspected following the routine pediatric examination in the delivery room and the nursery. However, after each positive roentgenogram, re-examination demonstrated crepitation of the fracture site. Even in the newborn, these fractures may be complete, with an overriding fragment (Fig. 9-21), but they should not be confused with congenital pseudarthrosis of the clavicle (see Fig. 9-25).

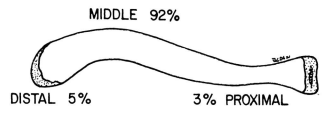

FIG. 9-16. Schematic showing usual areas of clavicular injury.

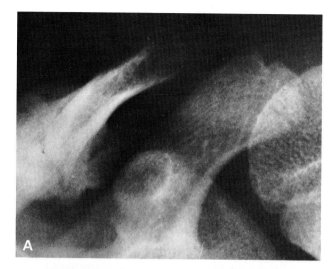

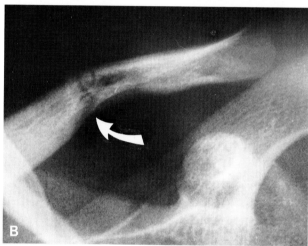

FIG. 9-17. *A,* Undisplaced fracture of clavicle with hypertrophic callus not diagnosed until three weeks after the injury. *B,* Questionable fracture in a child who fell on the shoulder. This is really the nutrient foramen (arrow).

Muscle function in the upper limb should be assessed by reflex stimulation to rule out associated brachial plexus paralysis. Occasionally, birth fracture of the clavicle may be accompanied by a physeal fracture of the upper humeral epiphysis. While this may not be seen on initial roentgenograms, massive subperiosteal new bone formation makes it evident. Such osteoblastic reaction may be confused with osteomyelitis.

In infants and young children, the patient again tends to be asymptomatic and there may be no clinical evidence of the injury until the child develops callus, which causes a marked swelling and disturbs the parents (Fig. 9-22). When fractures are complete, displacement and clinical appearance are typical. Fractures in the middle third will be clearly depicted in normal anteroposterior roentgenograms. However, demonstration of fractures of the medial and lateral ends of the clavicle often require special oblique, lateral, or posteroanterior views. In the adolescent, the diaphyseal fracture has a greater tendency to be comminuted.

Treatment

Birth fractures do not always require treatment, as they often are unrecognized, form callus rapidly, and become evident only when the mother notices the palpable mass of callus. Union usually occurs without any external immobilization, and malalignment corrects rapidly with growth in this age period. The infant should be handled gently, with no direct pressure being placed over the clavicle. If the fracture is painful, or there is pseudoparalysis, it is best to protect the arm by a splint for 2 to 3 weeks. Within a week, or at most 10 to 14 days, pain will subside and the fracture will begin to unite.

In general, children under six years of age with a fractured clavicle do not require formal, manipulative reduction. The massive callus formation will remodel and disappear, generally within six to nine months, a fact that should be impressed upon the parents so they are not disturbed by the clinical appearance. The child should be made comfortable by application of a figure-of-eight bandage (Fig. 9-23) and having the arm in a sling may also help. The bandage may be tightened slightly by the parents each evening to bring the fracture fragments back into reasonably anatomic position.[22,23] Immobilization should be required for three to four weeks. The axillary region as well as neuromuscular

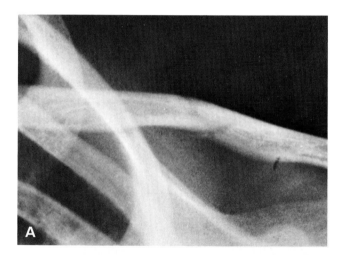

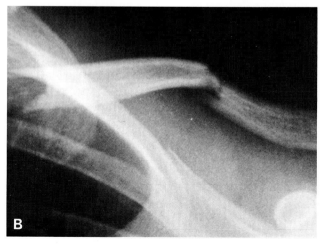

FIG. 9-18. *A,* Greenstick fracture. *B,* Complete fracture.

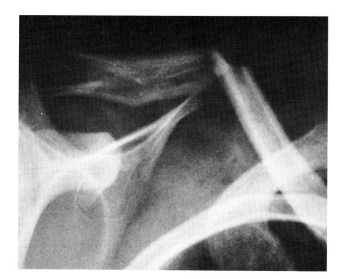

FIG. 9-19. Severely angulated fracture. Two weeks later this penetrated the skin (the adolescent patient decided to remove the clavicular strap and go skiing). The result was a superficial osteomyelitis with Staphylococcus epidermidis.

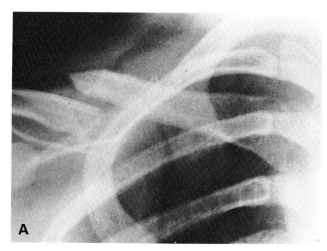

A

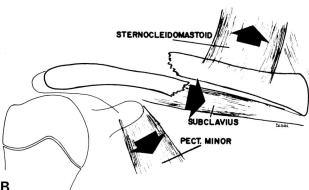

B

FIG. 9-20. *A*, Typical overriding of complete fracture. *B*, Schematic of muscle forces creating this displacement pattern.

and vascular function in the arm should be checked frequently by the parents. Professional re-evaluation at reasonable intervals is also advisable to rule out these problems.

As the child gets older, the capacity for complete remodeling, particularly of any significant angular deformity, lessens. This increases the desirability of reasonably accurate reduction. If the fracture is complete, markedly displaced, or overriding, closed reduction is necessary. While this may be done after local injection of procaine or lidocaine (Xylocaine), great care should be taken to avoid introduction of skin bacteria. The patient should sit, and the surgeon should be behind to pull the shoulders backwards while applying leverage between the scapula with his knee. The patient also can be placed recumbent with the back over a midline sandbag. The arm should be placed over the side, which generally will effect a gradual reduction. In older children who require closed reduction, plaster may be added to the figure-of-eight dressing to reinforce its stability.[24]

Fracture of the clavicle in a child who is forced to rest in bed because of other major trauma, may be managed more easily in the recumbent, supine position with a small sandbag or pillow placed between the scapulae so that the weight of the upper limbs gradually falls backwards and reduces the fracture. For comfort, a figure-of-eight bandage made of felt may also be applied. If significant cosmetic deformity is present, and one does not wish to undertake an open reduction, modified lateral arm skin traction may be used, with the shoulder at 90° of abduction and 90° of external rotation.

Open reduction of a fractured clavicle is generally contraindicated in children.[25] The only justification for explorative surgery is to repair damaged subclavian vessels or brachial plexus (Fig. 9-24). Vascular complication is suggested by a large, rapidly increasing hematoma. Surgical intervention in this case must be immediate, as the patient may die of extravasation or shock.[26,27]

Complications

The only acute vascular complication recorded in children is subclavian compression due to greenstick fracture with inferior bowing.[28] This is rapidly recognizable by the venous congestion and edema of the ipsilateral arm. An arteriovenous fistula has also been reported.[29]

The incidence of nonunion of all clavicular fractures, as reported by Rowe, ranges from 0.8% to 3.7%.[30] Nogi reported nonunion of the clavicle in a 12-year-old child.[31] The main differential diagnoses of discontinuity of the clavicle in children and adolescents include congenital pseudarthrosis, nonunion following fracture, birth fracture, cleidocranial dysostosis, and neurofibromatosis. Birth fractures usually can be distinguished by abundant callus formation and ultimate fracture healing.

Treatment of discontinuity of the clavicle in children seems to be well-defined. In the overwhelming majority of cases there is little functional impairment. Surgery is therefore of a cosmetic nature for the unsightly, enlarged, midclavicular mass. In patients whose presenting symptoms include pain, either at the nonunion site or with diffuse discomfort of the involved upper extremity, and limited function, surgery has succeeded in returning the patient to full, painless activity.

Osteomyelitis is a rare complication, and may result either from an open wound or hematogenous spread.

With anterior displacement, the periosteal sleeve may be pulled into the displaced region, effectively creating a membrane between the epiphysis, which is still in the joint, and the metaphysis. This increases the tendency to instability of the joint after closed reduction.

Pain and swelling usually are obvious if a sternoclavicular injury is present. Most of the injuries are anterior, with a mass evident over the sternoclavicular region. The sternal end of the clavicle may be sharply prominent and palpable immediately beneath the skin. The clavicular part of the sternocleidomastoid muscle is pulled anteriorly with the bone and is in spasm, causing the patient's head to tilt toward the affected side. Posterior displacements may cause intrathoracic problems, such as tracheal compression leading to dyspnea.[44-46]

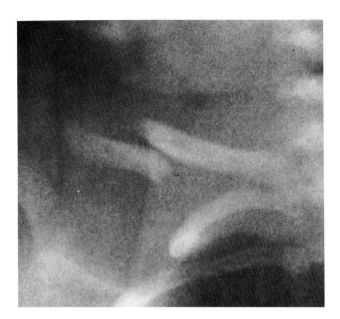

FIG. 9-21. Complete overriding fracture sustained during difficult delivery (see Fig. 9-25).

Congenital pseudarthrosis

Characteristically, this affects the right clavicle. The lesion is probably well-established at birth and results from a failure of normal ossification patterns.[32-34] Swelling is found at or soon after birth. The children do not have obvious histories of birth injuries and the limb is usually painless. The child may be reluctant to move the arm or unable to push it when crawling. The relationship of the two fragments is always the same, with the sternal fragment being larger and lying in front of and slightly above the shorter and deformed acromial fragment (Fig. 9-25).

Sternoclavicular Joint

Traumatic separation of the epiphysis of the sternal end of the clavicle is rare. Poland collected 6 cases.[35] Karlen reported a case in a boy 12 years of age.[36] Denham and Dingly reported 4 cases, all in children under 18 years of age.[37] Wheeler reported anterosuperior displacement in a 7-month-old girl.[38]

Because of late fusion of this epiphysis, physeal separation may occur even in young adulthood. This injury mimics a sternoclavicular dislocation, which cannot occur until the clavicle is mature. Any injury to this end of the clavicle in a child or adolescent must be treated as an epiphyseal separation.[39-43]

The stability of the sternoclavicular joint is contingent upon the joint capsule, the fibrocartilaginous disc, and the interclavicular and costoclavicular ligaments.[3] The chondroosseous configuration of the joint itself is unstable.

Sternoclavicular injury commonly is caused by indirect violence, such as a fall on or blow to the point of the shoulder, which drives the clavicle inward or forward. The injury occasionally may be produced by direct violence.

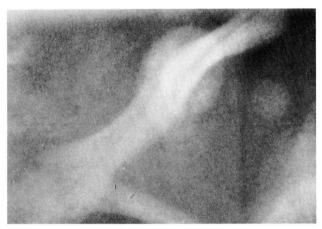

FIG. 9-22. Massive callus characteristically forms around these fractures in neonates and infants.

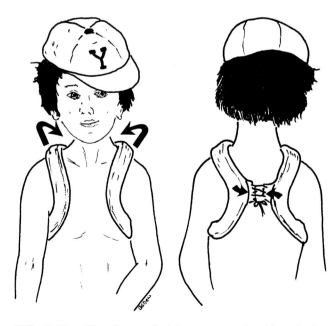

FIG. 9-23. The figure-of-eight support should pull the shoulders backward and should be tightened regularly.

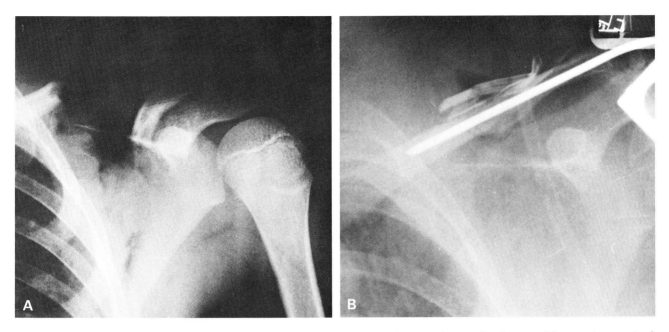

FIG. 9-24. *A,* Open clavicular fracture with avulsion of entire brachial plexus at the root level. Several large veins required ligation, but the artery was intact. *B,* After extensive debridement the clavicle was reduced and fixed with a medullary pin.

Anteroposterior roentgenograms may appear normal even if sternoclavicular injury is present. However, special oblique views will show the displacement of the sternal end of the clavicle (Figs. 9-26 and 9-27). If the injury occurs before ossification in the medial epiphysis, the condition is easily and often mistaken for true dislocation of the sternoclavicular joint.

Treatment consists of closed manipulative reduction and immobilization. Open reduction is indicated when closed manipulative reduction fails.[47] It is best to drill a Kirschner wire obliquely through the anterior cortex, across the epiphysis, and into the sternum to stabilize the fragments. The arm must be immobilized to minimize joint motion and stress. The wires can be removed in six weeks. Recent anatomic studies suggest that extensive capsular repairs may be unnecessary. Recurrent displacement is the only significant complication.

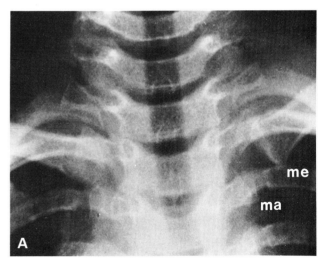

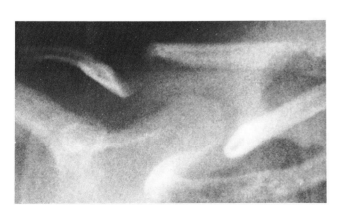

FIG. 9-25. Congenital pseudarthrosis in a two-month-old. This must be distinguished from a fracture.

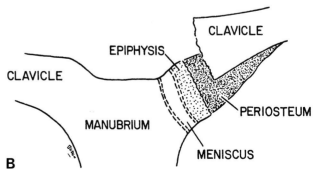

FIG. 9-26. *A,* Epiphyseal displacement (anterior) of the proximal clavicle in a four-year-old. Note the metaphysis, (me), and the manubrium (ma). *B,* Schematic of the injury pattern.

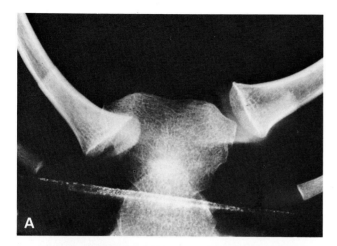

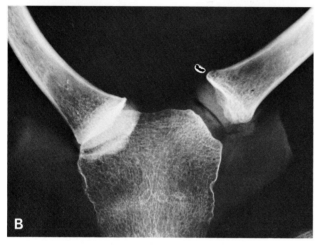

FIG. 9-27. Specimen radiographs showing, *A,* anterior and, *B,* posterior displacement of right clavicle.

Distal Clavicle

Fractures of the lateral third of the clavicle are infrequent, usually resulting from direct violence applied to the shoulder. This is usually a transverse fracture. If the conoid and trapezoid coracoclavicular ligaments are disrupted, displacement is more likely.

Children may sustain an often unrecognized injury to the distal clavicle which is analogous to a metaphyseal-epiphyseal fracture (Fig. 9-28). The coracoclavicular ligaments remain intact, so that there is little depression of the shoulder tip.[48] Marked anteroposterior instability may be present, suggesting that the injury is due to a backward blow on the shoulder. Again, as in the medial end, maintenance of reduction may be difficult and percutaneous Kirschner-wire fixation may be beneficial (Fig. 9-29).

Dislocations of the acromioclavicular joint are extremely rare in young children, primarily because the deforming forces that would cause such a separation in an adult result in a clavicular fracture in children, either at the distal end or at the midshaft.[49] However, with increased emphasis on contact sports during adolescence, acromioclavicular dislocation occurs more frequently (Fig. 9-30). Three types of acromio-

clavicular injury may occur: (1) ligamentous strain, (2) rupture of the acromioclavicular ligaments only; or (3) rupture of the entire ligament complex (acromioclavicular, conoid, and trapezoid). The severity of the injury determines the clinical presentation. There is discrete tenderness over the joint, and it is accentuated by motion. If separation is complete, the end of the clavicle may be prominent. The patient usually complains of pain upon all movement of the shoulder, particularly forward rotation. There is specific tenderness over the acromioclavicular joint. If the joint is dislocated, the upright, prominent, lateral end of the clavicle can be easily palpated.

Roentgenograms should be made with the patient standing, holding weights in each hand, and a central beam passing anteroposteriorly through the joint. In subluxation, the acromial process is depressed relative to the lateral end of the clavicle, whereas in dislocation, there is complete discontinuity of the articular end. Because the ends of the clavicle and acromion may be incompletely ossified, a normal cartilage space width may be misinterpreted as widening of the acromioclavicular joint. An associated fracture of the lateral end of the clavicle should be ruled out.

Treatment is contingent upon the degree of injury, although the general principle in children and adolescents is closed reduction. Sprains and undisplaced lateral clavicular fractures require symptomatic treatment with a sling. Subluxation caused by acromioclavicular ligament injury without concomitant conoid-trapezoid ligament damage can be treated with an adjustable strap going across the acromioclavicular joint. In complete dislocation, the same immobilization should be employed initially, but if the reduction cannot be maintained easily, open reduction should be considered. In open reduction, the capsule is repaired and the joint fixed with threaded wires, which are removed after four to six weeks. Because the adolescent is still undergoing skeletal maturation, *no* joint components should be resected as often advocated for comparable repairs in adults.

Scapula

Fractures of the scapula, which is highly mobile, extremely resilient, and well protected by bulky muscles, are extremely rare.[49a,50] Like the ribs, this thin bone is more resilient in the child than in the adult. The entire medial (vertebral) border is pliable hyaline cartilage. Fractures usually occur along the lateral margin, including the glenoid, coracoid, and acromion. However, many of these regions have secondary ossification centers that should not be confused with fractures (see Fig. 9-5).

Wilbur and Evans reported 40 cases of fractured scapulae.[50] The patients ranged in age from 3 to 80 years. The majority of the fractures were through non-articular regions and did not lead to significant problems. The authors felt that open reduction was indicated only when the glenohumeral joint was involved, an unlikely event in a child.

Fractures of the body of the scapula result from direct violence, such as a crushing injury, an auto accident, or a fall. The blade of the scapula is often comminuted, with the fracture lines running in various directions. At times there may be a small fracture along the scapular margins (Fig. 9-31). The spine of the scapula may be fractured along with the body of the scapula. The infraspinous portion is more fre-

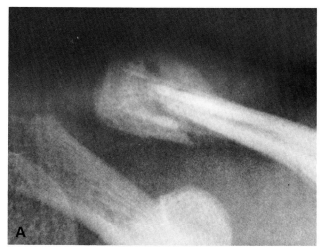

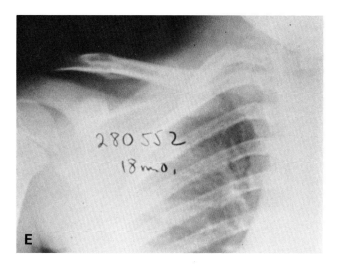

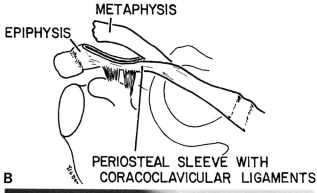

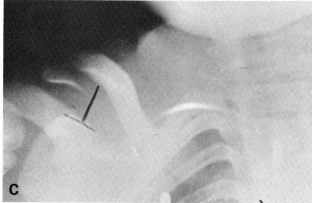

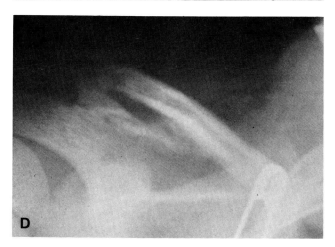

METAPHYSIS

EPIPHYSIS

PERIOSTEAL SLEEVE WITH
CORACOCLAVICULAR LIGAMENTS

FIG. 9-28. *A,* Epiphyseal fracture of lateral clavicle, with massive callus from metaphyseal periosteum (the child was not treated until four weeks after the injury). *B,* Schematic of the injury pattern. *C,* Distal clavicular fracture. Note separation of coracoid from proximal fragment. *D,* Appearance of *C,* one month later. *E,* Appearance of *C,* one year later.

quently fractured than the supraspinous. Usually, the fracture fragments are minimally displaced, if at all, as they are held together by the surrounding muscles. Because the mechanism of injury involves major trauma, coextensive crush injuries of the soft tissue of the thorax may be present, as well as multiple fractures of the ribs and spinal column, pneumothorax, and subcutaneous emphysema.

In order to adequately demonstrate the fractures, it is often necessary to obtain oblique or tangential views, in addition to the routine anteroposterior roentgenograms.

The primary objective of treatment is to make the patient comfortable. Usually, reduction of the fracture is unnecessary; simple immobilization of the entire arm and shoulder is sufficient. The scapula may be immobilized with a sling-and-swathe dressing.

Fractures of the scapular neck usually are caused by a direct blow to the front or back of the shoulder. The fracture line begins at the suprascapular notch and runs downward and laterally to the axillary border of the scapular neck, inferior to the glenoid, with the capsular attachments of the glenohumeral joint remaining intact. Displacement varies, but is usually insignificant.

Treatment should consist of support of the shoulder and arm in a sling-and-swathe dressing and onset of pendulum exercises about 14 days later, when the patient is comfortable. Markedly displaced fractures, which are extremely rare in children, should be treated with skeletal traction comparable to Dunlop's traction for a supracondylar fracture.

Fractures of the glenoid cavity are rare in children. They are produced by direct violence. They should be managed conservatively, unless a large displaced fragment is present, in which case skeletal traction should be attempted, and open reduction used as a last resort. The results of surgery are not overwhelmingly good, although again, much of the data are derived from treatment of this injury in adults.

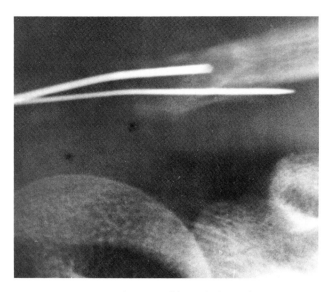

FIG. 9-29. Open reduction of lateral clavicular injury.

The acromium occasionally fractures from direct violence, or from indirect force transmitted vertically by the humeral head. Care must be taken in rendering the diagnosis, because the tip of the acromium forms a separate ossification center that is easily confused with a fracture line in an acutely traumatized patient (Fig. 9-32).

Fractures of the coracoid process are rare, and may be caused by sudden muscular action of the short end of the biceps and the coracobrachialis muscles, or by direct violence (Fig. 9-33). Closed reduction and conservative treatment are indicated. Again, great care must be exercised in roentgenographic diagnosis because of the variability of ossification patterns (Fig. 9-33).

Prior to epiphyseal closure, the coracoclavicular ligaments often are stronger than the epiphyseal plate, and an injury that would result in ligamentous disruption in an adult may only injure the physis of the coracoid process in a child. In addition, an accessory ossification center often develops as a shell-like, rounded ossification at the tip of the coracoid process. This area is the site of insertion of the coracoclavicular ligament. The conjoint tendon of the short head of the biceps and coracobrachialis, as well as the pectoralis minor, insert into the coracoid process anterior to the accessory physis. During adolescence, acromioclavicular separation may be accompanied by avulsion of a fragment of the coracoid epiphysis, rather than by disruption of the ligaments.[51] Montgomery reported two cases in which the coracoid epiphysis was avulsed, allowing an acromioclavicular separation, as the two ligaments went with the coracoid process. In one patient the coracoid process was reattached and the other was treated nonoperatively.[52]

Brachial Plexus

The incidence and long term problems of obstetric traumatic paralysis of the upper extremity have dramatically decreased due to recognition of cephalopelvic disproportion and improved means of managing the complication of Erb's palsy and the less frequent complications such as Klumpke's palsy. The majority of babies with brachial plexus injuries are products of prolonged or traumatic deliveries; 10% are breech births. Birth weight and general size are significantly greater.[53-55]

The diagnosis of brachial plexus injury is made easily in the newborn infant when one upper extremity is not moving actively and the passive range of motion is equal on both sides. If the active and passive motions are equally restrictive, injury to the proximal humeral epiphysis (the Putti-Scaglietti lesion) should be suspected and confirmed by roentgenographic examination, although it is often difficult to interpret these roentgenograms of the upper extremity.[56] All infants with suspected or proven Erb's palsy must be radiographed routinely to rule out concomitant osseous injury (see Chap. 10).

In newborns, it is often difficult to accurately localize the anatomic lesion. Overlap of innervation resulting in partial loss of motor power in the muscles innervated by the different trunks of the brachial plexus makes anatomic diagnosis difficult. However, such an accurate diagnosis probably has no real advantage, either for management or for prognosis in the neonate. Classification into upper (Erb), lower (Klumpke) or whole (Erb-Duchenne-Klumpke) types is useful only insofar as it quickly conveys a general picture of the probable pattern of involvement.

In the neonatal period, the degree of severity and the time at which endpoint spontaneous recovery can be expected are difficult to estimate. Some of the apparently more severely involved extremities make spontaneous recovery after many months. The maximum time of recovery ranges from 1 to 18 months.[58,59]

The roots most commonly injured are C5 and C6, as evidenced by weakness in the deltoid, biceps, brachialis, supinator, supraspinatous, infraspinatous, and subscapularis muscles. Less commonly, the wrist and finger extensors may be weak. Specific muscle testing is difficult in the neonate, but one should record gross movement of the shoulder, elbow, hand, and wrist. Total plexus involvement is the second most common injury. It is evidenced by a totally limp

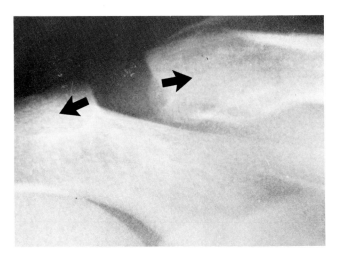

FIG. 9-30. Acromioclavicular separation (arrows) in a 14-year-old football player who landed on his shoulder during a tackle.

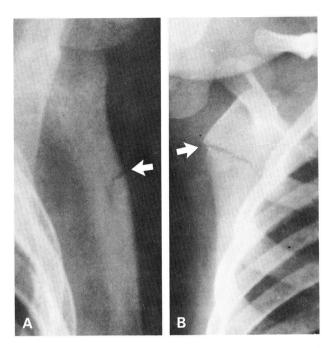

FIG. 9-31. Scapular fractures. *A,* Greenstick fracture of margin (arrow). *B,* More extensive fracture of subglenoid region (arrow).

arm, scapular winging, absence of the deep tendon reflexes in the biceps, triceps, and brachioradialis, absence of the grasp reflex, torticollis, facial palsy, Horner's syndrome from injury to the cervical sympathetic nerves, and diaphragmatic paralysis from phrenic nerve injury. The Moro reflex is absent in high brachial plexus injury. Injury to only the C7 and

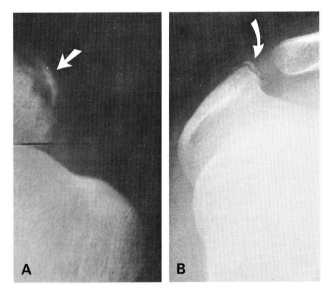

FIG. 9-32. *A,* Avulsion fracture of lateral tip of acromion (arrow). *B,* Avulsion of chondro-osseous segment of acromion at acromioclavicular joint (arrow). This is a variation of "A-C separation" in the adolescent.

C8 roots (Klumke's paralysis) results in weakness of the wrist and finger flexors and the intrinsic muscles of the hand.[57] The Moro reflex may be present, except for terminal fanning of the digits and flexion of the thumb and index finger. The grasp reflex is absent. Extensive sensory deficit implies a poor prognosis, but usually sensation is surprisingly intact.

Of far greater prognostic use is a clinical description, joint by joint, of the degree of involvement, particularly for patients whose care may not remain the responsibility of one physician from year to year. Such information allows an overall plan of management to be followed and ensures that a patient will not be left with a worthless hand or elbow, but a shoulder rendered nearly normal by successful surgery.

One should examine any infant with a brachial plexus injury at 4 to 8 week intervals to further evaluate the extent of the injury and the degree of recovery. A record should be made of the range of active and passive motion of the extremities and the gross reaction to pain. Neurologic examination of the upper and lower extremities should be repeated, since brain and spinal cord injury can also occur in these children. Edema, skin changes, and trophic ulcers should be noted, and two-point discrimination and proprioception determined in cooperative, older children.

Complete, spontaneous recovery of function is hoped for in all patients, but it is impossible to predict which patients will recover fully. A wide difference in the incidence of complete recovery has been reported; Wickstrom found an incidence of 13%, whereas Adler reported only 7%.[58,60] Regardless of the incidence of spontaneous recovery and the transience of the paralysis in some patients, contractures and deformities can occur rapidly.[61] Therefore, every child in whom birth palsy is diagnosed or suspected should receive early therapy. One should not await spontaneous recovery, since limitation of motion and deformity may persist, despite complete return of muscle power, if therapy is delayed.

Frequent, diligent, gentle exercise putting all the joints of the involved extremity through a full range of passive motion is the cornerstone of early management of the patient with obstetric palsy. Such therapy hopefully will prevent or decrease contractures. If some degree of paralysis persists, prevention of contracture will allow greater latitude in the choice of subsequent reconstructive procedures. As in deformities complicating poliomyelitis, it is a basic axiom of treatment that fixed deformity must be overcome before tendon or muscle transfers are performed in order to produce more normal function.

Braces, strapping, statue-of-liberty or other splints, or pinning the arm to the head of the crib have been recommended by many and still are mentioned in orthopaedic textbooks. These procedures are attractive because they supposedly prevent the most obvious deformity of an internally rotated and adducted shoulder.

The parents should be taught how to apply gentle motion to the shoulder, elbow, and wrist joints with each diaper change, and the physician should review the performance at each follow-up visit. The parents should hold the top of the shoulder and lift the patient's arm gently for effective, passive exercises at the glenohumeral joint. If there are supination contractures of the forearm or adduction contractures of the thumb, the parents should stretch them carefully. Occasionally, posterior plaster splints at the elbow and wrist may prevent palmar flexion contractures.

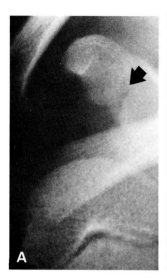
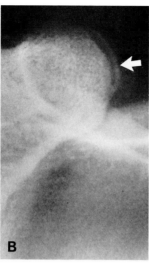

FIG. 9-33. *A,* Fracture through coracoid (arrow). *B,* Avulsion fracture of tip of coracoid (arrow).

The problems of later management and consequences of operative procedures to restore function are described well in articles by Adler and Wickstrom.[58,60] It is important to follow these children through to skeletal maturity, as their abnormally innervated muscle can lead to differences in the growth of the bones, particularly the shoulder and elbow (Fig. 9-34). Undoubtedly, these differences are due to abnormal growth stimulation from muscle imbalance.

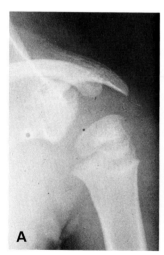
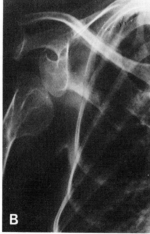

FIG. 9-34. Effect of Erb's palsy on proximal humeral development. *A,* At two years. *B,* At skeletal maturity (note pseudo-dislocation of proximal humerus due to laxity of the rotator cuff).

References

1. Ogden, J. A., Conlogue, G. J., and Bronson, M. L.: Radiology of postnatal skeletal development. III. The clavicle. Skeletal Radiol., *4:*196, 1979.

2. Fawcett, J.: The development and ossification in the human clavicle. J. Anat. Physiol., *47:*225, 1913.

3. Bearn, J. G.: Direct observations of the function of the capsule of the sternoclavicular joint in clavicular support. J. Anat., *101:*159, 1967.

4. Ogden, J. A., Phillips, S. B., and Conlogue, G. J.: Radiology of postnatal skeletal development. VI. The scapula. Skeletal Radiol., in press.

5. Phillips, S. B., Ogden, J. A., and Conlogue, G. J.: Morphogenesis of the human scapula. In preparation.

6. Klima, M.: Early development of the human sternum and the problem of homologization of the so-called suprasternal structures. Acta Anat. (Basel), *69:*473, 1968.

7. Ogden, J. A., et al.: Radiology of postnatal skeletal development. II. The manubrium and sternum. Skeletal Radiol., *4:*189, 1979.

8. McCally, W. C., and Kelly, D. A.: Treatment of fractures of the clavicle, ribs, and scapulae. Am. J. Surg., *50:*558, 1940.

9. Douglas, G. J., and Simpson, J. S.: The conservative management of splenic trauma. J. Pediatr. Surg., *6:*565, 1971.

10. Mishalany, H.: Repair of the ruptured spleen. J. Pediatr. Surg., *9:*175, 1974.

11. Zachary, R. B., and Emergy, J. L.: Abdominal splenosis following rupture of a spleen in a boy aged 10 years. Br. J. Surg., *46:*415, 1959.

12. Balfanz, J. R., et al.: Overwhelming sepsis following splenectomy for trauma. J. Pediatr., *88:*458, 1976.

13. Frieberger, R. H., and Mayer, V.: Ununited bilateral fatigue fractures of the first ribs. J. Bone Joint Surg., *46-A:*615, 1964.

14. Fisher, R. D., and Rienhoff, W. F.: Subclavian artery laceration resulting from fracture of the first rib. J. Trauma, *6:*579, 1966.

15. Galbraith, N. F., et al.: Fracture of the first rib associated with laceration of subclavian artery. J. Thorac. Cardiovasc. Surg., *65:*649, 1973.

16. Pierce, G. E., Maxwell, J. A., and Boggan, M. D.: Special hazards of first rib fractures. J. Trauma, *15:*264, 1975.

17. Calandi, C., and Bartolozzi, G.: On 110 cases of fracture of the clavicle in the newborn. Clin. Pediatr., *64:*541, 1959.

18. DeBlasio, A., and Iafusco, F.: Fracture of the clavicle in newborn infants. Pediatria (Napoli), *68:*815, 1960.

19. Farkas, R., and Levine, S.: X-ray incidence of fractured clavicle in vertex presentation. Am. J. Obstet. Gynecol., *59:*204, 1950.

20. Lehmacher, K., and Lehmann, C.: Clavicular fracture in newborn infants after spontaneous delivery in the occipital position. Z. Geburtshilfe Gynaek., *158:*134, 1962.

21. Nasso, S., and Verga, A.: La frattura della clavicola del neonato. Minerva Pediatr., *6:*593, 1954.

22. Billington, R. W.: A new plaster yoke for fracture of the clavicle. South. Med. J., *24:*667, 1934.

23. Gilchrist, D.: A stockinette-velpeau for immobilization of the shoulder girdle. J. Bone Joint Surg., *45-A:*1382, 1963.

24. Fitisenko, I.: On the treatment of clavicular fracture in children. Khirurgiia (Mosk), *39:*36, 1963.

25. Alkalaj, I.: Internal fixation of a severe clavicular fracture in a child. Isr. J. Med. Sci., *9:*306, 1960.

26. Dickson, J. W.: Death following fractured clavicle. Lancet, *2:*666, 1952.

27. The Death of Sir Robert Peal. Lancet, *2:*19, 1850.

28. Mital, M., and Aufranc, O.: Venous occlusion following greenstick fracture of the clavicle. J.A.M.A., *206:*1301, 1968.

29. Howard, F., and Shafer, S.: Injuries to the clavicle with arteriovenous complications. J. Bone Joint Surg., *47-A:*1335, 1965.

30. Rowe, C. R.: Symposium on surgical lesions of the shoulder. Acute and recurrent dislocation of the shoulder. J. Bone Joint Surg., *44-A:*977, 1962.

31. Nogi, J., et al.: Non-union of the clavicle in a child. A case report. Clin. Orthop., *110:*19, 1975.

32. Alldred, A. J.: Congenital pseudarthrosis of the clavicle. J. Bone Joint Surg., *45-B:*312, 1963.

33. Behringer, B. R., and Wilson, F. C.: Congenital pseudarthrosis of the clavicle. Am. J. Dis. Child., *123:*511, 1972.

34. Jinkins, W. J.: Congenital pseudarthrosis of the clavicle. Clin. Orthop., *62:*183, 1969.

35. Poland, J.: Traumatic Separation of the Epiphyses, London, Smith, Elder, and Co., 1898.

36. Karlen, M. A.: Traitmiento quirurgivo de la epifiseolosis clavicular. Bol. Soc. Cir. Uruguay, *14:*94, 1943.

37. Denham, R. H., Jr., and Dingley, A. E., Jr.: Epiphyseal separation of the medial end of the clavicle. J. Bone Joint Surg., *49-A:*1179, 1967.

38. Wheeler, M. E., Laaveg, S. J., and Sprague, B. L.: S-C joint disruption in an infant. Clin. Orthop., *139:*68, 1979.

39. Brooks, A., and Henning, G.: Injury to the proximal clavicular epiphysis. J. Bone Joint Surg., *54-A:*1347, 1972.

40. Lucas, G. L.: Retrosternal dislocation of the clavicle. J.A.M.A., *193:*850, 1965.

41. Nettles, J. S., and Linscheid, R. L.: Sternoclavicular dislocations. J. Trauma, *8:*158, 1968.

42. Paterson, D. C.: Retrosternal dislocation of the clavicle. J. Bone Joint Surg., *43-B:*90, 1961.

43. Tyer, H., Sturrock, W., and Callow, F.: Retrosternal dislocation of the clavicle. J. Bone Joint Surg., *45-B:*132, 1963.

44. Elting, J. J.: Retrosternal dislocation of the clavicle. Arch. Surg., *104:*35, 1972.

45. Ferry, A. M., Rook, F. W., and Masterson, J. H.: Retrosternal dislocation of the clavicle. J. Bone Joint Surg., *39-A:*905, 1957.

46. Kennedy, J. L.: Retrosternal dislocation of the clavicle. J. Bone Joint Surg., *31-B:*74, 1949.

47. Simurda, M.: Retrosternal dislocation of the clavicle—a report of four cases with a method of repair. Can. J. Surg., *11:*487, 1968.

48. Editorial: Internal fixation for fractures in childhood. Br. Med. J., *1:*1301, 1976.

49. Lazcano, M. A., Anzell, S. H., and Kelly, P. J.: Complete dislocation and subluxation of the acromioclavicular joint. End results in 73 cases. J. Bone Joint Surg., *43-A:*379, 1961.

49a. Imatani, R.: Fractures of the scapula: a review of 53 fractures. J. Trauma, *15:*473, 1975.

50. Wilber, M. C., and Evans, E. B.: Fractures of the scapula. An analysis of forty cases and a review of the literature. J. Bone Joint Surg., *59-A:*358, 1977.

51. Benton, J., and Nelson, C.: Avulsion of the coracoid process in an athlete. J. Bone Joint Surg., *53-A:*356, 1971.

52. Montgomery, S. P., and Lloyd, R. D.: Avulsion fracture of the coracoid epiphysis with acromioclavicular separation. J. Bone Joint Surg., *59-A:*963, 1977.

53. Babbitt, D. P., and Cassidy, R. H.: Obstetrical paralysis and dislocation of the shoulder in infancy. J. Bone Joint Surg., *50-A:*1447, 1968.

54. Chung, S. M. K., and Nessenbaum, M. M.: Obstetrical paralysis. Orthop. Clin. North Am., *6:*393, 1975.

55. Specht, E. E.: Brachial plexus injury in the newborn. Incidence and prognosis. Clin. Orthop., *110:*32, 1975.

56. Liebolt, F. L., and Furey, J. G.: Obstetrical paralysis with dislocation of the shoulder. J. Bone Joint Surg., *35-A:*227, 1953.

57. Klumpke, A.: Contribution a l'étude des paralysies radicularies du plexus brachial. Paralysies radiculaires totales. Paralysies radiculaires inférieures. De la participation des filets sympathiques oculo-pupillaires dans ces paralysies. Rev. Med., *5:*591, 1885.

58. Adler, J. B., and Patterson, R. L.: Erb's palsy. Long-term results of treatment in eighty-eight cases. J. Bone Joint Surg., *49-A:*1052, 1967.

59. Gordon, M., et al.: The immediate and long-term outcome of obstetric birth trauma. I. Brachial plexus paralysis. Am. J. Obstet. Gynecol., *117:*51, 1973.

60. Wickstrom, J., Haslam, E. T., and Hutchinson, R. H.: The surgical management of residual deformities of the shoulder following birth injuries of the brachial plexus. J. Bone Joint Surg., *37-A:*27, 1955.

61. Aitken, J.: Deformity of the elbow joint as a sequel to Erb's obstetrical paralysis. J. Bone Joint Surg., *34-B:*352, 1952.

10

Humerus

Anatomy

Proximal humerus

The contour of the neonatal proximal humeral physis has a transverse orientation with minimal elevation of the central region. However, during postnatal development, this physeal contour is progressively modified into a conical (pyramidal) shape, leading to the development of two major growth zones. One of these growth zones, located medially, under the humeral head that is subjected to compression stresses in most functional positions, and the other, a more lateral region, associated with the greater tuberosity is subjected to both compression and tension forces depending upon the position and functional activity of the various shoulder muscles (Figs. 10-1 to 10-4). The lateral portion of the physis should still be considered a compression-responsive structure, despite the application of compressive and tensile forces by portions of the rotator cuff, because its histologic structure is a columnar growth plate rather than the fibro-cartilaginous structural conversion that is seen in physes that are primarily traction-responsive, such as the tibial tuberosity (see Chaps. 4 and 19).

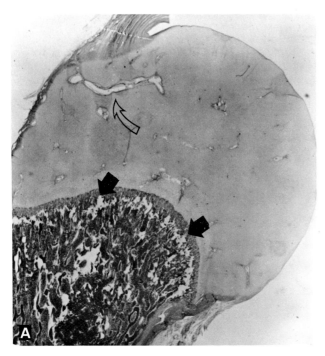

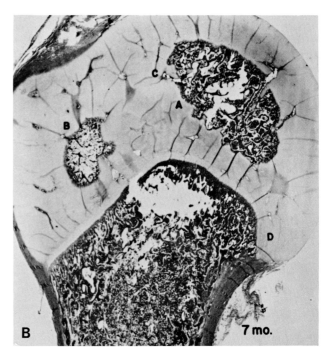

FIG. 10-1. Early development of proximal humerus. *A,* Neonatal humerus showing vascular cartilage canal penetrating from the greater tuberosity (open arrow). The preparation technique for this slide caused some separation through the metaphysis adjacent to the physis (solid arrows). This is the plane of separation in a birth injury. Such an injury invariably involves a type 1 growth mechanism fracture, rather than a shoulder dislocation. *B,* At seven months, secondary ossification centers are present in the capital humerus (A) and the greater tuberosity (B). A small vascular channel (C) enters the capital humeral center. Note how the medial physis curves distally at D, creating a contour similar to that of the early proximal femur.

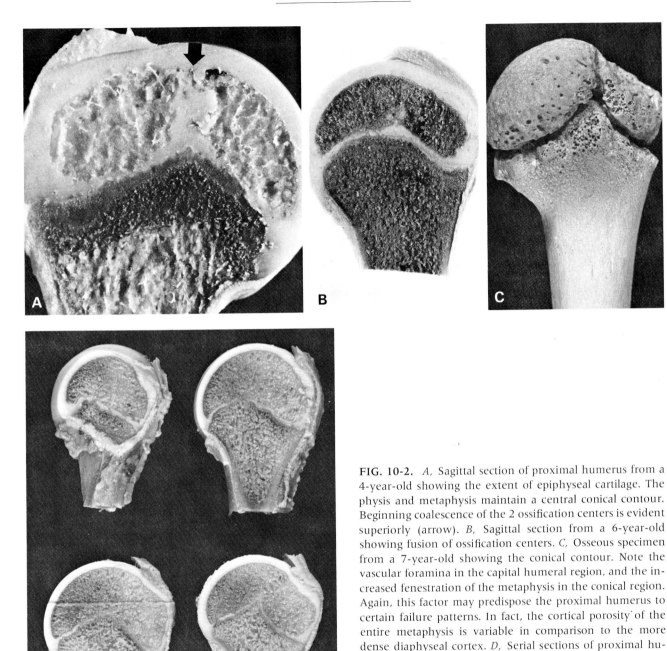

FIG. 10-2. *A,* Sagittal section of proximal humerus from a 4-year-old showing the extent of epiphyseal cartilage. The physis and metaphysis maintain a central conical contour. Beginning coalescence of the 2 ossification centers is evident superiorly (arrow). *B,* Sagittal section from a 6-year-old showing fusion of ossification centers. *C,* Osseous specimen from a 7-year-old showing the conical contour. Note the vascular foramina in the capital humeral region, and the increased fenestration of the metaphysis in the conical region. Again, this factor may predispose the proximal humerus to certain failure patterns. In fact, the cortical porosity of the entire metaphysis is variable in comparison to the more dense diaphyseal cortex. *D,* Serial sections of proximal humerus from a 12-year-old showing the variable contour of the physis depending upon the anteroposterior depth. This varied contour affects fracture patterns.

As the proximal humerus matures, the anatomic structure of the growth plate and contiguous metaphysis plays a major role in the overall resistive strength and patterns of fracture. The progressively conical apex has a posteromedial position that resists forces directed posteriorly and axially. The apex of the cone is medial to a plane drawn from the anterior to the posterior insertions of the rotator cuff musculature. This plane includes a small portion of the medial metaphysis anteriorly, but more of it posteriorly, and is probably a significant anatomic factor predisposing the proximal humerus to the relatively common type 2 growth mechanism fracture.

The epiphyseal ossification center is not usually present at

birth, except in its formative (pre-osseous) stage. However, approximately 20% of neonates have a radiographically evident epiphyseal ossification center. By four months, the ossification center is well-established. The ossification center in the greater tuberosity appears between 6 and 18 months and a third ossification center for the lesser tuberosity may appear later, although this structure is highly variable and frequently does not appear as an independent ossification center. The ossification centers of the greater tuberosity and humeral head begin to form osseous connections at the microscopic level as early as 10 to 14 months of age (see Fig. 10-2*A*), although this is extremely dependent upon individ-

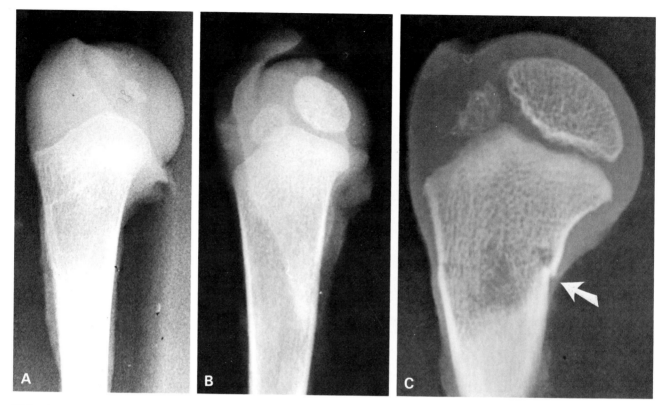

FIG. 10-3. Air-cartilage roentgenograms demonstrating cartilage as well as bone. *A,* Two months; *B,* seven months; *C,* three years. Also note the acute metaphyseal fracture (arrow).

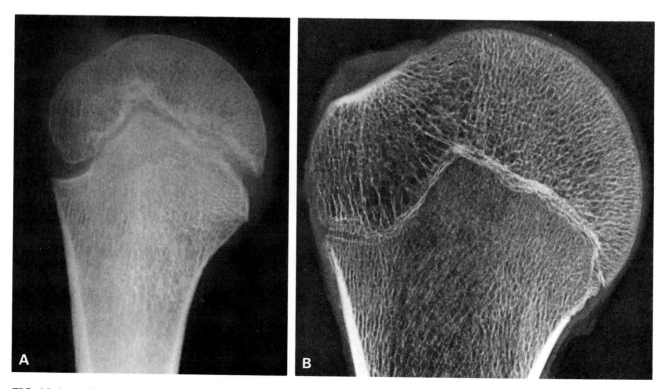

FIG. 10-4. *A,* Roentgenogram from a 13-year-old, showing sclerosis preceding final physeal closure. *B,* Slab section from a 15-year-old showing almost complete physeal closure with coalescence of subchondral plates.

ual rates of development. By 4 to 7 years, osseous coalescence of these two major centers is radiographically evident. The physis undergoes histologic closure at approximately 17 to 18 years in the female and 19 to 20 years in the male (see Fig. 10-4).

The periosteum plays a significant role in the strength of the proximal humeral growth plate even at an early age. Dameron found that the periosteum was thicker posteriorly than anteriorly and that this anatomic variation played a significant role in preventing posterior displacement of the metaphysis.[1] In contrast, displacement of the metaphysis was easily produced through the thinner anterior portion of the periosteum. This anatomic variation in thickness remains through skeletal maturity. When the periosteum gives way, it tends to disrupt lateral to the intertubercular groove under the long head of the biceps. The bicipital tendon thus appears to be a predisposing factor to the development of the medial metaphyseal fragment in type 2 injuries.

The proximal humeral physis is significant to both hu-

meral and overall arm length, contributing approximately 80% of the longitudinal growth of the humerus. Impairment of this normal growth process can have a major effect on the overall length of the involved limb.

Metaphysis and diaphysis

As a rough definition, the diaphysis extends from the upper border of the insertion of the pectoralis major to the supracondylar ridge (Fig. 10-5). This area has multiple muscular attachments, which, according to the level of fracture, may significantly affect the deformation of the fragments. The humeral shaft is roughly cylindrical in its upper half, becoming gradually broadened and flattened below.

The major nerves traverse the humeral shaft. The most serious potential injury is to the radial nerve, which lies in a shallow groove on the posterolateral surface of the shaft of the humerus. It traverses obliquely and laterally as it passes from the axilla to the anterolateral epicondylar region. It may either be injured acutely, or be subsequently entrapped in fracture callus. Such entrapment has been described even in greenstick diaphyseal fractures.[2,3]

A supracondylar process is a normal variation seen in approximately 1% of patients (Fig. 10-6). It is located 5 to 7 cm above the medial epicondyle. It may be connected distally with a tendinous band extending to the medial epicondyle and providing an anomalous insertion for the pronator teres. When this tendinous band is calcified, it outlines a supracon-

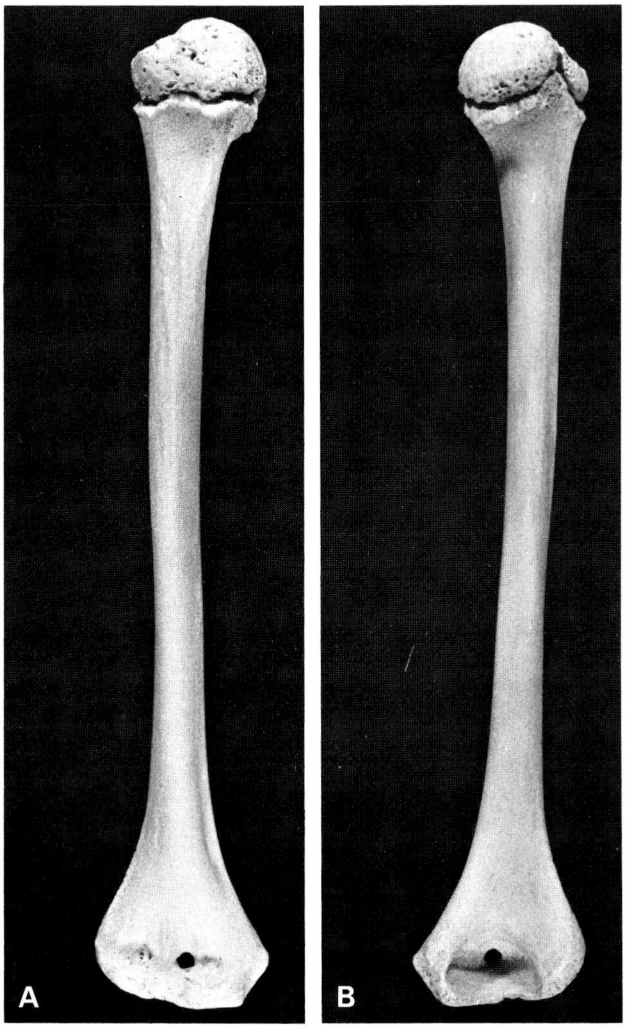

FIG. 10-5. *A,* Anterior and *B,* posterior views of humerus from a six-year-old child. Note the posterior direction (retroversion) of the humeral head, and the perforated supracondylar foramen.

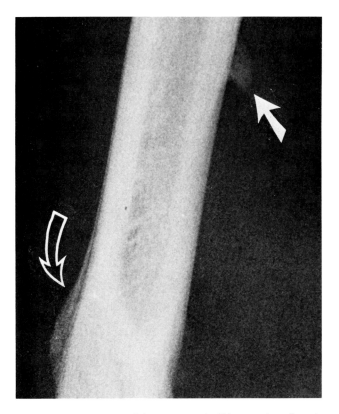

FIG. 10-6. Supracondylar process (solid arrow), a fortuitous finding in a patient with a dislocated elbow. Note the subperiosteal new bone along the posterior cortex (open arrow) consequent to periosteal stripping.

dylar foramen. When the median nerve and artery pass through this structure, sufficient compression may cause arterial or nerve dysfunction. On rare occasions, the supracondylar process may be fractured.[4,5]

Distal humerus

In the supracondylar region, the osseous septum separating the olecranon fossa from the coronoid fossa varies in thickness. Roentgenographically it casts a shadow of variable density (Fig. 10-7). Occasionally, there may be a complete perforation. The variability of the radiographic appearance must be considered when evaluating a patient.

Diagnosis of distal humerus injuries is rendered particularly difficult by the variable degree of secondary ossification (Figs. 10-8 to 10-13).[6,7,7a] Significant injury may occur with deceptively little roentgenographic evidence. The overall joint contours and separation of capitellar and trochlear surfaces are present at birth and do not change significantly with subsequent development. Disruption of these relationships, as with medial or lateral condylar fractures, may alter joint contours and mechanics. The ossification centers appear in the following sequence: capitellum (at 3 to 4 months), medial epicondyle (at 4 to 6 years), medial condyle (at 8 to 9 years), and lateral epicondyle (at 9 to 11 years).

The trochlear center is consistently irregularly ossified and always develops from several small foci (see Fig. 10-11). A small, medial accessory ossification center of the trochlea may appear after the major foci have fused. This may simulate a fracture fragment.

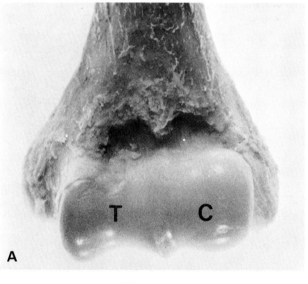

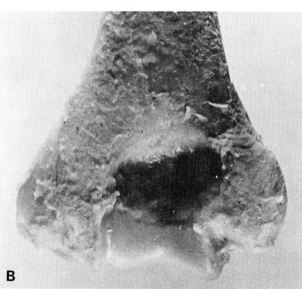

FIG. 10-7. Gross morphology of distal humerus from a six-year-old cadaver. *A,* Anterior view of trochlea (T) and capitellum (C). *B,* Posterior view of trochlea and olecranon fossa.

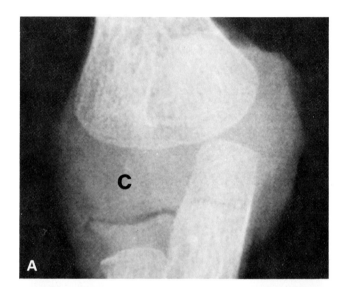

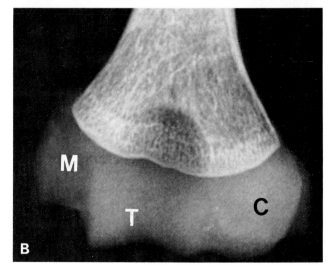

FIG. 10-8. Distal humeral development in a six-month-old baby. *A,* Intact elbow joint with air outlining the radiohumeral portions of the joint. Note the capitellum (c). *B,* Air-cartilage contrast to show cartilaginous epiphyseal contours. Note the medial epicondyle (M), the trochlea (T), and the capitellum (C).

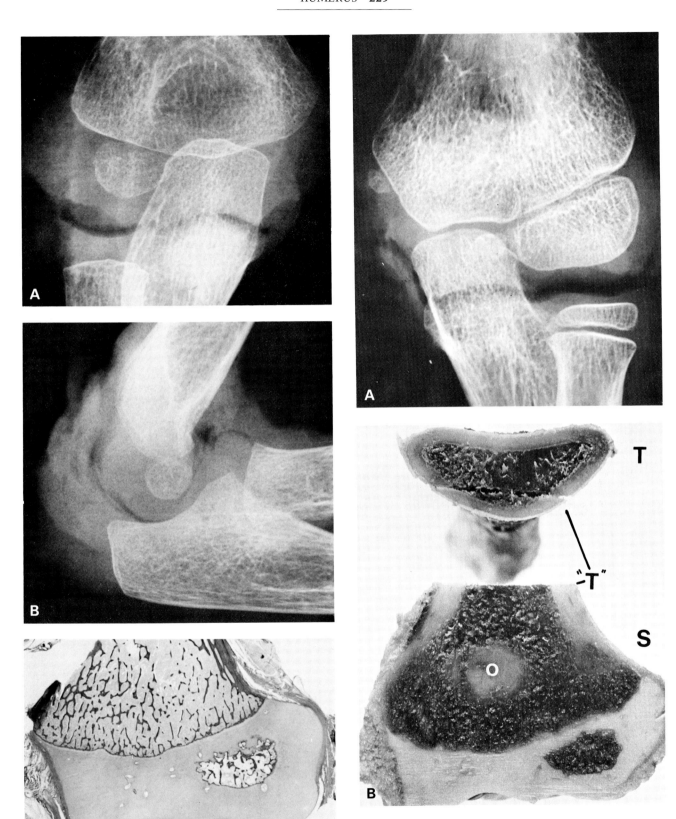

FIG. 10-9. Distal humeral development in a two-year-old. *A,* Reconstructed elbow showing chondro-osseous contours. *B,* Lateral view of *A. C,* Histologic section.

FIG. 10-10. Distal humeral development in a six-year-old. *A,* Air outlining joint and epiphyseal contours. *B,* Sagittal (S) section of chondro-osseous epiphysis and transverse (T) section of shaft at level of ("T"). Above the olecranon fossa (O), the anatomic configuration of the shaft is more stable than the transverse contour at the fossa.

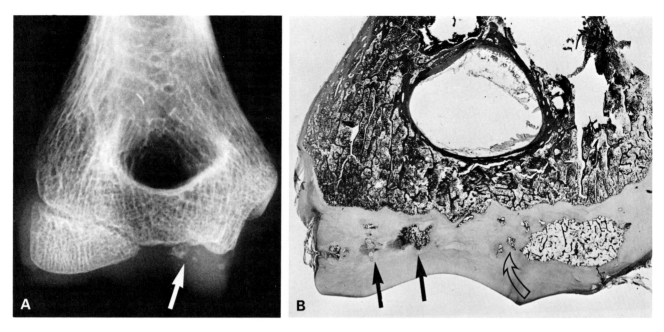

FIG. 10-11. Distal humeral development in an eight-year-old. *A,* Roentgenogram. Trochlear ossification is just beginning (arrow). *B,* Histologic section. Note the multifocal ossification of the trochlea (solid arrows) and the satellite ossification of the capitellum (open arrow).

The lateral epicondyle serves as the origin of the radial collateral ligament, the supinator, and the common extensor tendon. Irregular ossification is typical in the lateral epicondyle of the humerus, and it is often misdiagnosed as avulsion. Comparison to the opposite side is not helpful, since asymmetric ossification is relatively common. The ossification center for the lateral epicondyle on one side may appear several months after it appears on the contralateral side. The

lateral epicondyle does not fuse directly with the humeral shaft as the medial epicondyle does. Instead, it fuses first with the contiguous epiphyseal ossification center of the capitellum (see Fig. 10-13). Fusion with the capitellum occurs at 16 to 17 years. Then the combined mass fuses with the end of the humeral shaft.

The ossification center of the medial epicondyle appears at about 5 years of age and unites with the metaphysis be-

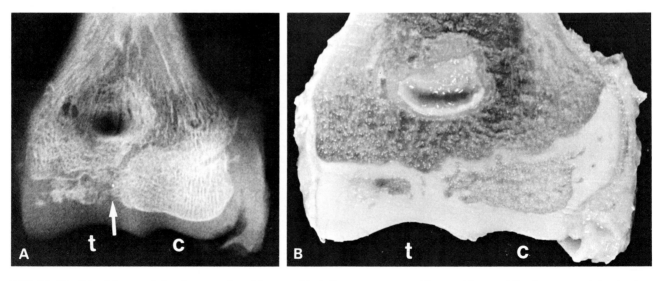

FIG. 10-12. Distal humeral development in a 10-year-old. *A,* Roentgenogram. The trochlear ossification center is beginning to coalesce with the multiple ossific foci and the capitellar ossification center (arrow). Note the trochlea (t) and capitellum (c). *B,* Sagittal section. Note the trochlea (t) and capitellum (c). The capitellar ossification center extends beyond the articular lip, separating these 2 regions. This anatomic factor undoubtedly causes propagation of lateral condylar fractures through the trochlear articular region.

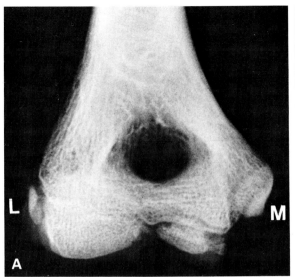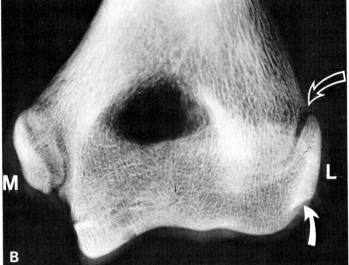

FIG. 10-13. *A,* Distal humeral development in a 12-year-old. *A,* Both epicondyles have developed secondary centers (lateral epicondyle = L; medial epicondyle = M). *B,* Distal humerus of a 14-year-old. The lateral epicondyle has fused with the capitellum (solid arrow), but not with the metaphysis (open arrow). (lateral epicondyle = L; medial epicondyle = M.)

tween 18 and 20 years of age. The common tendon of the flexor muscles of the forearm originates from the anterior aspect of the medial epicondyle, which also gives attachment to the ulnar collateral ligament of the elbow. The ulnar nerve runs in a groove along the posterior aspect of this epicondyle, an anatomic relationship responsible for the frequency of ulnar nerve injury in epicondylar fracture. The medial epicondyle is often considered an epiphysis that does not contribute to the longitudinal growth of the humerus. This is a misconception. This particular region initially develops as an integral part of the medial condyle. With growth, it becomes a functionally, though not anatomically, separate entity, and appears to be unassociated with the major histologic changes characteristic of a traction-responsive physis such as the tibial tuberosity. Injury to the medial epicondyle, if it occurs in a younger child, may lead to growth arrest because it causes disruption of the physis as it curves around the main portion of the condyle. The older the child at the time of a distal humeral injury, the less likely it is that any significant growth disturbance will follow.

The distal humerus has a normal forward angulation which is most evident when supracondylar or capitellar (lateral condylar) fractures are being evaluated (Fig. 10-14). Realignment of this anatomic configuration should be attempted, since misalignment may affect elbow mechanics.

Proximal Humerus

Glenohumeral joint dislocation

Anatomic structure and the extent of functional motion predispose the proximal humerus to epiphyseal separation in the child and adolescent in response to forces that would lead to glenohumeral dislocation in an adult. Rowe reviewed 500 cases of shoulder dislocation and found only 8 patients who were between the ages of 6 months and 10 years.[8] Al-

most 20% of the 500 cases occurred in the second decade of life, usually in the 17 to 20 year range (after skeletal maturity had been attained). Interestingly, Rowe described the highest recurrence rates in children rather than adults. He also showed that many young adults with habitual voluntary dislocation of the shoulder probably commenced the process during early adolescence, a time when the growth plate was undergoing normal physiologic closure and the laxity of the ligamentous structure around the shoulder was decreasing. The dislocation usually is anteroinferior (Fig. 10-15).

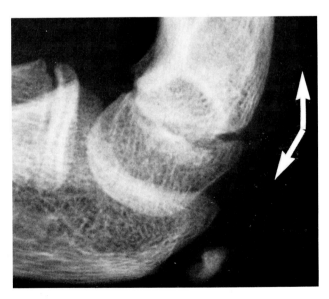

FIG. 10-14. Normal lateral view showing anterior angulation of the capitellum. This angulation must be restored in fracture reductions.

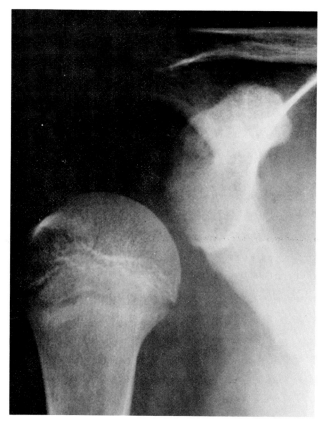

FIG. 10-15. Anterior view of glenohumeral dislocation in a 10-year-old.

Treatment of this injury is similar in adults and children. Longitudinal traction is applied to the arm, concomitant with countertraction. The arm initially is held in the internally rotated position. External rotation is applied gradually. Adequate muscle relaxation facilitates these maneuvers. Many children have generalized joint laxity, which makes reduction relatively easy. However, great care must be taken not to use undue force (particularly rotatory), since this may cause traumatic epiphysiolysis. The arm should be immobilized in a sling-and-swathe dressing. Pendulum exercises may be started at 10 to 14 days. Redislocation may occur.

Dislocation of the shoulder has also been described as a birth injury.[9] However, great care should be taken before rendering such a diagnosis, because the proximal humerus can be fractured easily at the junction of the growth plate and the metaphysis, an injury which leads to anteromedial displacement of the shaft and an apparent dislocation roentgenographically (Fig. 10-16). In actuality, the proximal humerus is still contained within the joint, while the metaphysis is laterally displaced. About 20% of newborns have an ossification center that is radiologically evident, and this assists in making a diagnosis. However, if there is any question, a shoulder arthrogram may be used to make a specific diagnosis. Fractures at this time in life are not inconsequential. Children sustaining these fractures should be followed closely throughout skeletal maturation so that growth abnormalities, such as humerus varus, can be detected.

Proximal humeral fracture

Since dislocation of the glenohumeral joint is an extremely rare injury prior to epiphyseal closure, fractures constitute the major injury to the proximal humerus.[10-20,22-26] Neer and Horwitz reported a 3% incidence of proximal humeral epiphyseal injuries in their series of epiphyseal fractures.[27] However, if metaphyseal fractures are also con-

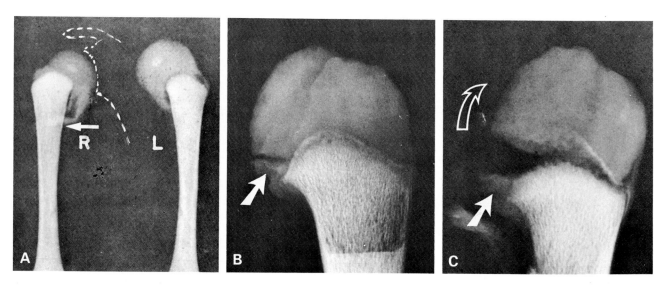

FIG. 10-16. *A,* Experimental attempts to create neonatal shoulder dislocation all caused lateral displacement of the shaft (arrow) relative to the glenohumeral joint (scapula indicated by dashes; R = right side; L = left side). *B-C,* The fracture line primarily traverses the metaphysis, but may include some of the medial epiphysis and physis (solid arrows), a factor that may explain humerus varus (see Figs. 10-34 and 10-35). The medial area probably sustains a type 5 injury. This injury is probably due to an adduction force (open arrow).

sidered (including the commonly encountered pathologic bone cyst fracture), then the incidence of proximal humeral injuries in children is probably reasonably comparable to the incidence in adults.

Injuries to the proximal humerus occur infrequently in the neonatal period, more frequently during the first decade, and quite frequently between 11 and 15 years. The oldest reported patient with a proximal humeral epiphyseal injury was a 23-year-old with pituitary dysfunction, although Poland mentioned the injury in a 25-year-old.[28-30] In most involved age groups, boys outnumber girls three or four to one.

Mechanism of Injury. In the perinatal period the usual mechanism of injury is a difficult delivery due to shoulder-pelvic disproportion (dystocia).[20,31-33] During infancy, the child may be injured by a fall or by catching the arm in the crib. The battered-child syndrome must also be considered, since injury to the proximal humerus is unusual (Fig. 10-17). The injury in later childhood and adolescence is associated with two major causal mechanisms. First, a falling child will throw the arm into an abducted, extended, and externally rotated position to break a fall. This transmits the force toward the shoulder joint, at which point the most structurally weak anatomic area fails, namely the metaphysis in the young child and the physis in the older child. Second, the child or adolescent may fall directly on the lateral side of the shoulder, in which case the major deforming force is imparted directly into the epiphysis and growth plate. After the initial deforming force ceases, maintenance or worsening of the deformity is contingent upon the interplay of the deforming muscular forces.

Pathologic Anatomy. Several types of fractures may be encountered. A type 1 physeal injury is characteristic of neonates, infants, and young children up to the age of four or five years (Figs. 10-17 and 10-18). In older children and ado-

lescents, the characteristic growth mechanism injury is type 2, with a posteromedial metaphyseal fragment attached to the physis (Figs. 10-19 and 10-20). Other types of physeal injury are encountered infrequently because of the mobility of the glenohumeral joint and the anatomy of the proximal humerus. In particular, since the humeral head is much larger than the associated glenoid, the mechanical forces that may be applied usually are not capable of introducing

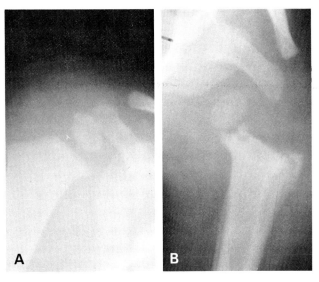

FIG. 10-17. Battered-child syndrome. *A,* Uninvolved shoulder. *B,* Contralateral shoulder with fracture of proximal humerus. Mild varus is already present, and significant growth abnormality is a distinct possibility. However, follow-up examination became impossible when the parents abruptly left the state.

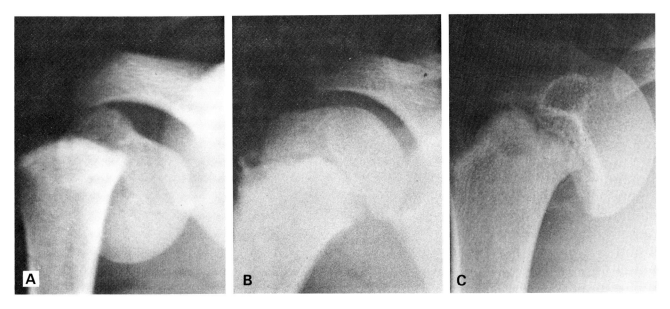

FIG. 10-18. Type 1 injury in a six-year-old. *A,* Displaced epiphysis. *B,* Reduced. *C,* Three years later, the child fell again and sustained another type 1 injury to the same shoulder.

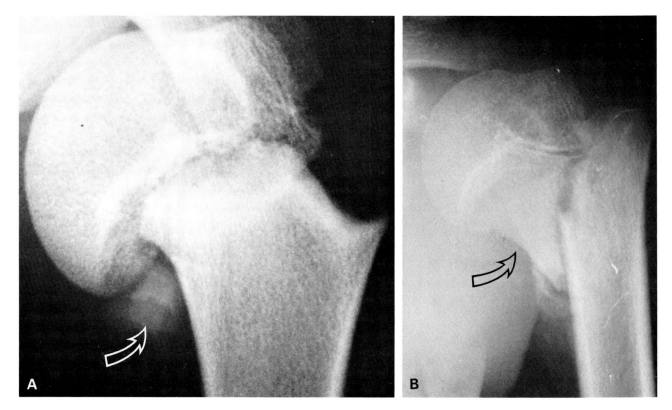

FIG. 10-19. Type 2 injuries. *A,* A small medial metaphyseal fragment (arrow). *B,* Large metaphyseal fragment (arrow), more characteristic of the injury in adolescence.

shear forces comparable to those that cause type 3 and 4 injuries in other epiphyseal regions. However, type 5 injuries may accompany type 1 or 2 injuries as a result of the adductive nature of the injury mechanism (see Fig. 10-16); this explains some of the growth abnormalities (e.g., humerus varus) and limb length inequalities that are discussed later in this chapter. Type 3 injuries may occur in the older adolescent undergoing closure of the growth plate (Fig. 10-21). Full closure of the proximal humeral growth plate may not occur until 19 or 20 years of age, and while the patient is going through the final stages of physiologic closure, injuries comparable to three or four fragment adult proximal humeral fracture patterns are more likely to be sustained.

In these aforementioned fracture types, partial displacement is more common than complete displacement. The fracture-producing mechanism and the deforming muscle forces usually cause an adduction deformity of the proximal fragment relative to the distal fragment, although abduction (valgus) angulation also occurs (Fig. 10-22).[35]

During the neonatal and early childhood periods, when children are more susceptible to type 1 than type 2 injury, the contour of the growth plate tends to be more transverse than conical. As the child grows, the underlying metaphyseal region assumes an increasingly asymmetric configuration, with the apex tending to be posteromedial. As this structure becomes more prominent, the older child becomes more susceptible to a type 2 rather than a type 1 injury (Fig. 10-23).

In type 2 injuries, the fracture begins in the lateral portion of the physis, propagates medially, and is continued into the metaphysis, leaving a variably-sized metaphyseal fragment. The periosteum tends to be stripped from the more lateral portions of the humeral metaphysis and to remain intact medially in the area of the metaphyseal fragment. The distal portion of the fracture may then be displaced through the rent in the periosteum (Fig. 10-24). The portion of intact periosteum extending from the metaphyseal fragment to the

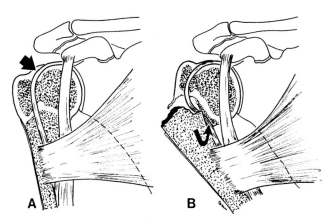

FIG. 10-20. Schematic of mechanism of medial fragment caused by path of the biceps tendon (long head). *A,* Normal anatomic relationships of long head (arrow). *B,* The tendon may be displaced behind the distal fragment (arrow), and this may prevent anatomic reduction.

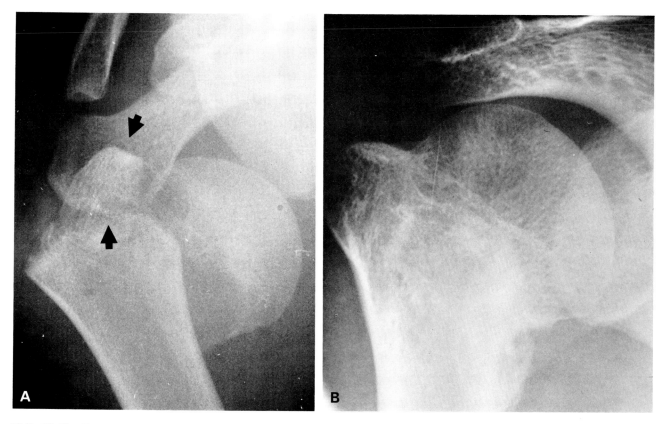

FIG. 10-21. Type 3B injury. *A,* Prereduction. Note the tuberosity fragment (arrows). *B,* Two years after closed reduction.

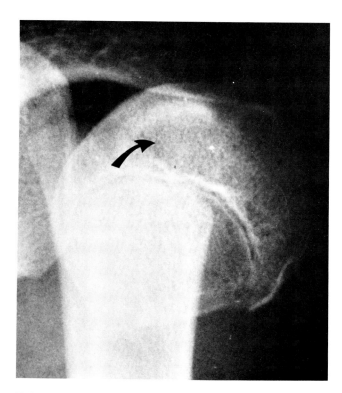

FIG. 10-22. Valgus deformation (arrow).

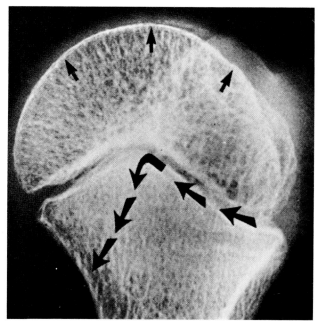

FIG. 10-23. Pattern of fracture propagation (arrows) due to conical nature of metaphysis and physis. The well-formed subchondral bone of the ossification center is evident (smaller arrows).

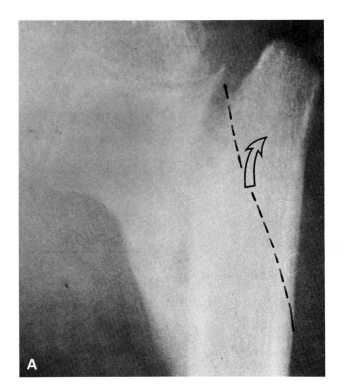

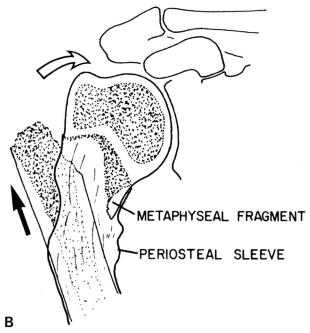

METAPHYSEAL FRAGMENT

PERIOSTEAL SLEEVE

B

FIG. 10-24. *A,* The distal fragment has probably displaced through a periosteal rent. *B,* Schematic of this injury.

more distal portions of the diaphysis tends to contract, making reduction difficult after a few days.[36] Periosteal continuity also allows some control over the formation of membranous new bone and callus. These anatomic findings are evident in Figure 10-25, which shows an open reduction. When the area of the fracture was explored, the periosteum was found to be lacerated along the course of the bicipital tendon. Posteromedially the periosteum was in continuity.

The periosteum was irregularly disrupted anterolaterally, but reasonably intact over the displaced metaphysis and diaphysis. The injury was completely extra-articular, and there was no evidence of blood within the glenohumeral joint.

As previously discussed, the degree of displacement of the fragments is contingent upon two factors—the deforming forces that cause the initial displacement, and muscle pulls

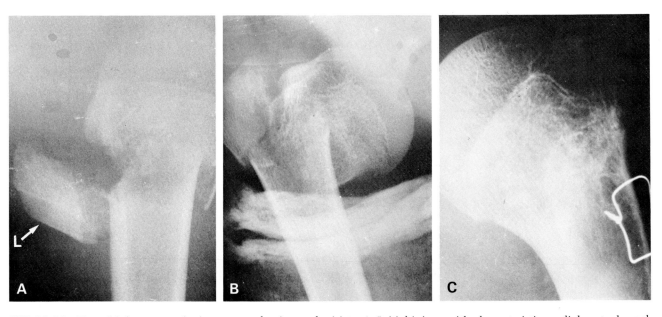

FIG. 10-25. Type 2 injury necessitating open reduction and wiring. *A,* Initial injury with characteristic medial metaphyseal fragment, but with additional free lateral metaphyseal fragment (L). *B,* Closed reduction was unsuccessful. *C,* Ten months after open reduction.

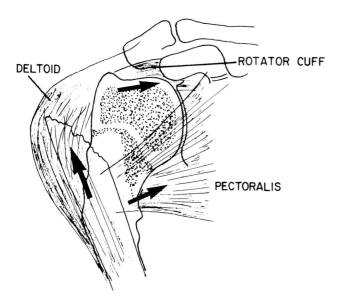

FIG. 10-26. Schematic of muscle pulls.

combined pulls of the pectoralis major, latissimus dorsi, and teres major muscles. Lateralization and cephalad displacement of the distal fragment tend to be accentuated by the pull of the deltoid (Fig. 10-26). When the fracture initially is minimally displaced, an inherent stability is imparted by the contour of the epiphyseal plate and the surrounding periosteum. This tends to negate any effect from muscle attachments. However, when the separation is grade 2 or 3, the fracture is less stable, and muscular deforming forces play a more dominant role, converting a partial displacement into a complete displacement.

Displacement is highly variable in injuries to the proximal humerus, and along with a patient's age and anticipated growth (Fig. 10-27), it is taken into account when deciding upon therapy. The younger the child, the less important aggressive, accurate correction of displacement is. However, as the child approaches adolescence, significant displacements become much less acceptable.

The main neurovascular bundle is anteromedial to the joint. However, the axillary nerve does course inferior to the glenohumeral joint, wrapping around it to supply the deltoid muscle. It is adjacent to the fragment of the metaphysis in a type 2 injury and near the apex of the injury in a type 1 injury. A complete or transient paralysis of the deltoid may accompany injury. However, since the mechanism of injury is often a direct fall on the shoulder, a contusion is possible to the nerve where it goes between the deltoid and the proximal humerus. Most of these neural injuries are transient, being due to contusion rather than disruption.[37]

Diagnosis. In the newborn period, diagnosis is often difficult. A neonate with a fracture consequent to a birth injury will have a relative "paralysis" (pseudoparalysis) of the arm, so the injury often is misinterpreted as a brachial plexus palsy. However, it is usually possible to stimulate the child to move the major part of the arm and forearm musculature. Confirmation of a fracture is possible by repeat films seven to

that either maintain displacement or worsen it. Displacement may be graded into three types: (1) displacement less than one-half the diameter of the metaphyseal shaft; (2) displacement greater than one-half the metaphyseal diameter; and (3) complete displacement. In grades 2 and 3 there usually is accompanying angular deformity in a varus position. When there is angular displacement, the epiphysis tends to be adducted and posteriorly displaced, while the remaining metaphysis and shaft are comparably adducted, but anteriorly displaced. While some displacement relates to the primary mechanism of injury, the epiphysis tends to be rotated into mild adduction and external rotation by the pull of attached muscles, while the shaft is drawn forward by the

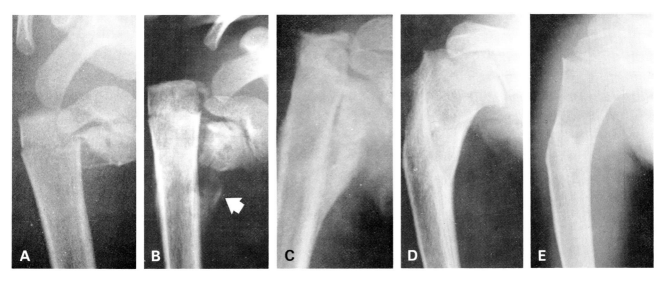

FIG. 10-27. *A,* Initial injury in a three-year-old, with medial displacement of the proximal fragment, and overriding. Multiple attempts at closed reduction under general anesthesia were unsuccessful. *B,* Four weeks later, new bone formation is evident in the periosteal sleeve (arrow). *C,* Eight weeks later, the medially displaced sleeve is filling. *D,* Four months post-injury, longitudinal growth and remodeling have taken place. *E,* Four years after the injury.

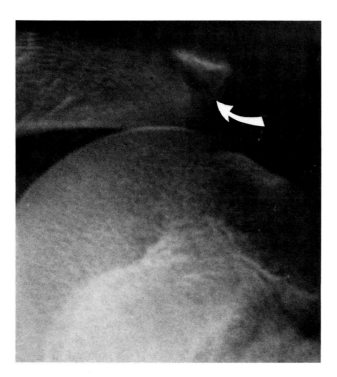

FIG. 10-28. Concomitant fracture of the proximal humerus and acromion (arrow).

ten days after birth, at which time metaphyseal callus is becoming evident. The type of trauma that causes a brachial plexus injury also may cause chondro-osseous injury.

Swelling and localized tenderness around the shoulder joint enhance the diagnosis of a shoulder fracture. Ecchymosis may appear two or three days after the injury. Since displacement is not a major part of these injuries, relative shortening of the arm is infrequent, although the presence of such a physical sign certainly helps in diagnosis. False motion and crepitus between the fracture fragments may be detected. However, searches for such findings should be held to a minimum, so as not to risk injury to the axillary nerve. Diagnosis is best made on the basis of roentgenographic rather than physical findings.

Roentgenographic Findings. The evidence for a fracture depends upon the age of the child, the extent of ossification of the humeral head and greater tuberosity, and the presence of any pathologic conditions. Pathologic changes are reasonably obvious in the adolescent, the age at which they are most likely to be encountered. Similarly, fractures of either the metaphysis or the growth plate tend to be reasonably obvious because of their characteristic anatomic changes, particularly the displacement and contiguous metaphyseal fragment. In the infant or young child, diagnosis is difficult because of the small amount of epiphyseal cartilage that has undergone ossification.

Other areas, such as the acromion, are often injured concomitantly (Fig. 10-28). Adequate radiologic evaluation must include the entire pectoral girdle.

Treatment. In general, treatment of injuries to the proximal humerus should utilize closed methods, with open reduction saved for extremely difficult cases and for older patients in whom initial non-operative methods are unsatisfactory. The fracture usually heals satisfactorily and eventually remodels, no matter how severe the displacement. However, the extent of remaining growth potential must always be kept in mind.

An effort should be made to bring the arm out to length by gentle longitudinal traction. The arm then should be placed in a comfortable position. Use of a general anesthetic is difficult to justify, because perfect anatomic reduction usually is not necessary. Furthermore, most series have shown that young children treated in a conservative fashion, with minimal efforts at reduction, even with significant displacement of the proximal humerus relative to the shaft, have virtually no significant long term abnormalities. Even in adolescents, it has been suggested that sufficient longitudinal growth and remodeling capacity remain to justify leaving the fragments overriding or in mild varus.

In older children and adolescents the fracture is generally a type 2 injury, usually accompanied by a grade 1 displacement. This fracture is stable, and manipulation is not necessary. In grade 2 and 3 injuries, in which angulation and displacement are greater, it is recommended that the humeral fragments be manipulated gently into a more acceptable position, although absolute anatomic reduction is still unnecessary.

The use of various anesthetic agents should be based on the experience of the surgeon and the cooperativeness of the patient. It may be better to perform such a reduction under a general anesthetic, since the use of an analgesic-amnesic agent (e.g., diazepam) may not allow enough muscle relaxation to gain an adequate reduction. The longer the time interval from injury to reduction, the greater the amount of soft tissue swelling and contractures (especially in the damaged periosteum) and the greater the amount of involuntary muscle activity that makes reduction increasingly difficult. Further, it is difficult to control the proximal epiphyseal fragment, since it is a relatively mobile structure, and almost impossible to stabilize completely during manipulation.

The arm should be brought into approximately 90° of abduction, flexion, and mild external rotation to accomplish the reduction. The arm then should be brought back into a position adjacent to the body. This will give an idea of the degree of stability of the reduction and whether it will be possible to treat the patient with shoulder immobilization. Whenever possible, the physician should avoid treatment in a forced abduction position, as this will increase the deforming forces applied through the pectoralis major and may affect the stability of the fracture. If there is any angular deformity, even in a grade 1 fracture, a gentle closed reduction can be attempted. Absolute anatomic reduction is again unnecessary, as remodeling will correct most grade 1 deformities.

The shoulder and arm should be immobilized by whatever method the physician prefers to use.[38] My preference is a stockinette shoulder immobilizer.

Should the fracture prove unstable, Nilsson and Svartholm have reported some success using a hanging cast with gradual spontaneous reduction of the displaced, angulated proximal fragment.[39] The shoulder may also be placed in a spica cast with the arm in abduction and forward flexion and neutral rotation (Fig. 10-29). Exact position may be determined using image intensification. The arm should be abducted

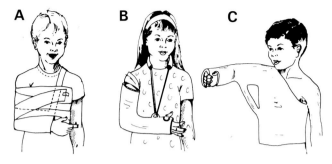

FIG. 10-29. Standard methods of treatment for various humeral injuries in children. *A,* Sling-and-swathe. *B,* Hanging long arm cast. *C,* Shoulder spica.

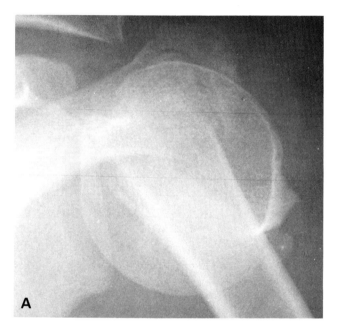

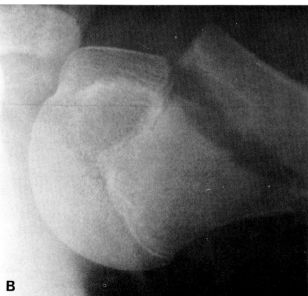

FIG. 10-30. *A,* Type 2 injury with displacement. *B,* Position after placement in traction.

only as far as necessary to ensure stability of reduction. Placement in the extreme positions (e.g., "Statue of Liberty") may cause problems such as incomplete brachial plexus palsy.

The patient may be placed in either skin traction or, if necessary, skeletal traction with an olecranon pin (Fig. 10-30). Tachdjian suggests that this method of treatment tends to stretch the capsule and subluxate the humeral head, rather than disengaging the fragments.[40] This has not been my experience, even after treating many cases by such a method.

Whether a sling, cast, or traction is chosen as the primary method of non-operative treatment, it is imperative that periodic roentgenograms be obtained, since the reduction may be lost anytime within the first three weeks. By the end of three weeks there usually is sufficient cartilaginous and ossifying callus to impart intrinsic stability. Solid union should be present by three weeks and certainly four weeks at the latest, and the child can then progressively be allowed out of immobilization. Early motion, the mainstay of therapy in adults, is relatively unnecessary in children.

Open reduction should be reserved for the older or difficult to treat patients in whom there is concern over persistent deformity and shortening. The inability to control fracture fragments because of severe multisystem injury, particularly head injury, is also an indication for open reduction. It has been suggested that the long head of the biceps may be caught between the fragments and impede adequate reduction. However, this condition is difficult to ascertain and should not be used as the primary indication for open reduction. A child whose presenting symptom many days after injury is a prominent segment of bone (the lateral metaphysis) is not necessarily a candidate for an operation either, since remodeling usually leads to the gradual disappearance of such a protuberance and improved shoulder abduction, if limitation was present.

Other than children with a head injury and uncontrolled rigidity, I have encountered few patients who seemed to fit the criteria for open reduction. One such patient had multiple injuries, including a Monteggia fracture-dislocation of the ipsilateral elbow. Following reduction of the elbow, he was placed in traction. What appeared to be a type 2 epiphyseal injury of the proximal humerus did not respond effectively (see Fig. 10-25). Because of inability to control the additional metaphyseal fragment, the injury was explored. The segment was a large portion of the anterolateral metaphysis that had fractured completely free from the remainder of the shaft and from the adjacent metaphyseal fragment, which was still attached to the epiphysis. The free fragment was completely denuded of all soft tissue attachments. The fragment was placed back in an anatomic position beneath the biceps tendon, which was preventing its reduction. Then it was stabilized with a wire suture. The patient has done well subsequently.

Results. Most authors feel these injuries heal well, even in instances of serious displacement, and that a normal shoulder may be expected at completion of skeletal growth.[41,42] However, Neer and Horwitz showed that the long term results are not as benign as most authors have described,[27] with a high incidence of longitudinal growth impairment being the main complication.

Complications. The usual problems encountered in adult shoulder injuries, such as joint stiffness, malunion, avascular necrosis, nonunion, myositis ossificans, and extra-articular calcification are extremely rare in children. The major complications in children are: (1) limb length inequality and (2) varus deformity. Mild angular growth deformities are more readily tolerated in this joint than any other because of the degrees of freedom of motion.

Neer found a large number of patients who had shortening whether associated with displacements of less than one-third the shaft diameter, or with total displacement.[27] This shortening appeared to affect mainly those patients sustaining their injury after the age of 11. Patients younger than 11 did not have major growth abnormalities, and in fact, appeared to make up initial shortening through a process comparable to femoral overgrowth. The same criteria appeared to apply to angular deformity; children over 11 had less correction and maintained some varus deformity. The major factor to consider in any decision for treatment thus appears to be the anticipated longitudinal growth in the physis.

Varus deformity complicating proximal fractures in adults is a well-acknowledged clinical occurrence, but it is virtually ignored as a significant complication during childhood.[43-45] Most authors state that such an angular deformity will correct spontaneously with subsequent growth. Similarly, varus deformity sustained during the neonatal period, when diagnosis of actual fracture is difficult, is also considered to have minimal long term consequences.

Of the fracture texts directed at children's injuries, only Blount mentions humerus varus as a possible long term consequence.[76] This condition probably develops gradually and not as a result of immediate rotation of the humeral head. It most likely occurs as a result of undetectable trauma to the medial side of the proximal humeral growth plate, eventually resulting in a significant radiologic deformity (Figs. 10-31 and 10-32). If a patient presents with such a severe deformity, he should be followed annually, because physeal fusion will eventually occur, and the apparent radiolucent defect (in reality filled with articular and epiphyseal cartilage) appears not to represent a major risk to fracture. If the abnormality is encountered at a relatively early age (before six or seven years of age), it may be possible to resect the osseous bridge. If any significant functional limitations occur, in the late adolescent period, acromionectomy may be more beneficial than a valgus osteotomy of the surgical neck.

An infrequent complication is injury to the circumflex or axillary nerve adjacent to the region of the fracture. This is usually a transient paralysis of the deltoid that resolves itself within a few weeks or months.

Diaphysis and Metaphyses

Fractures of the humeral diaphysis are relatively uncommon in children. Osseous injuries more frequently involve the metaphyseal ends, especially the distal metaphysis, with supracondylar fracture being one of the most common injuries to the developing skeleton.

Proximal metaphysis

The proximal metaphysis is highly susceptible to fracture in the 5 through 11 year range, during which period such

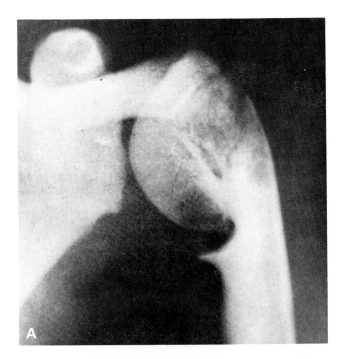

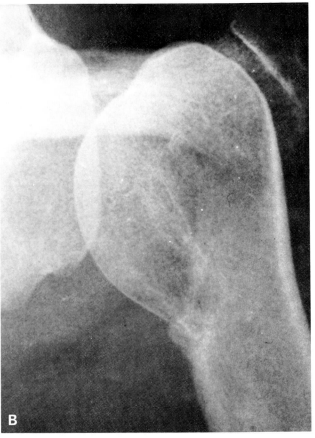

FIG. 10-31. *A,* Patient at eight years, showing a well-established humerus varus. She had sustained a fracture of the proximal humerus during birth.[43] *B,* This patient, now skeletally mature, has no functional limitation. Note how the radiolucent defect between the humeral head and the shaft has filled in completely.

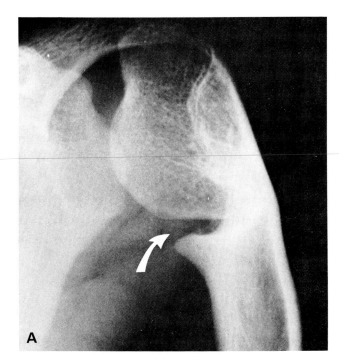

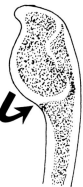

B   **HUMERUS VARUS**

FIG. 10-32. *A*, Roentgenogram of shoulder of a 12-year-old boy with humerus varus. The parents were told that the shoulder was "dislocated" during a traumatic delivery. The radiolucent gap (arrow) is filled with rotated articular cartilage. *B*, Schematic showing how cartilage fills the radiolucent gap. Some of this is undoubtedly articular cartilage that had inturned as the proximal physis and epiphysis progressively turned into varus.

injuries may be more frequent than proximal epiphyseal fractures. The susceptibility of the metaphysis to these fractures probably relates to structural changes and remodeling taking place in the cortex and spongiosa. Two basic fracture patterns occur: (1) transverse fracture with loss of cortical continuity (Figs. 10-33 and 10-34), and (2) torus fracture with maintenance of cortical integrity despite the buckling (Fig. 10-35).

Greenstick fractures are common, but seldom with significant angular deformity. These are torus-type fractures. Completely displaced metaphyseal fractures may be more difficult to manage than type 2 physeal injuries. The shaft may

penetrate the deltoid muscle and lie subcutaneously, making reduction difficult because of interposed muscle.

Treatment for undisplaced fractures is simple immobilization and inception of exercises when pain subsides. If the fracture is complete and displaced, manipulative reduction should be undertaken. However, repeated manipulation to attain anatomic reduction is probably unnecessary, since overgrowth will occur as it does in displaced proximal epiphyseal fractures. The periosteal sleeve will be relatively intact, and fill in with subperiosteal new bone (Fig. 10-36). Even if anatomic reduction cannot be attained, longitudinal alignment should be.

The use of a hanging cast may effectively align the fragments over a few days. Roentgenograms must be taken to assess the degree of correction or loss of alignment. Failure to monitor this may result in significant malunion (Fig. 10-37).

Fracture of the proximal metaphysis may lead to temporary ischemia of the juxtaphyseal bone, the mechanism of which is described in Chapters 2 and 4 (Fig. 10-38). However, the area is well vascularized, and quickly reestablishes the normal peripheral and central metaphyseal circulatory patterns. Because of the rapid rate of growth of the proximal humeral physis, the cartilage may become quite thick while the invasive metaphyseal circulation is being reestablished.

Pathologic fractures may be treated as metaphyseal fractures with immobilization in a sling for several weeks until the acute fracture healing is completed, at which time primary treatment of the cyst can be undertaken if necessary. However, treatment of the cyst with bone graft at the time of fracture is not absolutely contraindicated. The fractured region often has collapsed into a varus position, and while an attempt should be made to correct this, it is often difficult (see Chap. 8). Steroids should *never* be injected at the time of an acute pathologic fracture, as they may adversely affect the normal healing response.

Diaphyseal fractures

Diaphyseal injuries are relatively uncommon in children, the proximal and distal humeral chondro-osseous structures being more likely to fail. Significant segments of the periosteum remain intact, lessening degrees of displacement and facilitating treatment (Fig. 10-39). Transverse humeral shaft fractures generally result from a direct blow (tapping fracture), whereas spiral fractures are produced by twisting injuries, although muscular violence without an associated fall may also do this. These fractures may be treated easily by a number of methods.[47] As in the femur, bayonet apposition is satisfactory and approximately 1 cm of overgrowth may be expected. Angulation, which is commonly varus, should be kept at less than 20°. Complications are infrequent. The radial nerve may be injured, although much less commonly than with supracondylar fractures. Nerve injury is particularly likely to occur in fractures of the junction of the middle and lower thirds of the shaft. Furthermore, the nerve may become entrapped at the time of fracture between reduced fracture fragments, or subsequently in the developing callus.

Mechanism of Injury. Most fractures of the shaft of the humerus are caused by indirect violence, such as a twisting fall, rather than direct impact. This tends to cause oblique or comminuted fractures (Fig. 10-40). When the child lands on

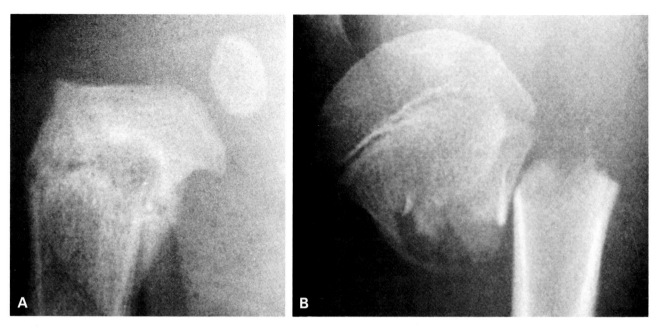

FIG. 10-33. *A,* Metaphyseal fracture in five-month-old child. Strong periosteal attachments maintain the alignment. *B,* Proximal metaphyseal fracture in a 12-year-old. This is anatomically comparable to a physeal fracture. The shaft is displaced anteromedially.

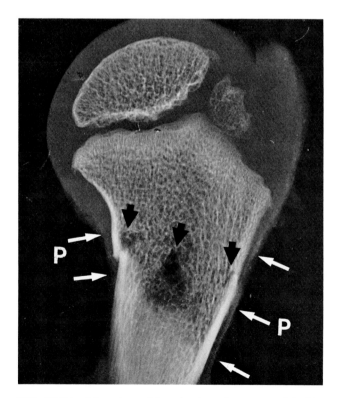

FIG. 10-34. Metaphyseal fracture in a three-year-old. This child had been fatally injured in an auto accident. The fracture (black arrows) crosses the metaphysis transversely, but the periosteum (P, white arrows) remained intact and prevented significant displacement. This fracture is primarily a compression failure, a mechanism that is more likely in a young child.

the elbow or hand with a twisting motion to the remainder of the body, incidence of spiral or oblique fractures is greater. Less commonly, athletic activities such as throwing a football, baseball, or javelin may also cause a similar spiral injury. However, if a child sustains an injury in such situations, the possibility of a pathologic fracture must be closely assessed. Transverse fractures tend to be associated more frequently with direct blows, often by landing on the upper arm or shoulder. In contrast to adults, segmental fractures are infrequent in children.

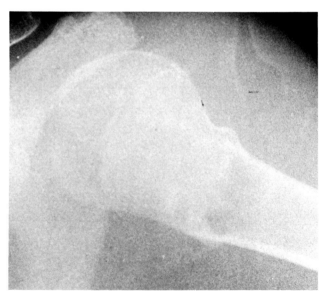

FIG. 10-35. Torus metaphyseal fracture in an 11-year-old.

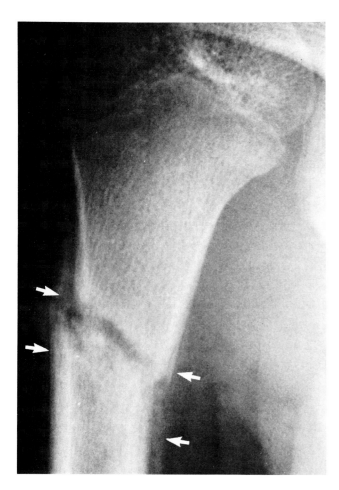

FIG. 10-36.   Fracture at metaphyseal-diaphyseal junction, with angular deformity. Early bone formation is confined by the intact periosteal sleeve (arrows).

Pathologic Anatomy.   The direction of displacement of fracture fragments is contingent upon the level of the fracture relative to the levels of muscular insertion, especially the deltoid muscle. Fractures involving the lower third of the shaft below the level of deltoid insertion generally exhibit anterolateral displacement of the proximal fragment due to the combined pull of the supraspinatus, deltoid, and coracobrachialis muscles. The distal fragment in these fractures usually is displaced proximally and medially by the spasm and contraction of the biceps and brachialis muscles (Fig. 10-41). If the fracture involves the diaphysis or metaphysis proximal to the insertion of the deltoid, but distal to the insertion of the pectoralis major, the deltoid muscle displaces the distal fragment laterally and upward. At the same time, the pectoralis major, latissimus dorsi, and teres major muscles, as well as the rotator cuff musculature of the shoulder joint, adduct and internally rotate the proximal fragment (Fig. 10-41).

The proximal humerus is usually retroverted relative to the supracondylar region. Therefore, when treating these injuries in children, particularly those with significant displacement, an attempt should be made to restore this normal anatomic configuration. Rotation does not correct itself following fracture. Therefore, it must be assumed that treatment of the arm with significant internal rotation of the lower fragment may, if the upper fragment is at all displaced or externally rotated, cause decreased retroversion and predispose the shoulder to subsequent subluxation anteriorly. However, since the more powerful forces deforming the proximal fragment tend to be those that represent the rotator cuff and internal rotators of the shoulder, it usually cannot be sufficiently internally rotated to have a major effect on the normal degree of retroversion.

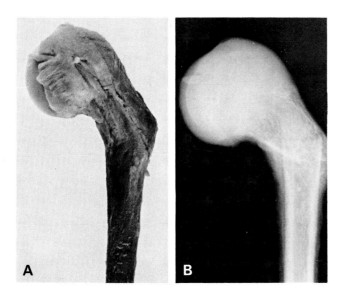

FIG. 10-37.   Malunion of proximal humeral fracture in a 10-year-old. *A*, Anterior view. *B*, Roentgenogram of specimen.

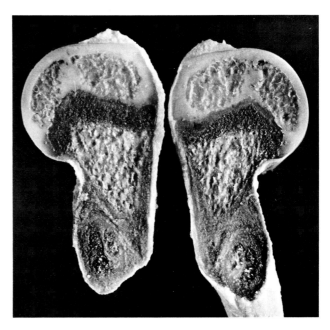

FIG. 10-38.   The specimen shown in Figure 10-37 was sectioned to produce these slabs. Note that little remodeling has taken place between the proximal and distal cortices. The darker metaphysis reflects temporary ischemia.

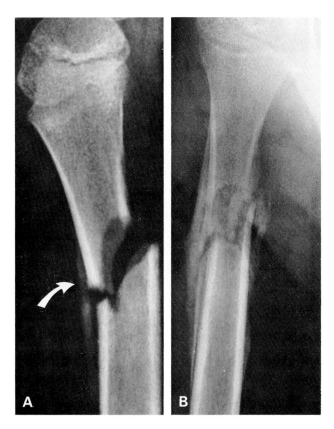

FIG. 10-39. Diaphyseal fracture. *A,* Three weeks after reduction, early bone formation is evident along the periosteal tube, which remained intact along one side of the fracture (arrow). *B,* At five weeks, extensive callus formation is evident along the side with intact periosteum, while the side with periosteal rupture shows much less formation of new bone.

Diagnosis. Clinical diagnosis is usually obvious because of deformity, local swelling, and pain. Roentgenographic studies will establish the pattern of fracture.

The close relationship of the radial nerve to the humeral shaft along the musculospiral groove makes it particularly vulnerable to injury, contusion as well as neurotmesis and axonotmesis. Further, injury to the nerves may occur consequent to their deformation by the fracture fragments, either during the original injury or during subsequent manipulation. A careful assessment of the nerve function, both sensory and motor, is absolutely essential. If the radial nerve is paralyzed, the dorsum of the hand between the first and second metacarpals commonly is anesthetic, and a variable amount of motor power is lost in the extensors of the wrist, fingers, and thumb, and in the forearm supinators.

Treatment. Treatment of children requires an appreciation that their normal state of activity is greater than an adult, and that once pain subsides, they will be less willing to be quiet and properly utilize such methods of treatment as hanging casts. If there is marked displacement of the fragments, the initial step must be reduction of the fracture, which should be accomplished by closed means, unless there is a compound injury, in which case primary treatment of the compound wound is indicated (see Chap. 6).

The initial reduction maneuver is application of downward traction to correct overriding, disengage the fracture fragments, and displace them from muscular interpositions. The proximal fragment needs to be put in continuity with the distal fragment. If the fracture is unstable, or if there is evidence of compounding, it is often easier to place the child in Dunlop's or side-directed 90°-90° traction (Fig. 10-42). Roentgenograms following reduction must be taken in both anteroposterior and lateral views. Overriding of 1 to 2 cm can be accepted, because the humerus exhibits overgrowth, similar to the femur. Angulation of 15° to 20° is the most that should be accepted. This is particularly true if the angulation is at the middle or lower third, because the bulk of the corrective growth occurs proximally, meaning that there will not be the same amount of remodeling in this area that

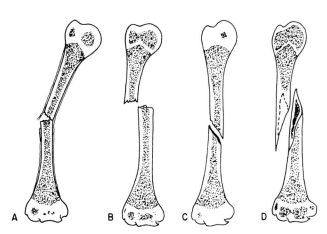

FIG. 10-40. Schematic of diaphyseal fracture patterns. *A,* Transverse, with some of periosteum intact; *B,* transverse, with complete periosteal rupture; *C,* oblique; *D,* spiral.

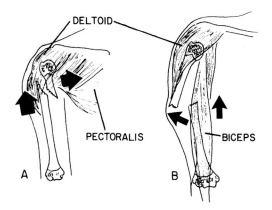

FIG. 10-41. *A,* Schematic of effects of muscle pulls on displacing fracture fragments when fracture is above the deltoid insertion. *B,* Schematic of effects of muscle pulls on displacing fracture fragments when fracture is below the deltoid insertion.

there would in an angularly displaced fracture involving the more proximal regions. In the more proximal regions, a 20° to 25° angular deformation is likely to be corrected by growth and remodeling. The only exception might be in the neonate, in whom fractures that seem innocuous initially may rapidly deform to significant malunion during treatment, but rapidly remodel.

In infants and young children, the fracture requires immobilization for four to six weeks, usually by the use of a modified Velpeau bandage or sling-and-swathe.[47,48] If the fracture is unstable, traction may be indicated. In smaller children, this probably can be accomplished with skin traction. In the older child, it may be necessary to use skeletal traction with an olecranon pin, especially if the fracture is extremely unstable or if there is any suggestion of neurovascular compromise. A shoulder spica may also be used in the older child with a relatively unstable fracture that can be reduced only in abduction.

It is possible that older children will cooperate enough to allow utilization of a device like the hanging cast. The supinating force of the biceps is lost by a fracture at this level, and the elbow joint is held in pronation by the unopposed action of the pronators. Since the joint is relatively fixed in pronation, attempts to place the forearm in supination may result in varus deformity at the fracture site. A collar and cuff should be attached to a plaster loop at the wrist and passed around the patient's neck. The cast should be light, so that excessive distraction of the fracture fragments will not occur, although continuity of at least some of the thick periosteum tends to prevent this. The forearm should be transverse to the longitudinal axis of the body when the patient is standing. The suspension collar should be adjusted in length to allow the arm to be in this position. The patient should sleep in a semi-recumbent position, rather than totally supine. As soon as pain subsides, the patient can be treated with range of motion (circumduction and pendulum) exercises.

Complications.   Malunion may result either if too much angulation is accepted, or if pathologic circumstances (e.g., cerebral palsy) are present. Since the humerus exhibits preferential proximal growth (80% of overall humeral length),

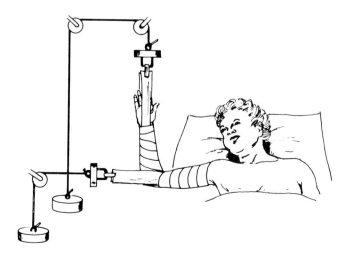

FIG. 10-42. Side-directed traction for humeral shaft fractures. Skin traction is usually sufficient.

angulation in the middle and distal thirds of the diaphyseal/metaphyseal shaft will have little likelihood of major correction. Furthermore, if malunion is at the level of the deltoid tuberosity, normal muscular forces may help maintain the deformity.

Radial nerve paralysis is rare in children.[49] Complete transsection of the nerve is extremely unlikely in a closed fracture. Nerve function is usually recovered rapidly and completely. If there is evidence of nerve compromise, the patient should be treated by traction to see if subsidence of edema will allow relatively rapid return of function. If the damage appears to be a major contusion of the nerve that will take a long time to recover, then the hand and wrist should be splinted in positions of function as part of the treatment. Follow-up should include electromyographic evaluation to determine the level and extent of injury and the chances for recovery. As long as continued improvement occurs, there is no indication for exploration. However, if the fracture has satisfactorily healed (three to four months) without any evidence of neurologic improvement, then exploration of the nerve and appropriate surgery is indicated. In some instances, the nerve is trapped in scar tissue or even in callus, and if so, it must be carefully removed and transposed to prevent recurrence of the injury. The radial or medial nerve may even be trapped by greenstick fracture.[50,51]

Distal metaphysis

Supracondylar humeral fracture is the most common type of elbow injury in the developing skeleton, accounting for approximately 50 to 60% of injuries to this area.[52-111] It occurs most frequently in children between the ages of three and ten years. It is associated with a high incidence of complications, both consequent to malunion resulting from inadequate reduction and maintenance, and consequent to selective growth mechanism injuries. Angular malunion has minimal chance of correcting spontaneously in the varus/valgus plane and must be corrected during reduction. However, anterior or posterior angulation usually will improve, if not correct itself completely. The potential for neurovascular compromise, both acute and chronic, may also lead to serious dysfunction in the forearm and hand.[5,17,35,41,42,61,73,80,82,83,90,92,98,99,112-135]

Classification. Supracondylar fractures can be classified into four types, with all basically involving the foraminal region (Fig. 10-43): (1) the flexion type (which probably accounts for 1 to 2% of these fractures); and the extension types (each representing about a third of the fractures) (2) pure extension; (3) extension-abduction, which is usually easy to treat, especially in traction, because the osseous instability lies on the lateral side where soft tissue stability is available and where traction tends to reduce the fracture; and (4) extension-adduction, which constitutes the source of most varus deformities, especially when the fracture line lies in the oblique plane and is comminuted on the medial side.

Pathologic Anatomy. *Extension Type.* Viewed from the sagittal plane, the fracture line traverses obliquely upward and backward. Viewed from the coronal (frontal) plane it usually appears transverse. The more transverse the fracture is in both planes, the more stable the injury. While the fracture is

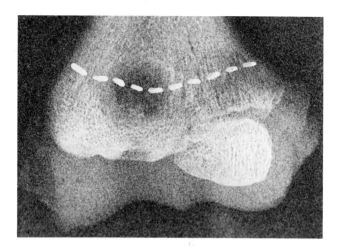

FIG. 10-43. Specimen of distal humerus showing characteristic region of fracture (dotted line) relative to the epiphyseal region and articular surface. Notice how the fracture traverses the supracondylar foraminal region.

often complete, greenstick injuries do occur (Fig. 10-44). The latter can be deceptive, impaction or widening may lead to acute, often unrecognized, cubitus varus (Fig. 10-45) or valgus (Fig. 10-46). The distal fragment may be displaced proximally and posteriorly by the transmission of the fracture force upward through the bones of the forearm. Internal rotation of the distal fragment is usually evident on the roentgenogram (Fig. 10-47).

The distal end of the proximal fragment projects anteriorly, and often pierces the periosteum as it is stripped from both the anterior surface of the lower fragment and the posterior surface of the upper fragment (Fig. 10-48). In severe displacement, the proximal fragment may penetrate the skin and create an open injury. The displacement of fracture fragments is somewhat limited by the extent of periosteal stripping, since this structure is rarely disrupted completely.[136]

There is considerable extravasation of blood from the open marrow cavity and disrupted periosteum, causing associated swelling and accumulation of fluid in the elbow region. Since this compartment is fairly tight, it is essential to closely observe the extent of swelling and decide whether surgical release is indicated. The nerves and blood vessels

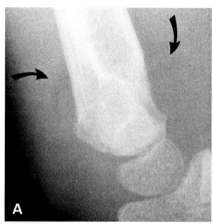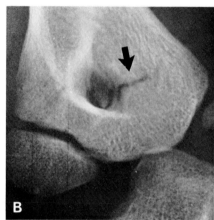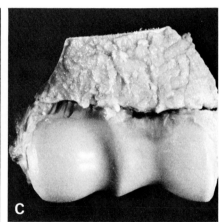

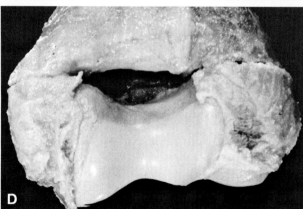

FIG. 10-44. Greenstick supracondylar fracture. *A,* Elevation of anterior and posterior fat pads (solid arrows) associated with minimal cortical disruption. *B,* Anterior view of greenstick injury. Note how the fracture goes into the supracondylar foramen (arrow). *C-D,* Anterior and posterior views of specimen to show how fracture involves both anterior and posterior fat pads.

may be contused, depressed, or lacerated by the osseous fragments or by the dissecting hematoma that infiltrates the antecubital region.

Flexion Type. The fracture line in the sagittal plane generally courses upward and forward, with the proximal fragment being displaced posteriorly and the distal fragment anteriorly and upward. Again, degrees of varus, valgus, tilting, and rotation may vary. The periosteum is stripped from the posterior surface of the distal fragment and from the anterior surface of the proximal fragment. Soft tissue swelling and damage are usually less extensive than they are in the extension type; and neurovascular complications are rare.

Displacement. In general, three main types of displacement may occur in a supracondylar fracture. The first is loss of the normal anterior tilt of the distal end of the humerus. This is usually a greenstick fracture and probably requires no reduction. In the second type, the distal fragment is displaced and tilted posteriorly. In addition, there may be some medial or lateral shift. In the third type, the distal fragment is completely displaced in a posterior direction with medial or lateral shift and usually some medial or lateral angulation.

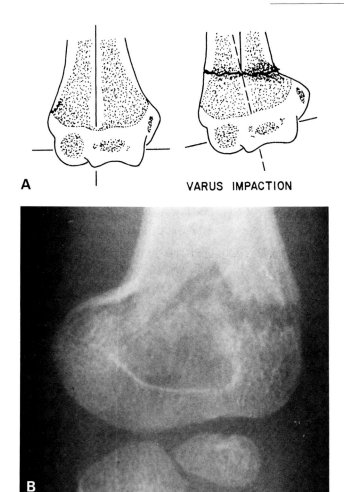

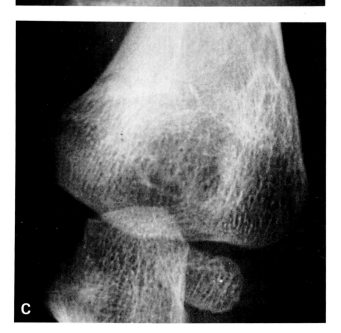

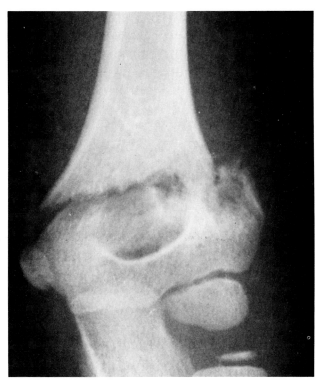

FIG. 10-46. Greenstick fracture with lateral compression leading to mild cubitus valgus.

FIG. 10-45. *A,* Schematic of greenstick fracture causing a medial trabecular/cortical compression leading to cubitus varus. This must be corrected with manipulation. *B,* Acute cubitus varus in a five-year-old. This was not corrected. *C,* Mild cubitus varus two years later.

The displacement may be such that the distal end of the shaft fragment projects through the skin or deep fascia. If it projects through the deep fascia, ecchymosis can be seen in the antecubital fossa, in addition to gross deformity and marked swelling. Early ecchymosis means that the deep fascia has been punctured and signifies that reduction of the fracture may be difficult owing to interposition of soft tissues.

Since the muscles around the elbow are ensheathed in dense fascia and reinforced by the lacertus fibrosis, these vessels are held down tightly as they traverse the antecubital fossa. If there is marked posterior displacement of the distal fragment, the neurovascular bundle is usually stretched over the distal end of the shaft fragment. This may occlude the venous and arterial blood supply by causing attenuation, direct compression, or irritation of the adventitia and sympathetic nerve fibers, and causing spasm at the level of or distal to the injury and even in the collateral circulatory branches (Fig. 10-49).

Graham studied adult cadavers to better comprehend the problems encountered in supracondylar fracture and found that: (1) soft tissue stability was provided on the lateral side of the fracture by expansion of the triceps, the brachioradialis, and the extensor carpi radialis longus. Soft tissue stability was *not* provided on the medial side. The expansion of the triceps provided some posterior soft tissue stability, but the muscle mass spanning the fracture site anteriorly was insufficient to provide soft tissue stability. Except for a few clinically insignificant fibers arising from the medial supracondylar ridge, the pronator teres arises only from the medial epicondyle and therefore is part of the forearm. However,

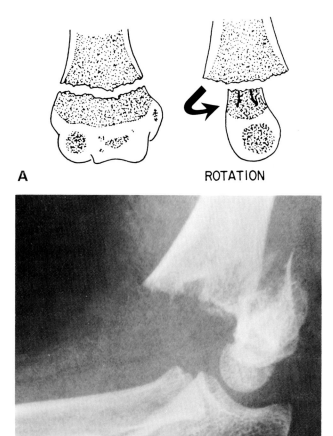

A   ROTATION

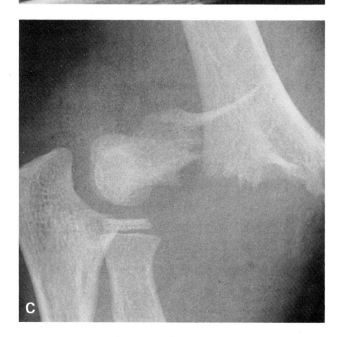

FIG. 10-47. *A,* Schematic of rotation. *B,* Roentgenograms of acute injury showing anteroposterior view of proximal fragment and lateral view of distal fragment and forearm with mild displacement. *C,* Significant rotation and posterolateral displacement of the distal fragment.

this muscle did not reliably influence rotation of the distal fragment.[137,138] Recent experimental work in primates suggests that muscular soft tissue and periosteal hinging have few effects on fracture stability.

When the fracture is forcibly rotated, the sharp corner of the proximal fragment may tear the periosteum, permitting gross displacement. The rent in the periosteum is "L" shaped and leaves $\frac{2}{3}$ of the periosteum around the fracture intact to form a useful hinge that may aid reduction. The periosteum may be stripped from the shaft for several inches depending upon the degree of displacement at the time of injury.

Rang's suggestion that the elbow has a fishtail shape and is extremely narrow at this point simply refers to that portion within the olecranon fossa (Fig. 10-50).[139] Actually, there are medial and lateral columns on either side of the supracondylar fossa (foramen). Instability accrues primarily from the obliquity of the fracture line.

Diagnosis. Supracondylar fractures usually are diagnosed by history, clinical findings, and roentgenographic studies. Swelling may be minimal if the injury is seen shortly after occurrence, or when displacement has been minimal. The more the displacement, the more swelling and deformity are likely to be evident. The forearm is usually held in pronation during examination. Note the degree of pronation or supination, as this may help in determining varus/valgus instability.

More important than examination of the fracture site is careful assessment of the neurovascular function in the injured limb. Any neurovascular deficit must be assessed completely and followed carefully. Failure to detect vascular injuries may be disastrous and lead to permanent deformity and disability of the forearm musculature.[140] Signs of vascular injury include pain, pallor, cyanosis, absence of pulse, coldness, or paralysis, any of which indicate the possibility of impending Volkmann's ischemia. Radial and ulnar nerve injuries are recognized relatively easily. Median nerve involvement is generally incomplete and often overlooked. It may result in loss of flexion of the distal interphalangeal joint of the index finger, loss of flexion of the interphalangeal joint of the thumb, or numbness of the tip of the index finger.

The arm also should be examined for possible concomitant fractures of the proximal or distal radius or proximal humerus.

Roentgenology. Roentgenographic examination confirms the diagnosis. The limb must be splinted adequately and comfortably before the patient is sent to the radiographic department. The limb should be immobilized in a simple splint in the deformed position it was in when the patient entered the emergency room. The elbow should be in some extension, although excessive flexion of the elbow should be avoided to minimize possible neurovascular compromise.

Instructions to the technician must indicate that true anteroposterior and lateral projections of the distal humerus and elbow joint be taken *without* specifically rotating the arm. If instructions are not given to move the entire upper extremity as a unit, the technician may simply rotate the arm at the fracture site and give two views of the distal fragment rotated 90°, while the proximal fragment remains the same. An anteroposterior view of the elbow will reveal whether the fracture line is transverse or oblique, and

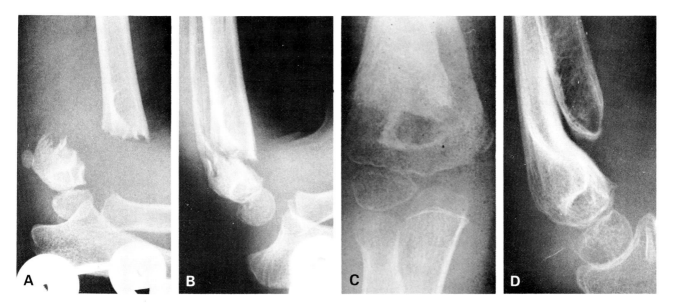

FIG. 10-48. *A,* Posterior displacement and overriding when first placed in traction. *B,* The distal fragment then settles into anatomic position. *C-D,* Further growth gradually corrects the deformity. Note the extensive posterior callus and complete lack of anterior callus.

whether the distal fragment is medially or laterally angulated. A lateral view of the elbow will show whether the distal fragment is displaced posteriorly or anteriorly, and the extent to which normal angulation is lost.

Radiographs should be taken before any cast is applied, because cubitus varus may occur even in this seemingly innocuous group of fractures if initial displacement is underestimated and treatment is perfunctory.

Treatment.   The direction of the fracture line is a major factor in success of treatment. Generally, fracture fragments separated by a long, oblique line are more difficult to reduce and more likely to slip after reduction than those separated by a relatively transverse fracture line.

Treatment of undisplaced or minimally displaced extension-type fractures consists of immobilizing the arm with the elbow flexed to 90° and the forearm in neutral position or pronation. This is continued for three to four weeks. However, follow-up roentgenograms should be taken after one week to be certain that the fracture has not displaced or angulated (especially varus).

Cubitus varus has been reported following minimally displaced fractures.[141] *One must always be cautious that a minimally displaced fracture is not of more magnitude than seemingly evident.* A feeling that no reduction is necessary may be inappropriate (see Fig. 10-45). If there has been compression on the medial side or widening laterally with an incompletely broken medial cortex, the fracture should be manipulated,

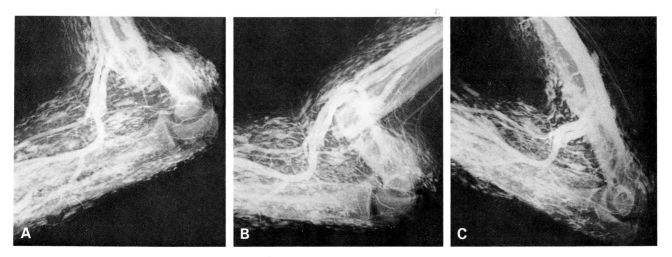

FIG. 10-49.   Injection of cadaver arm from adolescent showing kinking of vessels. *A,* Vascular relationships at 90° flexion. *B,* In extension, the artery may be traumatized by the proximal fragment or kinked by soft tissue attachments. *C,* In hyperflexion, the vessels may be compressed in the edematous antecubital region.

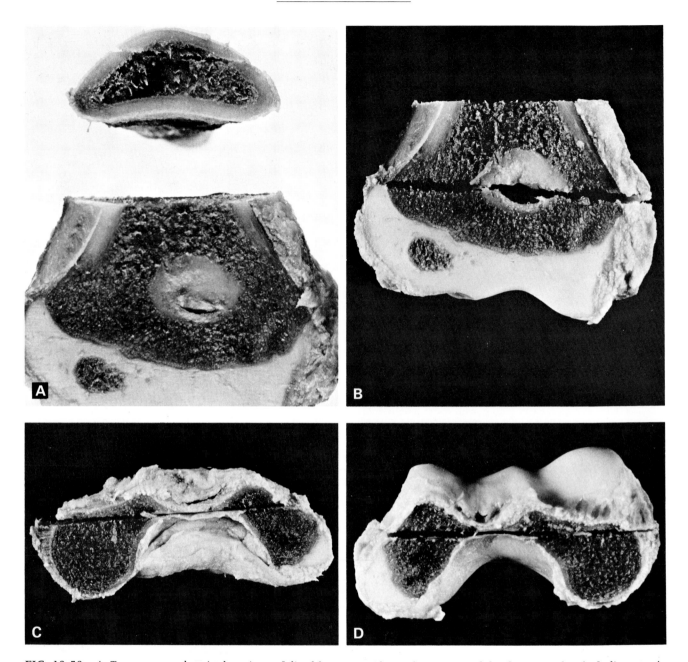

FIG. 10-50. *A,* Transverse and sagittal sections of distal humerus. Above the supracondylar foramen, the shaft diameter is wide. *B,* However, if a cut is made through the supracondylar foramen, the "bicolumnar" nature of this region becomes evident, as seen in *C,* looking proximally, and *D,* looking distally.

and medial or lateral tilting of the distal fragment corrected. The carrying angle of the elbow should always be matched to the normal side.

Compression forces from normal muscle tone and elasticity of soft tissues surrounding the fracture fragments may also tilt the distal fragment, even during immobilization. Even in the presence of mild medial or lateral displacement, these factors may further a deformity that is already present or has been unrecognized.

The moderately displaced extension type supracondylar fracture with some residual bone continuity should be treated by closed reduction under general anesthetic, pro-

vided there is minimal swelling and no neurovascular compromise. The techniques should be as follows (Figs. 10-51 and 10-52). Length should be restored first by traction and counter-traction with the elbow in extension, not hyperextension, to prevent excessive traction on the brachial vessels. Next, while maintaining traction, with the forearm pronated and the elbow in slight flexion, the posterior displacement of the distal fragment should be reduced. This is done by lifting it anteriorly and pushing the proximal fragment posteriorly. Then, lateral displacement should be reduced by pushing the distal fragment medially. Any rotational deformity should be corrected at this time. The elbow is then flexed to 90° to

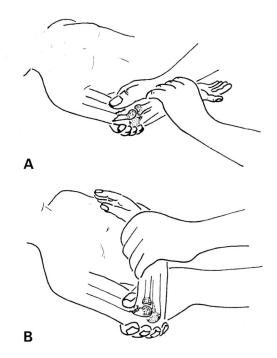

FIG. 10-51. Schematic of reduction utilizing flexion methods.

tighten the posterior hinge of the periosteum and maintain the reduction. In supracondylar fractures, the biceps loses its supinating action. Because of the broken continuity of the humerus, the unopposed action of the strong pronator teres muscle may swing the proximal radioulnar joint into pronation. Since the joint is fixed by the pronators, varus deformity of the fracture site may gradually result from unopposed muscular force, even in plaster.[142,143]

The direction of original displacement of the distal fragment is also considered when deciding the position in which the forearm is to be immobilized in the cast. If the distal fragment is displaced medially, the forearm should be pronated in order to tighten the medial hinge and close the fracture line on the lateral side, thus decreasing the tendency to cubitus varus deformity. If the distal fragment is displaced laterally, supination of the forearm will tighten the lateral periostal hinge and close the fracture line on the medial side, thus preventing cubitus valgus. In the posteriorly displaced fracture a posterior hinge of the periosteum is obvious. The use of the remaining, intact periosteal hinges to aid in and maintain reduction is the key to successful reduction.

The effect on the carrying angle caused by various types of displacement of the distal fragment was studied by Smith.[102] He simulated transverse supracondylar fractures in an articulated, adult upper extemity by osteotomy. Medial and lateral displacement of the distal fragment *without* concomitant angular deformity did not change the carrying angle. Internal rotation of the distal fragment also had no effect on the degree of the carrying angle.

The osseous relations of the medial and lateral epicondyles and the olecranon process can be assessed through the Lyman Smith triangle. With the elbow flexed to a right angle, the three osseous points make a fairly symmetric

equilateral triangle and tend to lie in a plane parallel to the plane of the posterior surface of the upper arm. In some children, the capitellum becomes quite prominent in 90° of flexion and disturbs the symmetry of the lateral segment of the triangle. When the elbow is in complete extension, the three osseous points are almost in a straight line.

Circulation must be assessed frequently, certainly several times within the first 48 hours after injury. The family should be instructed of the signs of circulatory compromise so that they can watch the child carefully at home. If there is a mildly displaced fracture, but a moderate amount of swelling with any suggestion of vascular compromise, the child should be hospitalized for observation and elevation of the extremity.

This displaced type of fracture should be reduced under general anesthetic because of the difficulty of reduction and the importance of obtaining reduction on the first attempt. Repetitive manipulations must be avoided because of the possibility of injury to vessels and nerves. Once the fracture has been reduced satisfactorily, the peripheral circulation must be assessed again. If it is normal, a long arm cast may be applied. The cast should not constrict the soft tissues of the antecubital area. A window should be cut in the region of the radial artery so the circulation can be checked.

About 120° of flexion may be necessary to ensure stability. The radial pulse may disappear for a few minutes after initial reduction. If the fingers remain pink, this may be satisfactory. But if the fingers become white, reduce the degree of flexion. If flexion to a right angle is not possible without circulatory impairment, check to see if the posterior displacement is corrected. If the moderately displaced fracture is anatomically corrected, but the vascular status remains questionable, three options are open: (1) fixing with percutaneous K-wires, (2) casting in this position, then increasing the flexion when the swelling is less, usually in three to seven days, or (3) placement in traction.

Roentgenograms in the anteroposterior and lateral projections determine the adequacy of reduction (Fig. 10-53). Any lateral or medial tilting must be corrected *completely*. Appositional alignments are less significant, as they usually correct spontaneously through extensive remodeling and have little or no effect on the carrying angle or the final range of motion of the elbow. Posterior angulation and flexion deformities are in the plane of motion of the elbow and usually correct themselves. However, rotation of the distal fragment is not corrected by remodeling, and may look unusual on the roentgenograms. While this rotation is well

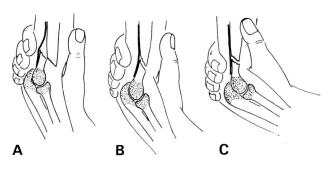

FIG. 10-52. Schematic of reduction utilizing extension methods.

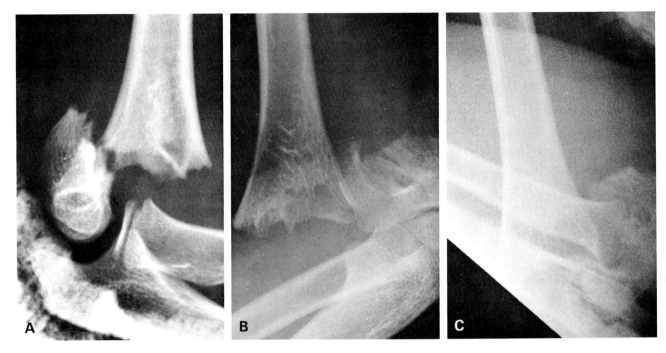

FIG. 10-53. *A,* Relative reduction with minimal overriding. This, however, has been incompletely corrected for rotation. *B,* Posterolateral fracture. *C,* Alleged reduction failed to correct the lateral displacement.

compensated clinically by the degree of rotation at the shoulder, this should not be an excuse for failing to observe and correct rotational malalignment as much as possible.

In the presence of marked swelling, closed reduction is carried out just as outlined, but the patient should be placed in Dunlop's skin or skeletal traction for several days until swelling subsides. If it is impossible to maintain adequate skin traction, it may be necessary to apply skeletal traction with a pin inserted through the proximal ulna. However, in general, skeletal traction should be reserved for a severely displaced fracture or one that cannot be reduced satisfactorily or proves unstable.

After swelling subsides, the arm may be removed from traction and immobilized. The overall degree of stability must be checked before and after application of the cast. Roentgenograms should be made at short intervals following the injury to check maintenance of reduction. These are best obtained 5 to 10 days following the injury and 3 to 4 weeks later. These roentgenograms are important, because muscular forces may reintroduce deformity in the first 10 to 14 days after injury, particularly if a crushing injury has occurred to the medial or lateral side with loss of cortical integrity.

Flexion Injury. The flexion type of injury usually is relatively simple to treat. Closed reduction is carried out by traction and flexion, followed by correction of the lateral tilting and displacement by manual pressure. The elbow then is immobilized in "extension," although 20° to 30° of flexion may be more comfortable for the patient.

Severe Displacement. A completely displaced supracondylar fracture is treated best by closed manipulative reduction, followed by either skeletal traction or some type of internal fixation (e.g., percutaneous pins), since these are unstable injuries.

The traction technique is as follows. Under general anesthesia the child's arm should be suspended by an assistant while the surgeon inserts a Kirschner wire through the proximal ulna about 2 to 3 cm distal to the tip of the olecranon process, and *beyond the physis.* Osseous landmarks about the elbow are carefully identified, and the wire is drilled from the medial to the lateral side to avoid tethering of the ulnar nerve. Since considerable swelling often is present, great care must be taken to insert the pin into metaphyseal bone (Fig. 10-54). The assistant should not flex the elbow acutely in an attempt to increase the prominence of the olecranon. A threaded Kirschner wire has less chance of becoming loose and causing skin tract infection, but it is more uncomfortable during removal.[129,144] As an alternative, there are screws available for placement directly into the olecranon.[141] The traction bow is then put in place.

Once the pin is in place, the surgeon must decide upon the most efficacious method of traction. Traction may be directed to the side (Fig. 10-55) or overhead (Fig. 10-56).[123,145,146] Each method has advocates. If used properly and diligently, neither method is inferior to the other. In setting up the traction, medial and lateral tilting of the distal fragment must be assessed and carefully corrected. Roentgenograms are made to determine the accuracy of reduction.

Lateral traction may be applied with the shoulder abducted 60° and the arm elevated 20° from the horizontal, a position that introduces maximum venous drainage of the upper limb and limits patient movement. The disadvantage of overhead traction is that it does not always provide optimum control of the proximal fragment as the patient moves about in bed. However, if the child is placed in overhead traction with his head against the headboard, he can only

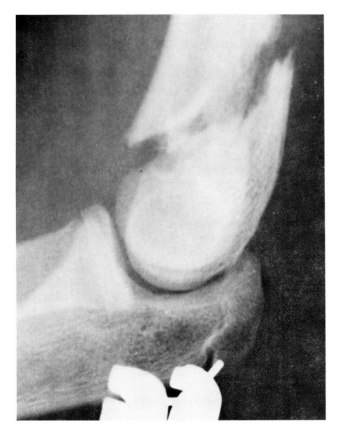

FIG. 10-54. The pin must be placed through the olecranon in a position that avoids the proximal physis. However, the pin must be placed in the bone. In this case, superficial placement in the subperiosteal space is evident. Because of swelling, easy palpation of landmarks is not always possible.

move downward and externally rotate, thereby minimizing rotational abnormality. It is possible for the child to force the elbow into acute flexion and cause circulatory embarrassment.[147] A 3 to 5 lb weight should be applied to the lateral traction bow and the forearm suspended. In fractures in which the proximal fragment is anteriorly displaced, a sling with a 1 lb weight is applied to the upper arm, pulling it posteriorly to try to reduce this angular displacement.[148]

The maintenance of reduction is determined by serial roentgenograms. The fracture should be removed from traction when it proves stable enough to be casted.

Rotation and varus or valgus deformities do not straighten spontaneously and may require remanipulation as late as three or four weeks after injury. If a deformity exists after this time, corrective osteotomy may be considered, but should be postponed until maximum improvement of function has been obtained. The functional result may be such that late osteotomy will be unnecessary.

Closed reduction may be performed, and percutaneous K-wires introduced, to prevent redisplacement, particularly when the elbow cannot be flexed beyond a right angle.[149,150] After the fracture has been reduced by closed methods, one K-wire is inserted through the medial epicondyle and another through the lateral epicondyle (Figs. 10-57 and 10-58). This is best done using the image intensifier. Transfixing

the ulna and condylar fragment by traversing the elbow joint is unnecessary (see Fig. 10-65) and may lead to stiffness.

Open reduction is indicated if the fracture is unstable or if there is significant neurovascular compromise. In the latter case, it may be necessary to either explore the artery or increase the amount of space through which the vessels traverse at the level of the lacertus fibrosus.[51,134,153,156-161] Open reduction with internal fixation has been condemned because it frequently causes elbow stiffness. However, a careful open reduction with minimal soft tissue dissection should not create more problems than multiple attempts at closed reduction. For older adolescents with T-shaped fractures, open reduction certainly may be indicated.

Hart described the operative management of difficult supracondylar fractures.[162] Conservative treatment was used for 138 of these, including 29 type 4 injuries (complete displacement). Operative treatment was used in only 15 cases, of which 13 were type 4. Indications for surgery were: (1) failure to secure an adequate primary reduction (4 cases); (2) primary reduction successful but not maintained

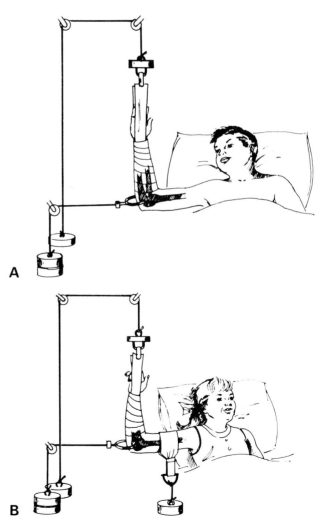

FIG. 10-55. A, Side-directed (Dunlop's) traction. Control of pronation and supination is not easy. B, Additional traction may be applied to the proximal fragment.

(8 cases); (3) circulatory insufficiency (1 case); and (4) neurologic findings or symptoms (2 cases).

A posterior approach may be used for open reduction.[163,164] The triceps aponeurosis is incised as an inverted "V" and turned distally. The ulnar nerve is isolated and protected. Kirschner wires then may be introduced retrograde through the fracture site into the medial and lateral epicondyles, emerging through the skin, but avoiding the ulnar nerve. Under direct vision, the fracture is reduced and the Kirschner wires passed into the proximal fragment. Rotational correction is checked before passing the second Kirschner wire. The assurance of a reduction would seem to make this method preferable to percutaneous pinning.

Results. The child should be allowed to set his own pace of rehabilitation, and determine his own physical limitations, if any. In virtually every instance, there will be no residual contractures. Weights and physical therapy should never be used to stretch the elbow into full extension.

Most minimally to moderately displaced fractures heal with no significant problems, and function is fully returned within three months. If displacement is severe, the recovery time is longer, but return of function is usually complete.

However, complete return of flexion may take from several months to several years because of prominence of the anteriorly directed metaphysis. Remodeling generally corrects this problem.[164a]

Complications. *Varus-Valgus.* The carrying angle is defined as the lateral angle that the longitudinal axis of the fully supinated forearm makes with the longitudinal axis of the upper arm when the elbow is completely extended, but not hyperextended. If the forearm is pronated or if the elbow is flexed, this carrying angle cannot be evaluated adequately.[165] However, if the flexed elbow is examined posteriorly and compared with the opposite normal elbow, changes in the carrying angle become apparent.

It is important to remember that the carrying angle is subject to considerable normal individual variation. Lyman Smith studied the angle in 150 normal children and found it averaged 6.1° in girls with a range of 0° to 12°, and 5.4° in boys with a range of 0° to 11°.[166] Some children (9%) have no carrying angle (cubitus rectus), and 48% have a carrying angle of 5° or less.

The complication of reversed carrying angle (gunstock deformity, cubitus varus) has two causes: (1) incomplete

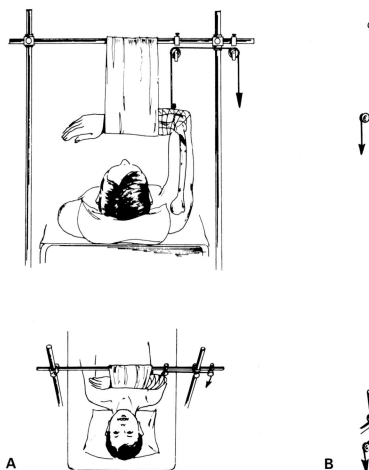

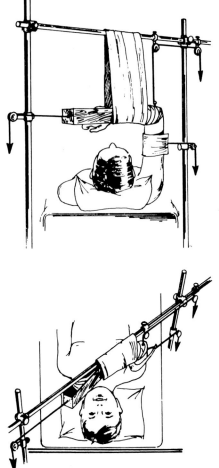

FIG. 10-56. *A,* Schematic of placement of patient in bed relative to overhead traction. *B,* Angulation of the traction may control rotation.

correction of deformity of the distal fragment at the time of original reduction (Fig. 10-59), or (2) growth disturbance of the trochlear physis. This reversed carrying angle rarely causes significant loss of elbow joint function, but may create an unappealing cosmetic deformity.[124,167-170]

The varus angulation may be mild, moderate, or severe (Fig. 10-60). Depending upon the age at time of injury, it may lead to deformation of the forearm as a secondary response.

If treated properly, varus should be minimum as an immediate complication.[171] However, this type of injury is a trap, particularly if there is minimal displacement (see Fig. 10-45). Immediate malunion or angular deformity after treatment is *always* due to malunion and *not* to a growth disturbance.

If the varus or valgus deformity of the elbow is severe and stable (i.e., not related to growth injury, but to static deformity from the original injury), correction may be indicated by supracondylar osteotomy of the humerus.[171a,172-174] The operative technique of the osteotomy is illustrated in Figures 10-61 and 10-62. If there has been injury to the nerve or perhaps involvement with the fracture callus, this can be corrected at the same time.

Corrective supracondylar osteotomy is not an easy operation. It is best to use a closing wedge osteotomy. However, care should be taken in placement of the wires, as false aneurysm formation, nerve injury, and bone infection have been reported.[40] Tachdjian advocates external pin fixation using the Roger Anderson device.[40] Langenskiöld has described the four-hole plate, and others have advocated a wire loop around two screws.[40]

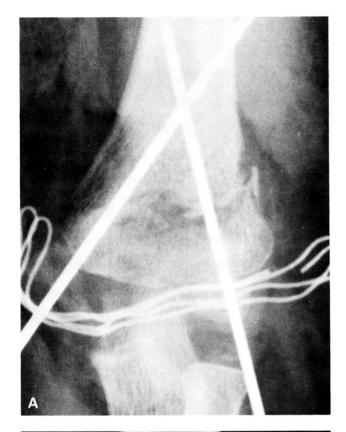

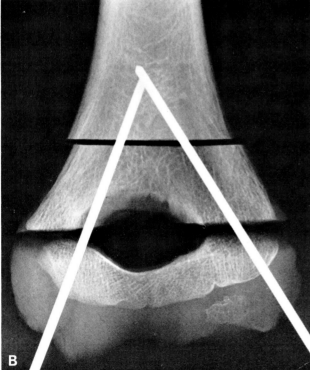

FIG. 10-57. Techniques of pin fixation. *A,* Open reduction allows anatomic restoration and accurate pin placement. *B,* Specimen showing proper pin placement: one in each osseous column medial and lateral to the supracondylar foramen.

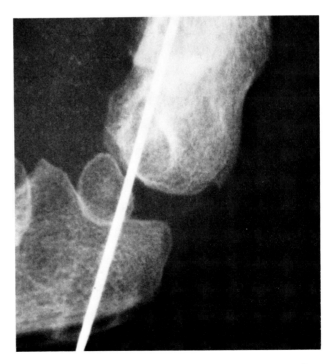

FIG. 10-58. Fracture fixed by a pin going through the olecranon, the joint, and the distal and proximal fragments. Note the reactive bone around the olecranon. This method is not recommended.

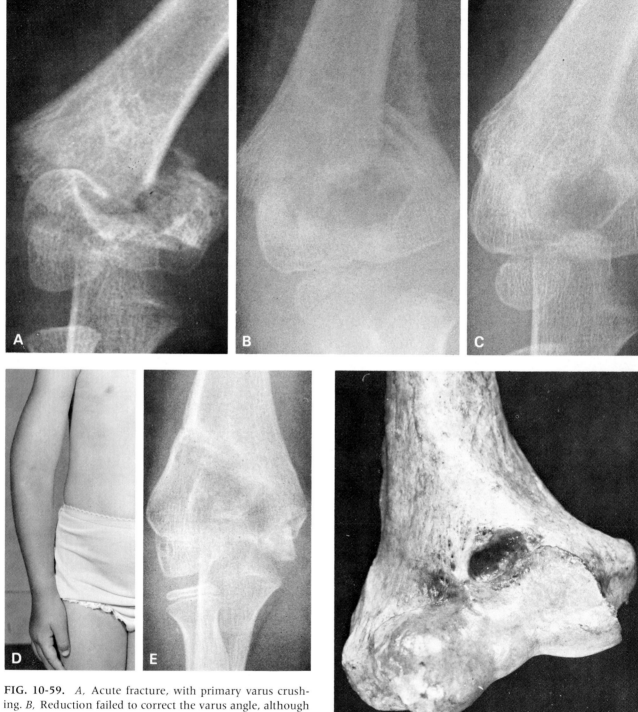

FIG. 10-59. *A,* Acute fracture, with primary varus crushing. *B,* Reduction failed to correct the varus angle, although the position appeared good from the lateral view. *C,* One year later, the varus has not corrected at all. *D,* Clinical appearance of the cubitus varus. *E,* Appearance after corrective osteotomy.

FIG. 10-60. Moderate varus deformity of distal humerus.

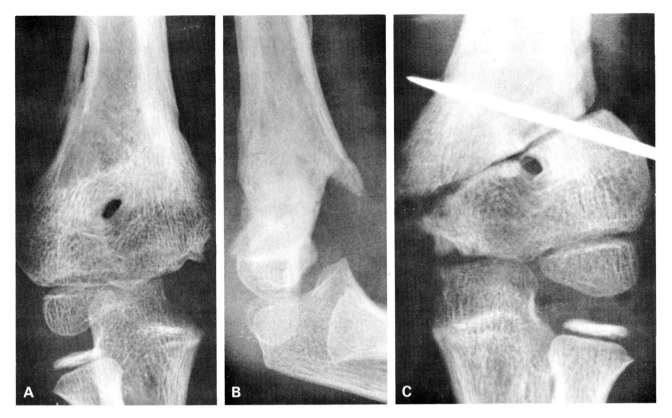

FIG. 10-61. *A-B,* Varus and hyperextension following supracondylar fracture. *C,* Closing wedge osteotomy with pin fixation.

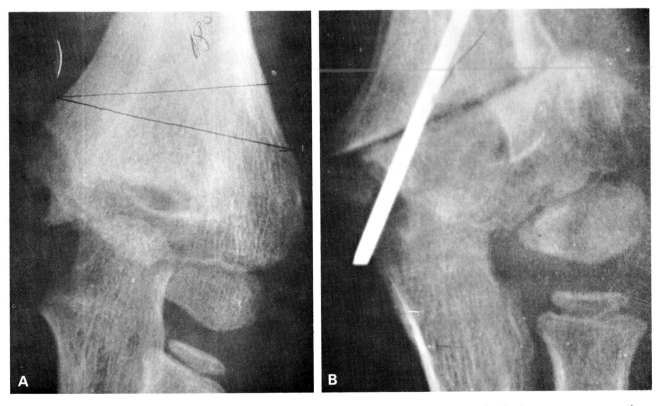

FIG. 10-62. *A,* The corrective osteotomy is properly outlined preoperatively. *B,* However, the final osteotomy was too close to the medial epicondyle, and the fixation pin should be in bone, not epiphysis.

Volkmann's Ischemia. As recognition of Volkmann's ischemia as a major complication of supracondylar humeral fractures has increased, its incidence has decreased.[50,99,175-177] The five classic warning signs of Volkmann's ischemia are pain, pallor (cyanosis), pulselessness, paresthesia, and paralysis. *The most important is pain.* Ischemia should always be suspected when increasing pain develops in the forearm following injury to the elbow and forearm. A characteristic physical finding is exaggeration of the pain upon passive extension of the fingers, followed by very taut, progressive swelling, and firmness of the lower compartment of the forearm. The radial pulse may be absent or present. The presence of a normal radial pulse does *not* absolutely rule out Volkmann's ischemia. There may be a varying degree of sensory loss, with the median nerve almost always involved and the ulnar nerve involved in many cases.

The pathophysiology is as follows. The ischemia initially produces anoxia in the muscles. The increasing intramuscular edema causes progressive increase in the intrinsic pressure within the muscles. Circular, unyielding dressings of the limb and limited expansion of the taut fascia around the muscles of the forearm increase the venous compression and intramuscular compression, further increasing the intrinsic pressure. Pressor receptors within the forearm compartment and within the muscle itself stimulate reflex vasospasm which subsequently affects all the vessels in the general area. This vasospasm further aggravates and worsens the initial vascular compromise, setting up a destructive ischemia/edema cycle.

If the process persists, the next stage is necrosis of muscle, with eventual secondary fibrosis and possible development of heterotopic calcification. The infarct is an ellipsoid shape along the axis of the distribution of the anterior interosseous artery. The flexor digitorum profundus and pollicis brevis muscles and the median nerve are the most commonly and severely affected. If, during the acute stage, the palmar compartment of the forearm is surgically exposed, the deep fascia will be taut, and spread widely when split. The muscles may be pale or blue-black from extravasation of blood resulting from the altered hemodynamics. The veins are always distended.

This circulatory embarrassment may occur if the brachial artery is caught and kinked at the fracture site (see Fig. 10-49); because the artery is contused and in spasm at the moment of fracture; because a tight encircling cast is compressing the brachial vessels; because there is rapidly progressive swelling in the taut fascial compartment; or because of subintimal hematoma.[131,178-180] Distal to the lacertus fibrosus, the brachial artery branches into the radial and ulnar arteries. The radial artery is superficially located, whereas the ulnar artery is situated more deeply, traversing deep to the pronator teres. The ulnar artery gives origin to the common interosseous artery, which divides into anterior and posterior interosseous branches. The flexor digitorum profundus and flexor pollicis longus receive their blood supply from the anterior interosseous artery. The median nerve is particularly vulnerable to damage because of its course deep to the lacertus fibrosus and through the substance of the pronator teres muscle.

The destructive processes of Volkmann's ischemia are progressive and generally reach a peak within 12 to 24 hours after the injury. At this time, decisions must be made whether to continue observation or consider surgical de-

compression. This can be assessed by placing a wick catheter in the muscles and evaluating at appropriate intervals to see if the pressure in the palmar (volar) compartment has increased. In 5 to 10 days the swelling and sensitivity will gradually subside, even if ischemia has been present, and the muscles of the flexor compartment will become hardened and elastic, with progressive fibrosis leading to contractural deformity with the elbow fixed, the forearm pronated, the wrist flexed, the metacarpal phalangeal joint hyperextended, and the interphalangeal joint flexed (Fig. 10-63).

In the acute ischemic stage, treatment must be immediate.[181] If the various signs and symptoms cannot be relieved within 6 to 12 hours by extension of the elbow, removal of tight encircling bandages, or reduction of the fracture, then arteriography should be considered. If the brachial artery is only in spasm, a stellate ganglion block may lead to relief. If this does not improve the situation, fasciotomy of the forearm and exploration of the brachial artery are indicated.

In this procedure, a longitudinal incision is made at the flexor crease of the elbow, medial to the biceps tendon. It is extended along the middle of the palmar surface of the forearm to the flexor crease of the wrist. Proximally, the incision may be extended to expose the brachial artery without crossing the flexor crease. The subcutaneous tissues are divided and the antebrachial fascia sectioned longitudinally throughout the entire length. The fascial sheath of each muscle (the epimysium or perimysium) is carefully divided from its lower to upper margin. However, muscle fibers should not be sectioned. Usually, circulation will return immediately, unless the muscles have already become gangrenous. If this still does not lead to improvement, the brachial artery should be explored. The fascia must be left open. Muscle edema may prevent approximation of the skin edges. In such an instance, the wound should be left open and closed several days later, after edema has subsided. Postoperatively, the wrist and hand must be splinted effectively to prevent deformation.

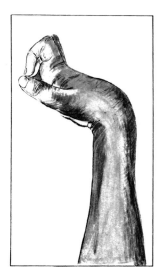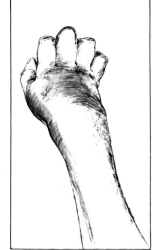

VOLKMANN'S ISCHEMIC CONTRACTURE

FIG. 10-63. Appearance of Volkmann's ischemic contracture.

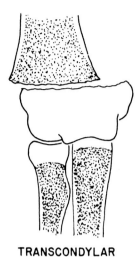

TRANSCONDYLAR

FIG. 10-64. Schematic of transcondylar fracture.

Treatment of established Volkmann's ischemia is contingent upon the severity of the deformity and the length of time since the original injury. Fasciotomy and epimysiotomy weeks or even months following the original injury have an uncertain efficacy. Within two to three months, the contracted flexor muscles in the forearm may be lengthened at their muscle junction, along with neurolysis of the median and ulnar nerves. In severe cases, it is possible to shorten both bones of the forearm to gain relative length of the contracted muscles.

Osseous Vascular Changes. Graham reported avascular necrosis of the trochlea in one child with hyperextension injury.[138]

Neurologic Complications. At any time, the radial, ulnar, or median nerve may be injured—at the time of fracture, during attempted reduction, or by compression from Volkmann's ischemia.[182-189] The radial nerve is the most commonly injured, because of its position relative to the fracture line and the musculospiral groove. Siris reported 11 nerve injuries in 330 supracondylar fractures (7 radial, 4 ulnar).[102] Serrill and Serrill-Dejerine found a nerve injury incidence of 7% (16 of 207) with 7 ulnar, 4 radial, 4 median, and 1 combined ulnar-median.[190]

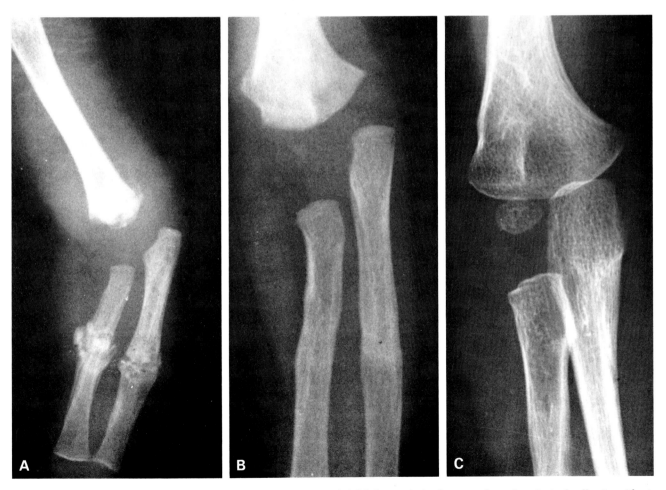

FIG. 10-65. Transcondylar fracture in infant. This was a case of child abuse. *A,* At three weeks, subperiosteal callus is evident at the transcondylar fracture, as well as the radius and ulna. *B,* Four months later, remodeling shows some medial displacement. *C,* Appearance of fracture one year later.

Elbow Dislocation. Failure to correct the normal anterior angulation of the entire distal epiphysis in hyperextension injuries, based on the assumption that this type of malunion will correct with time, may alter elbow mechanics. Recurrent posterior dislocation following supracondylar fracture has been reported infrequently.[191]

Distal Humerus

Entire epiphysis (transcondylar)

While transcondylar (physeal) injury is reportedly extremely rare, it may be much more common than is fully appreciated.[9,53,56,87,133,145,192-204] It is often misdiagnosed as a dislocated elbow because of difficulties in interpreting the roentgenogram, particularly in infants and young children. The entire distal epiphysis of the humerus is displaced posteriorly, laterally, or forward, depending on the mechanism of injury (Figs. 10-64 to 10-68). The violence may be direct or indirect. Separation of the entire distal humeral epiphysis is a relatively common injury in the battered-child syndrome.

These fractures may be difficult to diagnose as true transcondylar fractures. Their most important distinguishing feature is the normal relationship of the ossification center of the capitellum to the proximal radius. However, in the extremely small child this relationship may not be readily evident. A longitudinal line drawn through the shaft of the radius normally passes through the capitellum, but in dislocation of the elbow or radial head, it does not. This indicates some type of disruption of the radiohumeral joint. A type 2 physeal injury of the entire epiphysis must be differentiated from a fracture of the lateral condyle of the humerus, which is a type 3 or 4 physeal injury. In type 3 and 4 physeal injuries, the fracture fragment is often displaced by the pull of the common extensor muscles of the forearm, with subsequent loss of the normal relationship of the radial head. Epiphyseal separations usually occur medially, while elbow dislocations are usually lateral.

If the diagnosis cannot be made accurately, the child should be treated empirically. However, if there is any question, particularly regarding the possibility of deformity, then it is feasible to consider use of arthrography to help in the diagnosis of the injury.

Closed reduction is the initial treatment of choice. Reduction is performed by traction on the forearm, and most importantly, gentle correction of the medial displacement and varus tilt of the epiphyseal fragment. Since the cross sectional area at the physis (level of fracture) is greater than that in the supracondylar area, the tendency to tilt is less. Any malrotation should also be gently corrected. The elbow is flexed to 90° and the forearm pronated.

Since the distal epiphysis is usually displaced medially, the medial portion of the periosteal hinge remains intact, and by pronating the forearm, the intact periosteal sleeve may be used as a hinge in maintaining the reduction.

Corroborative roentgenograms must be taken to assure adequacy of reduction. A posterior splint is applied for three to four weeks. Admission to the hospital following reduction is essential to allow monitoring of the circulation.

When there is a delay between time of injury and medical care, there may be massive swelling about the elbow. This

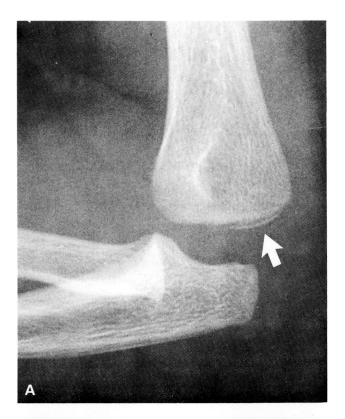

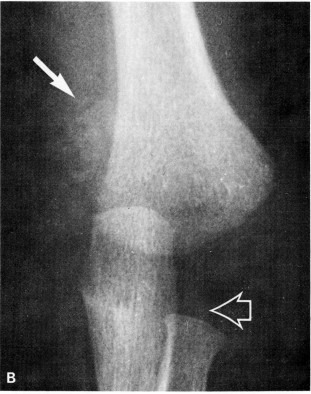

FIG. 10-66. Transcondylar fractures. *A,* Note the thin plate of metaphyseal bone. A further clue was a lateral view of the radius and ulna versus an AP of the humerus. *B,* Early ossification along medial side (solid arrow). Note the relatively medial shift of the radius and ulna (open arrow).

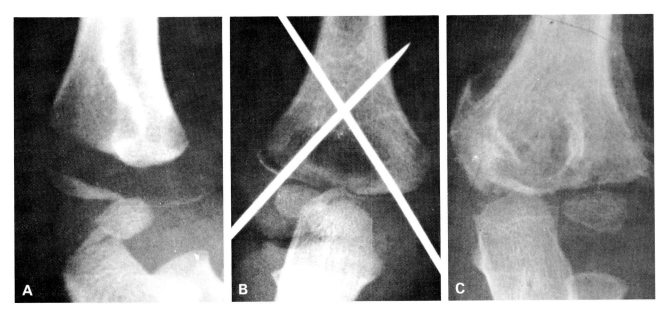

FIG. 10-67. *A,* Transcondylar fracture in two-year-old showing complete metaphyseal plate (arrow). *B,* This fracture was treated with open reduction and pin fixation (note air outlining capitellum). *C,* Appearance of fracture three months later.

may necessitate Dunlop traction following reduction to reduce the swelling.

Open reduction is rarely indicated. Holda used open reduction in four patients, but found that such an approach did not enhance the outcome.[196]

If the patient is not seen until several weeks have elapsed since the initial injury, no attempt at reduction should be made. Any residual deformity may be corrected by osteotomy.

Cubitus varus occurs less frequently in transcondylar fractures than in supracondylar fractures. Growth deformity due to premature epiphysiodesis has not been described. Neurovascular complications also appear infrequently.

In the case shown in Figure 10-69, apparently no reduc-

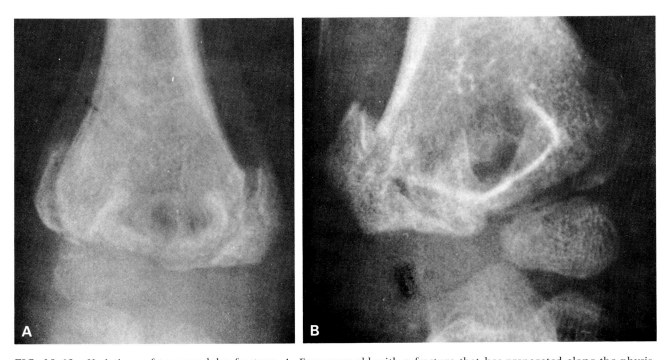

FIG. 10-68. Variations of transcondylar fracture. *A,* Four-year-old with a fracture that has propagated along the physis, curving proximally into metaphyseal bone at both epicondyles. *B,* Fracture leaving a thin plate of metaphyseal bone over the capitellum and subsequently propagating into the metaphysis above the trochlea. This is a type 2 injury.

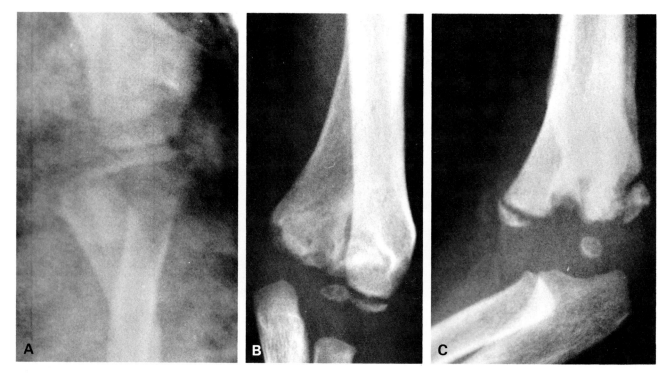

FIG. 10-69. Unusual transcondylar fracture in an infant (original films were unavailable). Note the massive subperiosteal new bone formation. Apparently, the fracture left the lateral epicondyle attached to the proximal fragment. *A,* Appearance early during the initial treatment. *B-C,* Large subperiosteal new bone segment medially, with irregular bone in region of presumptive lateral epicondyle.

tion was done. Several months later, anatomy is impossible to define accurately. The entire condylar unit apparently has shifted medially, forming a large area of new bone subperiosteally. Some of the lateral epicondyle was probably left behind, and has subsequently ossified.

Medial condyle

These injuries have been reported very infrequently.[122,141, 205-211] Potter described 2 cases in children aged 8 and 12; both were treated by open reduction.[210] This injury may sometimes be confused with displacement of the medial epicondyle, particularly if it occurs at a time when there is minimal ossification in the trochlea. Cauthey reported a case of displacement of the lower medial epiphysis of the humerus before development of the ossific nucleus in a 4-year-old girl.[208] Six months after the injury, the elbow was explored and it was found that not the medial epicondyle, but rather the entire medial condyle, was displaced. This was fixed with pins, but long term follow-up is not available.

These fractures are comparable to the lateral condyle fracture, with a type 4 being the most common pattern (Figs. 10-70 and 10-71). However, type 3 injuries also may occur. Epiphyseal propagation of the fracture probably remains within the trochlea. In some cases, particularly during adolescence, both the medial and the lateral condyles may be involved in a variation of an adult "T" fracture (Fig. 10-72).

These are unstable fractures involving physeal and articular disruption and should be treated with open reduction

and accurate restoration of the joint congruency. A posterior approach through or around the triceps, as discussed earlier in this chapter, is the most effective approach.

Significant complications have not been reported. However, extensive dissection of the fragment should be avoided, because this might predispose it to avascular necrosis of the trochlea. A neglected medial condyle fracture may go on to nonunion. Growth injury also may occur, leading to cubitus varus deformation.

Medial epicondyle

Fractures of the medial epicondyle usually occur between 7 and 15 years of age, constituting about 10% of all fractures of the elbow region in children.[121,212-215] This injury is unusual in younger children. The mechanism is usually a valgus strain of the joint, which produces traction on the medial epicondyle through the flexor muscles (Fig. 10-73). The epicondyle may be variably displaced, or even dislocated into the elbow joint due to the opening up of the joint by a marked valgus stress.[216,217] There may be displacement in association with posterolateral dislocation of the elbow; about half of the cases are associated with partial or complete dislocation of the elbow (see Chap. 11).

Classification. Several patterns of epicondylar fracture are possible (Figs. 10-74 to 10-77). Most common are pure type 1 or type 2. In reality, epicondylar fractures represent type 3 or type 4 injuries, because part of the fracture propagates through the epiphyseal cartilage between the epicondyle

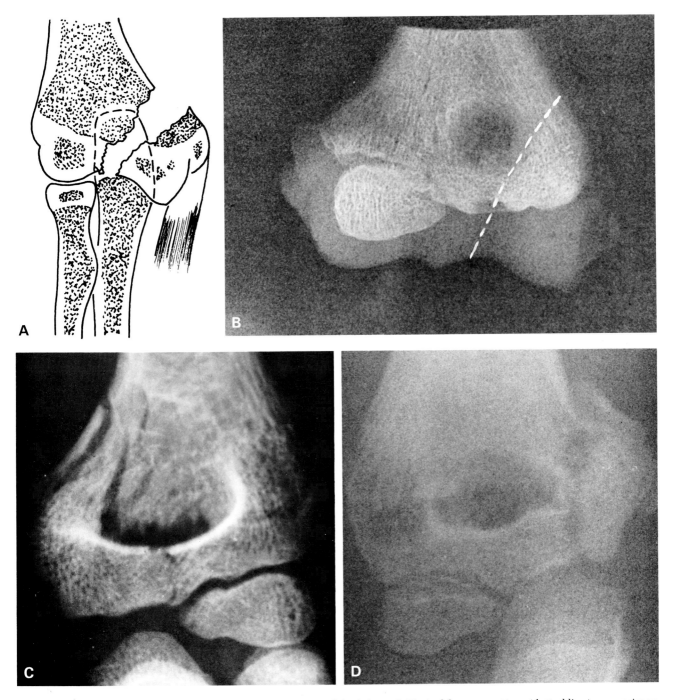

FIG. 10-70. Type 4 injury of medial condyle. *A,* Schematic of the injury. *B,* Typical fracture pattern (dotted line) on specimen roentgenogram. *C,* Greenstick medial condylar injury. *D,* Moderate displacement and rotation, comparable to lateral condylar injury. This osseous fragment is the metaphysis; trochlear ossification is not present.

and condyle and disrupts the normally continuous distal humeral growth plate.

Diagnosis. Physical findings depend upon the degree of displacement. The elbow usually is partially flexed for comfort. Motion is painful, particularly to a valgus stress or pronation of the forearm. The medial joint line is tender. There are some diagnostic problems. The unossified region in a

child less than five years of age is not easily diagnosed radiographically. Separation of the medial condyle may masquerade as an epicondylar separation.

The clinical signs of medial hematoma and pain may be more obvious than any radiographically evident separation of the epicondyle. The degree of displacement must be assessed as accurately as possible, and the presence of concomitant injury noted. Fracture of the radial neck may occur as a

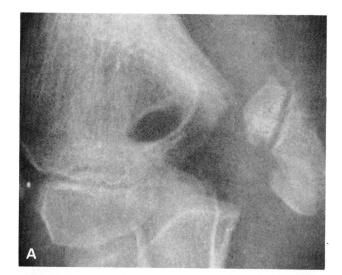

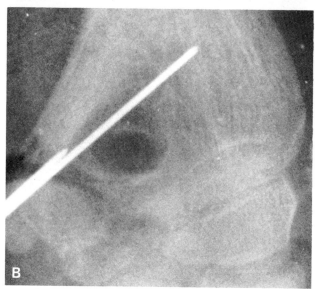

FIG. 10-71. *A,* AP view of type 4 injury with 90° of rotation of fragment. *B,* Appearance of this fracture following open reduction.

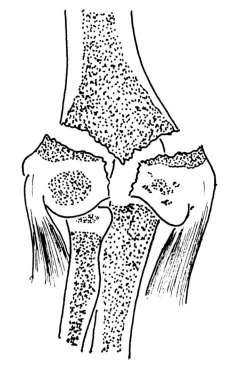

FIG. 10-72. Schematic of fractures involving both condyles, the analogue of an adult "T" fracture.

MEDIAL EPICONDYLE

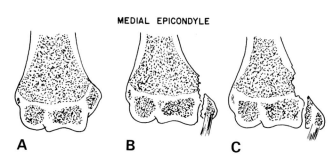

A   B   C

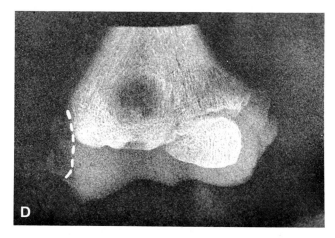

FIG. 10-73. Schematic of medial epicondylar injury. *A,* Normal. *B,* Type 3. *C,* Type 4. Flexor muscle mass tends to displace the fragment. *D,* Typical pattern of fracture (dotted line) depicted on specimen.

result of the injury mechanism (see Chap. 12). The ulnar nerve frequently is traumatized by the force and direction of displacement.

Roentgenograms may disclose the absence of the medial epicondyle from its normal position, or a widening of its physis compared to the physis of the opposite side. The displaced fragment may be seen in the lateral and posterior-oblique projections. If the diagnosis is in doubt, roentgenograms of the opposite elbow should be made in the same degree of rotation (remember, some asymmetry may be normal). When the medial epicondyle is displaced into the joint space, the articular cartilage space may be widened on the medial aspect. However, in a young child with a large mass of cartilage in the trochlear region, this is not as evident. When the elbow is dislocated posterolaterally, the medial epicondyle is usually located posterior to the trochlea.

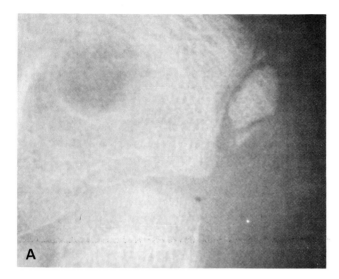

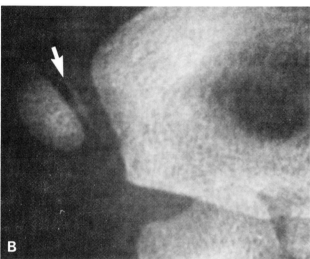

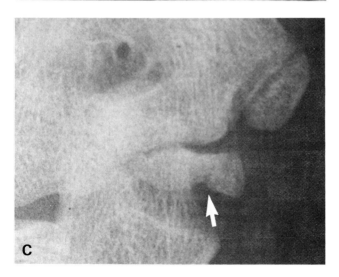

Treatment. If the medial epicondyle is minimally displaced, the joint should be immobilized for three weeks in a long arm cast with the elbow in moderate flexion and the forearm in pronation. If the epicondyle is moderately displaced, but the elbow is stable on valgus strain, treatment again should consist of simple immobilization in a long arm cast for three weeks. According to some authors, the functional result may be excellent, despite the fact that healing is by fibrous union.[121] Occasionally, the fragment may fail to heal and symptoms of ulnar nerve damage and irritation present themselves upon local pressure. If such symptoms supervene, the fragment should be excised. If closed treatment is chosen for any of the aforementioned, a roentgenogram of the elbow should be taken again in four or five days to see if the pull of the attached flexor musculature has caused subsequent displacement.

If the medial epicondyle is markedly displaced (i.e., more than 5 mm, and rotated 90°) or if the elbow joint is unstable on application of valgus strain, open reduction and internal fixation are indicated (Fig. 10-78).

According to Rang, the child should be operated on in a prone position. However, there is no reason why the child cannot have surgery in the supine position.[139] While a transverse incision may leave a cosmetically more acceptable scar, a longitudinal incision placed slightly posteriorly allows better visualization of the ulnar nerve, which should be exposed completely. There usually is significant hematoma throughout the subcutaneous tissue, and dissection must be carried out carefully down to the level of fracture. The joint hematoma should be evacuated. The ulnar nerve must be accurately identified and isolated. While Rang recommends ignoring the nerve by not dissecting it, my impression has

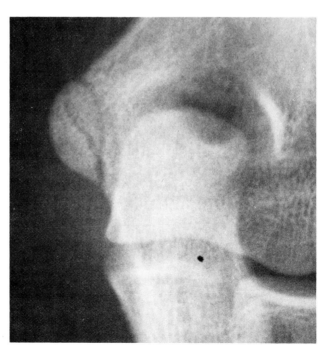

FIG. 10-74. *A,* Fragmented, undisplaced fracture of medial epicondyle. *B,* Displaced fracture showing small metaphyseal fragment (arrow). *C,* Propagation of fracture into medial condylar physis (arrow). This was an undisplaced "greenstick" injury.

FIG. 10-75. Medial epicondylar fracture in a 16-year-old girl. This originally was interpreted as a normal physis. However, it was really a fracture through the closing physis, analogous to a Tillaux fracture of the distal tibia.

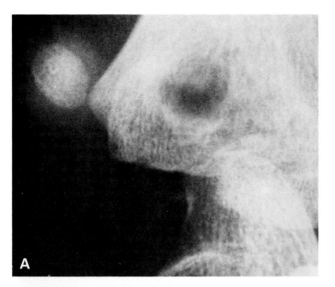

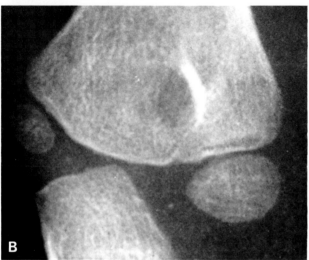

FIG. 10-76. *A,* Superior displacement. *B,* Inferior displacement.

been that significant swelling and contusion is present, and that a neurolysis and decompression of the tunnel in which the ulnar nerve traverses usually results in improved symptomatology in cases with mild to moderate preoperative ulnar compression symptoms. This procedure also allows evaluation of the nerve and, in virtually every case, a variable contusion of the nerve has been evident. This contusion explains some of the problems that develop as part of the normal healing phenomenon following closed reduction. To attribute all postoperative nerve injuries to surgical trauma is probably not totally accurate, inasmuch as these children are frequently operated on immediately after arrival at the hospital, sometimes without an adequate neurologic examination to thoroughly ascertain damage present preoperatively. Further, it might take a few days or at least a few more hours for the actual signs of neurologic damage from the contusion to develop. If the ulnar nerve has been displaced into the joint with the fragment, it must be extricated during open reduction.

The elbow should be flexed and held in neutral rotation to minimize traction in the flexor muscles. Rotation can be checked by lining up the flexor muscle fibers. The fragment is secured with Kirschner wires. Two wires lessen the chance for rotation. The arm should be placed in a cast and held for three weeks, at which time the pins are removed. Early motion is started, although sometimes it is necessary to immobilize the elbow for two more weeks.

Results. There are few reports chronicling long follow-up on cases of medial epicondylar fractures, and the choice of treatment is somewhat empiric.[121] Prior to 1950, the majority of patients were probably undertreated by closed reduction and pronation, with local pressure applied over the medial epicondyle. Fibrous union was common by such methods. However, elbow movement returned more slowly with such methods than it did following open reduction and many patients required late excision of the fragment because of discomfort due to the fibrous union.

Complications. Ulnar nerve paresis is a common complication of this injury, but it may not occur until several months or years after the initial injury. It is probably more common in moderately displaced fractures that are allowed to heal by fibrous union and then develop an irritative pseudarthrosis. Excision of the fragment and neurolysis are usually sufficient treatment in such cases. Translocation of the nerve anterior to the epicondyle may also be necessary.

This injury is not usually associated with any major growth problems, primarily because it tends to occur at a time when physiologic physeal closure is commencing. Therefore, premature epiphysiodesis generally does not result in any major growth deformity (see Fig. 10-84C). Full extension may be slow to return and incomplete when it does, although this occurs in only a few cases.

Nonunion of medial epicondylar fractures is not seen frequently, and rarely leads to pain. This is because most minimally displaced injuries heal satisfactorily after closed reduction, whereas most moderately to severely displaced fractures are now treated routinely with open reduction (which should be the procedure of choice for displaced epicondylar fractures). If the epicondyle is painful, excision of the fragment may be undertaken.

Lateral condyle

Fractures of the lateral condyle are relatively common and constitute approximately 10 to 15% of all fractures in the region of the elbow. They occur in children between the ages of 3 and 14 years, but seem to be most common between 6 and 10 years.[92,102,120,126,135,218-227,229-231]

Classification. While the injury normally is considered a type 4 physeal injury, it also may be a type 3 injury if there is minimal or no extension of the fracture into the metaphysis (Fig. 10-79). In most instances however, there is a thin plate of metaphysis where the fracture has propagated and therefore, by definition, a type 4 injury exists. The thin metaphyseal bone plate may be centrally located because of the "lappet" contour of the physis. The most important considerations are that this fracture is both an intra-articular injury, as well as a disruption of a major portion of the physeal growth mechanism of the distal humerus.

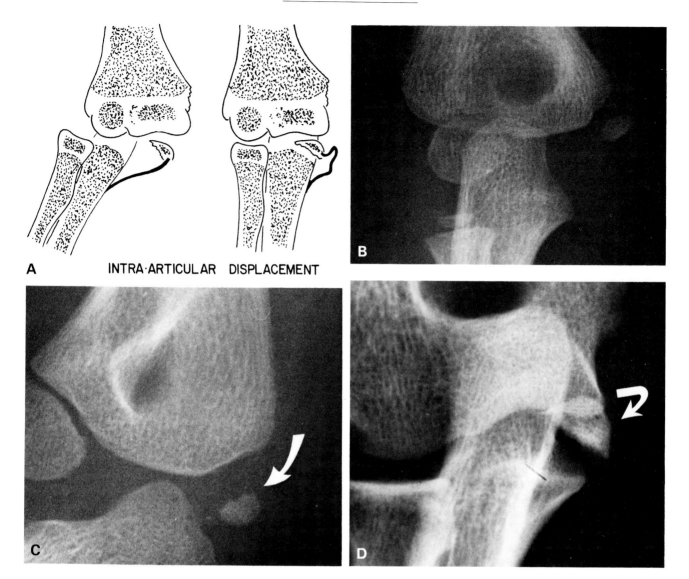

INTRA-ARTICULAR DISPLACEMENT

FIG. 10-77. *A,* Schematic of intra-articular displacement. *B,* Three-year-old child with pain over the medial epicondyle and apparent separation. *C,* Application of valgus stress pulled the epicondyle inferiorly. *D,* Fragment displaced into joint.

Another important concept is that the propagation of the fracture through the epiphysis rarely occurs exactly at the junction between trochlea and capitellum (see Fig. 10-79).

The condylar fragment usually includes: the physis and secondary ossification center of the capitellum, cartilaginous portions of the trochlea (including physis), the lateral epicondyle, and part of the lateral metaphysis with the radial collateral ligament and the common tendon of the extensor muscles attached to it. The fracture fragment may be undisplaced (Fig. 10-80), or variably displaced and rotated by the pull of the extensors of the wrist and fingers (Fig. 10-81).

The degree of the rotation of the fragment varies. It may be turned 90° so that the articular surface faces inward (toward the remaining trochlea), and the fracture surface laterally (Fig. 10-82). In its extreme form, it is rotated 180° around both horizontal and vertical axes, with the distal articular surface facing outward and the lateral surface inward. If left in these malrotated positions, the apposition of joint surface cartilage to the remaining fracture surfaces of me-

taphysis and trochlea invariably results in nonunion and a subsequent deformity, since the articular tissue is not associated with a normal process of ossification (see Chap. 2).

Less frequently, there may be a fracture through part of the capitellar ossification center (Fig. 10-83). In such fractures, only the capitellum and extreme lateral portions of the physis (especially epicondyle) are involved. The trochlea is not injured. Fractures of the lateral condyle of the humerus may also be associated with partial or complete medial dislocation of the elbow.

Pathomechanics. The fracture usually results from indirect violence, such as a fall on the outstretched hand with the forearm abducted and the elbow extended. The force is transmitted through the radius. The lesion also may be produced by a traction force that thrusts the elbow into a varus position (Fig. 10-84). In such instances, the fracture may begin at different points. When there is indirect force, as from a fall on the hand, the fracture may start as an intra-

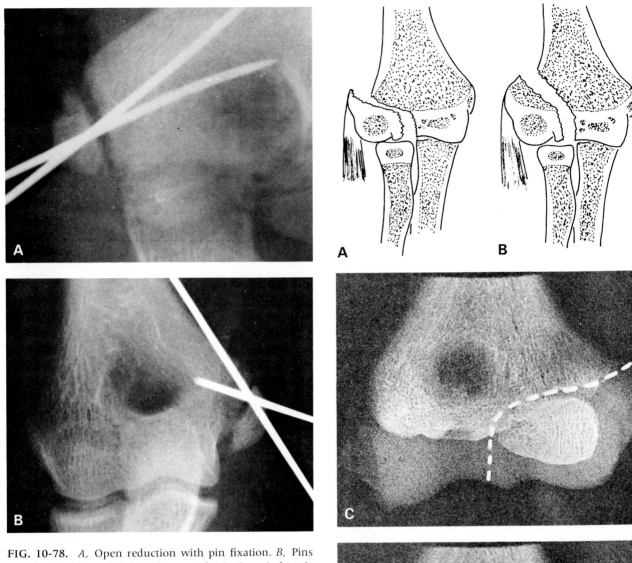

FIG. 10-78. *A,* Open reduction with pin fixation. *B,* Pins must be placed carefully into the metaphysis. One pin here is primarily in soft tissue.

articular fracture propagating toward the physis. In contrast, a varus stress to the region may be associated with disruption of the peripheral zone of Ranvier and propagation across the physis to the junction of the capitellum and trochlea. The biomechanics of the cartilage probably change because of the variable appearance and size of the capitellar and trochlear ossification centers.

Jakob produced this type of fracture experimentally by applying a varus strain to the extended elbow (see Fig. 10-82).[224] In this anatomic study, the only deforming force that produced a fracture of the lateral condyle was forced varus angulation with the elbow extended and the forearm supinated. This caused a fracture in 4 out of 7 elbows.[224] The children, all of whom had died from injury, were between 2½ and 10 years of age at the time of death. In one case, there was an associated transverse adduction fracture of the olecranon, not unlike that seen in the clinical situation (see Fig. 10-84).

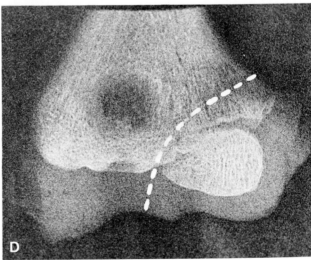

FIG. 10-79. *A-B,* Schematics of type 3 and type 4 lateral condyle fractures. Note how the fracture does not involve just the capitellum, but extends through part of the trochlear cartilage. *C-D,* Specimen roentgenograms depicting these two patterns.

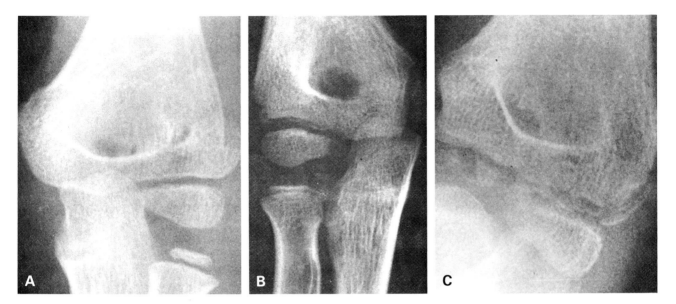

FIG. 10-80. Undisplaced fractures through the lateral condyle. *A,* A metaphyseal disruption should alert to condylar injury. *B,* A thin metaphyseal (juxtaphyseal) remnant indicates this condylar injury. *C,* Thin metaphyseal plate with propagation into the trochlear ossification center.

In three of the four elbows, the lateral condylar fragment was attached to the humerus by a substantial bridge of cartilage. When the arm was repositioned, this bridge acted as a hinge guiding the fragment back into position, preventing significant displacement, and maintaining an intact articular surface enclosing the fracture line. Whether this occurs in the clinical situation is difficult to say, but the use of arthrography may help to delineate this situation, particularly if there is any question about whether to go ahead with an open reduction. The trochlear ridge on the ulna behaves as a fulcrum for avulsion of the lateral condyle by the lateral fragment. The bone will separate, but some epiphyseal and articular cartilage may remain intact as a hinge. As soon as this hinge divides, the fracture becomes extremely unstable and the condyle can be easily displaced and rotated. The fracture reduces when the varus angulation is corrected. In essence, this is an incomplete type 3 or type 4 epiphyseal fracture. If deforming angulation is increased, the cartilage hinge may tear, which may lead to fracture displacement and dislocation of the elbow (type 4 injury).

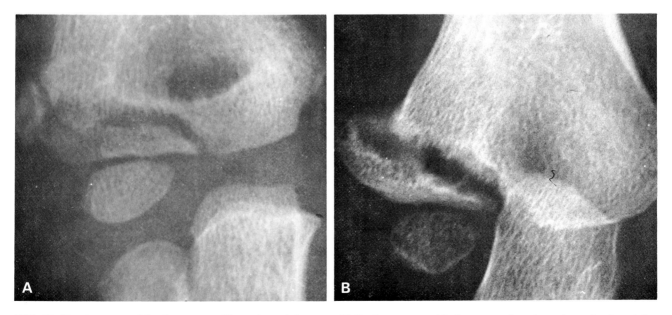

FIG. 10-81. Patterns of displacement of lateral condyle. *A,* Mild displacement, with fragmentation above lateral epicondyle. *B,* Wider separation and lateralization.

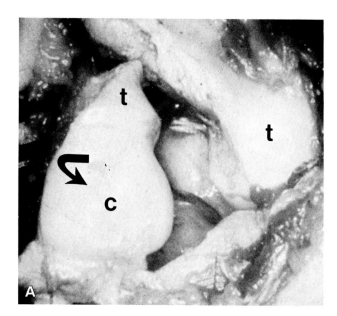

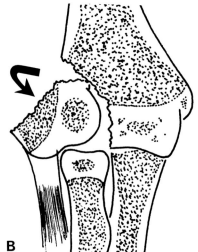

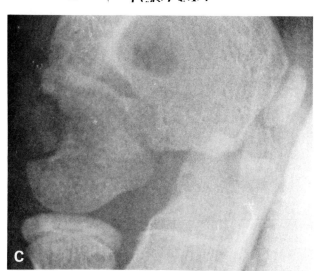

FIG. 10-82. *A,* Pathologic fracture in cadaver specimen. Note capitellum (c) and trochlea (t). *B,* Schematic, emphasizing fragment rotation. *C,* Clinical example.

Some of the blood supply to the lateral condyle enters by its soft tissue attachments, particularly posteriorly at the origin of the long extensor muscles.[130,232] However, important intracartilaginous vessels traverse from the trochlea to the capitellum and are disrupted by the transepiphyseal nature of the fracture. Extensive dissection during open reduction may jeopardize remaining vascularity beyond the initial traumatic disruption.

Diagnosis. These patients generally have severe pain following injury, with marked swelling, ecchymosis, and local tenderness over the lateral portion of the elbow. Rotation of the forearm is often unrestricted, especially in undisplaced fractures, but it may be quite painful. In most cases, the diagnosis can be confirmed by roentgenographic findings (see Figs. 10-80 and 10-81). However, sometimes only the oblique view will disclose either displacement or evidence of the undisplaced fracture line. A true lateral view, particularly when compared to the opposite side, may show a severe anterior/posterior tilt of the capitellum and should suggest the diagnosis.

Lateral condyle fractures are serious injuries. The displaced fragment is often diagnosed merely as a chip fracture on the outer margin of the elbow (i.e., the metaphysis) and not recognized as being half of the lower articular surface of the humerus (and epiphysis).

Grossly displaced fractures are usually obvious on radiographs, but hairline fractures are easy to miss. When there is clinical evidence of a fracture but no radiographic signs, further views should be taken, particularly obliques, until the fracture is evident. Even stress films may be used to show this. In the particularly young child, the ossification center may not be present, and the true nature of the injury may not be completely comprehended. An arthrogram may help (Fig. 10-85). The younger the child and the less well-developed the ossification centers, the greater the likelihood that this injury will be overlooked.

Treatment. The undisplaced fracture can be treated by immobilization in a long arm cast with the elbow in 90° of flexion and the forearm in full supination to minimize the pull of the extensor muscles. *However, even undisplaced fractures of the lateral condyle are unstable and may become displaced while immobilized.* In an undisplaced lateral condylar fracture, if the adjacent soft parts are intact, satisfactory outcome is usually assured. Repeat roentgenograms should be made within the first five to ten days to detect any subsequent displacement that may require open reduction (Fig. 10-86).

Even these undisplaced fractures must be considered unstable, as they tend to become displaced, *even with immobilization,* because of the pull of the common extensors. Since the fracture line crosses the physis, accurate anatomic reposition is imperative to decrease the likelihood of growth damage. Further, congruity of the joint must be restored.

Flynn emphasized that all minimally displaced fractures of the lateral condylar epiphysis should be watched closely for increasing displacement and for delayed healing.[128] They should be followed roentgenographically until it is certain that union is solid. Our experience showing that there is a small area of osseous fracture compared to a large surface area of cartilaginous fracture supports this concept. While a small amount of healing may occur bone to bone, the heal-

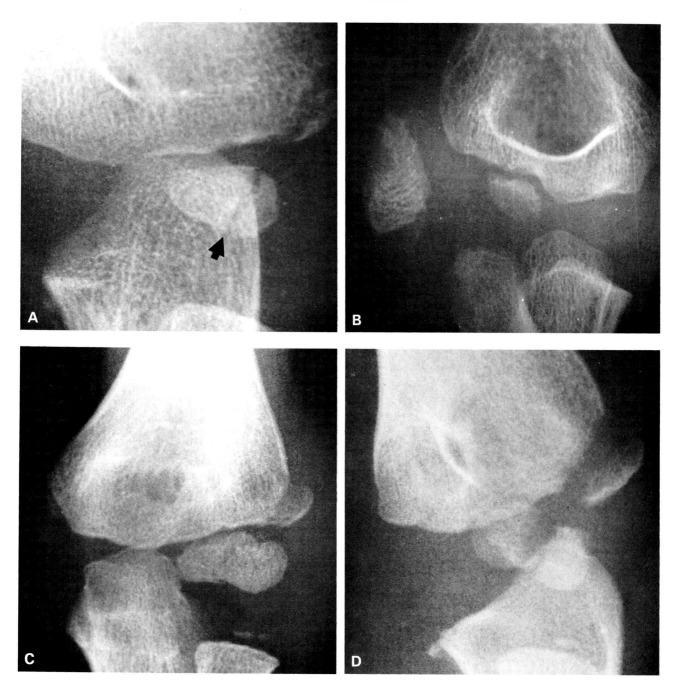

FIG. 10-83. Patterns of fractures through the capitellar ossification center. *A,* Undisplaced (arrow). *B,* Displaced. *C,* An oblique showed a metaphyseal fragment. *D,* Stress view showed extension into capitellum.

ing of the cartilaginous areas may take significantly longer (see Chap. 5).

Any evidence of acute or delayed displacement is an indication for open reduction and internal fixation (Figs. 10-87 and 10-88). This should be done by fixation across the entire epiphysis, as well as fixation of the fragments of the metaphysis if they are sufficiently large. If possible, pins crossing the growth plate should be avoided. While image intensification can be used, it is probably wiser to treat these with an open reduction, since part of the concept of reduction is adequate

restoration of the various articular surfaces. Further, any intra-articular fragments of cartilage or bone may be removed and the joint thoroughly irrigated.

Open reduction and internal fixation should be done under tourniquet with an incision made directly over the lateral condyle. The joint should be irrigated to obtain a clearer view of the articular surfaces. The fragment should be minimally dissected and freed of soft tissue attachments, but it should be visualized sufficiently to see if it is rotated in different planes. The periosteum may be herniated into the

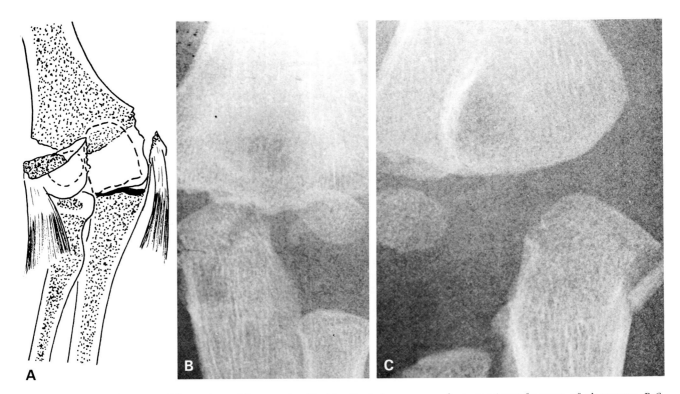

FIG. 10-84. *A,* Concept of formation of fracture by "locking" of olecranon and concomitant fracture of olecranon. *B-C,* Examples of injury pattern with concomitant olecranon and lateral condylar fractures.

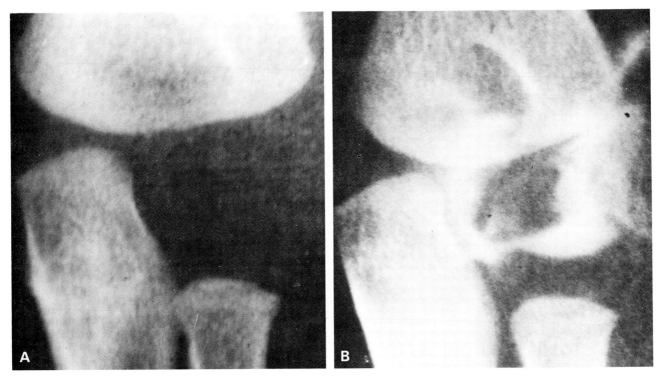

FIG. 10-85. *A,* In the young infant without capitellar ossification, diagnosis is impossible on standard films. *B,* Arthrography will help in diagnosis. The dye has surrounded the capitellar fragment.

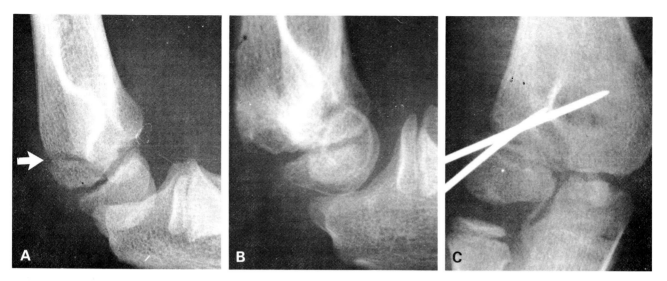

FIG. 10-86. *A,* Initially, the diagnosis was missed, but the lateral view shows an obvious injury (arrow). The AP view appeared normal. This is not a variation of ossification. Several days later, the fragment displaced (no treatment had been performed). *B,* This was treated with open reduction. *C,* Six months later, the fracture is healing.

region between the fragments. This should be removed. The fracture must be reduced anatomically, both at the fracture line in the metaphysis as well as at the joint surface. Failure to do so may create an abnormal elbow joint (Fig. 10-89). Kirschner wires, which should be smooth, should be placed across the region. Fluoroscopy, image intensification, or biplane radiographs should be taken to ensure reduction.

Conner and Smith described a series of cases treated by a new type of screw, the "Glasgow" screw, which is a coarse-threaded malleolar screw.[218] This type of device can be used only if the metaphyseal fragment is of adequate size. Under no circumstances should it be placed through the epiphysis or physis, as it undoubtedly will lead to premature growth arrest. Conner and Smith saw no cases of definite premature

epiphyseal fusion, but did note the occurrence of mild valgus deformities in two children, suggesting that the screw interfered with the growth plate.

In opening and reducing the fracture, one must not detach all the muscles from the lateral epicondyle, because these carry some of the blood supply to the condylar fragment. If detachment is undertaken, the condyle may undergo partial to complete aseptic necrosis and premature epiphysiodesis (Fig. 10-90).

The Late Case. A patient with a relatively undisplaced fracture with no clinical or roentgenographic union may not seek treatment until several weeks or months after injury (Figs. 10-91 and 10-92). Flynn reported a series of nonu-

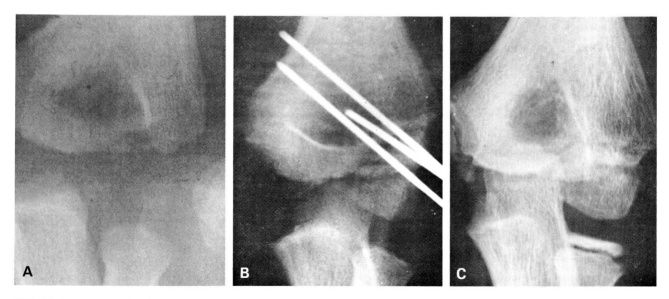

FIG. 10-87. *A,* Completely displaced and rotated capitellar fragment. *B,* Open reduction and pin fixation. *C,* Three years later.

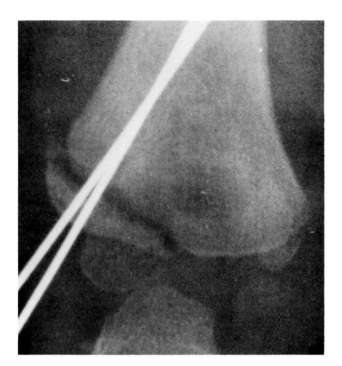

FIG. 10-88. Open reduction of type 4 injury. Large metaphyseal fragments are ideal for pinning without crossing the physis.

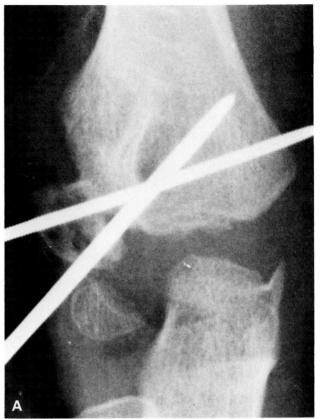

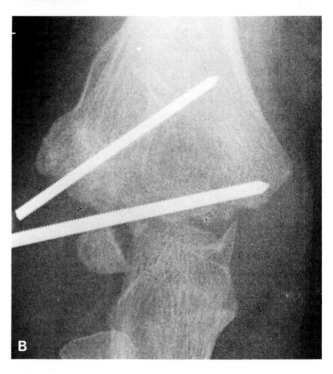

FIG. 10-89. Bad open reduction. *A,* Fragment not reduced. Also note the olecranon fracture. Unfortunately, neither the treating physician nor the radiologist recognized the inadequacy of this reduction, and it was left in this position. *B,* Healing took place in deformed position and resulted in a poorly functional elbow.

nited minimally displaced fractures.[126,128] He felt that in unrecognized fractures, the results of the nonunion were the symptoms that brought the child to the attention of the surgeon. Jeffrey pointed out that: (1) nonunion may originate in a fracture with relatively minor displacement and little or no rotation; (2) the orthopaedist may be unaware that union has failed; and (3) the nonunion may not be discovered until some later date.[224]

Flynn felt that early roentgenographic evidence of nonunion was seen best in the anteroposterior view as a "high collar-like projection" of the posterolateral metaphyseal fragment attached to the epiphysis (see Fig. 10-92).[128] There was lateral shifting and blunting of the fracture edges of the metaphyseal fragment, little or no callus formation, and a still distinct fracture gap. If this phenomenon is observed after the fifth week, it should be recognized as a delayed union. If it persists after the third month, nonunion is definite, and appropriate surgical treatment should be carried out.

This delayed union may respond effectively to pin stabilization, even several months after the injury. Minimal resection of fibrous callus is needed, and bone grafting may be unnecessary if the metaphyseal subchondral plate adjacent to the nonunion is fenestrated with two or three drill holes and the fragment immobilized by pin fixation.

Jakob found that the results of open reduction performed more than three weeks after the fracture are no better than those of no treatment at all.[224] Reduction may infarct the lateral condylar fragment by damaging the blood supply. The degree of displacement seems to be significant. The greater the displacement, the more likely surgery is to lead to complications.

Occasionally, a child seeks treatment several weeks after the original injury for a significantly displaced fracture of the lateral condyle. Should this be accepted or corrected? Late surgery often causes stiffness and avascular necrosis. Rang recommends a "hands-off" policy in any displaced fracture that has gone untreated for more than four weeks.[139] However, if it is still reasonably early (within a few weeks of the injury), open reduction, careful dissection, and anatomic reduction may still be recommended. It may be necessary to carefully curette some healing callus in order to get accurate anatomic reduction. Ununited fractures beyond a few weeks of age, in which nonunion is established, probably are difficult to treat by any method. However, an effort should be made to create bone-to-bone apposition of metaphyseal fragments.

Results. Flynn studied the healing responses of fractures with less than 4 mm of displacement, the majority of which were treated with closed reduction. He ascertained 3 patterns of healing.[126] The first type, which comprised almost half of the lesions, healed rapidly in 6 weeks with abundant callus and subperiosteal new bone. The second group (38%) healed slowly over 8 to 12 weeks, mostly by endosteal union with little peripheral callus. The remaining 13% had progressive displacement of the fragment in the plaster cast and required subsequent surgery to prevent nonunion. These elbows were salvaged with either fixation or bone grafting, sparing the physis of the condylar fragment. Flynn also noted that if the fracture was displaced less than 2 mm, union was usually adequate. If the displacement was 3 mm or greater, the incidence of delayed union, malunion, and nonunion was much higher.

Jakob reviewed 48 children, 20 with minimally displaced fractures, and 28 with displaced fractures requiring open reduction and internal fixation.[224] Four patients had a fracture line crossing the capitellar epiphysis and entering the joint lateral to the trochlea. The rest had injuries in which the fracture fragment included the capitellum and lateral part of the trochlea. Three of the patients developed avascular necrosis, and in two, the lateral part of the distal humeral growth plate closed prematurely.

Hardacre has demonstrated clearly that open reduction and internal fixation yield better results than traction or closed reduction in displaced fractures.[222]

Rang studied 27 patients whose original injury occurred between the ages of 4 and 8 years, and for whom the average follow-up was 6 years. The range of movement was normal in 24 of 27, with the remaining 3 losing no more than 10°. The carrying angle was normal in 26 of 27, but the lateral condyle had hypertrophied in 15 of 27, probably because of increased vascularity consequent to the injury.[139] The method of fixation was equally divided among pins and sutures, and this seemed to make no difference in the outcome. Several of the children showed radiographic evidence of mild growth abnormalities, although functionally there were no problems.

Complications. Severe and unrecognized injuries may go on to nonunion and marked elbow deformity (Fig. 10-93).[232a] Smith recently reported an 84 year follow-up of a patient with nonunion.[166] The functional disability was minimal, but complete ulnar nerve palsy was present.

Nonunion and growth arrests more commonly result from minimally displaced fractures than from markedly displaced

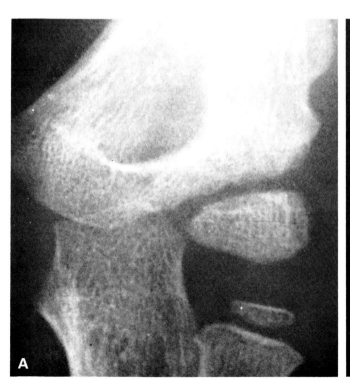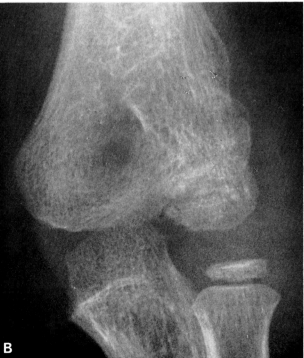

FIG. 10-90. *A*, Early avascular necrosis and growth slowdown following open reduction for fragment rotated 180°. *B*, The capitellum has fused to the metaphysis.

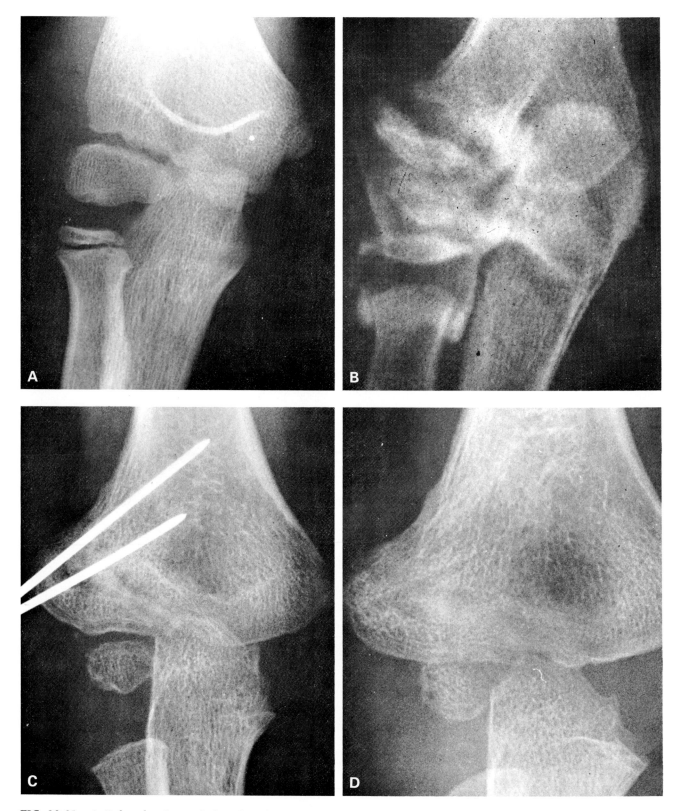

FIG. 10-91. *A,* Delayed union and clinical tenderness three months after lateral condylar fracture. *B,* Intraoperative stress arthrogram. *C,* Open reduction. *D,* Two months later, the fracture has healed.

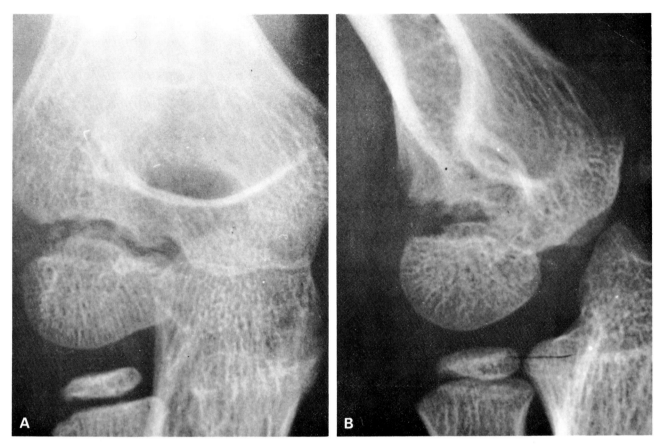

FIG. 10-92. Delayed union. *A,* Appearance five months after undisplaced fracture. *B,* Oblique view. Both views show absence of callus. The child was subsequently treated by excision of the fibrous nonunion and pin fixation. Healing was rapid.

and rotated fractures, probably because severe fractures are treated more adequately with surgery.[125-128]

Minimally displaced fractures may displace a few more millimeters by continued motion, but rarely rotate to the degree significantly displaced injuries rotate. The continual motion creates a bridge of fibrocartilage between the osseous and cartilaginous fragments.

Nonunion subsequently results in progressive cubitus valgus due to retardation and growth arrest of the lateral condylar physis and continued normal growth of the medial condylar region of the physis.

Suggested causes for delayed union and nonunion have included lack of immobilization, synovial fluid bathing the fracture, and soft tissue interposition. Continued motion is probably the most significant factor. In many cases, the fracture has been rotated 90° in at least one, if not two, planes, causing articular cartilage to appose epiphyseal cartilage or metaphyseal bone. Since it has been shown that articular cartilage does not ossify, even when transplanted into an epiphysis, it is unlikely that this cartilage will heal and fuse to the remaining portions of the distal humerus.[233]

Flynn was also emphatic in arguing that nonunion in a good position was acceptable, but that nonunion may become symptomatic, especially in athletic children.[128] Furthermore, careful distinction must be made between what is considered nonunion in good position and nonunion in poor position. Early surgery is recommended for established non-

union when the condylar fragment is in good position. If the united fragment is in poor position, unless the surgeon is skilled and familiar with the area, particularly the contours of the growth plate, it is advisable to either refer the patient to another surgeon or leave the fracture fragment as it is. An attempt to replace it anatomically may traumatize the physis of the fragment, and while the remainder of the elbow will continue to grow, the physeal plate of the fragment may close and growth potential will be lost, leading to valgus deformity and few benefits from this semiacute surgery.

Extensive bone grafting to obtain union before completion of growth is not recommended, because functional disability is not usually significant in the presence of nonunion. However, if the fracture has been treated by closed reduction, the presence of nonunion is a strong indication that the fragments have not been adequately stabilized or that they may have rotated 90° or 180°, and only seem to be reduced. In such a situation, open reduction and exploration are indicated, despite the fact that the fracture may be several weeks old. Surgery may reveal that there is a rotation or that there is unopposed tissue that can be removed with a firm reduction and Kirschner-wire fixation. Bone graft from the metaphyseal fragment to the remainder of metaphysis may be helpful.

A patient with established nonunion in which the epiphyseal cartilage plate of the condylar fragment is already closed is not a good candidate for surgery. Surgery may

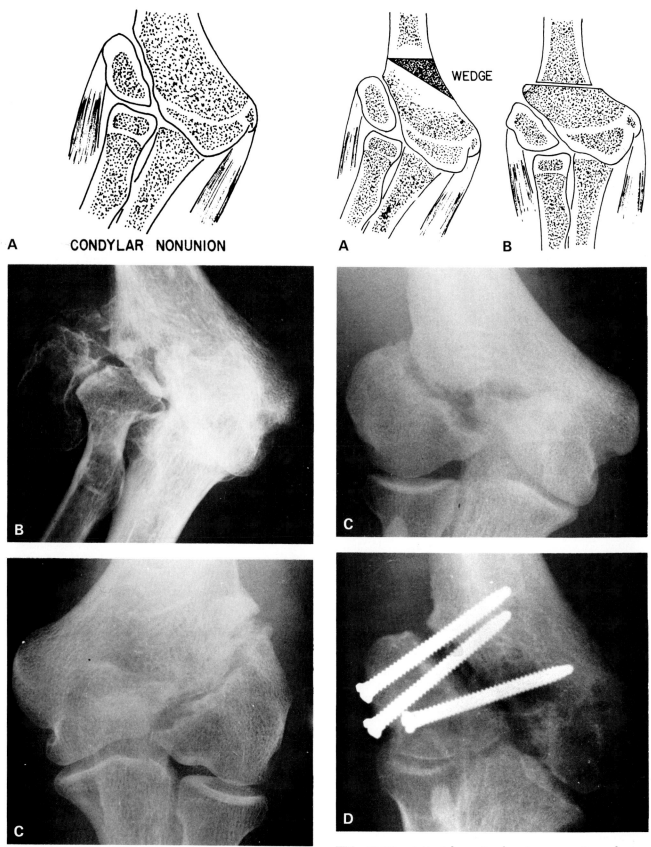

FIG. 10-93. *A,* Schematic of condylar nonunion. *B-C,* Adults with established condylar nonunion.

FIG. 10-94. *A-B,* Schematic showing correction of nonunion. *C,* Preoperative appearance. *D,* Postoperative appearance.

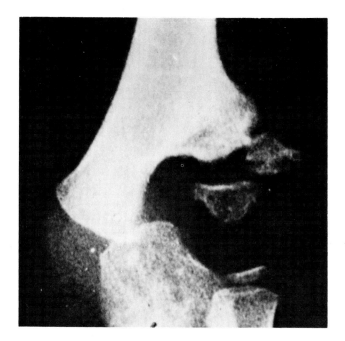

FIG. 10-95. Fishtail deformity.

achieve union, but the condyle will be unable to grow with the remainder of the elbow. Thus, surgery will not prevent recurrent valgus deformity and may not yield a satisfactory elbow. Such a patient may be better left untreated until growth is complete, with a later transfer of the ulnar nerve if tardy ulnar palsy occurs. In the adult, when the site of nonunion is painful, the fragment can be fixed or excised, but only after careful consideration of the effect it may have on the elbow. Excision of the fragment should never be done in the immature elbow because the same sequelae that follow excision of the radial head will ensue. Osteotomy of the distal part of the humerus at maturity may be necessary to correct deformity in some cases.

Lateral condylar fractures are generally type 4 injuries, with the majority passing through the cartilaginous trochlear epiphysis, and are likely to effect subsequent growth, although to a *highly variable* and *unpredictable* degree.[234] Because they do go through an area that will subsequently ossify, there may be premature fusion between the trochlea and capitellar ossification centers that will limit latitudinal development and osseous bridging across the physis. If the fracture involves the margins of the secondary ossification of the capitellum, the likelihood of subsequent growth arrest is greater. Should there be growth arrest, it will increase cubitus valgus deformity.

Malunion and premature growth arrest to the lateral condyle also cause progressive cubitus valgus. This deformity of the elbow may be corrected by an osteotomy of the distal humerus (Fig. 10-94). However, if this is done in the face of premature growth arrest, the deformity may recur because of the localized growth injury. If a specific localized defect can be observed, it may be possible to treat it with resection and fat interposition.

Wadsworth studied 28 children with fractures of the capitellum, 8 of which were undisplaced and 20 of which were displaced.[229,235] He found 6 cases of premature epiphys-

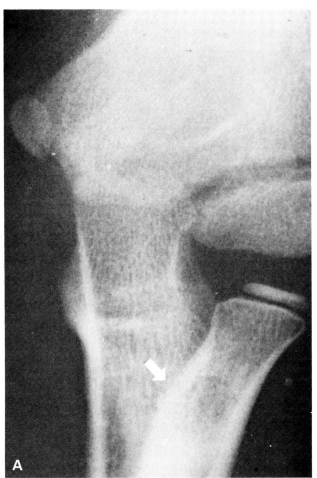

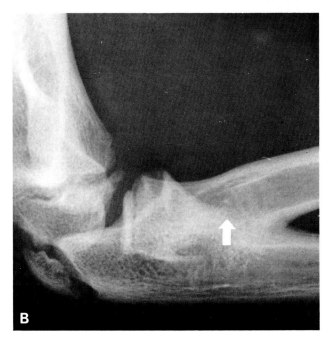

FIG. 10-96. Radioulnar synostosis (closed arrow in *A* and *B*). This was present prior to the lateral condylar fracture, and was probably a predisposing factor. *A,* Anteroposterior view. *B,* Lateral view.

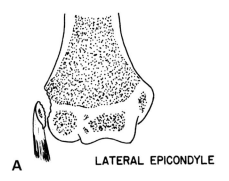

LATERAL EPICONDYLE

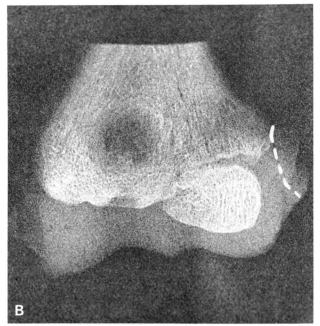

FIG. 10-97. *A,* Schematic of fracture of lateral epicondyle. *B,* Roentgenographic depiction in a specimen.

eal fusion, and distinguished 2 types. In the first, the capitellar secondary ossification center fused to the metaphysis, and in the second, the capitellum and the trochlea ossifications fused together, then fused subsequently to the metaphysis at the apex of the original fracture. Delayed union will result in prolonged hypermia and possible stimulation of growth on the lateral side of the elbow producing a cubitus varus. If there is damage to the growth plate, an osseous bridge inevitably forms across the plate. Besides the obvious premature growth arrest and fusion, an additional 11 of the remaining 22 patients had narrowing of the distal humeral epiphyseal plate, implying some loss of appositional growth.[229]

Growth of the distal humerus is a complex, but integrated process. In early development, the capitellar and trochlear regions are almost equal, but as the elbow grows, the trochlea becomes the dominant latitudinal growth region. Blockage of one or both areas by premature fusion adversely affects the integration of these growth mechanisms.

Another complication is poor articulation of the ulna with the trochlea, which impairs elbow movement.[92] Since the

fracture often extends through a significant portion of the trochlea, it is easy to understand how inadequate apposition of the joint surfaces creates this complication.

An infrequent radiologic finding is the "fishtail" deformity of the distal end of the humerus. This deformity is probably due to damage of the growth plate immediately adjacent to the fracture line (Fig. 10-95). Other authors have reported this abnormality and stated that it may produce cubitus valgus with limitation of movement or even progress to degenerative arthritis.[231,235] None of the three patients with this abnormality reported by Jakob had a deviation of the carrying angle nor did they lose any mobility of the elbow.[224]

This phenomenon may occur in well reduced as well as poorly reduced fractures, and it may be due to deficient development of part of the trochlea or to fibrous union not unlike that shown in Chapter 4, in which there is fibrocartilage rather than true hyaline cartilage. This deformity was always most marked when the capitellum had united in a rotational deformity and in cases with overgrowth of the lateral condyle.

Voshell excised a lateral condyle that was fractured, but left behind a portion of it, and the patient progressively regenerated a significant amount of this region as the epicondyle ossification center took over for the missing region.[236] However, this did not produce a roentgenographically normal elbow despite the allegations of the authors that this result was good.

Another reported complication of lateral condylar fractures is radioulnar synostosis (Fig. 10-96). However, great care should be taken in ascribing this particular deformity to the fracture. In the illustrated case, which was treated by closed reduction and cast immobilization, the possibility of pre-existent synostosis was not considered. However, careful history subsequently revealed that the patient had never been able to pronate or supinate. The synostosis undoubtedly had predisposed the condyle to fracture.

One of the more important complications of injury to the capitellar epiphysis is ulnar neuritis, which is usually tardy and usually associated with a progressive cubitus valgus.[132,237-239] Neuritis may be due to a simple compression by the band bridging the two heads of the flexor carpi ulnaris when the capacity of the cubital tunnel is less than normal. Additional factors leading to cubitus valgus can be premature fusion, malunion, nonunion, and avascular necrosis of the capitellum.

The ulnar nerve is repeatedly stretched by motion of the elbow at the apex of the deformity, as well as the increasingly valgus deformation, and may become progressively irritated in its course behind the medial epicondyle.[240] At the earliest signs of neuritis, either the ulnar nerve should be transferred anterior to the medial epicondyle or the epicondyle should be removed and the nerve allowed to move over the remaining area. However, use of the latter approach is contingent upon the degree of deformity and the age of the child; it should not be used prior to skeletal maturity.

Lateral epicondyle

The ossification center of the lateral epicondyle appears about the age of 12 and fuses with the lateral condyle at the age of 14. The lateral epicondylar center often is irregular and may be confused with a fracture. Injury to this particular epicondyle, compared to the medial epicondyle, is extremely

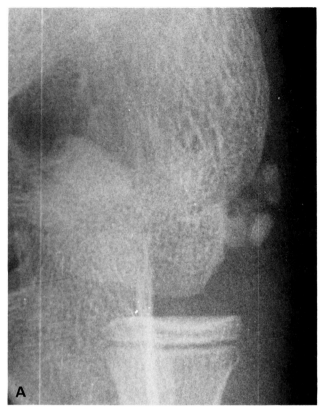

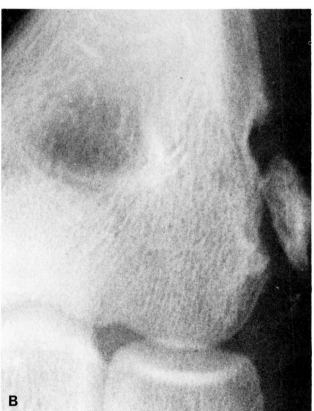

FIG. 10-98. *A,* Acute fracture of lateral epicondyle. *B,* Appearance of the fracture five years later, following skeletal maturation. A fibrous nonunion has occurred.

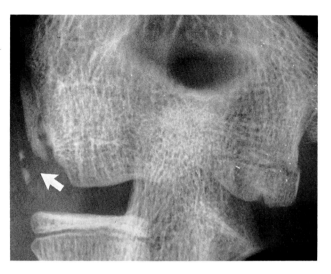

FIG. 10-99. Lateral epicondylar avulsion injury (arrow) in a 14-year-old boy who fell directly on his elbow. There was mild varus instability. The fracture was treated by closed reduction and immobilization at 90° of elbow flexion.

rare (Figs. 10-97 to 10-99). The injury may accompany elbow dislocation.

In most cases, there is relatively little displacement of the fragment. Immobilization of the elbow for three to four weeks may be sufficient. If the fragment is displaced more than three millimeters, open reduction should be considered. Since these injuries tend to occur only in children approaching skeletal maturity, the risk of associated growth arrest is minimal.

References

1. Dameron, T. B., Jr., and Reibel, D. B.: Fractures involving the proximal humeral epiphyseal plate. J. Bone Joint Surg., *51-A:*289, 1969.
2. Macnichol, M. F.: Roentgenographic evidence of median-nerve entrapment in a greenstick humeral fracture. J. Bone Joint Surg., *60-A:*998, 1978.
3. Wolfe, J. S., and Eyring, E. J.: Median-nerve entrapment within a greenstick fracture. J. Bone Joint Surg., *56-A:*1270, 1974.
4. Genner, B.: Fracture of the supracondyloid process. J. Bone Joint Surg., *41-A:*1333, 1959.
5. Kolb, L. W., and Moore, R. D.: Fractures of the supracondylar process of the humerus. J. Bone Joint Surg., *49-A:*532, 1967.
6. Silberstein, M. J., Brodeur, A. E., and Garviss, E. R.: Some vagaries of the capitellum. J. Bone Joint Surg., *61-A:*244, 1979.
7. Smith, M. G. H.: Osteochondritis of the humeral capitulum. J. Bone Joint Surg., *46-B:*50, 1964
7a. McCarthy, S. M., and Ogden, J. A.: Roentgenography of postnatal skeletal development. V. The distal humerus. Skeletal Radiol., in press.
8. Rowe, C. R., and Sakellarides, H. T.: Factors related to recurrences of anterior dislocations of the shoulder. Clin. Orthop., *20:*40, 1961.
9. Haliburton, R. A., Barber, J. R., and Fraser, R. L.: Pseudo-dislocation: an unusual birth injury. Can. J. Surg., *10:*455, 1967.

10. Austin, L. J.: Fractures of the morphological neck of the humerus in children. Can. Med. Assoc. J., *40:*546, 1939.

11. Bourdillon, J. F.: Fracture-separation of the proximal epiphysis of the humerus. J. Bone Joint Surg., *32-B:*35, 1950.

12. Butterworth, R. D., and Carpenter, E. B.: Bilateral slipping of the proximal epiphysis of the humerus. J. Bone Joint Surg., *30-A:*1003, 1948.

13. Campbell, J., and Almond, G. A.: Fracture-separation of the proximal humeral epiphysis. J. Bone Joint Surg., *59-A:*262, 1977.

14. Conwell, H. E.: Fractures of the surgical neck and epiphyseal separations of upper end of humerus. J. Bone Joint Surg., *8:*508, 1926.

15. Fraser, R., Haliburton, R., and Barber, J.: Displaced epiphyseal fractures of the proximal humerus. Can. J. Surg., *10:*427, 1967.

16. Friedlaender, H. L.: Separation of the proximal humeral epiphysis. Clin. Orthop., *35:*163, 1964.

17. Jeffrey, C. C.: Fracture separation of the upper humeral epiphysis. Surg. Gynecol. Obstet., *96:*205, 1953.

18. Lee, H. G.: Operative reduction of an unusual fracture of the upper epiphyseal plate of the humerus. J. Bone Joint Surg., *26:*401, 1944.

19. McBride, E. D., and Sisler, J.: Fractures of the proximal humeral epiphysis and the juxta-epiphyseal humeral shaft. Clin. Orthop., *38:*143, 1965.

20. Michel, L.: Le decollement obstetrical de l'epiphyse superieure de l'humerus. Rev. Orthop., *24:*201, 1937.

21. This reference has been deleted.

22. Sherk, H., and Probst, C.: Fractures of the proximal humeral epiphysis. Orthop. Clin. North Am., *6:*401, 1975.

23. Smith, F. M.: Fracture-separation of the proximal humeral epiphysis. Am. J. Surg., *91:*627, 1956.

24. Vivian, D. N., and Janes, J. M.: Fractures involving the proximal humeral epiphysis. Am. J. Surg., *87:*211, 1954.

25. Whitman, R.: A treatment of epiphyseal displacements and fractures of the upper extremity of the humerus designed to assure definite adjustment and fixation of the fragments. Ann. Surg., *47:*706, 1908.

26. Zanolli, R.: Fracture dell epifisi superiore del omero. Chir. Organi. Mov., *12:*445, 1928.

27. Neer, C. S., II, and Horwitz, B. S.: Fractures of the epiphyseal plate. Clin. Orthop., *41:*24, 1965.

28. Poland, J.: Traumatic Separation of the Epiphyses. London, Smith, Elder, and Co., 1898.

29. Robin, G. C., and Kedar, S. S.: Separation of the upper humeral epiphysis in pituitary gigantism. J. Bone Joint Surg., *44-A:*189, 1962.

30. Van Hove, R.: Decollement epiphysaire du coude: recul de trente-six ans. Acta Orthop. Belg., *17:*289, 1951.

31. Scaglietti, O.: The obstetrical shoulder trauma. Surg. Gynecol. Obstet., *66:*868, 1938.

32. Bonelli, A., and Schiavetti, E.: Considerazioni su alcuni aspetti delle fratture di gomito nel bambino. Chir. Organi. Mov., *52:*286, 1963.

33. Lemberg, R., and Liliequist, B.: Dislocation of the proximal epiphysis of the humerus in newborns. Acta Paediatr. Scand., *59:*377, 1970.

34. This reference has been deleted.

35. Levin, G. D.: A valgus angulation fracture of the proximal humeral epiphysis. Clin. Orthop., *116:*155, 1976.

36. Charry, V.: Un cas de fracture irreductible du col chirurgical de l'humerus chez un adolescent. Rev. Orthop., *24:*244, 1937.

37. Ciaramella, G., and Rulfoni, R.: Le complicazioni neurologiche nelle fratture dell'artro superiore. Chir. Ital., *14:*569, 1962.

38. Gilchrist, D.: A stockinette-velpeau for immobilization of the shoulder girdle. J. Bone Joint Surg., *45-A:*1382, 1963.

39. Nilsson, S., and Svartholm, F.: Fractures of the upper end of the humerus in children. Acta Chir. Scand., *130:*433, 1965.

40. Tachdjian, M.: Pediatric Orthopedics. Philadelphia, W. B. Saunders, 1972.

41. Aitken, A. P.: End results of fractures of proximal humeral epiphysis. J. Bone Joint Surg., *18:*1036, 1936.

42. Aitken, A. P.: Fractures of the proximal humeral epiphysis. Surg. Clin. North Am., *43:*1575, 1963.

43. Langenskiöld, A.: Adolescent humerus varus. Acta Chir. Scand., *105:*353, 1953.

44. Lucas, L., and Gill, J. H.: Humerus varus following birth injury to the proximal humerus. J. Bone Joint Surg., *29:*367, 1947.

45. Stropeni, L.: L'omero varo da rottura spontanea de cisti ossea metafisari. Chir. Organi. Mov., *12:*531, 1938.

46. Blount, W.: Fractures in Children. Baltimore, Williams & Wilkins, 1955.

47. Sarmiento, A., et al.: Functional bracing of fractures of the shaft of the humerus. J. Bone Joint Surg., *59-A:*596, 1977.

48. Astedt, B.: A method for the treatment of humerus fractures in the newborn using the S. von Rosen splint. Acta Orthop. Scand., *40:*234, 1969.

49. Holstein, A., and Lewis, G. B.: Fractures of the humerus with radial-nerve paralysis. J. Bone Joint Surg., *45-A:*1382, 1963.

50. Lipscomb, P. R., and Burleson, R. J.: Vascular and neural complications in supracondylar fractures of the humerus in children. J. Bone Joint Surg., *37-A:*487, 1955.

51. Weller, S.: Konservierte oder operative Behandlung von suprakondylaren Oberarmfrakturen. Aktuel. Traumatol., *2:*79, 1974.

52. Aebi, H.: Der Ellbogenwinkel, seine Beziebungen zu Geschlect, Korperbay und Huftbrate. Acta Anat., *3:*228, 1947.

53. Allen, P. D., and Gramse, A. E.: Transcondylar fractures of the humerus treated by Dunlop traction. Am. J. Surg., *67:*217, 1945.

54. Avellan, W. H.: Uber Frakturen des unteren Humerusendes bei Kindern. Acta Chir. Scand. [Suppl.], *27,* 1933.

55. Barac, M., Gujic, M., and Hranilovic, B.: Behandlungen der Bruche am distalen Teil des Oberarms. Hefte Unfallheilkd., *114:*26, 1974.

56. Basom, W.: Supracondylar and transcondylar fractures in children. Clin. Orthop., *1:*43, 1953.

57. Baumann, E.: Beitrage zur Kenntnis der Frakturen am Ellbogenbelenk. Unter besonderer Berucksichtigung der Spatfolgen. I. Allgemeines und Fractura supracondylica. Bruns Klin. Chir., *146:*1, 1929.

58. Baumann, E.: Die Behandlung von Oberarm bruchen mittels Vertikalextension. Beitr. f. Klin. Chir., *152:*260, 1931.

59. Beck, A.: Therapy of supracondylar fractures in children. Zentralbl. Chir., *60:*2242, 1933.

60. Bertola, L.: On supracondylar fractures of the humerus in childhood. Minerva Ortop., *10:*543, 1959.

61. Blount, W. P., Schulz, I., and Cassidy, R. H.: Fractures of the elbow in children. J.A.M.A., *146:*699, 1951.

62. Boyd, H. B. and Altenberg, A. R.: Fractures about the elbow in children. Arch. Surg., *49:*213, 1944.

63. Brewster, A. H., and Karp, M.: Fractures in the region of the elbow in children. An end-result study. Surg. Gynecol. Obstet., *71:*643, 1940.

64. Bristow, W. R.: Myositis ossificans and Volkmann's paralysis. Notes on two cases illustrating the rarer complications of supracondylar fracture of the humerus. Br. J. Surg., *10:*475, 1923.

65. Coventry, M. B., and Henderson, C. C.: Supracondylar fractures of the humerus—49 cases in children. Rocky Mt. Med. J., *53:*458, 1956.

66. Deutschlander, K.: Zur Behandlung der suprakondylaren Uberstreckungsbruchen des Oberarmes. Chirurg., *6:*733, 1934.

67. Divis, G.: Epiphyseolysis Humeri unter Betrachtlicher Dislokation des Gelenkskopfes: Unblutige Reposition Archiv. Orthop. Unfallchir., *25:*342, 1927.

68. Duben, W.: Frakturen des Ellenbogengelenkes. Kinderchirurg. [Suppl.], *B11:*736, 1972.

69. El-Sharkawi, A., and Fattah, H.: Treatment of displaced supracondylar fractures of the humerus in children in full extension and supination. J. Bone Joint Surg., 47-B:273, 1965.

70. Elstrom, J. A., Pankovich, A. M., and Kassab, M. T.: Irreducible supracondylar fracture of the humerus in children. A report of two cases. J. Bone Joint Surg., 57-A:680, 1975.

71. Fowles, J. V., and Kassab, M. T.: Displaced supracondylar fractures of the elbow in children. J. Bone Joint Surg., 56-B:490, 1974.

72. Gartland, J. J.: Management of supracondylar fractures of the humerus in children. Surg. Gynecol. Obstet., 109:145, 1959.

73. Griffin, P.: Supracondylar fractures of the humerus. Treatment and complications. Pediatr. Clin. North Am., 22:477, 1975.

74. Hart, V. L.: Reduction of supracondylar fracture in children. Surgery, 11:33, 1942.

75. Henrikson, B.: Supracondylar fracture of the humerus in children. A late review of end-results with special reference to the cause of deformity, disability and complications. Acta Chir. Scand. [Suppl.], 369, 1966.

76. Hesoun, P.: Die suprakondylare Oberarmfraktur im Kindesalter. Auswertung von 99 suprakondylaren Oberarmfrakturen aus den Jahren 1965 bis 1975. Unfallheilkunde, 79:213, 1976.

77. Hirt, H. J., Vogel, W., and Reichmann, W.: Die suprakondylare Humerusfraktur im Kindesalter. M.M.W., 118:705, 1976.

78. Hofmann, V.: Behandlung der suprakondylaren Humerusfraktur im Kindesalter. Zentralbl. Chir., 93:1678, 1968.

79. Holmberg, L.: Fractures of the distal end of the humerus in children. Acta Chir. Scand. [Suppl.], 103, 1945.

80. Infranzi, A., and Trillat, A.: Une nouvelle technique pour le traitement des fractures sus-condyliennes de l'humerus. Lyon Chir., 55:90, 1960.

81. Izadpanah, M.: Die modifizierte blountsche Methode bei suprakondylaren Humerusfrakturen im Kindesalter. Arch. Orthop. Unfallchir., 77:348, 1973.

82. Jensenius, H.: Efterundersogelse af fraatura humeri supracondylica hos born. Nord. Med., 37:19, 1948.

83. Judet, J.: Traitment des fractures epiphysaires de l'enfant par broche transarticulaire. Mem. Acad. Chir., 73:562, 1947.

84. Kutscha, E., Lissberg, K., and Rauhs, R.: Frische Ellenbogenverletzungen im Wachstumsalter. Hefte Unfallheilkd., 118:26, 1974.

85. LaGrange, J., and Rigault, P.: Fractures supracondyliennes. Rev. Chir. Orthop., 48:337, 1962.

86. Lawrence, W.: Supracondylar fractures of the humerus in children. A review of 100 cases. Br. J. Surg., 44:143, 1956.

87. Macafee, A. L.: Infantile supracondylar fracture. J. Bone Joint Surg., 49-B:768, 1967.

88. Madsen, E.: Supracondylar fractures of the humerus in children. J. Bone Joint Surg., 37-B:241, 1955.

89. Mann, T. S.: Prognosis of supracondylar fractures. J. Bone Joint Surg., 45-B:516, 1963.

90. Maylahn, D. J., and Fahey, J. J.: Fractures of the elbow in children. J.A.M.A., 166:220, 1958.

91. McDonnell, D. P., and Wilson, J. C.: Fractures of the lower end of the humerus in children. J. Bone Joint Surg., 30-A:347, 1948.

92. McLearie, M., and Merson, R. D.: Injuries to the lateral condyle epiphysis of the humerus in children. J. Bone Joint Surg., 36-B:84, 1954.

93. Mitchell, W. J., and Adams, J. P.: Effective management for supracondylar fractures of the humerus in children. Clin. Orthop., 23:197, 1962.

94. Mitchell, W. J., and Adams, J. P.: Supracondylar fractures of the humerus in children. A ten year review. J.A.M.A., 175:573, 1961.

95. Morger, R.: Verletzungen am kindlichen ellbogen. Z. Kinderchirurg., 11:717, 1972.

96. Palmer, E. E., et al.: Supracondylar fracture of the humerus in children. J. Bone Joint Surg., 60-A:653, 1978.

97. Prietto, C. A.: Supracondylar fractures of the humerus. J. Bone Joint Surg., 61-A:425, 1979.

98. Rosman, M.: A fracture board to facilitate the management of supracondylar humeral fractures in children. J. Trauma, 15:153, 1975.

99. Sabate, A. F., Rubio, I., and Olivares, M.: Desprendemientos epifisarios graves del cuello humeral. Barcelona Quirurgica, 18:329, 1974.

100. Salter, R. B.: Supracondylar fractures in childhood. J. Bone Joint Surg., 41-B:881, 1959.

101. Sandegard, E.: Fracture of the lower end of the humerus in children—treatment and end results. Acta Chir. Scand. [Suppl.], 89, 1943.

102. Siris, I. E.: Supracondyle fracture of the humerus. An analysis of 330 cases. Surg. Gynecol. Obstet., 68:201, 1939.

103. Smith, F. M.: Children's elbow injuries: fractures and dislocations. Clin. Orthop., 50:7, 1967.

104. Smith, L.: Supracondylar fractures of the humerus treated by direct observation. Clin. Orthop., 50:37, 1967.

105. Smith, R. W.: Observations on dysfunction of the lower epiphysis of the humerus. Dublin Quarterly J. Med. Sci., 9:63, 1850.

106. Sorrel, E., and Longuet, Y.: La voie trans-brachial anterieure dans la chirurgie des fractures supra-condyliennes de l'humerus chez l'enfant (indication et technique). Rev. Chir. Orthop., 32:3, 1946.

107. Sorrel, E.: A propos des fractures supracondyliennes de l'humerus chez l'enfant. Rev. Orthop., 32:383, 1946.

108. Staples, O. S.: Supracondylar fracture of the humerus in children. J.A.M.A., 168:730, 1958.

109. Thompson, V. P.: Supracondylar fractures of the humerus in children. J.A.M.A., 146:609, 1951.

110. Vahvanen, V., and Aalto, K.: Supracondylar fracture of the humerus in children. Acta Orthop. Scand., 49:225, 1978.

111. Virenque, J., and LaFage, J.: Les fractures supra-condyliennes du conde chez l'enfant. Resultats compares des traitments orthopedique et chirurgical, a propros de 163 observations. Ann. Chir., 21:544, 1967.

112. Klima, M.: Early development of the human sternum and the problem of homologization of the so-called suprasternal structures. Acta Anat. (Basel), 69:473, 1968.

113. Liebolt, F. L., and Furey, J. G.: Obstetrical paralysis with dislocation of the shoulder. J. Bone Joint Surg., 35-A:227, 1953.

114. Ogden, J. A., Phillips, S. B., and Conlogue, G. J.: Morphogenesis of the human scapula. In preparation.

115. Simurda, M.: Retrosternal dislocation of the clavicle—a report of four cases with a method of repair. Can. J. Surg., 11:487, 1968.

116. Specht, E. E.: Brachial plexus injury in the newborn. Incidence and prognosis. Clin. Orthop., 110:32, 1975.

117. Tyer, H., Sturrock, W., and Callow, F.: Retrosternal dislocation of the clavicle. J. Bone Joint Surg., 45-B:132, 1963.

118. Wilber, M. C., and Evans, E. B.: Fractures of the scapula. An analysis of forty cases and a review of the literature. J. Bone Joint Surg., 59-A:358, 1977.

119. Zachary, R. B., and Emergy, J. L.: Abdominal splenosis following rupture of a spleen in a boy aged 10 years. Br. J. Surg., 46:415, 1959.

120. Badger, F. G.: Fractures of the lateral condyle of the humerus. J. Bone Joint Surg., 36-B:147, 1954.

121. Bede, W. B., Lefebvre, A. R., and Rosman, M. A.: Fractures of the medial humeral epicondyle in children. Can. J. Surg., 18:137, 1975.

122. Dahl-Iverson, E.: Fracture condylienne humerale interne. Reduction simple, sanglante. Lyon Chir., 33:234, 1936.

123. Dodge, H. S.: Displaced supracondylar fractures of the humerus in children—treatment by Dunlop's traction. J. Bone Joint Surg., 54-A:1408, 1972.

124. Finochietto, R., and Ferre, R. L.: Fractures del codo. Cubito varo posttraumatico. La Prensa Med. Argent., 12:598, 1937.

125. Florio, L., and Maurizo, E.: Meccanismo di produzione delle fratture sovracondiloidee del'omero: contributo su 24 fratture rare. Arch. Putti Chir. Organi. Mov., 20:171, 1965.

126. Flynn, J. C., and Richards, J. F., Jr.: Non-union of minimally displaced fractures of the lateral condyle of the humerus in children. J. Bone Joint Surg., 53-A:1096, 1971.

127. Flynn, J. C., Matthews, J. G., and Benoit, R. L.: Blind pinning of displaced supracondylar fractures of the humerus in children. Sixteen years experience with long-term follow-up. J. Bone Joint Surg. 56-A:263, 1974.

128. Flynn, J. C., Richards, J. F., Jr., and Saltzman, R. T.: Prevention and treatment of non-union of slightly displaced fractures of the lateral humeral condyle in children. J. Bone Joint Surg., 57-A:1087, 1975.

129. Hoyer, A.: Treatment of supracondylar fracture of the humerus by skeletal traction in an abduction splint. J. Bone Joint Surg., 34-A:623, 1952.

130. LaGrange, J., and Rigault, P.: Fractures du condyle externe. Rev. Chir. Orthop., 48:415, 1962.

131. Montgomery, A. H., and Ireland, J.: Traumatic segmentary arterial spasm. J.A.M.A., 105:1741, 1935.

132. Mouchet, A.: Paralysies tardines du nerf cubital a la suite des fractures du condyle externe de l'humerus. J. Chir. (Paris), 12:437, 1914.

133. Omer, G. E., Jr., and Simmons, J. W.: Fracture of the distal humeral metaphyseal growth plate. South. Med. J., 61:651, 1968.

134. Ramsey, R. H., and Griz, J.: Immediate open reduction and internal fixation of severely displaced supracondylar fractures of the humerus in children. Clin. Orthop., 90:130, 1973.

135. Rohl, L.: On fractures through the radial condyle of the humerus in children. Acta Chir. Scand., 104:74, 1953.

136. Arnold, J. A., Nasca, R. J., and Nelson, C. L.: Supracondylar fractures of the humerus. The role of dynamic factors in prevention of deformity. J. Bone Joint Surg., 59-A:386, 1977.

137. Graham, H. A.: Supracondylar fractures of the elbow in children. Part I. Clin. Orthop., 54:85, 1967.

138. Graham, H. A.: Supracondylar fractures of the elbow in children. Part II. Clin. Orthop., 54:93, 1967.

139. Rang, M.: Children's Fractures. Philadelphia, J. B. Lippincott, 1974.

140. Ashbell, T. S., Kleinert, H. E., and Kutz, J. E.: Vascular injuries about the elbow. Clin. Orthop., 50:107, 1967.

141. Fahey, J., and O'Brien, E.: Fracture separation of the medial humeral condyle in a child contused with fracture of the medial epicondyle. J. Bone Joint Surg., 53-A:1102, 1971.

142. Eid, A. M.: Reduction of displaced supracondylar fracture of the humerus in children by manipulation in flexion. Acta Orthop. Scand., 49:39, 1978.

143. Ekesparre, W. V.: Treatment of supracondylar fractures of the humerus in the child. Ann. Chir. Infant., 11:213, 1970.

144. Carli, C.: Wire traction for supracondylar fracture of the elbow in children. Chir. Organi. Mov., 18:311, 1933.

145. Dunlop, J.: Transcondylar fractures of the humerus in childhood. J. Bone Joint Surg., 21:59, 1939.

146. Edman, P., and Lohr, G.: Supracondylar fractures of the humerus treated with olecranon traction. Acta Chir. Scand., 126:505, 1963.

147. Staples, O. S.: Complications of traction treatment of supracondylar fracture of the humerus in children. J. Bone Joint Surg., 41-A:369, 1959.

148. Hagen, R.: Skin-traction-treatment of supracondylar fractures of the humerus in children. Acta Orthop. Scand., 35:138, 1964.

149. Haddad, R. J., Jr., Saer, K. J., and Riordan, D. C.: Percutaneous pinning of displaced supracondylar fractures of the elbow in children. Clin. Orthop., 71:112, 1970.

150. Swenson, A. L.: The treatment of supracondylar fractures of the humerus by Kirschner-wire fixation. J. Bone Joint Surg. 30-A:993, 1948.

151. Bergenfeldt, E.: Uber Schaden an der Epiphysenfuge bei operativer Behandlung von Frakturen am unteren Humerusende. Acta Chir. Scand., 71:103, 1932.

152. Carcassone, M., Bergoin, M., and Hornung, H.: Results of operative treatment of severe supracondylar fractures of the elbow in children. J. Pediatr. Surg., 7:676, 1972.

153. Casiano, E.: Reduction and fixation by pinning "banderillero" style, fractures of the humerus in children. Milit. Med., 125:363, 1960.

154. This reference has been deleted.

155. This reference has been deleted.

156. Fowles, J. V., and Kassab, M. T.: Displaced supracondylar fractures of the humerus in children. A report on the fixation of extension and flexion fractures by two lateral percutaneous pins. J. Bone Joint Surg., 56-B:490, 1974.

157. Gruber, M. A., and Hudson, O. C.: Supracondylar fractures of the humerus in childhood. End-result study of open reduction. J. Bone Joint Surg., 46-A:1245, 1964.

158. Huegel, A., and Bijan, A.: Zur dringlichen primar-operativen Versorgung kindlicher suprakondylarer Oberarmfrakturen. Klin. Chir., 221:633, 1974.

159. Shifren, P. G., Gehring, H. W., and Iglesias, L. J.: Open reduction and internal fixation of displaced supracondylar fractures of the humerus in children. Orthop. Clin. North Am., 7:573, 1976.

160. Weiland, A. J., et al.: Surgical treatment of displaced supracondylar fractures of the humerus in children. J. Bone Joint Surg., 60-A:657, 1978.

161. Windfeld, P., and Pilgaard, S.: Osteosyntese af suprakondylare humerus frakturer hos born. Nord. Med., 66:1266, 1961.

162. Hart, G. M., Wilson, D. W., and Arden, G. P.: The operative management of the difficult supracondylar fracture of the humerus in the child. Injury, 9:30, 1977.

163. Alonso-Llames, M.: Bilaterotricipital approach to the elbow. Its application in the osteosynthesis of supracondylar fractures of the humerus in children. Acta Orthop. Scand., 43:479, 1972.

164. Arino, V. L., et al.: Percutaneous fixation of supracondylar fractures of the humerus in children. J. Bone Joint Surg., 59-A:914, 1977.

164a. Attenborough, C. G.: Remodeling of the humerus after supracondylar fractures in childhood. J. Bone Joint Surg., 35-B:386, 1953.

165. Klinefelter, E. W.: Influence of position on measurement of projected bone angle. A.J.R., 55:722, 1946.

166. Smith, F. M.: An eighty-four year follow-up on a patient with ununited fracture of the lateral condyle of the humerus. J. Bone Joint Surg., 55-A:378, 1973.

167. Bakalim, G., and Wilppula, E.: Supracondylar humerus fractures in children. Causes of changes in the carrying angle of the elbow. Acta Orthop. Scand., 43:366, 1972.

168. French, P. R.: Varus deformity of the elbow following supracondylar fractures of the humerus in children. Lancet. 1:439, 1959.

169. King, D., and Secor, C.: Bow elbow (cubitus varus). J. Bone Joint Surg., 33-A:572, 1951.

170. Langenskiöld, A., and Kivilaakso, R.: Varus and valgus deformity of the elbow following supracondylar fracture of the humerus. Acta Orthop. Scand., 38:313, 1967.

171. D'Ambrosia, R. D.: Supracondylar fractures of humerus-prevention of cubitus varus. J. Bone Joint Surg., 54-A:60, 1972.

171a. Alonso-Llames, M., Diaz Peletier, R., and Moro Martin, A.: The correction of post-traumatic cubitus varus by hemi-wedge osteotomy. Int. Orthop., 2:215, 1978.

172. El-Ahwany, M. D.: Supracondylar fractures of the humerus in children with a note on the surgical correction of late cubitus varus. Injury, 6:45, 1973–75.

173. Kagan, N., and Herold, H. Z.: Correction of axial deviations after supracondylar fractures of the humerus in children. Int. Surg., 58:735, 1973.

174. Milch, H.: Treatment of humeral cubitus valgus. Clin. Orthop., *38:*120, 1965.

175. Fevre, M., and Judet, J.: Traitement de sequelles de la maladie de Volkmann. Rev. Chir. Orthop., *43:*437, 1957.

176. Schink, W.: Die Fractura supracondylica humeri und die ischamische Kontraktur im Kindesalter. Chirung.,*39:*417,1968.

177. Wray, J.: Management of supracondylar fracture with vascular insufficiency. Arch. Surg., *90:*279, 1965.

178. Cregan, J. C. F.: Prolonged traumatic arterial spasm after supracondylar fracture of the humerus. J. Bone Joint Surg., *33-B:*363, 1951.

179. Spear, H. C., and Janes, J. M.: Rupture of the brachial artery accompanying dislocation of the elbow or supracondylar fracture. J. Bone Joint Surg., *33-A:*889, 1951.

180. Staples, O. S.: Dislocation of the brachial artery. A complication of supracondylar fracture of the humerus in childhood. J. Bone Joint Surg., *47-A:*1525, 1965.

181. Ottolenghi, C. E.: Prophylaxie du syndrome de Volkmann dans des fractures supracondyliennes du coude chez l'enfant. Rev. Chir. Orthop., *57:*517, 1971.

182. Bailey, G. G., Jr.: Nerve injuries in supracondylar fractures of the humerus in children. N. Engl. J. Med., *221:*260, 1939.

183. Holmes, J. C., Skolnick, M. D., and Hall, J. E.: Untreated median-nerve entrapment in bone after fracture of the distal end of the humerus: postmortem findings after forty-seven years. J. Bone Joint Surg., *61-A:*309, 1979.

184. Hordegen, K. M.: Neurologische Komplikationen bei kindlichen Suprakondylaren Humerusfrakturen. Arch. Orthop. Unfallchir., *68:*294, 1970.

185. Lugnegard, H., Walheim, G., and Wennberg, A.: Operative treatment of ulnar nerve neuropathy in the elbow region. Acta Orthop. Scand., *18:*176, 1977.

186. Post, M., and Haskell, S. S.: Reconstruction of the median nerve following entrapment in supracondylar fracture of the humerus. J. Trauma, *14:*252, 1974.

187. Spinner, M., and Schreiber, S.: Anterior interosseous nerve paralysis—a complication of supracondylar fracture of the humerus in children. J. Bone Joint Surg., *51-A:*1584, 1969.

188. Symeonides, P. P., Paschaloglou, C., and Pagalides, T.: Radial nerve enclosed in the callus of a supracondylar fracture. J. Bone Joint Surg., *57-B:*523, 1975.

189. Vanderpool, D. W., et al.: Peripheral compression lesions of the ulnar nerve. J. Bone Joint Surg., *50-B:*792, 1968.

190. Rettig, H.: Frakturen im Kindesalter. Munich, Verlag-Bergmann, 1957.

191. Levai, J. P., et al.: Un cas de luxation posterieure recidivante du conde liee a un cal vicieux de la palette humerale. Rev. Chir. Orthop., *65:*457, 1979.

192. Heuter, C.: Anatomische Studien an der Extremitatengelenken Neugeborner und Erwachsener. Virchows Arch., *25:*572, 1862.

193. Chand, K.: Epiphyseal separation of distal humeral epiphysis in an infant. J. Trauma, *14:*521, 1974.

194. Cothay, D. M.: Injury to the lower medial epiphysis of the humerus before development of the ossific center. J. Bone Joint Surg., *49-B:*766, 1967.

195. DeLee, J. C., et al.: Fracture-separation of the distal humeral epiphysis. J. Bone Joint Surg., *62-A:*46, 1980.

196. Holda, M. E., Manoli, A., and LaMont, R. L.: Epiphyseal separation of the distal end of the humerus with medial displacement. J. Bone Joint Surg., *62-A:*52, 1980.

197. Judet, J.: Traitment des fractures sus-condyliennes transversales de l'humerus chez l'enfant. Rev. Chir. Orthop., *39:*199, 1953.

198. Kaplan, S. S., and Reckling, F. W.: Fracture separation of the lower humeral epiphysis with medial displacement. J. Bone Joint Surg., *53-A:*1105, 1971.

199. Marmor, L., and Bechtol, C. O.: Fracture separation of the lower humeral epiphysis. Report of a case. J. Bone Joint Surg., *42-A:*333, 1960.

199a. LaGrange, J., and Rigault, P.: Les fractures de l'extremite inferieure de l'humerus chez l'enfant. Rev. Chir. Orthop., *48:*4, 1962.

200. Mauer, I., Kolovos, D., and Loscos, R.: Epiphyseolysis of the distal humerus in a newborn. Bull. Hosp. Joint Dis., *28:*109, 1967.

201. Mizuno, K., Hirohata, K., and Kashiwagi, D.: Fracture-separation of the distal humerus in young children. J. Bone Joint Surg., *61-A:*570, 1979.

202. Rogers, L. F., and Rockwood, C. A., Jr.: Separation of the entire distal humeral epiphysis. Radiology, *106:*393, 1973.

203. Siffert, R. S.: Displacement of the distal humeral epiphysis in the newborn infant. J. Bone Joint Surg., *45-A:*165, 1963.

204. Smyth, E. H. J.: Primary rupture of brachial artery and median nerve in supracondylar fracture of the humerus. J. Bone Joint Surg., *38-B:*736, 1956.

205. Chacha, P. B.: Fracture of the medial condyle of the humerus with rotational displacement. J. Bone Joint Surg., *52-A:*1453, 1970.

206. Ghawabi, M.: Fracture of the medial condyle of the humerus. J. Bone Joint Surg., *57-A:*677, 1975.

207. Ingersoll, R. E.: Fractures of the humeral condyles in children. Clin. Orthop., *41:*32, 1965.

208. Kilfoyle, R. M.: Fractures of the humeral condyles in children. Clin. Orthop., *41:*43, 1965.

209. Pollosson, E., and Arnulf, G.: Fracture du condyle interne-Reposition sanglante. Lyon Chir., *34:*337, 1937.

210. Potter, C. M. C.: Fracture-dislocation of the trochlea. J. Bone Joint Surg., *36-B:*250, 1954.

211. Speed, J. S., and Macey, H. B.: Fractures of the humeral condyles in children. J. Bone Joint Surg., *15:*903, 1933.

212. Hasner, E., and Husby, J.: Fracture of epicondyle and condyle of humerus. Acta Chir. Scand., *101:*195, 1951.

213. Higgs, S.: Fractures of the internal epicondyle of the humerus. Br. Med. J., *2:*666, 1936.

214. Roberts, N. W.: Displacement of the internal epicondyle into the elbow joint. Lancet, *2:*78, 1934.

215. Wilson, J. N.: The treatment of fractures of the medial epicondyle of the humerus. J. Bone Joint Surg., *42-B:*778, 1960.

216. Aitken, A. P., and Childress, H. M.: Intraarticular displacement of internal epicondyle following dislocation. J. Bone Joint Surg., *20:*161, 1938.

217. Patrick, J.: Fracture of the medial epicondyle with displacement into the elbow joint. J. Bone Joint Surg., *28:*143, 1946.

218. Conner, A. N., and Smith, M. G. H.: Displaced fractures of the lateral humeral condyle in children. J. Bone Joint Surg., *52-B:*460, 1970.

219. Crabbe, W.: The treatment of fracture-separation of the capitular epiphysis. J. Bone Joint Surg., *45-B:*722, 1963.

220. Fontanetta, P., MacKenzie, D. A., and Rosman, M.: Missed, maluniting, and malunited fractures of the lateral humeral condyle in children. J. Trauma, *18:*329, 1978.

221. Freeman, R. H.: Fractures of the lateral humeral condyle. J. Bone Joint Surg., *41-B:*631, 1959.

222. Hardacre, J., et al.: Fractures of the lateral condyle of the humerus in children. J. Bone Joint Surg., *53-A:*1083, 1971.

223. Holst-Nielsen, F., and Ottsen, P.: Fractures of the lateral condyle of the humerus in children. Acta Orthop. Scand., *45:*518, 1974.

224. Jakob, R., et al.: Observations concerning fractures of the lateral humeral condyle in children. J. Bone Joint Surg. *57-B:*430, 1975.

225. Kalenak, A.: Ununited fracture of the lateral condyle of the humerus. A fifty year follow-up. Clin. Orthop., *124:*181, 1977.

226. Kini, M. G.: Fractures of the lateral condyle of the lower end of the humerus with complications. A simple technique for closed reduction of the capitellar fracture. J. Bone Joint Surg., *24:*270, 1942.

227. Milch, H.: Fractures of the external humeral condyle. J.A.M.A., *160:*641, 1956.

228. This reference has been deleted.

229. Wadsworth, T. G.: Injuries of the capitular (lateral humeral condylar) epiphysis. Clin. Orthop., *85:*127, 1972.

230. Wilson, J. N.: Fractures of the external condyle of the humerus in children. Br. J. Surg., *43:*88, 1955.

231. Wilson, P. D.: Fracture of the lateral condyle of the humerus in childhood. J. Bone Joint Surg., *18:*301, 1936.

232. Haraldsson, S.: On osteochondrosis deformans juvenilis capituli humeri including investigation of the intra-osseous vasculature in distal humerus. Acta Orthop. Scand. [Suppl.], *38:*1959.

232a. Jeffrey, C. C.: Non-union of the epiphysis of the lateral condyle of the humerus. J. Bone Joint Surg., *40-B:*396, 1958.

233. McKibbin, B., and Holdsworth, F.: The dual nature of epiphyseal cartilage. J. Bone Joint Surg., *49-B:*351, 1967.

234. Magilligan, D. J.: Unusual regeneration of bone in a child. J. Bone Joint Surg., *28:*873, 1946.

235. Wadsworth, T. G.: Premature epiphyseal fusion after injury to the capitulum. J. Bone Joint Surg., *46-B:*46, 1964.

236. Voshell, A. F., and Taylor, K. P. A.: Regeneration of the lateral condyle of the humerus after excision. J. Bone Joint Surg., *21:*421, 1939.

237. Gay, J. R., and Love, J. G.: Diagnosis and treatment of tardy paralysis of the ulnar nerve—based on a study of 100 cases. J. Bone Joint Surg., *29:*1087, 1947.

238. Harrison, M. J. G., and Nurick, S.: Results of anterior transposition of the ulnar nerve for ulnar neuritis. Br. Med. J., *1:*27, 1970.

239. Holmes, J. C., and Hall, J. E.: Tardy ulnar nerve palsy in children. Clin. Orthop., *135:*128, 1978.

240. Adams, J., and Rizzoli, H.: Tardy radial and ulnar nerve palsy. J. Neurosurg., *16:*342, 1959.

11

Elbow

Anatomy

Much of the chondro-osseous anatomy of the elbow, particularly the variability of development of the epiphyseal ossification centers around it, is covered in Chapters 10 (Humerus) and 12 (Radius and Ulna). The development of these ossification centers may be irregular, and they must not be confused with acute fracture, osteochondritis, or elbow lesions encountered in adolescent athletes (Fig. 11-1).[1,2]

The elbow joint is a tightly constrained hinge joint. The ligaments attach to various points around the distal humeral metaphysis and epiphysis, particularly the epicondyles. In contrast, the distal attachments are to the ulnar and radial metaphyses (Fig. 11-2). Deforming forces tend to be transmitted away from the joint to the proximal third of the radial and ulnar shafts, or to the distal humerus. This usually results in radioulnar shaft, supracondylar metaphyseal, or transcondylar physeal fractures, rather than elbow joint dis-

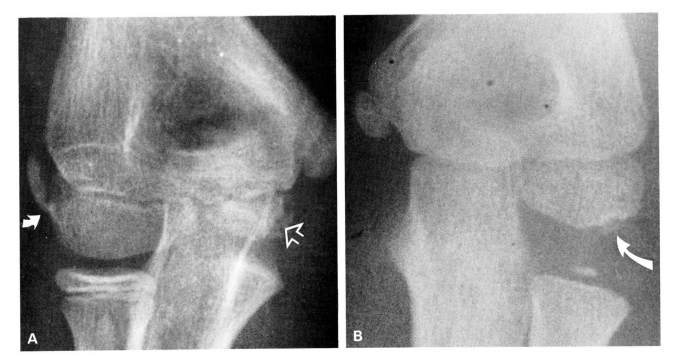

FIG. 11-1. *A,* Traumatized elbow of a 12-year-old girl with elbow pain. The trochlear ossification center is irregular (open arrow), but this is a normal developmental variation. The lateral epicondyle appears to be separating from the contiguous metaphysis. However, this is also a normal roentgenographic appearance. Further, this epicondyle is beginning to fuse with the capitellum (solid arrow), an occurrence which lessens the likelihood of avulsion during elbow dislocation. *B,* Injured elbow of a 6-year-old boy showing irregular ossification of the capitellum (arrow). This is a normal variant and should not be interpreted as a lateral injury or traumatic osteochondrosis. In an older child, similar roentgenographic findings might suggest Panner's disease.

283

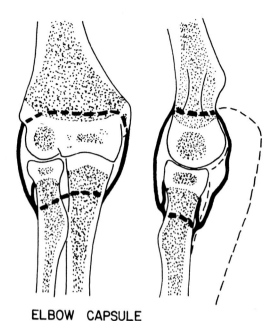

ELBOW CAPSULE

FIG. 11-2. Schematic of elbow capsular/ligamentous attachments in an eight-year-old. These attachments change slightly with chondro-osseous development. The medial and lateral capsules and ligaments are relatively tight in extension, but become relaxed in flexion. The anterior and posterior elements have more redundancy to allow for flexion and extension. The ulna is outlined by the narrow dashed line in the lateral view.

locations. While a roentgenogram in an infant or young child may show an apparent elbow dislocation (an easy interpretation if secondary ossification centers have not appeared), the elbow joint per se is really completely intact. Because distal humeral physeal failure (usually a type 1 injury) is more likely than ligamentous disruption in a young child, the entire elbow unit, including distal humeral epiphysis, radius, and ulna is displaced as an intact unit.

Dislocation

Dislocations, which probably constitute as much as 5 to 6% of all elbow injuries in children, appear to be the most common joint dislocations in children. They are increasingly frequent after 10 years of age. While the injury usually follows a fall on the outstretched hand with the elbow incompletely flexed, dislocation also may occur as a hyperextension injury.

The direction of displacement varies with the direction of the deforming force. Posterior displacement, usually accompanied by some lateral displacement, is most common. Rotatory luxation with total displacement of one forearm bone and part of the other may occur in the posterior type when only one collateral ligament is torn. Divergent dislocation of the radius and ulna is extremely rare in the child. Anterior dislocation is also rare.

The complex association of axial and rotatory forces causes not only capsular and ligamentous disruptions, but

also a wide variety of concomitant chondro-osseous injuries. Pure dislocation, unaccompanied by fracture, is unusual in children. Always look for an associated fracture. Frequently, there may be occult separation of the medial epicondyle. Less frequently, the lateral condyle or epicondyle may be fractured. Also, multiple injuries may occur in the same arm, with distal radioulnar fractures being relatively common (Fig. 11-3). Complete examination of the injured extremity and sufficiently detailed pre- and post-reduction films are essential to diagnosis of these associated injuries.

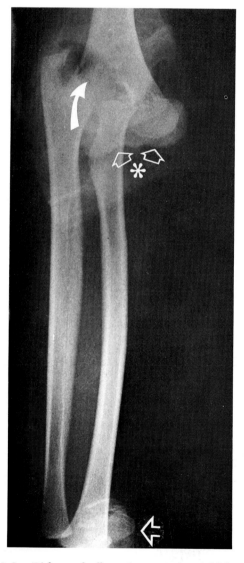

FIG. 11-3. Dislocated elbow in a ten-year-old boy. This roentgenogram focused on the compound injury with a total laceration of the brachial artery (also see Fig. 11-19). The solid arrow indicates the intra-articular air present because of the open wound. Note how the air-cartilage interface has outlined the cartilaginous components of the capitellum and trochlea (*, arrows). A concomitant fracture of the distal radius was also present (open arrow), but was barely visible on the roentgenogram, which had been centered specifically on the elbow region.

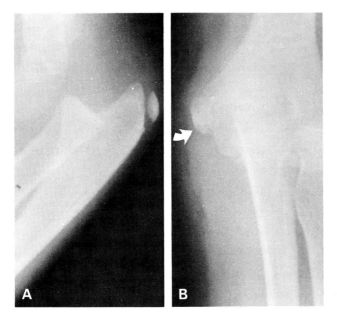

FIG. 11-4. *A,* Lateral and, *B,* anterior views of posterior dislocation in a nine-year-old. The medial epicondyle is fractured, but undisplaced (arrow).

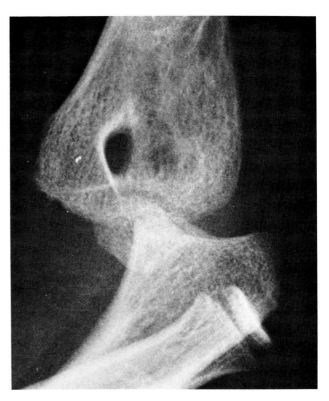

FIG. 11-5. Anterior view of posterior dislocation, without accompanying, roentgenographically obvious chondroosseous injury. If the medial epicondyle has not yet formed a secondary ossification center, diagnosis of injury must be conjectural, based on indications from clinical findings.

Dislocation of the elbow is unusual in children under one year of age. Instead, they usually sustain a fracture of the distal humeral physis; this leads to a complete posterolateral or posteromedial shift of the radiolucent distal humeral epiphysis that is easily misinterpreted as an elbow dislocation (see Fig. 8-3). Diagnosis must be accurate, since treatment of fracture and dislocation differ significantly.

Because of the hazard of concomitant neurovascular injuries, reduction frequently becomes an urgent matter.[3-8] The complete neurovascular status at and distal to the injured elbow must be routinely ascertained before reduction, particularly in view of the potential for entrapment of the median nerve or stretching of the ulnar nerves. The same, careful neurovascular evaluation must also be carried out after reduction.

Classification

Several types of elbow dislocation occur in children. They include: (1) posterior dislocation of the radius and ulna (Figs. 11-4 and 11-5); (2) posterior dislocation of the radius and ulna with fracture of the coronoid process (Fig. 11-6); (3) posterior dislocation of the radius and ulna with separation of part or all of the medial epicondyle (Fig. 11-7). The epicondylar fragment may completely displace into the elbow joint (Fig. 11-8); (4) posterior displacement of the radius and ulna with fracture of the radial head or neck (Fig. 11-9); (5) any elbow dislocation with a fracture of the olecranon (Fig. 11-10); (6) lateral dislocation of the radius and the ulna with fracture of the lateral epicondyle of the humerus (Fig. 11-11); (7) divergent dislocation of the proximal radius and ulna (Fig. 11-12);[8a] and (8) anterior or anterolateral displacement of the radius with a fracture of the upper third of the ulnar shaft and a Monteggia fracture dislocation (see Chap. 12).

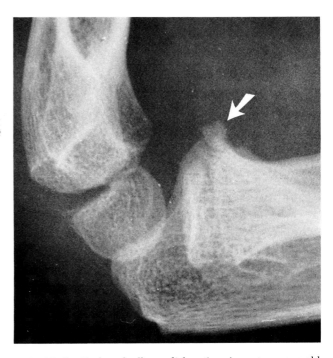

FIG. 11-6. Reduced elbow dislocation in a ten-year-old showing concomitant fracture of the coronoid process of the ulna (arrow).

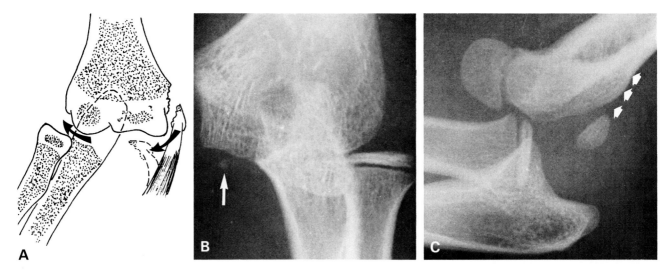

FIG. 11-7. *A,* Schematic of posterior dislocation with concomitant avulsion of medial epicondyle, which may be pulled into the joint. *B,* Posterolateral dislocation with small fragment of epicondyle (arrow). Such small fragments may be missed on initial evaluation. *C,* Posterior displacement of medial epicondyle. Posteromedial soft tissue attachments are still intact (arrows), and may allow satisfactory closed reduction without a need for pin fixation of the epicondyle.

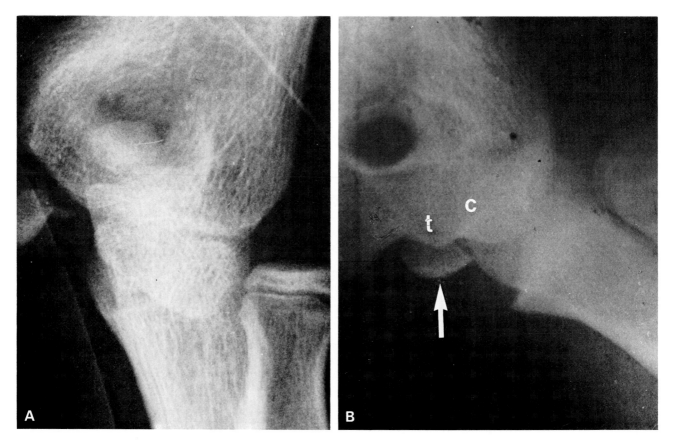

FIG. 11-8. *A,* Anteroposterior view showing moderate displacement of the medial epicondyle. This degree of soft tissue and chondro-osseous disruption may increase the likelihood of intra-articular entrapment following reduction. *B,* Severe posterolateral displacement with medial epicondylar avulsion. The epicondyle is pulled into the joint (arrow) and rests at the junction of the capitellum (c) and the trochlea (t). When reduction was attempted, the epicondyle was trapped in the joint. Open reduction was necessary.

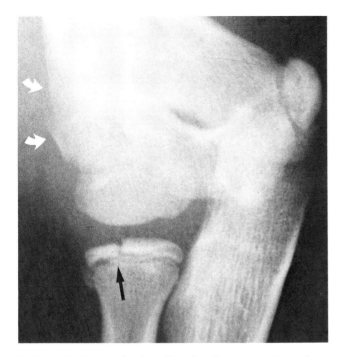

FIG. 11-9. Post-reduction film showing concomitant fracture of the radial epiphyseal ossification center (black arrow). Such a growth mechanism injury (type 4) is unusual in the radial head. The extent of medial ligamentous disruption is evidenced by the degree of cubitus valgus on this film. Lateral periosteal/ligamentous stripping has caused subperiosteal new bone formation (white arrows).

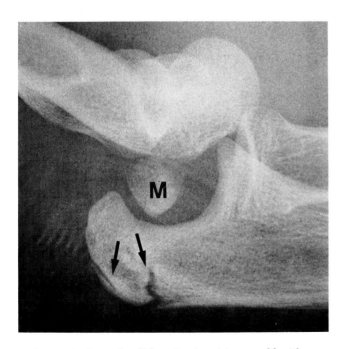

FIG. 11-10. Posterior dislocation in a 14-year-old with concomitant olecranon fractures (arrows). One fracture line initially involved the closing physis, but then extended into the joint. The medial epicondyle (M) has been displaced posteriorly.

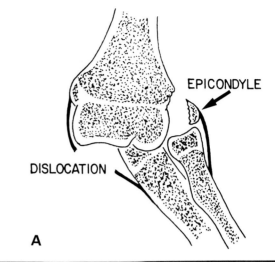

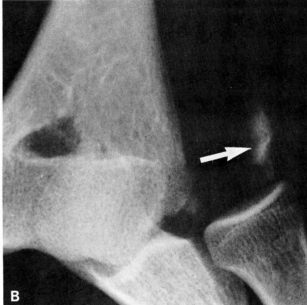

FIG. 11-11. A, Schematic of lateral displacement with concomitant fracture of the lateral epicondyle. B, Dislocation and lateral epicondylar fracture (arrow) in a 15-year-old girl.

Pathomechanics

Posterior dislocation usually results from a fall on the outstretched hand with the forearm supinated and the elbow extended or partially flexed. The force of the fall is transmitted along the forearm to the trochlear notch and the coronoid process. The coronoid process, which normally resists posterior displacement of the ulna, is easily deformed in children because it is incompletely ossified. The laterally sloping surface of the inner ⅔ of the trochlea converts the vertical thrust into a lateral rotation and partial valgus strain. The anterior capsule of the elbow joint is torn by the force of the impact as it is transmitted upward through the ulna and radius. The upper end of the ulna is displaced backward and then swung laterally. Collateral ligaments are stretched or ruptured. On the outer side of the joint, the lateral ligament

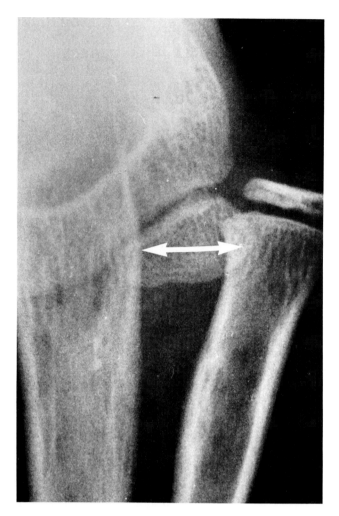

FIG. 11-12. Divergent dislocation. There is dislocation not only of the elbow joint, but also of the proximal radioulnar joint (arrow), leading to separation of the radius and ulna. This damages the annular ligament significantly and may require open reduction and repair of the ligament. This injury is analogous to a Monteggia injury.

and capsule are attenuated or stripped superiorly and the posterolateral capsule is torn, allowing the radial head to rotate backward from the capitellar surface (Figs. 11-13 and 11-14).

In simple posterolateral dislocations, damage also occurs to the medial side of the capsule, with considerable bruising and swelling often present on the medial side of the joint. The medial epicondyle may be detached in children, and the medial ligament stretched or ruptured. However, after reduction it is not always possible to strain the joint into valgus. This indicates that the ligaments retain relative continuity with the periosteum, even though the actual attachment may have been stripped from the bone.

The forearm bones may be laterally or medially displaced to varying degrees, depending on the extent of injury to the radial and ulnar collateral ligaments. Without damage to the ulnar collateral ligament, continued valgus stress may avulse the medial epicondyle, displacing this fragment along with

forearm bones (see Fig. 11-8). The lateral ligament may be torn at its upper attachment, but only rarely is there an accompanying detachment of a fragment of the lateral epicondyle. The posterior part of the capsule, particularly the part behind the lateral ligament, may be torn from its superior attachment (see Fig. 11-14).

The radius and ulna, being firmly bound by the annular ligament and interosseous membrane, are displaced posteriorly together. The coronoid process of the ulna becomes locked in the olecranon fossa of the posterior distal humerus.

Since most capsular damage, even when medial and lateral ligaments are involved, is anterior to the epicondyles, and since the medial epicondyle stays attached to the posterosuperior periosteal/perichondrial tissue (which may be stripped extensively from the distal humeral metaphysis), the ulnar nerve is rarely mobile enough to be displaced into the joint. Even when the epicondyle is displaced into the joint, the ulnar nerve usually stays attached to the soft tissue.

Anterior dislocation, which usually is caused by a direct blow or fall on the olecranon process, occurs infrequently in children.

Diagnosis

The presenting symptoms usually are a painful, swollen, deformed elbow that may be held in partial flexion and supported by the opposite hand because of extreme discomfort. Attempted motion of the elbow is usually painful and restricted, with marked muscle spasm. From an anterior view, the forearm appears shortened. Most physical findings are obscured by the marked soft tissue swelling. Again, as in assessment of injuries to the supracondylar region, it is imperative that the neurovascular function of the forelimb be closely assessed to determine damage to the brachial artery and the ulnar, radial, and median nerves.

The diagnosis is made most easily roentgenographically. Roentgenograms *always* must be made prior to treatment to rule out the presence of associated fractures of the epicondyles, coronoid process, proximal radius and ulna, or lateral condyle. Furthermore, an apparent dislocation may be found, upon clinical examination, to be a supracondylar or transcondylar fracture.

Treatment

Reduction of an acute posterior dislocation usually may be accomplished without general anesthesia. Associated fractures may occur, including separation of the medial epicondyle. Prior knowledge of lateral rotation and displacement is useful in the reduction, since initial hypersupination may be necessary to free the head of the radius and the coronoid process.

A gentle and effective reduction method is as follows. Place the patient in the prone position with the injured limb hanging over the edge of the table. The weight of the arm provides distal traction. Encircle the arm to give countertraction and push the olecranon downward and forward (Fig. 11-15). Following reduction, the elbow should be acutely flexed as much as swelling will permit without causing neurocirculatory impairment. An alternative method of reduction is hyperextension, subsequent downward traction

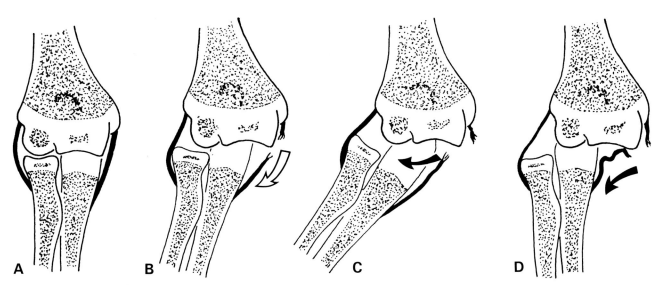

FIG. 11-13. Schematic of mechanics of elbow dislocation.

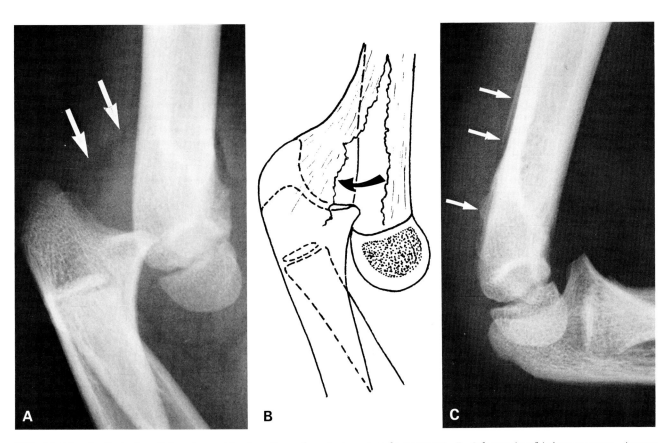

FIG. 11-14. *A,* Posterior dislocation with elevation of posterior capsule (arrows). *B,* Schematic of injury pattern. Arrow indicates posterior periosteal sleeve. *C,* Four weeks post-reduction, subperiosteal new bone is evident where the capsule/periosteal unit had been traumatically stripped.

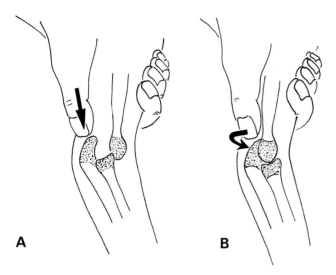

FIG. 11-15. Schematic of reduction utilizing elbow flexion. Posterior pressure is applied directly to the olecranon.

and final flexion (Fig. 11-16). Open reduction is indicated if closed reduction is unsuccessful, or in a chronic dislocation several days to weeks old.

In most cases, the presence of the epicondyle in the joint is an indication for open reduction in order to reduce the epicondyle satisfactorily and fix it with pins. The fragment must be removed from the joint or it impedes reduction and subsequent function.

Roentgenographic confirmation of reduction is essential, since swelling may lead to a false impression that complete reduction has been attained (Fig. 11-17).

Unreduced dislocations

Allende reported a series of chronic, untreated dislocations of the elbow.[9] He felt that any acute elbow dislocation that had not been reduced by 3 weeks could not be reduced satisfactorily by closed, manipulative reduction. He described 31 cases of chronic dislocations of the elbow in children and reported various operative methods of reduction.

The major problem is soft tissue contracture, particularly in the triceps, since the elbow has usually been held in extension.[9a] Often, it is impossible to reduce these adequately and still have full length in the triceps. The tendinous portion must be lengthened. There usually is fibrous pannus within the joint, and this has to be removed from the olecranon region to permit adequate reduction.

If the dislocation remains for several months to years, the distal humerus may progressively deform, as may the proximal radius and the ulna (Fig. 11-18). Undoubtedly, such deformations result from lack of normal joint reaction forces. The younger the child (i.e., the greater the amount of cartilage), the more likely it is that an alteration of morphology will occur. The longer the elbow remains dislocated, the greater the likelihood that reduction will be impossible owing to both altered morphology and soft tissue contractures.

Complications

Wheeler reported vascular complications in 8 of 110 elbow dislocations.[10] These are generally associated with more violent injuries, particularly open ones (Fig. 11-19). The severity of injury to the brachial artery can vary from simple contusion or spasm to laceration, rupture, or subintimal hemorrhage. Any discrete vascular injuries should be repaired, as indicated, following diagnosis by either direct observation (if the wound is compound) or arteriography.

Spear suggested that vascular injury was rare if a pure dislocation occurred, but that it became more likely if fractures were also present.[11] In one of the cases he cites, hemorrhage into the closed antecubital space produced sufficient tension to cause forearm ischemia.

Volkmann's ischemic contracture also may complicate posterior dislocation of the elbow when the brachial artery has been injured. Following closed reduction, depending upon the severity of the trauma and the extent of soft tissue swelling, it may be wise to admit the child to the hospital for observation for 24 to 48 hours.

Nerve injury is encountered more frequently than vascular injury. Wheeler reported neurologic complications in 24 of 110 elbow dislocations (3 times more neurologic complications than vascular complications were found in their study).[10] The ulnar nerve was involved in 16 of 24 patients,

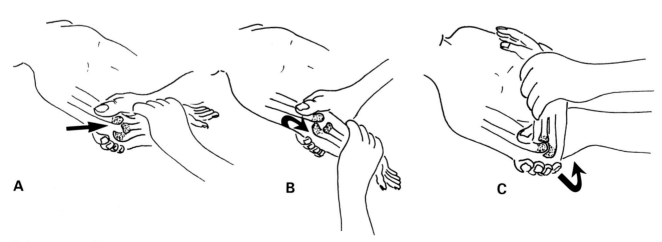

FIG. 11-16. Schematic of reduction utilizing mild elbow hyperextension.

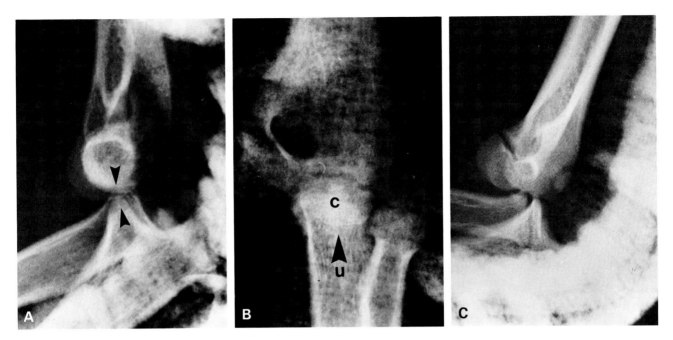

FIG. 11-17. *A,* Post-reduction film showing failure to obtain reduction. The distal humerus is locked on the coronoid process of the ulna (arrows). Subsequent closed reduction was successful. *B-C,* Anteroposterior and lateral films showing ulna (u, arrow) locked behind the capitellum (c). Apparent reductions must always be checked with post-reduction films, since soft tissue swelling may give a false impression of reduction.

the median nerve in 3, and both ulnar and median nerve in 4; the remaining patient sustained a brachial plexus injury. Treatment of neurologic complications should be conservative, as most cases recover spontaneously. The ulnar nerve, being rather firmly anchored in the medial epicondylar groove, is easily damaged in dislocations, particularly if the medial epicondyle is avulsed. Persistent ulnar nerve paralysis should be treated by neurolysis and, if necessary, anterior transposition. Most injuries are contusions or stretching injuries, with no gross disruption of nerve continuity. Rarely is the ulnar nerve displaced into the joint during reduction.

Intra-articular entrapment of the median nerve may occur during dislocation or reduction.[12] Since the medial epicondylar attachments are usually intact, it is assumed that the median nerve loops into the trochleoulnar joint through the torn medial capsule as the forearm is forced into valgus and extension during acute dislocation.[4] It is then trapped in this location during reduction by the flare of the medial condyle of the trochlea (Fig. 11-20). Speculation in another case is that the nerve entrapment was associated with avulsion of the medial epiphysis.[7] All nerves had good return of function after open reduction and removal of the nerve from the joint.[4] To avoid such a rare neurologic complication, Watson-Jones suggested gentle traction on the forearm while it is in the flexed position. He also recommended no hyperextension of the joint preliminary to reduction.[8] Hyperextension is a potentially dangerous reduction procedure, predisposing the median nerve to intra-articular displacement.

Heterotopic bone formation (myositis ossificans) occurs less frequently in children than in adults, but frequently enough to be of concern in children who dislocate the elbow.[13] If it occurs, it may restrict elbow motion. In one series, this complication occurred in 32 of 110 dislocations.

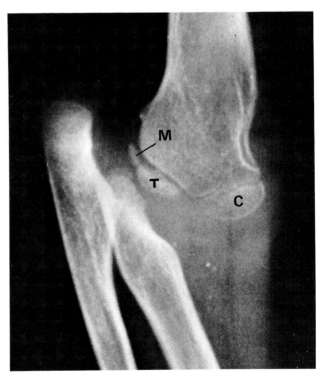

FIG. 11-18. Chronic elbow dislocation in a nine-year-old who had sustained an "injury" to the elbow four years earlier. This had never been treated. Lateral view shows posterior displacement of radius and ulna. Ossification is evident in the capitellum (C), trochlea (T), and medial epicondyle (M).

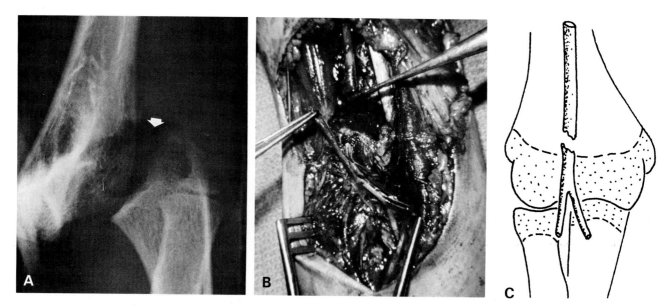

FIG. 11-19. *A*, Compound (open) dislocation of elbow. Note the air in the soft tissue (arrow). *B*, The brachial artery was transected by this injury. Each disrupted end is held by a pair of forceps. *C*, Schematic of injury, showing how arterial disruption was above the joint line, where the artery is relatively fixed by the lacertus fibrosis.

Formation of heterotopic bone usually occurs below the medial or lateral epicondyle along the course of the collateral ligaments (Fig. 11-21). It is generally evident within 3 to 4 weeks after initial injury. Bone also may form in damaged muscle (Fig. 11-22). Large deposits of bone may impair normal joint function. However, children show a predisposition to absorb ectopic calcification before it becomes mature bone, although this may not occur until 6 to 8 months postinjury. If surgical excision is necessary, the best results occur in skeletally immature patients.

An unusual complication of elbow dislocation is proximal radioulnar translocation (Fig. 11-23). During dislocation, the proximal radioulnar soft tissue interrelationships (especially the annular ligament) are apparently disrupted to the point that the two bones become disparate and cross (hyperpronation mechanism). This reversed anatomic relationship remains after reduction. The radial head then articulates with the trochlea, and the ulna with the capitellum. In the only reported case of this complication, an open reduction and restoration of anatomic relationships was undertaken. This required ulnar osteotomy. Ischemic necrosis of the proximal radial epiphyseal ossification appeared to complicate this open reduction.[8a]

Recurrent dislocation

Recurrent dislocation is a rare complication in children.[14] Osborne proposed that the pathologic defect was laxity of the posterolateral ligamentous capsular structures due to failure of spontaneous reattachment following the tear at the time of the original traumatic dislocation.[15] The pathologic defect causing recurrent dislocation appears to be failure of the posterolateral ligamentous and capsular structures that were torn or stretched at the time of dislocation to become reattached. The lateral epicondyle may also develop nonunion. This allows displacement of the radius from its normal articulation with the capitellum (Fig. 11-24). The intact lateral ligament normally would prevent this displacement, but if its superior attachments have been stripped or if it is more lax than normal, the head of the radius is no longer obliged to follow the curve of the capitellum, and at some point in extension, backward slipping of the radius may occur.

Not all patients with recurrent dislocation have complete dislocation. The radial head may subluxate into a capitellar defect or capsular pocket and be reduced easily by the pa-

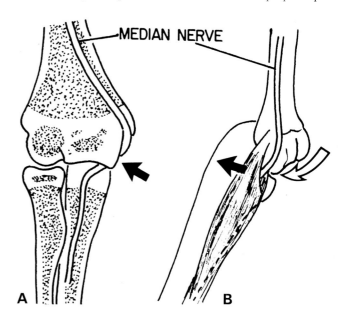

FIG. 11-20. Schematic of nerve entrapment. Even if the epicondyle is not damaged, hyperextension may allow the median nerve to translocate around the trochlea.

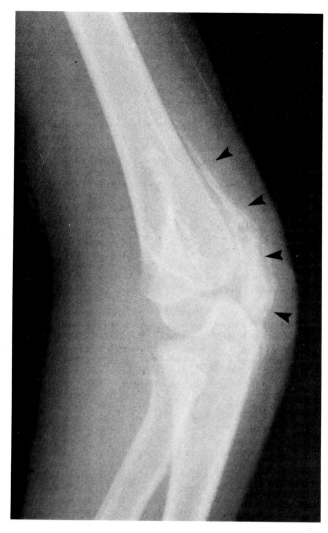

FIG. 11-21. Severe heterotopic ossification (arrows) in the posterior capsular, subperiosteal, and muscular regions following dislocation.

tient, who may complain only of a sensation of locking. Progressive damage to the osteochondral surfaces is often significant. As the head of the radius displaces backward, its edge can strike and abrade the posterolateral margin of the capitellum. An osteochondral fracture may occur. A permanent defect or crater in the posterolateral margin of the capitellum may result, and the edge of the radial head can be damaged. The ulna, especially the coronoid process, may be deformed, and the olecranon process may be deficient (Fig. 11-25). Anterior capsular instability may also contribute to chronic dislocation. Arthrography is useful in diagnosing the lesion, and it may adequately delineate the lesion.[16,17]

Trias strongly advocated the view that chondro-osseous changes, such as the purported congenital hypoplasia of the olecranon, were secondary to ligamentous instability, which was the primary cause of chronic dislocation.[18] However, the normal hyperlaxity of the ligaments of children may also be a significant causal factor.

If recurrent dislocation is infrequent, one should refrain from any operative treatment in childhood, since the normal process of growth is associated with gradual tightening of ligaments and may lead to improved overall stability. Operative treatment is indicated if dislocation recurs following minimal injury in the older child or adolescent. Reattachment of capsule and ligaments to the lateral epicondyle is the most important step in repair of this complication (Fig. 11-26). Other available methods include: (1) transfer of the bicipital tendon to the coronoid process of the ulna, reinforcing the joint anteriorly by an active tenodesis; (2) increase in the depth of the coronoid process by an intra-articular bone graft (which cannot be used effectively in the skeletally immature child in whom this area is still cartilaginous); and (3) repair or reinforcement of soft tissues around the elbow joint, using either fascial strips or tendon strips to reinforce the collateral ligaments.

Nursemaid's Elbow

This condition, which primarily involves the proximal radius and annular ligament, is discussed in Chapter 12.

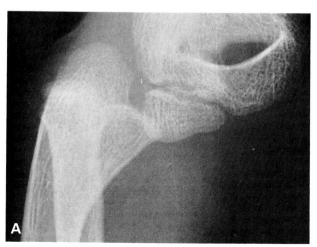
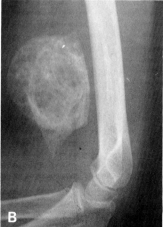
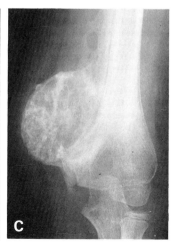

FIG. 11-22. *A,* Complete lateral dislocation in an eight-year-old. *B-C,* Extensive myositis ossificans in the biceps of this child five months later.

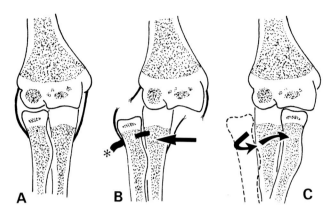

FIG. 11-23. Schematic of translocation of radius and ulna following dislocation, (* = disrupted annular ligament).

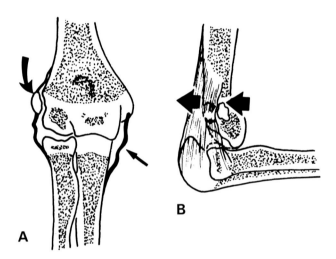

FIG. 11-24. Schematic of recurrent dislocation. *A,* The ligaments are attenuated (small arrow), and the lateral epicondyle does not reattach (large arrow). *B,* This allows chronic posterior displacement (arrows) and leads to progressive deformation of the capitellum and radial head.

Little League Elbow

Throwing a baseball, especially in the way required of juvenile pitchers, is a relatively abnormal activity for the developing arm, and puts an unusual, repetitious strain on the wrist, shoulder, and elbow. The elbow joint is whipped forcefully from acute flexion into complete extension with either pronation or supination of the forearm and ulnar flexion of the wrist, especially if a curve ball is thrown.[19] Throwing a curve ball puts additional traction strain on the medial epicondyle, which is the point of attachment of the pronator and flexor muscles of the forearm. The epiphyses are still open in children of the age groups involved in most organized baseball, so the epicondyle is often subjected to the repeated forceful pull of these muscles.[15] Little league elbow seems to reach its peak in boys at the age of 13 to 14 years.

Adams studied both elbows of 162 boys in the 9 to 14 year age group, dividing them into three categories: pitchers, nonpitchers, and a control group who had never played organized baseball.[20] Changes involving the medial epicondylar epiphysis and opposing articular surfaces of the capitellum and head of the radius in the throwing arm appeared to be directly proportional to the amount and type of throwing. The most striking changes were in the arms of pitchers. Some degree of accelerated growth, separation, and fragmentation of the medial epicondylar epiphysis was noted in the throwing arm of all eight pitchers in the study. Five cases of traumatic osteochondritis of the capitellum and the head of the radius were found. One case of juvenile osteochondritis of the head of the radius was also found among the pitchers. That these conditions develop only in the throwing arms leaves no doubt that the major cause is excessive, repetitious trauma.

Many coaches and managers argue that most sore arms are due to wrong throwing motions or failure to warm-up properly, which is often true in adults. In youngsters, however, regardless of the throwing motion, the nonunited epiphyses are subjected to the pull of the attached muscles. Structurally and histologically epicondylar epiphyses do not seem to be specifically adapted to excessive, forceful, traction stress, as is the tibial tuberosity. The opposing articular surfaces of the joint are also subjected to repetitive trauma from

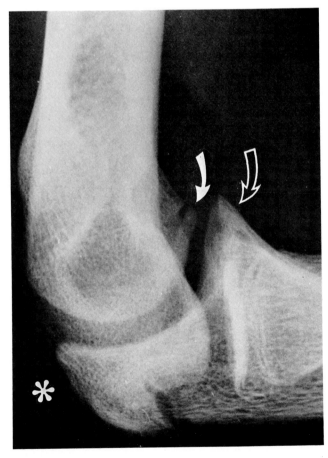

FIG. 11-25. Chronic elbow dislocation in a 15-year-old has resulted in overgrowth of the coronoid process (open arrow), irregularity of the contiguous trochlea (solid arrow), and insufficient development of the olecranon (*).

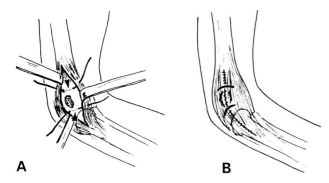

FIG. 11-26.   Schematic of repair for recurrent elbow dislocation.

excessive throwing. Trauma of this kind can eventually bring about osteochondritic changes, exfoliation of the cartilage, and cause loose bodies. Bone chips are commonly found in professional baseball pitchers, but were rarely seen in children before the advent of organized baseball.

Epicondylar trauma may occur without roentgenographically apparent separation; the diagnosis then must be made on clinical grounds. Demonstrable epicondylar separation may be associated with capitellar fragmentation of the ossification center or, in cases of violent motion, dislocation of the elbow joint. Soft tissue injury will be evident. Roentgenograms of the contralateral elbow are extremely helpful in diagnosing minimal separation. They should be obtained in every case, since the epicondyle tends to displace inferiorly, and sometimes enters the elbow joint. Epicondylar separation treated by closed reduction commonly heals by fibrous union, and consequently, roentgenographically demonstrable callus is not always encountered.

Treatment for these conditions is primarily preventive. The following recommendations are in order: (1) alert parents, coaches, administrators, and family physicians that these conditions do exist, and that the presenting symptoms of soreness or pain in this age group indicate "epiphysitis," and should *not* be treated as the muscle soreness routinely encountered in adult pitchers; (2) encourage youngsters to report elbow pain or soreness immediately, and reassure them that doing so does not always mean they cannot play baseball anymore; (3) discourage youngsters from excessive pitching practice, as successive throwing invites trouble rather than perfection; and (4) abolish curve ball throwing for younger age groups, as it not only places additional strain on the elbow, but also encourages excessive practice to perfect it.

Figure 11-27 shows a typical case of little league elbow in a 14-year-old. The patient had persistent pain and discomfort laterally, but did not seek medical care until the arm could not be fully extended. An arthrogram demonstrated defects in the articular cartilage. At arthrotomy, one fragment was found displaced toward the ulna, with the fragment relatively fixed by inflammatory fibrous tissue. Other small fragments were removed, and the defect of the capitellum was drilled to encourage development of fibrocartilaginous repair tissue.

Osteochondral Lesions

The pathogenesis of osteochondral lesions of the elbow still is not completely understood.[21,22] The sex and age of the patient and location and laterality of the lesion all suggest trauma as the cause. Underlying this are the possibilities that either the cartilage fails to ossify or the repair mechanisms in some patients are defective.

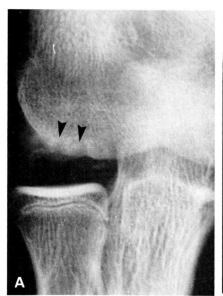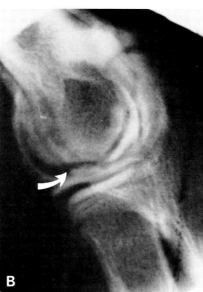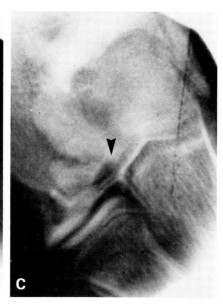

FIG. 11-27.   *A,* Irregularity of capitellum (arrows) in little league pitcher complaining of pain in elbow. Arthrography showed, *B,* a capitellar defect (arrow) and, *C,* a "loose body" (arrow). Surgery revealed that the "loose body" was interfering with complete pronation/supination, and it was fixed in position in the proximal radioulnar joint by scar tissue.

This condition is restricted essentially to males, and it involves the dominant elbow almost exclusively. The majority of patients are first seen when between 9 and 15 years of age, and they complain of dull ache, effusion, and restricted elbow extension.

The capitellum of the humerus consistently is involved; the radial head occasionally is involved. The earliest radiologic lesion is a faint radiolucency of the convexity of the capitellar epiphyseal ossification center adjacent to its radial articulation. Tomography may show the crater (see Fig. 11-27), which eventually will become apparent on plain radiographs. Arthrography may show the cartilage to be normal or irregular. The edges of this fossa are often ragged and sometimes faintly sclerotic. If the fragment is significantly displaced, it can be assumed to be free within the joint. However, if the osseous body is situated in the fossa, arthrography is helpful in determining its mobility and indications for surgery.

The prognosis for healing and recovery is good once any loose fragments have been removed. If all loose bodies are not removed, overgrowth, secondary reactive sclerosis, and cystic changes in the condyle may be seen, and similar findings may be apparent in the radial head, especially overgrowth of the radial head and neck. This latter pattern is often termed Panner's disease.

References

1. Gunn, G.: Patella cubiti. Br. J. Surg., *15:*612, 1927.
2. Zeitlin, A.: The traumatic origin of accessory bones at the elbow. J. Bone Joint Surg., *17:*933, 1935.
3. Cotten, F. J.: Elbow dislocation and ulnar nerve injury. J. Bone Joint Surg., *11:*348, 1929.
4. Mannerfelt, L.: Median nerve entrapment after dislocation of the elbow. J. Bone Joint Surg., *50-B:*152, 1968.
5. Matev, I.: A radiological sign of entrapment of the median nerve in the elbow joint after posterior dislocation. A report of two cases. J. Bone Joint Surg., *58-B:*353, 1976.
6. Pritchard, D. J., Linscheid, R. L., and Svien, H. J.: Intra-articular median nerve entrapment with dislocation of the elbow. Clin. Orthop., *90:*100, 1973.
7. Steiger, R. N., Larrick, R. B., and Meyer, T. L.: Median-nerve entrapment following elbow dislocation in children. J. Bone Joint Surg., *51-A:*381, 1969.
8. Watson-Jones, R.: Primary nerve lesions in injuries of the elbow and wrist. J. Bone Joint Surg., *12:*121, 1930.
8a. Harvey, S., and Tchelebi, H.: Proximal radio-ulnar translocation. J. Bone Joint Surg., *61-A:*447, 1979.
9. Allende, G., and Freytes, M.: Old dislocation of the elbow. J. Bone Joint Surg., *26:*691, 1944.
9a. Silva, J. F.: The problems relating to old dislocation and the restriction of the elbow movement. Acta Orthop. Belg., *41:*399, 1975.
10. Wheeler, D. K., and Linscheid, R. L.: Fracture-dislocations of the elbow. Clin. Orthop., *50:*95, 1967.
11. Smith, M. G. H.: Osteochondritis of the humeral capitulum. J. Bone Joint Surg., *46-B:*50, 1964.
12. Rana, N. A., et al.: Complete lesion of the median nerve associated with dislocation of the elbow joint. Acta Orthop. Scand., *45:*365, 1974.
13. Thompson, H. C., and Garcia, A.: Myositis ossificans: aftermath of elbow injuries. Clin. Orthop., *50:*129, 1967.
14. Osborne, G.: Recurrent dislocation of the elbow. J. Bone Joint Surg., *48-B:*340, 1966.
15. Godshall, R. W., and Hansen, C. A.: Traumatic ulnar neuropathy in adolescent baseball pitchers. J. Bone Joint Surg., *53-A:*359, 1971.
16. Eto, R. T., Anderson, P. W., and Harley, J. D.: Elbow arthrography with the application of tomography. Radiology, *115:*283, 1975.
17. Johanson, O.: Capsular and ligament injuries of the elbow joint. A clinical arthrographic study. Acta Chir. Scand. [Suppl.], *287,* 1962.
18. Trias, A., and Comeau, Y.: Recurrent dislocation of the elbow in children. Clin. Orthop., *100:*74, 1974.
19. Albright, J. A., et al.: Clinical study of baseball pitchers: correlation of injury to the throwing arm with method of delivery. Am. J. Sports Med., *6:*15, 1978.
20. Adams, J. E.: Injury to the throwing arm. Calif. Med., *102:*126, 1965.
21. Roberts, N., and Hughes, R.: Osteochondritis dissecans of the elbow joint. A clinical study. J. Bone Joint Surg., *32-B:*348, 1950.
22. Woodward, A. H., and Bianco, A. J., Jr.: Osteochondritis dissecans of the elbow. Clin. Orthop., *110:*35, 1975.

12

Radius and Ulna

Anatomy

Proximal aspect

The development of the proximal ulna sometimes makes interpretation of injury difficult. There are two functional prominences, the olecranon and the coronoid, with epiphyseal and articular cartilage between them (Fig. 12-1). It is important to remember that an epiphysis and physis are present under all of this articular cartilage, even though much of the region does not develop a secondary ossification center. The latter is primarily confined to the olecranon segment, although a small ossification center may develop in the coronoid. The distal portion of the proximal ulna and the coronoid process are formed mainly by the ulnar metaphysis, while the proximal portion is formed by the olecranon epiphysis (see Fig. 12-1). The secondary ossification center usually does not appear in the olecranon until about the tenth year (Figs. 12-1 to 12-3). This secondary ossification center is usually single, but may be bipartite or multipartite (Fig. 12-4). When bipartite, the accessory center is usually located near the tip of the olecranon. An unusual variation is a patella cubiti, which is a true sesamoid in the triceps tendon.

Radiographs of the elbow in children are notoriously troublesome, particularly those of young children with absent or incompletely developed secondary ossification centers. Single and multiple secondary ossification centers in the olecranon epiphyseal cartilage may simulate fracture fragments (see Fig. 12-4). The secondary ulnar centers are characteristically rough.

The anatomy of the proximal radius minimizes significant injury (Figs. 12-5 to 12-7). The disc-shaped head of the radius is *always* of greater diameter than the neck. Even in the nine-week embryo, the head and neck of the radius are well-defined, and the radial notch appears in the ulna. While not as marked during fetal life, the radial head, even within the first year, shows the same eccentric concavity and sharp anterolateral rim as in the adult (Fig. 12-8). Thus, nothing in the overall appearance of the fetal, neonatal, or postnatal radial head predisposes it to subluxation, as has been suggested (see section on ''Pulled Elbow'' in this chapter).

The plane of the articular surface is tilted relative to the longitudinal axis of the radius. This tilt varies depending upon the rotation. The exact degree of tilting and shifting can only be measured on those films taken at proper angles of the plane of angulation (see Fig. 12-7). Undoubtedly, the changing tilt affects the up- and down-sliding motion of the annular ligament. Since one of the problems of proximal radial fractures is increased angulation, during reduction one should remember that there normally is a slight tilt.

The epiphysis of the radial head and the sides are covered extensively by articular cartilage (see Fig. 12-5). The epiphyseal blood supply has a short intra-articular course along the metaphysis, which is surrounded by the annular ligament. This creates an intracapsular epiphyseal blood supply

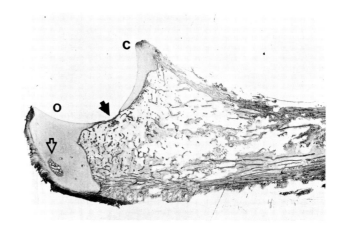

FIG. 12-1. Histologic section of proximal ulna of a five-year-old showing early development of secondary ossification center (open arrow). The well-formed subchondral metaphyseal plate predisposes the ulna to a fracture pattern leaving a thin layer of metaphyseal bone, rather than propagating through the physis. The solid arrow shows an attenuated central area of the articular surface which effectively separates the proximal ulnar epiphysis into olecranon (o) and coronoid (c) segments.

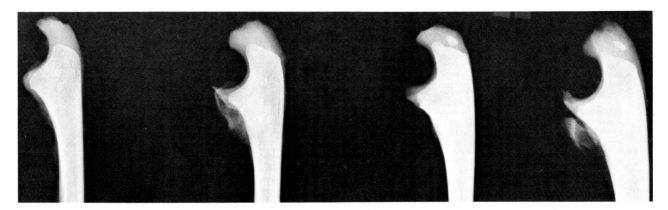

FIG. 12-2. Serial roentgenographic development of the proximal ulna at four, six, eight, and nine years. Note that an extensive cartilaginous olecranon is present in all four specimens, and that it continues along the articular surface to the coronoid process. All of this cartilage, from the coronoid process to the olecranon processes, comprises the composite proximal chondro-epiphysis. The specimen from the nine-year-old, while morphologically larger, had a smaller ossification center than the specimen from the eight-year-old, demonstrating variation in this region, much like the rest of the elbow epiphyses.

similar to that of the capital femoral epiphysis (Fig. 12-9). The blood supply may be damaged by epiphyseal or metaphyseal separation. Since the usual level of injury through the metaphysis is near the entry of the vessels, avascular (ischemic) necrosis must be considered a potential complication. However, more often there is hyperemia of the site, and a tendency to overgrowth of the radial head, rather than significant growth limitation.

The proximal radial epiphysis does not ossify until the fifth to seventh year and unites when the child is 16 to 18 years of age (see Figs. 12-6 and 12-7). It usually ossifies symmetrically. Because of the epiphyseal tilt, the ossification may be asymmetric and resembles a triangle rather than an ellipse. However, an angular shape may also indicate a problem of abnormal radiohumeral joint stress, such as a radioulnar synostosis or Panner's disease. Since many children with these conditions are not diagnosed until an episode of trauma, the physician should be aware of the potential problem.

The upper end of the ulna articulates with the trochlea of the distal humerus, and provides primary flexion-extension of the elbow. It also articulates with the head of the radius through an extension of the joint proximally on both the radius and ulna (Fig. 12-10). These radioulnar joints tend to be ignored articulations, but are especially important in the problems of Monteggia's injury, pulled elbow, and Galeazzi's injury.

The radial head is tightly constrained by the capitellar and ulnar articular surfaces. This anatomic construct permits rotation and flexion/extension, yet creates intrinsic stability. Both joint relationships must be disrupted during a Monteggia injury. The annular ligament hugs the radial metaphysis to the shaft of the ulna and the ulnar articular extension (Fig. 12-11). The annular ligament further restrains the radioulnar joint. This ligament has a certain degree of laxity that allows displacement in radial head subluxation, and may permit displacement of the radial head without significant tearing. However, the ligament is usually torn, rather than displaced, in most Monteggia injuries. The synovial recess extends under and just distal to the ligament.

The proximal radioulnar joint is most stable in supination because: (1) the radial head is not circular, but somewhat oval, and with the forearm in supination, the greatest diameter of the head comes in contact with the proximal radioulnar joint; (2) the margin of the radial head is not the same width around the head, such that in full supination the broadest portion of the margin of the radial head comes in contact with the proximal notch of the ulna, and gives the broadest articular contact; (3) in full supination the interosseous membrane is most taut; (4) the annular ligament is reinforced by the anterior and posterior components of the radial collateral ligaments; and (5) in full supination the anterior, thicker fibers of the quadrate ligament of Tenuce stabilize the radial head more strongly into the proximal radioulnar joint.[1-3]

The biceps inserts onto the radial tuberosity. This osseous enlargement becomes progressively prominent as the child grows. Evans stressed its potential use in assessing relative rotation of the proximal fragments in forearm fractures.[4-6] However, its usefulness is contingent upon it being developed sufficiently to allow roentgenographic evaluation. When the child is two to three years old there should be enough prominence for the tuberosity to be visible roentgenographically (Fig. 12-12), and this is the time when displaced forearm fractures become an increasing problem. Prior to this age range, forearm fractures are not as frequent and are generally undisplaced, the thick periosteal sleeve maintaining longitudinal continuity.

Diaphysis

The sagittal and coronal cross-sectional diameters of the radius and ulna change with age and the level observed. Proximally both have a circular appearance. However, for much of the diaphysis the two bones have a cam shape ("pear shape"). As such, rotational deformities may be detected by differences in the width of the apposed fragments.

The radius and ulna are bound together firmly by the interosseous membrane, which provides a hinge mechanism for integrated rotatory movements.[7] This interosseous liga-

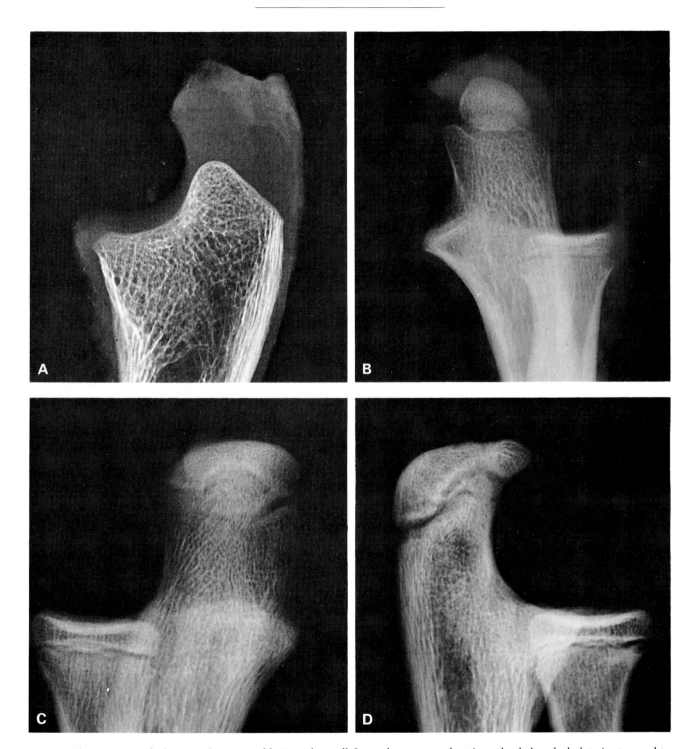

FIG. 12-3. *A,* Proximal ulna in a five-year-old. Note the well-formed, transversely oriented subchondral plate juxtaposed to the chondro-epiphysis. This influences the tendency to metaphyseal, rather than physeal injury. *B,* AP view of proximal ulna and radius in an 11-year-old. This view of the olecranon ossification center and physis is usually blocked by the distal humerus. It should not be misinterpreted as a fracture line. *C-D,* AP and lateral views of the proximal radius and ulna in a 14-year-old. The epiphyseal ossification centers are well developed.

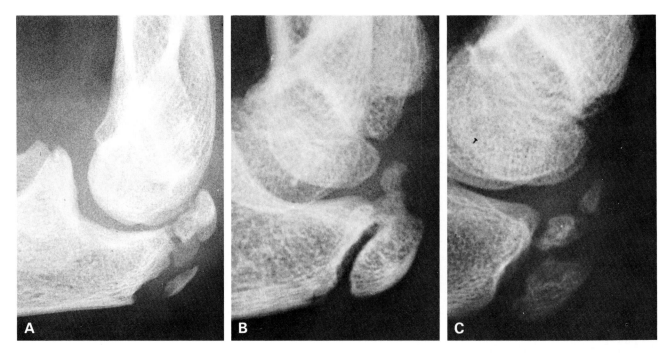

FIG. 12-4. Normal variations of formation of the olecranon secondary ossification center. These could easily be interpreted as a fracture during the evaluation of acute trauma. *A,* Large ossification center with superior irregularity. *B,* Large superior segments with smaller distal portion. *C,* Multifocal early ossification.

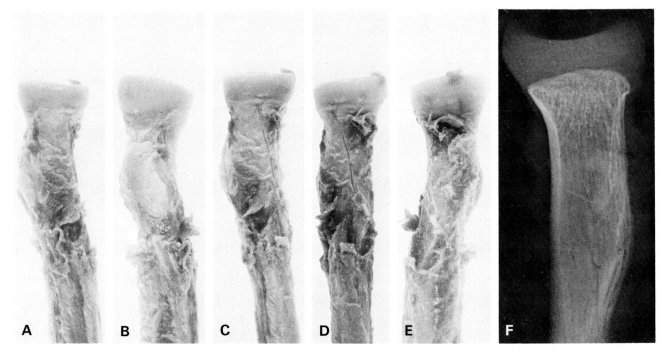

FIG. 12-5. *A-E,* Gross anatomic specimens of proximal radius from six-year-old child, ranging from, *A,* full supination to, *E,* full pronation. Articular cartilage covers the entire circumference of the radial head. Note how rotation (pronation-supination) affects the tilt of the radial articular plane relative to the longitudinal axis. Also note the contour differences as the head flares from the metaphysis. *F,* Roentgenogram of proximal radius from a 14-month-old child. Notice how the epiphyseal-metaphyseal contour near the bicipital tuberosity is less flared than it is on the opposite side. Undoubtedly, the flaring limits proximal excursion of the annular ligament. However, in forced pronation, the less flared portion is presented to the annular ligament, thus enhancing potential for partial annular ligament displacement.

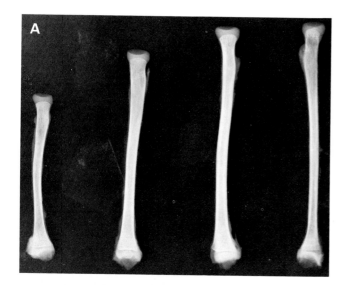

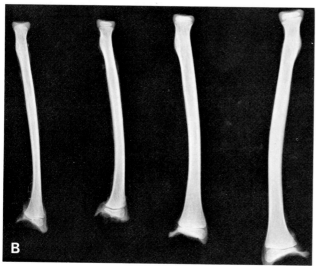

FIG. 12-6. *A,* Early development of radius. *B,* Anterior view of subsequent developmental pattern. Note that the proximal radius tilts relative to the longitudinal axis, and that the contours of the proximal epiphysis and metaphysis change. Undoubtedly, these morphologic factors play a role in the ease with which the annular ligament subluxates over the radial head in "nursemaid's elbow."

ment attaches along the tip of the "cam" of both the radius and the ulna. Correction of rotational deformity is directed at restoring the interosseous ligament mechanics, which are essential to pronation and supination. Specialized ligaments are present at each end. The annular ligament holds the proximal radioulnar joint together. The distal radioulnar and radiocarpal joints are connected by the dorsal and volar radiocarpal ligaments, as well as a meniscus bridging from the distal radius to the ulnar styloid.

Throughout the diaphyses, the radius and ulna exhibit gentle curves (Figs. 12-13 and 12-14). The radiologist and orthopaedist should be familiar with these patterns, as they allow one to detect excessive bowing (plastic deformation) without evident fracture. Such a pattern of deformation,

rather than complete fracture, is characteristic of these bones in infants and young children.

When these gentle curve patterns are present along the shafts of both the radius and the ulna, basic forearm rotation (supination-pronation) follows a relatively simple conical pattern when analyzed mathematically.[8] The essential feature is paired joint motion at the proximal and distal radioulnar joints. The mechanical axis of the forearm is a line connecting the rotational center of the proximal radius and the center of the distal ulna. This line is the stable leg of a right triangle, of which the hypotenuse is the radial longitudinal axis and the rotating leg is the transverse axis of the distal radius and the triangular ligament. Rotation of the radius about the ulna thus generates a volar-placed half cone (Fig. 12-15).

If the effective mechanical axis is disrupted, as in angulation of the radius, the ulna, or both, paired joint motion is disrupted, and a simple rotational cone is impossible. Radial angular deformity is more significant, since this bone essentially generates the rotational (half) cone. Angular deformity introduces nonaxial torsion of the segment distal to the fracture.

Normally, the ulna abducts during pronation and adducts during supination. Thus, there is some motion of the ulna relative to the radius during pronation and supination in that it does not remain totally stable and unmoving.[9]

When one or both of the forearm bones have been fractured, the direction and extension of displacement of the fragments are contingent upon the initial deforming force, the level of fracture, and the degree of muscle action. In the

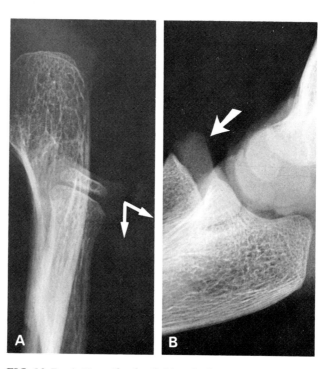

FIG. 12-7. *A,* Note tilt of radial head relative to longitudinal axis (arrows). The variability of this tilt in pronation and supination also undoubtedly affects susceptibility to radial head subluxation. *B,* The tilt may also be a factor in the ability to subluxate anteriorly (arrow).

lower end of the humerus and inserts on the lateral surface of the distal radius immediately above the styloid process. Depending upon the position of the arm, this muscle assists in pronation or supination, bringing it from either position to neutral. The extensors of the wrist and digits have less deforming influence on forearm fractures than does the brachioradialis. The extensors may act as a dynamic posterior splint when under tension. The extensor and abductors of the thumb are synergistic with the brachioradialis and tend to pull the distal fragment of the radius proximally. The powerful flexor muscles of the forearm tend to pull the distal fragments anteriorly and produce dorsal bowing of the radius and ulna.

In fractures involving the upper third of the forearm above the insertion of the pronator teres, the proximal fragment is usually supinated and flexed because of the relatively unopposed action of the biceps and supinator. The distal fragment is pronated by the action of the pronator teres and quadratus muscles. Therefore, to properly align the fracture, the distal fragment should be supinated.

In fractures of the middle third (i.e., below the insertion of the pronator teres), the proximal fragment of the radius is held in neutral rotation as the action of the supinator muscle is counteracted by the pronator teres. The proximal fragment is drawn into place by the action of the biceps. The distal fragment is pronated and drawn toward the ulna by the pronator quadratus. In achieving anatomic reduction, the distal fragment is brought into neutral rotation. Failure to correct excessive angular deformities in childhood fractures may limit normal rotational mechanics in adulthood.

Distal aspect

The distal radioulnar joint is a double-pivot joint that unites the distal ulnar epiphysis, the ulnar notch of the radius, and the distal radial epiphysis by the triangular (meniscal) cartilage.[10,11] The distal ulnar articular cartilage surface is

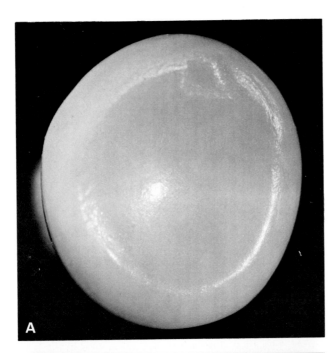

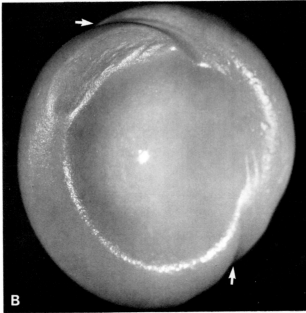

FIG. 12-8. *A,* Normal radial head showing slightly eccentric central depression. *B,* Effect of hyperpronation prior to fixation. The annular ligament partially displaced over the anterior margin and indented into the biologically plastic cartilage (arrows).

reduction and immobilization of these fractures, the origin, insertion, and action of the various forearm muscles must be considered. The biceps and supinator muscles insert into the proximal third of the radius, and are powerful supinators of the forearm. The pronator teres inserts into the middle third of the radius, while the pronator quadratus is located on the anterior aspect of the lower forearm and inserts into the distal third of the radius. The brachioradialis originates from the

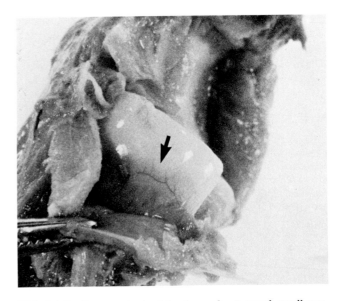

FIG. 12-9. Intra-articular blood supply. Several small vessels extend transversely and longitudinally (arrow) under the annular ligament, which has been pulled down.

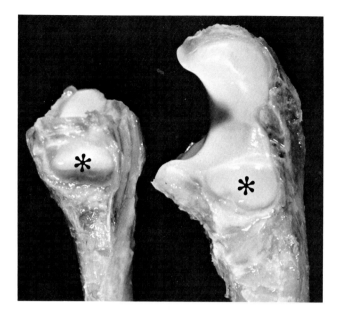

FIG. 12-10. Proximal and distal ulnae showing the articular surfaces (*) for the radius. These are important joints, and must be considered in evaluation and treatment of wrist and elbow trauma. These joints remain throughout skeletal maturation and the correct structural relationships are necessary for forearm rotation.

completely covered by this disc, so that the ulna never articulates directly with the proximal carpal row. The distal ulnar surface glides against the articular disc (triangular cartilage). The triangular cartilage attaches by a thick apex to the base of the ulnar styloid (Fig. 12-16). The thinner base of the triangular ligament is attached to the leading edge of the radius just proximal to the carpal articular surface.

The dorsal portion of the triangular fibrocartilage and the dorsal radiocarpal ligament tend to be taut in pronation. The slight dorsal displacement in pronation, with the ulnar styloid relatively fixed, explains the tendency of the fracture

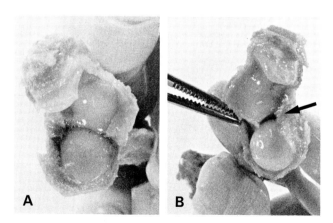

FIG. 12-11. A, Proximal radioulnar relationships in six-month-old. The bones are supinated. B, Pronation may "open" this joint (arrow).

through the ulnar styloid, even in children in whom the entity may not be recognized because the area is completely cartilaginous. As the area ossifies, nonunion becomes evident.

The distal radial ossification center appears at 6 to 12 months, while the distal ulna initially ossifies at 5 years of age (Figs. 12-17 to 12-19). The radial and ulnar centers then progressively expand. The radial center is initially spherical, but becomes triangulated. Physiologic epiphysiodesis occurs at 14 years in girls and 16 years in boys. The metaphyseal cortex changes significantly during development, as does the thickness of the hypertrophic zone of the physis. Both factors undoubtedly play a role in the age-related changing patterns of distal radial fractures.

The radial styloid is one of the last areas to ossify, and does so by the extension of the secondary center. Accessory bones have not been reported in the styloid. A fracture is more likely if a lucency is seen in this area. The ulnar styloid is the last region to ossify. A cartilaginous fracture of the ulnar styloid may accompany a distal radial fracture, and not become evident until a separate secondary center appears in the styloid. This is not a variation of ossification. A separate ossification center for the ulnar styloid is rare, but should not be mistaken for a fracture fragment.

Before and during adolescence many children show multiple longitudinal osseous striations in the physis between the metaphysis and the distal epiphyseal ossification centers, both radial and ulnar (Fig. 12-20). These striations represent calcification or ossification in the portions of cartilage contiguous to the channels of the transepiphyseal arteries. These calcifications have not been studied anatomically.

Fracture Incidence

Forearm fractures are common in children. Problems of treatment vary considerably with the age of the patient and the level and displacement of the fracture. Generally, there is less comminution, union is more rapid, and residual deformities tend to be corrected by subsequent growth compared to similar injuries in an adult.[12-20]

From the standpoint of age relationship to injury, the average ages for fractures are: 6.1 years in the upper third, 6.7 years in the mid-third, 6.9 years in the lower third, 8.5 years in the lower sixth, and 9.8 years for epiphyseal fractures. In Gandi's series, 20% were in children under 5 years of age.[21] The susceptibility of the lower radial epiphysis to injury about the age of 10 may be related to the increased growth rate that occurs about that time and consequent microscopic changes at the level of the epiphyseal plate.[22] Preliminary data in our skeletal development laboratory suggest changes in physeal thickness, the zone of Ranvier, and metaphyseal cortical density during these different age-susceptibility periods.

One series of 375 forearm fractures included 23 fractures of the radial head and neck, 8 fractures of the upper third, 28 fractures of the mid-third, 54 fractures of the lowest third, 195 fractures of the distal metaphysis, and 67 juxta-epiphyseal injuries.[23] Gandi studied over 1700 fractures of the forearm in children under 12 years of age.[19] The incidence of the fractures (excluding those of the olecranon and head and neck of the radius) showed 0.4% Monteggia fracture dislocations, 1% fracture of the upper third, 2.6% com-

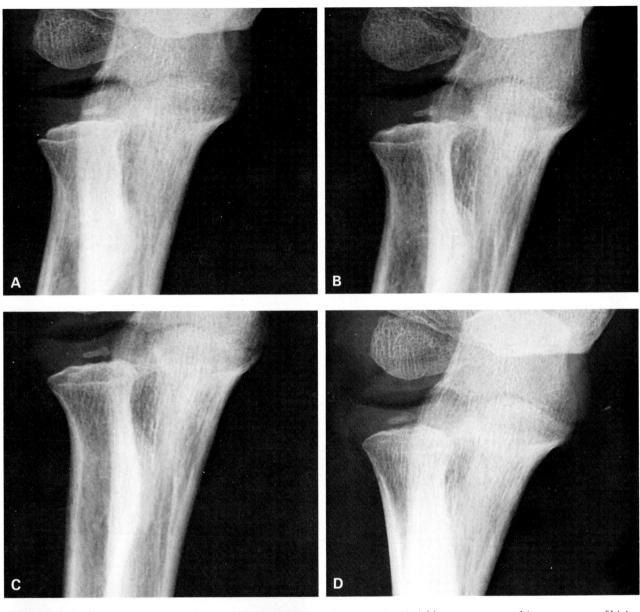

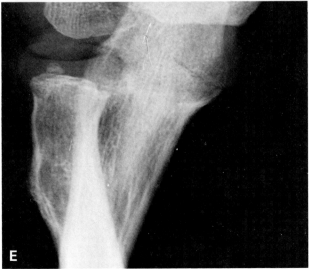

FIG. 12-12. Variable roentgenographic appearance of bicipital tuberosity in a six-year-old. *A*, Supination (0°); *B*, 45°; *C*, neutral (90°); *D*, 150°; *E*, pronation (180°).

plete fracture in the middle third involving both bones, 0.9% complete fracture of the middle third of both bones, 42% greenstick fracture in the lower third of one bone, 24.6% greenstick fracture of the lower third of both bones, 5.2% with complete fractures of the lower third of the radius, with or without complete or greenstick fracture of the lower third of the ulna, and 14% involving a fracture separation of the lower radial epiphysis. Bilateral fractures were seen in 12 patients.

Most fractures of the radius and ulna in children are either distal compression fractures or undisplaced angulated greenstick fractures, and present minimal problems in treatment. However, there tends to be complacency about reducing some deformities, and significant problems may occur if any

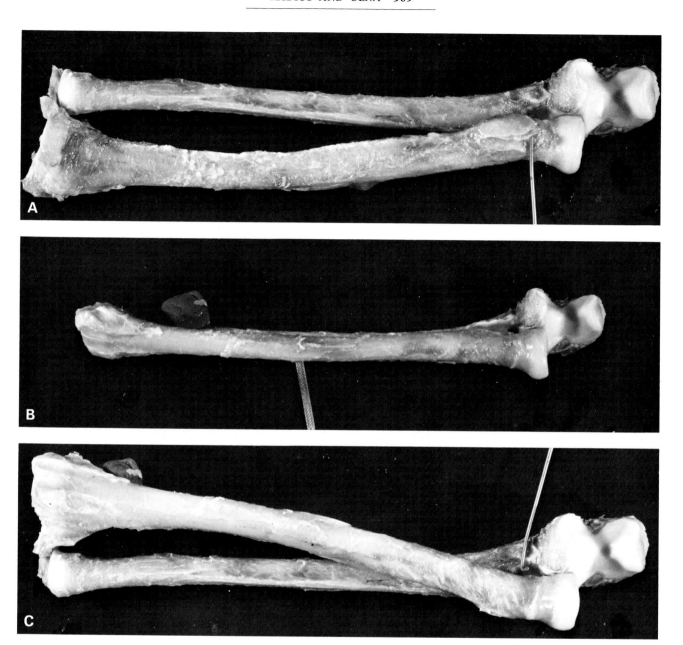

FIG. 12-13. Gross appearance of, *A*, supination, *B*, neutral, and, *C*, pronation in specimen from a six-year-old. In supination, the bicipital tuberosity (probe) faces anteriorly, while in pronation it rotates posteriorly. Again, note that in supination the radial "flare" is prominent, but it decreases in pronation. This lessens the mechanical block to proximal migration of the annular ligament.

bowing (plastic deformation) is allowed to remain, even in the undisplaced greenstick fracture. The goal of treatment of any radial or ulnar fracture must be restoration of full function as soon as possible, with prevention of loss of supination and pronation.

Rotational deformities should not exist at any forearm fracture site after manipulative reduction. Loss of pronation of up to 30° can be hidden by abduction of the shoulder. In contrast, loss of supination is not as easy to conceal.

Some authors have stated that angular deformity of up to 35° remodels in fractures of the distal third, but that over 15° of residual angulation in more proximal fractures proba-

bly leads to diminished function. Sharrard recommends open reduction in fractures of the middle third of the radius and ulna to prevent angular deformity, and suggests that *any* such deformity leads to some loss of rotation.[24]

Since the extent of correction of malunion depends on further longitudinal bone growth, it is influenced also by the distance of the fracture from the metaphysis. The closer the fracture to the metaphysis (especially the distal one), the greater the potential for spontaneous correction. The nearer to the midshaft, the more likely there will be a significant problem. Therefore, angulation in the midshaft of the bone should be accepted with caution.

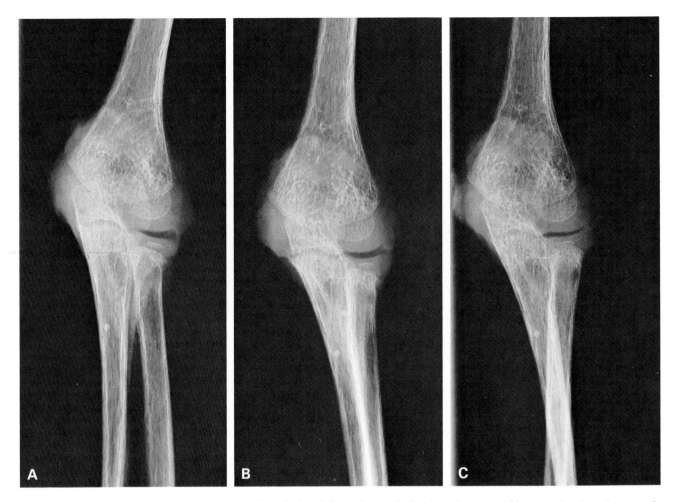

FIG. 12-14. Roentgenographic appearance of the shafts of the radius and ulna in a five-year-old. *A,* Supination; *B,* neutral; *C,* pronation. Note the difference in the "lateral" contour and the tilt of the radial epiphysis and metaphysis that are presented to the annular ligament in each position.

The usual outcome of forearm fractures in children appears to be complete functional recovery in most patients when manipulative closed reduction and immobilization are used. However, in one series conducted by Thomas,[23] fractures of the upper third showed unsatisfactory results in 50% of the patients, with the major problem being loss of supination and pronation, although the children did not complain of any significant functional disability.[23] Of this group, there were 28 patients with fractures in the middle third, 11 with unsatisfactory results at 4 months, but only 2 with unsatisfactory results at 4 years. At the end of 3 months, 45 children with fractures of the lower third were considered unsatisfactory, but by 4 years post-injury, there were only 3 children who had a measurable loss of rotation. Thomas stressed that those patients with a poorer outcome were all treated by open reduction and fixation.[23] In 67 patients with juxtaphyseal fractures, 5 developed a Madelung-type deformity, which was probably due to an unsuspected type 5 physeal injury. In one patient, a Darrach-type procedure was performed to relieve painful symptoms. To summarize, 65 patients failed to achieve satisfactory results at the end of 3 months, but by the end of 4 years, only 9 had any problems when judged by the same standards.[23]

Blount, Carr, and Tracey believe that open reduction is unnecessary.[14,25-27] Certainly, open reduction and internal fixation are seldom indicated, but they should not be discounted totally as treatment modalities when necessary. With the improved methods of internal fixation and anesthesia, there is an increasing tendency to use open reduction for young children and adolescents, a treatment that is extremely successful for forearm fractures in adults.

Refracture or a second fracture at the same site after an apparently solid union is relatively common in forearm fractures in children.[14] Bosworth encountered 6 cases in his study of 54 fractures.[28] In another series, refractures occurred in only 9 patients, representing 0.5%, at intervals varying from 2 to 6 months from the time of union.[21]

Olecranon Fractures

Fractures involving the olecranon are unusual in children.[29,30] Mahlahn and Fahey recorded only 19 cases in a series of 300 elbow fractures in children.[31] Newell reviewed 40 cases in children whose ages ranged from 15 months to 11 years.[30] He found that olecranon fractures

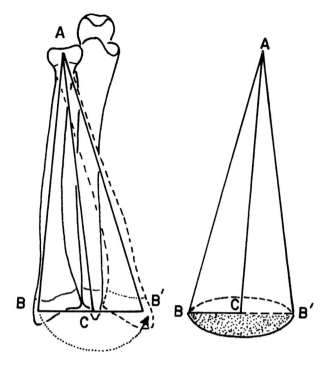

FIG. 12-15. Schematic of rotation of the radius on the ulna. The mechanical triangle of rotation (ABC) has an axis from the center of the radial head (A) to the ulnar styloid (C). The radial styloid (B) rotates around to a pronated position (B'), subtending a semicircular conical base.

were most common around the age of 5, while Mahlahn and Fahey found the average age to be 8½ years.

In a report of 24 cases of fractures of the radial neck in children, Jeffrey noted that 3 cases had associated olecranon fracture.[32] Of olecranon fracture cases, 10% have associated injury at the proximal end of the radius. Some cases are associated with fractures of the neck of the radius or with a fracture of the radial head. Dislocation of the radial head has also been reported. Hume described 3 cases of anterior dislo-cation of the head of the radius associated with undisplaced fracture of the olecranon in children.[33] Hume appears to be the first to describe this particular injury, although Speed suggested that a hyperextension injury to the elbow may cause displacement of the olecranon epiphysis associated with anterior dislocation of the radial head.[34]

Classification

The olecranon fracture is usually undisplaced, incomplete, and fractured approximately perpendicular to the long axis of the ulna, probably due to a locking into the olecranon fossa. The longitudinal split fracture, which appears in ap-proximately 10% of the adult cases, is atypical in children.

These fractures usually occur just distal to the olecranon physis (Fig. 12-21). Occasionally there may be a fracture through the cartilaginous-osseous junction in a child under the age of 10 when the olecranon ossification center has not as yet appeared. Often the fracture is incomplete and does not encroach upon the joint surface, since the fracture has not propagated through the hyaline and articular cartilage (Fig. 12-22).

Fractures of the coronoid process are uncommon (Fig. 12-23). These injuries have minimal displacement in the younger child; however, in children 10 to 12 years of age, the olecranon displaces more often (Fig. 12-24).

Mechanism

The total structure of the olecranon in a child differs sig-nificantly from that of an adult. The bone is more trabecular and fractures are often difficult to identify. Articular cartilage and epiphyseal cartilage layers are thick and permit osteo-chondral fractures. The transversely oriented subchondral bone of the metaphysis tends to direct fractures into the metaphysis rather than the physis.

In one series, 20 of the 33 children in whom the olecranon fracture was the only injury had a direct blow to the elbow from a fall, rather than a fall on the hand with hyperex-tended elbow.[30] This most likely caused an undisplaced frac-ture.

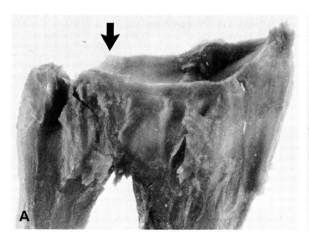
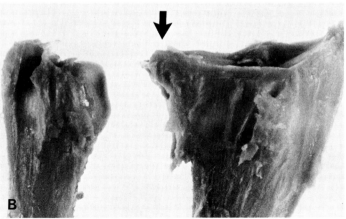

FIG. 12-16. *A,* Intact and, *B,* exploded views of the distal radius and ulna to show the triangular ligament or meniscus (arrows), and the way in which the ulna articulates with this ligament and the radius, but does not articulate directly with the carpus.

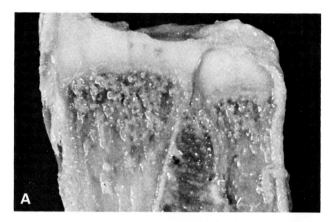

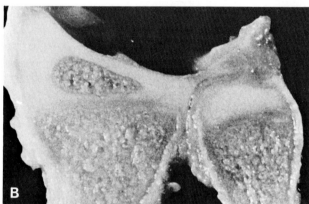

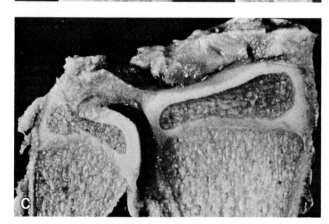

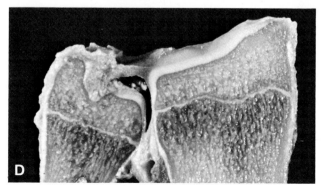

FIG. 12-17. Slab sections showing sequential development of the distal radius and ulna. *A,* Neonate; *B,* 1 year; *C,* 8 years; *D,* 12 years.

However, if the elbow is extended, the olecranon is locked in the olecranon fossa of the distal humerus. When a varus or valgus force is then applied (Fig. 12-25), the olecranon levers against the fossa margins and the deforming strain is absorbed by the metaphyseal region located at the level of the joint. With a valgus force, the radial head or medial epicondyle may also fracture.

Diagnosis

In most cases, the diagnosis is readily evident on the lateral film. However, if the fragments are undisplaced, or if the fracture is through the physeal-metaphyseal interface of an epiphysis with no secondary ossification center, the diagnosis must sometimes be empiric or based on careful examination. Palpation of the fracture gap may not be easy because of the degree of swelling.

Ossification variations may also affect interpretation of fractures.[30]

Treatment

Closed reduction seems to be the ideal initial method of treatment, especially since many olecranon fractures represent greenstick fractures with some cortical and epiphyseal integrity (especially if acquired by locking the olecranon during a varus or valgus stress). Since the fracture occurs in extension in this pathomechanism, the greenstick deformity may be hyperextended relative to the rest of the ulna, and should be pushed back with the elbow flexed. The elbow should then be splinted and a repeat roentgenogram taken to be sure the fracture fragments are still in continuity.

Although immobilization in plaster with the elbow at approximately 90° for 1 month is usually recommended, the results indicate that in the usual undisplaced, incomplete fracture, a period of 3 weeks in a sling may be the only treatment necessary. If closed reduction is impossible, or in cases of delayed diagnosis, open reduction may be necessary (Fig. 12-26).

The displaced olecranon fracture in childhood is a less frequent injury that is usually best treated by open reduction with internal fixation of the fracture, repair of the triceps aponeurotic tear, and external immobilization (Figs. 12-26 and 12-27). Methods of fixation include smooth pins or Kirschner wires transfixing the epiphysis to the metaphysis, and annular wire or suture fixation. Pins should be small and should be removed when healing is evident (at least 4 to 6 weeks, as this is a slowly growing physeal unit, and new formation of metaphyseal bone on the proximal side of the fracture is accordingly limited). Annular fixation has the advantage of avoiding the physis. The wire should loop through the triceps aponeurosis and a transverse tunnel in the metaphysis just distal to the joint to avoid physeal damage (see Fig. 12-26). Under no circumstances should a transfixation screw (e.g., Leinbach screw) be used, as it will permanently damage the physis.

Results

Olecranon fractures usually heal without any limitation of function or growth deformity, especially when a greenstick injury is involved. In displaced injuries healing may be delayed, especially if a thin layer of metaphyseal bone must be incorporated back into the main metaphysis.

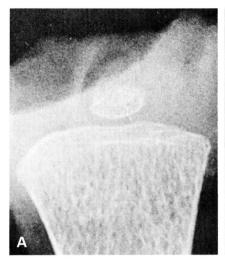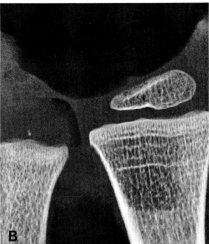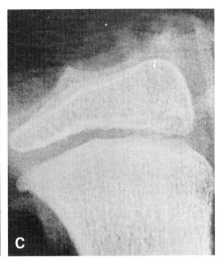

FIG. 12-18. Sequential roentgenographic development of the distal radius and ulna. *A,* One year; *B,* three years; *C,* seven years.

Complications

Growth arrest is unusual after an olecranon fracture, primarily because this region does not contribute significantly to the overall longitudinal growth of the ulna. However, in the young child, growth arrest could lead to disparate development of the proximal ulna relative to the proximal radius, and thereby affect varus or valgus and limit elbow function. One case, reported by Hume, developed significant myositis ossificans in the area where the radial head had been displaced.[33]

Proximal Radius

Proximal radius fractures are common injuries to the developing elbow.[36-46] Newman described 48 displaced radial neck fractures in children 4 to 13 years of age.[47] Length of follow-up varied from 6 months to 22 years, with an average of 4 years. In 2 children, the fracture occurred before ossification appeared and was recognized only by the displaced flake of metaphysis (Thurston Holland sign). In 38 cases, the pattern of injury was lateral or valgus angulation. In all cases, the angulation of the radial head was at least 30° from the normal axis. There was moderate displacement in 16 patients, and severe displacement in 32. Henrikson found 55 cases of fractures of the proximal radius, which included 50 cases of fracture of the neck and 5 cases of fracture through the epiphysis.[48]

In Jeffrey's article, 24 of 450 patients with radial head fractures fit into the children's group.[32] These patients could be classified into two subgroups: Group I, 22 cases with lateral tilting of the head of 30° or more caused by fracture separation of the epiphysis or a greenstick fracture of the neck with angulation, and Group II, 2 cases with posterior angulation.

O'Brien reviewed approximately 125 cases.[49] He found only 4 that he would classify as a true slip of the epiphysis (i.e., type 1 or 2 growth mechanism injury), feeling that most were fractures through the juxtaphyseal metaphysis.

There were 40 patients who had early closure of epiphysis, and increased carrying angles up to 25°, although none was severe enough to require osteotomy; 6 cases went on to proximal radiohumeral synostosis.

Fractures generally occur when children are around 10 to 13 years of age, with the range beginning at about 5 years, when the ossification center first appears. Whether these injuries occur before that time is difficult to ascertain because of the absence of the ossification center. Approximately 75% of the cases occur in children 9 years or older.

Multiple injuries may occur.[50,51] In one series, 11 of 38 patients had associated avulsion injuries of the medial side of the elbow; 5 had olecranon fractures, 4 had avulsed medial epicondyles, and 2 had ruptured medial collateral ligaments.[47,52] Other injury patterns include: (1) radial head dislocation and fracture, (2) rupture of the annular ligament, (3) elbow dislocation, (4) capitellar fracture, (5) dislocated radial head, (6) navicular fracture, and (7) radial nerve palsy. The wrist must be assessed carefully.

Classification

Proximal radius fractures include only those within the confines of the annular (orbicular) ligament. Fractures distal to the annular ligament are considered extra-articular and are a different type of injury.

Fractures of the proximal radius can be defined as: (1) mild, less than 30° of angular deformation; (2) moderate, 30 to 60° of angulation; and (3) severe, greater than 60° of angulation.

The fractures vary from classic type 1 or 2 growth mechanism injuries to fractures through the metaphysis with angular deformity (Figs. 12-28 and 12-29). The fracture line may appear to be through the epiphysis, but it actually is a compression of the epiphyseal head into the soft metaphyseal expansion of the narrow neck supporting the articular disc. Thus, they tend to be impaction or greenstick fractures.

A fracture of the neck of the radius must be differentiated from a true physeal or epiphyseal fracture of the head of the radius, which occurs infrequently in childhood and is more

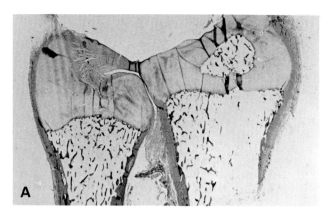

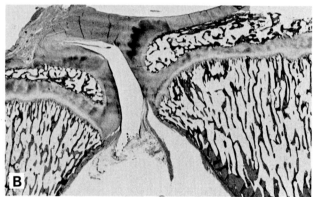

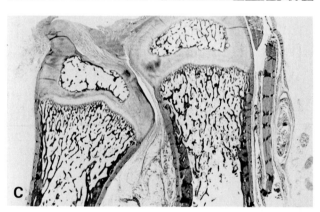

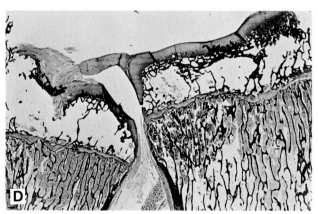

FIG. 12-19. Sequential histologic development of the distal radius and ulna. *A,* 1 year; *B,* 7 years; *C,* 7 years, ulna minus variant; *D,* 13 years.

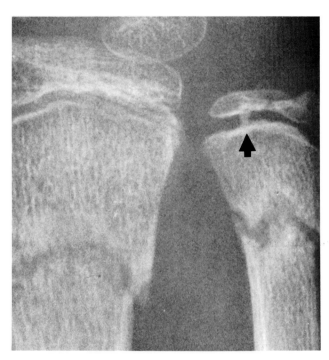

FIG. 12-20. Transphyseal longitudinal ossification patterns (arrow) in a 10-year-old.

likely in the child approaching skeletal maturity, much like the fracture of Tillaux. Most authors believe that physeal injuries are infrequent; McBride believes that a true slipped epiphysis is rare.[53] However, in a report of 34 cases, 50% were in the radial neck proper and 50% were type 2 fractures involving the proximal radial physis and metaphysis.[54]

Direct crushing of the radial head by a convex lateral condyle of the humerus may cause an intra-articular fracture of the proximal radial epiphysis. O'Brien reported several unusual variations of type 3 fractures (Fig. 12-30).[49] These are significant injuries and must be treated by open reduction and accurate anatomic reduction.

Pathomechanics

The normal carrying angle of the elbow makes valgus injury more likely in a fall on the outstretched arm. Anatomically, the position of the elbow determines whether the ulna will be fractured. In full extension, the ligaments around the elbow are tight and the olecranon keys into the olecranon fossa of the distal humerus, such that varus and valgus movements are minimized or prevented. In this position, a pure valgus force fractures the radial neck and the olecranon frequently sustains a concomitant oblique fracture (see Fig. 12-25). If there is some flexion, the olecranon is not firmly held within the olecranon fossa, and may rotate. Thus, a solitary fracture of the radial neck results from the force, and there may not be an accompanying injury of the ulna. If a child sustains a simple posterior dislocation of the elbow, and falls down landing on the injured elbow, a posteriorly displaced fracture of the radial neck may be produced.

The mechanism of injury of a fall on the outstretched hand drives the capitellum against the outer side of the head

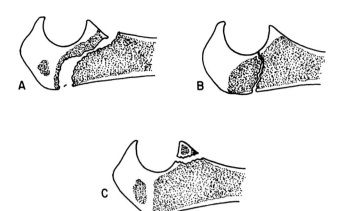

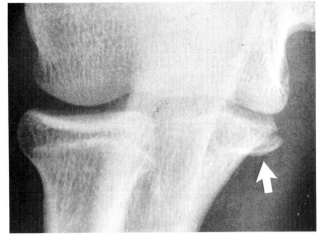

FIG. 12-21. Schematic of fracture patterns in the proximal ulna. *A,* Fracture through entire metaphysis. *B,* Fracture into the joint. *C,* Coronoid fracture.

FIG. 12-23. Avulsion fracture of coronoid process (arrow) in a 14-year-old girl.

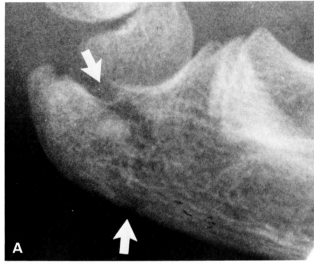

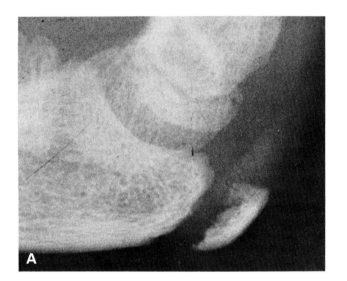

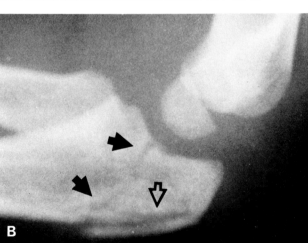

FIG. 12-22. Patterns of fracture within the metaphysis, most likely due to valgus force rather than avulsion. *A,* Mild displacement with comminution (arrows). *B,* Greenstick injury (solid arrows) with comminution of cortex (open arrow).

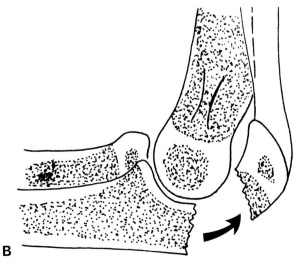

FIG. 12-24. *A,* Fracture of proximal ulna. The fragment is a portion of the metaphysis, not the secondary ossification center. *B,* Schematic of displaced fracture pattern.

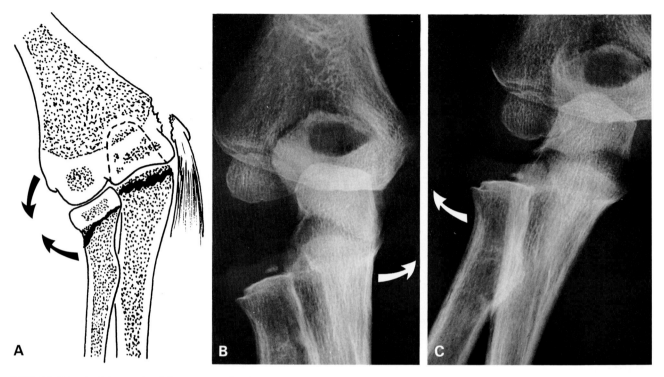

FIG. 12-25. *A,* Schematic of fracture mechanism. *B-C,* Roentgenograms showing how this olecranon pivots in the humeral fossa in, *B,* varus and, *C,* valgus deformations.

of the radius, tilting and displacing it outward. Such a mechanism implies a valgus strain on the elbow at the moment of injury. Accordingly, one may find an associated traction lesion on the inner side of the joint, which may take the form of a medial epicondyle avulsion or a rupture of the medial collateral ligament.

The direction of tilting of the displaced head of the radius relative to the shaft of the radius varies with the rotational position of the radius at the time of injury. Thus, if the forearm is supinated at the moment of impact, the displacement of the capital epiphysis is outward (lateral). This displacement is shown in the usual anteroposterior radiograph taken in supination. But if the forearm is in midposition, the adjacent posterior quadrant of the radial head is subjected to the greatest violence, and when the forearm is returned to a position of full supination, the head is tilted backward relative to the radial shaft.

According to Jeffrey, another mechanism of injury is when the patient first falls on his hand and sustains a temporary posterior dislocation or subluxation of the elbow joint.[32] The resulting upward force of the flexed elbow displaces the radial head posteriorly, almost 90°, by the impact against the inferior aspect of the capitellum. Spontaneous reduction of the elbow dislocation leaves the separated radial head beneath the capitellum. This form of injury is rare.[32,49,55]

Diagnosis

When injured, the elbow is usually held in moderate flexion with the forearm in neutral rotation. There may be local swelling and ecchymosis over the lateral aspect of the elbow. Pressure applied to the radial head and neck may elicit ten-

derness, although not in every instance, depending on the extent of injury. There may be occasional bony crepitus of the fragments when motion is attempted. Pain may be referred distally to the radial side of the wrist. Flexion and extension are restricted; pronation and supination are more painful and restricted.

Roentgenograms should be made in anterior and lateral views (Figs. 12-31 and 12-32). When the clinical findings are suggestive, but the roentgenogram inconclusive, it is best to make roentgenograms of the contralateral normal proximal forearm held in the same degree of flexion and rotation as the affected side; sometimes small metaphyseal fragments will be visible. It is also advisable to take several views of the proximal radius in various degrees of rotation, or evaluate the proximal radius under fluoroscopy. A dislocated proximal fragment may be projected into the shadow of the ulna; as a result, the structural and functional changes may be missed on routine films. In such cases, oblique or tangential projections may be useful. The maximum degree of the tilting of the radial head should be assessed. The fat pad sign may be the only indicator of an undisplaced injury.

Treatment

For the undisplaced or minimally displaced fracture of either the radial head or neck, treatment consists of simple immobilization of the elbow with a posterior plaster splint in 90° of flexion, and neutral rotation of the forearm for approximately 10 to 14 days. Movement should be started when the injury is no longer painful.[56] Early mobilization is recommended, but not used if there is residual pain at the fracture site to either motion or direct palpation. Initial

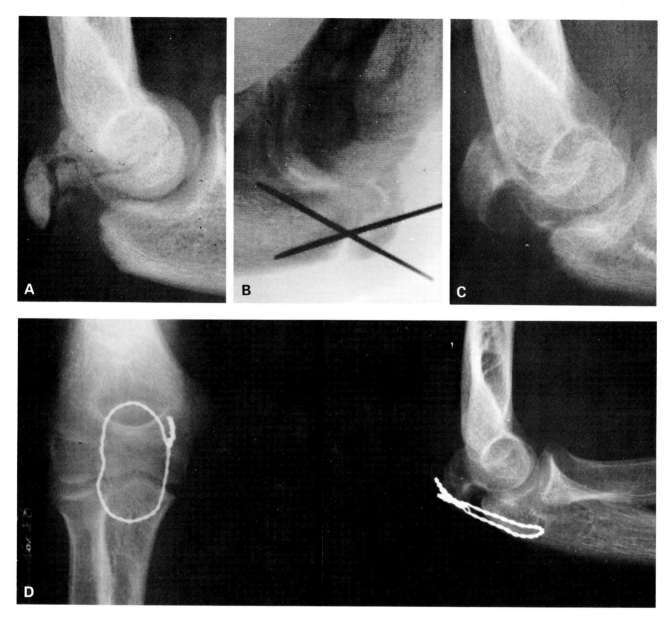

FIG. 12-26. *A*, Fracture of proximal ulna of a nine-year-old. The triceps has displaced the fragment. Closed reduction in extension failed to reduce the fragment. *B*, This fracture was fixed with crossed K- wires, which were removed six weeks later. *C*, Three days after removal of the wires, the fragment redisplaced during normal activity. *D*, This was fixed by cerclage wiring.

movements should include flexion-extension and prona-tion-supination exercises; the arm should be protected in a sling because of the normal state of activity of a child.

The aim of treatment is always restoration of the normal range of forearm supination and pronation; tilting of the radial head 20 to 30° may be compatible with this. However, this is not an excuse to leave this degree of angular deform-ity. Correction down to 30 to 40° of angular deformity is often advocated as acceptable for continuing with conserva-tive treatment. However, this may not improve with time and every attempt should be made to get a better degree of angular correction. Tachdjian believes that lateral tilting of up to 30° is acceptable, since there will be spontaneous cor-rection through remodeling;[57] however, this is less likely

with the older child because the proximal radius has much less growth potential than the distal physis. Further, in a crushing metaphyseal injury one cannot be certain about the possibility of a concomitant type 5 injury that may lead to the formation of an osseous bridge and cause further an-gular deformity or complete growth arrest. If the child is over 10 years of age, it is preferable to correct *any* angular deformity and tilting of the radial head to less than 10 to 15°. If improvement in the tilt to at least 10 to 20° cannot be attained, early open reduction is advocated. Remodeling is not extensive in this area, and permanent malunion may result.

Closed reduction is usually accomplished by partial to complete extension of the elbow to provide some fixation of

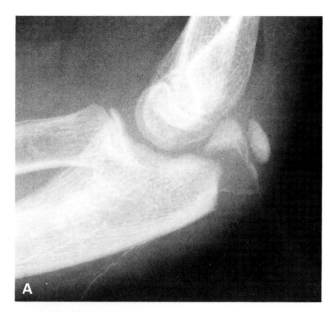

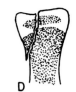

FIG. 12-28. Schematic of growth mechanism injuries. *A*, Type 1 transphyseal injury; *B*, Type 2; *C*, Type 3; *D*, Type 4.

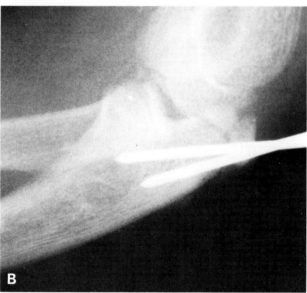

FIG. 12-27. *A*, Fracture of proximal ulna with triangular fragment and remnants of transverse subchondral plate. *B*, Post-reduction appearance.

in such a way that the thumb can be applied to produce a correction force. Firm digital pressure is applied in an upward and inward direction to complete the reduction. If roentgenography proves that the reduction is satisfactory, the arm should be immobilized in a posterior plaster splint.

In moderately displaced fractures (that is, 30 to 60° of angular deformity), closed reduction under general anesthesia is attempted first.[58] If satisfactory reduction is achieved, a long arm cast is applied with the elbow joint held at 70 to 90° of flexion, neutral rotation, and three-point fixation with the medial elbow as the fulcrum, and a slight varus stress applied to the cast to lessen pressure at the radiohumeral joint. Usually 3 to 4 weeks are sufficient to achieve healing. Remember, this area does not normally have a dense cortex and is not accustomed to assuming significant joint reaction forces, so it might collapse if the arm is used too soon. By 3 to 4 weeks, active protected range of motion and pronation-supination should be started. Repeat roentgenograms for the first 2 weeks to ensure maintenance of reduction. If reduction is not maintained, as occurred in 2 of 7 cases by Dougall and 3 of 34 cases by Jones, manipulation is repeated.[50,59]

Open reduction is undertaken when the radial epiphysis is displaced completely from the shaft or when manipulative reduction has been unsuccessful, and should be done as soon as possible after the injury, as extended periods of time may be associated with a higher incidence of myositis ossificans.[58,60]

the ulna relative to the humerus, followed by adduction of the forearm to correct or overcorrect the carrying angle and widen the radiohumeral articulation, a maneuver designed to create a space into which the displaced radial head may be reduced.[56] This position is held and the forearm rotated to bring the radial head into a position from which it may be pushed by direct pressure into correct alignment (Fig. 12-33). As a prelude to manipulation it is important to determine the direction of displacement of the radial head. Manipulative reduction is carried out with the forearm in the degree of rotation that brings the most prominent part of the displaced head farthest laterally. If this is done under image intensification, it is often possible to determine the position of supination or pronation that best emphasizes the fracture

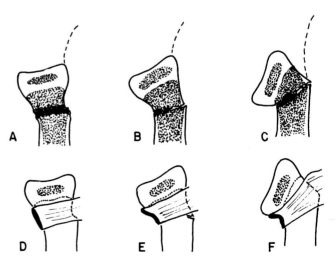

FIG. 12-29. *A-C*, Schematic of metaphyseal injuries showing patterns of angular deformation. *D-F*, Schematic of presentation of injury relative to annular ligament.

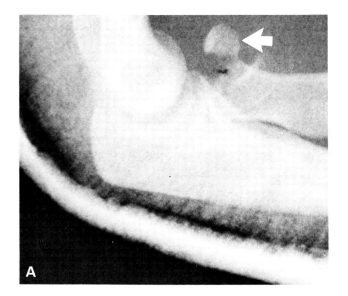

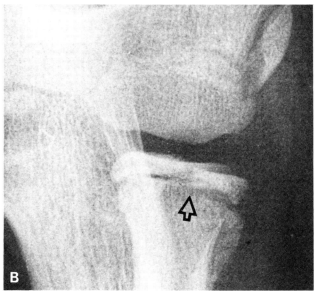

FIG. 12-30. *A,* Type 3 fracture (arrow) of the proximal radius in a 13-year-old girl during final stages of epiphysiodesis (similar to a Tillaux fracture). *B,* Type 4 fracture (arrow). Both of these fractures should be anatomically reduced.

Open reductions are carried out through a lateral approach. It may be possible to affect a reduction by remaining outside the annular ligament and applying pressure under direct vision. If this is not successful, the joint should be opened above the annular ligament to allow gentle replacement of the head on the neck. If possible, the annular ligament should not be divided. Internal fixation is usually unnecessary, except for an occasional suture.

Sectioning of the annular ligament is not performed unless it is absolutely necessary to achieve reduction. Every effort should be made to protect the annular ligament, but if it is damaged, it should be repaired. The forearm should be fully pronated and supinated to test the stability of the reduction.

Fixation can be accomplished by angular placement of wires in two points through the margin of the radial head down into the metaphysis, although Tachdjian recommends placing the wire through the capitellum into the center of the radial head and along the length of the radial shaft with the elbow flexed at 90° and the forearm in midrotation.[57] If it is possible to achieve fixation without violating the articular surfaces, I recommend peripheral placement of the fixation wires. The ends of the wires are left either subcuticular or penetrating the skin so that they can be easily removed, and bent 90° to prevent migration. A well-padded dressing is applied, followed by a posterior shell that can be converted after three to four days to a formal long arm cast when swelling has subsided. Other authors have recommended different methods of fixation. Key used sutures in the periosteum of the neck and sutured the annular ligament about it.[61,62] Reidy did not use any internal fixation except for an occasional suture.[9] O'Brien occasionally used a Kirschner wire.[49] Jones used Kirschner wires introduced behind and lateral to the lateral condyle of the humerus, crossing the radial head obliquely into the shaft.[59]

Care must be taken to protect the posterior interosseous nerve. This nerve may be exposed by separating the fibers of the supinator muscle with a blunt dissector. This wide exposure prevents neuropraxia of the posterior interosseous nerve and facilitates positioning of the radial head on its neck.

Even if it is completely separated, the radial head should be replaced anatomically (Fig. 12-34), since revascularization is the rule. Removal may result in significant relative deformities of growth rates between the radius and ulna.[63] Both the head and neck of the radius are poorly vascularized; their nutrition comes from the nutrient arteries and the periosteal veins. In cases with major dislocation of fragments, the periosteum may be completely severed. Extensive stripping of the periosteum should not be undertaken.

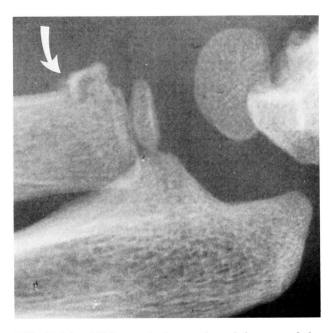

FIG. 12-31. Mildly crushed metaphyseal fracture of the proximal radius (arrow).

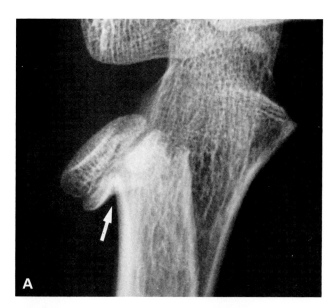

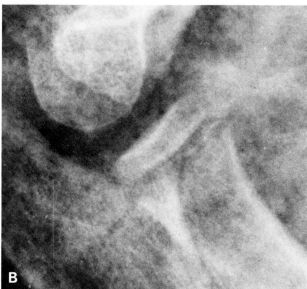

FIG. 12-32. *A*, Severely angulated proximal radial fracture. Notice the bent, but intact metaphyseal cortex (arrow). *B*, Appearance after closed reduction. See text for details.

In type 3 or 4 growth mechanism injuries, a closed reduction should be attempted first. Most of these injuries result in premature closure of the epiphysis and may accentuate some valgus, depending on the amount of remaining growth. Open reduction is frequently necessary.

In treating markedly displaced and fragmented fractures, many authors believe only two methods are likely to give satisfactory results—either excision of the capital fragment or open reduction. However, under no circumstances should one excise the radial head in a child, because marked growth disturbance may occur and the child may develop a Madelung-type deformity at the wrist, with marked radial deviation of the hand, depending on the amount of growth remaining. In a child approaching skeletal maturity, with a severely comminuted injury of the proximal radius, it is probably best to treat the child as an adult and excise the radial head.

If the fracture is diagnosed late, radial head tilting may be corrected by an opening wedge osteotomy and using a bone graft. If the patient is skeletally mature, the radial head may be excised, but only if warranted by the symptoms.

Results

Following this fracture, full return of supination and pronation may take several months, although there is little permanent disability. Restriction of motion of the elbow may occur; however, rotation of the forearm is most frequently affected. Pronation was limited in 21 elbows and supination in 14, with both motions being restricted in 13.[32] Flexion and extension, in contrast, were infrequently limited. According to Jeffrey, when the upper radial epiphysis has been completely displaced from the shaft, some permanent loss of movement is anticipated, even when accurate reduction has been secured by open operation.[32]

McBride reported 9 patients with a follow-up that ranged from 3 to 15 years.[53] In general, the results were good. He was negative about the results of open reduction in these injuries, but did recommend that after transsection of the annular ligament reduction could be maintained by a small Kirschner wire through the center of the head into the neck, and a good repair of the annular ligament. Two patients treated by open reduction went on to nonunion and eventually required resection of the radial head because of persistent pain.[53]

The carrying angle was increased 5 to 10° in 6 cases and 15 to 20° in 3, while 17 patients had no change in the carrying angle.[64] Only 2 patients showed an increased valgus of

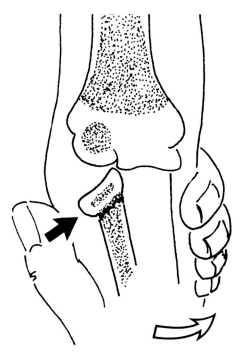

FIG. 12-33. Mechanism of reduction of radial head angulation.

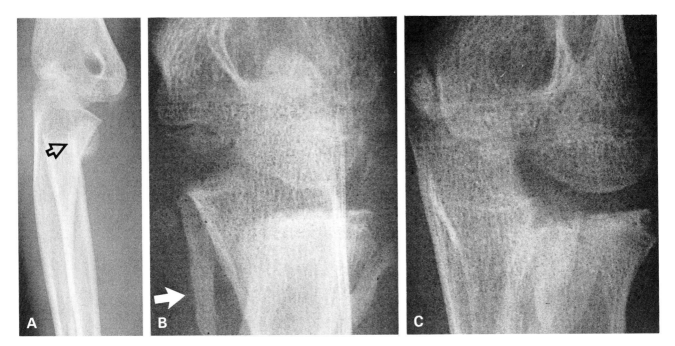

FIG. 12-34. *A,* Complete displacement of radial head (arrow). This was placed back on the shaft by open reduction. *B-C,* AP and oblique views showing ischemic necrosis and premature epiphysiodesis 18 months later. Ectopic bone is also evident (arrow).

more than 10° in the injured arm, as compared to the unaffected arm.[65] The carrying angle was increased in about 30% of the children due to premature closure of the growth plate of the radius. Nonunion is rare.

Complications

Key described a patient with an elbow dislocation with posterior displacement of the radius.[61] The patient was operated on 48 hours after the original injury. Roentgenograms showed an irregularity of the epiphyseal plate 13 months later. Since this child was still in active growth, it was possible that further deformity might result. There was also an indentation of the capitellum, suggestive of some irregular joint reaction forces across the radiohumeral joint. Wood reported 2 similar cases of posterior displacement of the epiphysis.[55] One patient was treated with open reduction and seen 6½ years later with good function and a normal radiograph. The second patient was also treated with open reduction, and when seen 2 years after injury, radiographs showed some distortion of the growth of the proximal end of the radius and some limitation of pronation and supination.

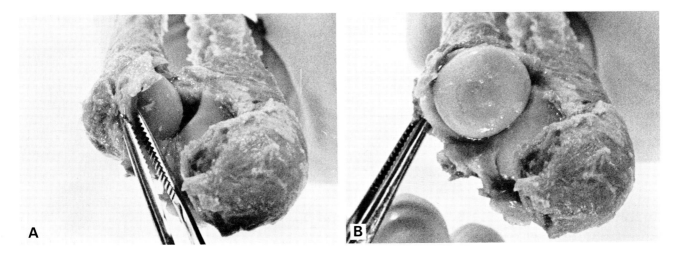

FIG. 12-35. Mechanism of pulled elbow. *A,* In pronation, the radial head subluxates away from the ulna, while the annular ligament displaces onto the radial head. *B,* With supination, the radial head relocates in the radioulnar joint, and the annular ligament relocates below the radial head.

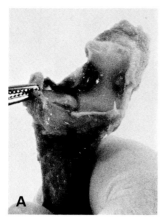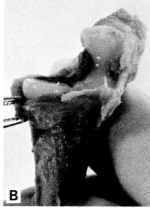

FIG. 12-36. Anatomy of pulled elbow. *A,* In pronation, the annular ligament slips up over the anterolateral radial margin. *B,* With supination, the higher, more flared side of the radial head forces the annular ligament back into anatomic position.

There is a slightly greater incidence of complications following open reduction than closed reduction.[65] Synostosis, though rare, is a hazard even of closed reduction, and may result in cubitus varus. Heterotopic ossification may also occur and reduce rotation, although Rang claims it is seen only after open reduction.[65] Early fusion and some deformity of the radial physis can also be expected.

Synostosis between the proximal radius and ulna has been reported.[49,50,66] Three cases in Henrikson's study developed synostosis between the radius and the ulna.[48] One developed a radioulnar synostosis consequent to the osteotomy.[53] Fielding reported a radioulnar cross-union following displacement of the proximal radial epiphysis in an 11-year-old boy who was treated with closed reduction.[66] Fibrous adhesions between the radius and ulna were also noted in one case by Jones.[59] These adhesions block rotation of the forearm.

Nonunion results from failure to achieve adequate reduction and maintain it. Premature fusion of the upper radial epiphysis occurs often in moderately and markedly displaced

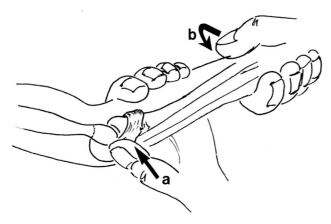

FIG. 12-37. Mechanism of reduction of pulled elbow. The thumb is placed directly over the radial head (a) while the forearm is rapidly supinated (b).

fractures, which may cause shortening of the radius and increased cubitus valgus, contingent upon the age of the child at the time of the injury and the severity of the cartilaginous damage. Premature fusion occurred in about one third of O'Brien's cases, but in none of them was the cubitus valgus severe enough to require osteotomy.[49]

Ischemic necrosis of the radial head occurred in 10% of the cases.[59] It does not appear relative to the degree of initial displacement, nor to the age at the time of injury. The results are poor.[59] Ischemic necrosis of the whole head is rare, even when the head is completely reduced. Partial ischemic necrosis is seen more frequently. Irregularity of the radial head and premature closure of the proximal radial physis are common (see Fig. 12-34). Premature fusion occurred in 11 of 30 cases.[9]

New bone formation and deformity of the radial head with enlargement occurs in some cases and may restrict elbow motion. O'Brien reported a notch in the radial neck in 6 of 125 cases, and believed it due to scarring and damage to the annular ligament.[49]

Pulled Elbow

One of the most common elbow injuries encountered in infants and young children is the "pulled" elbow.[31,67-92] This term is used to identify an entity in which the radial head is traumatically "locked" because of sudden traction on the hand or forearm when the elbow is extended and the forearm (hyper) pronated. This entity is described by various eponyms, including "nursemaid's" and "temper tantrum" elbow. It can also occur when pulling a child as he stumbles, when swinging him, or when forcefully pulling him away from something. It is one of the most common injuries to the elbow in children under 4 years of age, and rarely occurs after the age of 5, with peak incidence between 1 and 3 years. High incidences of this injury have been reported by Salter and Zaltz,[93] Griffin,[78] and Snellman.[90]

Pathomechanics

One of the early theories reported that the head of the radius was not fully developed, that the perimeter of the cartilaginous end was smaller than the neck, and thus not firmly held in place by the annular ligament. This is probably a misinterpretation of a statement by Pierseol.[94] Ryan examined the upper end of the radius in 15 fetal specimens and found that the radial head, even at birth, was definitely larger than the neck, and that the ratio of the two (head:neck) does not differ greatly from that of an adult.[94] This investigation was subsequently supported by Salter and Zaltz, who examined the proximal end of the radius in 12 child cadavers ranging in age from 2 days to 9 years.[93] In each specimen they found that the diameter of the radial head was larger than the neck by 30 to 60%, the ratio varying from 1.3 to 1 to 1.6 to 1. Thus the concept that the radial head is easily pulled through the annular ligament because it is smaller than the radial neck is erroneous. Similar unpublished studies in our skeletal developmental laboratory of 54 fetal specimens (3 fetal months to term), and 38 postnatal specimens support this observation that the radial head is *always* larger than the metaphysis (neck).

Stone studied the mechanism of injury in 12 anatomic specimens and was able to produce the lesion in 6 of the elbows.[95] He observed that the annular ligament slipped over the radial head only when the forearm was pronated. He also noted that the radial head was slightly oval, rather than circular, and that when the forearm was supinated, the anterior aspect of the radial head was elevated sharply from the neck. Salter and Zaltz also observed that the superior surface of the radial head, viewed from above, is slightly more oval than circular and with forearm supination the sagittal diameter of the radial head is consistently greater than the coronal diameter.[93]

My studies have shown that the plane of the articular surface is not completely perpendicular to the longitudinal axis of the radius. Laterally and posteriorly the radial head rises rather gradually, so that when traction is applied with the forearm in pronation, the annular ligament must lie over the less prominent (i.e., "lower") portion, which also has a straighter side angle relative to the longitudinal axis (see Fig. 12-7). The annular ligament may stretch and slip over a part of the head (Figs. 12-35 and 12-36; also see Fig. 12-8).

In full supination, the radius at the site of the annular ligament is outflared, so that it is difficult for the annular ligament to be displaced onto the epiphysis and further onto the joint. However, when the arm is fully pronated this portion of the metaphysis and epiphysis begins to assume a much straighter position that more easily allows the annular ligament to be displaced in a proximal direction.

McRae studied 25 stillborn elbows and concluded that a pulled elbow was caused by the annular ligament slipping partially over the radial head.[96] Salter and Zaltz anatomically duplicated the mechanism of displacement with sudden firm and steady traction on the extended elbow, first in supination and then in pronation.[93] They were not able to subluxate the radial head in any of the specimens when the traction was applied with the forearm in supination, but when traction was applied in pronation, a transverse tear was produced in the thin distal attachment of the annular ligament to the periosteum of the radial neck. Once this transverse tear occurred, the anterior portion of the radial head could escape under the anterior part of the annular ligament, which displaced over the radial head. Our studies show this displacement may occur even without tearing annular ligament attachments, and that the ligament may displace laterally or posteriorly. When the proximal edge of the annular ligament did not extend beyond the diametric (midportion) of the radial head, the interposed ligament could be repositioned in its normal site by simple supination in the forearm. In specimens from older children, this tear could not be produced because of thicker, stronger attachments.

Diagnosis

The clinical picture of pulled elbow is characteristic. The young infant or child suddenly refuses to move his arm and holds it slightly flexed and pronated. Parents often think the arm is paralyzed. The child's elbow is painful and he often admits to having felt a click when the injury occurred. He always holds the injured elbow with the forearm pronated and the elbow proximally flexed. On palpation one can elicit local tenderness over the radial head. Generally there is no restriction of flexion and extension, but the child resists supination.

Roentgenograms of the elbow are normal, with no displacement of the proximal radius from the capitellum. A roentgenogram is only useful for ruling out associated fractures, which are rare.

Treatment

Reduction is easily accomplished by rapid supination. This may be done inadvertently by the technician when taking radiographs. The preferred method of reduction is flexing the elbow to 90°, placing the thumb over the radial head and exerting mild pressure (Fig. 12-37). Using the other hand, the child's forearm is rapidly and firmly rotated into full supination. As reduction is achieved, a palpable, and sometimes audible, click can be felt in the region of the radial head. The child generally evinces instantaneous relief of pain, stops crying, and begins almost immediately to use the arm in a normal fashion. Immobilization other than the use of a sling for comfort is not necessary, unless this is a repeat occurrence.

If the subluxation is irreducible (a rare situation), open reduction is indicated. This may require dividing the annular ligament. However, using small nerve hooks to grasp the ligament within the joint and pulling it over the radial head allows reduction without transsection of the annular ligament.

Results

Restoration of motion and function is instantaneous. Recurrence of the injury is uncommon and probably occurs in less than 5% of cases.

Dislocation of the Head of the Radius

Congenital dislocation of the head of the radius with no other congenital abnormality in the elbow is rare (Fig. 12-38).[97-100] Wright suggested that some of the cases reported as congenital dislocations of the radial head were, in reality, caused by trauma and probably occurred during delivery.[101] In distinguishing between congenital and traumatic dislocations, one of the most reliable signs is the condition of the capitellum. If it is significantly underdeveloped, a congenital dislocation is more likely, although early postnatal subluxation or dislocation (i.e., infantile "nursemaid's" elbow) might lead to secondary joint deformation on both sides of the joint, just as in congenital hip disease. Confusion may arise when a child with a congenital or pathologic dislocation falls on his elbow. The ensuing radiograms may mimic an acute injury.

In congenital dislocation of the radial head, Bell Tawse believes that there is no capsular inclusion and that there is a poorly developed radial head with a convex shape.[102] Vesely explored the radial heads in two cases of congenital dislocation and described capsular distortion and displacement of the annular ligament.[100] These findings were similar to the case shown in Figure 12-38.

Caravias reported 3 cases of acute radial head dislocation that resembled those of a classic "congenital" dislocation of the head of the radius. The first case was treated with a closed reduction, but anatomic restoration was not attained. There was also a dislocation of the elbow in association with

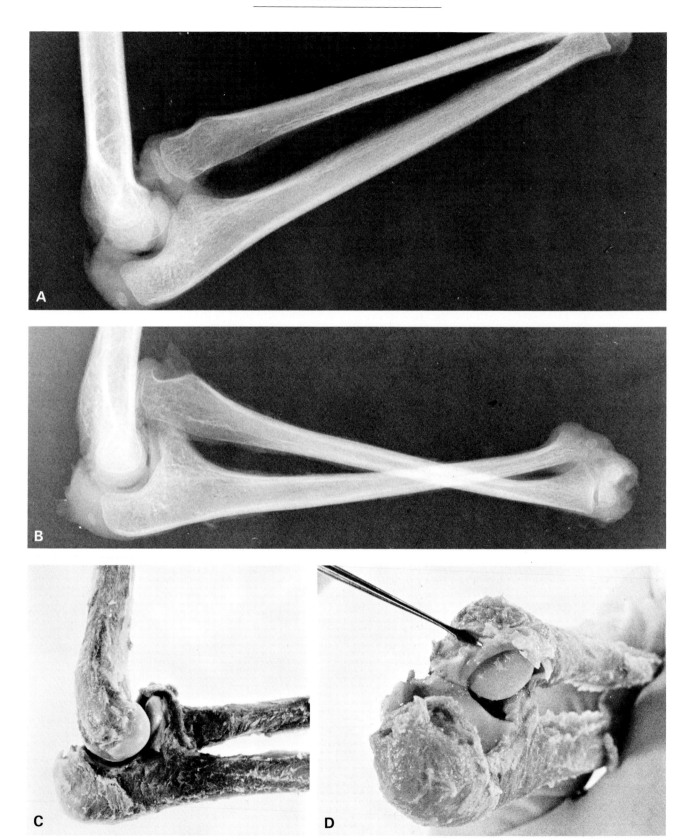

FIG. 12-38. "Congenital" subluxation of the radial head in cadaver specimens. *A,* Roentgenogram of right side. This side could be reduced in some positions. *B,* More severe involvement of the left side. This could not be reduced because of severe capsular distortion. *C,* Gross specimen of fracture shown in part *A,* after reduction. *D,* Annular ligament over radial head of specimen shown in *A.* After dissection freed this from the capsule, it could be reduced, intact, back around the metaphysis.

the neck fracture. In follow-up 4 years later, after skeletal maturation had been attained, the head of the radius was completely displaced from its radiohumeral articulation and angulated forward. His second case was a 36-year-old woman who had injured her elbow at the age of 5. The head of the radius was lateral to the capitellum, but not as high riding as some cases of congenital dislocation. His third case was a girl of 18 who apparently had a lesion that was first recognized when she was approximately 2 weeks old, although it had not been associated with any known birth trauma.[97]

Schubert described a case of a dislocated radial head in a newborn who was treated with the arm in supination; the infant had an uneventful recovery.[103] He also described a bilateral case, reported by Cockshott, of a 6-day-old baby with dislocations that seemed to reduce easily in full supination and dislocate in pronation. Further, one may question whether some congenital dislocations of the radial head are not the end result of a subluxation or dislocation of a newborn that was unrecognized. In support of this speculation, a 30% incidence of "dislocations" of the radial head in cases of Erb's palsy was reported by Aitken.[12] Possibly, in addition to the current concept that these dislocations are due to muscular imbalance, some radial head dislocations in Erb's palsy may be due to unrecognized accidental subluxation or dislocation in the newborn (i.e., neonatal "nursemaid's" elbow), or progressive post-natal displacement due to muscle imbalance.

Vesely also described isolated traumatic dislocations of the radial head in children.[100] He reviewed 17 cases and found 2 with concomitant fractures of the radial head; 13 of the dislocations were anterior, 3 were lateral, and 1 was posterior; 4 were treated with open reduction. Chronic dislocation developed in 2 cases, including 1 case that was not reduced until 8 months after the injury. A persistent synostosis at the superior radioulnar joint developed in 1 case.

Hamilton described a dislocation in a 9-year-old, but there is little written about the injury.[104] This injury should not be confused with nursemaid's elbow, which is rare over the age of 5 and generally is not due to a fall on the outstretched hand, but rather secondary to a traction force in the extended arm. The flexibility of the developing ulna allows some anterior bowing without fracture.

Neviaser and LeFevre also reported an isolated dislocation of the radius without ulnar fracture in a 7-year-old.[105] They treated the child with open reduction because of irreducibility and found a transverse tear in the anterior capsule, exactly where one might expect it if this were a mechanism somewhat similar to that of nursemaid's elbow. The proximal portion of the capsule was lying in the normal anatomic bed of the radial head precluding reduction. The constricting buttonhole effect of the tear was relieved by a capsular incision, and when the capsule was withdrawn from the joint, the radial head was easily reduced.

Lloyd-Roberts believes that many of these cases represent perinatal or infantile radial head subluxation that progressively deforms.[106] He believes that open reduction and reconstruction of the annular ligament are indicated to reestablish radiohumeral-radioulnar rotational mechanics. I have treated a similar case in a boy with generalized joint laxity. He was found to have sternoclavicular and radial head "dislocations" at birth, but no treatment was rendered. Figure 12-39 shows the roentgenographic appearance when

he was examined four years later. He lacked full rotation and was having elbow pain localized to the radial head. During the operation, the annular ligament was displaced over the radial head, similar to the case shown in Figure 12-28. The ligament segments were then dissected free anteriorly and posteriorly to the ulnar attachments. The ligament was then divided laterally, displaced to its anatomic position around the neck, and repaired. The capitellum was mildly deformed and permitted some continued subluxation. The reduction was maintained with a pin for six weeks. He has complete flexion and extension six months postoperatively, but has a mild subluxation in full pronation.

Monteggia Lesions

Classically, this injury involves a fracture of the proximal third of the ulna in association with anterior dislocation of the radial head, but the injury must be suspected whenever there is an apparent injury (bowing or fracture) *anywhere* along the course of the ulna without an obvious associated fracture of the radius.[35,54,102,107-113,113a,114-127]

The level of the fracture of the ulna varies. In approximately 66% of the cases it is located at the junction of the proximal and middle thirds of the shaft, in 15% it is located in the middle third, and in the remainder it is equally distributed between the distal third of the ulnar shaft and the olecranon process. The ulnar fracture may be greenstick (Fig. 12-40), and the apparent mildness of the injury may prevent accurate interpretation of the actual severity. Fractures of both bones of the forearm with anterior dislocation of the radial head may also occur.

Theodorou described 3 cases that were interesting because the radial head dislocation was associated with the fracture of the distal radius and ulna, a combination not usually found in adults.[92] Because of the mechanism of falling injury, wrist injuries often accompany Monteggia fracture-dislocations, and it is imperative that the wrist be accurately assessed at the same time the elbow and midforearm are being roentgenographically examined.

The age of incidence has been reported from 2 months to 14 years, but the injury occurs most frequently between 7 and 10 years.

Classification

There are basically three types of Monteggia fractures: type 1 (extension type), in which the head of the radius is dislocated anteriorly with volar angulation of the fractured shaft of the ulna (Fig. 12-41), type 2 (flexion type), in which the radial head is dislocated posteriorly with dorsal angulation of the fractured shaft of the ulna (Fig. 12-42), and type 3, in which the radial head is dislocated laterally along with the fractured shaft of the ulna (Fig. 12-43). Some authors also describe a type 4, which is essentially a type 1 pattern, except that there is also a fracture through the radius in its proximal third.

There are equivalents to type 1, such as dislocation of the head of the radius without any evident fracture of the ulna, which may occur because of the capacity of the ulna to elastically or plastically deform, with variable return to its original shape (see Fig. 12-40).

The type 2 injury, with posterior dislocation of the radial

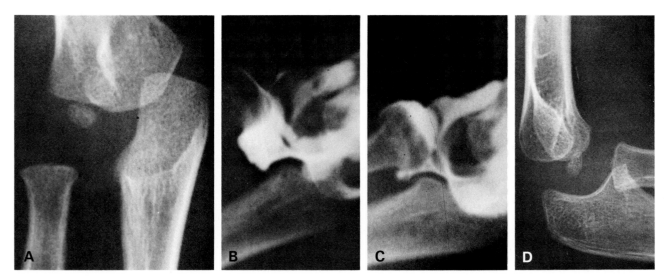

FIG. 12-39. *A,* Appearance of elbow in four-year-old boy with "congenital" dislocation of the proximal radius. *B,* Arthrogram showing maximum displacement. *C,* Arthrogram of "reduction," which was incomplete because of soft tissue interposition. The patient subsequently underwent exploratory surgery. The annular ligament was displaced completely over the radius, sitting in the space between the radius and the ulna. This was dissected free of the capsule, divided, and reattached in anatomic position. *D,* Appearance six months later.

head, is commonly associated with a fracture of the radial head and is found primarily in adults, although it may occur in children. Penrose described this type of injury as a variation of posterior dislocation of the elbow.[128]

The type 3 Monteggia lesion with lateral dislocation occurs in both children and adults and has a higher incidence of radial nerve injury. Wise reported a case of lateral dislocation of the head of the radius associated with incomplete fracture of the olecranon that produced varus deformity in a 7-year-old boy, a fracture Wise considered an unusual

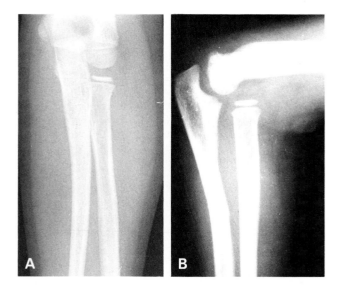

FIG. 12-40. *A,* Be wary of the normal-appearing view. *B,* In the lateral view the Monteggia injury is evident. The ulna had only a greenstick deformation.

Monteggia fracture.[129] Beddow and Wright described similar cases.[101,130]

In one series, type 1 was the most common (85%), type 2 (10%), and type 3 (5%).[5] Bado described an incidence of 1.7% in 3200 forearm fractures, with 57% being type 1, 15% type 2, 19% type 3, and the others scattered through the various equivalents of type 4 and subtle variations of the previous types.[107]

Pathomechanics

When a patient falls forward on his outstretched hand the forearm is usually pronated, and at the moment of impact his hand becomes relatively fixed to the ground. Because of the downward momentum of the falling body, a rotation force is added when twisting of the trunk causes external rotation of the humerus and ulna. If this force continues until the normal limit of pronation at the proximal radioulnar joint is reached, something must give. The ulna is liable to fracture. At the same time, the radius is forced into extreme pronation and lies across the ulna at the junction of the upper and middle thirds. Evans believes that as the ulna fractures, the two bones come in contact and at that point a fulcrum is formed over which the upper end of the radius is forced forward.[5] As the pronation force continues, the radius is either levered forward out of the superior radioulnar joint, or is fractured in its upper third. However, it is not necessary to have contact, since hyperpronation places the radial head and radiocapitellar morphologic relationships in a position whereby the annular ligament can be displaced and allows dislocation (Fig. 12-44).

Speed reported that a direct blow over the posterior aspect of the proximal ulna could produce this injury.[34] This hypothesis was accepted until evidence gained from 18 cadavers and clinical observations suggested hyperpronation as a mechanism of injury. Speed stated that the bicipital tuberos-

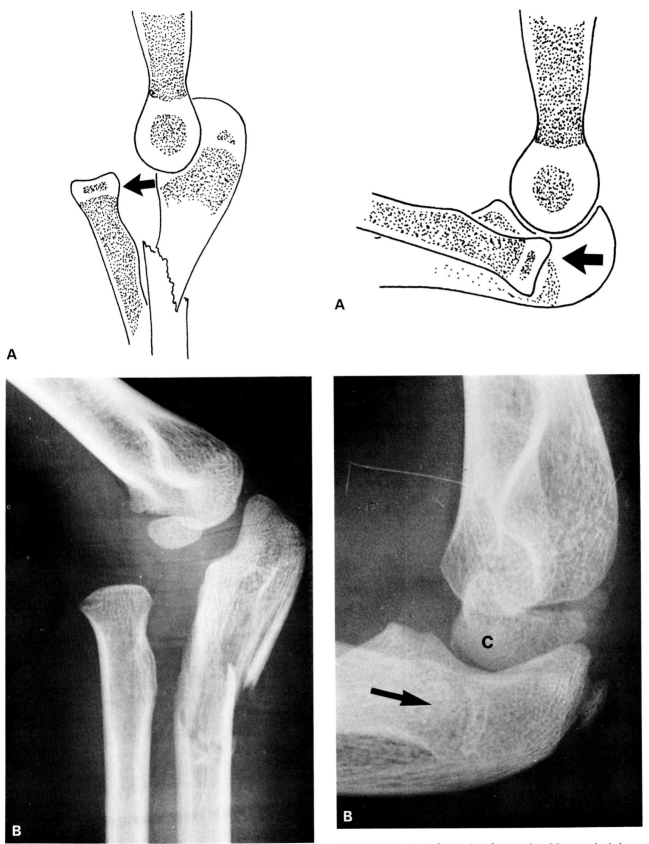

FIG. 12-41. *A,* Schematic of anterolateral Monteggia injury. *B,* Roentgenographic appearance.

FIG. 12-42. *A,* Schematic of posterior Monteggia injury. *B,* Roentgenographic appearance. Arrow shows radius pointing away from capitellum (c).

ity was most posterior in hyperpronation, and that this position made the radius subject to the greatest force from the biceps tendon during violent contraction of the muscle. Just as Evans, who produced 12 anterior Monteggia lesions by pronation in 18 cadavers, so Penrose was able to produce a posterior Monteggia alone by weakening the proximal anterior ulna.[5,128]

Both hypotheses were challenged by Tompkins, who presented evidence that hyperextension with the forearm in a neutral position was also an acceptable pathomechanism for type 1 injuries.[131] He based this on clinical and radiologic examinations of the acutely injured patient that showed type 1 Monteggia lesions with the forearm in neutral or slightly supinated position. In compound type 1 fractures, the proximal ulnar fragment usually penetrates the palmar skin on the ulnar side of the forearm, a phenomenon anatomically impossible if the forearm is in hyperpronation due to blockage by the radius. Biomechanical investigations of the moments and components of force suggest, theoretically at least, that with the hand fixed in pronation with the elbow in full extension or hyperextension, contraction of the biceps tends to pull the head of the radius more securely into the lesser sigmoid notch. Neutral position of the forearm tends to lift the radius out of the annulus.

Evans showed that in the anterior Monteggia injury, forced hyperpronation first ruptures the capsular and annular ligaments, then fractures the shaft of the ulna, and finally rotates the head of the radius so that it lies in front of the capsule.[5] Having prevented the reduction of the radial head, the interposed capsule would then act as a mechanical block to full flexion.

Because of the ease with which the radial head is often reduced in children, especially if treated early, and the excellent long-term results, it is feasible that the annular ligament is not disrupted longitudinally, but that it tears transversely along its more distal insertion and is incompletely herniated into the joint, much as the mechanism in a nursemaid's elbow in a younger child.

In a greenstick ulnar injury the most probable mechanism is a fall on the outstretched hand during which the forearm is supinated as it might be if the child were falling backward. The direction of the angulation of the ulna is determined by the exact direction of the fall, which may produce a varus, valgus, or hyperextension strain in the forearm.

Diagnosis

For practical purposes, there never is an isolated fracture of the ulna. The radius should be closely examined clinically and roentgenographically for injury to the proximal radiohumeral joint. Some fractures in Evans' series were greenstick, and the mildness of this injury may have prevented accurate interpretation of the actual severity.[5] Wright also reported the complication of greenstick ulnar fracture with Monteggia injury or displacement of the superior radial epiphysis.[101]

Any discussion must emphasize that a *fracture of the ulna with angulation or overriding without an accompanying fracture of the radius makes dislocation of the radial head suspect until proved otherwise.* Such proof can be obtained by including the elbow in all radiographs of suspected fractures of the ulna. In children, it is significant that a high percentage of ulnar fractures may be greenstick or even excess bowing, lulling one into a

false sense of security regarding possible subluxation or dislocation of the proximal radius. Further, it is often difficult to distinguish the exact location of the radial head, since it may not be ossified in many children. Great care must be taken not to miss this particular diagnosis.

A patient with a Monteggia injury usually holds his elbow partially flexed, with the forearm in pronation. Any rotation of the forearm or flexion-extension of the elbow is painful and restricted. The dislocated radial head may be palpable. However, in the presence of soft tissue swelling or deformity of the forearm or elbow, a dislocated radial head can be difficult to demonstrate clinically.

Roentgenograms of the forearm must include both the elbow and wrist in order to rule out injuries at both the proximal and distal end of the radial head. Normally the longitudinal axis of the radius should pass through the ossification center of the capitellum of the humerus. If it does not, then the radial head is subluxated or dislocated (see Figs. 12-41 to 12-43). A line drawn through the long axis of the radius should pass through the capitellum in all views. The radial head may be displaced anteriorly, laterally, or occasionally posteriorly.

If the roentgenographic beam is centered over the midforearm, as it often is, the elbow is included on the edge of the radiograph, especially if the ulna is fractured at mid or distal shaft. Distortion may make the radiohumeral relationship seem normal. The fractured ulna may be the predominant clinical and radiographic finding that focuses attention to the ulna lesion alone. Accurate AP and lateral views must be *centered on the elbow.*

Treatment

The anterior Monteggia dislocation is reduced as follows. The forearm is placed in full supination and longitudinal traction is applied. The elbow is gently flexed 90 to 120° to relax the biceps. The radial head is repositioned by direct manual pressure anteriorly. The angulated ulnar shaft is reduced by firm manual pressure, which is not difficult, once the radial head has been repositioned. Following reduction, the radial head is usually stable, as long as the elbow is kept in acute flexion and the annular ligament is in its normal position (see Fig. 12-44).

Tompkins pointed out that the ulnar fracture tends to develop an increased radial bow during immobilization.[131] This is caused by the normal slight bowing of the ulna and the contraction of the flexor muscles in the forearm. Therefore, Tompkins recommends immobilizing the forearm in neutral rotation or only slight supination, with the cast carefully molded over the lateral side of the ulna at the level of the fracture. As long as the elbow is in acute flexion of 110° or more, the biceps is relaxed and it is unnecessary to keep the forearm in full supination to maintain the reduction.

A posterior Monteggia fracture is reduced by applying traction to the forearm with the elbow in full extension. The radial head is reduced manually and the posterior angulation of the ulnar fracture anatomically aligned. The arm should be casted in almost full extension.

Once one believes that reduction of the radial head is complete, the elbow should be flexed, extended, and then flexed again. If there is no interposition of the annulus, the radial head should remain reduced, especially if the reduced ulnar fragments are also reasonably stable. In children, it is head. Interposition may be of three types: partial, in which portions of the ligament are interposed between the radial head and the ulna; complete, in which the radial head pulls out of the ligament, leaving it intact, an injury that accounts for the majority of failures of reduction; and fragmentary, in which osteocartilaginous fragments are present, most frequently associated with type 2 lesions. Open reduction of the radial head and repair of the annular ligament always carry the risk of subsequent ectopic ossification.

Although closed reduction of the radial head displacement may be successful (Fig. 12-47), open reduction may be necessary for the accompanying ulnar injury.

Immobilization is maintained until there is union of the ulna, which ordinarily requires 6 to 10 weeks, depending on the patient's age. The patient's elbow is then progressively mobilized. Emphasis should be on flexion-extension exercises for a week, followed by supination-pronation exercises.

Late Case

Bell Tawse reported six children with undiagnosed Monteggia fractures.[102] These patients all developed malunited fractures of the ulna with persistent dislocation of the radial head, restricted flexion, and increased cubitus valgus. *All these children originally had greenstick fractures of the ulna.* Five were treated successfully by open reduction and reconstruction of the annular ligament. One patient had recurrence of the dislocated radial head. In instances where the diagnosis was delayed or missed, open surgery was necessary to reduce the radial head (Fig. 12-48).

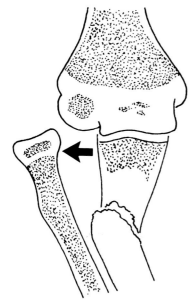
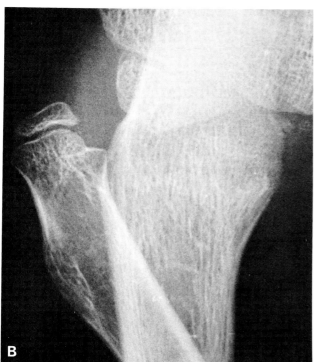

FIG. 12-43. *A,* Schematic of lateral Monteggia injury. *B,* Roentgenographic appearance.

more important to reduce the radial dislocation accurately than to gain absolute anatomic reduction of the ulnar fracture, because remodeling corrects minor angulations of 5 to 10°. Confirming roentgenograms should be taken at weekly intervals to ascertain that the radial head does not redislocate.

Occasionally, open reduction is necessary, particularly when one is unable to replace the radial head into its normal position (Figs. 12-45 and 12-46). Interposition of the annular ligament frequently prevents reduction of the radial

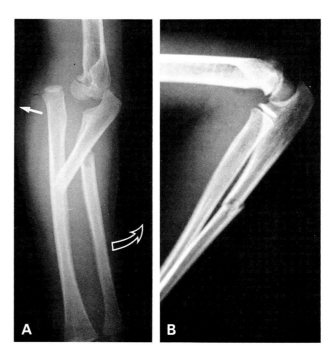

FIG. 12-44. *A,* Midshaft ulnar fracture associated with proximal radial dislocation. As the distal radius and ulna displace dorsally (open arrow), the radial head levers out anteriorly (solid arrow). *B,* Closed reduction of the radial head eased closed reduction of the ulnar fracture.

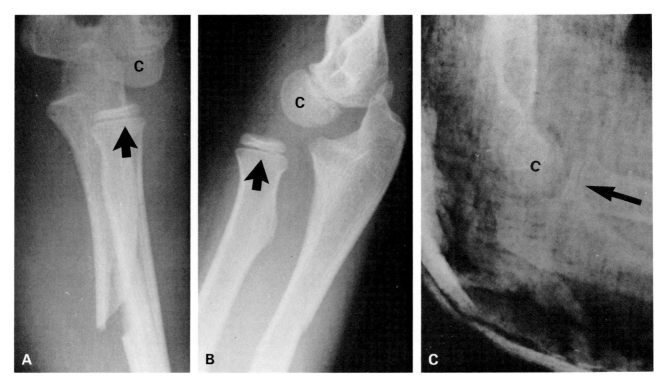

FIG. 12-45. *A-B,* Original injury. Closed reduction was unsuccessful. Note that the axis of the radial shaft (arrow) does not point to the capitellum (c). *C,* This injury was subsequently treated by open reduction and removal of the herniated annular ligament from the joint. Removal was accomplished by a nerve hook without transection of the ligament. Note how the longitudinal axis (arrow) of the radius is now directed at the capitellar ossification center (c).

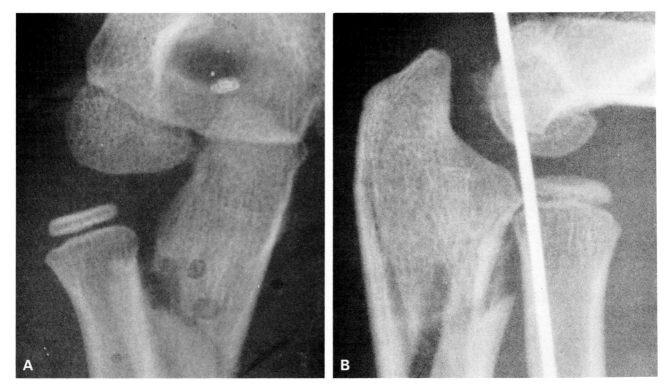

FIG. 12-46. *A,* Monteggia injury. *B,* Post-reduction and internal fixation with a threaded wire. This type of fixation is unacceptable. A smooth wire should be used.

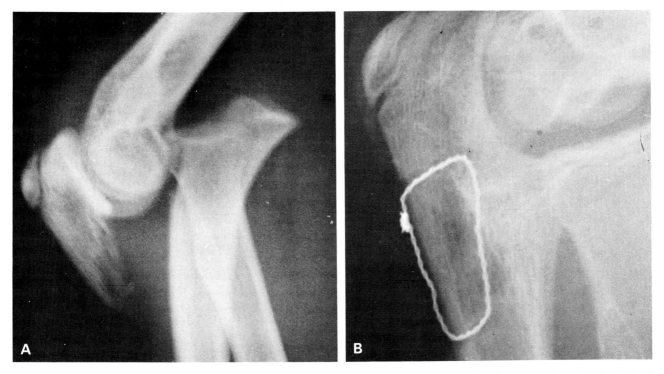

FIG. 12-47. *A,* Anterior Monteggia injury accompanying a proximal ulnar fracture. *B,* The ulna was reduced and stabilized with a tension wire, while the radius was reduced without opening the joint.

Bell Tawse suggested an easily attained method of treating the unreduced, late dislocation without having to divide the ulna.[102] He constructed a new ulnar ligament by turning down a slip of the triceps tendon, leaving it attached to the ulna, passing it around the neck of the radius, and securing it through a drill hole in the ulna. However, accurate dissection of the damaged or displaced annular ligament may allow direct repair (Fig. 12-48). The radioulnar joint, as well as the radiohumeral joint, must be accurately reduced. The arm should be held in extension and supination for six weeks after open repair.

If reduction of the radial head is difficult because ulnar angulation has caused shortening, it is better to lengthen the proximal ulna with an oblique (overlapping) osteotomy, rather than shortening the radial neck.

If more than three months have elapsed, the possibility of heterotopic ossification causing ankylosis or fibrosis of the elbow following surgery may be real. In a child, a dislocated radial head should never be resected since it may cause cubitus valgus, prominence of the distal end of the ulna, and radial deviation of the head. Removing the radial head must be deferred until the completion of skeletal growth, and then only if symptoms or decreased function make it necessary.

Results

In most reported series, children have no sequelae from the Monteggia lesion; major complications generally occur in adult patients. There are no significant problems of healing of the ulnar fracture in children. There is full return of elbow function; redislocation of the radial head is rare.

Complications

Complications, although infrequent in children, may include: (1) Chronic dislocation and malposition as result of misdiagnosis, which represents the most frequent complication (incidence ranging from 16 to 50%). (2) Recurrent dislocation of the radial head after initial closed reduction. (3) Posterior interosseous nerve neuropathy, which is most common in type 3, but has also been reported in types 1 and 2. Spontaneous recovery is generally expected in all patients and exploration should not be attempted prior to 6 weeks following occurrence of the injury. (4) Fracture of the radial head may occur in type 2 lesions, and may lead to premature epiphysiodesis of the proximal radial physis. If the fractured radial head is displaced in the child, it should be reduced, transplanted, and kept in place, as it is inappropriate to remove the radial head in a child. (5) Distal radioulnar joint disturbance may occur, but is not believed to be significant. (6) Compound wounds frequently cause complications. (7) Myositis ossificans. (8) Radiohumeral ankylosis. (9) Radioulnar synostosis.

According to Thompson, the development of myositis ossificans is commonly associated with dislocation of the elbow, rather than just the radial head.[126] The only case in Vesely's series was one in which there had been an open reduction.[11] The time lapse between injury and operation has been implicated as a predisposing factor in the formation of myositis ossificans. The subsequent resolution of myositis ossificans is influenced by the patients' age.

Spinner described 3 cases of posterior interosseous nerve palsy that was a complication of Monteggia fractures in children.[132] The posterior interosseous nerve is the motor

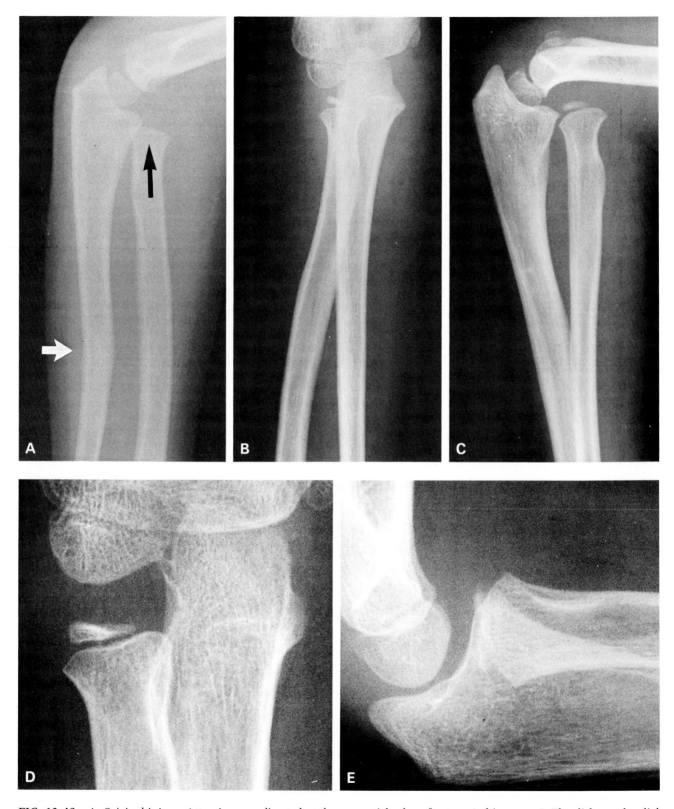

FIG. 12-48. *A,* Original injury. Attention was directed at the greenstick ulnar fracture (white arrow). The dislocated radial head was missed (black arrow). *B-C,* Two years later, a secondary ossification center has developed in the proximal radius, but not in the normal side. This may be due to injury-induced hyperemia. Open reduction and internal fixation were performed. The annular ligament, which was torn, displaced, and scarred, was dissected sharply from the anterior and posterior capsules. It was anatomically intact on the ulna. The damaged ends were repaired, restoring it to an annular configuration. *D-E,* Appearance six months after operation. The radius is stable and there is full return of motion.

branch of the radial nerve. In 25% of all individuals, the nerve lies in direct contact with the radius during its passage to the supinator, and in 30% a marked fibrous arch is formed in the muscle insertion, by which the nerve is held close to the bone. This is an area that can easily be injured in dislocation of the radius. The area where the nerve passes around the head of the radius is most susceptible to a traction or compression type of injury. With a radial head dislocation, a lesion in continuity is created at this level. Two of Spinner's cases were transitory, with neuropraxia-type lesions.[132]

Morris reported a case in which the radial head dislocation was irreducible because of entrapment of the radial nerve between the radial head and the ulna.[133] Stein described posterior interosseous nerve compression at the proximal edge of the supinator muscle through the fibrous arch of Frohse.[134] Guardjian and Smathers illustrated an anterior dislocated radial head that caused direct pressure on the radial nerve.[132] Jessing described nerve injuries in 6 of 14 patients.[135] There were 3 children in his series. One of them had a type 1 lesion with complete paralysis of the deep branch of the radial nerve. Beginning functional improvement was evident 8 weeks after the injury. Bado's 55 cases included 4 with radial nerve injuries, 2 with ulnar nerve injuries, and 1 with ulnar and median nerve injury.[107]

Chronic dislocation may be compatible with normal use of the elbow (Fig. 12-49). Many patients have no symptoms and are able to use the arm in all sports and activities.

Diaphysis

Diaphyseal injuries are common in children.[8,25,26,136-143] The severity may vary from pure bowing to greenstick to complete displacement. The level of fracture varies. In children there is a greater tendency for the radius and ulna to fracture at the same level, rather than at significantly different levels. The thick periosteum allows maintenance of some continuity, even when both bones are displaced. This highly osteogenic tissue also creates excellent healing of both fractures by closed means. Only when the adolescent is approaching skeletal maturity does the periosteum lose some of this function, increasing the risk of delayed union or nonunion.

Classification

These fractures follow many patterns. There may be simple plastic deformation (bowing), greenstick injury, or complete fracture. The bones may be angulated or displaced, with or without significant overriding. The bones may be fractured at different levels, or only one bone may be fractured (however, look carefully for bowing or greenstick failure of the seemingly noninjured one).

Plastic deformation is an infrequent failure pattern affecting small tubular bones like the fibula, radius, and ulna (see Chaps. 3 and 4), and is often difficult to diagnose. Due to microstructural failure, permanent deformation may be introduced (Figs. 12-50 and 12-51). More often there is definite evidence of the greenstick injury. Cortical failure may be minimal. The radius often sustains a greenstick failure while the ulna undergoes plastic deformation (Fig. 12-52). The ulna may also sustain a greenstick fracture without apparent radial injury (Fig. 12-52). Both bones may sustain greenstick injuries (Fig. 12-53).

Angular deformation varies. The radius may deform 30° to 40° without ulnar injury (Fig. 12-54). The periosteum is disrupted on the tension failure side in such angulation, but is usually intact along the compression side, a factor to be considered in any manipulation. Even if both bones are fractured, only one may be angulated. Angulation varies from mild to severe. Similarly, overriding varies significantly.

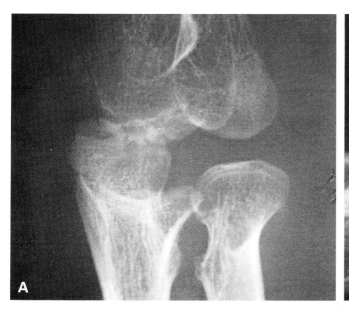
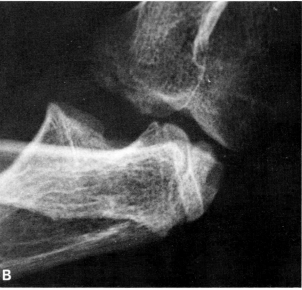

FIG. 12-49. *A,* AP and, *B,* lateral views of chronic posterior dislocation two years after original injury (a greenstick ulnar fracture). The patient lacked full extension by 10°. Note the capitellar and radial head deformities. The family refused treatment.

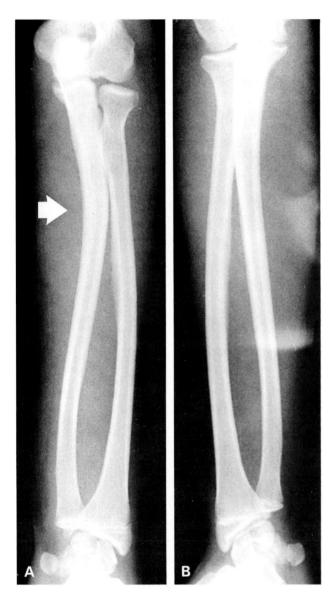

FIG. 12-50. *A,* Plastic deformation of ulna (arrow). *B,* Contralateral side. This girl lacks full supination and pronation.

Diagnosis

Roentgenograms should include both the wrist and elbow joints to be certain that there is no dislocation of either the proximal or distal radioulnar joints. It is feasible to have a Monteggia injury with a fracture of the radius or plastic deformation of the ulna, as well as the classic injury of a fracture of the ulna. Roentgenograms should be true anteroposterior and lateral views, since nonstandard angles and degrees of rotation complicate interpretation.

The radius is a curved bone that is cam-shaped in cross section at several levels. Malrotation of the radius can be recognized by a break in the smooth curve of the bone or a difference in the width of the cortices of the apposed fracture fragments. In fractures of the forearm, palmar or flexor bowing (that is, of the apex) is usually a sign of pronation deformity, while dorsal or extensor bowing (at the apex) usually signifies a supination deformity.

Evans drew attention to the bicipital tuberosity roentgenographic sign.[4] The problem in the younger child is that the region of the tuberosity often is minimally developed, and may not suffice as an accurate indicator as much as it does in an older child or adult. The tuberosity normally lies medially when the forearm is fully supinated (i.e., it faces the ulna). It lies posteriorly in the midposition, and laterally in full pronation (see Fig. 12-12). If there is any question about this, a similarly rotated view of the normal, uninvolved arm can be obtained. The estimated degree of rotation proximally can be used as a guideline to determine the best position in which to place the distal fragments.

In young children, child abuse must be considered as part of the differential (Fig. 12-55), especially when the fracture already had callus or when metachronous fractures are present.

Neurovascular injury

Nerves and blood vessels are seldom injured in children's forearm fractures. There is a tendency to overlook the possibility of damage to the nerves in the forearm. The median nerve is protected from the radius by intervening layers of muscles. The ulnar nerve is close to bone and occasionally may be damaged, especially in open fractures near the lower end. Warren described 2 cases of anterior interosseous nerve

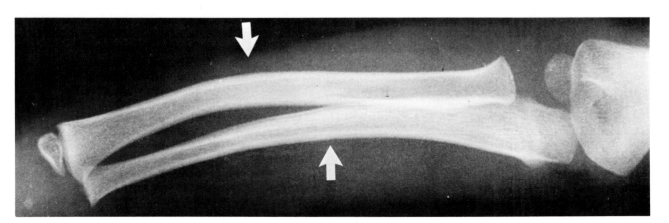

FIG. 12-51. Greenstick bowing of both bones (arrows) in a four-year-old.

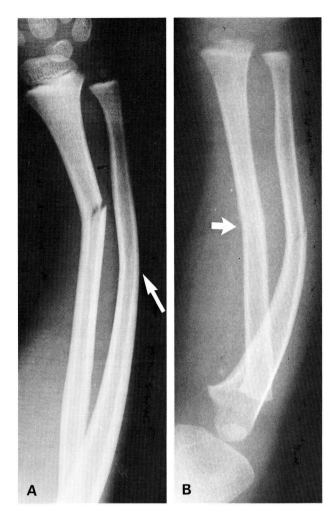

particularly when complete, tend to allow dissipation of intracompartmental pressure into the more superficial areas, and throughout other compartments. Care must be taken to watch for increased pressure in the anterior compartment. Monitoring of pressure with a wick catheter may be necessary.

Rotation

Before discussing treatment, it is essential to consider rotation (supination-pronation), since restoration of this anatomic function is the most important aspect of treatment. Forearm rotation has a range of 180°.[10,145,146] The vertically paired proximal and distal radial ulnar joints move synchronously. Normal radial bowing is essential to the rotational axis of the radius about the ulna and must be maintained in any reduction. Failure to do so disrupts the rotational cone (Fig. 12-56; also see Fig. 12-15).

Although a child may functionally adapt to a decrease in motion up to 50%, forearm fractures must be treated in a manner that avoids, as much as possible, any significant loss of the normal range of supination and pronation.[147]

Loss of rotation is a common problem after forearm fractures, no matter what the level of fracture.[108,148] Knight and Purvis found residual rotational deformity between 20 and 60° in 60% of their patients. Evans found malrotation deformity of more than 30° in 56% of the cases.[4,6] The distal fragment is usually pronated, so that supination is primarily affected (see Fig. 12-56).

FIG. 12-52. *A,* Radial greenstick and ulnar plastic failure pattern. Ulnar failure is proximal (arrow) to the radial fracture. *B,* Ulnar greenstick fracture with barely discernible radial injury (arrow). This was a hyperpronation injury.

palsy.[144] In both cases, there was a complete, but temporary, paralysis of the flexor pollicis longus and index finger segment of the flexor digitorum profundus. Both patients made a full spontaneous recovery without any need for exploration of the nerve. The anterior interosseous nerve branches from the median nerve just distal to the neck of the radius and passes along with the anterior interosseous vessels, down the interosseous membrane along the radius. Because of its proximity to the radius, it is subject to injury in a displaced forearm fracture.

Davis and Greene reported 6 nerve injuries: 4 median, 1 ulnar, and 1 posterior interosseous. All cleared spontaneously within three weeks, suggesting that all were neuropraxia.[17] This is particularly important in distal third fractures when adequate assessment of the median nerve must be carried out. Although infrequent, the median nerve may be traumatized as the distal fragment is dorsally displaced and the forearm shortened.

Despite the presence of closed fascial spaces in the forearm, the risk of ischemic contracture is low. The fractures,

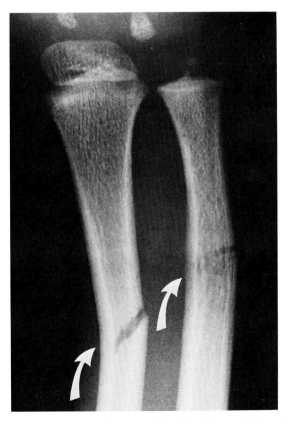

FIG. 12-53. Greenstick injury of both radius and ulna. The lateral cortex is intact on both (arrows).

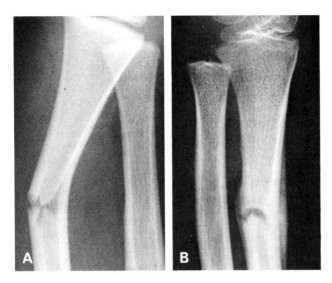

FIG. 12-54. *A,* Angulated radial fracture with intact inner cortex. *B,* Similar patient following correction of the angulation. Note that subperiosteal bone formation is better along the "compression" side, where there was cortical integrity. The initial angulation and hematoma elevate the periosteum.

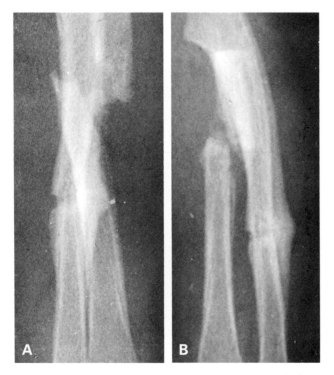

FIG. 12-55. *A,* AP and, *B,* lateral views of greenstick fractures of radius and ulna of an abused infant. The radial angulation probably should have been corrected. However, the patient was not seen until seven weeks after the injury was inflicted. There is new bone along the concavity, indicating some early "realignment." The radial fracture is significantly displaced and is developing a pseudarthrosis. Even in young children, fracture of both bones of the forearm may not be an innocuous injury.

Rang produced fractures in cadavers to determine the effects of various degrees of angular malunion: 10° of malrotation limited rotation by 10°, while 10° of malunion limited rotation by 20°, because of variable widening and narrowing of the interosseous membrane during the rotatory movements.[65] Bayonet apposition did not limit rotation. Pure narrowing of the interosseous space was important in proximal fractures. Narrowing impeded rotation by causing the bicipital tuberosity to impinge on the ulna. Malalignment of the fractures of the ulnar metaphysis increased tension on the articular discs so that the head of the radius was not free to rotate.

Christensen tried to find out why there is a diversion of opinion in the literature concerning immobilization of the forearm to insure the separation of the radius and ulna to prevent cross union.[7] He studied 36 cadaver forearms. The smallest interosseous distance was in pronation. The greatest distance was in midposition, closely followed by a few degrees in supination. The widest base was in the middle third of the forearm. He further showed that the interosseous membrane was taut in 30° of supination, but became increasingly relaxed in further supination or pronation.

It is possible to recognize these rotational deformities and correct them when treating the fracture. The variability of supination and pronation of the proximal and distal fragments is demonstrated at this time. If the upper part of the arm lies in supination, and the distal part looks as if it is pronated, then supination should be the major reduction direction to get the fracture back to anatomic position. Infrequently, the fracture reduction is sufficiently stable to allow testing of range of movement. Of course, full range of movement indicates an accurate reduction. The determination of

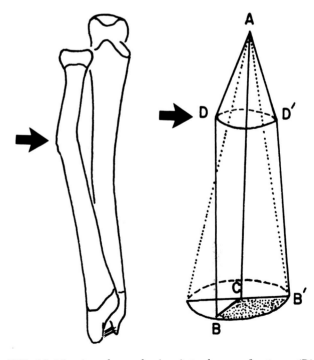

FIG. 12-56. Angular malunion introduces a frustrum (D) into the normal cone of rotation, thereby limiting the area (stippling) of the cone base. In this example, residual pronation of the distal radius restricts full supination.

the correct rotational position in which to immobilize fractures of both bones of the forearm is important to prevent a corresponding limitation of rotational movement.

Significant rotational deformity can be created at the time of reduction of complete fractures if they are manipulated improperly. It is further probable that the major cause of deformity has resulted from the universal application of the principles advocated by Evans.[6] The concept of pronating all distal third fractures, supinating all proximal third fractures, and leaving middle third fractures in neutral has been repeatedly recommended as the proper method of reduction since Evan's original article on the rotatory nature of forearm fractures. The "rule of the thirds" should not always be applied rigidly to these fractures. Reduction of the complete distal third fracture by forcible pronation may, in fact, result in malrotation of the fracture site, the one deformity that does not correct itself with growth, regardless of the age of the child.

Accurate reduction of the jagged bone ends is best accomplished when the rotational deformity is corrected. Even a small inaccuracy may prevent the interlocking of the bone ends upon which stability in plaster depends. The orthodox position in which to immobilize these fractures is that of full supination for the upper third, and midposition (neutral rotation) for fractures of the middle and lower thirds. These positions are based upon the anatomic arrangement of the pronators and supinators in the forearm. However, it is unreasonable to suppose that all fractures at a given level present the same degree of rotational deformity. Other factors may also be involved, such as variations in the direction and leverage of muscle pull with varying degrees of angulation of the fragments, variations in the tension of the biceps with flexion and extension of the elbow, and the effect of the interosseous membrane. The position, with respect to rotation, in which such fractures should be immobilized is governed by the degree of rotation of the upper radial fragment, the upper fragment of the ulna being stable because of the type of elbow articulation.

Although remodeling often corrects 30 to 40° of angular displacement of a metaphysis in a child with a growth left, remodeling does not do anything more than round off the ends of malunited fractures of the diaphysis, and never corrects rotational deformity accompanying the malunion. Always remember that angular fractures of the forearm are

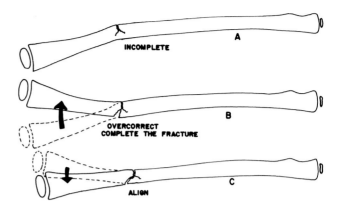

FIG. 12-57. Schematic of completion of the fracture in greenstick injuries of the radius and ulna.

associated with some degree of rotational deformity. Any loss of motion due to midshaft or proximal fractures tends to be permanent.

Treatment

In treating fractures of the radius and ulna in children, longitudinal (axial) and rotational alignment are the most important goals of reduction. Reduction is more difficult when the radial fracture is proximal to the ulnar fracture. These fractures may be more difficult to hold with the elbow in flexion; sometimes they are more stable in extension. Overriding can be accepted.

Blount advocated completion of the greenstick fracture(s), maintaining that failure to do so predisposed to later displacement.[14] Other authors found that reangulation may be prevented by placing the arm in the correct degree of pronation or supination and holding this position in plaster. In general, greenstick fractures should be slightly over-corrected by slow manipulation to take the plastic deformation out of the fracture (Fig. 12-57). Over-correction completes the fracture and is usually accompanied by an audible crack. If this is not done, the deformity may reappear, even in plaster (Fig. 12-58). This applies primarily to midshaft fractures.

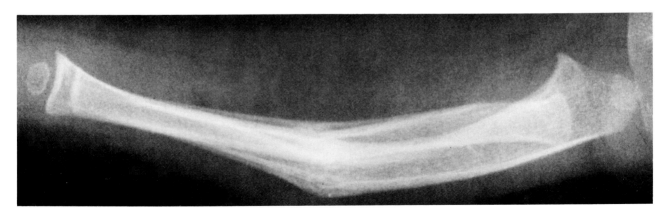

FIG. 12-58. Residual angular malunion complicating greenstick fractures in which the injury was not "completed."

Complete fractures of the radius and ulna can be troublesome and the following guidelines should be used: (1) Good reductions must be attained and held with a well-molded cast. (2) Cortical apposition, even if bayonet, is adequate, if rotation is correct, if the interosseous space is preserved, and if there is no angulation. (3) Immobilize the fracture in the position—*any position*—in which the alignment is correct and reduction feels stable. (4) Minor improvements can and should be made up to three or four weeks, when the fracture is "sticky"; do not be afraid to remanipulate. (5) Be prepared to carry out open reduction and internal fixation, even in children under the age of ten, rather than accept a poor position. However, skin traction is a method that can be used to try to attain a reduction in the first few days after significant injury, subsequently attempting another closed reduction. (6) Always warn the parents about the possibility of remanipulation and growth deformity.

The method of reduction advocated for complete fractures of the radius alone, or the radius and ulna together, precludes the possibility of a rotational deformity. After satisfactory anesthesia has been administered to provide adequate muscle relaxation, the arm may be suspended by finger traps and a counterweight of 10 to 15 lbs across the upper arm. Several minutes should elapse to allow the fracture to be brought out to length and to correct the overriding of the distal fragment, although a toggle maneuver is often necessary to connect the cortices. After length has been restored in this fashion, the fracture should be allowed to seek its own level of rotation, rather than manipulating the distal fragment into any preconceived position of theoretically correct rotation. With the forearm suspended in finger-tip traction, the two fragments usually fall spontaneously into correct rotational alignment. The position that such a fracture usually assumes is neutral or slight pronation.

No rotatory manipulation of the fracture should be done once the overriding has been corrected and the cortices engaged. A check can be taken to see if there is adequate rotational correction by assessing the width of the cortices of the two fragments. This complication is easily recognized by the disparity of width between the two fracture fragments. Remodeling may correct the cortical width difference, but it does not correct the rotational deformity.

The width of the interosseous space can be restored by manual pressure to the soft tissues between the bones, provided there is no excessive swelling. If swelling is present, then attempts to reduce the fracture should be deferred several days, and overhead traction used, until there is a subsidence of soft tissue swelling. When traction is maintained, a long arm cast is applied with the elbow in 90° of flexion and the forearm fully supinated. The cast must be molded well over the palmar aspect of the radius. Again apply pressure to the interosseous space while the plaster is setting.

Failure to restore normal alignment, both with regard to longitudinal as well as rotational deformation, may cause restriction of pronation and supination of the forearm after fracture healing. Bayonet or side-to-side apposition with some overriding is acceptable, provided that the ulna and radius do not deviate toward one another and that the interosseous space is maintained (Figs. 12-59 and 12-60). However, reduction of one bone with continued overriding of the other is not an acceptable reduction. To determine this, it is best to obtain true anteroposterior and lateral films. Any obliquity in the film may be deceptive as far as the degree of deformation.

It has been standard teaching that fractures of the uppermost third of the radius and ulna be immobilized in full supination, because the proximal fragment may be pulled into supination by the biceps and supinator muscles.[150-152] Pollen suggests that this route is a mistake, and in cases when the fully supinated position was used, there was a significant incidence of malunion.[153] Pollen states that in full pronation the brachioradialis muscle acts as a bowstring to increase the dorsal tilt of the distal fragment, and tends to cause angulation or redisplacement.[153] However, flexing the wrist may counteract this deformity. An accurate study of the radiogram is required to decide whether these are pronation or supination injuries, and the degree of rotation should be assessed in order to decide the position of greatest stability. Gainor and Hardy recommended immobilizing these fractures in full extension in order to control rotation.[154] Manipulation under fluoroscopy is often helpful to determine positions of stability.

These fractures must be maintained in an immobilized position in a well-molded cast with three-point fixation (Fig. 12-61) for longer than most children's fractures (in the realm of 6 to 8 weeks), in order to allow satisfactory callus formation. The cast should be changed as necessary to com-

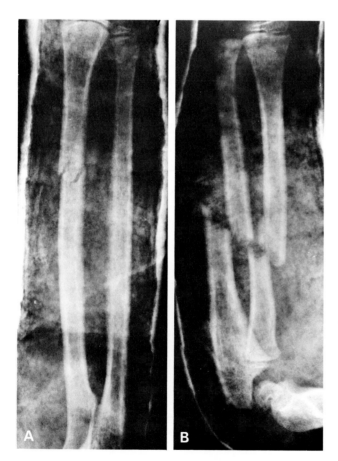

FIG. 12-59. Satisfactory reduction of both bones. *A,* The AP view shows longitudinal alignment and good maintenance of the interosseous space. *B,* The lateral view shows mild overriding, but again, adequate longitudinal alignment.

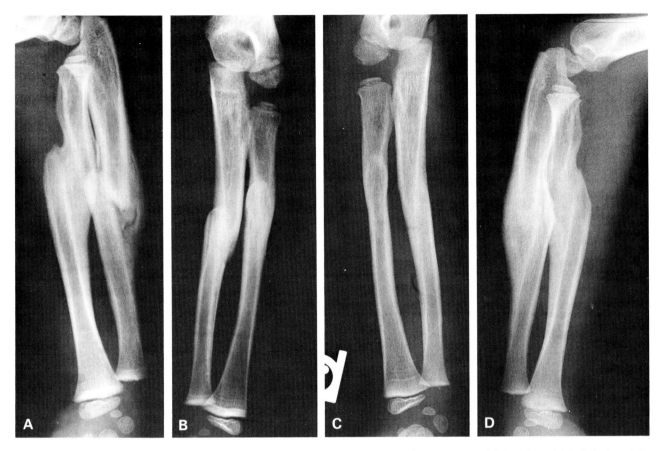

FIG. 12-60. *A-B,* Appearance 4 months after injury of displaced, overriding fractures in a child with multiple injuries. *C-D,* Appearance 16 months later. Extensive remodeling has occurred.

pensate for decreased swelling, which lessens the external fixation.

Since deformation and angular malalignment may occur at a much later time after the initial injury, it is imperative that serial roentgenograms be taken to detect any loss of position. If closed manipulation is unsuccessful, immediate open surgical reduction is not indicated, except in the older child who is close to skeletal maturity. A well-padded cast that acts as a compression dressing may be applied and combined with elevation. The fracture should be remanipulated 5 to 7 days later. Skeletal traction can also be applied.

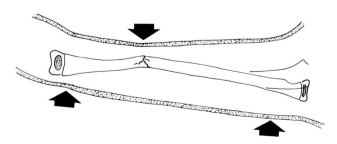

FIG. 12-61. Principle of three-point fixation of the greenstick fracture to prevent reangulation while in the cast.

Open reduction of both bone fractures in young children is infrequently indicated. There is a feeling that open reduction is forbidden in children, but not all fractures of both bones can be managed by closed reduction (Figs. 12-62 to 12-64). Internal fixation is preferable to malunion. Teenagers with high oblique fractures are likely to require open reduction.

Results

In a series of 88 greenstick fractures described by Davis and Green, the only complication was recurrent palmar angulation of the fracture during the period of healing.[17] Recurrent palmar angulation was seen in 8 patients; it was encountered in 3 patients during the first 3 weeks and they were remanipulated. Beyond this time period, remanipulation is decreasingly successful. They did not find any complications in the cases of torus fracture, although Hughston has described that complication. Of greenstick fractures of the distal third of the radius and ulna, there were 8 complications in 62 patients, all developed recurrent palmar angulation between 15° and 30°. This loss of position, which resulted in up to 30° of palmar angulation, occurred within the first week in 5 patients who were all improved by remanipulation. Gradual increase in angulation over 4 to 6 weeks may occur in these patients, but usually does not increase beyond 15°.

children and adolescents are increasingly susceptible to this complication. The radius usually unites, albeit delayed, while the ulna develops a nonunion (Fig. 12-65). This should be treated with compression plating and localized bone grafting. Extensive bone grafting is usually unnecessary once the fracture is immobilized.

Angular union (malunion) is also infrequent (Fig. 12-66). When present, it should be allowed to mature and then be treated by corrective osteotomy.

Synostosis may occur, especially when the fractures are at the same level (Fig. 12-67). Removal of the synostosis is not easy, and should not be attempted until the process is mature (approximately 6 months). Interposition of soft tissue, fat, muscle, or silastic membrane may prevent recurrence.

Allowing children out of immobilization too early may result in a fracture through the original fracture and new callus (Fig. 12-68). One way to prevent this is graded mobilization. At 4 to 6 weeks the long arm cast is converted to a short arm cast. This allows elbow movement and limited supination-pronation, and begins to stimulate some corrective remodeling of trabecular and cortical bone.

In one series, 3 of the 547 fractures were open. One of these was a small puncture wound, which was subsequently complicated by gas gangrene, even though adequate debridement had been carried out at the time of presentation.[17]

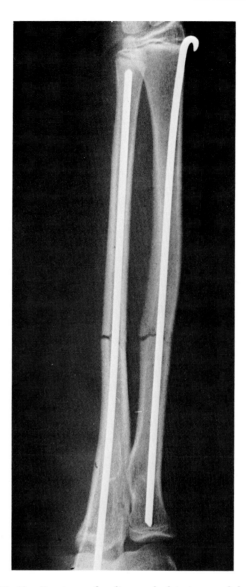

FIG. 12-62. Fracture of radius and ulna in an adolescent. These fractures were treated with Rush rods. However, if this technique is used, it is recommended that the ulnar rod be placed through the proximal metaphysis if this region is still functional. In this patient, the proximal radius and ulna had undergone physiologic epiphysiodesis. The distal ends were still functional, and rod placement in the radial metaphysis did not interfere with growth.

During the first decade of life, there usually is complete correction of angular deformity up to 20 to 25°, but above this age, or this degree of malposition, the power of correction is decreased or is incapable of preventing residual angular problems.[155]

Complications

Complications are infrequent, but often difficult to manage.

While delayed union or nonunion is rare in young children because of the highly osteogenic periosteum, older

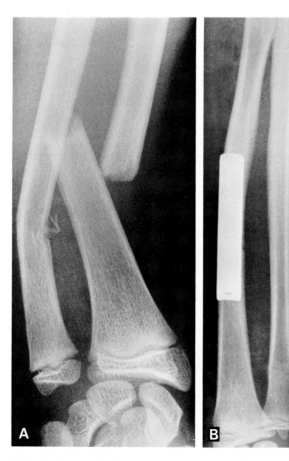

FIG. 12-63. *A*, Radial fracture combined with torus injury to ulna in an 11-year-old. Closed reduction was impossible. *B*, A tubular plate was applied.

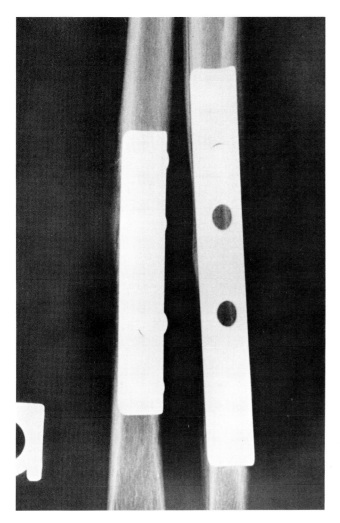

FIG. 12-64. Bilateral plating of both bones in a 12-year-old.

Distal Radial and Ulnar Metaphyses

These fractures are the most common injuries to the developing skeleton.[156] Yet despite their frequent occurrence, treatment and results are often less than ideal.

Classification

The most frequent type of fracture is greenstick injury, which may take several forms. A torus fracture is a variably evident buckling of the cortical bone of the radius, with minimal evidence of trabecular disruption (Fig. 12-69). A diagnosis must often be made in a film taken several weeks after the original injury because the original roentgenogram did not disclose the injury. This is a type 8 growth mechanism injury that results in temporary ischemia of the metaphysis distal to the fracture and subsequent sclerosis during revascularization (see Chap. 4). The ulna may be uninvolved or may sustain variably severe injury. The other pattern is a classic greenstick injury with buckling of the volar cortex, angulation, and dorsal loss of cortical integrity (Fig. 12-70), which may also be associated with a crushing injury with

some cortical displacement. An unusual injury is longitudinal splitting of the cortex (Fig. 12-71).

In a more severe greenstick injury, the fracture may be dorsally angulated with disruption of the volar cortex and an intact, but deformed, dorsal cortex (Fig. 12-72). The fracture may also exhibit complete loss of cortical integrity. If undisplaced, the periosteal sleeve is usually intact and imparts a significant degree of stability.

In the most severe injury pattern, the distal fragments are displaced dorsally and radially with varying degrees of overriding (Fig. 12-73). The fracture of the radius is usually complete, although fractures of the ulna may be complete and similarly displaced, greenstick, or minimally involved with injury to the styloid process, similar to a Colle's fracture in an adult.

Pathomechanics

In a greenstick injury, the impact of indirect violence of a fall on the outstretched hand coupled with a rotational strain crumples the distal cortex, but the palmar cortex re-

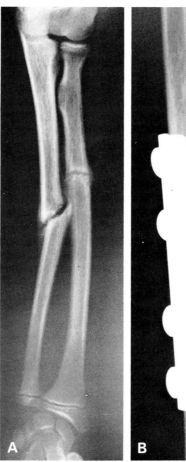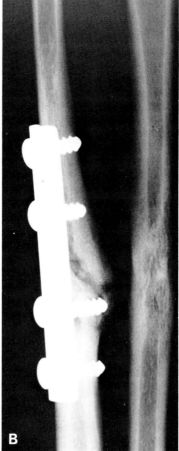

FIG. 12-65. *A,* Delayed union and malunion of ulna with delayed union of radius. The radius had healed by four months after the injury. *B,* One year later, the patient still had a tender ulnar malunion, and she was treated by a compression plate. Four weeks postoperatively, the fracture is healing. Note that the radius has healed well.

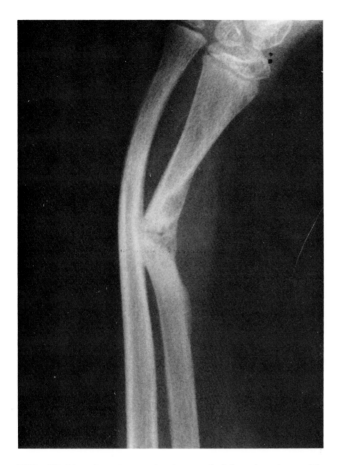

FIG. 12-66. Angular malunion and delayed union with accompanying severe plastic deformation of the ulna. Correction required osteotomy of both bones.

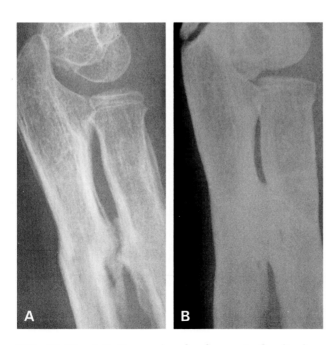

FIG. 12-67. *A-B,* Progressive development of radioulnar synostosis complicating proximal third fractures of both bones.

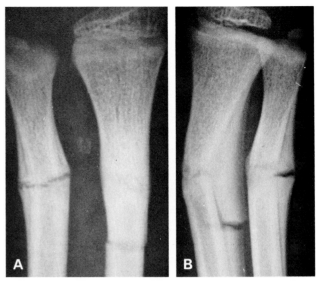

FIG. 12-68. Refracture following injury to the distal third. The ulna has fractured through the callus at the level of the original injury, while the radial callus has fractured proximal to the original injury. *A,* AP view. *B,* Lateral view.

mains intact. The distal fragment in a torus fracture may be angulated dorsally or may be displaced minimally. Because the greenstick injury absorbs a large amount of energy that is not dissipated by a complete cortical fracture or displacement of fragments, the compression force may be transmitted into the physis as a type 5 injury, which is difficult to diagnose at the time of original injury, but must be sought in the follow-up.

Even when there is no displacement of the radial fracture, the ulnar styloid is often fractured (Fig. 12-74). This occurs because of the integrated relationship of the distal radius and ulna through the triangular cartilage (see Figs. 12-17 and 12-19).

Diagnosis

The diagnosis is usually clinically evident. The child presents with a painful, swollen wrist. If there is dorsal displace-

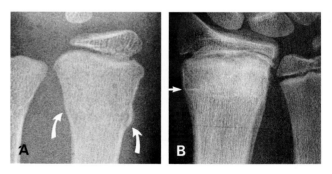

FIG. 12-69. *A,* Typical distal radial torus fracture (arrows). *B,* Similar injury in an older child. There is mild sclerosis in the distal metaphysis, and subperiosteal new bone proximal to the fracture. The ulnar styloid is fractured. The fracture itself is still minimally evident (arrow).

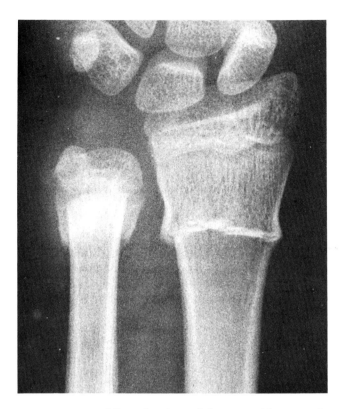

FIG. 12-70. Buckling of entire radial cortex with concomitant ulnar fracture. Cortical integrity and overlap are present on the dorsal (compression) side. In this patient the ulna was intact.

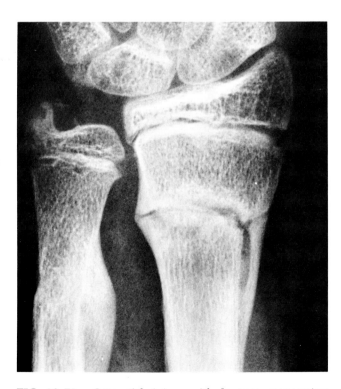

FIG. 12-71. Greenstick injury with fracture propagation along the longitudinal axis.

ment, the classic "silver fork" deformity is evident. Roentgenography confirms the injury in most instances; however, in some cases initial roentgenograms may not show any evidence of injury. In these cases, the diagnosis must be made empirically, on the basis of clinical findings.

Neurovascular status should be assessed carefully. In the dorsally displaced fracture, the median nerve is particularly susceptible to acute injury from the fracture fragment as well as more chronic injury from the swelling and compromise of the tunnel by displacement of soft tissue and skeletal elements.

Treatment

A torus fracture is an undisplaced injury that usually involves only the distal metaphysis and does not necessitate reduction, merely immobilization in a well-fitting plaster cast for 3 to 4 weeks. Hughston advocates using a cast that includes the wrist and elbow; he believes that if this type of cast is not used, there may be angulation during the healing process.[155]

Many of the authors cited by Önne and Sandblom define the angular deformity of the distal third fractures, but do not define an absolute number to use as a guideline.[157] If the angle exceeds 25 to 30° in infants, or 15° in children beyond their second year, closed reduction with completion of the fracture by reversal of the deformity is indicated. Similar to greenstick fractures of the midshaft, torus fractures may deform because of powerful muscles that act across the wrist, coupled with intrinsic deforming plasticity in the remaining intact bone.

A greenstick fracture of the radius at the junction of the metaphysis and diaphysis with some supination is common, and has a bad reputation because angulation tends to recur, even after reduction. The forearm should be held in full pronation in an above-elbow cast with three-point fixation. If the deformity is severe, it may be necessary to complete the fracture, as previously described for midshaft. However,

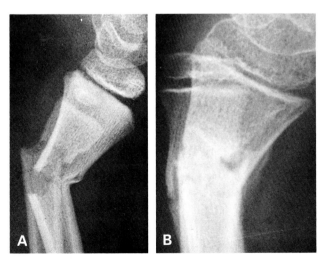

FIG. 12-72. Angular deformity after distal radial fracture. A, Moderate deformity of radius and ulna. B, Mild angular deformity of radius with possible dorsal displacement of the ulna (Galeazzi's injury).

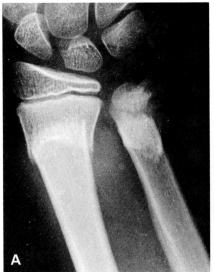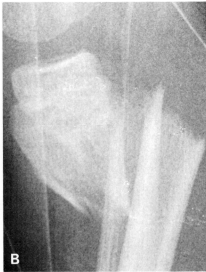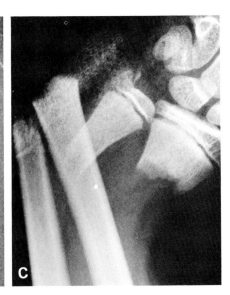

FIG. 12-73. Displaced fractures. *A-B,* AP and lateral views of characteristic dorsal displacement with minimal varus-valgus angular deformity. *C,* Severe displacement and angular deformity.

casting in full pronation with an above-elbow cast allows the intact periosteum to lock the fracture in place and full pronation stops a supine deformity from developing. Pollen advanced a different approach. He considers that the brachioradialis is the primary deforming force. In pronation the brachioradialis displaces the fragment, whereas in supination the pull of the brachioradialis holds the reduction. However, a position should be used that does not emphasize full supination or pronation.

Complete fractures should be reduced with a general anesthetic, since relaxation is an *essential* part of the reduction, and can rarely be obtained without complete muscular relaxation.[158] The technique of reduction is to recreate and overexaggerate the deformity (Fig. 12-75). First, the extremity is subjected to longitudinal traction in the line of the deformity, with counter-traction at the elbow. The surgeon pushes the fragments into normal position between his thumb and fingers. The soft tissues between the distal radius and ulna are pressed to restore the width of the interosseous space. It is desirable to achieve anatomic alignment in the longitudinal and rotational directions, but the cortices may overlap in the lateral view. However, bayonet apposition should not be accepted (Fig. 12-76). Encroachment on the interosseous space by the fragments should be corrected, as it may restrict the rotation of the forearm, although with growth there may be sufficient remodeling to overcome this. Minimal overriding can be remodeled; marked overriding may occasionally require skeletal traction through the metacarpals for correction.

An above-elbow cast can be applied for immobilization, and should be maintained for 6 weeks. Again, it is imperative to check the injury at intervals to assess any subsequent redisplacement.

An open reduction is rarely indicated in children. In my experience, this has been necessary in only 4 cases in over 300 examples of this injury. In these cases the pronator quadratus had been ripped with the proximal fragment of the radius herniated through the muscle, and it was impossi-

ble, except under direct vision, to free the fragments and replace them on the palmar side of the forearm, since the muscle had been displaced onto the dorsal aspect of the proximal fragment.

A totally unstable distal radial fracture in a child who is approaching skeletal maturity can probably be treated more like an adult fracture with open reduction and internal fixation with plates. However, every attempt should be made to avoid open reduction in these injuries.

Treatment Problems

These fractures may appear simple and easy to treat. However, they are more difficult to adequately take care of than can be appreciated initially, and are often mismanaged be-

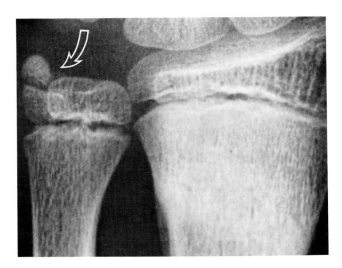

FIG. 12-74. Example of ulnar styloid nonunion (arrow). This accompanied a torus radial injury.

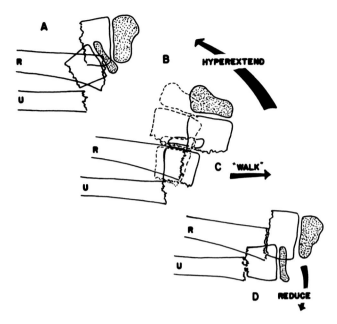

FIG. 12-75. Schematic of method of reduction of dorsally displaced distal radial or radioulnar fractures. *A,* Initial deformity. *B,* Hyperextend the distal unit. *C,* Push or "walk" the fractured ends until they lock. *D,* Bring the wrist back to its neutral position. While complete anatomic reduction is not essential, longitudinal and rotational alignments must be attained and maintained.

cause of certain concepts. The following are areas that lead to poor results.

Failure to Attain Adequate Initial Reduction. The more accurate the initial reduction, the less the potential for loss of alignment. Reduction of displaced, overriding fractures of the distal forearm is particularly difficult in the presence of marked local swelling. Unless there is neurovascular compromise, there is no emergency in treating these fractures. Apply compression with a plaster splint and admit the child

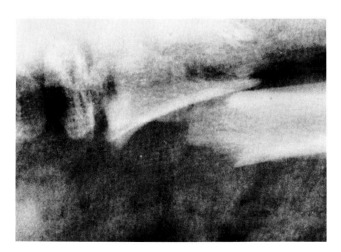

FIG. 12-76. Unacceptable reduction of distal radioulnar fracture.

to the hospital for elevation of the extremity and an adequate reduction once the swelling has receded. General anesthesia is less traumatic on patients, as the fracture can be manipulated under optimal conditions and frequently with the use of an image intensifier.

Failure to Immobilize the Forearm in a Position of Stability. The degree of rotation of the forearm in which fractures of the radius and ulna should be immobilized has been the subject of some controversy. The forearm should be immobilized in that position of rotation (i.e., supination, pronation, or neutral) in which reduction is most stable. This can be determined best by using an image intensifier, which unfortunately is not always available. A standard routine has been full pronation in lower third fractures, which should only be approached as a relative guideline and not an absolute indication for positioning the wrist and forearm. If the reduction is stable, full supination is recommended to allow the radius and ulna to parallel each other. If an adequately wrapped cast is maintained during this period, the pull of the muscles should not cause malalignment of the satisfactorily reduced, stable fracture. Stability of reduction can be determined clinically and by a roentgenographic examination.

Failure to Break the Cortex Completely in Angulated Greenstick Fractures. This problem is one of the most common pitfalls. To merely straighten the bone is not sufficient. The intact cortex must be completely broken. Further, in some instances when there is no apparent fracture of the ulna there may be significant greenstick bowing, in association with the complete fracture or a true greenstick fracture of the radius. These fractures are deceptive, and it is imperative that the fracture of the radius be completed in this instance, since the intrinsic plastic deformation of the ulna makes it bow the radius if the fracture is not completed.

Loose Cast. In order to maintain reduction, fixation must be secure. As swelling around the fracture site subsides and muscles atrophy, the cast becomes loose and the fracture fragments may become displaced or misaligned. A loss of position can occur as late as 3 to 4 weeks following reduction. A loose cast can be detected in the roentgenogram, as can the possibility of angular deformation. It is important that the fracture be roentgenographed within a week after initial reduction. If there is any evidence of loosening of the cast or beginning angular deformity, particularly toward the original deformity, the cast should be removed and replaced with a snug, well-fitting, three-point-fixation cast. The type of cast is, of course, the preference of the individual surgeon. One cannot overemphasize the importance of a snug, but not constricting, cast in preventing loss of alignment and frequent cast changes as necessitated by the subsidence of swelling.

Displaced fractures of the radius and ulna should always be immobilized in a sturdy long arm cast that extends from the upper arm to the metacarpal heads, with the elbow in 90° of flexion. Stiffness of joints from prolonged immobilization is generally not a problem in children. In unstable fractures of the distal third of the radius, the plaster should include the proximal phalanges to immobilize the metacarpophalangeal joints. Secure fixation of the proximal phalanx is particularly important; otherwise children tend to use the thumb and fingers, and may, through muscle action, cause deformation.

Failure to Detect and Correct Loss of Position. The fracture must be roentgenographed at appropriate intervals. By 10 to 14 days there is some radiolucent callus beginning to accumulate, and this may enhance the stability of a rereduction. Adequate roentgenograms are essential. In particular, anteroposterior and true lateral views must be obtained, since oblique views are misleading and may make the fracture appear more or less deformed than it actually is.

Results

In general, the results of treatment of this fracture are good to excellent. Since most are undisplaced greenstick injuries, there is minimal rotational or angular deformity requiring extensive remodeling. Even in displaced fractures, the results are good when a satisfactory reduction has been attained. Problems arise when the fracture reangulates, or when the fracture is left dorsally displaced.

Complications

A high incidence of complications is seen in complete fracture of the distal third of the radius and ulna. Of 47 patients in one series, 22 had complications that included angular deformity, rotational deformity, gas gangrene, median nerve injury, and refractures, while in another series, recurrent dorsal angulation at the fracture site was the most common complication, occurring in 43 of 547 patients.[17] The incidence of this complication in greenstick fractures of the distal third of the radius alone or that of the radius and ulna together is 10%, and in complete fractures of the distal radius and ulna it was 25%.[17] An intact ulna apparently helps to stabilize a complete fracture of the distal radius alone, for the incidence of reangulation of this fracture pattern was only 10%. This significant difference and incidence of reangulation between greenstick and complete fractures of the distal third suggests that breaking the intact cortex, thereby converting the greenstick distal fracture into a complete fracture, may not be the best method of reduction. As seen radiographically, greenstick fractures appear to be angulated, and several authors have advocated breaking the intact cortex to remove the potentially deforming force. I agree with this concept, and believe that greenstick fractures can be satisfactorily managed by the technique of converting the greenstick fracture into a complete fracture. However, Evans pointed out that the apparent angulation deformity seen in greenstick fractures in children was usually a rotational deformity. More recently, Rang has emphasized this concept, which can easily be proved clinically by rotating the forearm under an image intensifier, and observing that the apparent angulation disappears as the forearm reaches the proper plane of rotation. Rotational correction may be easier and more efficacious than trying to convert the greenstick fracture into a complete fracture. Evans showed that distal third greenstick fractures are reduced easily by maximum pronation of the forearm.[4]

Circulatory impairment, and its major form of Volkmann's ischemia, may occur in fractures of both bones of the forearm when the forearm is swollen, or when a displaced fracture is present that requires repeated manipulation. The more extensive the soft tissue trauma, particularly from a direct blow or wringer injury, the more likely the possibility of enough swelling to create forearm compartment problems. Wick catheter monitoring should be considered.

One of the least recognized complications is delayed union, nonunion, or overgrowth of the ulnar styloid, which represents a type 7 growth mechanism injury (Fig. 12-77). This injury occurs because of the anatomic relationships, especially the triangular cartilage. The injury often occurs through a completely cartilaginous styloid, making diagnosis roentgenographically difficult. Subsequently, as the styloid ossifies, the nonunion becomes evident. Nonunion probably occurs because of the difficulty of epiphyseal cartilage healing and chronic tensile stresses. Önne found two cases with follow-up problems relative to the ulnar styloid with pain on maximal supination due to a pseudarthrosis of the styloid process, or a fibrous union between the styloid and remainder of the ulnar secondary ossification center.[157] These fractures usually heal rapidly with extensive callus formation. However, severe periosteal injury or possible vascular disruption may be associated with delayed healing. The child must be protected until the fracture is completely healed.

Disruption of the periosteum may not heal completely. A fragment that is displaced beyond the confines of the periosteum may not remodel completely and may lead to formation of an exostosis (Fig. 12-78).

In the series described by Davis and Greene, of the 16 distal third greenstick fractures that reangulated, the majority were treated initially in neutral rotation, and only 2 were reduced in pronation.[17] It appears that although reduction of a greenstick fracture of the distal third by pronation of the forearm does not entirely eliminate the possibility of reangulation, recurrent palmar angulation is less likely to occur if this method of reduction is used. Palmar angulation probably is not of significant consequence in a child under 10, since the growing bone adequately remodels the deformity. In the child over 12, angulation cannot be accepted because of the limited amount of remodeling. The most difficult clinical problem then arises, which is how much angulation is acceptable in the child between the ages of 10 and 12.

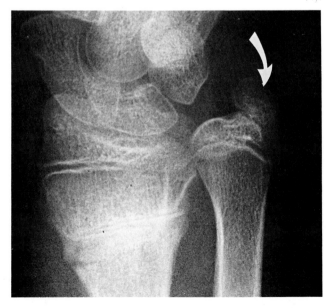

FIG. 12-77. Hypertrophic overgrowth of ulnar styloid fracture (arrow).

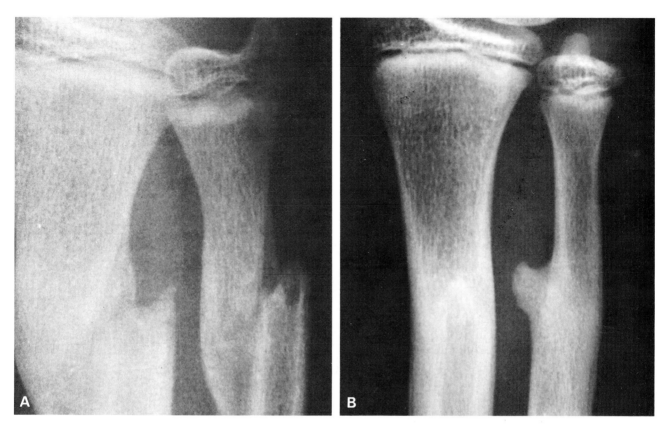

FIG. 12-78. *A,* Distal radioulnar fractures treated closed and left with side-to-side apposition. *B,* Extensive remodeling has taken place 16 months later, but a residual exostosis has formed. This was removed.

There were 36 fractures with significant deformities in Gandi's series.[21] He believed that angulation as great as 35° in the distal third of the radius would correct within 5 years, but emphasized that knowing that bone has this "correcting power" is not an excuse for leaving the fracture unreduced or not attempting to secure an adequate reduction (Fig. 12-79). However, at the same time, these results suggest that there is no justification for carrying out repeated manipulations or open reduction of such fractures. Despite reassurance, parents naturally are anxious if there is a clinical deformity when the plaster is removed, and they require an answer to the question of how long it will persist. It appears that most deformities of the distal third of the radius correct fully in 5 years (Fig. 12-80). There should be a reluctance to accept an angular deformity greater than 20° in a child over 10 years old who has less capacity for full correction, particularly if a girl who undergoes early fusion at 12 to 14 years of age.

Compound open fractures that involve the distal radius are relatively common, especially if the mechanism of injury is a fall on the wrist. If this occurs in dirt, the risk of contamination with soil microorganisms is significant (this may include Clostridia). These injuries must be treated aggressively with debridement and left open to heal by secondary granulation or subjected to delayed closure. Even with appropriate treatment, osteomyelitis may supervene (Fig. 12-81). Failure to fully appreciate the severity of such open injuries may lead to significant damage and loss of cartilage and bone (Figs. 12-82 and 12-83).

Distal Radial Epiphysis and Physis

This type of fracture is probably the most common injury to the growth mechanisms and constitutes about 50% of all physeal injuries.[12,13,77,159-161] It is common between the ages of 6 to 10 years.

Classification

Virtually every type of growth mechanism injury may affect the distal radius (Fig. 12-84). The distal ulnar physis is less frequently involved. Because of the crushing, twisting nature of many of these injuries, localized physeal damage (type 5) may occur, and is probably more frequent than realized.

Type 2 injuries are the most common and are usually associated with posterior (dorsal) displacement of the metaphyseal fragment and may be accompanied by a fracture through the ulnar styloid (Figs. 12-85 and 12-86).

Type 1 injury patterns are the next most common (Figs. 12-87 and 12-88). The epiphysis may be significantly displaced (Fig. 12-89). Type 3 and type 4 injuries may also occur, but are infrequent (Fig. 12-90). Type 7 injuries may involve the radial styloid (Fig. 12-91).

The radial fracture may be associated with a greenstick fracture of the metaphysis of the ulna, separation of the distal ulnar epiphysis, or fracture of the tip of the ulnar styloid process. The ulnar injury usually does not involve the growth plate itself.

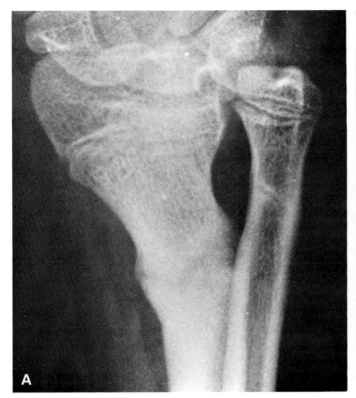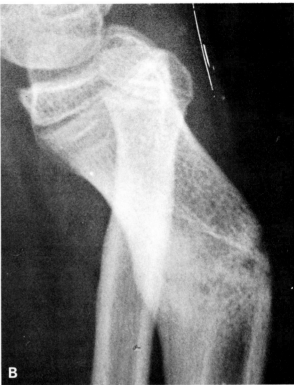

FIG. 12-79. *A,* AP and, *B,* lateral views of residual malunion in a 12-year-old girl. Insufficient growth was left in the distal radius following a fracture 8 months previous to this film. The radius was left angulated, resulting in decreased rotational capacity and relative ulnar lengthening. A corrective osteotomy will be necessary.

Pathomechanics

Distal radial epiphysis and physis injuries usually result from a fall on the outstretched hand. The forces are dorsally and longitudinally displaced, and produce a combination of impaction and shearing at the level of the growth plate (Fig. 12-92). Because of the triangular ligament, the ulnar styloid is frequently fractured. The shearing forces of hyperextension and supination displace the distal radial epiphysis dorsally. The periosteum strips from the dorsal metaphysis, but remains attached to the physis and epiphysis. If the transverse vector is greater and more shearing is present, the likelihood of growth damage decreases. However, when the longitudinal vector increases, the tendency for crushing of the physis and the potential rate of growth disturbance increase.

Ryan reported 5 cases of fractures of the distal radial epiphysis due to weightlifting in adolescent males.[94] Of these patients, 2 sustained bilateral fractures. All had been executing the military press at the time of injury.

Diagnosis

The fracture is usually dorsally displaced and the child presents with the classic "silver fork" deformity with pain and swelling. There are rarely signs of neurologic or vascular deficiency, but they must be adequately sought, as they do sometimes occur. Finger motion, though painful, is usually present and may appear normal. Sometimes only pain and swelling are present, with seemingly normal roentgenographic findings.

Roentgenograms establish the diagnosis, which is best visualized in the lateral projection. Often the dorsal metaphyseal fragment is small, but is pathognomonic of the injury, even if there is no plate displacement.

Treatment

The injury usually is easily reduced by direct pressure (under appropriate anesthesia). Wrist flexion does not help to hold reduction, because the wrist joint easily flexes to 80° before the capsule tightens enough to exert any influence on the distal fragment. This is an intolerable position. Therefore, leave the wrist in a neutral position once an epiphyseal separation has been reduced, and count on three-point molding of the cast. Following closed reduction, immobilization is maintained for 3 to 4 weeks.

Repeated forceful manipulations must be avoided because of the potential for damage to the physis. Malposition does not persist, as has been well demonstrated by Aitken.[12,13] Within a maximum period of 2 to 3 years, but more usually within 6 months, the distal radial epiphysis assumes its normal relationship to the radial metaphysis through remodeling and longitudinal growth. New subperiosteal bone forms on the dorsum and side of the distal radius (Fig. 12-93), and the palmar portion of the metaphysis is gradually absorbed. If repeated attempts at general closed reduction fail, it is wise

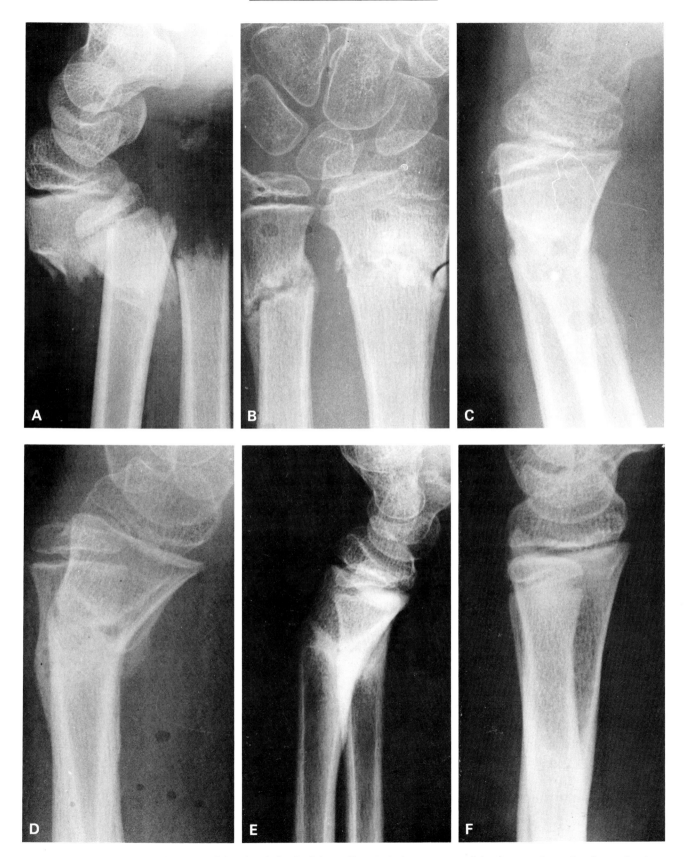

FIG. 12-80. *A,* Displaced fracture of the distal third of the radius. *B-C,* Appearance of the fracture 3 weeks after reduction. *D,* However, at 6 weeks there was further angulation. *E,* One year later remodeling is evident. *F,* Three years later, the malunion is fully corrected.

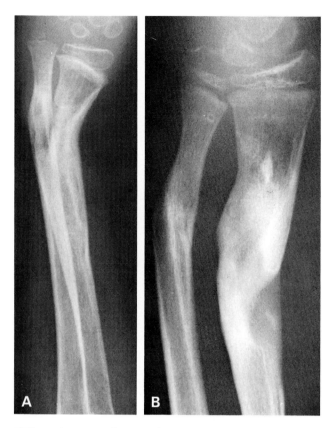

FIG. 12-81. *A,* Malunion after a compound fracture treated with open reduction. *B,* Two years later, the angular malunion is markedly improved and the sclerotic bone at the sites of the fracture and the osteomyelitis are remodeling.

to leave the epiphysis partially displaced and count on extensive metaphyseal remodeling, rather than risk growth plate injury.

Closed reduction is accomplished readily in most instances due to the type 1 and type 2 lesions with an intact dorsal periosteum. Rarely are these totally displaced, as in the comparable fractures of the distal metaphysis. In spite of the usual ease of reduction, it is not always possible to fully reduce the dorsal displacement. However, repeated forceful manipulations are not necessary, provided that approximately 50% apposition of the fragments has been attained. Repeated manipulation may even be harmful by further traumatizing the epiphysis (type 5 crush). Bragdon showed a case of premature closure of the distal radius consequent to forceful, repetitive manipulation.[159]

Open reduction of the markedly displaced epiphysis is usually not indicated; however, type 3 or type 4 injuries require open reduction (Fig. 12-94).

Results

In general, results are good to excellent. These injuries tend to occur in older children, and if growth arrest supervenes, the amount of remaining growth may not be enough to cause significant angular deformity or ulnar overgrowth. Functional limitation is minimal within a few weeks.

Complications

Sterling and Habermann reported a case of post-traumatic median nerve compression in a 10-year-old boy,[162] who had immediate improvement in many of his symptoms following initial reduction. However, the initial sensory decrease took several more days to return to normal. The boy did not require an open reduction or carpal tunnel release. The association of the median nerve compression and Colle's fractures in adults is well-known, but there have been few reports of this associated phenomenon in children.[163,164] In the case reported by Sterling and Habermann, they were able to reduce the symptoms with the fracture reduction. However, in one of my cases, traction and elevation after reduction did not relieve the symptoms and exploration and carpal tunnel release were finally necessary. The median nerve was obviously contused. It appears that carpal tunnel anatomic relationships do not change significantly with age. Consequently, compression of the median nerve in the carpal tunnel can occur at any age. It is important to carefully examine and recognize the condition of the median nerve prior to reduction.

Of 53 fractures of the distal radial epiphysis, only 1 patient in the Davis-Greene series had a growth disturbance.[17] They showed that during the first decade of life, there usually was complete correction of angulation up to 20 to 25°, but above this age, or this degree of malposition, the power of correction was decreased or was incapable of preventing residual angular problems.

A Madelung-type deformity may appear, although this does not radiographically resemble the true deformity (Fig. 12-95). The occurrence of 3 cases of Madelung-like deformity due to premature fusion of the distal radial epiphysis suggests that this fracture is not without complications.[23,165]

The distal end of the radius is a classic, although fortunately infrequent, site for growth disturbance due to crushing of the plate (type 5 injury) (Figs. 12-96 to 12-99). The distal ulna may also be involved and this may be due to a localized type 5 injury, which initially may be diagnosed as a sprain because there is no significant fracture evident radiographically.

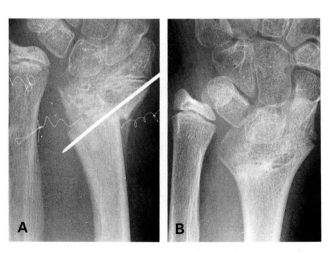

FIG. 12-82. *A,* Compound fracture of distal radius. This was immobilized with a K-wire. *B,* Infection caused consequent growth deformity.

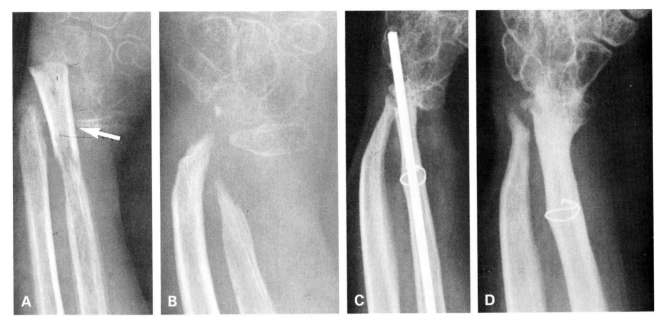

FIG. 12-83. *A,* Severe compound, comminuted injury. The distal radial fragment (arrow) sequestrated and had to be removed. *B,* Subsequent deformity. *C,* A year later, the radius was fused to the carpus. *D,* Eight months after fusion.

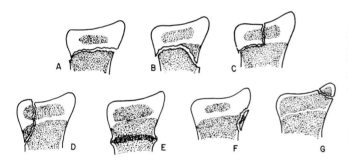

FIG. 12-84. Schematic of growth mechanism injuries.

Occasionally, longitudinal forces of the impact may crush some of the germinal cells of the physis, producing a localized type 5 physeal injury (see Fig. 12-98). This crushing injury cannot be detected immediately, but is often evident 6 to 12 months following injury. If caught early, the possibility of resection of the osseous bridge can be considered (see Fig. 12-99).

Önne found that two cases had follow-up problems relative to their ulnar styloid, having pain on maximal supination due to a pseudarthrosis of the styloid process or at least a fibrous union between the styloid and remainder of the ulnar secondary ossification center.[157] This fracture was

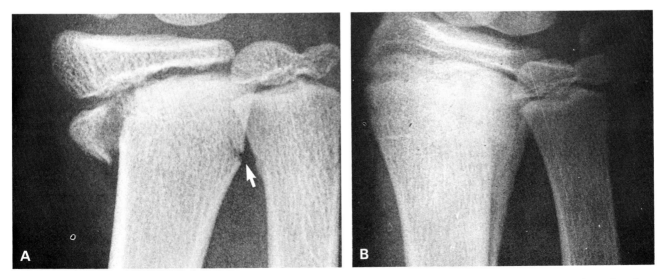

FIG. 12-85. *A,* Type 2 injury of the distal radius. Notice additional injury in opposite cortex (arrow). *B,* Extensive subperiosteal new bone due to stripping of the periosteum, which is densely attached to the epiphysis and physis.

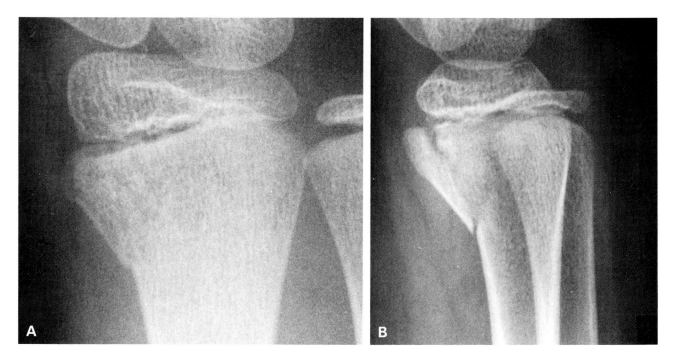

FIG. 12-86. Type 2 injury. *A,* AP shows minimal metaphyseal injury. *B,* Lateral view shows more extensive cortical disruption. The possibility of a type 4 injury complicating the type 2 injury must be considered.

completely nondemonstrable roentgenographically at the time of the original injury because of the extent of cartilage in that area. One should be careful to consider the possibility of an ulnar styloid fracture, even when ossification does not extend out to that region. The patient should be warned about it and follow-up roentgenograms taken to see whether it is present as ossification progresses into the region.

An exostosis may form (Fig. 12-100), which is probably due to localized type 6 damage to the periphery of the physis.

Distal Ulna

Injuries to the distal ulnar physis are unusual, but may lead to significant deformity (Figs. 12-101 to 12-104). Most of these injuries accompany distal radial fractures. Most often the distal ulnar injury is a type 7 (styloid) injury; however, they may also occur as solitary lesions.

Closed reduction should be used whenever possible. However, if significantly displaced, open reduction may be necessary (see Fig. 12-104). Growth arrest with creation of an ulnar minus variant may occur.

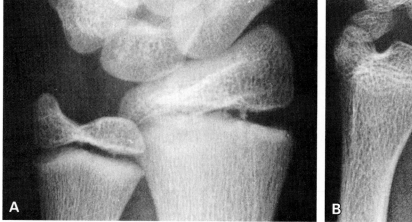
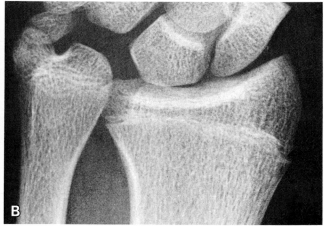

FIG. 12-87. *A,* Distal radial fracture (type 1). This fracture is open on the "radial" side and compressed on the "ulnar" side. Such a fracture must be watched closely for growth arrest. *B,* Two years later, the patient, who did not have proper follow-up examinations, returned complaining of pain over the ulnar styloid. The distal ulna had overgrown, while the distal radius closed prematurely. An ulnar styloid nonunion is evident. There was no indication of the ulnar injury in the initial film.

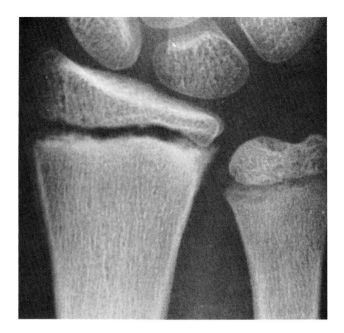

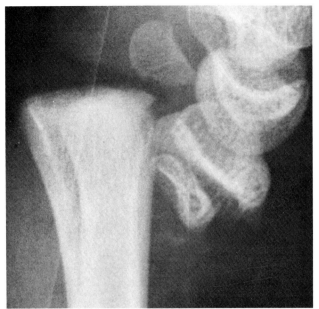

FIG. 12-88. Type 1 injury. Mild displacement with widening of physis.

FIG. 12-89. Dorsally displaced physeal injury.

Galeazzi's Fracture-Dislocation

The Galeazzi injury is a fracture of the shaft of the radius with an associated dislocation of the distal radioulnar articulation. This definition does not include those rare injuries in which there is a fracture of the radial neck and head associated with the dislocation of the distal radioulnar joint (Essex-Lopresti fractures).

Mikic described 125 patients, including 14 children with the classic lesion and 25 patients with a special type with fractures of both bones as well as dislocation of the distal radioulnar joints.[166] Of the children in Mikic's series, there was only 1 patient under 10 years of age and 13 patients between 10 and 16.

The involved children were all associated with subperiosteal, frequently greenstick-type fractures with angular displacement. Most of the time the dislocation of the distal radioulnar joint was evident clinically and roentgenographically (Fig. 12-105). However, sometimes the ulnar head was only subluxated, which was more evident clinically than roentgenographically.

The distal radioulnar joint is stabilized by various struc-

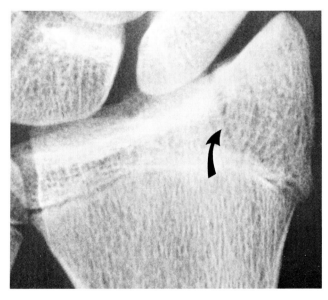

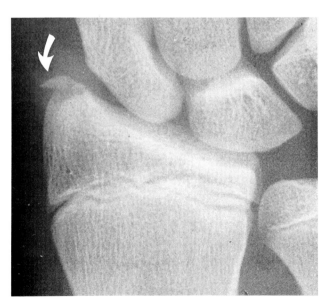

FIG. 12-90. Undisplaced type 3 injury (arrow).

FIG. 12-91. Type 7 injury of radial styloid (arrow).

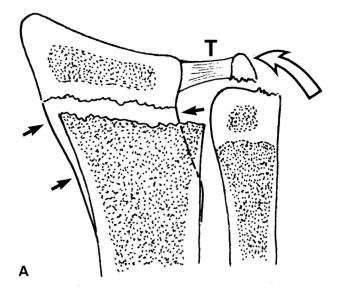

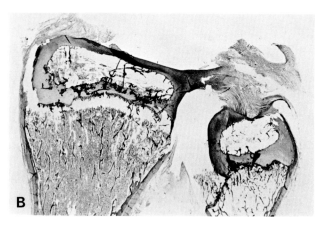

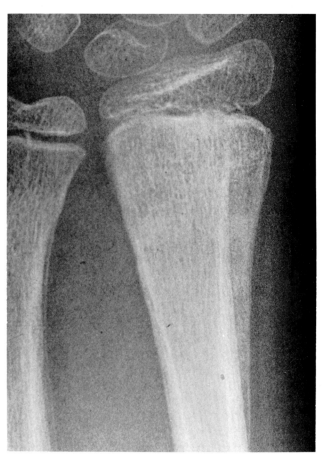

FIG. 12-93. Extensive subperiosteal new bone formation following a type 2 injury.

FIG. 12-92. *A*, Schematic of distal radial fracture. The periosteum (solid arrows) strips away and may be used to stabilize the reduction. The triangular cartilage (T) causes avulsion of the ulnar styloid (open arrow). *B*, Histologic specimen showing fracture of distal radius.

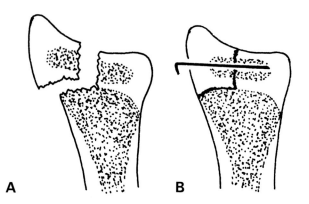

FIG. 12-94. *A*, Type 3 injury of distal radius. *B*, Recommended transverse pin placement.

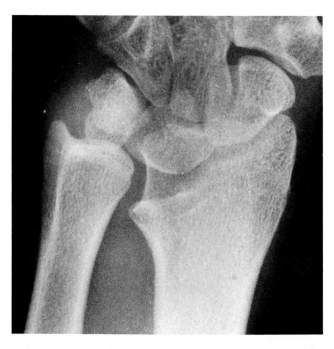

FIG. 12-95. Localized growth arrest with Madelung-like deformity.

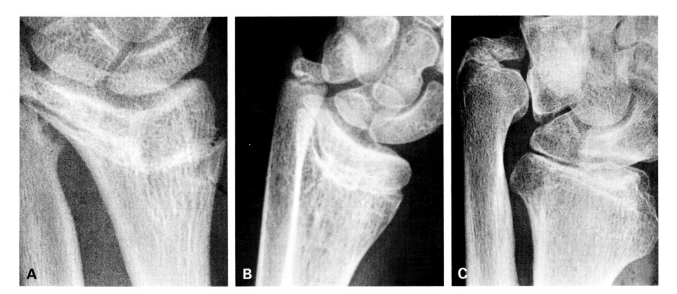

FIG. 12-96. *A,* Premature arrest of entire distal radius following type 2 injury. Note the styloid nonunion. *B,* Growth arrest of "radial" side of distal radius, with continued growth on the "ulnar" side. *C,* Complete growth arrest of the distal radius with overgrowth of the distal ulna.

tures, such as the ulnar collateral ligament, the anterior and posterior radioulnar ligaments, and the pronator quadratus. But the most important stabilizing force is the triangular fibrocartilage (Fig. 12-106). There can be no dislocation of the distal radioulnar joint without some rupture of this strong intra-articular fibrocartilaginous ligament. The specific function of the triangular fibrocartilage is to limit the rotational movements of the radius and ulna relative to one another. Avulsion of the ulna styloid process can be equivalent to rupture of the triangular fibrocartilage and was noted in 31.2% of the patients in Mikic's series.

There is disagreement as to the exact mechanism producing the Galeazzi injury. Most probably the mechanism is a fall on the outstretched hand combined with extreme pronation of the forearm. The forces are thought to cross the radiocarpal articulation, initially producing the dislocation and forced shortening of the radial shaft as the displacement discontinues. Dislocation of the distal ulna causes a tearing of the triangular fibrocartilage, which then loses its stabilizing influences on the wrist. Rotational stresses on the forearm would also seem to be essential for dislocation of the distal radioulnar joint. It has been demonstrated clinically and experimentally that a tear or detachment of the triangular articular disc is the first step to dislocation and occurs at the extreme of pronation and extension of the wrist.

Although the diagnosis of the Galeazzi fracture-dislocation should not be difficult, it is often missed or misdiagnosed. The radial fracture is always noted, but the disruption

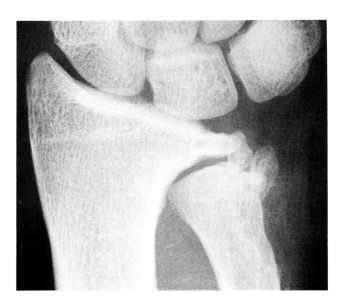

FIG. 12-97. Growth disruption of radioulnar joint. Premature growth arrest of ulna has caused angular deformity of distal radius.

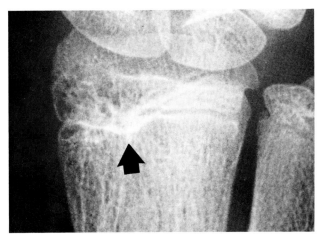

FIG. 12-98. Localized osseous bridge (arrow) following type 1 injury.

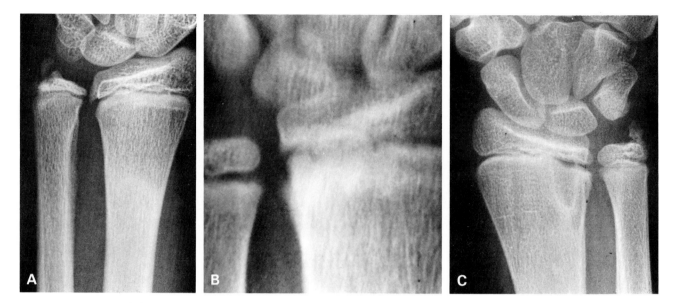

FIG. 12-99. *A,* Narrowing of middle physis. *B,* Tomography showed an osseous bridge. *C,* This was resected and replaced with fat. Growth has continued without bridge reformation months later. The fracture of the ulnar styloid is finally healing.

of the distal joint can be overlooked and the ulnar head may seem to protrude and be slightly more mobile than usual. Every roentgenographic examination of an isolated fracture of the radius must include the inferior radioulnar joint. Mikic advocated the use of arthrography to ascertain the presence of the Galeazzi lesion.[166] However, a positive arthrogram showing passage of contrast medium from the wrist into the inferior radioulnar joint cannot be specifically diagnostic of a triangular disc rupture because there may be a perforation in the normal disc. However, this perforation is

usually present in older patients and not in younger ones and arthrography probably can be used diagnostically in younger patients (Fig. 12-107).

In Mikic's group, 12 patients were treated nonoperatively.[166] In all cases, adequate stable reduction was easily achieved by manipulation, probably because most of the fractures were subperiosteal (greenstick). In 9 patients the results were excellent, and only in a 15-year-old boy did redisplacement of the radial fragments with palmar angulation occur. Closed reduction failed in 1 patient and he was

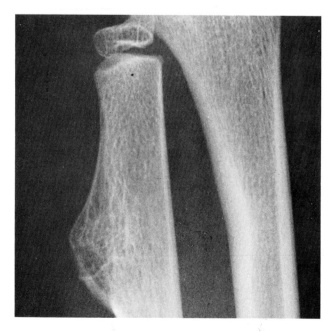

FIG. 12-100. Ulnar exostosis following an injury that occurred three years previous to this film.

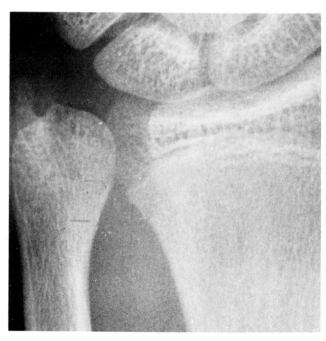

FIG. 12-101. Premature closure of distal ulna.

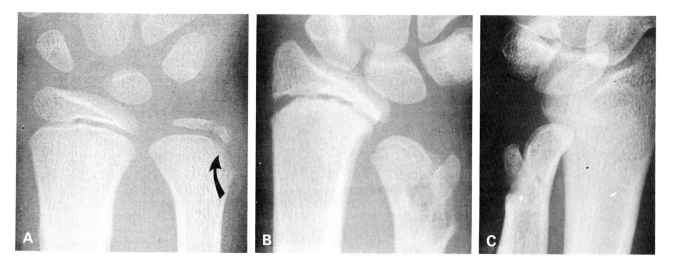

FIG. 12-102. Growth deformity, probably due to type 4 ulnar injury (original films unavailable). *A,* Six months; *B,* Two years; and *C,* Four years after the injury.

subsequently treated with internal fixation and had a fair result. In one 16-year-old boy, percutaneous rush-rod pinning yielded an excellent result. The patient shown in Figure 12-107 was treated by resection of the triangular cartilage.

References

1. Kaplan, E. B.: Surgical approach to the proximal end of the radius and its use in fractures of the head and neck of the radius. J. Bone Joint Surg., 23:86, 1941.
2. Spinner, M.: The arcade of Frohse and its relationship to posterior interosseous nerve paralysis. J. Bone Joint Surg., 50-B:809, 1968.
3. Spinner, M., and Kaplan, E. B.: The quadrate ligament of the elbow—its relationship to the stability of the proximal radio-ulnar joint. Acta Orthop. Scand., 41:632, 1970.
4. Evans, E. M.: Rotational deformity in the treatment of fractures of both bones of the forearm. J. Bone Joint Surg., 27:373, 1945.
5. Evans, E. M.: Pronation injuries of the forearm with special reference to the anterior Monteggia fracture. J. Bone Joint Surg., 31-B:578, 1949.
6. Evans, E. M.: Fractures of the radius and ulna. J. Bone Joint Surg., 33-B:548, 1951.
7. Christensen, J. B., Cho, K. O., and Adams, J. P.: A study of the interosseous distance between the radius and ulna during rotation of the forearm. J. Bone Joint Surg., 45-B:778, 1965.
8. Burman, M.: Primary torsional fracture of the radius or ulna. J. Bone Joint Surg., 35-A:665, 1953.
9. Reidy, J. A., and Van Gorder, G. W.: Treatment of displacement of the proximal radial epiphysis. J. Bone Joint Surg., 45-A:1355, 1963.
10. Salter, N., and Dareus, H. D.: The amplitude of forearm and of humeral rotation. J. Anat., 87:407, 1953.
11. Vesely, D. G.: The distal radio-ulnar joint. Clin. Orthop., 51:75, 1967.
12. Aitken, A. P.: Further observations on the fractured distal radial epiphysis. J. Bone Joint Surg., 17:922, 1935.
13. Aitken, A. P.: The end results of the fractured distal radial epiphysis. J. Bone Joint Surg., 17:302, 1935.
14. Blount, W. P.: Forearm fractures in children. Clin. Orthop., 51:93, 1967.
15. Buck, P., Folscheiller, J., and Jenny, G.: Uber die Behandlung

16. Dau, W.: Behandlung von Unterarmbrüchen im Kindesalter. Chir. Praxis, 4:485, 1966.
17. Davis, D. R., and Green, D. P.: Forearm fractures in children. Pitfalls and complications. Clin. Orthop., 120:172, 1976.
18. Koncz, M.: Spät-ergebnisse bei Unterarmfrakturen im Kindesalter. Arch. Orthop. Unfallchir., 76:300, 1973.
19. Lindholm, R., Puronvarsi, U., Lindholm, S., and Leiviskä, T.: Vorderarmschaft-brüche bei Kindern und Erwachsenen. Beitr. Orthop. Traumatol., 7:369, 1972.
20. Steinert, V.: Unterarm-frakturen im Kindesalter. Beitr. Klin. Chir., 212:170, 1966.
21. Gandhi, R. K., Wilson, P., Mason Brown, J. J., and MacLeod,

von 376 Vorderarmschaft-brüchen bei Kindern. Hefte Unfallheilkd., 89:51, 1976.

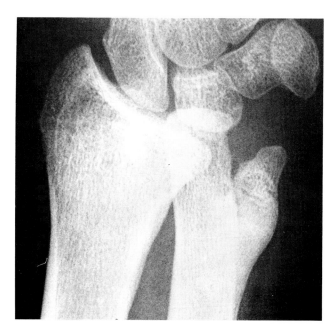

FIG. 12-103. Growth arrest of styloid, with continuing growth of the rest of the ulna.

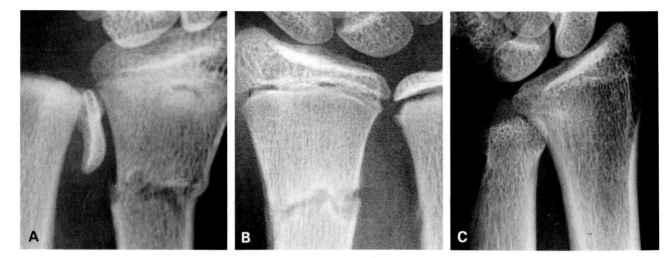

FIG. 12-104. *A,* Type 1 injury of distal ulna associated with radial metaphyseal fracture. *B,* The fracture was treated with open reduction and a transphyseal fixation pin. *C,* The patient came back three years later because of wrist pain. The ulnar physis had closed prematurely and the radial articular surface was deformed angularly.

W.: Spontaneous correction of deformity following fractures of the forearm in children. Br. J. Surg., *50:*5, 1963.

22. Alexander, C. J.: Effect of growth rate on the strength of the growth plate shaft junction. Skeletal Radiol., *1:*67, 1976.

23. Thomas, E. M., Tuson, K. W. R., and Browne, P. S. H.: Fractures of the radius and ulna in children. Injury, *7:*120, 1975.

24. Sharrard, W. J. W.: Paediatric Orthopaedics and Fractures. Oxford, Blackwell, 1971.

25. Blount, W. P.: Fractures of the forearm in children. Indust. Med. Surg., *32:*9, 1963.

26. Blount, W. P., Schaeffer, A. A., and Johnson, J. H.: Fractures of the forearm in children. J.A.M.A., *120:*111, 1942.

27. Carr, C. R., and Tracy, H. W.: Management of fractures of the distal forearm in children. South. Med. J., *57:*540, 1964.

28. Bosworth, B. M.: Fractures of both bones of the forearm in children. Surg. Gynecol. Obstet., *72:*667, 1941.

29. Grantham, S., and Kiernan, H. A.: Displaced olecranon fracture in children. J. Trauma, *15:*197, 1975.

30. Newell, R. L. M.: Olecranon fractures in children. Injury, *7:*33, 1975.

31. Mahlahn, D. J., and Fahey, J. J.: Fractures of the elbow in children. J.A.M.A., *166:*220, 1958.

32. Jeffrey, C. C.: Fractures of the head of the radius in children. J. Bone Joint Surg., *32-B:*314, 1950.

33. Hume, A. C.: Anterior dislocation of the head of the radius associated with undisplaced fracture of the olecranon in children. J. Bone Joint Surg., *39-B:*508, 1957.

34. Speed, J. S., and Boyd, H. B.: Treatment of fractures of the ulna with dislocations of the radius. J.A.M.A., *115:*1699, 1940.

35. Hunt, G. H.: Fracture of the shaft of the ulna with dislocation of the head of the radius. J.A.M.A., *112:*1241, 1939.

36. Ellman, H.: Anterior angulation deformity of the radial head. J. Bone Joint Surg., *57-A:*776, 1975.

37. Judet, J., Judet, R., and Lefranc, J.: Fracture du col radial chez l'enfant. Ann. Chir., *16:*1377, 1962.

38. Mouchet, A.: Fractures of the neck of the radius. Rev. Chir. [Orthop.], *22:*596, 1900.

39. Murray, R. C.: Fractures of the head and neck of the radius. Br. J. Surg., *28:*109, 1940.

40. Schwartz, R. P., and Young, F.: Treatment of fractures of the head and neck of the radius and slipped radial epiphysis in children. Surg. Gynecol. Obstet., *57:*528, 1933.

41. Speed, K.: Fractures of the head of the radius. Am. J. Surg., *38:*157, 1924.

42. Speed, K.: Traumatic lesions of the head of the radius. Surg. Clin. North Am., *4:*651, 1924.

43. Stankovic, P., Emmerman, H., Burkhardt, K., and Kurtsch, U.: Die Frakturen des proximalen Radius im Kindesalter. Z. Kinderchir. Suppl., *16:*77, 1975.

44. Vahvanen, V., and Gripenberg, L.: Fracture of the radial neck in children. Acta Orthop. Scand., *49:*32, 1978.

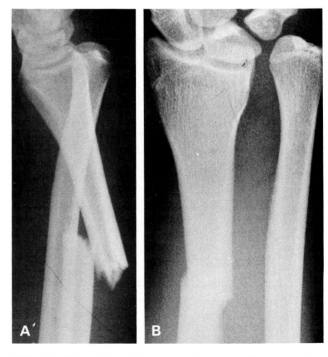

FIG. 12-105. *A-B,* Galeazzi's injury complicating radial fracture in a 15-year-old girl. *A,* Lateral view. *B,* AP view.

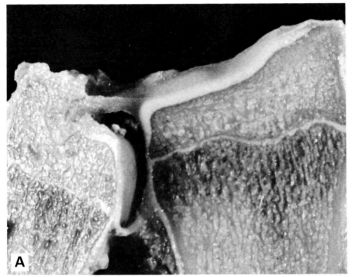
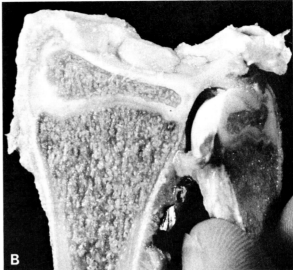

FIG. 12-106. Re-creation of Galeazzi's injury in specimens, showing how the ulna rotates out from under the triangular cartilage. *A,* Beginning rotation. *B,* More pronounced rotation.

45. Van Arsdale, W. W.: On subluxation of the head of the radius in children—with a resume of one-hundred consecutive cases. Ann. Surg., *9:*401, 1889.
46. Vostal, O.: Fractures of the neck of the radius in children. Acta Chir. Orthop. Traumatol. Cech., *37:*294, 1970.
47. Newman, J. H.: Displaced radial neck fractures in children. Injury, *9:*114, 1977.
48. Henrikson, B.: Isolated fractures of the proximal end of the radius in children. Epidemiology, treatment and prognosis. Acta Orthop. Scand., *40:*246, 1969.
49. O'Brien, P. I.: Injuries involving the proximal radial epiphysis. Clin. Orthop., *41:*51, 1965.
50. Dougall, A.: Severe fractures of the neck of the radius in children. J. R. Coll. Surg. Edinb., *14:*220, 1969.
51. Manoli, A.: Medial displacement of the shaft of the radius with a fracture of the radial neck. J. Bone Joint Surg., *61-A:*788, 1979.
52. Dunlop, J.: Separation of medial epicondyle of humerus. Case with displaced upper radial epiphysis. J. Bone Joint Surg., *17:*584, 1935.

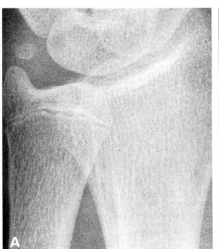
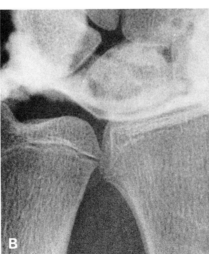
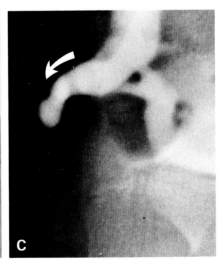

FIG. 12-107. *A,* Premature growth arrest of distal radius one year after bilateral type 1 injuries. The ulnar styloid exhibits nonunion. This patient subsequently had her wrist "twisted" and had chronic, unremitting pain for three months prior to this film. *B,* An arthrogram was performed. Dye surrounds the styloid ossicle, but the triangular cartilage is intact. *C,* Extrusion of dye through capsular defect (arrow). Exploration showed that the triangular cartilage was subluxated from the ulnar articular surface. There was extensive synovitis. This was felt to be an incomplete Galeazzi's injury. Treatment consisted of excision of the triangular cartilage and the styloid fragment, and capsular repair. Eight months after treatment the patient was asymptomatic.

53. McBride, E. D., and Monnet, J. C.: Epiphyseal fractures of the head of the radius in children. Clin. Orthop., 16:264, 1960.
54. Bryan, R. S.: Monteggia fracture of the forearm. J. Trauma, 11:992, 1971.
55. Wood, S. K.: Reversal of the radial head during reduction of fracture of the neck of the radius in children. J. Bone Joint Surg., 51-B:707, 1969.
56. Goldenberg, R. R.: Closed manipulation for the reduction of fractures of the neck of the radius in children. J. Bone Joint Surg., 27:267, 1945.
57. Tachdjian, M.: Pediatric Orthopedics. Philadelphia, W. B. Saunders, 1972.
58. Patterson, R. F.: Treatment of displaced fracture of the neck of the radius in children. J. Bone Joint Surg., 16:695, 1934.
59. Jones, E. R. L., and Esah, M.: Displaced fractures of the neck of the radius in children. J. Bone Joint Surg., 53-B:429, 1971.
60. Svinukhov, N. P.: The outcomes of operative treatment of fractures of the neck of the radius in children. Orthop. Travmatol. Protez., 26:13, 1965.
61. Key, J.: Survival of the head of the radius in a child after removal and replacement. J. Bone Joint Surg., 28:148, 1946.
62. Key, J. A.: Treatment of fractures of the head and neck of the radius. J.A.M.A., 96:101, 1939.
63. Lewis, R. W., and Thibodeau, A. A.: Deformity of the wrist following resection of the radial head. Surg. Gynecol. Obstet., 64:1079, 1937.
64. Perrin, J.: Les fractures du cubitus accompagnées de luxation de l'extrémité superieur du radius. Paris, Thése de Paris, G. Steinheil, 1909.
65. Rang, M.: Children's Fractures. Philadelphia, J. B. Lippincott, 1974.
66. Fielding, J. W.: Radio-ulnar crossed union following displacement of the proximal radial epiphysis. J. Bone Joint Surg., 46-A:1277, 1964.
67. Anderson, S. A.: Subluxation of the head of the radius, a pediatric condition. South. Med. J., 35:286, 1942.
68. Beagel, P. M.: "Slipped elbow" in children. J. Maine Med. Assoc., 45:293, 1906.
69. Bourquet: Mémoire sur les luxations dites incomplètes de l'extrémité. Rev. Med. Chir. Soc. Med. Nat. Iasi, 15:287, 1854.
70. Boyette, B. P., Ahoskie, N. C., and London, A. H., Jr.: Subluxation of the radius, "nursemaid's elbow." J. Pediatr., 32:278, 1948.
71. Broadhurst, R. W., and Buhr, A. J.: The pulled elbow. Br. Med. J., 1:1018, 1959.
72. Caldwell, C. E.: Subluxation of the radial head by elongation. Cincinnati Lancet Clinic, 66:496, 1891.
73. Corrigan, A.: The pulled elbow. Med. J. Aust., 2:187, 1965.
74. Costigan, P. G.: Subluxation of the annular ligament at the proximal radioulnar joint. Alberta Med. Bull., 17:7, 1952.
75. Cushing, H. W.: Subluxation of the radial head in children. Boston Med. Surg. J., 114:77, 1886.
76. Davis, J. H.: Subluxation of the radial head in children (nursemaid's elbow). Med. Times, 13:1379, 1965.
77. Gardner, J.: On an undescribed displacement of the bones of the forearm in children. London Med. Gaz., 20:878, 1837.
78. Griffin, M. E.: Subluxation of the head of the radius in young children. Pediatrics, 15:103, 1955.
79. Hart, G. M.: Subluxation of the head of the radius in young children. J.A.M.A., 169:1734, 1959.
80. Hutchinson, J., Jr.: On certain obscure sprains of the elbow occurring in young children. Ann. Surg., 2:91, 1885.
81. Kanter, A. J., and Bruton, O. C.: Subluxation of the head of the radius. Am. Practitioner, 31:39, 1952.
82. Lindeman, S. H.: Partial dislocation of the radial head peculiar to children. Br. Med. J., 2:1058, 1885.
83. McVeagh, T. C.: The slipped elbow in young children. Calif. Med., 74:260, 1951.
84. Magill, H. K., and Aitken, A. P.: Pulled elbow. Surg. Gynecol. Obstet., 98:753, 1954.
85. Matles, A. L., and Eliopoulous, K.: Internal derangement of the elbow in children. Int. Surg., 48:259, 1967.
86. Moore, E. M.: Subluxation of the radius from extension in young children. Trans. N.Y. Med. Assoc., 3:18, 1886.
87. Silquini, P. L.: La pronazione dolorosa. Minerva Ortop., 14:481, 1963.
88. Silver, C. M., and Simon, S. D.: Subluxation of head of the radius in children. R.I. Med. J., 43:722, 1960.
89. Smith, E. E.: Subluxation of the head of the radius in children. Ohio State Med. J., 45:1080, 1949.
90. Snellman, O.: Subluxation of the radial head in children. Acta Orthop. Scand., 28:311, 1959.
91. Sweetman, R.: Pulled elbow. Practitioner, 182:487, 1959.
92. Theodorou, S. D.: Dislocation of the head of the radius associated with fracture of the upper end of the ulna in children. J. Bone Joint Surg., 51-B:700, 1969.
93. Salter, R., and Zaltz, C.: Anatomic investigations of the mechanism of injury and pathologic anatomy of "pulled elbow" in children. Clin. Orthop., 77:134, 1971.
94. Ryan, J. R.: The relationship of the radial head to radial neck diameters in fetuses and adults with reference to radial-head subluxation in children. J. Bone Joint Surg., 51-A:781, 1969.
95. Stone, C. A.: Subluxation of the head of the radius—report of a case and anatomical experiments. J.A.M.A., 1:28, 1916.
96. McRae, R., and Freeman, P.: The lesion in pulled elbow. J. Bone Joint Surg., 47-B:808, 1965.
97. Caravias, D. E.: Some observations on congenital dislocation of the head of the radius. J. Bone Joint Surg., 39-B:86, 1957.
98. Green, J. T., and Gay, F. H.: Traumatic subluxation of the radial head in young children. J. Bone Joint Surg., 36-A:655, 1954.
99. Storen, G.: Traumatic dislocation of the radial head as an isolated lesion in children. Acta Chir. Scand., 116:144, 1959.
100. Vesely, D. G.: Isolated traumatic dislocations of the radial head in children. Clin. Orthop., 50:31, 1967.
101. Wright, P. R.: Greenstick fracture of the upper end of the ulna with dislocation of the radio-humeral joint or displacement of the superior radial epiphysis. J. Bone Joint Surg., 45-B:727, 1963.
102. Bell Tawse, A.: The treatment of malunited anterior Monteggia fractures in children. J. Bone Joint Surg., 47-B:718, 1965.
103. Schubert, J. J.: Dislocation of the radial head in the newborn infant. J. Bone Joint Surg., 47-A:1019, 1965.
104. Hamilton, W., and Parkes, J. C., II: Isolated dislocation of the radial head without fracture of the ulna. Clin. Orthop., 97:94, 1973.
105. Neviaser, R. J., and LeFevre, G. W.: Irreducible isolated dislocation of the radial head. Clin. Orthop., 80:72, 1971.
106. Lloyd-Roberts, G. C., and Bucknill, T. M.: Anterior dislocation of the radial head in children. J. Bone Joint Surg., 59-B:402, 1977.
107. Bado, J. L.: The Monteggia Lesion. Springfield, Charles C Thomas, 1962.
108. Bado, J.: The Monteggia lesion. Clin. Orthop., 50:71, 1967.
109. Boyd, H. B., and Boals, J. C.: The Monteggia lesion. Clin. Orthop., 66:94, 1969.
110. Boyd, H. B.: Treatment of fractures of the ulna with dislocation of the radius. J.A.M.A., 115:1699, 1940.
111. Boyd, H. B.: Surgical exposure of the ulna and proximal third of the radius through one incision. Surg. Gynecol. Obstet., 71:87, 1940.
112. Bruce, H., Harvey, J. P., Jr., and Wilson, J.: Monteggia fractures. J. Bone Joint Surg., 56-A:1563, 1974.
113. Creer, W. S.: Some points about the Monteggia fracture. Proc. R. Soc. Lond., 40:241, 1947.
113a. Cunningham, S. R.: Fracture of the ulna with dislocation of the head of the radius. J. Bone Joint Surg., 16:351, 1934.
114. Curry, G. J.: Monteggia fracture. Am. J. Surg., 73:613, 1947.
115. Duverney, J. G.: Traité des Maladies des Os. Paris, De Bure l'aine, 1751.

116. Eady, J. L.: Acute Monteggia lesions in children. J. S. C. Med. Assoc., *71:*107, 1975.

117. Eady, J. L.: Acute Monteggia lesions in children. Orthop. Digest., *4:*15, 1976.

118. Fournier, D.: L'Oeconomic Chirurgical, 250, Paris, Francoise Clouzier & Cie, 1671.

119. Guistra, P., Killoran, P., and Furman, R.: The missed Monteggia fracture. Radiology, *110:*45, 1974.

120. Kini, M. G.: Dislocation of the head of the radius associated with fracture of the upper third of the ulna. Antiseptic, *37:*1059, 1940.

121. Monteggia, G. B.: Instituzione Chirurgiche, 2nd ed. Milan, G. Maspero, 1813–1815.

122. Naylor, A.: Monteggia fractures. Br. J. Surg., *29:*323, 1942.

123. Poinsot, G.: Dislocations of the head of the radius downward (by elongation). N. Y. State J. Med., *41:*8, 1885.

124. Smith, F. M.: Monteggia fractures; analysis of 25 consecutive fresh injuries. Surg. Gynecol. Obstet., *85:*630, 1947.

125. Solcard, R.: Fractuare de Monteggia vicieusement consolidée avec synostose radiocubitale. Rev. Chir. Orthop., *19:*36, 1932.

126. Thompson, H. A., and Hamilton, A. T.: Monteggia fracture; internal fixation of fractured ulna with intramedullary pin. Am. J. Surg., *73:*579, 1950.

127. Van Santvoordt, R.: Dislocation of the radial head downward. N. Y. State J. Med., *45:*63, 1887.

128. Penrose, J. H.: The Monteggia fracture with posterior dislocation of the radial head. J. Bone Joint Surg., *33-B:*65, 1951.

129. Wise, A.: Lateral dislocation of the head of the radius with fracture of the ulna. J. Bone Joint Surg., *23:*379, 1941.

130. Beddow, F. H., and Corkery, P. H.: Lateral dislocation of the radiohumeral joint with greenstick fracture of the upper end of the ulna. J. Bone Joint Surg., *42-B:*782, 1960.

131. Tompkins, D. G.: The anterior Monteggia fracture. J. Bone Joint Surg., *53-A:*1109, 1971.

132. Spinner, M., Freundlich, B. D., and Teicher, J.: Posterior interosseous nerve palsy as a complication of Monteggia fractures in children. Clin. Orthop., *58:*141, 1968.

133. Morris, A. H.: Irreducible Monteggia lesion with radial-nerve entrapment. J. Bone Joint Surg., *56-A:*1744, 1974.

134. Stein, F., Grabias, S. L., and Deffer, P. A.: Nerve injuries complicating Monteggia lesions. J. Bone Joint Surg., *53-A:*1432, 1971.

135. Jessing, P.: Monteggia lesions and their complicating nerve damage. Acta Orthop. Scand., *46:*601, 1975.

136. Bagley, C. H.: Fractures of both bones of the forearm. Surg. Gynecol. Obstet., *42:*95, 1926.

137. Crowe, J. E., and Swischuk, L. E.: Acute bowing fractures of the forearm in children: a frequently missed injury. A. J. R., *128:*981, 1977.

138. Hogstrom, H., Nilsson, B. E., and Willner, S.: Correction with growth following diaphyseal forearm fracture. Acta Orthop. Scand., *47:*299, 1976.

139. Lorthior, J.: Traitment des fractures chez l'enfant. Acta Orthop. Belg., *31:*611, 1965.

140. Moesner, J., and Ostergaard, A. H.: Diaphysefrakturer hos born. Nord. Med., *75:*355, 1966.

141. Rydholm, U., and Nilsson, J. E.: Traumatic bowing of the forearm. Clin. Orthop., *139:*121, 1979.

142. Thorndike, A., Jr., and Simmler, C. L., Jr.: Fractures of the forearm and elbow in children. N. Engl. J. Med., *225:*475, 1941.

143. Wilson, J.: Fractures of the forearm. Pediatr. Clin. North Am., *14:*664, 1967.

144. Warren, J. D.: Anterior interosseous nerve palsy as a complication of forearm fractures. J. Bone Joint Surg., *45-B:*511, 1963.

145. Patrick, J.: A study of supination and pronation with special reference to the treatment of forearm fractures. J. Bone Joint Surg., *28:*737, 1946.

146. Ray, R. D., Johnson, R. J., and Jameson, R. M.: Rotation of the forearm. An experimental study of pronation and supination. J. Bone Joint Surg., *33-A:*993, 1951.

147. Undeland, K.: Rotational movements and bony union in shaft fractures of the forearm. J. Bone Joint Surg., *44-B:*340, 1962.

148. Daruwalla, J.: A study of radioulnar movements following fractures of the forearm in children. Clin. Orthop., *139:*114, 1979.

149. Knight, R. A., and Purvis, G. D.: Fractures of both bones of the forearm in adults. J. Bone Joint Surg., *31:*755, 1949.

150. Ashhurst, A. C., and John, R. L.: The treatment of fractures of the forearm with notes of the end results. Episcopal Hosp. Rep., *1:*224, 1913.

151. Destot, E.: Pronation and supination of the forearm in traumatic lesions. Presse Med., *21:*41, 1913.

152. Destot, E.: De la perte des mouvements de pronation et de supination dans les fractures de l'avant bras. Lyon Méd., *112:*61, 1909.

153. Pollen, A.: Fractures and Dislocations in Children. Baltimore, Williams & Wilkins, 1973.

154. Gainor, J. W., and Hardy, J. H., III: Forearm fractures treated in extension. Immobilization of fractures of the proximal bones of the forearm in children. J. Trauma, *9:*167, 1969.

155. Hughston, J. C.: Fractures of the forearm in children. J. Bone Joint Surg., *44-A:*1678, 1962.

156. Levinthal, D. H.: Fractures of the lower one third of both bones of the forearm in children. Surg. Gynecol. Obstet., *57:*790, 1933.

157. Önne, L., and Sandblom, P.: Late results in fractures of forearm in children. Acta Orthop. Scand., *98:*549, 1949.

158. Finsterbush, A., et al.: Recent experiences with intravenous regional anesthesia in limbs. J. Trauma, *12:*81, 1972.

159. Bragdon, R. A.: Fractures of the distal radial epiphysis. Clin. Orthop., *41:*59, 1965.

160. Eichler, J.: Spätschäden an den Radioulnargelenken nach unterarmverletzungen am wachsenden. Skeletal Chir. Praxis, *4:*437, 1966.

161. Grimault, L., and Leonhart, E.: Dé collement epiphysaire de l'extrémities inferieure du radius. Rev. Chir. [Orthop.], *12:*261, 1925.

162. Sterling, A. P., and Habermann, E. T.: Acute post-traumatic median nerve compression associated with a Salter II fracture dislocation of the wrist. Bull. Hosp. Joint Dis., *34:*167, 1963.

163. Abbott, L. E., and Saunders, J. B.: Injuries of median nerve in fractures of the lower end of the radius. Surg. Gynecol. Obstet., *57:*507, 1933.

164. Meadoff, N.: Median nerve injuries in fractures in the region of the wrist. Calif. Med., *70:*252, 1949.

165. Ranawat, C. S., DeFiore, J., and Straub, L. R.: Madelung's deformity. An end-result study of surgical treatment. J. Bone Joint Surg., *57-A:*772, 1975.

166. Mikic, Z.: Galeazzi fracture-dislocations. J. Bone Joint Surg., *8:*1071, 1975.

13

Wrist and Hand

Anatomy

The changing osseous anatomy of the hand and wrist (Fig. 13-1) is probably better known than the remainder of the child's developing skeleton, primarily because this region has been evaluated frequently for skeletal aging. However, virtually all studies are based upon cumulative roentgenographic data, and have little actual anatomic substantiation.

Prenatally the carpal bones assume their basic shape as a cartilaginous anlage. During postnatal development there are minimal changes in the contours of the cartilaginous components. Little ossification is present at birth. Each primary ossification center gradually proceeds from a relatively small, central focus (or foci) out to the peripheral contours. The osseous contours are variable and changing and do not always reflect the actual contour of the still-to-be-ossified cartilaginous precursor. Longitudinal growth deformity in the distal radius or ulna, or abnormal muscle forces exerted across the wrist may cause mild to moderate structural changes in the cartilaginous portions of the carpal bones. Ossification simply follows any pre-existent cartilaginous deformation.

The scaphoid is the largest bone in the proximal carpal row; ossification begins between the ages of 5 and 6 and is complete by 13 to 15 years of age (see Fig. 13-1). Before ossification is complete, the scaphoid is almost entirely cartilaginous circumferentially, which increases the cushioning effect during trauma, thus lessening susceptibility to fracture throughout skeletal maturation. The retrograde blood supply of the scaphoid is such that waist fractures endanger the vascularity of the proximal pole and ischemic necrosis may accompany nonunion, although to a much lesser extent in children than in adults.

The lunate may develop two ossification centers early in its development. These subsequently fuse, although they may persist as separate ossicles. Sometimes the lunate fuses incompletely with adjacent carpals to give rise to a spurious "fracture line" at the site of fusion. Binuclear ossification has also been described for the multangular and semilunar bones. The pisiform, the smallest carpal bone and the last to ossify, often does so from several small foci (Fig. 13-2). Irregular or multifocal ossification should not be misinterpreted as chondro-osseous trauma.

In the basal phalanx of the thumb, and in the proximal and middle phalanges of the other fingers, small, sharply defined linear "defects" are frequently visible on routine radiographs. These are the diaphyseal nutrient foramina, which are less frequent in the distal phalanges (except the thumb). These defects should not be confused with incomplete cortical fractures.

Epiphyses are located at the proximal *and* distal ends of each phalanx. However, only one epiphysis in each phalanx and metacarpal eventually forms a secondary ossification center. In such areas, the associated physis is transversely oriented. This secondary center forms in the proximal epiphysis of each phalanx. In contrast, the secondary centers of the metacarpal epiphyses are distal, except for the thumb, in which it is proximal. At the opposite end of each of these developing bones the epiphyseal cartilage is rapidly replaced by endochondral ossification until only a thin layer of cartilage exists. This layer is comprised of articular cartilage, germinal epiphyseal cartilage, and a slow-growing, spherical physis that contributes little to longitudinal growth, but does allow continued hemispheric growth of the end of the bone as the joint enlarges.

Sometimes there may be an apparent epiphysis at each end of a metacarpal. Extra or false (pseudo) epiphyseal ossification centers may appear in the distal first metacarpal (Fig. 13-3), or in the proximal epiphyseal cartilage of the second, third, fourth, and fifth metacarpals. The first metacarpal is more frequently involved than other areas. While Caffey believes that the term pseudoepiphysis is a misnomer and that there is no such anatomic entity, Haines has shown histologically that there is such a structure, which results when metaphyseal ossification mushrooms into that region (see Chap. 2).[1,2] Solitary involvement should not be misinterpreted as a fracture line, or be indicative of any systemic disease. However, if several pseudoepiphyses are present, they may indicate underlying illness or dysplasia; particularly, hypothyroidism (cretinism) may be associated with these developmental chondro-osseous variations.

Functional anatomy relative to fracture care

Proper hand splinting following fracture is extremely important, even in a child who is not as likely to develop complications from inappropriate splinting compared to an adult.[3] Stiffness and swelling after injury often last several months, even when the injury does not primarily involve the skeleton (e.g., dorsal-surface contusion). Because of the overall amount of ligamentous laxity usually present, permanent contractures are not as common a problem in children as they are in adults. Further, injuries to the hand produce bleeding and swelling in the surrounding soft tissues. The inflammatory process, an essential part of healing in the early stages, creates adhesions between the complex gliding tissue planes. These adhesions are inevitable and necessary for complete healing, and their formation cannot be prevented. Their effect may be minimized by appropriate positioning during treatment, as well as controlled mobilization.

The classic "position of function" for the hand that is described in most textbooks is better termed the "ready to grasp position," or the "position of rest" (Fig. 13-4). However, even children's fingers may become stiff in this position. In view of today's better concepts of hand rehabilitation, this is not an optimal position.

It is well recognized that the metacarpophalangeal joint is a biaxial, ball-and-socket joint. In acute flexion, the collateral ligaments are under the greatest length and tension because of the eccentric origin of the ligament on the metacarpal, and the flare of the metacarpal head. If the metacarpophalangeal joint drifts into extension due to edema of the fingers, it may remain in relative extension when the collateral ligaments become stiff in this shortened abnormal position. Therefore, the position of function for the metacarpophalangeal joint in the injured hand appears to be full flexion of 90° (see Fig. 13-4).

However, the ligamentous morphology is completely different in the proximal interphalangeal joint. This is a hinge joint without significant lateral motion capacity. The volar plate is less mobile than that in a metacarpophalangeal joint. It is attached firmly to the base of the middle phalanx, although its attachment to the neck of the proximal phalanx is loose. The volar plate may fold upon itself like an accordion. If left in the flexed position, portions of the volar plate may become adherent to each other, which leads to a stiff joint. The checkreins appear to be the primary pathologic structure causing middle joint (PIP) contracture.[4] The collateral ligaments of the proximal interphalangeal joint are under the greatest tension (length) in approximately 15° of flexion when the fibers are riding lightly over the lateral aspect of the condyle of the proximal phalanx.[5] Consequently, splinting proximal interphalangeal joints must be diligently performed in 15° to 20° of flexion to prevent shortening of the collateral ligaments and volar plate.

Thus, the true "position of safety" would be the intrinsic-plus position, with 90° of flexion at the metacarpophalangeal joints and almost complete extension in the proximal interphalangeal joints (see Fig. 13-4). The thumb is best held in the widely abducted, opposed position.

Incidence

Due to the activity level of children, the hand is one of the most frequent areas of trauma, although not necessarily specific chondro-osseous injury.[6-28] Hand fractures are relatively common in children, and phalangeal fractures and dislocations are most common. Probably the hand fracture that occurs most often is a crush injury to the distal phalanx at the fingertip. However, even fractures of the phalanges in children, which may not seem like major injuries, may have serious consequences because of aberrant growth (Fig. 13-5). Carpal injuries and multiple unstable fractures of the metacarpals are rare in children. Unfortunately, many of these fractures are often treated by guidelines for comparable adult injuries.[29]

Children's ligaments are strong and resilient. Since they are stronger than the associated physes, sudden extension of a ligament at the time of injury generally results in separation of the physis, rather than a tear in the ligament. To a lesser extent, this is also true of fibrous joint capsules. Injury mechanisms that result in a torn ligament or dislocation in an adult's hand often produce traumatic separation of the physis in a child's hand.

Other than open crush injuries of the tips of the fingers, children usually sustain less serious open fractures; nonunion is extremely rare. Fracture healing is rapid in children, about half the time of fracture healing in adults.

The largest series of hand fractures in children was reported by Leonard and Dubravicik.[30] They collected a series of 276 fractures, 41% of which were physeal fractures. However, these children's hand fractures only constituted 0.45% of their overall practice. Of these fractures, 10% required open reduction for adequate restoration of normal anatomy.

Bora reviewed 100 patients with epiphyseal fractures of the hand, 90 of which were closed fractures and 10 of which were open fractures.[30] Of the 90 closed fractures, 80 were treated successfully with closed manipulation. The remaining 10 required anesthesia and pin fixation. Seven of these ten were treated with reduction and percutaneous pin fixation, while three required an open reduction (two of these latter three were old fractures that had healed in an unacceptable, malaligned position).

Radiology

Roentgenograms, in at least two planes (anteroposterior and lateral), are imperative to adequately assess any fracture. It is essential that a true lateral view of the involved digit be obtained. Superimposition of other fingers in the lateral view may obscure significant details. The fourth and fifth metacarpals can be brought into lateral view with 10° of supination, and the second and third metacarpals can be brought into lateral view with 10° of pronation. Perhaps the most common cause of missed or improper diagnosis of fractures in children's fingers is the failure to obtain a true lateral view of the involved finger. Additional oblique views may also be necessary to properly evaluate joint injuries, particularly to assess small, juxta-articular fractures.

The presence of foreign bodies in all open or penetrating wounds should be suspected in children. Roentgenograms cannot be relied upon to visualize foreign bodies because wood splinters, most types of glass, and other foreign contaminants, especially biologic materials, may not be radiopaque.

General Treatment Guidelines

Initial evaluation and primary care of the injured hand are critical. One of the greatest pitfalls in treating these injuries is that primary focus is on the fracture and more subtle, but

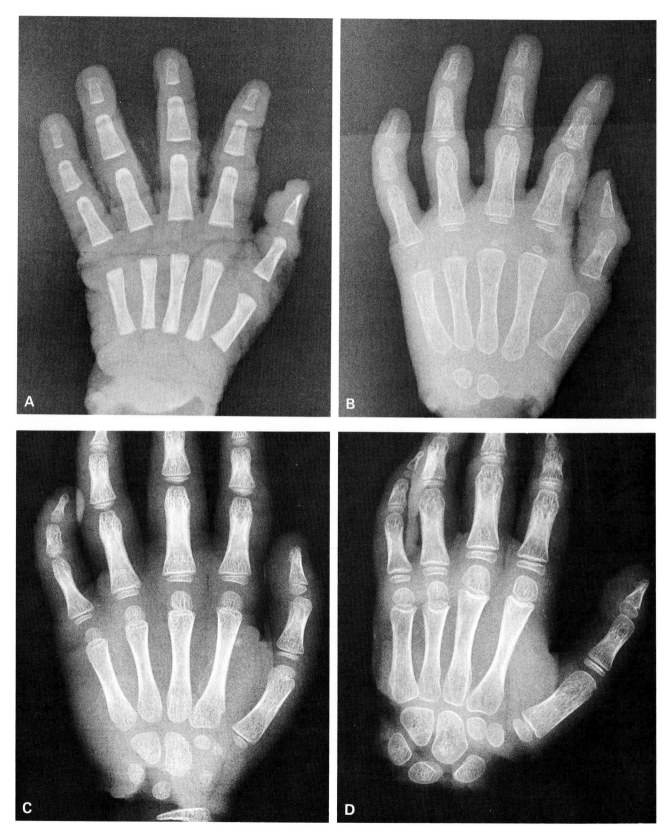

FIG. 13-1. Sequential development of the wrist and hand. *A-B,* Early development. Note the variable development of the secondary ossification centers of the metacarpals. *C-E,* Later developmental sequence. *C* and *E* have pseudoepiphyses of the distal first metacarpal. Also note that the carpal navicula does not completely ossify until late in skeletal maturation, a factor that may minimize fracture during childhood and adolescence.

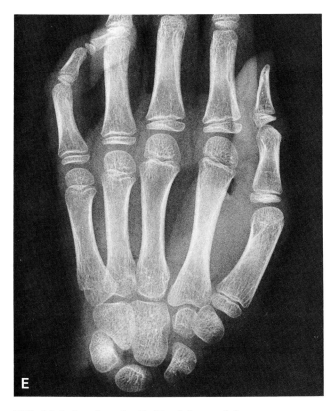

FIG. 13-1 Continued. *E,* Hand from adolescent.

often more significant, damage to soft tissues is often overlooked. Both open and closed injuries must be examined meticulously for injury to adjacent tendons, nerves, and blood vessels. Maximum functional recovery must be the goal of treatment in every hand injury.

Immobilization of a child's hand always presents a challenge. Well-fitting plaster casts and splints are notoriously difficult to apply in the small child. Bulky, soft dressings may be used for immobilizing the infant's hand. In older children, plaster gutter splints incorporating an adjacent normal digit may be used to help control rotational deformity. Mold the splint in the "intrinsic plus" position. Another important principle is to never immobilize a solitary finger in a child. When a single finger is immobilized, there is an increased possibility that angulation will develop by the time the cast or splint is removed.

Placing the fingers on a banjo splint, in which the fingers are pulled straight and divergent, is condemned. Wrapping the hand around a gauze bandage over which all the fingers stiffen in a poor functional position is also a poor practice. Finally, the universal splint is mentioned only to be condemned. Because of the ease with which the hand can slip backward, the universal splint causes fingers to assume a position that can only do harm.

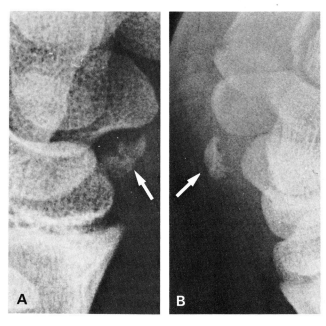

FIG. 13-2. *A,* Multifocal ossification of the pisiform (arrow) in a ten-year-old girl. *B,* Irregular ossification of margin (arrow) of primary ossification center of pisiform in a ten-year-old boy. In both cases (*A* and *B*), there was trauma to the wrist and pain along the joint. However, chondroosseous fracture of this bone (similar to tibial spine avulsion) is an unlikely injury pattern.

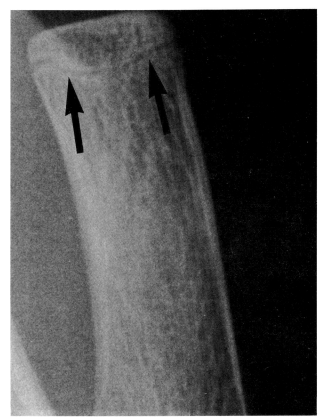

FIG. 13-3. Pseudoepiphysis of the thumb in a six-year-old. Note how the lucency extends across most of the transverse diameter of the shaft (arrows). Metaphyseal ossification "mushrooms" into the cartilage and leaves peripheral cartilage remnants that appear roentgenographically like peripheral physeal cartilage during physiologic epiphysiodesis.

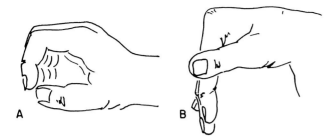

FIG. 13-4. *A*, Classic position of function. *B*, More appropriate "intrinsic plus" position of function for treating (splinting) hand injuries in children.

Closed phalangeal fractures in children are usually treated by simple methods, with a return to normal or almost normal function expected. It is the exceptional case that requires open reduction. The most common exception is a fracture through the neck (distal end) of the phalanx with subluxation or dislocation of the head of the phalanx in relation to the more distal phalangeal base.

Most fractures in the hand can be treated adequately with closed reduction and immobilization for a maximum of three weeks. Because immobilization is more difficult in children, Kirschner-wire fixation is important, particularly for stabilization.

Adequate anesthesia for reduction of the little finger may be obtained with a block of the ulnar nerve at the wrist, including the dorsal sensory branch. However, this or more extensive nerve blocks are often difficult to achieve in children.

Fractures of the phalanges and metacarpals heal rapidly, and remodeling of angulation deformity often occurs in fractures in the metaphyseal region. Little remodeling can be expected in fractures distant from the epiphyseal end containing the secondary ossification center. For example, in the distal end of a phalanx, growth is primarily from a spherical rather than a transverse physis, which is nonlongitudinal growth (see Chap. 4).

In fractures of the metacarpals and phalanges it is important to recognize and correct *rotational* malalignment. Remodeling does *not* correct rotational deformity, and for this reason it is imperative to reduce all fractures of the phalanges and metacarpals in perfect rotational alignment. This is not always easy, since subtle degrees of malrotation that are not recognized during the period of immobilization may result in significant functional impairment after full range of motion has been regained. The best way to monitor rotational alignment is to carefully study the planes of the fingernails in the splint, comparing the injured digit to the adjacent normal fingers and to the counterpart in the opposite hand (Fig. 13-6). Assessing malrotation of the thumb is more difficult, but not as important to correct during treatment.

Wrist Joint Injury

Injury to the wrist joint is unusual prior to skeletal maturity. Except in the child with significant ligamentous laxity (e.g., Larsen's or Ehlers-Danlos syndromes, or homo-

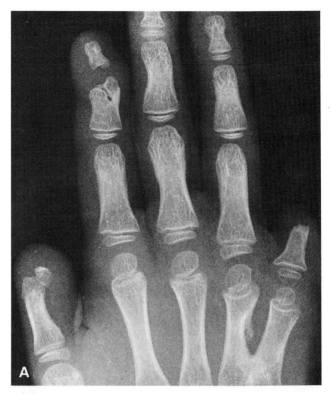

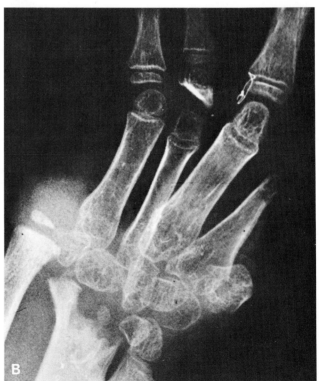

FIG. 13-5. *A*, Early growth abnormalities following severe compound hand injury caused by a firecracker. There is exostosis formation in the proximal phalanx of the thumb, a split middle phalanx in the index finger, and synostosis of the fourth and fifth metacarpals. *B*, Multiple deformities of hand, wrist, and distal radius due to a compound injury caused earlier in childhood by a lawnmower.

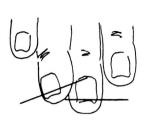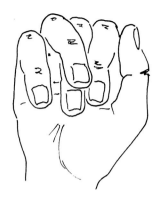

FIG. 13-6. The fingernails should be reasonably coplanar and all the flexed fingers should be almost parallel. In malrotation, whether involving a metacarpal or phalanx, the uniform plane of the fingernails is disrupted, and the involved digit overlaps the normal digits.

cysteinuria), subluxation or dislocation of the carpus is almost nonexistent. Instead, because of the density of ligamentous and capsular attachments from the carpus into the distal radial and ulnar epiphyses, injurious forces will likely cause distal radioulnar epiphyseal and metaphyseal fracture-dislocations.

However, the wrist joint capsule may be damaged during a fall, and because of the proximity of extensor tendon compartments, a communication may develop and lead to progressive symptoms of chronic, painful tenosynovitis (Fig. 13-7). These may be accurately diagnosed by wrist joint arthrography and subsequently treated by operative closure of the capsular defect.

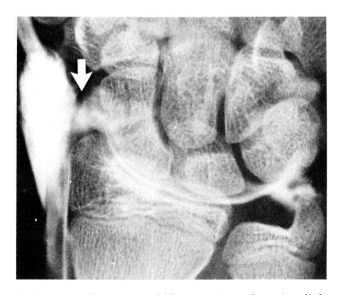

FIG. 13-7. This 10-year-old boy ran into a fence in a little league baseball game, sustaining a wrist injury. Roentgenography was unremarkable. However, he experienced severe pain for 14 months. This arthrogram shows communication of the wrist joint with the thumb extensor/abductor compartments (arrow). Closure of the capsular defect brought total symptomatic relief.

Carpus

Injuries of the carpus, particularly of the carpal scaphoid, are rare in children (Figs. 13-8 and 13-9). It has been suggested that the cartilaginous covering of the juvenile bones imparts a certain resilience that renders the osseous centrum less liable to fracture than the adult.

Fracture of the scaphoid is the most common injury of the carpal bones in the child. The vulnerability of the scaphoid to fracture appears to be greatest between the ages of 15 and 30 years. During the preceding 5 years, from the ages of 10 to 15, the ossific nucleus gradually enlarges to conform to the contours of the adjacent bones (see Fig. 13-1). The youngest reported patient with scaphoid fracture was 9 years of age.[18] Grundy reported 8 scaphoid fractures in patients between the ages of 10 and 15.[32] The usual mechanism of injury is dorsiflexion.

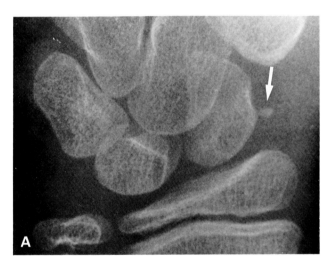

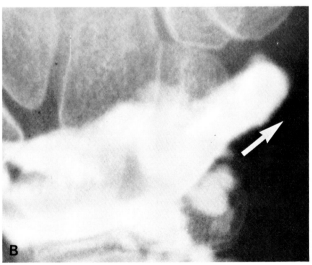

FIG. 13-8. *A,* Chondro-osseous avulsion fracture (arrow) of the carpal navicula in an 11-year-old. *B,* An arthrogram showed a diverticulum near this fracture (arrow). At surgery, the capsule was damaged and a nonunion was evident. The small fragment was removed and the capsule reattached to the navicular perichondrium.

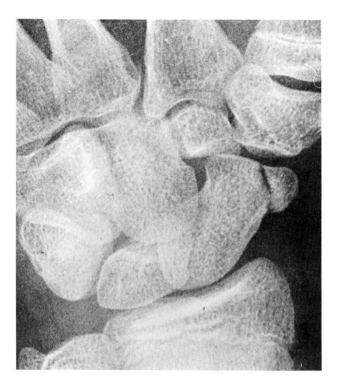

FIG. 13-9. Distal carpal navicula fracture in a 14-year-old.

Mussbichler reviewed over 3000 examinations of the hand and wrist in children and believed that injuries of the scaphoid were relatively common in children. Of those patients, he found 107 with roentgenologic evidence of damage to the carpal bones, 100 of which had a fracture through the scaphoid.[18] These included 15 injuries through the waist, 33 distal, and 52 avulsions of the radial-dorsal aspect. There were no fractures through the proximal part of the bone. Avulsion with detachment of small fragments from the dorsal-radial surface of the scaphoid constituted over 50% of Mussbichler's material and must be regarded as typical of childhood injury (Fig. 13-10). The fragments were clearly seen when the wrist was placed in extreme pronation so that the fracture surface was in a projection tangential to the beam. All patients responded to conservative treatment.

One of the major concerns in adult navicular fractures is ischemic necrosis.[31] This does not appear to be a significant complicating factor in children's fractures. Grundy reported irregularity of the radial margin of the navicular at the site of the healed fracture in four cases.[32] However, this might have been a change consequent to the injury and not necessarily indicative of any vascular complications.

Mussbichler described two instances of nonunion, both of which were neglected (untreated) cases.[18] Eight patients with navicular fractures were reported by Southcott, all of which had established nonunion with average follow-up of almost four years.[23] Prior to their reports, Southcott found no report of nonunion of fracture of the carpal scaphoid in children. However, nonunion, with or without radiologically evident avascular necrosis, can occur in children. All nonunions were grafted with autogenous bone which led to good clinical and radiologic results. The authors concluded

that nonunion in children is best managed by bone grafting through the volar approach.[23]

Traumatic carpal instability in the young child presents problems of diagnosis and management. Only one case has been described, that of a seven-year-old girl with scapholunate dissociation.[33] The original injury apparently occurred when the girl was only three months old. Instability may be difficult to diagnose early because of variable degrees of carpal ossification. The scaphoid and lunate do not ossify until four years of age. An arthrogram may be useful.

Even when scapholunate dissociation is suspected and treated by immobilization, the outcome is uncertain. Once the collapse is established, treatment should be based on the patient's symptoms and skeletal maturity. In long-term treatment, a protective orthosis should be used. Any operative treatment should be directed toward achieving a stable, painless wrist. In a young child, another important treatment goal must be to prevent the development of structural deformities. As long as these bones have a significant amount of cartilage, remodeling may occur (biologic plasticity).

Thumb

Dislocation

Dislocation of the thumb often involves the metacarpophalangeal joint (Fig. 13-11). This is frequently caused by the child's hand catching in a washing-machine roller, a mechanism that may also cause a childhood Bennett's fracture.

The metacarpal head is often pushed through the thumb musculature, especially the flexor pollicis brevis, and may also buttonhole through the joint capsule (Fig. 13-12). Such

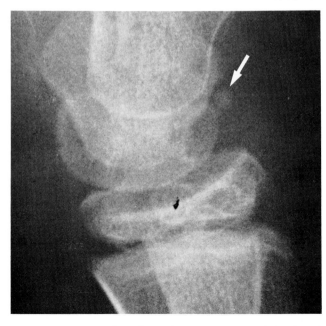

FIG. 13-10. Typical avulsion fracture (arrow) of the dorsal radial navicular surface in a 12-year-old.

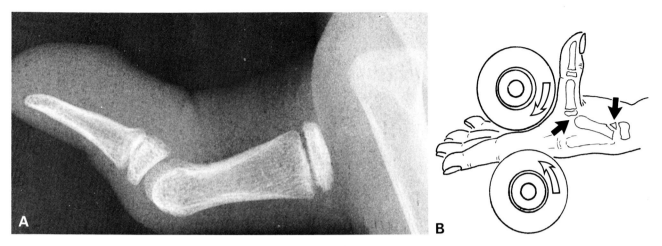

FIG. 13-11.   *A*, Typical metacarpophalangeal dislocation of the thumb in a five-year-old. *B*, Mechanism of either MCP dislocation or Bennett's fracture when the hand is caught in machine rollers.

structures may partially entrap the metacarpal head. However, unlike digital metacarpophalangeal dislocations, complete encirclement of the metacarpal neck does not occur, thereby increasing the likelihood of closed reduction. The intrinsic muscles retain their insertion with the sesamoids and serve to guide the plate palmarward, keeping it from being irreducibly displaced into the joint. The sesamoids, which may not be roentgenographically evident in younger children, indicate the position of the palmar (volar) plate.[34]

Initial treatment should be closed reduction, which is usually successful. Reduction may be simplified by initially flexing the metacarpal into the palm to reduce intrinsic muscle tightness, while concomitantly applying longitudinal traction. Flexion with continued traction completes the reduction. However, if capsular or muscular interposition is present, an open reduction may be necessary. Because the course of the digital nerves of the thumb may be altered (displaced) by the traumatic anatomy, care must be taken to adequately visualize these prior to, as well as following, reduction.

Collateral ligament tears of the thumb

Gamekeeper's thumb or collateral ligament injury of the metacarpophalangeal joint occurs from partial or total disruption of the ulnar collateral ligament in the adult. In a child, ulnar and radial collateral ligament "tears" of the thumb are usually type 3 chondro-osseous injuries (Fig. 13-13). These corner fractures of the epiphysis are equivalent to collateral ligament injuries in adults. If the articular surface is involved, these fractures should be accurately corrected by open reduction and buttress pinning.

Fractures

Fractures of the thumb sometimes represent unique problems. The base of the proximal phalanx and that of the thumb metacarpal are common sites of epiphyseal injury. A closed injury at the metacarpophalangeal joint that results in ulnar or radial instability of the proximal phalanx on the metacarpal is probably an epiphyseal fracture of the proxi-

mal phalanx, rather than the ligamentous injury commonly seen in the adult. Stress views may be necessary to delineate the fracture.

The proximal phalanx usually sustains a physeal fracture (Figs. 13-13 and 13-14). This fracture may be a type 1, 2, 3, or 4 injury, depending upon the mechanism and degree of skeletal maturity. There is usually associated radial angulation. Treatment for types 1 and 2 injuries is closed reduction with adduction to correct the radial angulation. Types 3 and 4 usually require open reduction and accurate restoration of joint surface anatomy.

The proximal phalanx may also sustain a distal fracture (Fig. 13-15). This may be a difficult injury to handle, despite its innocuous appearance. Delayed union may occur, especially if the original injury is not splinted, and may necessitate open reduction and temporary pin fixation. Remodeling

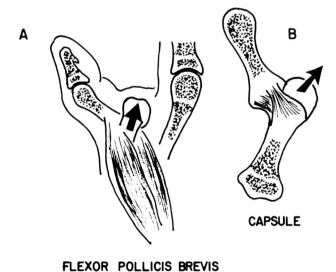

FIG. 13-12.   Schematic of displacement of metacarpal head through, *A*, flexor pollicis brevis or, *B*, capsule.

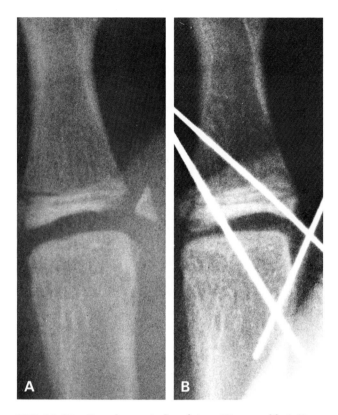

FIG. 13-13. Gamekeeper's thumb in a 12-year-old. *A,* Type 3 avulsion fracture with rotation of the fragment. *B,* This was treated by multiple K-wires which fixed the fragment and buttressed and immobilized both the fragment and the phalanx.

is not extensive in this end of the bone and malunion may result in permanent deformity.

Fractures of the distal phalangeal epiphysis are relatively common (Fig. 13-16). These are often crushing injuries associated with open fracture, and must be handled carefully so as not to lose soft tissue or cause complicating osteomyelitis, which could result in premature epiphysiodesis in a young child. The flexor tendon attaches to the volar (palmar) shaft surface, while the extensor slip primarily attaches into the epiphysis. Accordingly, the epiphysis may retain a normal relationship to the proximal phalanx, while the remainder of the distal phalanx is flexed. This angular deformity must be corrected during closed reduction. Open reduction may be necessary for a type 3 injury, the pediatric analogue of "mallet finger."

Bennett's Fracture. Impacted fractures of the base of the thumb are commonly seen in children.[11,20] Bennett's fracture in children is usually a physeal injury, with the most frequent being a type 2 injury (Figs. 13-17 and 13-18). The anterior oblique ligament that anchors the palmar lip of the metacarpal to the trapezium is quite strong. The two primary variables of childhood Bennett's fracture are the size of the metaphyseal fragment and the amount of displacement of the shaft from the epiphysis. The base of the metacarpal is pulled medially by the abductor pollicis longus, which inserts at the base, while the insertion of the adductor distally

further levers the base radially (abduction). However, the periosteal sleeve is usually intact along one or more sides, and may be used for stabilization during reduction.

Minimally displaced fractures require only cast protection. In a young child, up to 30° of angulation may be acceptable at the base of the thumb, although reduction to a lesser degree of malalignment should be attempted (see Fig. 13-17). Angulation over 30° must be corrected by manipulation. Pressure is applied to the base of the thumb, and counterpressure is placed over the head of the metacarpal. The common error is to hyperextend the metacarpal joint by applying pressure too far distally, which does nothing to correct the deformity. The parents must be warned that a bump will remain for a year or so, but that the bone straightens with time.

Occasionally, a complete displacement may buttonhole through the periosteum. Although a closed reduction may look easy and is worth attempting, many of these injuries require open reduction to maneuver the metaphysis back into position through the periosteal tear.

Radial displacement of the thumb may be corrected by manipulation and cast immobilization. Ulnar displacement, however, usually defies attempts at closed reduction and frequently requires open reduction with Kirschner-wire fixation (see Fig. 13-18). Even if an ulnar displacement can be treated by closed reduction, a fracture of this type must be followed closely because redisplacement may occur in the cast.

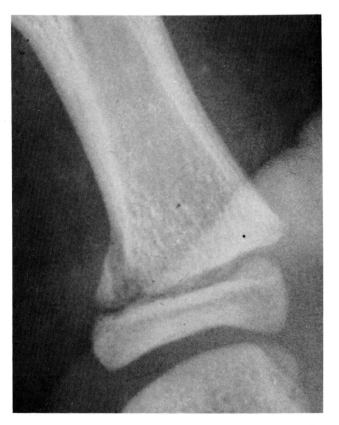

FIG. 13-14. Type 2 fracture of proximal phalanx. The Thurston Holland fragment is usually on the radial side. Radial angulation of the rest of the thumb is common.

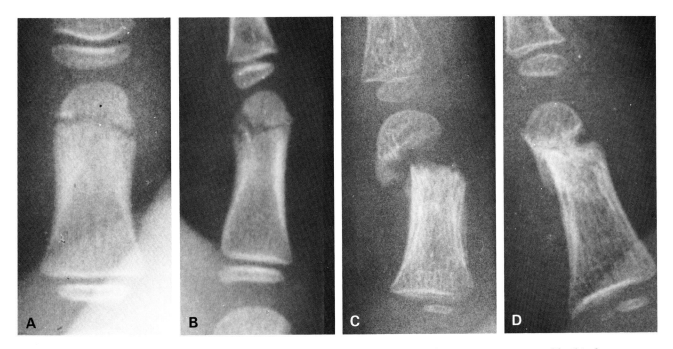

FIG. 13-15. *A-B,* AP and lateral views of fracture of distal end of proximal phalanx in a seven-year-old. This fracture was undisplaced and healing was uneventful. *C,* However, a similar injury in a four-year-old had this appearance seven weeks after injury (splinted for two weeks, with no roentgenogram at the time of splint removal). The child was subsequently treated by open reduction. *D,* Three weeks after open reduction and fixation, the fracture shows osseous healing.

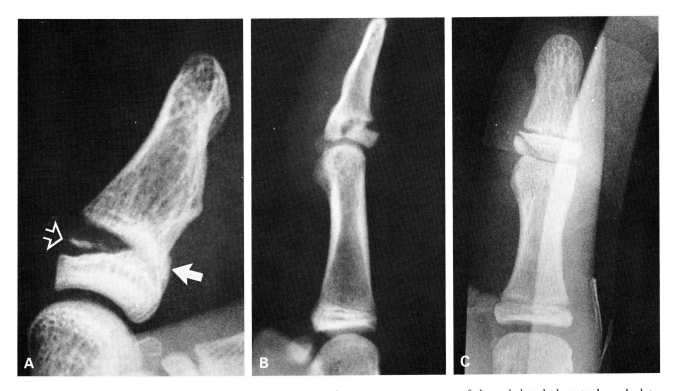

FIG. 13-16. *A,* Type 2 fracture of distal phalanx. Notice the transverse remnant of the subchondral metaphyseal plate (Werenskiöld fragment) on the tension failure side (open arrow), and the Thurston Holland fragment on the compression failure side (closed arrow). *B,* Type 3 injury pattern. *C,* Type 7 injury confined to the secondary ossification center.

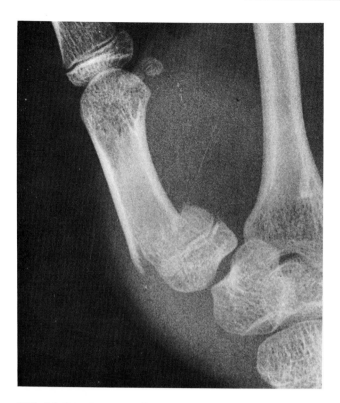

FIG. 13-17. Bennett's fracture leaving ulnar metaphyseal fragment and adduction angulation of the rest of the thumb.

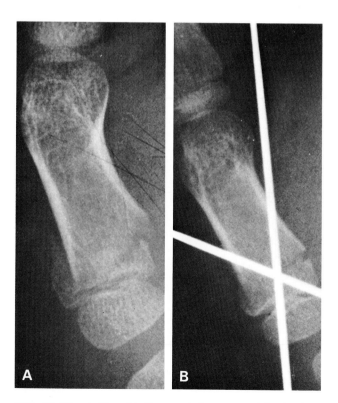

FIG. 13-18. *A*, Unstable Bennett's fracture with both ulnar and radial metaphyseal fragments. *B*, Closed reduction was combined with percutaneous pinning.

Metacarpals and Phalanges

Interphalangeal dislocations

Dislocations frequently involve the proximal interphalangeal joints (Fig. 13-19). These hinge joints allow only flexion and extension. The accessory fibers on the volar plate and the two quadrilateral collateral ligaments form three sides for each joint. The thickest portion of the collateral ligament reinforces the insertion of the volar plate into the base of the middle phalanx. In a dislocation, two of the three sides are usually disrupted. Following relocation, a collateral ligament usually heals with little difficulty.[19] However, in children, a collateral ligament may occasionally be avulsed and does not become affixed to the chondro-osseous structures. Abundant callus may be laid down and a tumorlike mass may develop on the side of the finger. If this occurs it may be necessary to remove this surgically.

Ligaments and capsular structures around the joints in the child are strong in comparison to the physis, and injuries that would frequently cause a dislocation in an adult result in an epiphyseal fracture in a child or adolescent. For this reason it is important to obtain roentgenograms of any joint injury prior to and after reduction (see Fig. 13-19).

In most interphalangeal dislocations, reduction is easily accomplished by closed manipulation. The correct technique for closed reduction is to hyperextend the joint and then *push* the distal bone over into the reduced position from above. One should *not* apply traction to a dislocated finger joint and attempt to *pull* the distal bone back into position as this may possibly entrap soft tissue within the joint, preventing reduction. After reduction, it is imperative to check the stability of the collateral ligaments; occasionally one of these may be torn at the time of initial displacement. However, remember that joint laxity is common in children. Compare the motion to the contralateral digit. If the joint is stable after reduction, which it usually is, allow immediate protected motion of the finger by taping it to an adjacent normal digit (dynamic splinting). An acceptable alternative is to immobilize the finger for 10 to 14 days in the aforementioned functional position.

Metacarpophalangeal dislocations

Anyone treating hand injuries in children should be aware that there is a specific type of dislocation of the metacarpophalangeal joint that is, with rare exception, irreducible by closed means—the so-called complex metacarpophalangeal dislocation.[3] This dislocation cannot be reduced because the volar plate becomes entrapped between the base of the proximal phalanx and the head of the metacarpal (Fig. 13-20). The physician should not have to wait for multiple attempts at closed dislocation to fail before concluding that the dislocation is irreducible, because definite clinical and radiographic clues exist. First, displacement of the phalanx on the metacarpal is not at 90° (as it generally is in a simple interphalangeal dislocation), but is more nearly parallel, with only slight displacement and minimal angulation (Fig. 13-21). Second, there is dimpling of the palmar skin. In the index finger (the most common site of complex dislocation), the dimple is difficult to visualize because it lies within the proximal palmar crease; but in the thumb, the dimple is readily seen in the thenar eminence. Finally, widening or

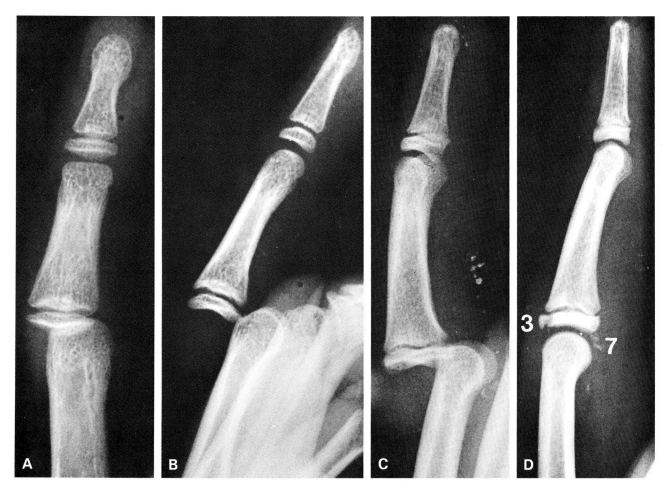

FIG. 13-19. *A-B*, AP and lateral views of dislocation of proximal interphalangeal joint. *C*, Seemingly simple PIP dislocation. *D*, However, post-reduction films of the fracture shown in *C* showed type 3 dorsal (3) and type 7 volar (7) epiphyseal ossification center fractures.

lateralization of the joint space radiographically suggests a complex dislocation because of interposition of the volar plate within the joint.

Reports of dislocations of the metacarpophalangeal joints in children are rare, with the exception of the thumb.[15,17,35-37] Baldwin reported four cases, three of which involved children; three were index metacarpophalangeal joint dislocations and the fourth involved the little finger, which presented similar anatomic and clinical problems.[35]

Forced hyperextension of the proximal phalanx of the index finger, usually from a fall on the hand, results in the metacarpal head being pushed through the palmar (volar) capsule. The fibrocartilaginous palmar plate is torn loose at its weakest point of attachment, the membranous attachment to the metacarpal. The metacarpal head is displaced toward the palm, while the palmar plate remains attached to the phalanx and is folded into the joint, where it becomes wedged between the metacarpal head and the base of the proximal phalanx. The phalanx is dislocated dorsally on the metacarpal head, which is forced through the transverse metacarpal ligament to become fixed between this ligament and the longitudinal portion of the superficial palmar fascia. The flexor tendons are displaced ulnarward and the lumbri-

cal tendons radialward, with both lying dorsal to the displaced metacarpal head (Fig. 13-22).

When the fifth finger is involved, because of the more distal course of the long flexor tendons to the little finger, these tendons are displaced radially, and trap the metacarpal head on that side, while the tendon of the abductor digiti quinti is the lateral trapping element (see Fig. 13-22). The fibrocartilaginous plate and the superficial transverse ligament, as in the index finger, form the floor and roof of the trap.

The palmar fibrocartilage is a rectangular reinforcement of the palmar capsule present in both metacarpophalangeal and interphalangeal joints. At the metacarpophalangeal joint, the capsule is loosely attached to the tissues proximal to the head of the metacarpal and is firmly attached to the base of the proximal phalanx. When the finger is hyperextended, the proximal attachment of the palmar fibrocartilage of the metacarpal ruptures and the proximal phalanx subluxates or dislocates dorsally, depending on the degree of hyperextension. As the phalanx is displaced, the fibrocartilage attached to the base is interposed between the metacarpal head and the phalanx (see Fig. 13-20).

Whether in the adult or the child, these cases usually re-

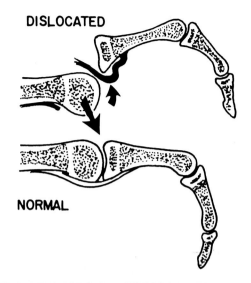

DISLOCATED

NORMAL

A

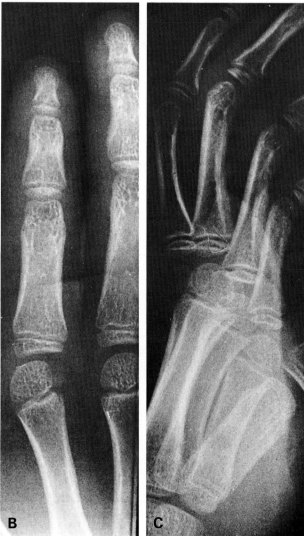

B

C

FIG. 13-20. *A*, Schematic of interposition of palmar (volar) plate dorsal to the dislocated metacarpal head. *B-C*, AP and lateral views of index metacarpal dislocation in a six-year-old.

quire open reduction. A reduction can be easily attained through a palmar approach, once the fibrocartilaginous plate has been incised, although an attempt should be made to reduce it prior to plate incision. The dorsal approach should *not* be used.

While extensive release of the various ligaments and tendons is advocated by Kaplan, particularly in delayed reduction, similar excessive transsection probably is not necessary in the child because of normally increased laxity of ligamentous structures.[37] Only enough fibrocartilaginous plate or ligament should be incised to effect a reduction. If reduction has been delayed longer than three to four weeks, the ulnar collateral ligament of the metacarpophalangeal joint must sometimes be excised through a separate dorsal incision before reduction can be accomplished.

This reduction is stable and wire fixation is not necessary. In fact, it may be harmful. Follow-up films in one reported case showed a defect of the head of the phalanx at the site of insertion of the K-wire, with shortening of the epiphysis.[35]

Metacarpals

Fractures. Fractures of the metacarpal shaft are less common in children than in adults (Fig. 13-23). The same principles apply to these fractures in both children and adults. Most fractures are correctly treated in a simple fashion. Overtreatment leads to complications. The dorsal "bowing" of metacarpal fractures is easily corrected by relaxing the wrist extensors, the long finger flexors, and the interosseous muscles. If the hand is properly positioned on the splint, these fractures heal with little difficulty.

Transverse fractures of the metacarpals are usually the result of direct blows. They angulate dorsally because of the original deformation and the palmar force subsequently exerted by the interosseous muscles. Oblique fractures of the metacarpal shafts result from a torque force with the finger acting as the long lever, and they tend to shorten and rotate, rather than angulate. Fractures of the third and fourth metacarpals tend to shorten less because of the tethering effect of the deep transverse metacarpal ligament, while fractures of the second and fifth metacarpals have more pronounced shortening and rotation.

Brown described a boy who sustained multiple trauma with a fracture through the neck and epiphysis of the third metacarpal,[38] which appeared to be a type 2 injury. He was treated by simple splinting. Three years later, he was seen for reinjury to the hand and roentgenograms showed a slowdown in growth of the third metacarpal. Figure 13-24 shows a similar case with antecedent injury to the third metacarpal head, with subsequent premature epiphysiodesis. This complication may involve the ring finger, leading to the short ring metacarpal syndrome. Figure 13-25 shows a similar fracture of the distal metacarpal of the index finger, with accompanying diaphyseal fractures of the long and ring fingers. Normal physeal closure had already commenced and the patient did not develop any deformity of the metacarpal head.

Fractures of the distal fifth metacarpal are relatively common, particularly during adolescence. These injuries may be metaphyseal or physeal injuries (Fig. 13-26). Correction of the angular deformity is necessary, as remodeling may not correct malunion, particularly in the patient close to skeletal maturity.

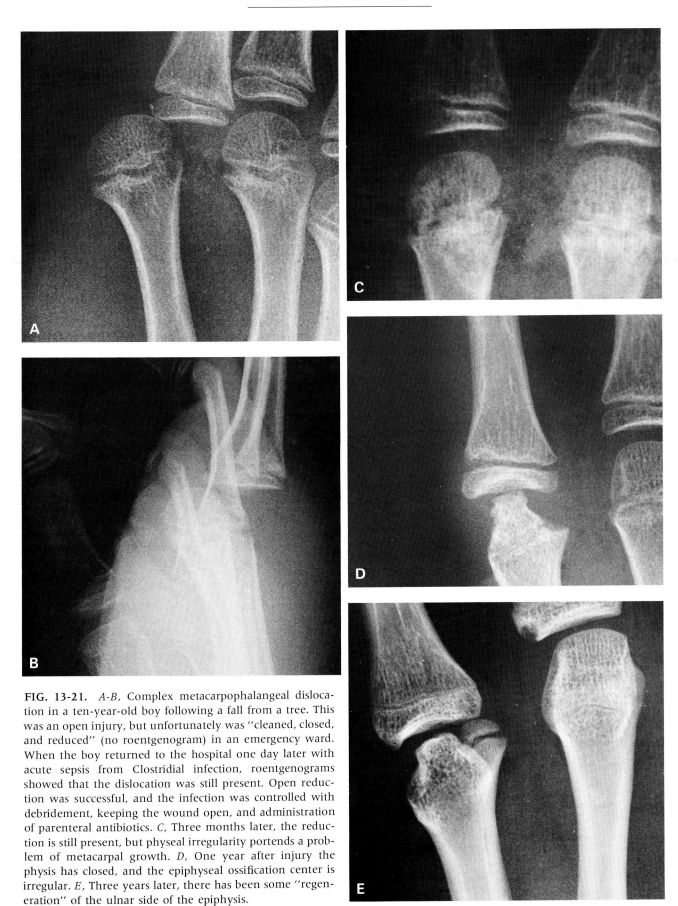

FIG. 13-21. *A-B*, Complex metacarpophalangeal dislocation in a ten-year-old boy following a fall from a tree. This
was an open injury, but unfortunately was "cleaned, closed,
and reduced" (no roentgenogram) in an emergency ward.
When the boy returned to the hospital one day later with
acute sepsis from Clostridial infection, roentgenograms
showed that the dislocation was still present. Open reduction was successful, and the infection was controlled with
debridement, keeping the wound open, and administration
of parenteral antibiotics. *C*, Three months later, the reduction is still present, but physeal irregularity portends a problem of metacarpal growth. *D*, One year after injury the
physis has closed, and the epiphyseal ossification center is
irregular. *E*, Three years later, there has been some "regeneration" of the ulnar side of the epiphysis.

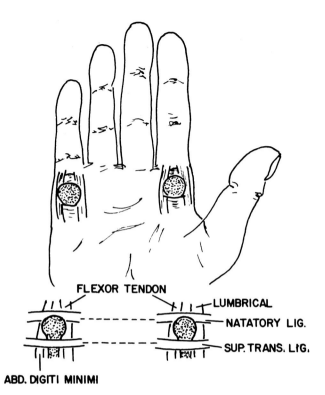

FLEXOR TENDON

LUMBRICAL

NATATORY LIG.

SUP. TRANS. LIG.

ABD. DIGITI MINIMI

FIG. 13-22. Schematic of structures involved in complex metacarpophalangeal dislocations of the index and little fingers.

An unusual pattern of metacarpal fracture is the split metacarpal head. If there is significant disruption of the articular surface in this type-4 growth mechanism injury, open reduction and accurate joint surface restoration are necessary.

Phalanges

Leonard and Dubravicik described 263 phalangeal fractures in children:[30] 75% were treated by simple external immobilization; 15% required manipulative reduction under anesthesia; 10% required open reduction. Epiphyseal separations or fractures through the metaphysis formed the largest group of this series, representing 41%; seven open reductions were necessary for these. Only 26% were shaft injuries. Eight diaphyseal fractures necessitated open reduction and internal fixation, the main indication being marked displacement with comminution and instability. The authors found that in those instances where there had been sufficient angulation to warrant surgical intervention, it was necessary to immobilize the fracture for about six weeks, as the distal fragment was relatively avascular and healing was slow. Using small Kirschner wires for internal fixation did not interfere significantly with the ultimate function of the interphalangeal joints or cause degenerative arthritis or epiphyseal arrest in the transfixed joints.

Some displacement of phalangeal fractures in children can be accepted as long as the fragments are aligned. Even mild angulation of a fracture in the plane of motion of a hinge joint often disappears, particularly if the apex is toward the flexor side. In children, angulation of a phalangeal fracture within a plane of motion of the joint often corrects itself.

Malrotation at the fracture site is the most frequent complication of phalangeal fractures, which must be avoided by careful attention to anatomic detail. When the fingers are flexed they do not remain parallel as they do in full extension, but rather point toward the region of the scaphoid tubercle. However, they do not actually converge upon a single fixed point, as is sometimes depicted (see Fig. 13-6). When the finger is only semiflexed, it helps to use the planes of the fingernails as an additional guide. The development of rotatory malalignment is primarily due to three contributing factors. These are failure (1) to recognize the rotation deformity, (2) to properly reduce the fracture, and (3) to properly immobilize the fracture.

A true lateral roentgenogram of the phalanx should show an image of a single condyle if the two are properly superimposed. However, when rotation exists, the shaft may be seen in the lateral position, but the head will be in an oblique position. This is not always easy to assess in children because of the variable degrees of ossification.

Malrotation in a finger is especially disabling. The fingers become entangled when flexed. Malrotation does not show easily on a radiograph and remodeling does *not* occur. Occasionally minimal congenital deformities of the phalanges may be present, so that the opposite normal hand must be checked and observed for rotation.

Correcting malrotation in a fresh fracture is relatively easy, but if the fracture heals with malrotation, an osteotomy is necessary to correct the position. Most malrotations occur in the proximal phalanx. If an osteotomy is necessary, a useful technique was described by Lewis and Hartman.[39] With this technique it is easy to control rotation of the phalanx with a long osteotomy.

Treatment can be varied. In general, if the injured finger is taped to the adjacent finger, certain criteria must be met: the fracture must be stable, and there must be adequate long term follow-up.

Fracture of the Proximal Portion of the Proximal Phalanx. Fractures of the proximal phalangeal growth region are relatively common (Fig. 13-27). The fracture-failure pattern frequently leaves not only the classic Thurston Holland metaphyseal fragment, but also a transverse plate of metaphyseal subchondral bone (Werenskiöld fragment). Types 3 and 4 growth mechanism fractures may also occur (Fig. 13-27). Since the mechanism is often a fall, open injuries are also relatively common (Fig. 13-28).

Coonrad focused attention on the poor results obtained in 41 children with impacted fractures of the proximal third of the proximal phalanx of the finger.[40] An impacted fracture of the proximal phalanx in the finger usually angulates toward the palm (Fig. 13-29), and if a significant degree of deformity remains, digital flexion and extension are limited. The fracture angulates toward the palm because the intrinsic muscles flex the proximal fragment, while the long extensor tendon causes shortening by axial pull. If the displaced or impacted fracture is allowed to heal at an angulation of 25° or more, the extensor tendon and its expansion over the proximal phalanx become shortened and exert a tethering effect on the bone. The oblique fibers of the retinaculum are at a mechanical disadvantage as they pull volar to the axis of rotation of the proximal interphalangeal joint. An uncorrected angulation of 22° or more in an older child may result in a disability similar to that in an adult.[40]

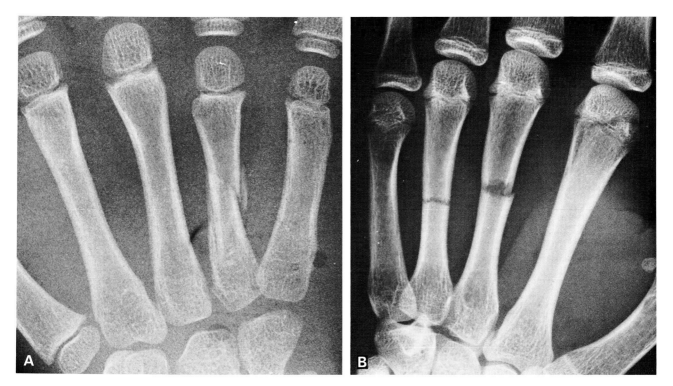

FIG. 13-23. *A*, Diaphyseal fracture of fourth metacarpal. *B*, Undisplaced transverse diaphyseal fractures of the third and fourth metacarpals.

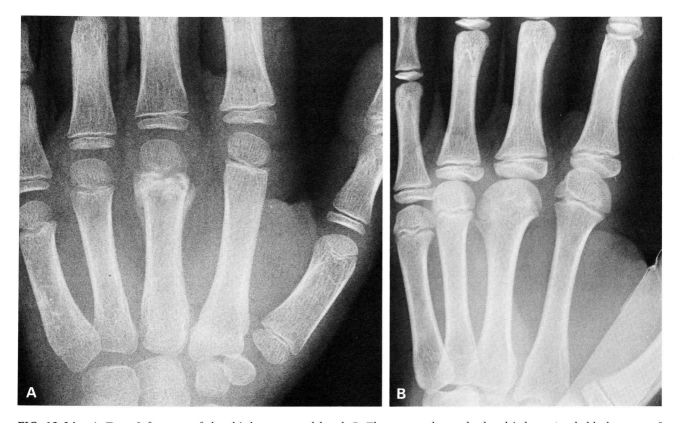

FIG. 13-24. *A*, Type 2 fracture of the third metacarpal head. *B*, Three years later, the head is large (probably because of hypervascularity following the injury), but the physis has closed, and this will lead to shortening.

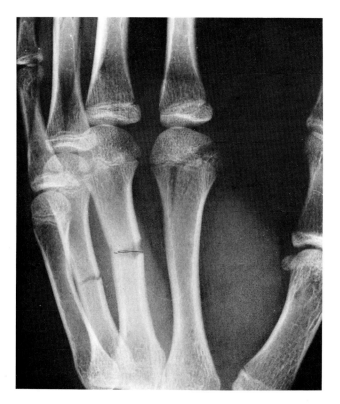

FIG. 13-25. Transverse diaphyseal fractures of the third and fourth metacarpals with concomitant type 4 fracture (split fracture) of the second metacarpal head.

The most common cause of angular malunion in this type of fracture is immobilization of the digit in insufficient flexion at the metacarpophalangeal and proximal interphalangeal joints. Extension permits a loss of reduction. A true lateral roentgenogram rather than an oblique view should be obtained for evaluating angulation in these patients, both before and after reduction. If these fractures heal in an abnormal position, an opening wedge osteotomy of the proximal phalanx could be done to correct the deformity. As emphasized previously, the majority of these complications can be prevented by proper splinting techniques.

Von Raffler described an unusual, irreducible juxtaepiphyseal fracture of the little finger due to interposition of the flexor tendon.[41] On open reduction, it was found that the flexor tendon had displaced onto the dorsal surface of the shaft (Fig. 13-30).

Cowen and Kranick reported a badly angulated type 2 injury of the proximal phalanx of the little finger that was irreducible by closed methods because the distal fragment was trapped in a buttonhole rent in the periosteum of the fractured phalanx and the dorsal hood simulated a "Chinese finger trap."[43] This injury was treated by open reduction.

Open reduction and internal fixation of these proximal phalangeal fractures may be required in the following situations: (1) when closed methods have failed to correct rotation; (2) when open fractures have to be reduced; (3) when the articular congruity of small articular fractures has to be restored; and (4) when widely displaced fractures are irreducible because of secondary soft tissue interposition.

Extra-Octave Fracture. A frequent fracture of the proximal phalanx involves the fifth digit (Fig. 13-31). This is often referred to as the "extra-octave" fracture. The mechanism of injury and the age of the patient may result in a greenstick fracture of the ulnar cortex. Treatment must restore rotational and angular malalignment.

As with most type 2 epiphyseal fractures, closed reduction usually gives a satisfactory result, but the problem in this specific fracture is that the epiphysis of the proximal phalanx lies proximal to the web. It is difficult to gain adequate purchase of the proximal fragment while manipulating the distal fragment into anatomic alignment. A pencil placed in the web space will serve as an effective fulcrum to bring the digit radialward (Fig. 13-32). A more effective method is to flex the metacarpophalangeal joint greater than 90°, which tightens the collateral ligaments and provides purchase on the proximal (epiphyseal) fragment. Reduction is then easily accomplished by adducting the distal fragment across the palm. If the ulnar cortex is incompletely fractured (greenstick), overcorrection and completion of the cortical fracture are essential. The intact periosteal sleeve on the ulnar side of the bone generally prevents overreduction and provides stability in the reduced position.

These fractures are difficult to keep controlled, and once the fracture is reduced, the little finger must be splinted to the adjacent uninjured finger. Protection of the reduction for three weeks in an ulnar gutter splint incorporating the adja-

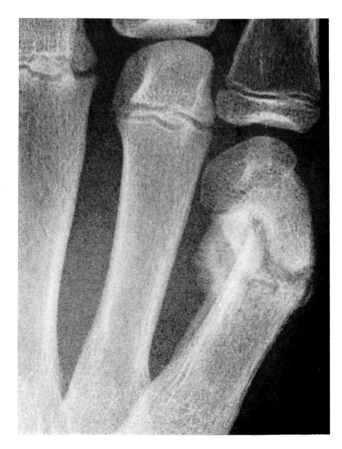

FIG. 13-26. Metaphyseal fracture of fifth metacarpal. Angulation was not corrected, and has led to malunion.

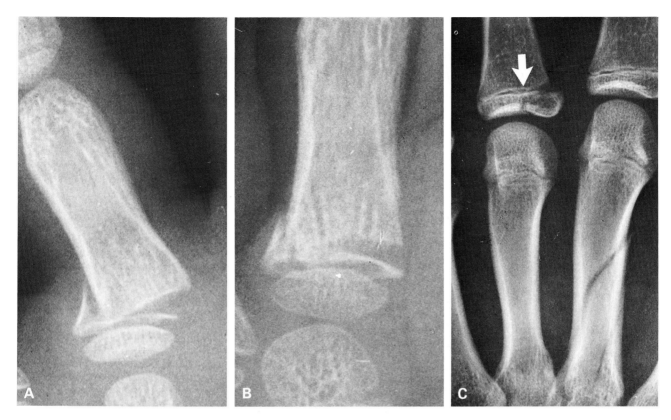

FIG. 13-27. *A*, Angulated (ulnarward) type 2 fracture of the proximal phalanx of the ring finger. As is typical of many of these injuries, there is transverse failure across the entire metaphyseal subchondral plate, rather than just across the physeal cartilage. *B*, This fracture was reduced to a more appropriate alignment. *C*, Type 3 fracture of proximal phalanx of ring finger (arrow), with concomitant metacarpal fracture in long finger.

cent ring finger is advisable. Because of the pull of the abductor digiti quinti minimi muscle, these fractures tend to drift and become redisplaced. Rarely, open reduction with pin fixation is required.

In a severe fracture the epiphysis may remain in place, while the remainder of the phalanx is totally dislocated palmarward (Fig. 13-33). Open reduction may be necessary in this fracture pattern.

Fractures of the Phalangeal Neck. Closed phalangeal fractures are common. Usually the phalanx is not locked into position. Such injuries can be treacherous. This is a classic "booby-trap" fracture in the hand, which is transverse through the neck of either the proximal or middle phalanx, with dorsal displacement of the distal fragment (Fig. 13-34).

Reduction is easy, but redisplacement in the splint or cast is likely to occur. The problem in recognizing this complication is that it is difficult to visualize the bone clearly on the postreduction lateral views because of superimposition of the other fingers in the splint. The resulting loss of reduction causes an unacceptable deformity, and late treatment of the healed, displaced fracture (even as early as three weeks after injury) is difficult. Early open reduction or closed reduction and percutaneous pinning of the fracture generally yield better results than attempts to correct the malunion later.[44]

The problem of adequate visualization of the fracture in the splint can be overcome by using a single laminographic cut in the lateral view at a measured distance to coincide with the long axis of the injured finger. The 90° rotation of the supracondylar phalangeal fracture can easily be missed. It is essential that an adequate lateral roentgenogram be taken to thoroughly delineate this.

In the series reported by Leonard, there were 38 phalangeal neck fractures (15% of the entire series) and 9 of these necessitated surgery.[30] Fractures of the phalangeal neck in children must be handled carefully.

Dixon and Moon reported treating five cases of an unusual phalangeal fracture through the neck of the proximal phalanx of the finger or thumb with 90° of rotation of the condylar fragment and entrapment by the capsule and collateral ligaments.[45] Lack of recognition and treatment of this fracture may result in permanent impairment of a child's digit (Fig. 13-35).

In children, the volar plate can roll on itself, causing a 90° rotation of the condylar fragment, which is then entrapped by the capsule and collateral ligaments (Fig. 13-36). This fracture may be easily overlooked, owing to a lack of finger deformity and obscure roentgenographic findings. However, early recognition and reduction are important because surgery is usually necessary. An untreated fracture proceeds to malunion and results in permanent disability of the hand.

The usual mechanism of injury seems to be hyperextension. Lack of tendon insertion into the distal aspect of the proximal phalanx easily allows rotation of this fragment.

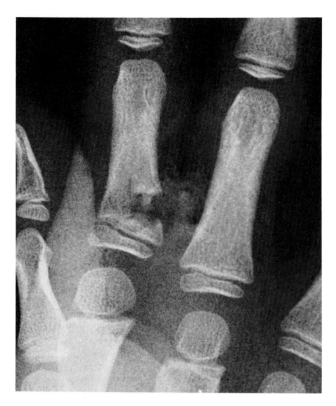

FIG. 13-28. Open metaphyseal fracture of the proximal phalanx of the index finger.

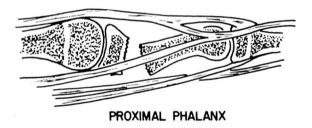

PROXIMAL PHALANX

FIG. 13-29. Schematic of proximal phalangeal growth mechanism fracture.

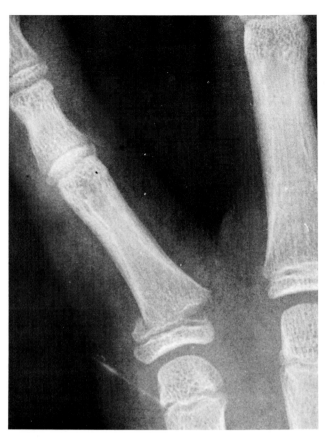

FIG. 13-31. Type 2 fracture of the fifth proximal phalanx, with concomitant ulnar deviation. Note the transverse metaphyseal fragment, which is characteristic of this type of injury when it occurs in the small longitudinal bones. This greenstick injury is often referred to as the "extra octave" fracture. Reduction must overcorrect and complete this fracture, or recurrent angular deformity may occur even while the fracture is immobilized.

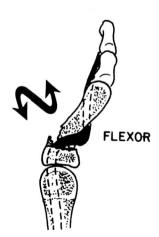

FLEXOR

FIG. 13-30. Schematic of injury described by von Raffler.[41] The flexor tendon looped onto the dorsal surface and then back to the palmar surface. Open reduction was necessary.

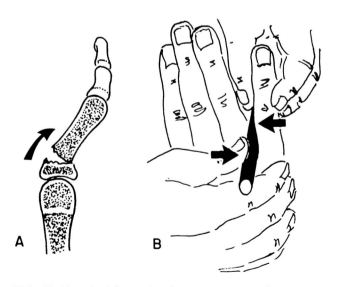

FIG. 13-32. *A,* Schematic of "extra octave" fracture. *B,* Method of reduction utilizing pencil in the four-fifths web space.

Leonard described a similar type of flexion injury that required open reduction, and stated that one cannot expect correction of angulation over 25° in a child's fracture, even if the angulation is in the plane of joint motion, particularly since there is limited longitudinal growth contribution in the involved nonepiphyseal end of the phalanx.[44]

Fracture of the extreme distal part of any phalanx in a child may be treacherous. The cartilage cap of the phalanx, even though it has no epiphysis in the classic sense, may occasionally be separated from the phalanx just like an epi-

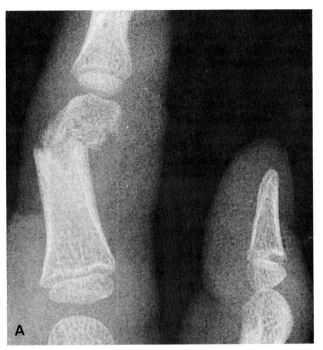

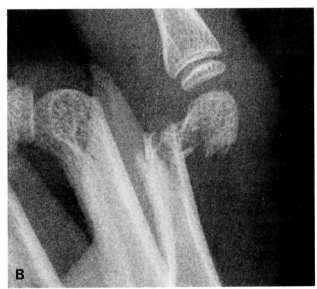

FIG. 13-34. A, Fracture of the distal end of the proximal phalanx. B, The lateral view reveals a major problem: dorsal displacement of the epiphyseal end.

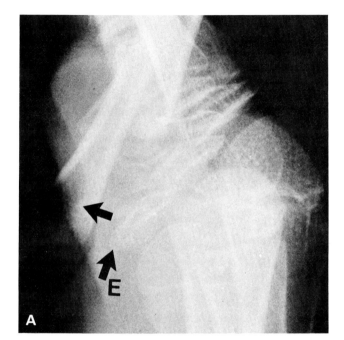

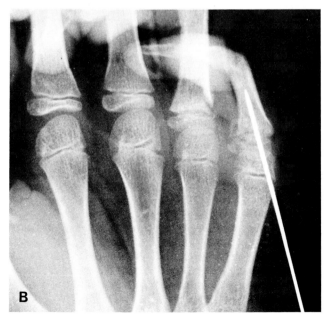

FIG. 13-33. A, Severe "extra octave" fracture with complete volar displacement of phalanx (arrow), while epiphysis (E, arrow) stays in the joint. B, Open reduction was necessary.

physeal injury. This is not immediately obvious at the time of injury, but with the passage of time, subperiosteal new bone forms and may explain the prolonged stiffness or rotation in the phalanx. If the angulation of the fracture is in the plane of motion of the hinge joint, the angulation will disappear to a remarkable degree, particularly if the apex is toward the flexor side. However, if there is angulation of the phalanx in a medial or lateral plane and nothing can be seen on roentgenographic examination, these fractures should be opened and the cartilaginous cap replaced and fixed with Kirschner wires.

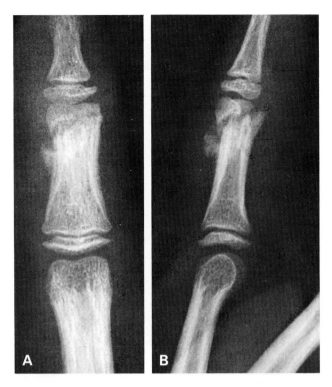

FIG. 13-35. *A-B*, Anterior and lateral views of condylar fracture of the middle phalanx.

Condylar Fracture. A fracture that virtually always demands internal fixation is a displaced fracture of one or both condyles of the proximal phalanx at the level of the PIP or DIP joint. This rule applies to children as well as adults, whether the fracture involves the nonepiphyseal or epiphyseal end (Fig. 13-37). Although less common than in the adult, displaced intra-articular fractures in the child should be treated by open reduction and internal fixation if anatomic restoration cannot be achieved by closed manipulation.

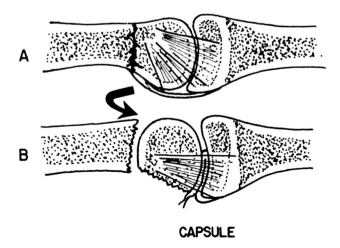

CAPSULE

FIG. 13-36. Schematic of rotation of fragment sometimes accompanying these fractures.

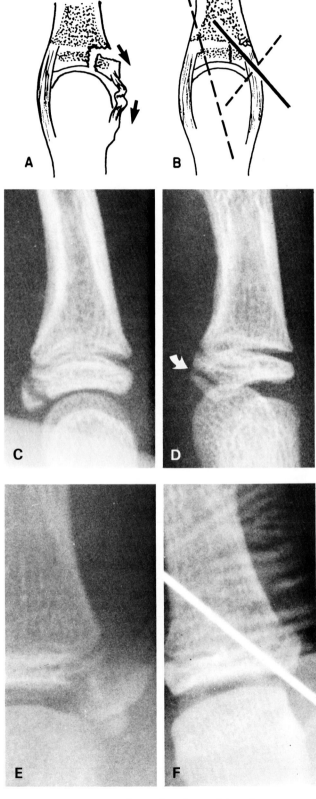

FIG. 13-37. *A-B*, Schematic of condylar fracture and method of pinning. Dashed lines represent potential courses for buttress pins. *C-D*, Types 3 and 7 (arrow) condylar fractures of the proximal phalanx. *E-F*, Type 3 condylar fracture treated by open reduction.

Intercondylar fractures in children are treated exactly as they are in adults. Displaced T-fractures of the distal end of a phalanx require open reduction and internal fixation with Kirschner wires. When 30% of a joint surface is involved, or if there is instability of the joint, it must be opened.

When pin fixation becomes necessary, healing of the fracture may be delayed. Therefore, Kirschner wires should be left in place for at least six weeks. Epiphyseal avascular necrosis has never been described. Stiffness after injury is not a problem in children, since they usually regain complete mobility.

Fracture of the Middle Phalanx.   The middle phalanx is injured much less commonly, and deforming musculotendinous forces are different (Fig. 13-38). The important forces are the insertion of the central slip onto the dorsal aspect of the proximal middle phalanx and the insertion of the flexor digitorum sublimus palmar along the shaft. The central slip extends the proximal phalanx, particularly if it is a more proximal or epiphyseal type of injury. If the fracture is proximal to the sublimus, the distal fragment tends to be flexed. If the fracture is distal to the sublimus tendon, then the proximal fragment is flexed and the distal fragment hyperextended.

Fractures of the middle phalanx may be undisplaced or angulated. If the fracture site is distal to the insertion of the flexor superficialis tendon, it can usually be treated by manual traction and flexion of the distal fragment (contrary to the general treatment rules). The extensor tendon pulls the distal fragment into extension, while the flexor superficialis causes flexion of the proximal fragment, producing an overall volar angulation.

Fracture of the middle phalanx proximal to the insertion of the flexor superficialis tendon may also be treated closed as long as the following principle is recognized: The central slip of the extensor tendon extends the proximal phalanx; the flexor superficialis flexes the distal fragment, producing dorsal angulation of the fragments; therefore, these fractures must be reduced and held in complete extension.

Fractures of the shaft of the middle phalanx heal correctly as long as the position of immobilization is recognized and maintained. Immobilization for up to five to seven weeks may be required, even in a child.

Mallet Finger.   Mallet finger deformities in children are different from those in adults, although the treatment is similar. In children, this is generally an epiphyseal injury with avulsion of a portion of the epiphysis.[22,27] In the small child, the deformity is usually a displaced type 1 or 2 epiphyseal fracture at the base of the distal phalanx (Fig. 13-39). In the adolescent, the injury is likely to be a type 3 or type 7 growth mechanism injury, which splits the epiphysis.

The deformity usually results from the end of the finger being forcibly flexed, while the extensor tendon is taut, as in catching a ball or striking an object with the finger extended.

The lateral radiograph is important because rupture of the extensor tendon is uncommon in childhood. The flexor digitorum profundus tendon flexes the metaphysis, into which it is inserted, while the extensor tendon, which inserts into the epiphysis, maintains the epiphysis in the extended position. The proximal epiphysis may be rotated significantly. Sometimes the proximal epiphysis is not ossified, a finding

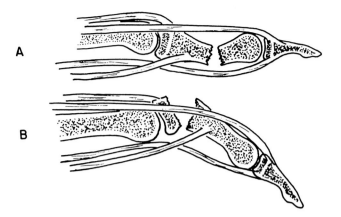

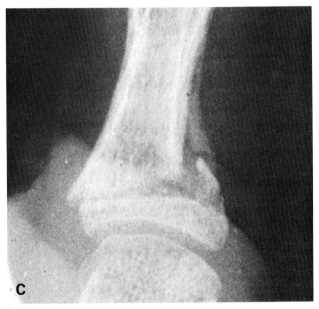

FIG. 13-38.   *A-B*, Schematics of variable effects of tendons on deformation of fracture fragments in middle phalangeal injury. *C*, Typical type 2 injury of middle phalanx.

that may lead to diagnostic difficulties and delay in treatment.

Methods of treatment should be directed at mild hyperextension. This can be accomplished with small splints fashioned out of aluminum or even a safety pin with a small piece of tape over the tip joint to provide three-point fixation. However, commercially available "stack" splints are best (Fig. 13-40). If anatomic reduction cannot be achieved with closed reduction, open reduction and internal fixation may be required (Fig. 13-40). In many children, this is an intra-articular or intraepiphyseal type 3 injury and warrants open reduction as the initial treatment.

Failure to reduce the fragments may result in significant malunion with exostosis formation and joint dysfunction (Fig. 13-41).

Since mallet finger injuries are often due to crushing, which causes extensive soft tissue damage, the possibility of infection is high and the use of any type of fixation should be done judiciously. Of five patients in whom K-wire fixation was used, three developed infection; one of these patients

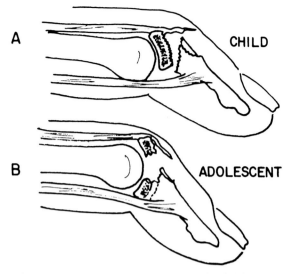

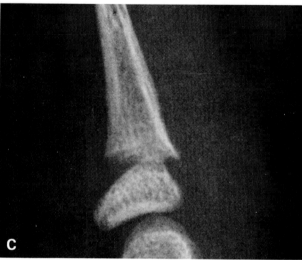

FIG. 13-39. *A-B*, Schematic of types of "mallet finger" epiphyseal injury in the child and adolescent. *C*, Typical appearance of type 1 injury in a five-year-old.

developed osteomyelitis, which eventually led to amputation of the finger.[46]

When treating the open mallet finger deformity there is a great temptation to remove the partially avulsed nail. If this is done, an easily treated injury may be converted into one that can be troublesome and may involve a long period of disability. To effect successful and stable reduction, the nail should be replaced under the proximal nail fold and a slight hyperextension force applied to the distal phalanx. Removing the nail makes the reduction more unstable. A small splint can then hold the distal interphalangeal joint in hyperextension for three weeks. In most instances, internal fixation with Kirschner wires is unnecessary and can lead to complications. Union becomes solid with no deformity.

Fractures of the Distal Phalanx. These are common injuries, probably accounting for the bulk of hand fractures in children. The extensor and flexor tendons that insert in the base of the distal phalanx, play no role in displacing fractures of the distal phalanx, except for the aforementioned dorsal avulsion injury (mallet finger). Radiating fibrous septae form a dense meshwork and probably stabilize these fractures, effectively preventing major amounts of displacement. The majority of these injuries occur from crushing, and therefore are accompanied by extensive soft tissue damage and subungual hematoma (Fig. 13-42).

Treatment of nondisplaced fractures should be directed toward soft tissue damage. Splints must be applied with care because of the amount of swelling. Evacuating the subungual hematoma generally gives marked relief of pain. This is best done by burning a hole in the nail with a hot paper clip, although small, high-speed sterile drills are available. Use care not to damage the lunula, as this may lead to permanent deformity of nail growth. Transverse angulated fractures must be reduced and held with either an external splint or percutaneous pinning with smooth Kirschner wires.

Fractures of the distal phalanx that result from crush injuries usually are comminuted and frequently are associated with "bursting" skin lacerations. These wounds should not be closed tightly, but cleansed thoroughly and covered with a soft dressing. Sutures should be used sparingly, if at all, and only to grossly reapproximate loose flaps of skin. If the fingernail is intact, it should be left undisturbed, for it provides some support for the fractured bone.

Fingertip injuries in children are generally easier to treat than similar injuries in adults because the regeneration capacity of local tissues in children is greater. Loss of skin only, with intact underlying subcutaneous tissue, is usually managed best by careful neglect (that is, by allowing the wound to heal by secondary intention). All that is required is initial debridement and cleansing of the wound, applying a bulky compressive dressing for the first 24 hours to control bleeding, and then small dressings to keep the wound clean (a small adhesive strip with a gauze pad usually suffices after the first few days). The finger can be soaked daily when the child is bathed, and then the wound redressed. Good results with maximum preservation of length and good sensibility can be achieved by using this technique, even in injuries in which there is a rather sizable loss of skin. If the tip of the distal phalanx is protruding slightly, the same plan of management can be carried out if the bone is rongeured at a level beneath the soft tissue at the time of initial debridement.

These injuries cause more parental concern than is usually justified. When an open fracture includes portions of skin and fat that are only partially attached, but of questionable viability, the tissue should not be removed. Bits of tissue that one suspects would not heal in an adult may go on to complete healing in a child. Regenerative potential in the child is remarkable. Often, even when the injury has caused complete amputation and the pieces are missing, regeneration occurs and the tip of the stump becomes covered with surprisingly good tissue.[14,21] In general, one should save as much tissue as possible and use "skillful neglect;" the outcome may be pleasantly surprising.

Thompson advocated using the cross-finger flap for treating avulsions of the fingertip.[47] Several authors recommend using the cross-finger flap in all fingertip injuries in children seven to eight years of age or older, but do not recommend it in younger children because immobilization is "more difficult in the younger age group." This does not appear totally appropriate. Thompson made the following conclusions

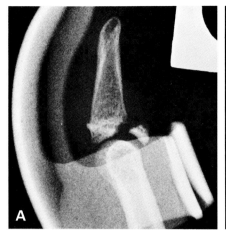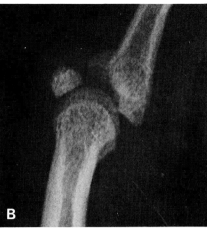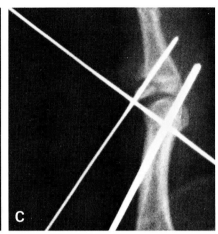

FIG. 13-40. *A*, Treatment of type 3 epiphyseal injury by standard techniques failed to correct the anatomic position of the fracture, despite DIP hyperextension. *B*, Similar adolescent type 3 "mallet finger." *C*, This fracture was treated by open reduction and buttress pinning.

based on 75 children with 79 operative procedures over 10 years: (1) Following cross-finger pedicle grafts, the lack of tactile sense with stereognosis and disability due to altered sensation is not as common in children as in adults. (2) From the cosmetic standpoint, the pedicle flap and its donor site were not entirely satisfactory. (3) The contour and color of the graft tip were less than ideal. (4) Index neglect was encountered in 20% of the children, but the middle finger was trained to compensate for this disability. (5) There was no postoperative joint stiffness. (6) Spread scars and interrupted suture scars were noted on the abdomen at the donor site of full-thickness free grafts. (7) The accepted indications for cross-finger pedicle flap should be modified in children to include all age groups; in children, the procedure has been associated with better clinical results than in adults.

Nailbed Injuries. Probably one of the most frequently neglected injuries in both children and adults is that involving the nailbed, where inadequate initial treatment may result in permanent residual deformity.[48] Lacerations of the nailbed should be sutured as carefully as lacerations of the skin. Although not all late deformity is preventable because of the crushing nature of the injury, it probably can be minimized by meticulous operative repair of the lacerated nailbed with fine absorbable suture material (5-0 or 6-0 plain or chromic catgut).

Traumatic avulsion of the fingernail in skeletally immature patients should arouse the physician's suspicion of associated bone injury. Enger reported a case of traumatic avulsion of the fingernail associated with injury to the epiphyseal plate of the distal phalanx.[46] Lateral roentgenograms frequently reveal fracture of the distal phalangeal epiphyseal plate.

Avulsion of the nail and frequently associated lacerations of the nailbed are probably produced by protrusions of the phalangeal fragment. The presence of fracture of the epiphyseal plate in association with avulsion of the nail and laceration of the nailbed has important therapeutic implications, because this becomes an open fracture. Simple reduction must also be accompanied with strong appreciation for

the open injury. Enger described two cases, both of which developed osteomyelitis and premature closure of the distal phalangeal epiphysis.[46] One was a type 1 and the other a type 2 physeal injury, both of which supposedly have a rare occurrence of premature epiphysiodesis.

The following treatment is recommended for nailbed injuries. When the attachment of the fingernail is nearly completely avulsed, the nail should be removed. If only the proximal portion is avulsed, a small proximal portion should be removed, leaving the remainder of the nail to act as a stent. After meticulous debridement and irrigation, a small drain should be inserted through the lacerated nailbed, and the epiphyseal separation reduced and maintained by splinting. Oral antibiotics should be used for at least two weeks. Since a high percentage of infections of the hand are due to Staphylococci resistant to penicillin, appropriate synthetic penicillins such as dicloxacillin sodium should be used. Cephalosporins may also be used, since they have also been

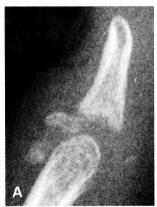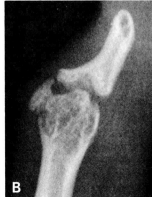

FIG. 13-41. *A*, Fragmented injury of entire epiphysis in an adolescent. *B*, Exostosis formation following non-operative treatment. This has caused a flexion deformity and impaired joint function.

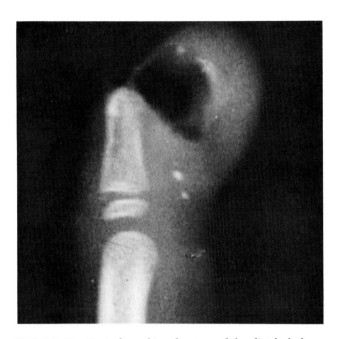

FIG. 13-42. Typical crushing fracture of the distal phalanx with an open injury and separation of volar soft tissue from the bone.

shown to decrease the infection rate after open fractures.[49] The drain should be removed after several days and splinting maintained for four to six weeks.

Amputations. Partial amputations of the fingertip in which the tip is dangling from a narrow bridge of skin should not be removed in the child. Even when the chances of survival of the tip are unlikely, it should be loosely approximated and given an opportunity to heal. There is little lost if the tip does not survive, and the remarkable healing capacity in a child sometimes results in a pleasant surprise. If the tip does become necrotic, it is best to allow it to demarcate spontaneously, as long as it is clean and free of drainage.

The completely amputated fingertip that is picked up at the scene of the accident and brought in separately with the child may, in some instances, warrant replantation. Although mere replacement of the tip with skin sutures usually is not successful, the rare survival that occurs may justify the attempt. Great advances in microvascular surgical techniques have made replantation of entire digits a clinical reality, *although not all amputations are suitable for replantation.* If the primary care physician sees a patient with a completely amputated digit, the patient should be referred to a surgeon *experienced* in microsurgical techniques as soon as possible. The digit should be wrapped in a sterile gauze pad soaked in Ringer's lactate, placed in a plastic bag, and *cooled* on ice. It should *not* be frozen, nor should the vessels be cannulated or irrigated.

Amputations at more proximal levels through the distal phalanx or distal interphalangeal joint usually require more sophisticated treatment in the operating room, and many different techniques for closure and coverage of these amputations have been described.

Principles of replantation, particularly relating to digital injuries, are discussed in Chapter 6. The specific problem of replanted or transplanted epiphyses and their subsequent capacity for growth are discussed in Chapter 4.

Autoamputation. Children with sensory neuropathy syndromes often have severe hand involvement because of inadvertent self-mutilation (Fig. 13-43). Lack of sensation may result in injuries, especially thermal injuries, which cause skin breakdown and exposure of the chondro-osseous elements. Many of these children have mild mental retardation and may chew their fingers, further exposing bone.

Treatment must always be directed at obtaining soft tissue healing without complicating infection. Because of the "chewing" mechanism, cellulitis from micro-organisms such as anaerobic Streptococcus is just as significant a possibility as staphylococcal osteomyelitis. These wounds should never be closed; allow granulation and spontaneous epithelialization.

Repetitive infection of the bone (chronic osteomyelitis) may require amputation. In a child, such procedures are done best at a joint, but this principle should be applied less rigidly to a child's hand. Remove only as much bone as necessary to control infection and assist in soft tissue coverage.

Repetitive trauma may lead to chronic epiphysiolysis or crushing injury to the physis, either of which may cause premature growth arrest, which only compounds the functional loss of the hand and wrist. Since these children cannot perceive pain, the parents should be taught to look for signs of swelling or erythema, especially about the wrist, so that roentgenograms may be taken to evaluate the presence of a fracture. Treatment (immobilization) lessens the likelihood of repetitive epiphysiolysis, which has a much higher incidence of premature growth arrest.

Thermal Injuries

The hand is often the site of major thermal injury, which may involve either cold (frostbite) or heat (burn). Primary management is generally directed toward obvious soft tissue damage (see Chap. 4). However, long-term effects on the chondro-osseous elements may occur, and should be of sufficient concern to warrant annual roentgenograms. The middle phalangeal physes seem particularly susceptible to premature growth arrest (Fig. 13-44), whether the thermal injury is excess heat or cold.

Tendon Injuries

Recognizing tendon lacerations is more difficult in the small child than in the adult because of problems of accurate physical examination. Precise testing of specific tendon function requires considerable skill and patience when examining a small child, and it may be virtually impossible in the painful hand of a frightened, injured child. In such a situation, the best information can usually be gleaned by careful, surreptitious observations, specifically looking for a digit that is held in an atypical position, or one that does not move in normal synchrony with the other digits. Sometimes absence of specific muscles can be seen by the lack of normal retraction response to gentle pin-prick examination. The slightest suspicion of tendon laceration demands thorough exploration under tourniquet control and adequate anesthesia, be-

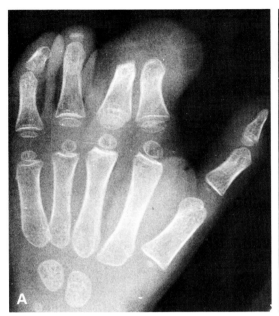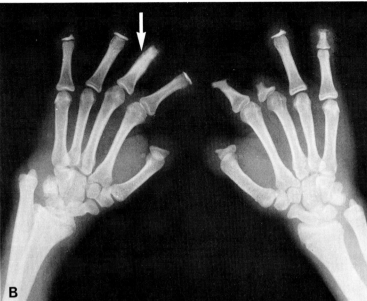

FIG. 13-43. *A*, Autoamputation of index and long fingers resulting from chronic chewing of the fingers in a five-year-old boy with Rothmund-Thompson syndrome. *B*, A 13-year-old with congenital sensory neuropathy. There had been intermittent fingertip infections, primarily from burns and cuts, from 3 years of age. The long finger of the right hand exhibits sclerosing osteomyelitis in the remaining phalanx (arrow). The distal radius of the same hand has fused prematurely, leading to marked overgrowth of the ulna.

cause this is the only sure way to identify tendon injury. In most hospital settings, this is done best in the operating room, where proper facilities are available for tendon repair.

Although concepts regarding repair of some types of tendon injuries are controversial, current thinking is that best results are likely to be achieved in children with primary repair of all lacerated tendons in clean wounds. This includes lacerated flexor tendons in so-called "no-man's land," that portion of the flexor apparatus between the proximal palmar crease and the proximal interphalangeal joint, in which both flexor tendons lie within a common sheath. Repairs of flexor tendons, especially within these tendon sheaths, are technically difficult in the adult and considerably more so in the diminutive structures of the child's hand.[50] Consequently, primary repair of flexor tendons, especially in no-man's land, demands meticulous technique, proper instruments, magnification, and most importantly, the skills of a surgeon experienced in the techniques of tendon surgery.

Nerve Injuries

Recognizing nerve injuries in children is even more difficult than recognizing tendon injuries. Diagnosis of a lacerated digital nerve is almost impossible to make in the small child by physical examination alone, and even injury to the major nerves in the forearm may be difficult to demonstrate objectively.[16,51] The size and location of the skin laceration give little aid in the diagnosis, for a penetrating wound may extend a great distance from the point of injury, and a small, benign-appearing skin laceration often masks rather extensive underlying soft tissue injuries. A tiny puncture wound

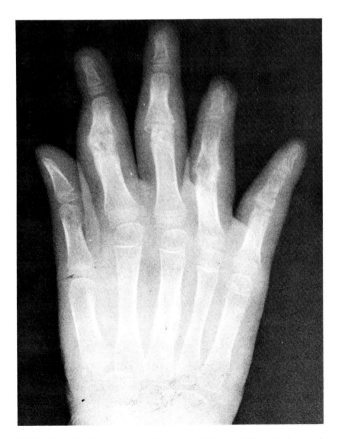

FIG. 13-44. Premature closure of the middle phalangeal physes following a thermal injury.

in the palm is often overlooked as the point of injury that results in a digital nerve laceration.

Since primary repair of lacerated nerves in clean wounds is likely to give the best results, recognizing these injuries when the child is first seen is important. It is imperative that all penetrating wounds with any possibility of nerve laceration be explored under appropriate conditions. This does not mean with a probing hemostat into a bloody field in a wriggling, unanesthetized child, but rather under adequate anesthesia and tourniquet control. Repair of a lacerated nerve should be done in the operating room under appropriate magnification.

References

1. Caffey, J.: Pediatric X-ray Diagnosis. 6th Ed. Chicago, Yearbook Medical Publishers, 1972.
2. Haines, R. W.: The pseudoepiphysis of the first metacarpal in man. J. Anat., *117:*145, 1974.
3. Green, D. P., and Terry, G. C.: Complex dislocation of the metacarpophalangeal joint-correlative pathological anatomy. J. Bone Joint Surg., *55-A:*1480, 1973.
4. Watson, H. K., Light, T. R., and Johnson, T. R.: Checkrein resection for flexion contracture of the middle joint. J. Hand Surg., *4:*67, 1979.
5. Kucynski, K.: The proximal interphalangeal joint: anatomy and causes of stiffness in the fingers. J. Bone Joint Surg., *50-B:*656, 1968.
6. Bora, F. W., Jr., Nissenbaum, M., and Ignatius, P.: The treatment of epiphyseal fractures of the hand. Orthop. Digest, *5:*11, 1976.
7. Ehalt, W.: Uber die Bruche des ersten Mittelhandknochens und ihre Behandlung. Arch. Orthop. Unfallchir., *27:*515, 1929.
8. Flatt, A. C.: The Care of Minor Hand Injuries. St. Louis, C. V. Mosby, 1959.
9. Freilinger, G.: Zur Handchirurgie heim Kleinkind. Z. Klin. Med., *11:*212, 1964.
10: Green, D. P.: Hand injuries in children. Pediatr. Clin. North Am., *24:*903, 1977.
11. Griffiths, J. C.: Bennett's fracture in childhood. Br. J. Clin. Pract., *20:*582, 1967.
12. Kleinert, H. E., Grooper, P. T., and Van Beck, A.: Trauma of the hand. Curr. Probl. Surg., *15:*1, 1978.
13. Knorr, P.: Entwicklungsstorungen nach Hand-und Fingerfrakturen im Kindesalter. Ph. D. Dissertation, University of Leipzig, 1969.
14. Metcalf, W., and Whalen, W. P.: Salvage of the injured distal phalanx. Clin. Orthop., *13:*114, 1959.
15. Milch, H.: Subluxation of the index metacarpophalangeal joint. J. Bone Joint Surg., *47-A:*522, 1965.
16. Moberg, E.: Evaluation of sensibility in the hand. Surg. Clin. North Am., *40:*357, 1960.
17. Murphy, A. F., and Stark, H. H.: Closed dislocation of the metacarpophalangeal joint of the index finger. J. Bone Joint Surg., *49-A:*1579, 1967.
18. Mussbichler, H.: Injuries of the carpal scaphoid in children. Acta Radiol. [Diagn.] (Stockh.), *56:*361, 1961.
19. Patel, M. R., et al.: Transverse bayonet dislocation of proximal interphalangeal joint. Clin. Orthop., *133:*219, 1978.
20. Ryba, W.: Die Bennettfraktur bei Jugendlichen. Z. Kinderchir., Suppl. *3:*394, 1967.
21. Sandzen, S. C.: Management of the acute fingertip injury in the child. Hand, *6:*190, 1974.
22. Seymour, N.: Juxta-epiphyseal fracture of the terminal phalanx of the finger. J. Bone Joint Surg., *48-B:*347, 1966.
23. Southcott, R., and Rosman, M. A.: Non-union of carpal scaphoid fractures in children. J. Bone Joint Surg., *59-B:*20, 1977.
24. Steinert, V., and Knorr, P.: Mittelhand und Fingerfrakturen im Kindesalter. Zentralbl. Chir., *96:*113, 1971.
25. Stelling, F. H., III: Surgery of the hand in the child. J. Bone Joint Surg., *45-A:*623, 1963.
26. Strickland, J. W.: Bone, nerve, and tendon injuries of the hand in children. Pediatr. Clin. North Am., *22:*451, 1975.
27. Wakefield, A. R.: Hand injuries in children. J. Bone Joint Surg., *46-A:*1226, 1964.
28. Wood, V. E.: Fractures of the hand in children. Orthop. Clin. North Am., *7:*527, 1976.
29. Jones, E. R. L., and Esah, M.: Displaced fractures of the neck of the radius in children. J. Bone Joint Surg., *53-B:*429, 1971.
30. Leonard, M. H., and Dubravicik, P.: Management of fractured fingers in the child. Clin. Orthop., *73:*160, 1970.
31. Taleisnik, J., and Kelly, L. J.: The extraosseous and intraosseous blood supply of the scaphoid bone. J. Bone Joint Surg., *48-A:*1125, 1966.
32. Grundy, M.: Fractures of the carpal scaphoid in children. Br. J. Surg., *56:*523, 1969.
33. Gerard, F. M.: Post-traumatic carpal instability in a young child. J. Bone Joint Surg., *62-A:*131, 1980.
34. Eaton, R. G.: Joint Injuries of the Hand. Springfield, Illinois, Charles C Thomas, 1971.
35. Baldwin, L. W., et al.: Metacarpophalangeal-joint dislocations of the fingers. J. Bone Joint Surg., *49-A:*1587, 1967.
36. Becton, J. L., et al.: A simplified technique for treating the complex dislocation of the index metacarpophalangeal joint. J. Bone Joint Surg., *57-A:*698, 1975.
37. Kaplan, E. B.: Dorsal dislocation of the metacarpophalangeal joint of the index finger. J. Bone Joint Surg., *39-A:*1081, 1957.
38. Brown, J. E.: Epiphyseal growth arrest in a fractured metacarpal. J. Bone Joint Surg., *41-A:*494, 1959.
39. Lewis, R. C., and Hartman, J. T.: Controlled osteotomy for correction of rotation in proximal phalanx fractures. Orthop. Rev., *2:*11, 1973.
40. Coonrad, R. W., and Pohlman, M. H.: Impacted fractures in the proximal portion of the proximal phalanx of the finger. J. Bone Joint Surg., *51-A:*1291, 1969.
41. von Raffler, W.: Irreducible juxta-epiphyseal fracture of a finger. J. Bone Joint Surg., *46-B:*229, 1964.
42. Meadoff, N.: Median nerve injuries in fractures in the region of the wrist. Calif. Med., *70:*252, 1949.
43. Cowen, N. J., and Kranick, A. D.: An irreducible juxta-epiphyseal fracture of the proximal phalanx. Clin. Orthop., *110:*42, 1975.
44. Leonard, M. H.: Open reduction of fractures of the neck of the proximal phalanx in children. Clin. Orthop., *116:*176, 1976.
45. Dixon, G. L., and Moon, N. F.: Rotational supracondylar fractures of the proximal phalanx in children. Clin. Orthop., *83:*151, 1972.
46. Enger, W. D., and Glancy, W. G.: Traumatic avulsion of the fingernail associated with injury to the phalangeal epiphyseal plate. J. Bone Joint Surg., *60-A:*713, 1978.
47. Thompson, H. G., and Sorokolit, W. T.: The cross-finger flap in children. A follow-up study. Plast. Reconstr. Surg., *39:*487, 1967.
48. Ashbell, T. S., Kleinert, H. E., and Putcha, S. M.: The deformed fingernail: A frequent result of failure to repair nail bed injuries. J. Trauma, *7:*177, 1967.
49. Patzakis, M., Harvey, J., and Ivler, D.: The role of antibiotics in the management of open fractures. J. Bone Joint Surg., *56-A:*532, 1974.
50. Bell, J. L., et al.: Injuries to flexor tendons of the hand in children. J. Bone Joint Surg., *40-A:*1220, 1958.
51. Harrison, S. H.: The tactile adherence test estimating loss of sensation after nerve injury. Hand, *6:*148, 1974.

14

Spine

Anatomy

The patterns of spine injury in children, especially in the cervical region, undoubtedly relate to changing anatomy. Compared to the rest of the body proportions, the skull of the developing child is relatively large at birth. With development, the ratio decreases so that less relative mass or potential angular momentum is presented to the cervical spine. The skull (occiput) articulates horizontally with the atlas, a situation not present in most mammals. The occipitoatlantal joints are relatively tightly constrained, allowing flexion and extension, but virtually no rotation. In addition to the two occipitoatlantal articulations, there are four atlantoaxial joints with a reasonably contiguous and common synovial lining—one between the anterior arch of the atlas and dens, one between the transverse ligament and dens, and two between the lateral masses (Fig. 14-1).

The dens is tightly applied to the anterior arch of the atlas by the thick, transverse ligament and its various ramifications. The transverse ligament is primarily responsible for the stability of the central atlantoaxial joint. The axis is further connected to the occiput by the (1) alar or check ligaments, (2) the apical dental ligament, (3) the tectorial membrane, and (4) the cruciate ligament. The transverse portion of the cruciate ligament is the most important mechanically.

The atlantoaxial relationship is a unique joint in man because the articular surfaces are convex with a horizontal orientation. This combination permits maximal mobility and rotation with minimal cost of stability. However, this is a joint that may be disrupted in children because of the intrinsically higher degree of ligamentous laxity. The possible movements are extension, forward flexion, and rotation. Rotation is limited to approximately 45°, although the defined range is from 22° to 58°.[1,2]

Separate ossification centers are present in the lateral masses of the atlas. A third center for the anterior arch is ossified in only about 20% of infants at birth, and may not be seen until one year of age (Figs. 14-2 and 14-3). This particular ossification center may be bifid, but not always symmetrically so. Posterior ossification may be incomplete, which may result in a mild spina bifida. These ossification variations and synchondroses should not be confused with traumatic disruption of the ring. The diameters of the C1 canal

reach "adult" size by three to four years of age, at which point little growth occurs in C1.

In the axis, the usual ossification pattern pertains in the centrum and neural arches. According to Freiberger, ossification of the dens begins in the fifth fetal month with 2 longitudinal primary ossification centers,[3] which are usually fused at birth. A separate ossification for the tip of the dens does not appear until the child is about 6 to 7 years old; this ossiculum terminale fuses with the rest of the bone at 12 years (Figs. 14-4 to 14-6).

The dens is separated from the body of the axis by a region of growth cartilage. This cartilage begins to disappear when the child is 5 to 7 years old. Ewald described the histologic appearance of this region in a 2-month-old infant, finding "no evidence of an epiphyseal plate but rather areas of cartilage with advancing zones of endochondral ossification above and below."[4] Based on Ewald's observations, the so-called plate was not an epiphyseal line, but only related cartilage that gradually ossified as the bone grew in from either side.

However, it is extremely important to realize that this is not only a bipolar growth zone responsible for longitudinal

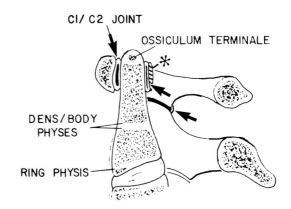

FIG. 14-1. Schematic of relationship of C1 and C2 in the immature stage. Note the joints anterior and posterior to the dens, as well as the horizontal joints (arrows). The asterisk marks the transverse ligament.

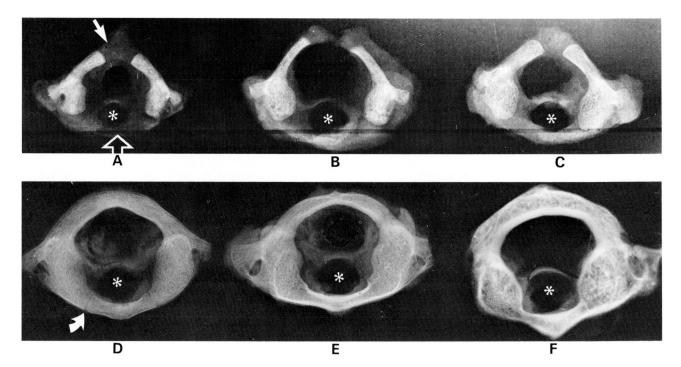

FIG. 14-2. Early development of C1: *A,* at birth; *B,* 3 months; and *C,* 7 months. The solid arrow (in *A*) points to the posterior synchondrosis, while the open arrow points to the unossified anterior arch. The asterisks mark the locations of the dens, with transverse ligament intact. Subsequent maturation of C1 is shown in 3 specimens from cadavers aged *D,* 7; *E,* 9; and *F,* 12 years. All show comparable shapes and cervical canal size. The arrow (in *D*) shows the anterior closing synchondrosis.

growth of the upper part of the C2 centrum and lower part of the dens, but it is also located below the level of the articular facets, within the eventual C2 vertebral body (see Figs. 14-4 to 14-6). It is also histologically continuous with the neurocentral synchondroses of the centrum and posterior elements of C2. A "ghost" of this structure may remain for several years and should not be confused with a fracture. In children, dens fractures extend through this growth mechanism, and thus are partially within the body of C2, a factor

that enhances healing. In contrast, the fracture level in the adult is usually several millimeters higher, at the articular level (Fig. 14-7).

Schiff and Parke, in a study of the arterial supply of the dens, concluded that the epiphyseal plate effectively prevented vascularization of the dens by direct or osteal extension of vessels from the centrum of the axis.[5] The circulation must enter the dens from two areas. At the upper end, near the ossiculum terminale, there are soft tissue attachments

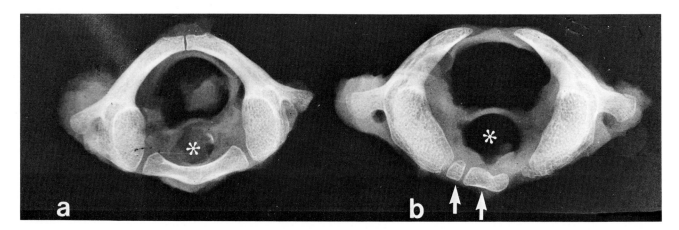

FIG. 14-3. Variation in anterior development of C1 in two 3-year-olds. *a,* Normal development, with posterior synchondrosis and anterior arch with two synchondroses. *b,* Widened posterior region, and irregular ossification centers in the arch (arrows). Asterisks mark the location of the dens, with transverse ligament intact.

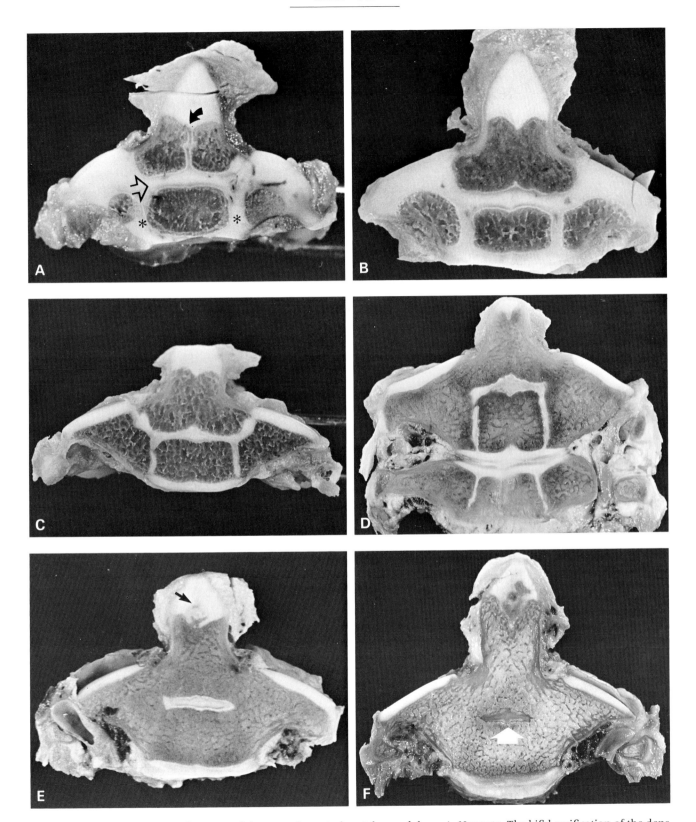

FIG. 14-4. Morphologic development of the second cervical vertebra and dens. *A,* Neonate. The bifid ossification of the dens is evident (solid arrow). There is considerable cartilaginous continuity throughout the centrum, the posterior elements and the dens (open arrow). The asterisks indicate the neurocentral synchondroses between the centrum and the posterolateral elements. *B,* 3 months. The dens ossification centers have coalesced. The neurocentral synchondroses separate the centrum from the posterolateral elements. *C,* 1 year. *D,* 3 years. The dens has fused to the lateral elements. *E,* 7 years. The ossiculum terminale is beginning to form (arrow). *F,* 9 years. The ossiculum terminale is more evident.

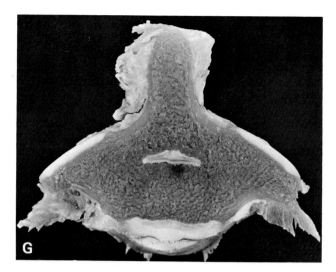

FIG. 14-4. (Continued). *G,* 12 years. The ossiculum has fused to the rest of the dens. In *E, F,* and *G* notice the remnant of the growth cartilage between the dens and centrum (arrow in *F*). This can create a radiolucent cleft that is easily mistaken for a fracture.

that allow penetration of vessels. However, the distal end is supplied by vessels entering just medial to the facet joints. These must go toward the dentocentral synchondrosis, and up into the main portion of the dens, which is almost totally free of soft tissue attachments, as it must serve in a rotatory capacity. This latter circulation is not damaged in childhood fractures, but may be cut off in an adult fracture because of the difference in the fracture planes mentioned previously.

The lymphatic drainage of these joints is primarily into the retropharyngeal glands, and ultimately into the deep cervical glands. Both sets of glands also drain the nasopharynx.

This is significant in C1, C2-C3, and C3-C4 subluxation secondary to pharyngitis.[6]

The third through seventh cervical vertebrae, as well as the thoracic and lumbar vertebrae, exhibit a common ossification pattern. One ossification center develops in each of the two neural arch cartilage centers, while one ossification center generally forms in the vertebral centrum (Fig. 14-8). The position of the two neural arches and single vertebral centrum ossification center is such that the cartilage separating them, the neurocentral synchondrosis, is slightly anterior to the anatomic base of the pedicles. This synchondrosis disappears between the ages of 3 and 6 years as osseous bridges form. The ossified portions of each neural arch fuse with each other posteriorly by 2 to 4 years of age. Prior to this time, they produce radiolucent lines on the frontal projection of the spine and should not be confused with congenital abnormalities (e.g., spina bifida) or trauma.[7] Thus, spinal canal diameters reach maturity long before longitudinal growth of the centrum ceases.

The normal planes of the articular surfaces may change with growth. However, there are no studies of the extent to which they change angulation. Preliminary data concerning the cervical spine show that the lower cervical spine facets change from 55° to 70°, whereas the upper cervical spine (i.e., C2-C4) may have initial angles as low as 30°, which gradually change to approximately 60° to 70° (Fig. 14-9).[8] This angulation variation is probably a major factor in the pseudosubluxation of infants and young children.

Similarly, development of the upward curve of the lateral margins of the cervical vertebral centra varies considerably with age. This region, sometimes referred to as the joint of Luschka, does not exist as a rigid structure in the infant and young child. However, by 7 to 10 years of age the marginal ossification has progressed sufficiently to begin formation of this structure. This is another developmental anatomic factor affecting mobility and fracture pattern susceptibility in the immature cervical spine.

Secondary ossification centers appear at the tips of the spi-

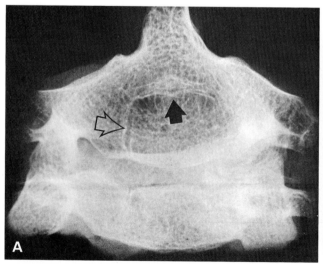

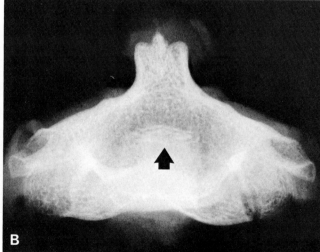

FIG. 14-5. Roentgenograms of C2. *A,* Three years. There is no ossiculum terminale. The neurocentral (open arrow) and dentocentral (solid arrow) synchondroses are closing. *B,* Nine years. The ossiculum in this specimen was fusing to the dens. The dentocentral growth plate remnant is evident (arrow).

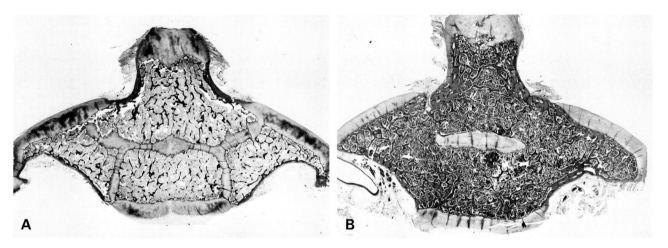

FIG. 14-6.   Histologic specimens. *A*, One year. *B*, Seven years.

nous, transverse, and mammillary processes about the time of puberty. Secondary ossification also appears at this time in the cartilaginous ring apophysis within the vertebral end plate (Fig. 14-10). This ring is involved in the vertical growth of the vertebral body. These secondary ossification centers fuse with the vertebral body in the third decade, usually by 25 years of age.

Individual vertebral bodies enlarge circumferentially by the process of perichondral and periosteal apposition, and grow vertically by endochondral ossification, with the cartilage in the vertebral end plates functioning similarly to other growth plates (Fig. 14-11). It has been said that the ring apophysis does not contribute to vertical growth of the vertebral body. However, it would be expected that this particular structure does, because it represents a secondary ossification center like that in a long bone. However, it does not form a discrete plate (secondary ossification center), as seen in most other mammalian species (Fig. 14-12). Instead, an incomplete epiphysis and ossification center are present.

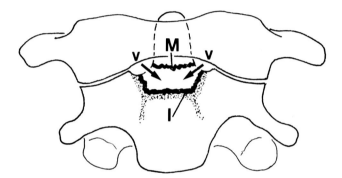

FIG. 14-7.   Schematic of dens fracture patterns in the mature (M) and immature (I) dens. Note the vascular entrance points (V), and how the childhood fracture pattern (I) does not interfere with the dental blood supply, whereas the adult fracture pattern (M) does. The neurocentral and dentocentral synchondroses are stippled.

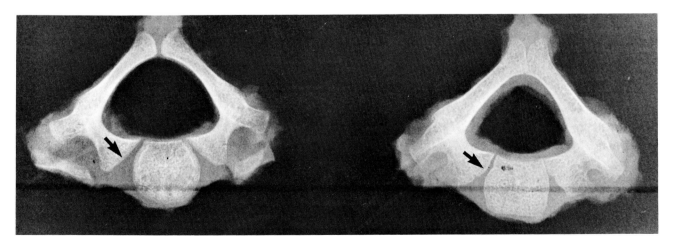

FIG. 14-8.   Representative cervical vertebrae at 7 (left) and 15 (right) months, showing location of the 3 growth regions—the posterior one at the spinous process and 2 anterior ones at the neurocentral synchondroses (arrows). These growth regions allow diametric increase in spinal canal diameter.

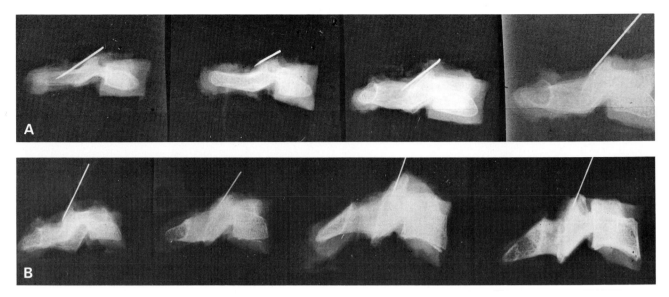

FIG. 14-9. Changes in angulation of the articular facet plane in the cervical spine from birth to 10 years. The pins follow the articular plane. *A* shows the C3 vertebra, which has a less acute angle than C7, which is shown in *B*. This may be a major factor in allowing subluxation of the second, third, and fourth cervical vertebra.

Values for the normal ratio of vertebral body height to sagittal diameter, and of vertebral height to disc space height, have been developed by Brandner.[9] Normal weightbearing appears to control vertical growth and keeps it in the normal relationship to anteroposterior diameter. In patients who do not have normal upright or walking posture, such as early quadriplegia secondary to trauma, the vertebral body grows disproportionately in height with the result that the vertebral bodies are tall and thin with biconvex end plates and decreased disc space height.[10]

Normal anteroposterior and lateral alignment of the spine are contingent upon the chondro-osseous anatomy, the truncal musculature, and the effect of gravity.[11] At any specific level of a motion segment where injury occurs, stability depends primarily upon the interrelationship between the anterior and posterior chondro-osseous and ligamentous columns (Fig. 14-13). In a traumatized spine, the degree of damage to one or both columns determines the overall stability in the acute and chronic phase. It is often difficult to accurately assess the amount of stability in the adult spine. It is even more difficult to assess the degree of stability of the cartilaginous portions of the immature spine. The goal of treatment, whether operative or non-operative, is still the same: that of spinal stability. Failure to do so may result in increasing deformity.

Studies of Incidence and Outcome

Spinal fractures in children have distinct differences in natural histories compared to adults. These differences result from the child's inherent ability to withstand trauma and the potential for growth and development subsequent to the discrete injury, a major factor that can dramatically improve or worsen the initial post-injury result. The principal differences observed in children are the relatively benign clinical course, the gradual restoration of the vertebral body height

when anteriorly wedged, and the development of progressive spinal deformity when there is either end plate injury or paralysis.

Fractures, dislocations, and fracture-dislocations of the spine in children and adolescents are relatively uncommon.[12-16] Accordingly, knowledge about spinal injuries has been obtained primarily from experience with the adult population. Few reports concerning comparable injuries in children exist, and those that do pertain almost exclusively to the cervical spine.

Henrys reviewed 1299 vertebral spine traumatic lesions; among these there were 631 cervical lesions, of which only 12 were in children under 15 years of age (1.9%).[17] The incidence of osseous injuries in the 6- to 15-year age group may reflect the fact that the cervical spine begins to gradually acquire the adult feature of reduced flexibility.

Fractures of the lower cervical and thoracolumbar spine and spinal cord injuries are less common in children than in adults. Only 5% of traumatic paraplegia occurs in children. The decreased frequency of concomitant spinal cord injuries does not mean that childhood back injuries should not be taken seriously. The child's spine is more mobile than the adult's, so that force is more easily dissipated over a greater number of segments. Dislocation of the spine is rare in children because the ligaments are generally stonger than the bone.

The line of the growth plate may mimic a fracture, or it may cause special types of fractures. This is a problem particularly in the dens. Separation of the epiphyseal end plates of a vertebral body usually represents a type 1 injury (Fig. 14-14), which may be an extremely unstable fracture that is accompanied by a certain degree of lateral or posterior disruption.

Rang reviewed 86 cases and found that trauma of the spine falls into 3 basic groups: (1) cord injury without fracture; (2) cord injury with fracture or dislocation; (3) fracture or dislocation alone (no neurologic injury).[18] Interestingly,

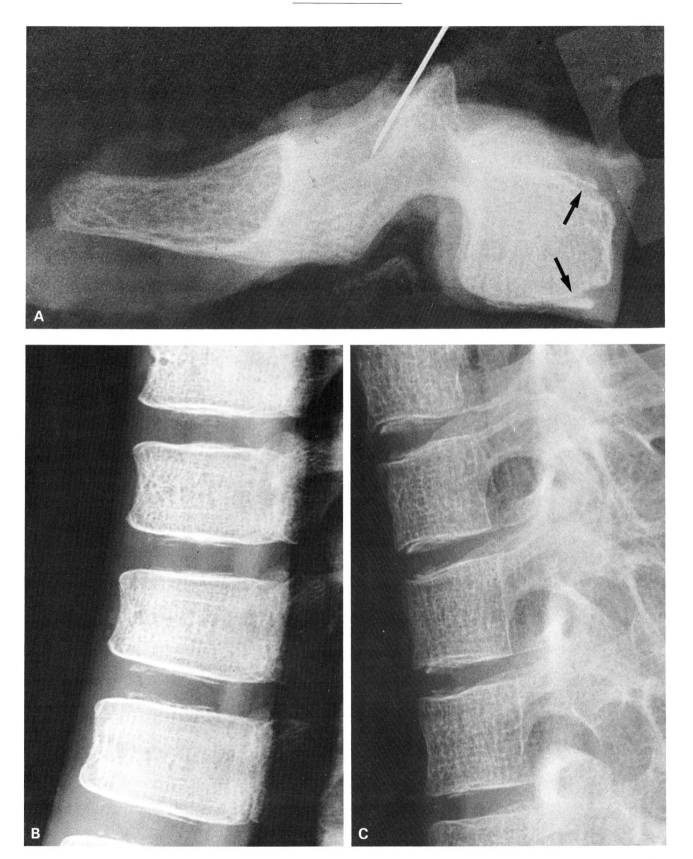

FIG. 14-10. *A,* Ring apophyses of C7 in a 12-year-old (arrows). *B-C,* Thoracolumbar development. *B,* 7 years. Note the greater degree of ring apophyseal maturation in the upper thoracic spine. *C,* 14 years. Note the more extensive development of ring ossification.

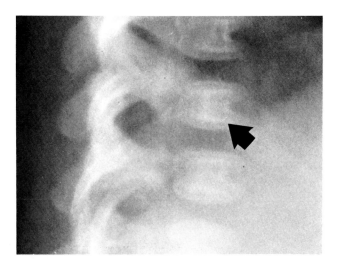

FIG. 14-11. Vertebra with vertebra (arrow). This process is the spinal analogue of the Harris growth arrest line.

that could be demonstrated radiographically. The frequent lack of radiographic findings in the young child is probably due to the elasticity of the osteocartilaginous spine and supporting ligaments.

Fracture-dislocation usually results from severe violence and accounts for the most severe neurologic complications.[20] Of the 6 patients with fracture-dislocations reported by Henrys, 5 developed neurologic complications and 1 died. Of the 6 patients, 3 underwent surgical fusion.[17]

Hubbard reviewed 42 cases of spinal injury, ranging in age from 17 months to 17 years;[21,22] two thirds were stable and one third was unstable. None of the patients with stable injuries had evidence of neurologic trauma. Of the 14 unstable lesions, 8 suffered neurologic damage; 6 to the spinal cord and 2 to a nerve root. All cases were of immediate onset, with the exception of 1 patient who sustained injury to the nerve roots 2 days after the initial trauma from a redislocation at the L2-L3 level. Of the 8 who suffered neurologic damage, 4 occurred with cervical injury, 3 from thoracolumbar injury, and 1 from injury in the lumbar region. Interestingly, radiographs obtained 6 months after injury revealed scoliosis in every case with a stable thoracic, thoracolumbar, or lumbar injury associated with hyperflexion force. However, the scoliosis was only slightly progressive and measured less than 10°, eventually becoming balanced with time. With unstable injuries, abnormal alignment was often present on the initial radiograph and tended to progress unless early surgery was performed.

In the adult, spinal deformity can be considered a preventable complication of fractures and fracture-dislocations of

cord injury without fracture, which is extremely rare in adults, represented about one quarter of all injuries in children with neurologic damage.

Melzak reported only 29 cases of spinal cord trauma in children less than 13 years of age among 4500 patients admitted to the National Spinal Cord Injury Center at Stoke-Mandeville Hospital.[19] Of the 29 cases, 16 had no fracture

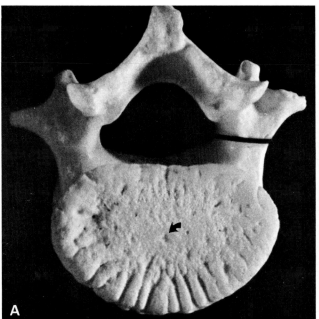

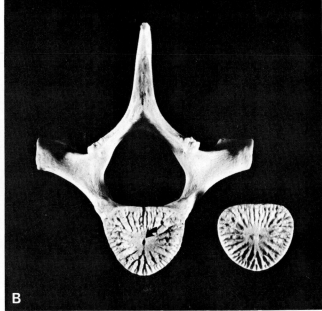

FIG. 14-12. Comparison of metaphyseal undulations in A, seven-year-old human and, B, adolescent dolphin thoracic vertebrae. The latter species forms a complete end plate, whereas the former species forms an incomplete marginal plate (ring). Asymmetric undulation in the human may be a factor in the development of scoliosis. In B, the matching complete end plate (secondary, or epiphyseal, ossification center) is adjacent to the centrum. Also note the central remnant (ghost) of the notochord (arrows) in each.

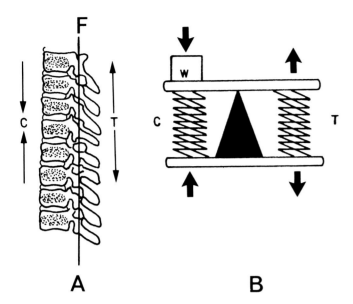

FIG. 14-13. Schematic of spine mechanics. *A*, Representative spine segment. The main compression forces (C) are anterior, while the main tension forces (T) are posterior. The facet joints act as the level fulcrum (F) for each motion segment. *B*, If weight (W) is applied, it must be equilibrated by both the compression (C) and tension (T) forces.

the axial skeleton. In the child, a different situation arises, since damage to end plate growth mechanisms may not be obvious and may lead to subsequent deformity during different periods of growth. Whether dealing with acute injury or progressive secondary changes due to growth deformity, associated morbidity may significantly limit the ultimate physical and neurologic rehabilitation of the spine-injured child and adolescent, months or even years following the original injury. The complex reconstructive surgery that is often required to correct deformities and relieve symptoms is not without potentially serious risk to the patient. These risks must be considered before entering into surgical approaches in skeletally immature children.

Factors that are responsible for spinal deformity may be either intrinsic (osteogenic, chondrogenic, discogenic), extrinsic (neurogenic, myogenic, iatrogenic), or combined. The intrinsic factors are the necessary growth mechanisms of the developing spine, while the extrinsic factors have a role in relative capacities of the intrinsic factors to develop normally.

In Hubbard's study, the clinical picture for patients with stable injury was characteristically benign and not associated with the long-term problems, strongly suggesting that treatment for longer than one month is probably not required.[21] The absence of spontaneous interbody fusion, and the discovery of only one patient with subsequent disc narrowing probably related to a healthy intervertebral disc and its inherent stability to withstand stress.

The most important finding in Hubbard's paper was the tendency to restoration of vertebral body height in the thoracolumbar fractures; however, Blockey did not see this occur in the cervical fractures.[21,23] There probably is a differ-

ence in the growth capacity in the cervical spine versus the thoracolumbar spine during adolescent growth spurts that may be a major factor in this tendency of one region to restore height and not the other. It appears likely that the cervical vertebrae reach approximate adult height sooner than the vertebrae in lower regions.[8]

Injury without fracture or open injury may result in concussion, contusion, or infarction of the cord, and probably often represents anterior spinal cord damage. The mechanism of injury is a matter of conjecture. A displaced type 1 injury of a cartilaginous end plate may spring back into position, but it is difficult to assess how real this particular problem is. This injury may heal without any radiographic signs. Another possible mechanism for this particular injury of the young spine is that the excessive mobility may stretch the spinal cord over a hyperextended or hyperflexed region and contuse the anterior portion of the cord, similar to the mechanism in the more rigid spine of an adult. Significant traction, particularly in a breech delivery, may be the most common mechanism of birth paraplegia. Burke reviewed 7 children with complete paraplegia who had no radiographic signs of injuries and found associated rib fractures in 3, a fractured transverse process in 1, and a slight forward subluxation of L2 and L3 in another.[24] Paraplegia was spastic in 5 of the children and flaccid in 2.

Infarction results in complete, permanent, flaccid paraplegia below the midthoracic level.[25] In one patient described by Rang,[18] arterial damage was confirmed as the cause of paraplegia. The blood supply of the thoracic cord depends significantly on the artery of Adamkiewicz. Anastomosis of these vessels between the first and eleventh intercostal arteries is poor, and may result in infarction of a major portion of the cord. Because the whole cord is malfunctioning, the paraplegia is flaccid, in contrast to spastic paraplegia, which is produced by a segmental lesion.

In thoracic injuries, prognosis for recovery is essentially nonexistent. The majority of injuries are fracture-dislocations, and it may be assumed that the cord is severely damaged or transsected initially. Cervical injuries show considerable variation in the extent of initial damage. In 1 series there were 31 such children,[18] 3 of whom died. However, most of the patients survived long enough to be admitted to the hospital with presenting symptoms of incomplete hemiplegia (almost 50%).

In complete cord lesions, with or without fracture, the incidence of spinal deformity, either lordosis, kyphosis, or scoliosis, is higher when the lesion is high (i.e., upper thoracic or cervical). There is muscle imbalance; the onset of paraplegia is early in life and laminectomy is often performed. Bracing is difficult and spinal fusion is usually required. Since progressive angular kyphosis may damage cord functions in partial lesions, early fusion is indicated. In extensive thoracic and lumbar lesions it may be necessary to use Dwyer as well as Harrington instrumentation.

Evaluation for injury may be the first indication of a congenital deformity (Fig. 14-15). In the illustrated case of a child sustaining a hyperflexion injury, there was concern that the wedging was traumatic. However, a bifid, deformed vertebral body was found on CAT scan, with no evidence of posterior disruption. Children and adolescents with Klippel-Feil syndrome may develop neck pain during sports, which may lead to an initial diagnosis of congenital spine deformity (Fig. 14-16).

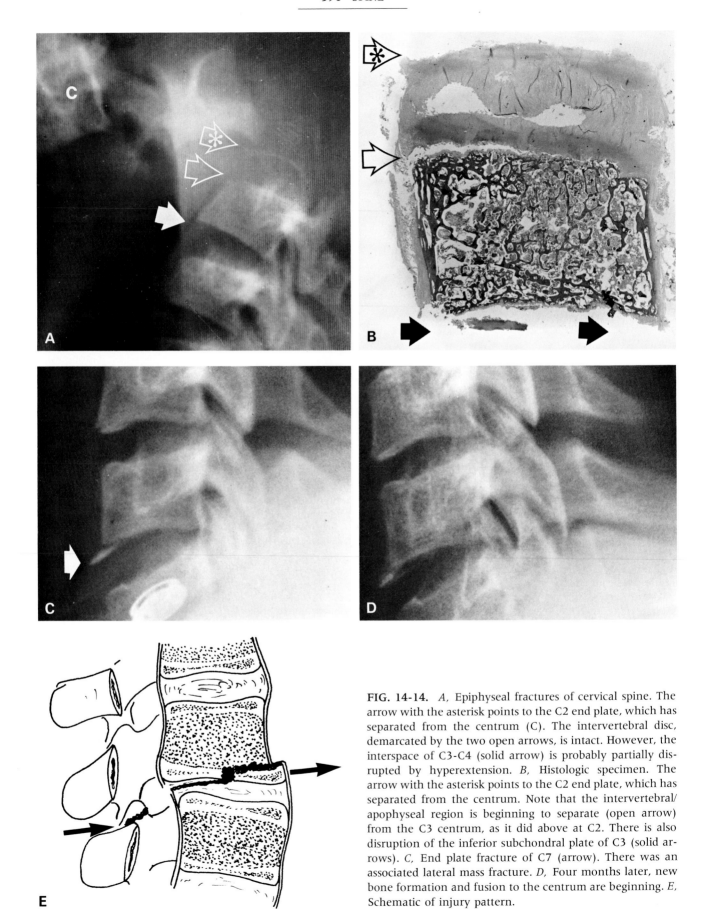

FIG. 14-14. *A,* Epiphyseal fractures of cervical spine. The arrow with the asterisk points to the C2 end plate, which has separated from the centrum (C). The intervertebral disc, demarcated by the two open arrows, is intact. However, the interspace of C3-C4 (solid arrow) is probably partially disrupted by hyperextension. *B,* Histologic specimen. The arrow with the asterisk points to the C2 end plate, which has separated from the centrum. Note that the intervertebral/apophyseal region is beginning to separate (open arrow) from the C3 centrum, as it did above at C2. There is also disruption of the inferior subchondral plate of C3 (solid arrows). *C,* End plate fracture of C7 (arrow). There was an associated lateral mass fracture. *D,* Four months later, new bone formation and fusion to the centrum are beginning. *E,* Schematic of injury pattern.

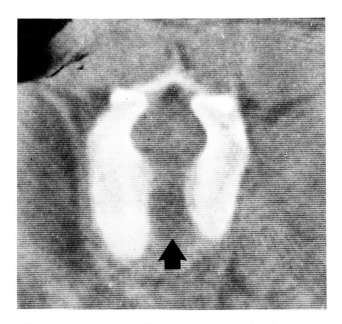

FIG. 14-15. Ten-year-old boy with back pain after hyperflexion injury. Lateral view showed apparent wedging, which suggested a compression fracture. The AP view showed widening of the pedicles and a central lucency. CAT scan showed a bifid vertebral body (arrow). The ligament had been strained, but no fractures occurred. The "compression" was part of the congenital deformity.

Pathomechanics

Yates showed that trauma to the cervical spine at birth could result in damage to the cervical portions of the vertical artery.[26] There was evidence of distortional trauma, but no evidence of major fracture or dislocation to the cervical spine. The lesions were considered under four main groups: (1) extradural, dural, subdural, and subarachnoid hemorrhage; (2) tears and hemorrhages in the nerve roots and spinal ganglia; (3) evidence of hemorrhage around one or both of the vertebral arteries in the form of a crescentic, adventitial hematoma or massive hemorrhage encircling the vessel; and (4) spinal cord lesions that consisted of contusion and bilateral necrosis of the lateral columns. Jones postulated that vertebral artery hemorrhage may be an important cause of perinatal mortality and morbidity, and that many cases of cerebral palsy alleged to be caused by anoxic spells may be explicable on the basis of vertebral artery trauma and ischemic cerebral, cerebellar, and cord damage at birth.[27]

Aufdermaur observed 12 out of 100 spinal injuries in subjects between the ages of stillborn and 18 years of age who were examined after death.[28-30] Each of the spines was completely dissected for evaluation. He also removed 20 intact spines from juveniles of similar age groups who had died, and subjected these to mechanical stress. One frequent finding was the tendency for the injuries to occur through the region of the subcondylar plate and hypertrophic cartilage, like the lesion shown in Figure 14-14 of a 14-year-old boy who was instantly killed in an automobile accident. Aufder-

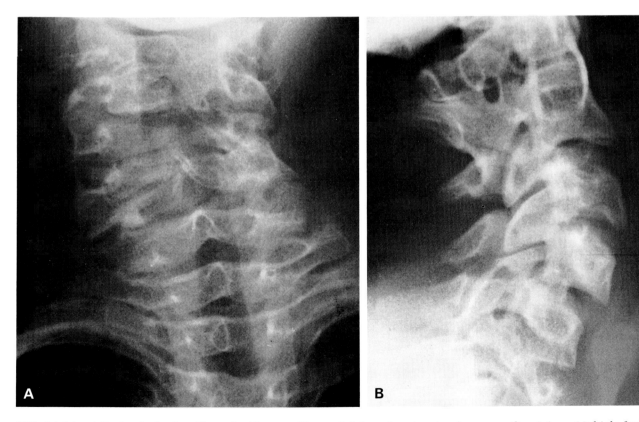

FIG. 14-16. *A-B,* Cervical spine films of a 12-year-old complaining of neck pain after a wrestling injury. Multiple fusions indicate Klippel-Feil syndrome.

maur believed that since there was a high likelihood of growth mechanism injury, the most likely radiographic sign would be widening of the intervertebral space.[30]

Aufdermaur's cases involved injuries to the following: the cervical spine (7 cases), the thoracic spine (4 cases), and the lumbar spine (1 case).[30] In 10 instances the injury occurred in traffic accidents, and in 2 instances the spine was hyperextended during childbirth. Clinically, a spinal fracture was suspected only once. In the other 11 cases, the spinal injury was noted first at necropsy. In all cases, death occurred within 1 to 1½ days of the accident. In 9 of the cases, the spinal injuries did not contribute to death. However, 3 cases were associated with significant cervical, epidural, and subdural hematomas and associated brain injury probably related to the cause of death. In 2 of the cases, there was also rupture of the anterior longitudinal ligament. In 3 cases, the supraspinous and intraspinous ligaments, the ligamentum flavum, and the capsules of the posterolateral joints were also ruptured, in addition to the rupture of the cartilaginous end plate and the longitudinal ligaments. Histologically, the fracture lines involved the layers of the growth zone almost exclusively. These layers were split in irregular, wavy lines. There were 4 patients with multiple cartilage plate injuries. The top plate was injured in 12 patients, and the base plate in 6 patients. Histologic findings were similar for cervical, thoracic, and lumbar vertebrae.

Damage to the end plate may not be evident in initial films. However, type 5 compression injuries may occur and lead to disparate growth across the "ring" apophysis, and major disruption of the disc and end plates may lead to a "traumatic bar" several years after the accident (Fig. 14-17).

Spinal injury prior to complete vertebral growth may lead to unequal growth and progressive deformity. Theoretically, premature asymmetric epiphyseal closure, like that seen in some types of epiphyseal injuries in the appendicular skeleton, is responsible for the unequal growth. With lateral wedge compression fractures in children, mild scoliosis is the rule and significant nerve progression is the exception. Horal showed that the residual of adolescent-incurred anterior wedge compression fractures was difficult to find radiographically at follow-up (some averaging 16 years), and concluded that unequal growth that resulted from an epiphyseal injury was rare.[31] Osseous bridging may also occur (see Fig. 14-17).

Deformation of a vertebral body invariably results in angular deformity. The most frequent deformities are kyphosis, scoliosis, and kyphoscoliosis, which results from a combination of the two. More than 30% loss in anterior height has the potential for increasing late deformity, since there is unrecognized disruption of the posterior elements (i.e., the interspinous ligaments). Alterations in vertebral body shape and deformities below the site of injury are usually the result of unequal pressure during normal epiphyseal growth that results from neuromuscular imbalance.[32]

Experimental cord injury

Wagner subjected the spinal cord of cats to controlled trauma and found that the first evidence of injury is hemorrhage in the gray matter.[33] The amount of hemorrhage varied with the magnitude of the injury. The vascular damage caused by the trauma and the hemorrhagic infarction that ensued were responsible for the parenchymal changes in

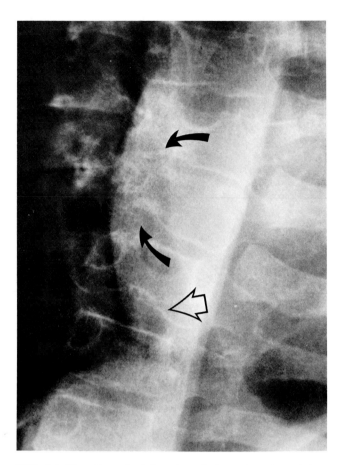

FIG. 14-17. Growth deformity of thoracic spine at ten years. When the original injury occurred at two years of age, roentgenograms reportedly showed a normal spine, although the child was rendered completely paraplegic. The fifth through seventh vertebrae seem to be fusing and slowing in growth on the lateral side (solid arrows), while the base plate of T7 is exhibiting a central growth arrest (open arrow).

gray and white matter. The myelinated axons were not exclusively associated with distortion of the tissue. The edema that occurred after the trauma was possibly an alternative to the mechanical injury, although the vascular damage caused some of the changes in the white matter. Animals studied several days to weeks after the injury showed some reparative responses with compound, granular cells in areas of cystic necrosis. In the animals that received the most trauma and that were observed up to four months after injury, there was dense fibrosis and adherence of the leptomeninges to the cord, with obliteration of the subarachnoid space. This confirmed what has been described clinically as the constrictive stage of adhesive spinal arachnoiditis. Such a reaction has been observed post mortem in patients with spinal cord injury, and has been produced experimentally by injecting blood into the cerebrospinal fluid.

This study emphasized that injury to the spinal cord severe enough to cause paralysis occurs at the instant of initial impact and that the cord undergoes pathologic changes due to hemorrhage and ischemia that have little relation to external pressure on the spinal cord.[33] Basic studies such as this explain why decompressive laminectomy is of *no* value in reversing complete lesions of the spinal cord.

Diagnosis

Vertebral or spinal cord damage should be suspected in the unconscious child with an injury that can cause flexion or rotation of the spine, in the awake child who complains of loss of sensation or motor power below a transverse level of the body, and in the injured child who complains of localized vertebral pain or tenderness, or pain radiating along radicular distribution. This must be done without moving possible areas of spinal column instability. Intubation in a child with a cervical spine injury is best accomplished by the nasotracheal route, and tracheostomy may be indicated if intubation cannot be accomplished without extending or manipulating the neck.

Remember that spinal shock and the resulting loss of sympathetic vasomotor tone may complicate the general evaluation and mimic the symptoms of shock from internal bleeding. Rapid restoration of normal blood pressure is essential to preserve cord function and can be accomplished by vasoconstrictors or blood volume expanders. A subsequent drop in blood pressure suggests blood loss rather than loss of vasomotor tone, and the source should be searched for in the abdominal cavity, thoracic cavity, pelvis, or fractured extremity. Abdominal reflexes may be absent, and guarding or complaining of abdominal pain may not occur in the patient with a high cord lesion.

Diagnosis includes the accurate evaluation of the level and extent of injury to both chondro-osseous and nervous system tissues. Early assessment is important, since it is the baseline against which the effectiveness of therapeutic manipulation or complications is evaluated.[34] Early assessment is composed of inspection and palpation, determination of neurologic function, and radiographic examination.

Inspection may reveal associated soft tissue injury. Abrasion of the face suggests cervical hyperextension injury, while abrasion of the upper neck may indicate flexion of the dorsal spine. Palpation may reveal a local area of tenderness. The presence of a palpable gap is indicative of disruption of the posterior ligaments and a potentially high degree of instability. Neurologic evaluation is of primary importance, since damage to the spinal cord is the main complication. Of the 18 patients reported by Henrys, 7 showed neurologic injuries.[17] Of subluxations of C1 and C2, 2 resulted in decerebration, and 1 patient with subluxation of C1-C2 presented with a transient parasthesia of the left arm, which was secondary to a football injury.

Detailed neurologic examination must be repeated frequently, since worsening neurologic patterns may require aggressive action, and improvements may encourage waiting. Motor function in the awake, cooperative patient should be described such that subsequent observers may be able to readily assess improvement or gradual loss of neurologic patterns. Loss of deep tendon reflexes generally parallels loss of motor function. In the unconscious patient, facial grimacing when in pain, in the absence of withdrawal of the extremities and loss of deep tendon reflexes, suggests cord injury. In the cervicodorsal region, the spinous process lies about 2 segments above the corresponding spinal segment (i.e., the spinous process of C6 overlies the C8 cord level). In the dorsolumbar region, as many as 11 spinal segments can lie between the spinous processes of T10 and L1. Radiographs should be obtained in accordance with neurologic findings.

Complete loss of motor and reflex function present immediately following injury and associated with sensory loss is generally consistent with motor level and involves all sensory modalities, including deep pain. In the Brown-Séquard syndrome, loss of touch and proprioception occurs on the same side as the motor loss. Analgesia occurs on the contralateral side, and because of the manner in which pain fibers cross the sensory level for pain, may be two or three levels below the motor level.

In the anterior spinal artery syndrome, touch and proprioception are preserved, although there is loss of all other long tract functions. This apparent anomaly occurs because the posterior cord (i.e., dorsal and dorsolateral columns) is supplied by branches of the posterior spinal artery. Preservation of touch and proprioception has no predictive value for motor recovery.

Preservation of sacral sensation is seen occasionally in central cord injuries due to the peripheral location of the sacral portion of the spinothalamic tract. Its predictive value is questionable, even in children in whom recovery potential is often remarkable.

In contrast, preservation of patchy areas of pin sensation or the appreciation of deep pain indicates that motor loss may be secondary to spinal shock. Spinal shock remains a misunderstood phenomenon. Deep tendon reflexes cannot be elicited and there is flaccid paralysis below the level of the lesion. Sphincter tone generally is little affected, and there is complete urinary retention.[35] If the injury is not too severe, reflexes return, voluntary micturition is reestablished, and motor recovery begins within hours or days of injury. If the cord injury is severe, recovery of reflexes is accompanied by reflex facilitation that may occur within hours or days, unaccompanied by any evidence of sensation or voluntary motor activity. In the infant, the reflex activity of the isolated cord may be almost indistinguishable from normal motor function.

Pain in a root distribution, often accompanied by sensory dysfunction, reflex loss, and motor weakness, is generally a reliable indicator of the level of injury. Since recovery of function is more likely following decompression, early diagnosis of root entrapment is essential. The value of functional recovery in any of the roots of the brachial plexus cannot be overemphasized, especially in the child.

A common situation in which spinal injury may be overlooked is the head-injured child. Any severe head trauma caused by rotation, flexion, or extension force directed against the head is capable of causing cervical spine injury, and failure to adequately immobilize the unconscious patient may lead to irreversible spinal cord damage. Unconscious patients with facial injuries, or patients who are vomiting may have to be transported on their side to prevent aspiration of blood or vomitus. These patients often require support of the cervical area by manual or halter traction, which is applied to the head. A neutral spine position generally is adequate, and in the case of a suspected cervical spine injury, the head should be supported laterally to prevent rotation or sideways motion. In lower spine injury, a small support under the affected area or lumbar lordotic curve may be required to support the spine in a neutral position without stress being applied to the point of injury.

Roentgenographic evaluation

Radiographic evaluation must be accomplished with regard for potentially severe and unstable injuries and must include prior adequate immobilization of the spine. Radiographs must show the exact nature of the lesion. The area of involvement, as suspected or defined by neurologic examination, must be included on the films. One of the most frequent errors in evaluating suspected injury of the cervical spine is failure to obtain good visualization of the C7-T1 vertebral bodies and posterior elements. Anteroposterior and lateral tomograms may be helpful; obliques may be necessary. A CAT scan may also be indicated to look at soft tissue injuries.

The normal spine in children differs considerably from that in adults, especially in the cervical region. Lack of awareness of the normal roentgenographic appearances may lead to misdiagnoses in pediatric patients. Common transient developmental features and more unusual normal variants may be mistaken for spinal trauma in children.[9] The multiplicity of the primary and secondary ossification centers and their intervening synchondroses are often mistaken for evidence of fracture or avulsion fragmentation.[36] In young children, the lateral thoracic or lumbar spinal radiograph may occasionally show a vertically oriented, lucent cleft. This may represent the more anteriorly placed neurocentral synchondrosis. A similar cleft may also represent a bifid vertebra (see Fig. 14-15). Morphologic variations in the lumbosacral region are common. Lumbarization of the first sacral segment to form a sixth lumbar vertebra or bilateral or unilateral fusion of L5 to the sacrum are often seen. Incomplete osseous fusion of the neural arch of L5 or S1 (or both) is high in children, with a level of 58% in some populations.[7] A gradual decrease in these values occurs throughout childhood, but remains high, even in adolescence.

The following areas are of major concern: (1) variations due to displacement of vertebra that may resemble subluxation. Marked anterior displacement of the second or third cervical vertebra resembling a true subluxation is extremely common in up to 20% of children between one and seven years of age. Less frequently, similar displacement can be seen between the third and fourth cervical vertebrae. In lateral roentgenograms, overriding of the atlas on the dens and apparent widening of the space between these two structures occur in about 20% of normal children.[37,38] Both appear to be suggestive of, but do not necessarily indicate, ligamentous injury. (2) Variations of curvature of the cervical spine that may resemble spasm and ligamentous injury. Absence of uniform angulation between adjacent vertebrae, and absence of a flexion curvature of the spine between the second and seventh cervical vertebrae seen on lateral roentgenograms made with the cervical spine in flexion. (3) Variations related to skeletal growth centers resembling fractures. The basilar cartilaginous plate of the dens frequently persists until the age of five years or older and may resemble an undisplaced fracture (see Fig. 14-4). Normal anterior "wedging" of the immature vertebral body can produce the appearance of a compression fracture. Spinous process secondary centers may be confused with avulsion fractures.

Apparent subluxation of C2 and C3 occurs in 19% of nor-

mal children, and there is no lordosis in the cervical spine in about 15%.[39] Absence of uniform angulation, absence of cervical lordosis, and absence of flexion curves have also been reported in a high percentage of normal, asymptomatic children.

In the young child, radiologic diagnosis is further complicated by the relative elasticity of the cartilaginous spine and supporting ligamentous structures, which may allow severe cord damage in the absence of radiographic evidence of fracture or dislocation. Burke reported 7 children (13 months to 12 years of age), and noted that 5 of the younger children sustained flexion-rotation injuries with a preponderance of dorsal spine involvement and extensive longitudinal traction injury extending over several levels.[24] Even in the 3 children in whom vertebral injury could be radiographically demonstrated, actual spinal cord involvement extended several segments above the osseous involvement.

Hyperextension injuries often reduce spontaneously, especially in the resilient spine of a child. The only indication of such an injury may be a small chip of bone pulled away from the anterior-inferior edge of the ossifying vertebral centrum at the point of separation of the end plate, anterior longitudinal ligament, and annulus (see Fig. 14-14).

Naik measured the sagittal and interpedicular diameters of the cervical spinal canal on radiographs of normal infants.[40] He assessed the difficulties in obtaining accurate measurements and mentioned a new method for measuring the sagittal diameter. Naik's values can be consulted for the interpretation of trauma, although the main reason was to assess possible congenital defects.

There are many congenital malformations of the cranial vertebral junction that should not be confused with traumatic lesions. Anomalies characterized by single or multiple ossification centers must be differentiated from traumatic fragmentation. Well-marginated, distinct ossification centers may be seen anterior to the dens above or below the arch of the atlas. There may be unilateral or bilateral clefts in the ring of the atlas, usually in the posterior arch, but rarely in the anterior arch. These clefts vary from small defects (spina bifida occulta) to agenesis of half or even the entire posterior ring.

In children, one may observe a V-shaped cleft within the tip of the ossified dens (see Fig. 14-4), which frequently contains a round ossification center. This variant, sometimes termed a bicornuate dens, represents incomplete fusion of the two lateral ossification centers that enclose the normal ossiculum terminale. Although these centers usually fuse completely in the adult, the lines of fusion may be demarcated by clefts throughout development. There may also be failure of osseous union of a normal ossiculum terminale with the dens.

A spectrum of anomalies may be associated with hypoplasia of the dens: hypoplasia with an os odontoideum, simple shortening of the dens owing to failure of development of the distal ossification center, and total agenesis of the dens. In the past, os odontoideum was thought to represent an unfused, deformed dens that failed to unite with the body of C2. However, this theory neglects the fact that the base of the normal dens is always lower than the plane of the C1-C2 joints, although the os odontoideum complex has a protrusion extending above the articular facets. The os odontoideum may also be considered a hypertrophic remnant of the proatlas associated with hypoplasia of the dens in the absence of the distal ossification center.

Subluxation

The fulcrum of the normal cervical spine in children under the age of eight years is at C2-C3 rather than C5-C6 as in the adult.[41-43] A flexion film of the cervical spine frequently shows the second segment misaligned relative to the third, which is termed pseudosubluxation and is usually a normal finding in children (Fig. 14-18). Failure to recognize this normal variation is responsible for many erroneous ideas regarding the relationship of subluxation of the cervical spine to streptococcal sore throats and peritonsillar abscesses. This normal variation in patients causes a major diagnostic problem when the finding is noted in patients who have suffered neck trauma.

Subluxation of the cervical vertebrae without associated fracture of spinal cord injury occurs more frequently in children than in adults. Anterior unilateral displacement of the atlas upon the axis is the most common pattern. Many of these cases appear to occur spontaneously, and although local infection has been cited as a predisposing factor, the high incidence of upper respiratory infection in the age group most frequently encountered (6 to 12 years) makes this relationship difficult to establish.[44,45]

The facet joints of the upper cervical vertebrae are more horizontal than those of the lower cervical vertebrae, and this variation is more pronounced in the younger child (see Fig. 14-9). Some laxity of the transverse ligament must occur for the atlas to slide forward on the axis. Although asymptomatic cases in children have been reported in which the distance between the anterior arch and dens is in excess of 3.5 mm, most agree that 3.0 mm is the upper limit of normal for children.[46-48]

Hypermobility of the cervical spine in young children may be noted at the C2-C3 and C3-C4 levels on lateral roentgenograms taken with the neck in full flexion.[44,45] Anterior subluxation of up to 4 mm may occur as a normal variant. The diagnosis should be made only when the radiographic finding of subluxation is accompanied by clinical evidence of muscular spasm and pain, generally with limitation of lateral extension of the neck. Evidence of soft tissue swelling with anterior tracheal displacement is sometimes present, and laminography may be helpful in demonstrating fractures not readily apparent on the plain films.

Bailey noted that infants and children should show a normal step-off of as much as 2 to 3 mm at the level of the second and third cervical vertebrae.[39] Similarly, the gap between the posterior portion of the anterior arch of the adolescent and the anterior portion of the dens may increase with motion. In normal adults it does not usually move more than 2 mm, but in normal children a 5-mm excursion may be perfectly normal in flexion. Furthermore, when the neck is in extension, the arch may appear to move posteriorly and may seem to lie on top of the dens.

Children who have normal pseudosubluxation and normal vertebral epiphyses do not require extensive and aggressive treatment. An awareness of the normal anatomy of the pediatric cervical spine helps prevent overtreatment. Seemingly positive radiographic findings must be accompanied by appropriate physical signs to warrant prolonged traction, casting, or surgery, under the misconception that serious or true injury exists.

Donaldson presented 37 cases of acquired torticollis and found rotatory subluxation of the first and second cervical vertebrae in some of these cases.[49] Dunlap's study reported

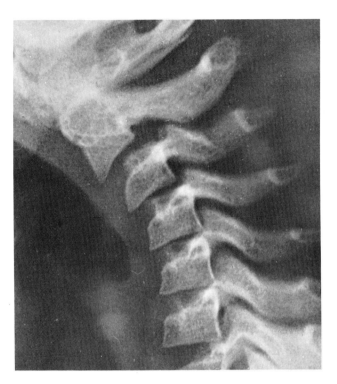

FIG. 14-18. Pseudosubluxation in a normal child. The C2-C3 joint is most involved. Notice the differences in the planes of the facet joint surfaces of C3-C4 versus C6-C7.

12 children between the ages of 3 and 8, only 1 of whom had an actual traumatic injury.[50] Altogether they reviewed 47 children and found 5 with marked subluxation of the second on the third cervical vertebrae and 3 with borderline dislocations. They believed that children with these normal variations should not be subjected to extensive orthopaedic treatment unless there is a supporting history of sufficient injury to the neck, and clinical examination bears out the probability that these are traumatic subluxations.

Differentiation of a traumatic subluxation from an inflammatory subluxation constitutes a major diagnostic problem.[51] Grisel's syndrome (atlantoaxial dislocation or subluxation in children) infrequently follows a major injury, and more often is associated with the hyperemia and local edema that follows pharyngitis, otitis, tonsillar abscesses, osteomyelitis, tuberculosis, and tumors, which may permit stretching of ligaments, so that even normal neck motion produces atlantoaxial displacement.[6,52]

Treatment

A number of unique problems are encountered in the treatment of infants, children, and adolescents with major spine and spinal cord injuries. In any closed, non-operative treatment regimen the spine must be reduced and then adequately protected from redisplacement or increasing deformity during the period of physiologic consolidation of the anterior or posterior columns. Treatment used in adults for external stabilization, operative stabilization, and anatomic reduction are often not directly applicable in children because of the difference in skull, spine, skin, musculature, and ligamentous stability, all of which must be considered when treating significant spinal chondro-osseous injury.

Unstable fractures must be treated with traction and, if necessary, internal fixation. Since ligamentous rupture is less frequent, most fractures stabilize by osseous healing. For cervical injuries, persistent deformity is corrected by skull traction; in thoracic and lumbar injuries, fusion may be needed for growth displacements. Instability complicating congenital anomalies may require fusion.

Laminectomy has been used frequently, but indiscriminately, and in general it is *not* indicated. However, laminectomy may be indicated if there is a discrete myelographic or CAT scan block, or by worsening neurologic signs. Iatrogenic disorders include removal of important posterior elements, such as extensive laminectomy, which becomes a major factor in post-traumatic kyphotic deformity. This is an ill-conceived and ill-advised operation as an isolated procedure and, except for a rare instance, has no place in the emergency management of closed spinal injuries.

Specific aspects of treatment are discussed in the sections on anatomic regions and chronic problems.

Specific Injuries

Cervical region

As mentioned previously, the cervical region appears to be the commonly involved spinal component injured in the skeletally immature patient. Fractures and dislocations of the upper cervical spine, in particular, occur with a greater incidence in children than in adults. Lesions of the atlas and axis were noted in 16% of cervical spine injuries in adults, whereas they comprise almost 70% of cervical spine injuries in children.[53]

Injury occurs at all levels in the cervical spine; the only striking feature is that locked facets, so common in adults, are not seen in children. An underlying congenital bone abnormality (e.g., Klippel-Feil syndrome) must be recognized as a predisposing cause of injury. Certain congenital deformities, such as Down's syndrome, may also enhance the risk of instability.[54]

Neonatal Injury. The youngest patients with upper spine lesions have been newborns in whom autopsy has revealed atlanto-occipital and atlantoaxial dislocation, fracture of the dens, and transsection of the cord. These injuries occur as obstetric complications. The upper cervical spine is not resistant to major torsional stresses under these circumstances, and injury occurs proximal to the tethering of the large brachial nerve roots. The heavy infantile head is poorly supported by cervical musculature, and the upper cervical spine is highly vulnerable to repeated shaking, such as might occur in the battered-child syndrome.

Birth trauma probably is one of the most common causes of spinal cord injury in children. Most injuries involve breech extraction and sustained laceration of the spinal cord without any roentgenographically evident injury to the spine.[55-61,61a] Spinal cord injury can also occur as a result of an accident in the neonatal phase or a difficult cephalic delivery. In the young infant, the vertebral column is extremely elastic, certainly more so than the spinal cord, which is tethered by nerve ends and blood vessels. During delivery it is possible to prolong longitudinal traction sufficiently to distract the neck without producing any permanent injury to chondro-osseous structures or dura, yet go beyond the tensile strength of the spinal cord, which can tear within the intact dura and spinal column.

Ligamentous laxity permits a longitudinal force to separate adjacent vertebral bodies sufficiently so that breech deliveries may cause total anatomic transsection of the cervical cord without apparent fracture-dislocation of the spine. The cervical musculature, so important to the stability and alignment of the adult cervical spine, is still not fully developed in the infant. Thus, distracting and displacing forces at the time of injury are less likely to be checked by the patient. After injury, protective muscular splinting is less effective.

These infants have difficult diagnostic patterns. Presenting symptoms may be a fever of unknown origin due to loss of temperature-regulating mechanisms. Reflex movements may be mistaken for voluntary movements. These infants may have respiratory distress due to paralyzed intercostal muscle function. Typically, if the child has had a cord transsection, painful stimuli above the level of the transsection does not induce movement in the limbs affected below the cord transsection. Stimulation below the sensory level elicits reflex withdrawal, but does not produce any irritable response in the infant.

Clinically, there are two primary neurologic syndromes seen in infants who sustain major cervical cord injury at birth. The first type is secondary to complete disruption of the spinal cord, and clinical signs seen immediately after birth include a completely flaccid, areflexic infant with spinal shock. Within a few weeks to several months, they lose the flaccidity and areflexia, and become hyper-reflexic and hypertonic. The second type of neurologic syndrome is seen in the infant who remains flaccid, rather than becoming spastic or hyper-reflexic. This syndrome probably results from further damage to the lower cord by the disruption of the vascular supply, which leads to anoxia and infarction.

Occipitoatlantal Dislocation. Rotatory subluxation or dislocation, rather than fracture of the atlantoaxial articulation, is the most common type of lesion in children with injuries to the atlas and axis. In adults, the steep inclination of the atlanto-occipital joint provides considerable stability. However, the relatively small size of the occipital condyles, the large joint space of the atlanto-occipital joints, and the relatively horizontal plane of these joints in children make the relationship between the atlas and occiput less stable, particularly in extension injuries. Congenital defects may also predispose to injury.[62] Spontaneous, nontraumatic occipitoatlantal dislocations have been reported secondary to various inflammatory diseases.

In children, the occipital condyles are small and the plane of the occipitoatlantal joint is almost horizontal. The steep inclination of the occipitoatlantal joint develops with aging. Because of this, dislocation without fracture may be possible in children, but does not appear possible in adults.

In children, the diameter of the cervical portion of the spinal canal is approximately 22 mm at the first cervical vertebra. The major changes of growth occur in the surrounding bones. The susceptible areas of neurologic dysfunction associated with occipitoatlantal injury are the caudal cranial nerves, the brain stem, the proximal portion of the spinal cord, and the upper three cervical nerves.

Total dislocation of the atlanto-occipital articulation is a rare, usually fatal injury with transsection of the medulla oblongata or the spinal medullary junction.[63] There is gross displacement of the occipital condyles from the superior facets of the atlas along with retropharyngeal swelling (Fig. 14-19). The relationship of the dens to the basiocciput, and the posterior arch of the atlas to the posterior rim of the foramen magnum are grossly distorted. Either the medulla oblongata or the spinal-medullary junction may be severed. The occipitoatlantoaxial ligaments are strong and fracture usually precedes ligamentous rupture.

Respiratory embarrassment, cranial nerve and upper cervical nerve involvement, and long-tract signs have been described. Most injuries of this type are instantly fatal, but even autopsy information of the anatomic lesion is sparse.[63] Evarts found only two patients who had recovered from this dislocation.[64]

There is little information available regarding the clinical course of patients who sustain this injury. One patient, a 6-year-old child, demonstrated great irregularities in pulse and respiration. When the head was extended, these disappeared. After recovery there were no neurologic sequelae. Gabrielson reported a case of partial dislocation in which the patient survived. This patient demonstrated some cranial nerve dysfunction, as well as some long-tract signs, but the only residual neurologic deficit was anesthesia over the distribution of the greater occipital nerve.[65] Evarts described a case of traumatic occipitoatlantal dislocation in which the patient, an 11-year-old boy, survived.[64] The case reported by Evarts demonstrated acute respiratory distress, stridor, and palsy of the sixth left cranial nerve, the left ninth cranial nerve, the left tenth cranial nerve, and both twelfth cranial nerves. He also had a left hemiparesis. Thus, he had both brain stem and cord involvement. A partial left lateral rectus paresis and a positive left Babinski persisted.[64] It is evident that with occipitoatlantal dislocation, a wide spectrum of neurologic abnormalities may be encountered from minimal involvement of the brain stem or proximal spinal cord to sufficient dysfunction resulting in immediate death.

Conservative management has succeeded in younger children, although surgical fusion was required in older children because of the difficulty in obtaining and maintaining reduction. The initial treatment of this dislocation is to relieve the respiratory distress by performing a tracheostomy, or by cervical traction. Care must be taken not to distract or increase the displacement with cervical traction. Monitoring the occipitoatlantal relationship with roentgenograms is vital. The patient should also undergo an occipitocervical fusion as early as possible.[66] The patient described by Evarts was eventually treated one month after the injury with a posterior spine fusion from the occiput to C3.[64]

Atlas Fractures. Statistics of atlas fractures in children are lacking. Weiss reported an atlas fracture in a 12-month-old child consequent to an automobile accident.[67] Indirect trauma usually causes these injuries. The overhanging occiput and multiple muscle layers protect the atlas, and fractures of this structure usually require axial transmission force through the skull to concentrate stresses directly on the atlantal components. Blows on the head by objects soft enough not to fracture the skull (e.g., falling into sand) may

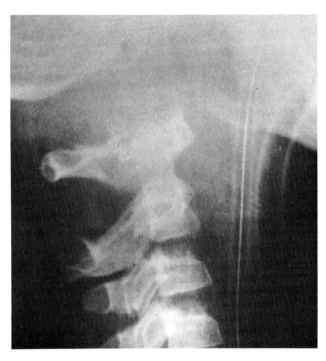

FIG. 14-19. Atlanto-occipital dislocation in a 14-year-old.

produce axial compression of the atlas by forcing the occipital condyles downward into the lateral masses of the atlas. If the lower cervical spine remains sufficiently rigid, the lateral masses displace centrifugally, albeit minimally (Figs. 14-20 and 14-21). The force may also comminute the lateral masses and detach or rupture the transverse ligament. Axial compression of the skull and cervical spine with hyperextension of the head can also shear the posterior arch of the atlas at its weakest point where it is grooved by the vertebral arteries just behind the lateral masses. Detachment of the posterior arch and atlas leaves it subjected to upward displacement by the posteroinferior oblique muscles, but the lateral masses are not displaced because they remain securely attached to the anterior arch.

Because of the oblique inward orientation of the occipital condyles, downward displacement of the skull has a bilateral chisel-like effect that causes a bursting fracture with variable displacement of the lateral masses of the atlas. Usually there is disruption of the atlas ring anteriorly and posteriorly. If the force is applied eccentrically there may only be single fractures. Spinal cord damage is uncommon in this injury.

Patients usually complain of a sense of instability, severe suboccipital discomfort, and pain, which may be the only symptoms. Pharyngeal soft tissue swelling and fat pad displacement are not usually prominent features.

Because of difficulties in visualizing this region in routine roentgenographic projections, other radiographic methods may be needed. CAT scanning, in particular, allows an excellent way of visualizing the entire ring, and is helpful in determining the extent of healing in follow-up evaluation (Fig. 14-21).[68]

Treatment should consist of a Minerva cast for approximately six months, followed by a cervical brace. Serial CAT scans allow assessment of progressive healing of the injury.

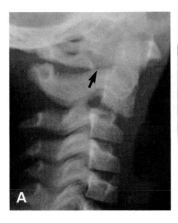
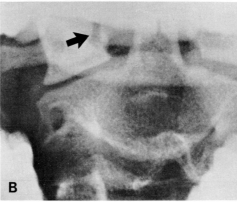
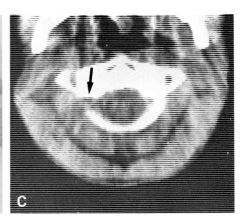

FIG. 14-20. C1 fracture. *A-B,* Lateral mass fracture (arrows) is evident on lateral and open mouth views. *C,* CAT scan shows the fracture clearly (arrow).

Subluxation of the Atlantoaxial Joint. Isolated atlantoaxial subluxation or dislocation is secondary to rupture of the transverse ligament or to inflammation such as tonsillitis, pharyngitis, or juvenile rheumatoid arthritis. Traumatic rupture of the transverse ligament is rare because the more vulnerable dens usually fails before the ligament.[69] In atlantoaxial dislocation, the atlas slides anteriorly, which increases the distance between the anterior arch of the atlas and dens. The maximum normal distance in flexion or neutral position in children is 3 mm, grading down to 2 mm at skeletal maturation. Pathologic inflammation produces increased laxity of the ligaments. There may be rotatory as well as anterior displacement.

The presenting symptom of patients with atraumatic subluxation is usually an isolated complaint of torticollis. Radiographic studies should be obtained in any youngster whose cervical spasm and pain do not remit rapidly with conventional therapy. In the most common type, anterior unilateral displacement, the head may be turned away from the affected side and neck movements are limited. Signs and symptoms of cord compression are infrequent. I have seen

one child who presented with infrequent apneic spells, and the diagnosis of severe atlantoaxial subluxation was made during pneumoencephalography.

Dewar and others described a condition of rotational strain of the atlantoaxial joint from comparatively minor injuries.[70] On rotation of the head, instead of the atlas moving on the axis, the two moved together. Fielding and Hawkins described 17 cases of irreducible atlantoaxial subluxation.[1] The striking features were delayed diagnosis and persistent clinical and roentgenographic deformities. All the patients presented with torticollis and restricted, often painful neck motion, and 7 young patients had longstanding deformity and flattening of one side of the face. They felt cineroentgenography was particularly helpful in making diagnosis.

Excessive mobility of the atlas and axis has also been reported.[1,71-74] This mobility may exist as an independent abnormality or it may exist with other regional malformations, such as Klippel-Feil syndrome.[75-80] The abnormally mobile atlantoaxial joint associated with a hypoplastic dens does not necessarily give rise to symptoms in the upper part

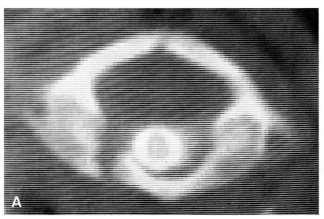
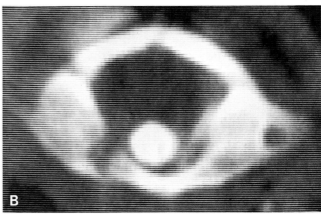

FIG. 14-21. Eight-year-old with neck pain following a fall on his head. *A,* CAT scan showed anterolateral and posterior fractures. *B,* Follow-up three months later showed healing of the posterior injury, and beginning osseous bridging of the anterior fracture.

of the cervical spine. Due to the absence of the dens, this excess mobility may be compatible with minimal, if any, risk, with the exception of acute trauma.

Rotatory subluxation of the atlantoaxial joint is a relatively common problem, particularly in a child with an upper respiratory infection, and differs from the fixed pattern mentioned previously. Associated hyperemia softens ligaments that support the upper cervical spine and makes the atlantoaxial joint unstable. Subluxation is produced by twisting the neck suddenly or rotating it beyond its normal range. The child presents with painful torticollis accompanied by marked spasm of the sternocleidomastoid muscle. He may support his head with his hands or may prefer to be recumbent. There is local tenderness of the atlantoaxial joint when the posterior aspect of the neck is palpated. Neurologic examination must rule out intraspinal lesions.

Rotatory fixation of the atlantoaxial joint may occur with a minor accident, such as a blow to the head or an automobile collision. The child complains of pain and stiffness in the neck and may have occipital neuralgia and torticollis.

Open mouth AP roentgenograms show that the dens is asymmetrically placed between the lateral articular masses of the atlas. Diagnosis is confirmed by a further open mouth view taken in various degrees of rotation. Roentgenograms disclose persistent asymmetry of the atlantoaxial joint in the open mouth view (Figs. 14-22 and 14-23) and may be the only evidence of this injury. It cannot be emphasized too strongly that correct diagnosis of traumatic displacement depends upon the analysis of a pair of true right-angle films of the atlas. The crucial observation on the lateral film is the distance of the dens from the anterior arch of the atlas. Overriding of the articular surfaces of the atlas is not signifi-

cant, since it can be produced by changing the angulation of the roentgenographic beam.

Rotatory deformities of the atlantoaxial joint are usually temporary and easily correctible. Treatment consists of continuous traction with a head halter. The subluxation may be reduced spontaneously within a few days, and the muscle spasm then subsides. In some cases, gentle reduction should be attempted, but only with the patient fully awake. One should never attempt to reduce this lesion with the patient under general anesthesia. After reduction the patient should be supported with a cervical collar, brace, or cast, depending on the etiology and severity of the injury.

In more severe injuries, treatment includes skull or halter traction followed by atlantoaxial arthrodesis, if necessary. Of 13 patients so treated, 11 showed good results, 1 showed fair results, and there was insufficient follow-up of the other patient. One other patient died while in traction as the result of cord transsection that was produced by further rotation of the atlas and the axis (despite traction).[81]

Only one reported patient sustained complete dislocation of C1 and C2 with no radiographic evidence of fracture and no neurologic deficit. Conservative treatment with a Minerva jacket in the reduced position failed and the patient underwent fusion of C1 and C2 three months after the original injury with satisfactory results. This patient was a seven-year-old and there was no long term follow-up.[17]

Dens Fracture. Fracture of the dens is rare in children who are less than 7 years old, and extremely rare in children less than 3 years of age.[17,82-84] Blockey and Purser reported 5 children less than 7 years old with fracture of the dens (2 of their own cases and 3 from literature).[23] Anderson, in a large series of dens fractures (60 patients), reported 5 between the ages of 3 and 6 years.[84] More recently, Gropper reported 5 children between 16 months and 5 years.[84] Although there is a high incidence of nonunion in adults, it is difficult to state how frequently this complication occurs in children.[85]

Cases of congenital absence of the dens have been reported frequently, and in some cases there were reports of trauma prior to definitive diagnosis. Other reports describe the disappearance of the central portion of the dens in the child.[56,86-88] In these cases, roentgenograms made shortly after injury revealed no fracture, whereas abnormalities were found when these patients were re-evaluated. Seimon's patients were 22 and 35 months old at the time of their injuries.[89]

Gwinn and Smith reported 27 cases of acquired and congenital absence of the dens.[90] In more than half of these patients there had been some antecedent trauma. Associated abnormalities of the cervical spine were present in 5 cases. Gillman described a case of congenital absence of the dens that was discovered after the patient sustained a head injury.[91] Freiberger suggested that not all cases of absence of the dens were congenital, but that some may be acquired due to unsuspected trauma.[3]

In most instances of dens fracture in children there is major trauma and most of these fractures are diagnosed readily on the basis of early roentgenograms (Figs. 14-24 to 14-26). However, swelling or widening of the retropharyngeal soft tissue space may be the only diagnostic sign in some young children.

There is a difference in the levels at which the axis fractures in the adult and in the young child (see Fig. 14-7). The

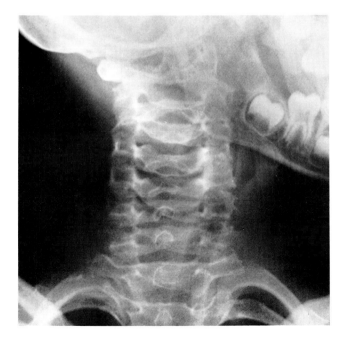

FIG. 14-22. Rotatory subluxation of C1 on C2 in a seven-year-old. This was gently "unlocked" by controlled traction with the patient awake. AP view of spine contrasts with lateral view of skull.

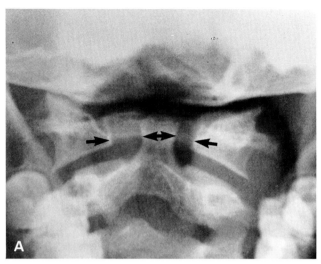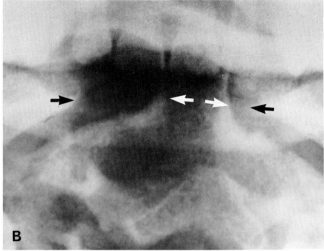

FIG. 14-23. Rotatory subluxation of C1 on C2 showing asymmetric dens—C1 distances. *A,* Mild rotation. Note widening on right (arrows). *B,* Moderate rotation. Note increased distance between dens (white arrows) and C1 (black arrows) on right side.

lateral radiograph shows that in the adult the fracture line usually lies at or above the level of the upper articular facets, whereas in the young child, the fracture line is well below the facets, in the body of the bone. In the lateral film, displacement of the dens can be recognized; the fracture line can be seen, but not the epiphyseal line. This means that it is likely that the fracture line propagates through the region of the epiphyseal plate, although it may involve bone on the dens side compatible with a type 1 or 2 growth mechanism fracture. Blockey believed that the dens fracture in young children was always an epiphyseal separation, which is probably a valid opinion.[23]

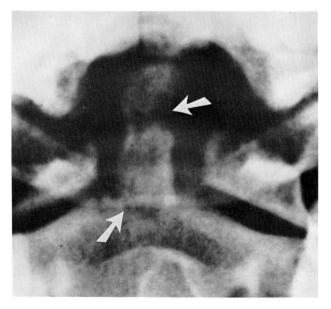

FIG. 14-24. Fracture of mid-dens as well as dentocentral interval (arrows).

Without question, this region is a bipolar growth plate. Ewald incorrectly stated that although the injury was considered an epiphyseal separation in the older literature, it cannot be considered a classic separation through the zone of hypertrophy "because there is no linear epiphyseal plate at that level."[4] However, it is likely that the fracture occurs through the primary spongiosa (the dens analogue of metaphyseal bone), like the type 2C injury of the phalanx, which is due to the increased amount of transversely oriented septae in this region. Blockey showed radiographs of thin sections of the dens and adjoining body of the axis and illustrated that the cortex is thinner with less cancellous trabeculation in the lower part at its junction to the body.[23] This is the site that appears to be the main area of fracture in the older child and young adult.

There is no diagnostic clinical syndrome for a dens fracture. The symptoms and signs may be so few and so indefinite that the diagnosis is missed. The immediate pain usually is severe and often referred to the occipital region; it may be accentuated in any attempt to move the head. The classic picture is of the child supporting his head with his hands in order to prevent the slightest movement. The neck may be held twisted to an acute torticollis or there may be a subluxation between C1 and C2. Displacement may be trivial. There may be little pain, but usually there is some stiffness in the neck.

According to Blockey, the most common neurologic complication is damage to the greater occipital nerve, giving referred pain to the occiput.[23] Obviously, the most serious complication is the immediate damage and potential for chronic damage to the spinal cord or medulla oblongata. One of the children in Blockey's series has pyramidal signs with absence of the abdominal reflexes and extensor plantar responses. None of these cases was associated with delayed onset paraplegia, although this was reportedly a potential complication in the adult.

Seimon presented two patients with dens fractures and described what he considered an important diagnostic clinical sign.[89] In each instance, injury to the cervical spine was suspected from the description of the trauma mechanics, but initial roentgenograms failed to reveal any fracture. The patients were comfortable when lying supine and when fully erect. Each child strongly resisted any attempt to extend his neck. This symptom was a valuable clinical sign when injury to the dens was suspected.

Open mouth views are significant, but lateral or AP tomography is also helpful (see Figs. 14-24 and 14-25). Care must be taken not to misinterpret the closing dentocentral synchondrosis as a fracture (see Fig. 14-5; also see Fig. 14-26).

Treatment in most cases should be conservative with strict bed rest, initial cervical traction, and a subsequent simple collar. With markedly displaced lesions, with or without neural deficit, treatment may have to be modified. Manipulation and the Minerva cast have been used, as well as skeletal traction followed by a halo cast. In older children and teenagers, the synchondrosis at the base of the dens is fused with the body of the axis, and injuries are the same as those of an adult. In general, basilar and apical fractures heal well when reduced and stabilized, whereas fractures of the dens above the level of the atlantoaxial articular facets tend to remain unstable and often require fusion.

The anteriorly displaced dens in younger children can usually be reduced easily by gentle manipulation into extension. The patient can be maintained with halo skeletal traction, tongs, and halter traction or Minerva jacket. The ease of reduction, stability with traction or plaster support, early callus formation, and prompt healing in most cases offer good prognosis in these patients, and surgical reduction or fusion rarely is necessary. The large size of the cervical canal relative to the spinal cord size at this level almost always contraindicates laminectomy. Furthermore, the level of fracture, which can often be through the body rather than the area of the synchondrosis, predisposes to more rapid healing in a child than in an adult.

Like epiphyseal separations in other parts of the body, the separated dens is purported to unite readily. In the 2 cases reported by Blockey, union occurred in 7 and 13 weeks and, at the end of 3 years, the clinical and radiologic appearances were normal.[23] This is in contrast to cases reported by others in which minimal to no evidence of a fracture was found, and eventuated in nonunion. These fractures in children above the age of 7 closely resembled those of adult type fractures.

Although there is a high incidence of pseudarthrosis or avascular necrosis in adults, this does not seem to be a serious complication in skeletally immature patients. Undisplaced fractures at the base of the dens within the substance of the body of the axis have a satisfactory potential for healing and can probably be treated conservatively. Fractures higher in the dens and displaced fractures, particularly those displaced posteriorly, have a much higher pseudarthrosis rate and usually require some type of fusion after reduction.

Price described an established nonunion in a four-year-old; it would seem that the disappearance of the central portion of the dens in acquired absence is a further example of nonunion and fibrous replacement of the bone.[84] Certainly, an untreated fracture through a cartilaginous plate in a mobile area of the body, such as the dens, may demonstrate all of the features of nonunion, especially if inadequately immobilized. If not seen radiographically, it does not necessarily mean that there is a loss of all tissue with a cystic defect. In a child, roentgenograms should be obtained about four months after suspected or definite dens fracture in order to demonstrate whether union has occurred or whether unforeseen problems have arisen.

In three reported cases in which injury of the dens was not recognized and treated, resorption of the basilar portion of the dens occurred, which produced the appearance of absence in one instance, and the appearance of an os odontoideum in the other two.[1] Thus, late atlantoaxial instability may complicate even a minimally displaced dens fracture, and follow-up must be accurate and maintained until the child stops growing.

Fractures of the Body and Neural Arches of the Axis. These fractures, compared to dens lesions or atlas fractures, are rare, and generally heal satisfactorily with non-operative treatment; however, congenital pseudarthroses may complicate diagnosis (Fig. 14-27).

Cervical Fracture-Dislocation. The remainder of the cervical spine, with the exception of pseudosubluxation, is less frequently involved in trauma. Compression fractures of the cervical spine centra are unusual in children.[92]

There usually is an associated disruption of the posterior ligaments that allows displacement. Posterior ligament disruption can often be recognized pre- or post-operatively from a lateral roentgenogram that demonstrates widening of the spaces between the posterior spinous processes.[93] At times this may be evident only with application of longitudinal traction; therefore, a lateral roentgenogram made with the patient in traction may be necessary to accurately diagnose whether the posterior ligaments are intact after injury to the immature cervical spine.

In younger children, reduction of a cervical fracture-dislocation with halter or skeletal traction usually suffices, and surgical stabilization is rarely necessary. This generally means 6 to 8 weeks in skeletal traction and a further 6 to 8 weeks in a brace or cast. Skeletal traction by any one of several devices is often difficult to maintain in young children because of the thin outer table of their skulls.[94] Using tantalum wire threaded between burr holes, as suggested by Matson, can be effective in treating children under 3 years of age.[95] The halo cast in small children has the advantage of rigid external fixation coupled with ease of application and ample surgical approach. Its use in 6 children aged 3½ to 10 years appears to be without significant complication.[96]

With either tongs or halo cast, meticulous attention to the sites of pin insertion is necessary to prevent superficial infection. Periodic roentgenograms of the skull are necessary for early detection of penetration of the inner table or osteomyelitis. Complaints of local pain should always suggest penetration of the inner table.

Stability is restored by ligamentous and chondro-osseous healing if the neck is held in reduced position. If subsequent roentgenographic examination suggests recurrent displacement, a two- to three-level *posterior* fusion with wires and bone grafts secures fixation in most instances. In young adolescents, spontaneous fusion at the fracture site is less likely, and in this age group fusion may be needed more often than in adults. The disturbance of the growth of the anterior centrum coupled with the disruption of the posterior ligaments may cause these injuries to remain unstable. Without fusion,

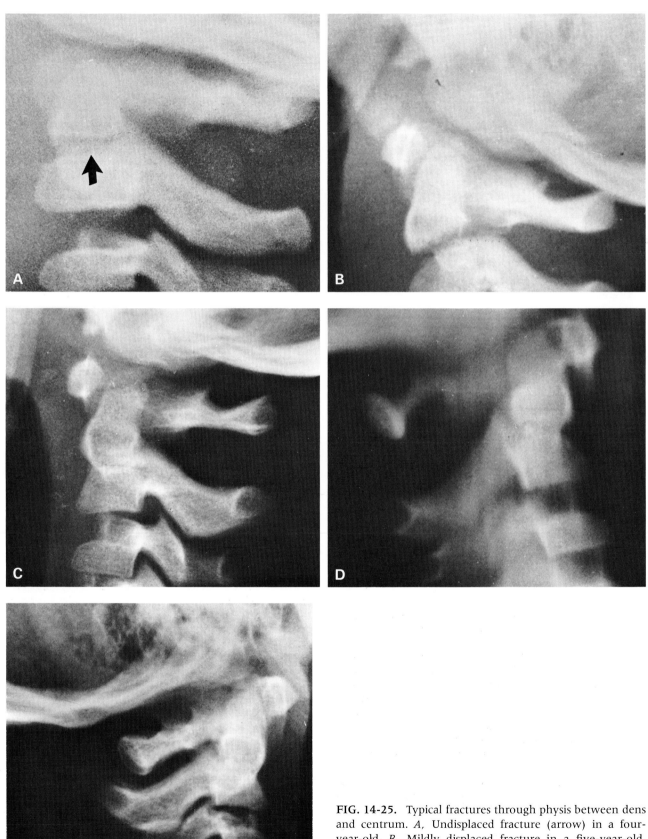

FIG. 14-25. Typical fractures through physis between dens and centrum. *A,* Undisplaced fracture (arrow) in a four-year-old. *B,* Mildly displaced fracture in a five-year-old. *C,* Fracture shown in *B* was treated by traction and healed rapidly. *D,* Slightly displaced fracture in a three-year-old. *E,* Appearance five years later of fracture shown in *D.*

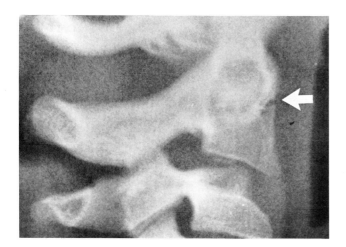

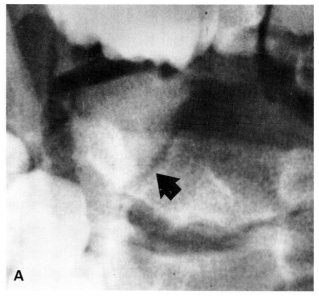

FIG. 14-26. Apparent fracture of dens (arrow). This is really the dentocentral synchondrosis remnant. The absence of retropharyngeal swelling should lead one to suspect a structural variation, not trauma.

these patients can possibly develop severe kyphotic deformities, thus worsening the neurologic deficit.

There are several ways that fracture dislocations of the cervical spine can be treated surgically. Controversy still surrounds the subject of whether decompression is useful. Decompression probably is *not* a significant factor in eventual restoration of function.

Restoring normal alignment is one major goal of treatment and stability is another. Non-operative treatment with skeletal traction and halo apparatus usually takes 8 to 12 weeks.[97] The addition of the posterior decompressive laminectomy, which is frequently done to relieve pressure in the damaged spinal cord, involves removing posterior ligaments and increases the degree of instability that may have been caused initially by the injury, leading to progressive angular deformity, with no documented evidence of significant restoration of neuromuscular function.

Stauffer and Kelly reported a series of 16 young patients treated by anterior dowel interbody fusion for fracture-dislocation of the cervical spine.[98] All 16 had post-operative instability with recurrent angular deformity and were shown to have disruption of the posterior ligaments. Of these patients, 3 had progressive neurologic deficit posteriorly. Stauffer and Kelly believed that anterior fusion should *not* be performed as the primary surgical treatment for fractures of the cervical spine in children, even when evidence of disruption existed.

There are several techniques of anterior interbody fusion, most of which were originally developed for treating degenerative cervical spine disease.[99,100] *These techniques are contraindicated in young children* (Fig. 14-28). Posterior approaches are more appropriate in the skeletally immature patient (Figs. 14-29 to 14-31).[101]

Combined anterior and posterior fusion have also been advocated. However, when the injury is primarily posterior, and the anterior longitudinal ligament is intact, as it usually is in the young child (in whom it is a thick structure), it probably is unwise to remove this ligament because it is the final stabilizing structure in a posterior to anterior disruption.

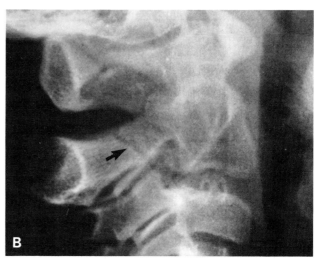

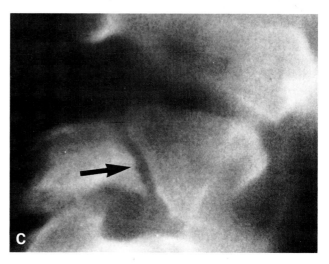

FIG. 14-27. *A-B,* Fracture of pedicle and lateral mass (arrows) of C2. *C,* Seemingly comparable case. However, this linear defect was present bilaterally and probably represented a congenital defect (arrow).

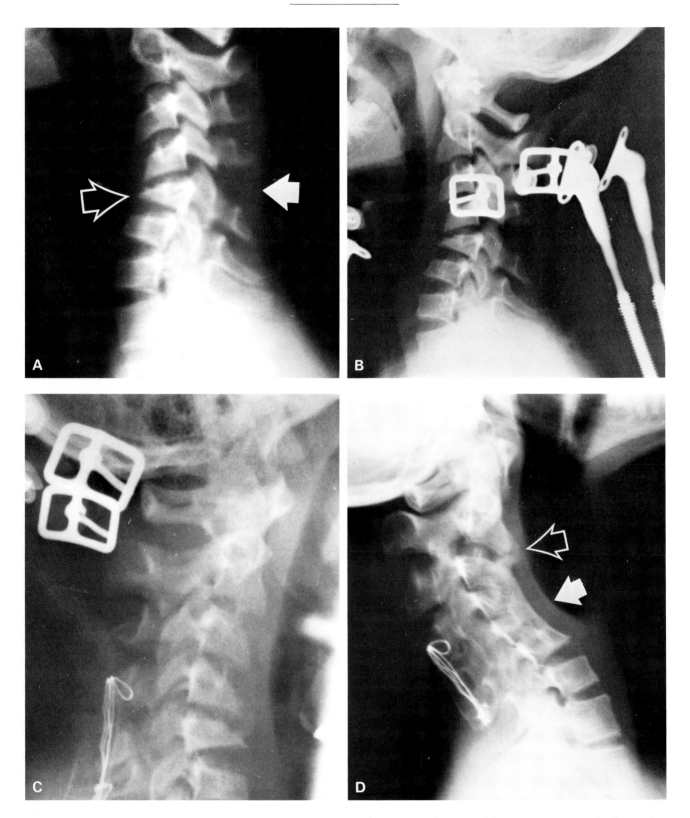

FIG. 14-28. *A,* Compression fracture of C5 (open arrow). Note the posterior widening (solid arrow), suggesting both anterior and posterior injury. *B,* Initial treatment in a brace failed to correct the deformity. *C,* This was then correctly stabilized by posterior interspinous wiring. *D,* However, it was felt that anterior fusion was also indicated. This procedure was not appropriate in such a skeletally immature individual. Surgical elevation of the anterior longitudinal ligament and the anterior vertebral cartilage to expose the incompletely developed central ossification caused fusion not only of C4 through C6 (solid arrow), but also of C2 and C3 (open arrow), leading to a major growth abnormality.

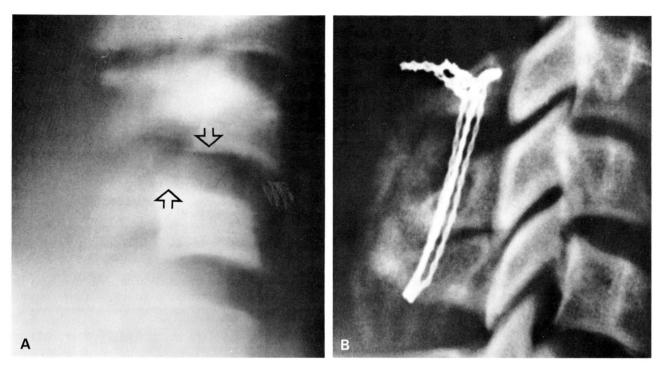

FIG. 14-29. *A,* Tomogram showing subluxation (arrows) of C4 on C5 following a hyperflexion injury. *B,* This was reduced and held by posterior interspinous wiring and bone graft.

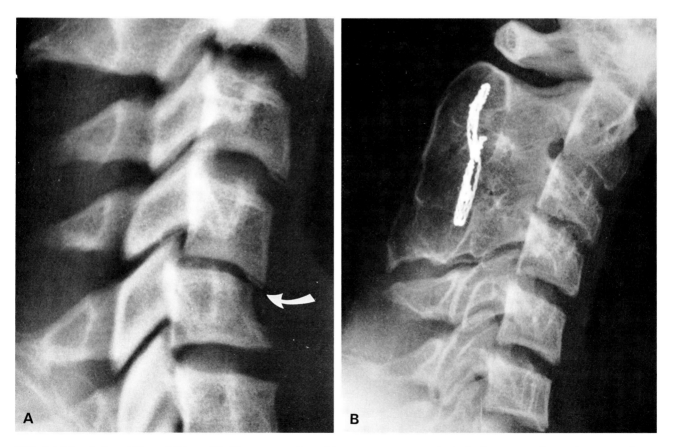

FIG. 14-30. *A,* Instability of C4 on C5. Note narrowing of interspace (arrow). *B,* A similar case with involvement of two intervertebral levels was treated by wiring of three spinous processes.

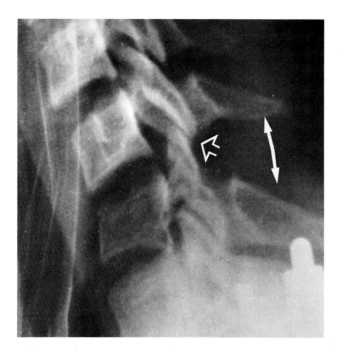

FIG. 14-31. C6-C7 disruption in automobile accident victim who had undergone previous Harrington instrumentation to T1 for scoliosis. Closed arrows show widening of spinous processes; open arrow shows facet joint disruption.

Treatment for fractures and fracture-dislocation of the cervical spine below the axis in children usually should *not* include laminectomy. As noted, the spinal cord injury frequently extends over several levels and decompression of one or two segments is inadequate unless there is active progression of the neurologic deficit. In addition, the multiple level laminectomy has adverse consequences from the standpoint of cervical spine stability in children, resulting in severe swan-neck deformity (Fig. 14-32).[102] If laminectomy has been performed, the facet joints should be stabilized subsequently with wiring and bone graft (Fig. 14-33).

Thoracic region

Injury to the vertebral elements in the thoracic region is rare. The intrinsic elasticity of the region, coupled with the protective effect of the rib cage to prevent excessive translational movements, minimize the abnormal stresses necessary to cause fracture or dislocation. In the thoracic region, especially in younger children, injury to the spinal cord occurs more often without associated vertebral fracture (Fig. 14-34). The thoracic cord appears more susceptible to injury because of its relatively narrow canal and potentially tenuous blood supply.

A relatively rare cause of thoracic spinal cord dysfunction in a child is blunt trauma to the abdomen. This usually relates to interference with the abdominal aorta and its branches, particularly the artery of Adamkiewicz, which arises at T11 (usually from the right side), and is a particularly important feeder to the spinal cord. Most patients with this condition have complete and permanent interruption of cord function.

Wedge fractures of the vertebral bodies, usually of minor degree, are relatively common (Figs. 14-35 and 14-36). As opposed to adults, the intrinsic elasticity in children allows these injuries to occur without major damage to the posterior elements, thus causing an intrinsically more stable injury. The posterior and anterior longitudinal ligaments are usually intact.

Ruckstuhl described a series of 26 children and adolescents with a total of 65 vertebral fractures.[103] Most of the fractures occurred in the midthoracic spine, and generally involved several vertebral levels. Fractures of the vertebral body with sagittal wedge deformity alone had a better prog-

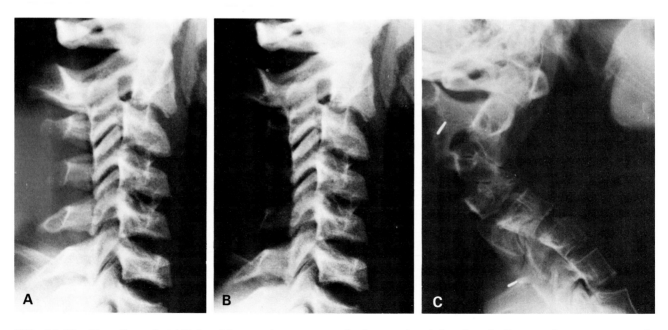

FIG. 14-32. Resection of stabilizing fulcrum elements may lead to major deformity. *A,* Preoperative appearance. *B,* Appearance after performance of a multiple laminectomy. *C,* Swan-neck deformity four years later.

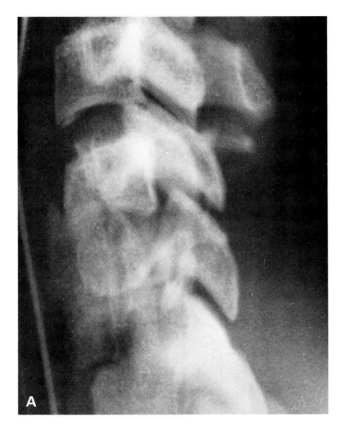

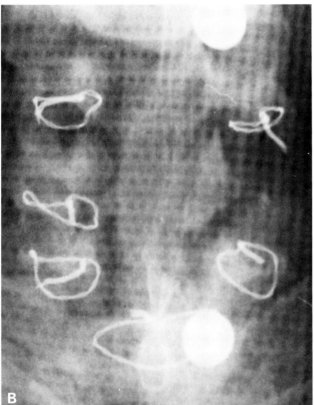

FIG. 14-33. *A,* Similar decompressive laminectomy. *B,* This was treated by immediate facet wire stabilization and bone graft.

nosis than those with concomitant sagittal frontal wedge deformities. Those in the first group tend to correct themselves partially or completely during subsequent growth, but improvement in the wedge deformity is present in only about one third of the patients in the second group. When the end plates were fractured there was no correction, and there was a distinct lack of vertebral growth. Severe destruction of the cartilaginous end plates and intervertebral disc led to a fusion of the corresponding segments, and an increase in wedge deformity was observed twice. Slight axial deviations of the intervertebral discs following vertebral body fractures were compensated for during growth in most cases. In comminuted fractures, the axial deviation is persistent, but could be compensated for by the adjacent segments of the spine. Unstable fractures were found difficult to control even with a Milwaukee corset.

The most common mechanism of injury causing unstable fractures in the thoracolumbar or lumbar spine is a rotation or flexion-rotation force. The majority of these injuries result from vehicular accidents. Falls from a height and sporting accidents are less common causes. Inability to walk and moderate to severe back and abdominal pain are common. Lower extremity pain, with or without neurologic symptoms, occur in at least half of the patients. Abrasions and contusions of the back are often present and are important in determining the mechanism of injury. For example, a patient complaining of back pain with an abrasion over the scapula probably has sustained trauma transmitting a rotation force to the spine. Palpation of the back may reveal muscle spasm.

Injuries secondary to flexion-rotation result in classic fracture-dislocations of the thoracolumbar and lumbar spine (Figs. 14-37 and 14-38). Anteroposterior and lateral roentgenograms show fractures of the articular processes, a lateral shift of the spinous process, increased interspinous distance, and forward displacement of the superior vertebral fragment.

Injury secondary to hyperflexion results in an anterior wedge compression fracture of the vertebral body. Most of these fractures occur in the combined thoracic and lumbar areas more commonly than fractures localized only to the lumbar spine. In children, compression of two or more vertebrae occurs more frequently than a single vertebral compression.

The presence of a healthy intervertebral disc in combination with well-mineralized bone is likely responsible for the finding of multiple anterior compression fractures. When normal disc turgor is present, the force applied to the spine can be transmitted from one vertebral body to the other. The "normal" intervertebral disc also might explain the rarity of the disc space narrowing and the absence of spontaneous interbody fusion in this group of children.

Physical examination commonly fails to reveal decreased mobility or abnormal neuromuscular findings. On inspection, spinal deformity is rare, although scoliosis, excessive lordosis, and kyphosis may be seen following severe compression fractures. When present, these deformities are usually seen in children who are past puberty at the time of injury. Whether this is a direct result of the injury or represents a variation seen in the normal population has not been determined.

Inspection of the back frequently reveals abrasions and contusions, which give a clue to the mechanism of injury.

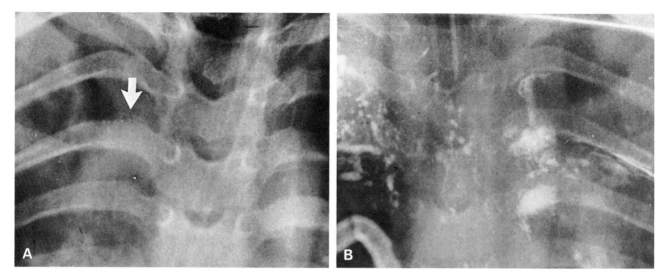

FIG. 14-34. Three-year-old child struck by a car. He was rendered paraplegic immediately. *A,* Initial roentgenogram did not show a major spinal fracture. However, careful observation along the ribs suggested avulsion fractures at the costotransverse junctions (arrow). *B,* Myelography showed extravasation of dye along the disrupted spinal nerve roots.

Palpation often elicits tenderness of the paravertebral musculature and spinous processes; however, a palpable widening of the interspinous distance does not occur. Neurologic symptoms and objective neuromuscular findings are typically absent. Excluding rib fractures, associated injuries are not helpful in diagnosis and often contribute to a delay in treatment.

Careful neurologic evaluation determines the presence of spinal cord or nerve root injury. Since the end of the spinal cord lies opposite the lower border of the first lumbar verte-

bra, fractures below this level only cause nerve root injury. With fractures at the thoracolumbar region, however, special attention is needed to determine whether complete or incomplete division of the spinal cord, with or without nerve root involvement, has occurred. Complete loss of voluntary power, and loss of sensation in all areas supplied by the sacral segment in association with a bulbocavernosus or anal skin reflex, indicate a complete division of the spinal cord.

Anterior-posterior radiographs almost always reveal scoliosis following a hyperflexion injury. The scoliosis is typically

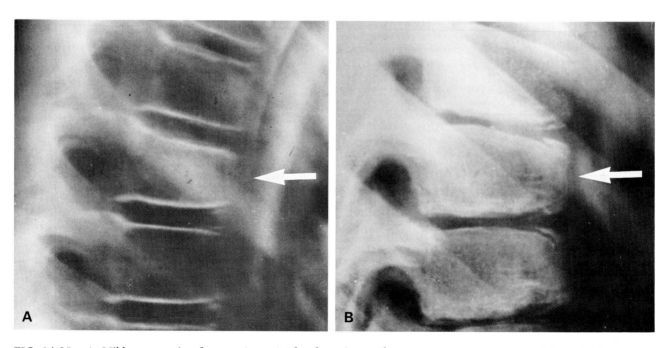

FIG. 14-35. *A,* Mild compression fracture (arrow) of a thoracic vertebra. *B,* Appearance one year later, with beginning reconstitution of anterior height (arrow).

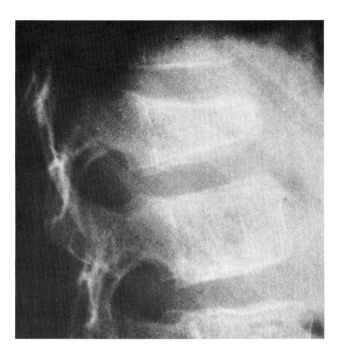

FIG. 14-36.   Crush fracture of T12.

a balanced thoracolumbar curve with the apex at the fractured area. The deformity is less than 10° and only slightly progressive.

Instability of the spine after injury depends upon the degree of damage to the posterior elements—osseous, ligamentous, or both. If these posterior structures remain intact, the fracture is probably stable. When fracture of the articular processes or rupture of the posterior ligaments occurs, the injury is potentially unstable. A fracture is grossly unstable when the posterior elements are completely disrupted and vertebral body displacement and dislocations are present by roentgenographic examination.

Simple bed rest is indicated, since most children with hyperflexion compression fractures are asymptomatic within a few weeks. If concern exists regarding the degree of vertebral compression, the development of ileus, or the care of associated injuries, treatment is best accomplished in the hospital. Reduction by postural or operative methods is not necessary, since these methods have been shown to make no significant difference in the end result. External support is generally not needed. Activity is initiated and gradually increased, depending upon the patient's symptoms. Traumatic ileus may accompany even minor injury.

Initial treatment of thoracic injury should consist of bed rest until the patient has complete relief of pain. Spica cast immobilization for two months should follow. Prognosis is excellent for full recovery. Early spinal fusion is rarely necessary in this region in a child, but should be considered in those cases with some residual instability.

Follow-up through spinal skeletal maturity is imperative to assess potential delayed development of scoliosis or kyphosis due to end plate damage (type 5 physeal injury). An acquired "bar" may form and lead to a situation analogous to an uncompensated congenital scoliosis (see Fig. 14-17).

In patients with unstable injuries, with or without paralysis, this same potential for growth and development, com-

bined with the instability of the fracture, can lead to a rapidly progressive spinal deformity.

Follow-up radiographs following compression fractures of the immature spine show varying degrees of restoration of vertebral body height. The extent of restoration is directly related to the severity of the fracture and the age of the patient at the time of injury. In children under 10 years of age with moderate compression injuries, reconstitution of the vertebral body is generally complete. Indeed, repair infrequently leads to vertebral body overgrowth. Children with severe fractures, or those injured when older, usually show some permanent asymmetrical wedging of the vertebral bodies with concave end plates, and deformity of the anterior contour of the bodies.

Although many varied and subtle differences exist between the child's and the adult's response to spinal trauma, the primary differences result from the presence of epiphyses and normal intervertebral discs. The ability of the immature spine to remodel the vertebral body and produce overgrowth is unique in some instances. This process appears to be limited to the portion of the body injured and is not associated with posterior element overgrowth. This restoration or increase in the growth of the vertebral body height is probably the result of an increase in the local vascularity, which stimulates epiphyseal growth. Undoubtedly, this process is responsible for the virtual absence of kyphotic deformity in patients with multiple thoracic compression fractures.

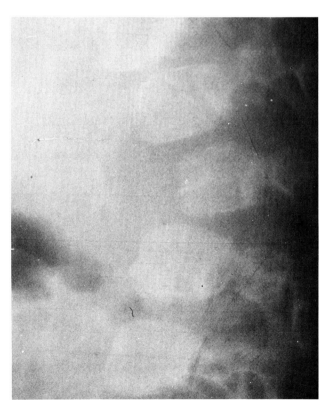

FIG. 14-37.   Hyperflexion injury in a three-year-old with generalized ligamentous laxity. T12 is anteriorly subluxated on L1. In contrast, L1 is posteriorly subluxated on L2. All four facet joints from T12 to L2 are displaced.

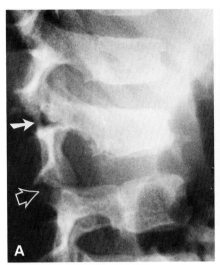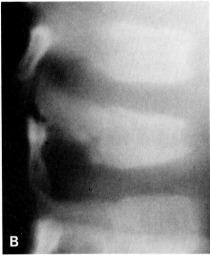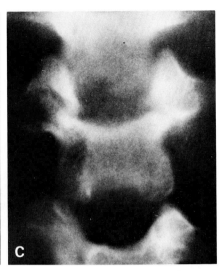

FIG. 14-38. *A*, Hyperflexion injury in a four-year-old. T12 is anteriorly crushed, but more importantly, it has a posterior (pedicle) fracture (solid arrow) as well as facet disruption (open arrow). *B*, Lateral tomogram shows the fracture and dislocation. *C*, The anterior tomogram accentuates disruption of both facet joints.

Lumbar region

The lumbar region is infrequently involved in significant injury, at least until the adolescent period, when the developing spine assumes more of the biomechanical characteristics of the adult spine. Minor and moderate wedge fractures may be seen at all levels (Figs. 14-39 and 14-40). The region is capable of greater translation and fracture-dislocation is more common (Figs. 14-41 and 14-42), thus increasing the likelihood of significant spinal cord injury.[104] Physeal (end plate) fractures may involve the lumbar spine during adolescence.[105]

Burst fractures may occur in the lumbar area. The mechanism of injury is a compression force transmitted directly along the line of the vertebral bodies. One of the end plates is ruptured, and the disc is forced into the body of the vertebra, causing it to burst. The posterior elements usually remain intact; therefore, this fracture is stable. A fragment of the vertebral body or disc extending posteriorly, compromising the spinal canal, can cause neurologic damage (Figs. 14-41 and 14-42).

Lumbar injuries may be associated with lap seat belts. Tension stress is primarily responsible for these injuries. Since the fractures are characterized by disruption of the posterior elements, they are potentially unstable. Injuries that are secondary to tension result in longitudinal separation of the posterior elements. Minimal, if any, anterior compression of the involved vertebral body occurs. Lateral or forward displacement of the superior vertebral fragment or vertebra is also common. Typically the injury is localized between the first and third lumbar vertebrae. The history and physical examination do not vary significantly from those of patients with flexion-rotation injuries with one exception—abdominal contusion caused by a seat belt, which can lead to a temporary paralytic ileus.

Isolated fractures that involve the neural arch, facet, or transverse process account for the remainder of stable injuries. The most common mechanism of injury is a direct blow.

Facet and neural arch fractures are best treated with an external support until evidence of healing is obtained by clinical and radiographic evaluation. With fractures of the transverse process, external support may or may not be used, dependent on the patient's discomfort with activity.

Postural reduction is the best method of initial treatment. Pillows, sandbags, pelvic slings, and various traction techniques can be used, depending upon the availability of equipment and the type of fracture.

The effect of initial treatment on the injury must be carefully and frequently assessed by neurologic and radiographic examination. Changes are made in the patient's posture until reduction is achieved. If reduction of the fracture is not adequate by postural methods, gentle manipulation with or without anesthesia is indicated. If the fracture remains unreduced following manipulation, open reduction must be considered.

Patients with minimal or no neurologic injury can usually be fitted with external supports and allowed to ambulate if acceptable reduction has been maintained for a period of 3 to 6 weeks. Paravertebral callus, when seen on roentgenographic examination, is helpful in determining the stability of the fracture and the time when external supports may be discontinued. Most fractures become intrinsically stable at 12 weeks; flexion and extension films should be obtained at this time.

In prepubertal children, supports should be well-padded, removable, and utilized until the majority of spinal growth has occurred (14 years in girls and 16 years in boys). This approach usually prevents progressive spinal deformity.

If non-operative treatment fails because of gross instability or progressive spinal deformity results, operative fusion is indicated. The surgical procedure—anterior, posterior, or combined—as well as the type of internal fixation utilized, is best determined on an individual basis, and with consideration of the skill of the surgeon.

Unstable lesions must be fused and intrinsically stabilized when necessary with compression or distraction rods (Fig.

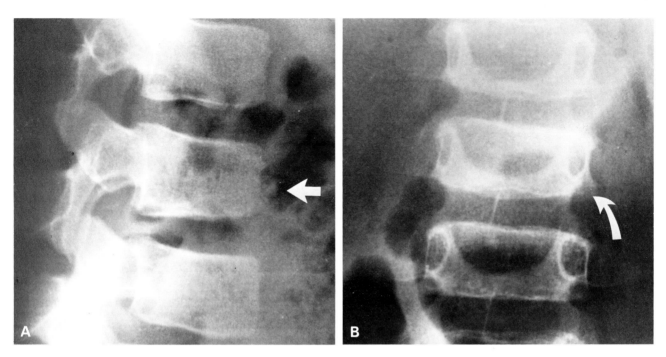

FIG. 14-39. *A,* Lateral view of mild compression fracture of L.2 (arrow). *B,* Anteroposterior view showing asymmetric crush (arrow). This may lead to asymmetric growth and scoliosis.

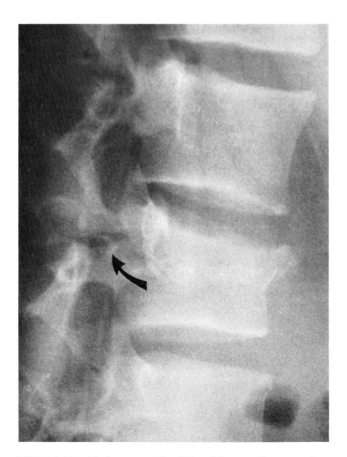

FIG. 14-40. Moderate crush of L3, with posterior extension (arrow).

14-43). Any nerve root impingement must be released by appropriate decompression of the neuroforamina. Post-operative immobilization in a spica cast that includes at least one leg is imperative. Close follow-up of possible growth deformity is essential, particularly if the child is just entering the adolescent growth spurt.

The decision regarding whether or not internal fixation by either bone graft, wire, plates, rods, or some combination of these methods is indicated depends on many factors, among them the degree of instability, malalignment, and the necessity for decompression of the spinal canal or removal of bone fragments. Fracture dislocations at the dorsolumbar junction are always highly unstable, and it is generally agreed that early fusion is the treatment of choice in these cases.[13] Whether or not early operative intervention has any role in the treatment of injuries believed to be total and complete at impact remains controversial. Operative intervention is always indicated when there is progression of the neurologic deficit associated with partial cord injury.

Patients with significant residual neurologic deficit, with or without severe spinal deformity, continue to require special care in order to obtain maximal independence in the community. Physical findings of decreased mobility and neuromuscular abnormalities are directly proportional to the extent of the residual structural and neurologic damage.

Lumbosacral region

The regions of major motion capacity change—thoracolumbar and lumbosacral junction—may be sites of increased susceptibility to injury, often seemingly innocuous at onset. This is especially true at the lumbosacral junction, where anatomic variations may predispose to debilitating pain.

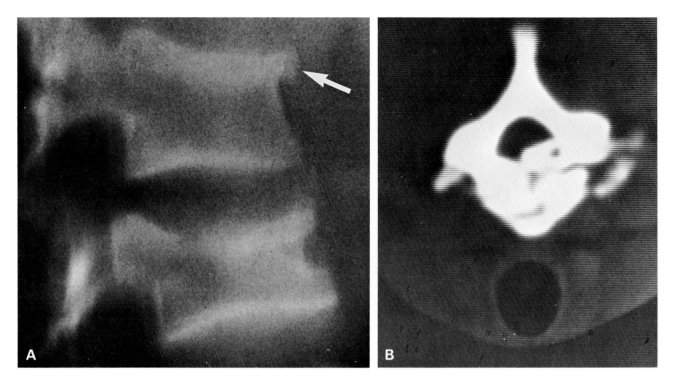

FIG. 14-41. *A,* Mild crush of superior plate of L2 (epiphyseal injury—arrow) and a more severe crush of L3 with posterior displacement of fragment. *B,* CAT scan shows fragmentation of body and extrusion of posterosuperior fragment into the spinal canal.

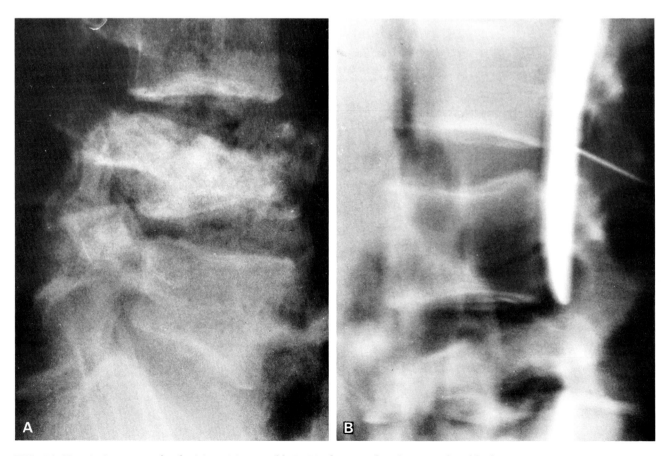

FIG. 14-42. *A,* Severe crush of L4 in a 14-year-old. *B,* Myelogram showing complete block.

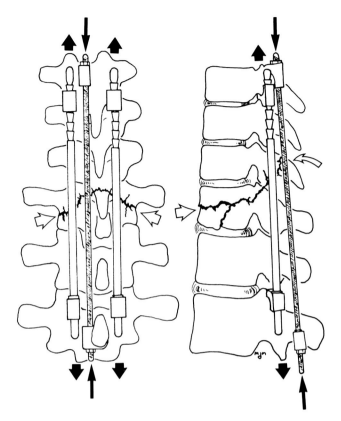

FIG. 14-43. Schematic of compression/distraction rod stabilization of severe lumbar fractures. This method may be used in adolescents.

A rare injury involves facet dislocation at the L5-S1 junction.[106] This pattern is usually associated with cervical injury, but may also occur in the thoracolumbar junction and lumbar vertebrae. The cervical facet obliquity predisposes to subluxation, but the lumbar facets are more vertical. Disruption of part of the facet joints by fracture probably contributes to the injury mechanism. Rolander pointed out that experimental end plate fractures are extremely difficult to visualize.[105]

A somewhat controversial topic is "traumatic" spondylolysis.[107] Wiltse believes that most, if not all, cases of spondylolysis represent a stress fracture through the pars interarticularis (Fig. 14-44).[68] Jackson and Wiltse described the condition in young athletes (adolescents).[108] In a study of 100 female gymnasts, 11 had radiologically evident spondylolysis, 6 of whom also had at least a grade one spondylolisthesis (Fig. 14-45). Of the 89 without radiologic disease, 19 had episodic lumbar pain. Low back pain in any young athlete should be a warning sign. A negative lumbosacral spine series (which must include oblique views) does not necessarily rule out a developing pars defect. A [99m]technetium bone scan is a valuable tool for diagnosing these lesions. If spondylolysis is present, restriction of vigorous athletic activity is essential until the lesion has healed.

Scheuermann's disease

The exact etiology of this disease, which primarily affects the thoracic spine more than the lumbar spine and may lead to significant kyphosis, is unknown.[109] Alexander recently proposed that the disease is a traumatic stress spondylodystrophy sequential upon traumatic growth arrest and end plate fractures (perhaps single and microscopic) that occurs during the heightened vulnerability phase of the adolescent growth spurt.[110] Once one fracture has occurred, an insidious compounding of the deformity ensues, with adjacent vertebrae being affected by abnormally applied static loads, which causes pathologic stress failure that increases in the anterior region (Fig. 14-46). He further believes that this anterior growth failure and irregular ossification is like the Osgood-Schlatter lesion, although I think the lucency and metaphyseal cyst of Legg-Calvé-Perthes disease might be a more appropriate analogy. Treatment should be symptomatic for mild deformity and a Milwaukee brace used for more severe deformation.

Disc herniation

Acute herniated discs are unusual in children under 16 years of age (Fig. 14-47).[111-115] Trauma appears to play an important etiologic role in lumbar disc herniation in the child or adolescent. This may involve contact sports, a fall, or an automobile injury. Noncontact sports, such as weight-

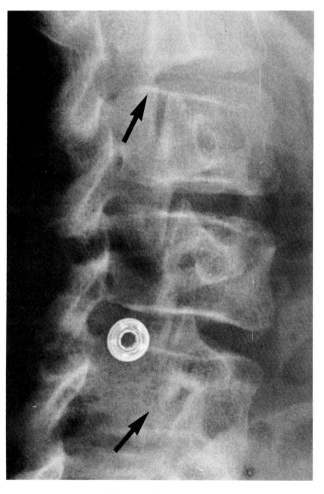

FIG. 14-44. Spondylolysis of L3 and L5 (arrows) in a young gymnast.

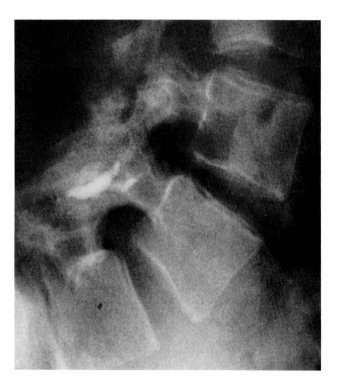

FIG. 14-45. Increased lumbosacral angle in a 12-year-old boy with grade 1 spondylolisthesis, which was due to a congenital deficiency of the sacral spinous processes.

lifting, have also been implicated.[116] There may be an accompanying fracture of a portion of the vertebral end plate (Fig. 14-48) due to the dense attachments of the annulus, and this structure rather than the disc may be the actual cause of any block.[116] It is uncommon for children with lumbar disc (or end plate) protrusions to have the usual signs and symptoms associated with the comparable adult disease. Low back pain, limitation of motion on forward flexion, a peculiar gait, and limitation of straight-leg raising are outstanding signs. Pain is not a prominent complaint and neurologic findings are rare. Be aware of congenital deformities of the posterior elements.

Sacrum and coccyx

These injuries are infrequent and are usually produced by direct violence. They are difficult to recognize radiographically because of the patterns of ossification in the region. Treatment should be symptomatic. Separation of the sacroiliac joint is covered in Chapter 15.

Late Sequelae

The late onset of progressive neurologic deficit is associated generally with extension of a post-traumatic syringomyelia, or the development of a kyphosis or scoliosis with associated cord injury.[15] Both lesions are surgically correctable, and early diagnosis is indicated to avoid further extension of an already disabling injury.

The effects of acquired neuromyogenic disorders, which

have to be considered in pathogenic mechanisms, are determined by the level and degree of spinal cord injury and the age of the patient at the time of injury. The relentless progression of spinal deformity in the untreated pediatric patient with acquired paraplegia exemplifies the effects of asymmetric muscle tension and spasm, fascial contraction, chronic posturing, and gravity on the unsupported growing spine. Almost any combination of deformities is possible. Pelvic obliquity, which may result from contracture above and below the pelvis, makes treatment even more difficult.

Deformity, per se, is not an indication for surgery except in an immature patient with a progressive post-traumatic deformity despite bracing, or a deformity greater than 40°.[99] The goals of surgical treatment are to prevent increasing deformity and its sequelae, to relieve the symptoms of mechanical instability, to improve spinal alignment through correction of the deformity, and to reverse or at least halt increasing neurologic dysfunction.

In scoliosis due to acquired paraplegia, the principles and techniques of Harrington instrumentation are applicable. If there is also pelvic obliquity and lumbar kyphosis or lordosis, the fusion mass must extend proximally at least two levels above the injury and distally as an intertransverse process fusion of the sacrum. Harrington instrumentation may have to be supplemented with Dwyer instrumentation. It may be necessary to release lumbodorsal fascia, the ilio-tibial band, or periarticular hip joint contractures pre-operatively.

The patient with loss of sensation following cord injury is uniquely vulnerable to the development of decubiti. Irreversible local necrosis may be seen after only three to four hours. The use of an alternating air, egg shell, or other mattress designed to distribute pressure areas is helpful in preventing decubiti, but the single most important factor is frequent turning and good skin care.

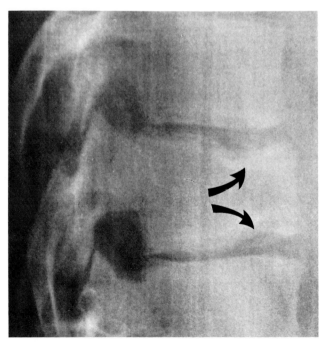

FIG. 14-46. Scheuermann's disease of vertebral end plates (arrows).

myelotomy and section of the anterior roots have not been consistently useful in this condition.[119,120] No pharmacologic agent is yet available that has proved to be useful in the more difficult cases. Variable success has been reported with a variety of agents in the less severe forms of the disorder.

Physical therapy is aimed at maximizing function by preventing contractures, and by the use of braces and assistive devices. In general, physical therapy should be combined with a program of occupational therapy aimed at making the child independent in the activities of daily life. Early enrollment in a rehabilitation program is instrumental in the child's rapid return to his family and community.

Obvious causes of treatment failure include incomplete reduction, incorrect assessment of stability with resultant insufficient quality and duration of spinal orthotic protection, and neglect of patients with skeletally stable injuries, but a cord deficit.

Growth Problems

Although injury to the vertebral column that results in cord damage is not common in the young child or adolescent, when it does occur the problems of continuing growth upon subsequent behavior of the fractured vertebral column must be considered. The normal growth rate slows to a steady rate after the age of three until the growth spurt of puberty. Griffiths followed a boy who initially had a cervical injury at the age of eight years with an incomplete Brown-Séquard lesion.[121] His initial injury was a flexion type with fractures through the vertebral bodies of C3, C4, and C5. Approximately two years later, he began to show evidence of a kyphotic deformity. Four years after the injury, his gait pattern was deteriorating and both of his legs showed increasing spasm. Again, a further degree of kyphosis was noted. Surgery was refused. Post-mortem examination showed well-preserved discs spaced with no evidence of anterior callus formation compatible with an attempt at spontaneous fusion. On the basis of the experience in this case,

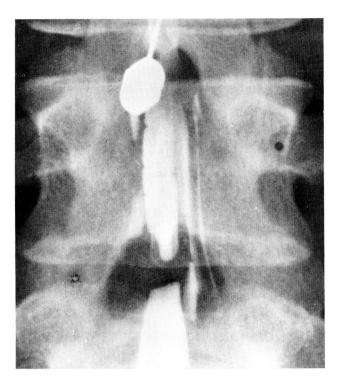

FIG. 14-47. Positive myelogram for herniated disc in a 13-year-old girl who had acute onset of back pain without any radiculopathy.

Development of a decubitus may delay rehabilitation by weeks or months. The injury frequently occurs in the first few hours after admission when the attention of the medical and nursing staff may be directed to other matters. Early and continued attention to this important parameter of nursing care provides incalculable benefit for long term management of these patients.

Spinal cord injury associated with spinal shock always produces urinary retention and overdistention, which can be avoided by using an indwelling catheter. Recovery from spinal shock is accompanied by the development of autonomic micturition. If urinary tract infection has been avoided and sphincter tone remains intact, i.e., the level of injury is above S2, then intermittent catheterization has proved to be a valuable means of achieving social continence. The older, paraplegic child can be instructed in self-catheterization. For the quadraplegic and younger paraplegic, instructing a family member, usually the mother, has been accomplished with relative ease. The low rate of urinary tract infection associated with intermittent catheterization has been well documented.[93] Pharmacologic and surgical methods are available that increase bladder capacity without causing loss of external sphincter tone.[117,118] Such procedures may enable the child to attend a full day of school without undue concern. Bowel control is relatively easy to accomplish by means of diet and the use of suppositories. The complication of flexor spasm frequently seen in patients with high cord injury is due to facilitation of local reflexes. Overflow into visceral channels may also produce a "mass reflex" phenomenon. This remains one of the least understood areas of spinal cord injury management. Dorsal

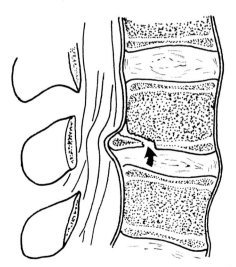

POSTERIOR DISPLACEMENT

FIG. 14-48. Schematic of posterior epiphyseal injury that may mimic a disc.

Griffiths subsequently treated fractures with an anterior cervical fusion when he confronted them in the young adolescent. However, I would strongly disagree. Posterior fusion is a more appropriate approach in the skeletally immature individual. The posterior elements are relatively mature in midchildhood, whereas the anterior end plates may grow until late adolescence.

Scoliosis following hyperflexion injury is probably also due to open epiphyses. The development of scoliosis is most likely related to unequal compression of the vertebra body end plates. This probably causes an incomplete cessation of longitudinal growth or asymmetric stimulation of epiphyseal growth. These processes can continue for approximately one year. This finite slowing or stimulation of osseous development in the patient who has a stable spinal fracture without neuromuscular deficit also explains why it is only mildly progressive.

Following management of the acute spinal cord injury episode, the orthopaedist's primary concern should be preventing subsequent spinal deformity (see Fig. 14-17). In a detailed review of 64 juvenile patients who were followed for more than 6 months after injury, spinal deformity, scoliosis, kyphosis, or lordosis were noted in approximately 91% of the patients. The experience was that girls up to 12 years and boys up to 14 years who had cervical or thoracic injuries developed significant spinal deformity with pelvic obliquity. This can lead to loss of sitting balance, requiring use of the upper extremities for trunk support, pressure sores on the ischium, and subluxation or dislocation on the high side of the pelvis. Children with lumbar lesions were less apt to develop spinal deformity. The majority of the scoliotic patients had complete lesions and almost all those with incomplete lesions had minimal return of function. Scoliosis was the most frequent primary spinal deformity noted. Kyphosis, when present, was generally thoracolumbar, and lordosis was either thoracolumbar or lumbar. Pelvic obliquity did not accompany primary kyphosis or lordosis. When seen with the scoliosis, it frequently was severe and impaired sitting balance. Non-operative treatment of spinal deformity employing external support should be initiated when the potential for spinal deformity exists. In young children, this would be prior to radiologic evidence of fixed deformity.

In addition to treating the deformity, bracing improves function by restoring sitting balance and freeing the upper extremities for activities other than trunk support. Any orthoses must be well padded to protect the anesthetic skin, easily removable to allow frequent skin checks, and easily adjustable to allow for growth. Campbell and Bonnett found that a modified Milwaukee brace was the best orthosis for this and used it in all patients with spinal lesions above T10.[122] For the levels below T10 they used a removable axillary-level, high-body jacket. Non-operative treatment was more apt to be successful in the older child with a scoliotic deformity that was subtle than in the patient with only kyphosis. Failure was seen in the uncooperative patient and those with moderate or severe spasticity.

When there is radiologic evidence of progressive spinal deformity in the growing child receiving non-operative treatment, surgery should be considered. Of the patients in the Rancho study who were skeletally immature and had complete or incomplete lesions, 50% required surgery.[122] For scoliosis, posterior spinal fusion with Harrington instrumentation was the surgical procedure of choice. Uniformly the fusion must extend to the sacrum to prevent pelvic obliquity, which is a consistent finding in those patients with fixed scoliosis. Instrumentation of the lumbosacral joint with either the transsacral bar or enlarged sacral alar hook was desirable. The Rancho study stated a preference for the sacral hook. Because of problems with correction of deformities, they also recommend pre-operative halo-femoral traction. Pseudarthroses were common, indicating the need for extensive lateral exposure and decortication to the tips of the transverse processes. They also used Knodt rods when operating on extremely small children in whom Harrington instrumentation was not satisfactory.

In progressive kyphosis, when the deformity exceeds 60° and appears rigid, they recommend anterior spinal fusion at the apex of the deformity followed several weeks later by a posterior spinal fusion with Harrington instrumentation with compression rods.[117] This decision was based upon the frequent observation of loss of correction or pseudarthroses at the apex of the kyphotic deformity when one procedure alone was relied upon. Progressive lordotic deformity, which generally includes the lumbosacral joint, can be satisfactorily corrected and stabilized employing posterior spinal fusion with Harrington instrumentation. However, when lordosis is severe or greater than 100°, rigid anterior spinal fusion with the Dwyer method is probably a better approach, but it must be appended with a posterior fusion, since anterior extension to the sacrum is not possible.

Great care must be taken to carefully observe the hips so that subluxation or dislocation does not occur. Myelotomy may be beneficial in relieving some of the spasticity that contributes to these structural contractures.[119]

References

1. Fielding J. W., and Hawkins, R. J.: Atlanto-axial rotatory fixation. J. Bone Joint Surg., *59-A:*37, 1977.
2. Penning, L.: Normal movements of the cervical spine. A.J.R., *130:*317, 1978.
3. Freiberger, R. H., Wilson, P. H., and Nicholas, J. A.: Acquired absence of the odontoid process. J. Bone Joint Surg., *47-A:*1231, 1965.
4. Ewald, F. C.: Fracture of the odontoid process in a seventeen-month-old infant treated with a halo. J. Bone Joint Surg., *53-A:*1636, 1971.
5. Schiff, D. C. M., and Parke, W. W.: The arterial supply of the odontoid process. J. Bone Joint Surg., *55-A:*1450, 1973.
6. Grisel, P.: Enucléation de l'Atlas et Torticollis Nasopharyngren. Presse Med., *38:*50, 1930.
7. Sutow, W. W., and Pryde, A. W.: Incidence of spina bifida occulta in relation to age. Am. J. Dis. Child., *91:*211, 1956.
8. Ogden, J. A.: Postnatal development of the cervical spine. Presented at Eastern Orthopaedic Association, 1979, 1981.
9. Brandner, M. E.: Normal values of the vertebral body and intervertebral disc index during growth. A.J.R., *110:*618, 1970.
10. Carpenter, E. B.: Normal and abnormal growth of the spine. Clin. Orthop., *2:*49, 1961.
11. Johnson, R. M., et al.: Some new observations on the functional anatomy of the lower cervical spine. Clin. Orthop., *111:*192, 1975.
12. Forsyth, H. F.: Extension injuries of the cervical spine. J. Bone Joint Surg., *46-A:*1792, 1964.
13. Holdsworth, F.: Fractures, dislocations and fracture-dislocations of the spine. J. Bone Joint Surg., *52-A:*1534, 1970.
14. Sherk, H. H., Schut, L., and Lane, J. M.: Fractures and dislocations of the cervical spine in children. Orthop. Clin. North Am., *7:*593, 1976.

15. Taylor, A. S.: Fracture-dislocation of the cervical spine. Ann. Surg., 90:321, 1929.

16. Vigoroux, R. P., et al.: Injuries of the cervical spine in children. Neurochirurgie, 14:689, 1968.

17. Henrys, P., Lyne, E. D., Lifton, C., and Salciccioli, G.: Clinical review of cervical spine injuries in children. Clin. Orthop., 129:172, 1977.

18. Rang, M.: Children's Fractures. Philadelphia, J. B. Lippincott, 1974.

19. Melzak, J.: Paraplegia among children. Lancet, II:45, 1969.

20. Schneider, R. C., Cherry, G., and Pantek, H.: The syndrome of acute cervical spinal cord injury. J. Neurosurg., 11:546, 1954.

21. Hubbard, D. D.: Injuries of the spine in children and adolescents. Clin. Orthop., 100:56, 1974.

22. Hubbard, D. D.: Fractures of the dorsal and lumbar spine. Orthop. Clin. North Am., 7:605, 1976.

23. Blockey, N. J., and Purser, D. W.: Fractures of the odontoid process of the axis. J. Bone Joint Surg., 38-B:794, 1956.

24. Burke, D. C.: Spinal cord trauma in children. Paraplegia, 9:1, 1971.

25. Ahmann, P. A., Smith, S. A., Schwartz, J. J., and Clark, D. D.: Spinal cord infarction due to minor trauma in children. Neurology, 25:301, 1975.

26. Yates, P. O.: Birth trauma to vertebral arteries. Arch. Dis. Child., 34:436, 1959.

27. Jones, E. L.: Birth trauma and the cervical spine. Arch. Dis. Child., 45:147, 1970.

28. Aufdermaur, M.: Zur Pathogenese der Scheuermannschen Krankheit. Dtsch. Med. Wochenschr., 89:73, 1964.

29. Aufdermaur, M.: Zur pathologischen Anatomie der Scheuermannschen Krankheit. Schweiz. Med. Wochenschr., 95:264, 1965.

30. Aufdermaur, M.: Spinal injuries in juveniles. Necropsy findings in twelve cases. J. Bone Joint Surg., 56-B:513, 1974.

31. Horal, J., Nachemson, A., and Scheller, S.: Clinical and radiological long-term follow-up of vertebral fractures in children. Acta Orthop. Scand., 43:491, 1972.

32. Roaf, R.: Vertebral growth and its mechanical control. J. Bone Joint Surg., 42-B:40, 1960.

33. Wagner, F. C., VanGilder, J. C., and Dohrmann, G. J.: Pathologic changes from acute to chronic in experimental spinal cord trauma. J. Neurosurg., 48:92, 1978.

34. Bedbrook, G. M.: Pathologic principles in the management of spinal cord trauma. Int. J. Paraplegia, 4:43, 1966.

35. Head, H., and Riddoch, G.: The automatic bladder, excessive sweating and some other reflex conditions in gross injuries of the spinal cord. Brain, 40:188, 1917.

36. Afshani, E., and Girdany, B. R.: Atlanto-axial dislocation in chondro-dysplasia punctata. Radiology, 102:399, 1972.

37. Hinck, V. C., and Hopkins, C. E.: Measurement of the atlanto-dental interval in the adult. A.J.R., 84:945, 1960.

38. Hohl, M., and Baker, H. R.: The atlanto-axial joint. J. Bone Joint Surg., 46-A:1739, 1954.

39. Bailey, D. K.: The normal cervical spine in infants and children. Radiology, 59:712, 1952.

40. Naik, D. R.: Cervical spinal canal in normal infants. Clin. Radiol., 21:323, 1970.

41. Swischuk, L. E.: Anterior displacement of C2 in children: physiologic or pathologic. Radiology, 122:759, 1977.

42. Teng, P., and Papatheodorou, C.: Traumatic subluxation of C2 in young children. Bull. Los Angeles Neurol. Soc., 32:197, 1967.

43. Townsend, E. H., Jr., and Rowe, M. L.: Mobility of the upper cervical spine in health and disease. Pediatrics, 10:567, 1952.

44. Sullivan, A. W.: Subluxation of the atlanto-axial joint: sequel to inflammatory processes of the neck. J. Pediatr., 35:415, 1949.

45. Sullivan, C. R., Bruwer, A. J., and Harris, L. E.: Hypermobility of the cervical spine in children: a pitfall in the diagnosis of cervical dislocation. Am. J. Surg., 95:636, 1958.

46. Cattell, H. S., and Filtzer, D. L.: Pseudosubluxation and other normal variations in the cervical spine in children. J. Bone Joint Surg., 47-A:1295, 1965.

47. Jackson, H.: The diagnosis of minimal atlanto-axial subluxation. Br. J. Radiol., 23:672, 1950.

48. Locke, G. R., Gardner, J. I., and VanEpps, E. F.: Atlas-dens interval (ADI) in children. A study based on 200 normal cervical spines. A.J.R., 97:135, 1966.

49. Donaldson, J. S.: Acquired torticollis in children and young adults. J.A.M.A., 160:458, 1956.

50. Dunlap, J. P., Morris, M., and Thompson, R. G.: Cervical spine injuries in children. J. Bone Joint Surg., 40-A:681, 1958.

51. Jacobson, G., and Bleeker, H. H.: Pseudosubluxation of the axis in children. A.J.R., 82:472, 1959.

52. Hanson, T. A., Kraft, J. P., and Adcock, D. W.: Subluxation of the cervical vertebra due to pharyngitis. South. Med. J., 66:427, 1973.

53. Funk, F. J., and Wells, R. E.: Injuries to the cervical spine in football. Clin. Orthop., 109:50, 1975.

54. Semine, A. A., Ertel, A. N., Goldberg, M. J., and Bull, M. J.: Cervical-spine instability in children with Down's Syndrome (Trisomy 21). J. Bone Joint Surg., 60-A:649, 1978.

55. Allen, J. P., Myers, G. G., and Condon, V. R.: Laceration of the spinal cord related to breech delivery. J.A.M.A., 208:1019, 1969.

56. Bresnan, M. J., and Abrams, I. F.: Neonatal spinal cord transection secondary to intrauterine hyperextension of the neck in breech position. J. Pediatr., 84:734, 1974.

57. Crothers, B., and Putnam, M. C.: Obstetrical injuries of the spinal cord. Medicine, 6:41, 1927.

58. Hellstrom, B., and Sallmander, V.: Prevention of spinal cord injury in hyperextension of the fetal head. J.A.M.A., 204:1041, 1968.

59. Hoffmeister, H. P.: Beitrag zur wirbelsäulenverletzung beim Neugeborenen. Geburtshilfe Frauenheilkd, 24:1085, 1964.

60. Shulman, S. T., Madden, J. D., Esterly, J. R., and Shanklin, D. R.: Transection of spinal cord. A rare obstetrical complication of cephalic delivery. Arch. Dis. Child., 46:291, 1971.

61. Towbin, A.: Spinal injury related to the syndrome of sudden death ("crib death") in infants. Am. J. Clin. Pathol., 49:562, 1968.

61a. Gaufin, L. M., and Goodman, S. J.: Cervical spine injuries in infants. Problems in management. J. Neurosurg., 42:179, 1975.

62. Martel, W., Uyham, R., and Stimson, C. W.: Subluxation of the atlas causing spinal cord compression in a case of Down's syndrome with a manifestation of an occipital vertebra. Radiology, 93:839, 1969.

63. Bucholz, R. W., and Burkhead, W. Z.: The pathologic anatomy of fatal atlanto-occipital dislocations. J. Bone Joint Surg., 61-A:248, 1979.

64. Evarts, C. M.: Traumatic occipito-atlantal dislocation. Report of a case with survival. J. Bone Joint Surg., 52-A:1653, 1970.

65. Gabrielson, T. O., and Maxwell, J. A.: Traumatic atlanto-occipital dislocation. A.J.R., 97:624, 1966.

66. Ehalt, W.: Uber die Bruche des ersten Mittelhandknochens unde ihre Behandlung. Arch. Orthop. Unfallchir., 27:515, 1929.

67. Weiss, M. H.: Hangman's fracture in an infant. Am. J. Dis. Child., 126:268, 1973.

68. Wiltse, L. L., and Jackson, D. W.: Treatment of spondylolisthesis and spondylolysis in children. Clin. Orthop., 117:93, 1976.

69. Carlioz, H., and Dubousset, J.: Severe atlas-axis instabilities in childhood. Rev. Chir. Orthop., 59:291, 1973.

70. Dewar, F. P., Duckworth, J. W. A., Wright, T. J., and Worsman, G.: Subluxation of the atlanto-axial joint in rotation. J. Bone Joint Surg., 46-B:778, 1964.

71. Balau, J., and Hupfauer, W.: The differential diagnosis of injuries of the atlanto-axial joint in childhood. Arch. Orthop. Unfallchir., 78:343, 1974.

72. Berkheiser, E. J., and Seidler, F.: Non-traumatic dislocations of the atlanto-axial joint. J.A.M.A., 96:517, 1931.

73. Marar, B. C., and Balachandran, N.: Non-traumatic atlanto-axial dislocation in children. Clin. Orthop., 92:220, 1973.

74. Sherk, H. H.: Lesions of the atlas and axis. Clin. Orthop., 109:33, 1975.

75. Beighton, P., and Craig, J.: Atlanto-axial subluxation in the Morquio syndrome. J. Bone Joint Surg., 56-B:478, 1973.

76. Dawson, E. G., and Smith, L.: Atlanto-axial subluxation in children due to vertebral anomalies. J. Bone Joint Surg., 61-A:582, 1979.

77. Dzentis, A. J.: Spontaneous atlanto-axial dislocation in a mongoloid child with spinal cord compression. J. Neurosurg., 25:458, 1966.

78. Finerman, G. A., Sakai, D., and Weingarten, S.: Atlanto-axial dislocation with spinal cord compression in a mongoloid child. A case report. J. Bone Joint Surg., 58-A:408, 1976.

79. Sherk, H. H., and Nicholson, J. T.: Rotatory atlanto-axial dislocation associated with ossiculum terminale and mongolism. J. Bone Joint Surg., 51-A:957, 1969.

80. Sherk, H. H., and Nicholson, J. T.: Cervico-occuloacusticus syndrome. Case report of death caused by injury to abnormal cervical spine. J. Bone Joint Surg., 54-A:1633, 1972.

81. Nicholson, J. T.: Surgical fixation of dislocation of the first cervical vertebra in children. N.Y. State J., 56:38, 1956.

82. Bhattacharvya, S. K.: Fracture and displacement of the odontoid process in a child. J. Bone Joint Surg., 56-A:1071, 1974.

83. Griffiths, S. C.: Fracture of the odontoid process in children. J. Pediatr. Surg., 7:680, 1972.

84. Sherk, H. H., Nicholson, J. T., and Chung, S. M. K.: Fractures of the odontoid process in young children. J. Bone Joint Surg., 60-A:921, 1978.

85. Michaels, L., Prevost, M. J., and Crang, D. F.: Pathological changes in a case of os odontoideum (separate odontoid process). J. Bone Joint Surg., 51-A:965, 1969.

86. Fielding, J. W.: Disappearance of the central portion of the odontoid process. J. Bone Joint Surg., 53-A:1228, 1971.

87. Mouradian, W. H., et al.: Fractures of the odontoid: a laboratory and clinical study of mechanisms. Orthop. Clin. North Am., 9:985, 1978.

88. Stillwell, W. T., and Fielding, J. W.: Acquired os odontoideum. Clin. Orthop., 135:71, 1978.

89. Seimon, L. P.: Fracture of the odontoid process in young children. J. Bone Joint Surg., 59-A:943, 1977.

90. Gwinn, J. L., and Smith, J. L.: Acquired and congenital absence of the odontoid process. A.J.R., 88:424, 1962.

91. Gillman, E. L.: Congenital absence of the odontoid process of the axis. J. Bone Joint Surg., 41-A:345, 1959.

92. Norton, W. L.: Fractures and dislocations of the cervical spine. J. Bone Joint Surg., 44-A:115, 1962.

93. Frankel, H. L.: The development of intermittent catheterization and treatment of the bladder in acute paraplegia. Proc. 18th V. A. Spinal Cord Injury Conference, Washington, D. C.: U.S. Government Printing Office, 1972.

94. Crutchfield, W. J.: Skeletal traction in treatment of injuries to the cervical spine. J.A.M.A., 155:29, 1954.

95. Matson, D. D.: Spinal Cord Injury in Neurosurgery of Infancy and Childhood. 2nd Ed. Springfield, Charles C Thomas, 1969.

96. Kopits, S. E., and Steingass, M. H.: Experience with the "halo-cast" in small children. Surg. Clin. North Am., 50:935, 1970.

97. Papavasiliou, V.: Traumatic subluxation of the cervical spine during childhood. Orthop. Clin. North Am., 9:945, 1978.

98. Stauffer, E. S., and Kelly, E. G.: Fracture-dislocation of the cervical spine. J. Bone Joint Surg., 59-A:45, 1977.

99. Holmes, J. C., and Hall, J. E.: Fusion for instability and potential instability of the cervical spine in children and adolescents. Orthop. Clin. North Am., 9:923, 1978.

100. Roy, L., and Gibson, D. A.: Cervical spine fusions in children. Clin. Orthop., 73:146, 1970.

101. Murphy, M. J., Ogden, J. A., and Southwick, W. O.: Spinal stabilization in acute spine injuries. Surg. Clin. North Am., 60:1035, 1980.

102. Cattell, H. S., and Clark, G. L.: Cervical kyphosis and instability following multiple laminectomy in children. J. Bone Joint Surg., 49-A:713, 1967.

103. Ruckstuhl, J., Morscher, E., and Jani, L.: Behandlung und prognose von wirbelfrakturen im kindes—und jugendalter. Chirurg, 47:458, 1976.

104. Nykamp, P. W., et al.: Computed tomography for a bursting fracture of the lumbar spine. J. Bone Joint Surg., 60-A:1108, 1978.

105. Rolander, S. D., and Blair, W. E.: Deformation and fracture of the lumbar vertebral end plate. Orthop. Clin. North Am., 6:75, 1975.

106. Zoltan, J. D., Gilula, L. A., and Murphy, W. A.: Unilateral facet dislocation between the fifth lumbar and first sacral vertebrae. J. Bone Joint Surg., 61-A:767, 1979.

107. Ferguson, R. J., McMaster, J. H., and Stanitski, C. L.: Low back pain in college football linemen. J. Sports Med. Phys. Fitness, 2:63, 1974.

108. Jackson, D. W., Wiltse, L. L., and Cirincione, R. J.: Spondylolysis in the female gymnast. Clin. Orthop., 117:68, 1976.

109. Schmorl, G., and Junghanns, H.: The Human Spine in Health and Disease. New York, Grune & Stratton, 1959.

110. Alexander, C. J.: Scheuermann's disease. A traumatic spondylodystrophy? Skeletal Radiol., 1:209, 1977.

111. Billot, C., Desgrippes, Y., and Bensahel, H.: La hernie discale lombaire chez l'enfant. Rev. Chir. Orthop., 66:43, 1980.

112. Carcassonne, G.: Sciatique de l'enfant. In Entretien de chirurgie infantile. Paris, Expansion Scientifique Française, 1977, p. 151.

113. Key, S. A.: Intervertebral disc lesions in children and adolescents. J. Bone Joint Surg., 32-A:97, 1950.

114. Pasquier, J.: Calcification due disque intervertebral de l'enfant. Ann. Chir., 16:249, 1975.

115. deSeze, S., and Levernieux, J.: La sciatique des adolescents. Etude sur 52 obserrations. Rev. Rhum. Mal. Osteoartic., 24:270, 1957.

116. Lippitt, A. B.: Fracture of a vertebral body end plate and disc protrusion causing subarachnoid block in an adolescent. Clin. Orthop., 116:112, 1976.

117. Kilfovle, R. M., Foley, J. J., and Norton, P. L.: Spine and pelvic deformity in childhood and adolescent paraplegia. A study of 104 cases. J. Bone Joint Surg., 47-A:659, 1965.

118. Lapides, J. L.: Neurogenic bladder: principles of treatment. Urol. Clin. North Am., 1:81, 1974.

119. Laitmen, L., and Singounas, E.: Longitudinal myelotomy in the treatment of spasticity of the legs. J. Neurosurg., 35:536, 1971.

120. Munro, D.: The rehabilitation of patients totally paralyzed below the waist: anterior rhizotomy for spastic paraplegia. N. Engl. J. Med., 233:453, 1945.

121. Griffiths, G. R.: Growth problems in cervical injuries. Paraplegia, 12:277, 1974.

122. Campbell, J., and Bonnett, C.: Spinal cord injury in children. Clin. Orthop., 112:114, 1975.

15

Pelvis

Anatomy

The pelvis is initially formed from 3 primary centers of ossification in the ischium, pubis, and ilium, all of which converge within the acetabulum to form the triradiate cartilage (Figs. 15-1 and 15-2). The triradiate cartilage may be considered the composite epiphysis of these 3 contributing areas. These particular chondro-osseous interrelationships allow integrated growth of the acetabulum commensurate with spherical growth of the capital femur. During adolescence, secondary centers of ossification develop within the "arms" of the triradiate cartilage (Figs. 15-3 and 15-4). This modified growth region normally undergoes epiphysiodesis at approximately 16 to 18 years of age. Damage to the triradiate growth mechanism can lead to severe deformities of the acetabulum (e.g., miniacetabulum), especially if such an injury occurs in a young child.

The anatomic os acetabulum, which appears within the triradiate cartilage at about 12 and fuses at 18 years, must be contrasted with the radiographic os acetabulum, which is a normal secondary center at the superior margin of the acetabulum (Figs. 15-4 and 15-5). This is rarely avulsed because of the confluence of the original tissues comprising the acetabular hyaline cartilage (in which the ossification occurs) and the fibrocartilaginous rim.

The ischium and pubis also have interposed cartilage within the inferior ramus (Figs. 15-6 and 15-7). Fusion of this region normally occurs between 4 and 7 years. Fusiform enlargement of the ischiopubic junction during physiologic fusion is often evident radiographically. This enlargement has been variably described as normal, an osteochondrosis, or even a stress fracture. In children in the 6-to-10-year range, this area should be considered a normal variation of skeletal maturation. It should not be misinterpreted as a healing fracture, since the appearance may be suggestive of callus formation or reactive new bone caused by osteomyelitis or neoplasia. However, in the older or symptomatic child, particularly with pain in the groin region, any apparent increased bone formation in the ischiopubic junction should be considered a possible stress fracture.

The normal, maturing ischial tuberosity may look irregular and be mistaken for fracture, infection, or tumor, especially if the patient presents several weeks following injury with apparent excessive reactive bone.

The growth and development of the iliac apophysis have been detailed by Risser and Caffey.[1,2] Secondary centers of

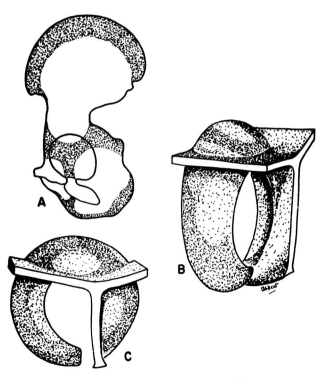

FIG. 15-1. *A*, Schematic composition of the pelvis in a neonate (also see Fig. 15-2). Stippled areas represent the epiphyseal cartilage analogues (including the triradiate cartilage). *B-C*, Isolated cartilage schematics (oblique and posterior) showing continuity of acetabular and triradiate cartilage.

423

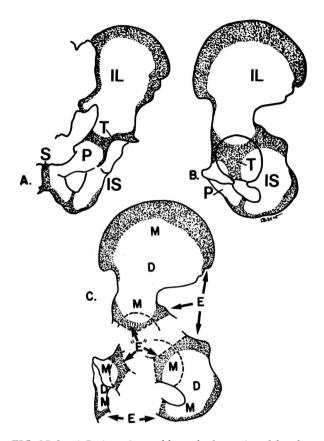

FIG. 15-2. *A-B,* Anterior and lateral schematics of developing pelvis showing areas of bone (white) and cartilage (stippled). Note: Ilium (IL); ischium (IS); pubis (P); symphysis pubica (S); and triradiate cartilage (T). *C,* Exploded view emphasizing the analogy of each component bone to a long bone and showing how several "epiphyses" fuse to form the triradiate cartilage. Similar "epiphyseal" fusions form the ischiopubic junctions and the symphysis pubica. Note: Epiphysis (E); metaphysis (M); diaphysis (D).

ossification appear along the anterolateral iliac crest at approximately 13 years (Fig. 15-8). Posterior advancement continues toward the posterior iliac spine. Fusion occurs by 15 to 17 years, although complete fusion may be delayed until age 25. Alternatively, after the ossification center first appears, separate ossification may proceed from a posterior center, with the central portion being ossified at a later date as the 2 centers grow toward each other.

There may be a secondary center of ossification at the anteroinferior iliac spine that appears between 13 to 15 years and fuses between 16 to 18 years of age. This is more common in males than females, and may be contiguous with secondary ossification extending from the acetabular margin.

The symphysis pubis also represents a growth region that may be injured, not unlike epiphyseal fractures of the long bones. The normal endochondral ossification process may be associated with an irregular, undulated appearance that should not be confused with trauma (Fig. 15-9). Apparent roentgenographic widening of the symphyseal region is variable and depends upon the degree of maturation of cartilaginous into osseous tissue.

History and Incidence

The pelvis of the child differs from that of the adult in that the bones are less brittle and the cartilage and joints (sacroiliac, symphysis pubis, triradiate, and ischiopubic) more pliant. The greater volume of cartilage provides a buffer for energy absorption. Fractures are uncommon.[3-5] However, when they do occur, the contiguous radiolucent cartilage may be damaged, either at the time of injury or later, particularly if the fracture heals in such a way that abnormal forces result in altered growth. For example, the triradiate cartilage may be damaged (most likely a type 5 injury), leading to acetabular maldevelopment and a situation comparable to congenital hip dysplasia (Fig. 15-10). A displaced fracture of the ischiopubic ring (essentially reversing an innominate or similar pelvic osteotomy) may lead to uncov-

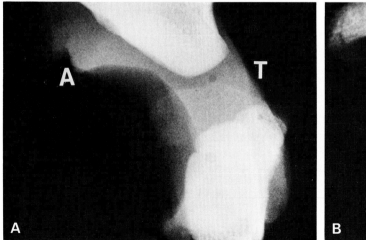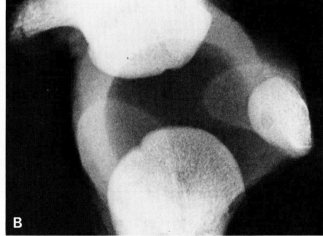

FIG. 15-3. Early development patterns of the triradiate cartilage. *A,* Duplication of standard anterior view of acetabular segment and composite bones from the pelvis of a stillborn neonate. Note the extent of the acetabular (A) and triradiate (T) cartilage. *B,* Direct view of acetabulum to show the true appearance of the triradiate cartilage.

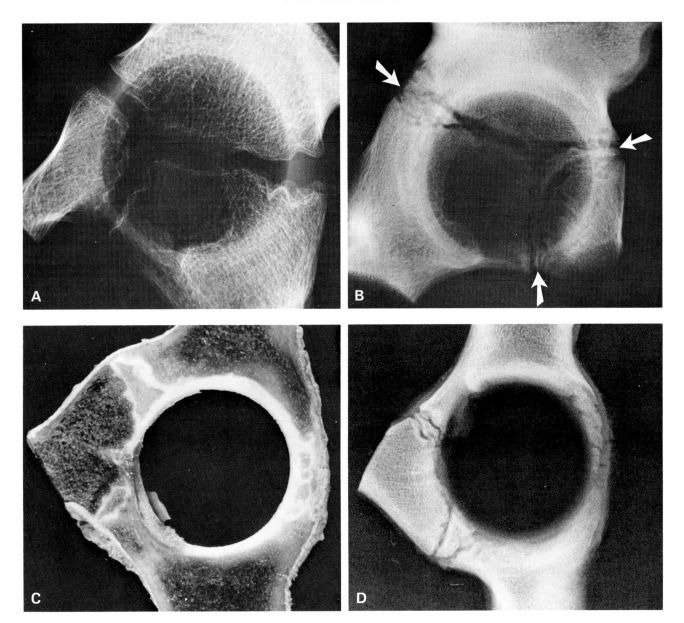

FIG. 15-4. Later development of the triradiate cartilage. *A,* 12 years of age: prior to the development of the secondary ossification center. *B,* 14 years of age: with development of secondary ossification centers in the arms of the triradiate cartilage (arrows). *C-D,* Serial sections (slab and roentgenogram) of specimen shown in part *B.*

ering of the femoral head with subsequent capital femoral subluxation. The presence of growth cartilage along several pelvic margins allows avulsion fractures (types 3, 4, and 7 growth mechanism injuries). These fractures can be considered comparable to epiphyseal-physeal injuries in a long bone, and are subject to all the potential acute and long term complications. Leg length discrepancy may be a problem when a hemipelvis is shifted superiorly (Fig. 15-11), which may lead to scoliosis in the adolescent period. Distortion of the pelvic ring theoretically could lead to eventual obstetric difficulties.

Fractures of the pelvic components must be placed in proper perspective. In the initial phase the orthopaedist must be more acutely aware of potential injury to the intra-pelvic and intra-abdominal visceral and vascular contents, rather than the obvious osseous injuries.[5-10]

In a child, the developing chondro-osseous pelvis is more resilient than in an adult, and therefore affords less rigid protection to the viscera, which, because of immature fibrous capsules and stroma, may be damaged more easily than comparable adult organs. The juvenile pelvis may undergo considerable elastic and plastic distortion without actual fracture; therefore, organ damage may occur with little roentgenographic evidence of chondro-osseous trauma. The identification of a pelvic fracture in a child, particularly if displaced, assumes even more clinical significance. The array of injuries, other than genitourinary, is roughly proportional to the severity of the pelvic fracture.

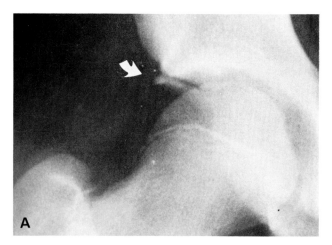

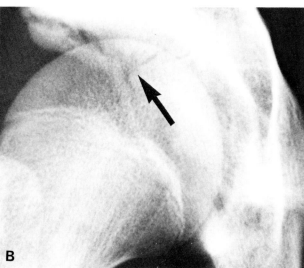

FIG. 15-5. Normal peripheral acetabular ossification characteristic of adolescence. *A,* Beginning formation of peripheral ossification along superior rim (arrow). This should not be confused with an avulsion fracture of the adjacent anterior/inferior spine. *B,* Complete rim ossification with posterosuperior continuity to the triradiate cartilage ossification (arrow).

Quinby reported 20 pediatric patients with fractures of the immature pelvis who were treated during an 11-year period.[11] There were 6 girls and 14 boys, with an average age of 8 years (ranging from 2 to 13 years). Of these patients, 19 were involved in vehicular accidents and 1 fell from a roof. They were divided into 3 treatment groups: Group 1 (6 patients) did not require laparotomy, the pelvic fractures were relatively mild and essentially undisplaced (including one mild separation of the sacroiliac joint), and none showed clinical shock or required blood transfusion; Group 2 (9 patients) all underwent laparotomy for visceral injuries accompanying the pelvic fractures. All but 1 of the patients with organ lacerations were in this group and 1 of these patients died; Group 3 (5 patients) all had massive retroperitoneal and pelvic hemorrhage with severe pelvic fractures. All group 3 patients had extensive disruption of the sacroiliac

joint and were in clinical shock. Of these patients, 1 died during laparotomy while an attempt was made to control hemorrhaging. There were 2 who died within 24 hours of surgery, and another who died 36 hours post-operatively. The amount of blood replacement from admission to either death or recovery was 3500 to 8000 mm, which represented 175 to 400% of the estimated volumes. Vascular injuries were combined arterial and venous, and both specific and diffuse. Of these children, 4 had no femoral pulse. In all cases there was injury to the primary branches of the iliac artery in relationship to the grossly disrupted sacroiliac joint. There also was diffuse bleeding from injured muscle and bone. Thus, of 20 patients, there were 5 deaths: 1 from associated brain injury, 3 from uncontrolled major vascular lacerations, and 1 from a mixture of possible causes, but primarily hemorrhage.

Shock appears to accompany only severe pelvic fractures, and certainly is hemorrhagic rather than neurogenic (see Chap. 7). Massive replacement transfusion and temporary postponement of laparotomy until the circulatory-volume status is stable are strongly recommended. A delay in the repair of visceral or arterial injuries is probably less serious than the crisis of cardiac arrest during an exploratory operation performed while the general circulation is in a state of

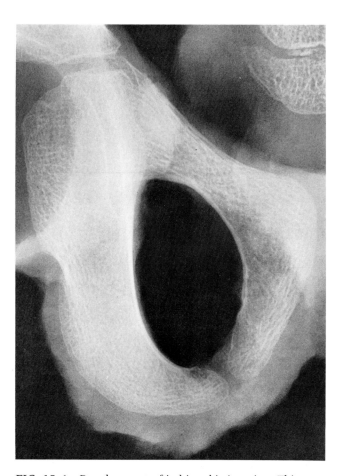

FIG. 15-6. Development of ischiopubic junction. This anatomic section from a six-year-old shows continuity of cartilage in the ischiopubic junction, with cartilage along the ischium, pubis, and symphysis.

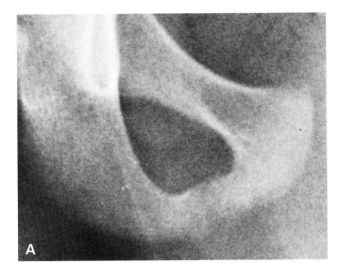

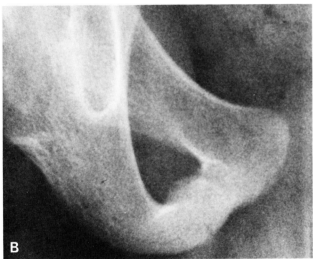

FIG. 15-7. Progressive development of the ischiopubic junction, which is initially cartilaginous, then, *A,* ossifies progressively, and, *B,* forms a fusiform enlargement and gradually remodels.

precarious stability. The sacroiliac region seems to be the point where the vessels and nerves are most susceptible to major laceration, and if this area is disrupted there should be concern for laceration of vessels up to the size of the iliac artery (see Fig. 15-11). Poorly responsive shock in the presence of a rapidly enlarging lower abdomen should be cause for immediate surgical exploration, rather than delay. It is a good surgical principle not to disturb stable retroperitoneal hematomas, regardless of their size, but rather to control the visceral or vascular lacerations.

When the sacroiliac joint is separated and pulses in one leg are absent, a major branch of the internal iliac artery probably has been disrupted. The child generally is in profound shock and requires rapid transfusion of blood in massive quantities. This type of injury has a high mortality rate. The importance of concealed hemorrhage from fractures of the pelvis cannot be overstated.

Sources of external hemorrhage should be sought around the urethral meatus, vagina, and anus. Abdominal and rectal examinations are essential. Pulses in the lower extremities must be examined beginning at the groin, and as reasonable a neurologic examination as possible should be performed, depending on the level of consciousness of the patient. Sacral sensation in particular should be tested.

Hemorrhage may be intraperitoneal or extraperitoneal. Intraperitoneal bleeding often necessitates control by laparotomy. Extraperitoneal bleeding is more difficult to control, especially with explorative surgery and attempts to ligate vessels. If surgery is undertaken, packing should be tried first. Arteriography may also be beneficial. Ring et al., have used arteriography to localize the site of hemorrhage.[12] An arterial catheter may be inserted as close to the site of hemorrhage as possible. An autologous clot may be injected. This appears to be successful and should be considered when appropriate facilities are available.

Many nerve injuries are missed because detailed initial neurologic examinations are neglected or cursory. The lumbosacral plexus is closely related to the sacroiliac joint and there may be some neural disruption when the joint is dislocated and widely separated. The lumbosacral trunk, the superior gluteal nerve, and the obdurator nerve may be stretched or even disrupted. Intrathecal rupture of the roots of the cauda equina may be produced by traction.

Reed reviewed 84 cases of pelvic fractures in children with over 80% being due to vehicular accidents;[13] 39% were classified as unstable. The most frequent type of pelvic fractures were diametric fractures in which there was a fracture of the ilium or sacrum, or a sacroiliac separation combined with a pubic fracture anteriorly on the same or opposite side. However, many diametric fractures in children probably are not truly unstable, because the posterior fractures are often undisplaced or incomplete epiphyseal separations with a certain degree of soft tissue (periosteal) stability. The others, most of which were pubic fractures, were stable. There were 16 patients with associated visceral injuries; 18 had transient microhematuria, but none had significant injuries to the genitourinary tract. There were 11 who had gross hematuria, and all had major injuries to the lower urinary tract or the kidney. Two patients had severe intracranial injuries. One third of the patients sustained fractures of other bones, the most common being the femur and the skull. Of the children, 5% (4 cases) had acetabular fractures, all of which represented separations of the innominate synchondrosis (triradiate cartilage).

Most children require only bed rest for treatment. Closed reduction is rarely necessary, and open reduction is rare. Associated injuries require more treatment than the fracture itself.

Diagnosis

Accurate diagnosis of pelvic injuries is difficult if based solely on clinical findings. Most children have multiple trauma. Variable levels of consciousness may limit response to pain. Physical examination should include pelvic compression, which may elicit pain. Posterior subluxation of the ilium on the sacrum at the sacroiliac joint is generally missed because the patient is supine. It may not be possible to examine the region carefully, particularly when there are multiple associated injuries.

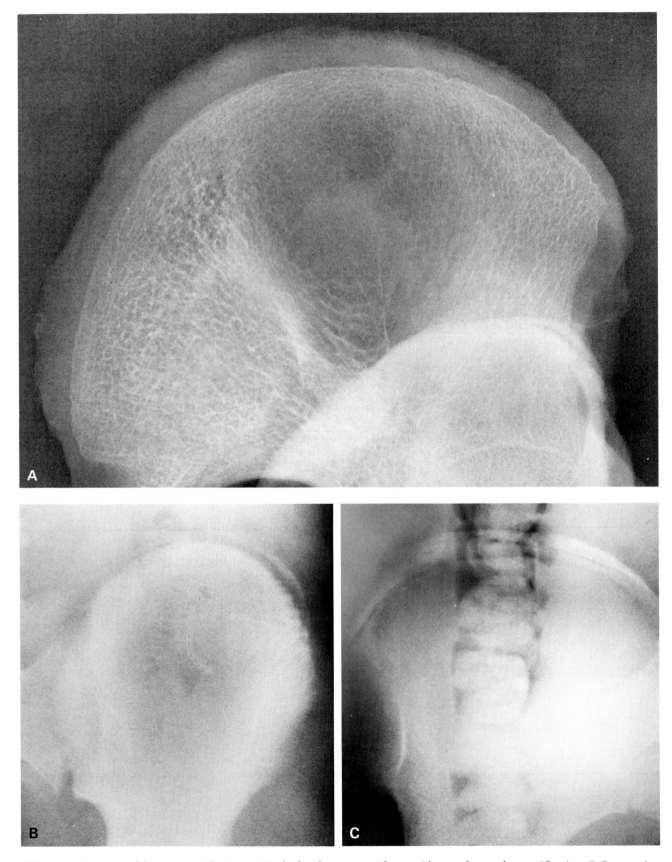

FIG. 15-8. Patterns of iliac crest ossification. *A,* Early development, with no evidence of secondary ossification. *B,* Progressive ossification toward anterior and posterior regions. *C,* Mature appearance in late adolescence, just prior to epiphysiodesis.

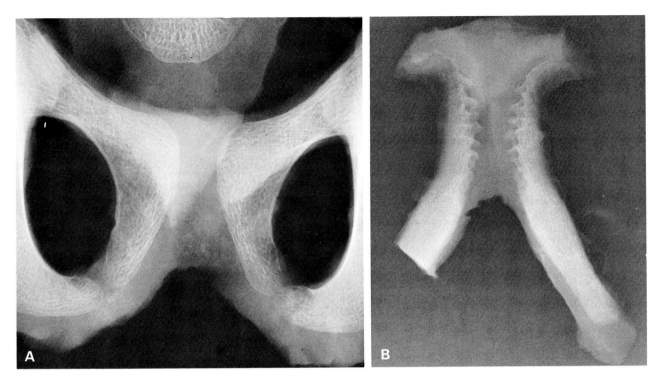

FIG. 15-9. Development of symphysis pubis. *A,* Early appearance in six-year-old showing extent of normally radiolucent cartilage, and how this is continuous with the ischiopubic cartilage. *B,* Slab specimen from 14-year-old, showing the normal undulated appearance that progressively develops.

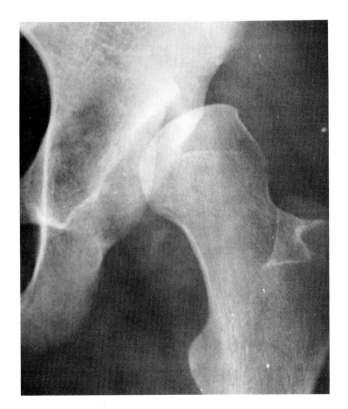

FIG. 15-10. Triradiate injury in a five-year-old. At skeletal maturity the acetabulum is shallow and the femoral head slightly deformed.

Adequate radiographic examination is critical. A gonad shield should not be used, as it may obliterate areas that have to be critically evaluated. The anteroposterior view of the pelvis that adequately demonstrates the pelvic ring is not always acceptable for determining fracture details because of the normal lumbar lordosis. The best view in the anteroposterior position is an oblique, depending on how much curvature there is in the spine. An inlet or downshot view is taken 30° off the vertical with the cone aimed distally to demonstrate bursting of the ring.

Types of Pelvic Fractures

Fractures of the pelvis may be classified basically into 4 groups: (1) isolated peripheral fractures with continuity of the pelvic ring, (2) unstable fractures with disruption of the pelvic ring, (3) intra-articular fractures of the acetabulum (especially involving the triradiate cartilage), and (4) avulsion fractures resulting from muscular violence. The most common fracture, comprising almost 50%, is a ramus fracture, with most being unilateral and primarily in the superior (pubic) ramus. The basic types are shown schematically in Figures 15-12 to 15-15.

Few pelvic fractures in children are seriously displaced, and most appear stable, including diametric fractures in which the posterior fractures tend to be incomplete. This stability may be the result of the relatively thick periosteum in children. Many of these injuries are analogous to epiphyseal injuries and have intrinsic stability because some of the periosteum is intact.

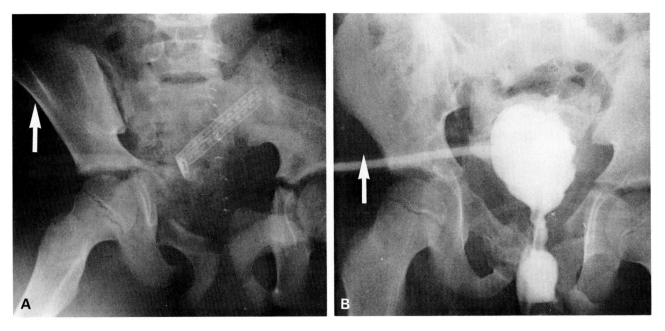

FIG. 15-11. *A,* Upward displacement (arrow) of hemipelvis associated with fractures of four rami and separation of symphysis. *B,* Significant upward displacement (arrow) of hemipelvis due to inferior fractures and sacroiliac separation. There was hypotension and incomplete loss of L5, S1, and S2 nerve function. The bladder is elevated by a retropubic hematoma. Rather than risk further neurologic loss or vascular disruption, no attempt was made to reduce this acutely, or more gradually, through skeletal traction.

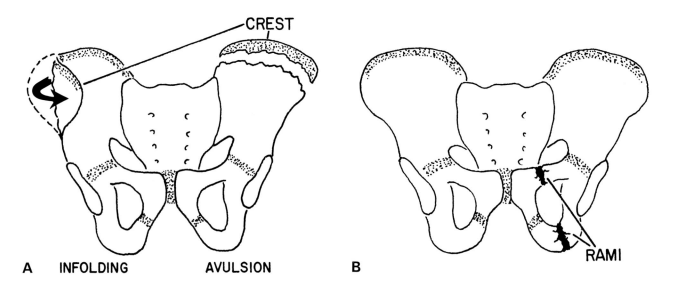

FIG. 15-12. Stable fracture patterns. *A,* Infolding of the iliac wing. This is analogous to a type 4 injury and may cause irregular crest development. Type 1 or type 2 injuries of the iliac crest may occur, although these avulsion patterns are unusual. Direct contusion (type 5 injury) may also occur. *B,* Fractures of the ischiopubic rami rarely displace in a child. In fact, the chondro-osseous fracture response in a child may allow fracture of only one ramus, an extremely unusual injury in the adult. However, one should always look for an accompanying disruption of either the sacroiliac joint or symphysis pubis.

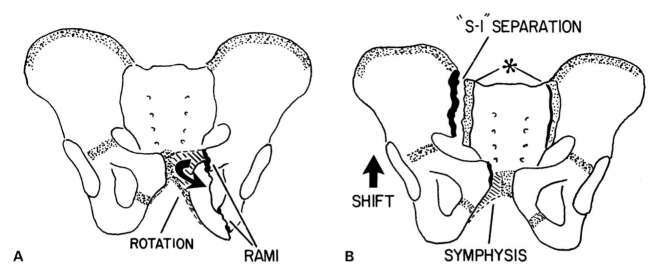

FIG. 15-13. Unstable fracture patterns. *A,* Rami fractures may be accompanied by displacement of the medial ischiopubic fragment from the symphysis (stippled area) and periosteum (lined area). The fragment is externally rotated, hinging at the fracture site. This is a type 1 growth mechanism fracture. If the fragment is not reduced, the relatively intact periosteal tube will produce bone (membranous, and some endochondral) to fill the defect. *B,* Malgaigne fracture of the immature pelvis. The true sacroiliac joint (*) is intact, but a chondro-osseous separation (type 1 injury) occurs on the iliac side, mimicking a sacroiliac disruption radiographically. The inferior disruption may be a type 1 symphysis-ischiopubic separation or fracture of the rami. However, soft tissue (periosteal) constraints generally limit the degree of displacement.

Stable pelvic ring fractures

The following pelvic ring fractures are considered stable fractures: (1) Wing of the ilium (Fig. 15-16), which may be displaced outward and downward. Pull of muscles on this fragment may be reduced by abduction (gluteus medius and

tensor) and flexion (sartorius and rectus). (2) The ischiopubic rami (Figs. 15-17 to 15-20). If one ramus is fractured, or both rami are fractured on the same side, the patient can usually be treated symptomatically. If only one ramus is fractured, always remember to look carefully for concomitant injury completing the fracture through the entire pelvic ring. This evaluation is particularly important at the sacroiliac joint. However, since the pelvic components are most resilient in the child, a solitary ramus fracture is possible,

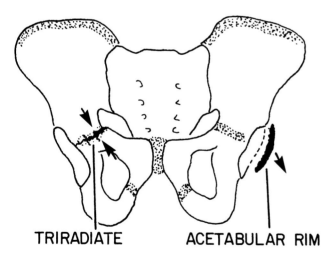

FIG. 15-14. Crush injury (type 5) to the triradiate cartilage (left). Mild translation may also occur (type 1 injury), although a significant crushing component is undoubtedly present. The ossifying region of the acetabular rim may be avulsed (right). This may occur prior to ossification, as an accompaniment to hip dislocation. However, diagnosis is extremely difficult in such a situation, and an avulsion should not be confused with normal ossification patterns.

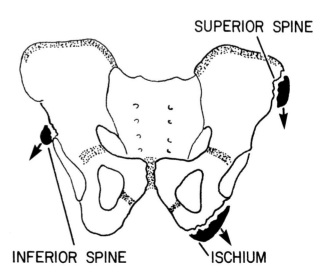

FIG. 15-15. Avulsion fracture patterns of those regions of the ilium and ischium that normally develop secondary ossification centers.

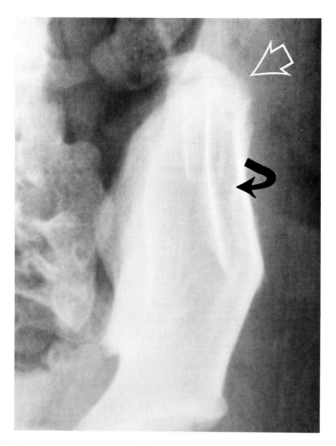

FIG. 15-16. Fracture of iliac wing, with infolding of anterior portion (black arrow) and some comminution of superior metaphyseal region (white arrow).

whereas the adult invariably completes a fracture through contraposed portions of the ring. (3) A separation of the symphysis. Always remember the changing size of this region with growth. Frequently, any injury to this area must be based on physical examination, as there is little radiographic evidence. These separations represent physeal injuries.

Oblique views may be useful for diagnosing some pubic fractures. Inlet views obtained by angling the cone 25 to 45° caudal and other projections (e.g., Judet views) may provide important information about fragment displacement.

Function is minimally impaired. The basic pelvic ring is usually undisplaced. Comfort is the primary treatment goal, which is best attained by bed rest (frequently mandated by accompanying injuries). Closed or open reduction is rarely necessary, particularly in the younger child, because of the extent of remodeling that occurs and the possibility of damaging intrapelvic structures.

Unstable pelvic ring fractures

Several patterns of unstable pelvic ring fractures may be encountered. (1) Separation of the symphysis pubis, accompanied by partial disruption at the sacroiliac joints (Fig. 15-21). The ring is disrupted and opened anteriorly at the symphysis. The posterior separation at the sacroiliac joint may be either an avulsion of the anterior capsule of the joint or an epiphyseal iliac fracture. Comparable epiphyseal separation at the sacrum is unlikely because of developmental patterns of the sacrum. The supine position aggravates the deformity, and it may be more comfortable to lie the child on his side. Frequently, placement of a pelvic sling is beneficial for the symptoms. This allows control of pelvic diastasis, as the straps may be crossed to increase compression. Compression

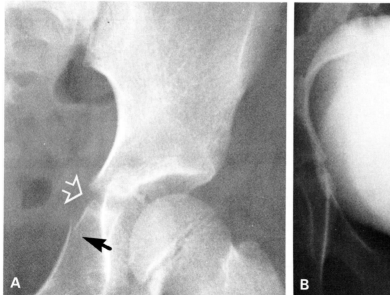
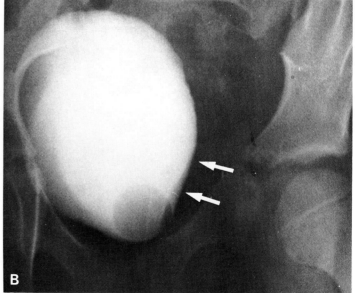

FIG. 15-17. *A,* Fracture of superior pubic ramus (solid arrow). The triradiate region (open arrow) also appeared offset. However, this appearance proved to be a variation due to projection. Three years later, no evidence of triradiate growth injury was present. *B,* A Foley catheter was inserted, and dye injected, which showed significant displacement (arrows) of the bladder by a retropubic hematoma.

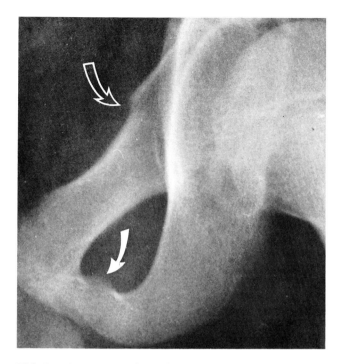

FIG. 15-18. Fracture through superior ramus (open arrow) in an eleven-year-old. The apparent inferior ramus fracture (solid arrow) was really the closing ischiopubic synchondrosis.

immobilization, either with a sling or spica should be maintained for 6 to 8 weeks, depending on the age of the child, to ensure adequate ligamentous union at the symphysis and to prevent late spreading. (2) Fractures of the anterior arch (Figs. 15-22 to 15-24). Crush injuries in the anteroposterior direction may cause fractures of both rami bilaterally to give a floating segment. In the child a variation of this injury is fracture of both rami, but with an ipsilateral separation of the bone from the symphyseal cartilage (Fig. 15-23). Disruption of the symphysis pubis is usually associated with separation of bone (i.e., metaphysis) away from the cartilage and thick periosteal sleeve, which may all fill in by endochondral bone formation (Fig. 15-24). The segment may displace posteriorly, superiorly because of the rectus abdominus muscles, or inferiorly because of the adductors and hamstrings. A pelvic sling should not be used as it may cause inward compression of the iliac wings. These children must be rested supine, and should be in a semi-Fowler's position to relax the abdominal and adductor muscles. Treatment must be maintained for 3 weeks, depending on the degree of displacement. Disruption of this region must be carefully assessed, particularly with regard to urethral and bladder injuries (Fig. 15-25). Thickened periosteum may not be damaged completely at all the fracture sites, so major displacement is uncommon in children. (3) Vertical shear. In this fracture, the ring is broken both in the front and back, the free pelvic segment is displaced by spasm of the muscles whose origin is fixed to the floating piece (e.g., the psoas, adductors, gluteus maximus, or lateral abdominal muscles). If upward dis-

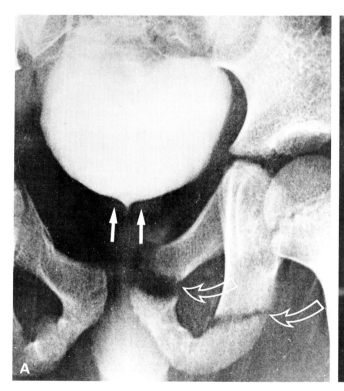

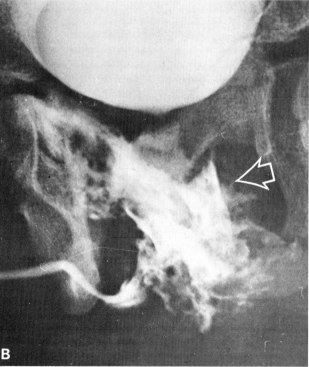

FIG. 15-19. *A,* Severe unilateral fractures involving both rami (open arrows) and extending toward the symphysis. Filling of bladder showed functional ureters and significantly elevated bladder (solid arrows) due to a hematoma behind the symphysis. Voluntary micturition was impossible. *B,* Retrograde injection of dye showed extravasation (arrow) where the urethra had been disrupted from the bladder.

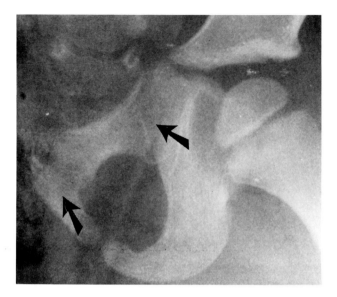

FIG. 15-20. Fractures through both sides of pubic ramus (arrows) accompanied by mild sacroiliac separation. The ischiopubic junction was not disrupted.

placement is marked, leg length discrepancy may result (see Fig. 15-11). Such fractures are treated best by skeletal traction using a Steinman pin through the distal femoral metaphysis. However, multiple system injury may preclude this method, since rigorous attempts at reduction may precipitate further retroperitoneal hemorrhage or nerve damage (traction or avulsion) and are contraindicated. Traction of 10

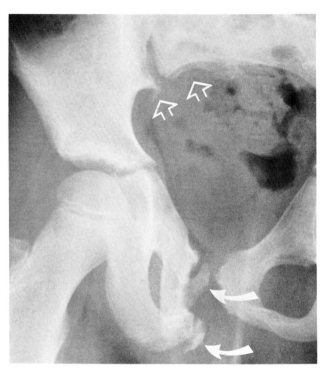

FIG. 15-21. Separation of right sacroiliac region and ipsilateral separation of symphysis. This roentgenogram was taken three months after the injury occurred and shows subperiosteal new bone at the sacroiliac joint (open arrows) and subperiosteal and endosteal bone at the symphysis (solid arrows).

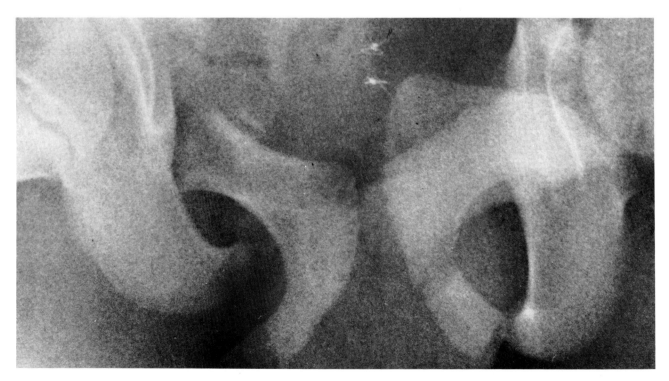

FIG. 15-22. Fractures of all four rami, creating a free-floating fragment. There is also a type 1 separation of the left side of the symphysis.

to 15 lbs may be necessary to reduce the fracture. After achieving reduction, which is usually within a week, the position should be held. Maintain counter-traction to prevent the child from inadvertently placing the injured leg in relative abduction. Open reduction is rarely indicated. (4) Bucket handle injury in which the pelvic ring is broken in front and back, and the floating pieces rotated so that the iliac crest is displaced medially and the ischial tuberosity is displaced laterally. This may be combined with some vertical shear. This type of injury, in effect, causes the reverse of an innominate osteotomy and thereby "uncovers" the femoral head. Again, this should be treated by skeletal traction if possible. It is important to reduce this deformity, since the uncovering, particularly in the young child (even up to 8 or 9 years of age), may cause relative or actual dysplasia of the acetabulum by the time growth is complete. (5) Lateral compression. Lateral crushing injury folds the wing of the pelvis, hinged posteriorly on the sacroiliac joint or hinged anteriorly at the pubis. However, the free fragment may be driven centrally. Traction frequently can be applied through the hip joint and proximal femur to try to reduce this over a period of time. This may take approximately 1 week and should be followed by bed rest. Open reduction may be indicated, particularly in the small child in whom skeletal traction is not feasible.

Management Guidelines

Complications

Osseous Damage. Pelvic fractures may be accompanied by other skeletal injuries. In particular, fractures of the proximal femur and hip dislocation may occur since many of the injuries are caused by direct blows. Such injuries must not be overlooked during the initial evaluation.

Vascular Damage. The most important aspect of pelvic fractures is the possibility of damage to viscera or major vessels. The osseous damage usually assumes secondary importance until these soft tissue injuries are completely evaluated and treated, as necessary. Massive retroperitoneal bleeding following pelvic fracture continues to produce high morbidity and mortality in victims of blunt trauma. Although less common in children, it still represents a significant potential complication.

Braunstein described autopsy studies of 200 consecutive fatally injured pedestrians; 90 (45%) were found to have pelvic fractures.[6] In 21, the only important injuries were to the pelvic area, which were accompanied by significant retroperitoneal bleeding. The hemorrhage accompanying pelvic fracture was either the direct cause of death or contributed substantially to the fatal outcome. In contrast, in a similar study of 500 pedestrians who did not succumb to their injuries, only 20 (4%) sustained pelvic fractures.

Barlow described a 7-year-old child who had lost over half of his blood volume into the hematoma.[14] The possible consequences of allowing continued rapid retroperitoneal blood loss, such as intraperitoneal rupture with exsanguination, prolonged jaundice, renal failure, coagulopathy, and prolonged ileus should be avoided.

Localization of the source of hemorrhage is often difficult. The magnitude of blood loss often goes unrecognized. Oper-

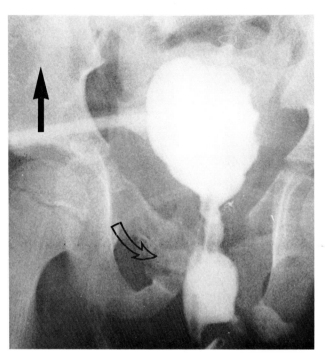

FIG. 15-23. Fractures of symphysis and ramus (open arrow) showing disruption of urethra with extravasation of dye. The entire right hemipelvis was displaced upwardly (solid arrow).

ative attempts at stemming this hemorrhage are frequently unsuccessful because identification of the primary bleeding site is difficult. Opening the peritoneum when tamponade has occurred, or will occur, may increase blood loss substantially. In addition, if the hemorrhage eventually is controlled, the risk of later sepsis is enhanced. Success with internal iliac artery ligation has also been variable. In fact, the morbidity of retroperitoneal exploration and arterial ligation may outweigh the risk of non-operative management with continued blood replacement.

Certain types of fractures have been correlated with specific vascular injuries. Lacerations or avulsions of common external iliac vessels are associated with disruption of the ilium or separation of the sacroiliac joint. In children, in whom sacroiliac luxation may be relatively common, disruption of the posterior pelvis has been associated with avulsion of the superior gluteal artery.[11]

Angiographic evaluation of bleeding, associated with pelvic fracture and treatment by selective embolization of clotted blood to sites in the vicinity of the fractures (usually branches from the obdurator artery along the pubic rami) have recently been described in adults.[15] This technique has been successful, and may be considered a non-operative approach to massive pelvic hematomas when contrasted with the hazards and limited success of surgical exploration. The technique involves arterial catheterization performed by the Seldinger technique on the side opposite the trauma. A flush aortogram is performed with the catheter at the level of the renal arteries. Visualization of the urinary tract is also obtained. Selective celiac axis arteriogram then follows to evaluate liver and spleen and rule out any bleeding in these areas. For embolization, the catheter is advanced just proxi-

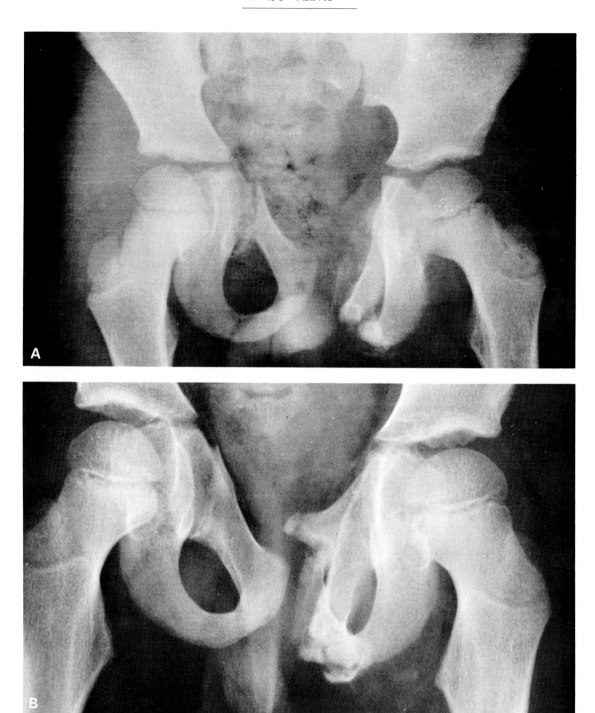

FIG. 15-24. *A,* Four weeks after multiple trauma caused a right-sided Malgaigne injury and subperiosteal rotational displacement of the contralateral rami, there is new bone formation. *B,* Two months later, significant membranous bone is filling the periosteal tube along the displaced ramus.

mal to the obdurator artery, and pieces of Gelfoam (mixed with contrast material) or autologous clot may be hand-injected into the obdurator artery under fluoroscopic control.

Margolies noted that hemorrhage after pelvic fractures was traditionally attributed to disruption of multiple pelvic veins.[15] However, recent evidence suggests that laceration of small arterial branches at the fracture site is more likely to be the major source of bleeding in pelvic fractures. The bleeding usually originates from branches of the obdurator artery that supply the pubic rami.

Bowel Damage. Injury to the bowel is an uncommon complication of pelvic fracture, and probably occurs in less than

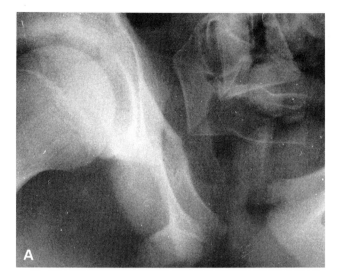

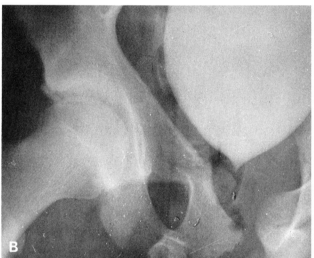

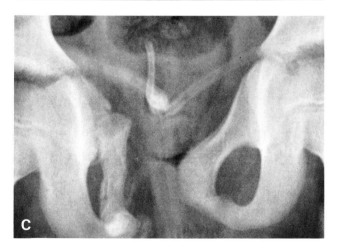

FIG. 15-25. *A,* Open fracture—separation of ischiopubic region from symphysis. *B,* During exploration of bladder, the fragment was easily rotated back into the subperiosteal tube. *C,* However, because of the open injury, and need for staged urethral surgery, skeletal fixation was not undertaken. The fragment subsequently displaced owing to muscle pulls.

3% of the cases, although a reactive ileus is common. Paralytic ileus frequently accompanies these injuries and a nasogastric tube should be used while this complication is present.

Entrapment of bowel between osseous fragments of the pelvis has been reported.[16,17] Everett described a 5-year-old boy who sustained a fractured pelvis with dislocation of the left sacroiliac joint.[18] The child subsequently developed evidence of small bowel obstruction, and at exploration apparent fracture-separation of the sacroiliac joint was a type 1 growth mechanism injury in which the cartilage at the sacroiliac joint, which is in continuity with the iliac crest, had retained normal continuity while the osseous portion of the ilium had totally separated away, allowing elements of small bowel to herniate through this area into the subcutaneous region.

In the long term, if there is severe disruption of the anterior ring, especially when it is rotated and disrupted by a symphysis pubis diastasis, the inguinal ligament may be disrupted and a hernia may develop. Similarly, disruption along the region of the iliac crest may lead to a lumbar or abdominal hernia.

Neurologic Damage. Although nerve injury may occur at several levels, it is infrequent when the sacroiliac region is separated. The nerve roots may be stretched or avulsed at the foramina. Injury to the sciatic nerve as it courses past the acetabulum is unusual, primarily because these injuries usually leave an intact periosteum that protects the nerve. Some degree of sciatic nerve function may be permanently lost.

Children with residual nerve damage, no matter what the final level, may have major problems with recurrent fractures, Charcot-like joints, and soft tissue contractures. Relative osteoporosis may significantly weaken the metaphyseal areas, predisposing to growth mechanism fractures (see Fig. 7-9).

Urologic Damage. Disruption of the symphysis or displaced fractures of the pubic rami are most likely to cause injury to the bladder and urethra, and complete urologic evaluation with urethrograms, cystograms, and intravenous pyelograms may be required (see Figs. 15-11, 15-17, 15-19, 15-23, and 15-25).

Suprapubic tenderness may be associated with contusion or tear of the bladder wall. A catheter should be placed through the urethra. If this proves difficult, suspect a tear of the urethra. Should the catheter enter the bladder without difficulty, then a major urethral injury can usually be excluded. If the urine that is drained is bloodstained, a cystogram may be performed by simply injecting some dye into the bladder through the catheter, looking for extravasation of the dye beyond the bladder outline. Detailed management of major urinary tract injuries, either bladder or urethral tears, should be left to the discretion of the urologic surgeon. If it is necessary to make a suprapubic approach to visualize the urethra for placement of a stent, it may be possible to concomitantly perform a better reduction of the fracture fragment. However, metallic fixation should not be used, since there is a high risk of bladder infection in the early post-injury course. Osteomyelitis by hematogenous or direct spread is a complication to be avoided.

Obstetric Damage. The possibility of an obstetric problem in the future has been posed. Pollen showed that a crush injury of the lateral pelvic wall in a 13-year-old girl narrowed the left pelvic outlet and was due to a central fracture-dislocation at the acetabular level.[19]

Acetabular Fractures

These fractures are often associated with dislocations of the hip in the adult.[20] However, because of the structure of the child's acetabulum, particularly the pliable cartilaginous components such as the labrum, dislocations of the hip usually occur without concomitant acetabular fracture. In the older child, posterior dislocation because of the position of the hip is more likely to displace an acetabular fragment than the less common anterior dislocation. This is also dictated by the relative extent of the posterior and anterior walls. The acetabular fracture that accompanies a hip dislocation must be reduced as accurately as possible, since this is an intra-articular injury in the child. Whether there are intra-articular fragments is not always easy to tell, as portions of the radiolucent cartilage may be displaced into the joint, particularly when involving separation of the acetabular labrum away from the main hyaline cartilage. Any suggestion of limitation of motion or failure to attain complete concentric reduction should make one suspicious of this. An arthrogram is often diagnostically beneficial. Oblique roentgenograms with the pelvis rotated 45° (both right and left obliques) must be taken to reveal the posterior acetabulum in profile. Depending on the age of the patient, the os acetabulum must be considered as a source of a roentgenographic "fracture" (see Fig. 15-4). Large superior fragments should be viewed with caution and must be followed carefully through skeletal maturity lest they lead to subsequent acetabular dysplasia and hip subluxation.

When compared to other portions of the pelvis, it is infrequent that the femoral head is driven centrally into the pelvis in children prior to adolescence, probably because of resiliency. Watts described total dislocation of the acetabulum through the triradiate cartilage anteriorly and the sacroiliac joint posteriorly in a 12-year-old child; this was successfully treated by open reduction and internal fixation.[21]

A series of fractures of the acetabulum over a 20-year period comprised 0.3% of the admissions to a hospital for orthopaedic trauma.[22] Of 107 acetabular fractures, 11 were in the 12 to 19 age group. Therefore, these patients did not have sufficient growth left to manifest major growth disturbances. Only 5 of 107 patients had injury to the sciatic nerve.

Treatment of a patient with a fractured acetabulum is determined by the general condition and associated injuries. Most authors have advised conservative treatment, although Judet has recommended surgical repair (series only included adults).[23] From this series, it appeared that conservative treatment was better for inner-wall or posterior acetabular fractures. Patients with superior fractures had poor results whether treatment was non-operative or operative. The most important factor seems to be re-establishment of the superior dome and extraction of any loose fragments of bone or muscle that may be herniated into the defects, thereby reconstituting a normal femoral head-acetabular relationship. The future of the hip depends primarily on the condition of the weightbearing portions of the acetabulum and femoral head, the potential for development of ischemic necrosis, an accurate femoral-acetabular relationship, and intrinsic stability of the joint.

Ljubosic described 13 patients with premature closure of the triradiate cartilage consequent to obvious and occult injury to the acetabulum.[24] Additional case reports have also been described, but none of the reported patients had significant pain in the hip upon completion of skeletal maturation, although 1 did have some pain with exertion at extremes of motion during physical examination.[25,26]

Blair reported a patient who was originally injured at the age of 4 when he sustained a fracture of the left femur, right pubis, and the diastases of the pubic symphysis, the right sacroiliac joint, and the left triradiate cartilage.[27] Premature bridging was present in the horizontal arm of the triradiate cartilage 2 months after the injury.[27] At 14 years the patient was having significant pain in the hip, and evaluation showed subluxation of the hip. By the age of 16, the pain had worsened and he underwent Chiari osteotomy.

Rodrigues noted growth arrest following injury to the triradiate cartilage, causing a miniacetabulum.[28] This has also been reported by Hallel and Salvati, and has been experimentally created.[29] Figures 15-26 and 15-27 show representative cases with injury to the triradiate cartilage. Potential injury may only be suggested contingent upon the degree of trauma and possible limitation of movement. The diagnosis is most often made retrospectively.[24-26] Narrowing of the triradiate cartilage and displacement are difficult to detect roentgenographically, especially when other pelvic components are damaged. In Figure 15-26A subperiosteal new bone along the inner table on either side of the triradiate cartilage strongly suggested injury. Fortunately, growth arrest did not occur. However, in Figures 15-26B and C, a child with significant triradiate cartilage damage had complete arrest. Since this is relatively pliable cartilage, injury potential is increased when ischiopubic or symphyseal disruption is transmitted to the rest of the pelvis. The adult would probably yield at the sacroiliac joint, but the child may also fail at the triradiate cartilage, making this a childhood variation of the Malgaigne injury.

The major problem these children subsequently have is disparate growth of the acetabulum and femoral head. The femoral head continues to grow, while the normal mechanism of concomitant hemispheric expansion of the acetabulum is removed. Growth may only occur at the margin, and this becomes increasingly subjected to pathologic pressure from the femoral head causing eversional deformation, not unlike that seen in congenital hip disease (see Fig. 15-27).

Reconstructive surgery may be necessary in many of these children, and must be individualized to the specific injury, concomitant pelvic deformation from other factors, and degree of anticipated growth. Shelf procedures may offer an answer in many of these cases.

Hallel and Silvati have experimentally caused this type of injury by placing an intrapelvic bone block across the triradiate cartilage.[29] Ljubosic found that roentgenographically evident bone bridge extending from the ilium to the pubis may be present as early as 3 weeks after injury, but he also found that the absence of a medial bone bridge did not exclude the possibility of delayed closure several years later.[24] In all of these cases, when the patient is young, acetabular dysplasia and hemipelvic disproportion are the ultimate consequence (see Figs. 15-26 and 15-27; also see Fig. 15-10).

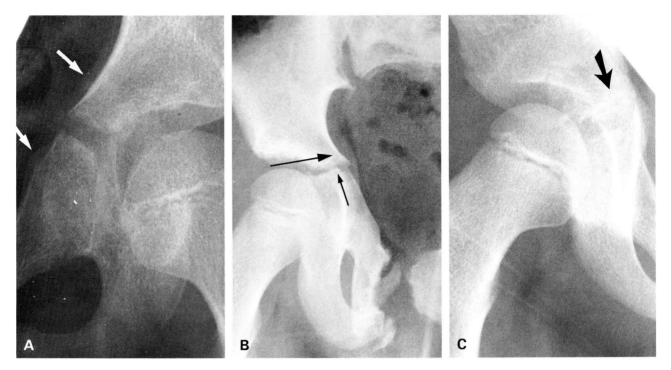

FIG. 15-26. *A,* Subperiosteal hemorrhage along the inner table (arrows) raises the possibility of triradiate fracture. Widening of the triradiate cartilage also suggests this injury, especially in an adolescent. *B,* Crush injury to right triradiate (arrows). *C,* Subsequent closure (arrow) of triradiate cartilage.

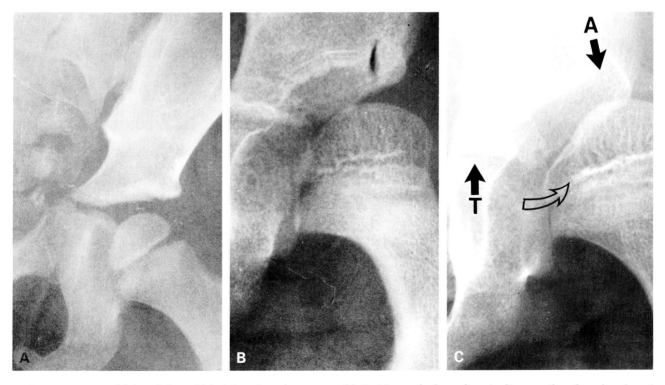

FIG. 15-27. *A,* Multiple pelvic and hip injury in a three-year-old. *B,* 16 months later the triradiate cartilage has closed, and significant deformity of the proximal femur is developing. Undoubtedly, this will lead to severe deformity as the child continues to grow. *C,* 26 months later, the proximal femur is beginning to lateralize (arrow). The triradiate cartilage (T) is completely closed. The acetabulum (A) is beginning to exhibit a superior deformity.

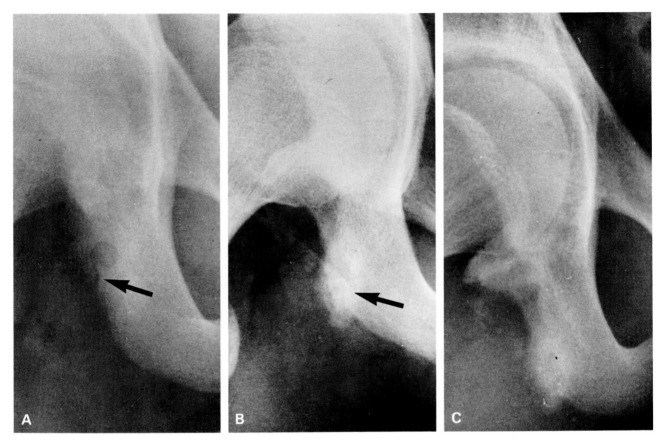

FIG. 15-28. *A,* Appearance of ischial tuberosity following "split" injury during water-skiing. Note the small linear crack which is suggestive of a fracture (arrow). *B,* Three weeks later, the presence of some reactive bone (arrow) confirms the diagnosis. *C,* Four months later, the area is beginning to remodel.

The consequences of this pathologic development of the acetabulum are not well understood. Many of the patients with traumatic acetabular dysplasia and subluxation of the femur, which usually is deformed in consequence, may have no symptoms. However, the case reported by Blair suggests that long term follow-up to skeletal maturity is necessary since the subluxating hip may eventually develop a problem.[27] In fact, one must consider the possibility of doing some type of pelvic osteotomy in the young child before the adolescent growth spurt, as a possible means of improving the overall congruency of the hip components. Disabling pain and incongruency may even require arthrodesis.[30]

Avulsion Fractures

These injuries probably represent the most common types of pelvic chondro-osseous injury, especially in the adolescent athlete.[31] Most avulsion fractures can be treated by bed rest, muscle relaxants, and cessation of athletic activity for 2 to 3 weeks. These regions may be avulsed prior to the appearance of the secondary ossification (which frequently does not appear until late adolescence). In the absence of definitive radiologic diagnosis the injury must be strongly suspected clinically and treatment instituted toward the presumptive injury. Several weeks later the diagnosis may be confirmed by the appearance of callus (Fig. 15-28). Because of the thick periosteum and perichondrium, these fractures are usually not significantly displaced. Post-injury muscle function generally is not impaired by eventual healing in a mildly displaced position, even if a fibrous, rather than osseous, union results due to the persistent tensile forces. Significant displacement, which is much less common, may cause functional insufficiency of the involved muscles and may require open reduction for optimal muscle function. Complications are unusual, since these are usually associated with seemingly minor athletic stress, rather than major trauma.

Iliac crest

Butler and Eggert reported a fracture of the iliac crest as a case of "hip pointer."[32] Hip pointer is defined in the standard nomenclature of athletic injuries as an "iliac crest contusion." Their patient sustained a direct blow to the crest from a football helmet. The fracture took several months to heal sufficiently to allow participation in contact sports.

Clancy and Foltz reviewed iliac crest apophysitis and believed that it was a significant cause of disability in the adolescent athlete.[33] They reported 13 cases of anterior iliac crest apophysitis and 3 cases of stress fractures of the anterior iliac apophysis in adolescent runners. The duration of symptoms had ranged from 1 to 36 weeks and initial roentgenographs often did not demonstrate significant injury. There were 4 patients who received local injections of steroid, which they felt did not affect the length of time of healing. However, such injections are contraindicated, since a fracture requires an appropriate inflammatory response to heal effectively (see Chaps. 4 and 5). Patients treated by bed rest and discontinuation of their normal athletic activity had complete relief of symptoms within 4 to 6 weeks, and were able to resume training programs at that point. There were 5 other adolescent track athletes in their series who had posterior iliac crest apophysitis with pain localized at the posterior iliac crest. This could be duplicated by resistance to abduction with the hip flexed with the patient lying on the unaffected side.

Roentgenograms are frequently unremarkable. One must seek subtle differences in contour or physeal width (Fig. 15-29).

Godshall reported a case of a 14-year-old boy with incomplete avulsion fracture of the iliac epiphysis due to a sudden severe contraction of the abdominal muscle associated with abrupt directional changes while running.[34] Godshall was unable to find any comparable cases, although he subsequently saw a 16-year-old boy with a similar injury and felt this particular condition in adolescent athletes could be confused with the "hip pointer" or a contusion of the iliac crest. If an immature athlete sustains a twisting injury with resultant pain in the region of the iliac crest, roentgenograms of good quality that may require special oblique projections should be obtained of both iliac crests for comparison, since developmental variation of the epiphysis may cause confusion. To avoid the risk of further avulsion and more serious damage, crutches should be used for 5 to 7 days and then physical activities should be limited for approximately 4 weeks.

Injury through growth cartilage may occur in major and minor trauma. Everett has described avulsion of a nonossified iliac crest, through the physis, resulting in intestinal obstruction due to a lumbar hernia.[18] Damage to the crest may lead to severe growth discrepancy (Fig. 15-30).

Iliac spines

The anterosuperior spine serves as the attachment of sartorius, and the anteroinferior spine as the attachment of the rectus femoris. Both are major hip flexors and can be under extreme force during athletic activity. The anterosuperior spine is injured more often than the inferior (Figs. 15-31 to 15-34).[10,35-37,37a] The classic case is of a 15-year-old sprinter who feels a sudden, sharp pain in the groin upon leaving the starting blocks. Usually the avulsed spine does not separate completely from the remainder of the pelvis (Fig. 15-31), although in rare instances it may be displaced several centimeters (Figs. 15-32 and 15-33). Hamsa described a displaced superior iliac spine that had led to formation of long osseous bar extending down from the pelvis.[31]

Treatment should be rest, minimal weight bearing with use of crutches, and discontinuation of athletic activities for 4 to 6 weeks. If a significant separation has occurred, open reduction may be indicated.

Irving reported two cases of exostosis formation after traumatic avulsion of the anteroinferior iliac spine.[38] This particular injury is much less common compared to other avulsion fractures around the pelvis (Fig. 15-34). These lesions should not be considered myositis ossificans.

Ischial tuberosity

This particular injury was reviewed in detail by Milch.[39] Hamada and Rida also present an excellent review.[40] The typical patient is a young athlete. This area can be avulsed (Fig. 15-35) and may lead to nonunion, although not necessarily symptomatic (Fig. 15-36; also see Fig. 15-28).

DePalma reported ischial apophyseolysis in brothers.[43] Interestingly, the left side was involved in both cases. Both fractures appeared while participating in athletics. One brother also had an early slipped capital femoral epiphysis.

The striking feature of ischial apophysiolysis is that the lesion is often diagnosed only after a considerable time pe-

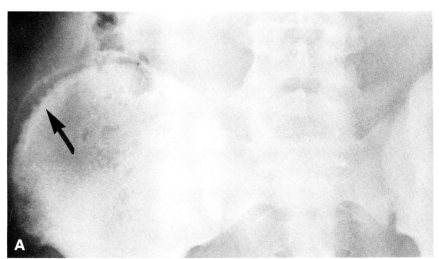
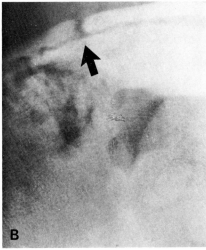

FIG. 15-29. Adolescent complaining of groin and anterior thigh pain after a football tackle. *A,* There is mild separation of the iliac ossification center on the right side (arrow). *B,* Fracture through crest ossification (arrow) following direct blow to the pelvic rim.

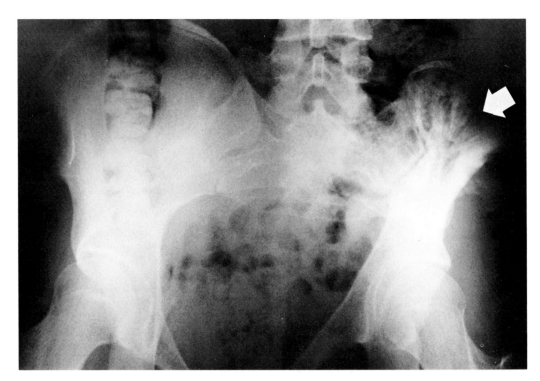

FIG. 15-30. Adolescent who had sustained injury to the left pelvis as a small child. The left hemipelvis is hypoplastic (arrow) and the entire pelvis is rotated, with displacement of the symphysis. The injury appeared to involve a portion of the crest; the acetabulum formed reasonably normally.

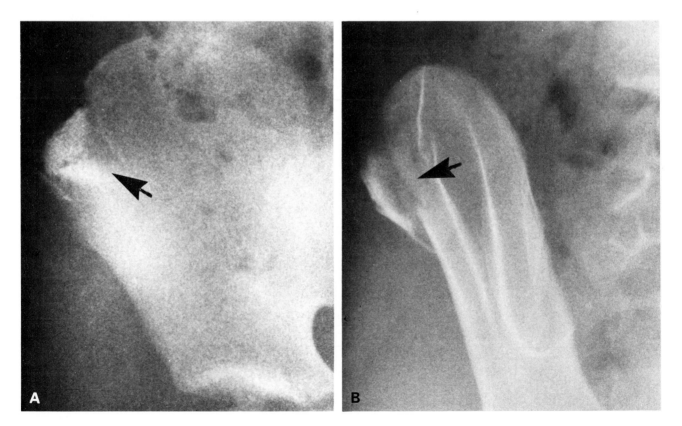

FIG. 15-31. Fractures of superior iliac spine. *A,* Undisplaced fracture (arrow) following direct blow. *B,* Avulsion (arrow) following direct blow.

riod (many months) has elapsed. In these delayed cases, the precipitating injury is not considered significant by either the patient or the physician.

From an anatomic standpoint, an avulsion is likely to be partial. The ischial tuberosity is roughly divisible into two portions, one for the insertion of the hamstrings and the other for the insertion of the adductor magnus. Thus, a high hurdler could produce a different pattern of injury from a dancer doing a split.

The mechanism of injury appears to be the action of hip flexors on the pelvis, transmitted across the femoral head as a fulcrum, which tends to elevate the ischium. This elevation is counteracted by the hamstring muscle, which pulls downward and laterally, a force neutralized by the sacrosciatic ligaments. Therefore, the degree of displacement of the ischial apophysis depends on the amount of tearing of these ligaments. Most authors agree that the most favorable conditions for the injury are when a powerful muscle contraction takes place in the hamstrings with the pelvis fixed in flexion and the knee in extension. This commonly is attained in hurdling and gymnastics, and as in the boy shown in Figure 15-28, who was injured during waterskiing.

Diagnosis often is difficult in these children. Figure 15-28 shows absence of any significant area, although the small crack, coupled with the history, should make one suspicious. Yet later, the diagnosis was obvious with formation of new bone.

Treatment may be divided into three categories contingent upon the diagnosis.[44] (1) Cases of apophysiolysis uniformly do well on a rest and protective program. Ideally, osseous union should be demonstrable by roentgenograms before strenuous exercises are permitted. Milch's excellent study indicated that this may require from two to four years in the younger age groups.[39] Failure to follow a protective program could result in avulsion fracture of the apophysis from a subsequent injury. The possibility of contralateral involvement should always be kept in mind. (2) Cases of avulsion fracture should be treated as a fracture and reduced anatomically, either by closed or open reduction. Open reduction seems to carry with it the most chance of success, depending upon the size of the actual fragment (see Fig. 15-36). An attempt at closed reduction probably is worthwhile and may be possible with direct pressure over the tuberosity. Open reduction of an avulsion fracture is a relatively straightforward procedure for an experienced surgeon. Attachment can be made with screws. (3) Chronic injuries (Fig. 15-37). These probably can be relieved best, when symptomatic, by excision of the ununited fragment and repair of the tendinous origin of the hamstrings.

An untreated avulsion fracture has two possible outcomes. It may unite spontaneously or may form a fibrous union with subsequent enlargement of the tuberosity.[45] The symptoms in the latter case are all similar: inability to sit comfortably on the enlarged, ununited tuberosity, and pain with associated discomfort in the back or limb especially while undergoing excessive activity.[46] The subsequent enlargement of the tuberosity may be irregular enough to suggest a tumor, and a diagnosis of osteogenic sarcoma or Ewing's sarcoma has been rendered in many cases. Sciatic-type pain is not a general feature of the older chronic lesions, and if this symptom is confronted, one should effectively rule out a herniated intervertebral disc before attributing neurologic symptomatology to this lesion.

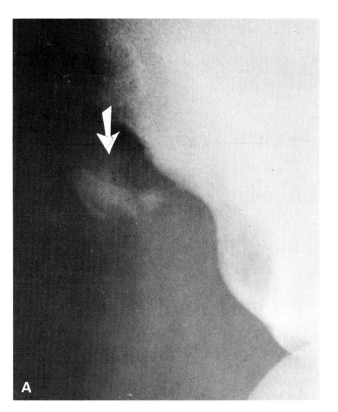

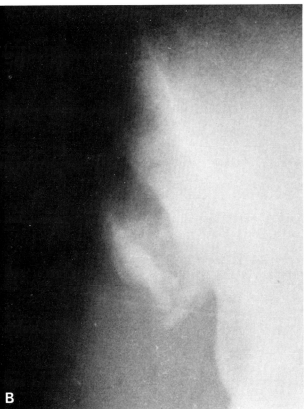

FIG. 15-32. *A,* Avulsion injury of superior iliac spine (arrow) in 14-year-old sprinter who sustained tear coming out of starting blocks. *B,* Appearance 7 weeks later with callus formation.

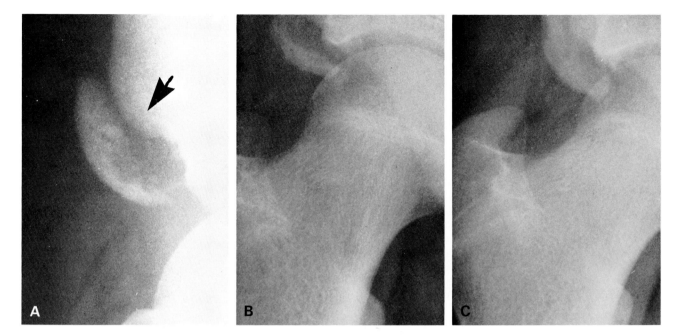

FIG. 15-33. *A,* Avulsion of inferior iliac spine (arrow). *B,* Avulsion of combined inferior spine and acetabular rim ossification center. *C,* Four months later, extensive healing of the fracture shown in *B* is evident.

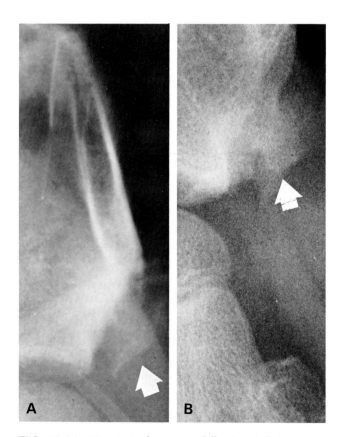

FIG. 15-34. Exostosis formation following inferior spine injury in six-year-old. *A,* A healing fracture (arrow) is evident three weeks after injury. *B,* Eight months later a prominent exostosis (arrow) has formed from callus in the space between the ilium and the avulsed spine.

References

1. Risser, J. C.: The iliac apophysis: an invaluable sign in the management of scoliosis. Clin. Orthop., *11:*111, 1958.
2. Caffey, J.: Pediatric X-ray Diagnosis. 6th ed. Chicago, Yearbook Medical Publishers, 1972.
3. Dunn, A. W., and Morris, H. D.: Fractures and dislocations of the pelvis. J. Bone Joint Surg., *50-A:*1639, 1968.
4. Heiss, W., Daum, R., and Fischer, H.: Bechenfraturen bei Kindern und Jugendlichen. Hefte Unfallheilk., *124:*283, 1975.
5. Schmidt, H. D., and Hofmann, S.: Die Problematik schwerer Bechenfrakturen im Wachstumsalter. Hefte Unfallheilk., *124:* 286, 1975.
6. Braunstein, P. W., et al.: Concealed hemorrhage due to pelvic fracture. J. Trauma, *4:*832, 1964.
7. Ger, R., Condrea, H., and Steichen, F. M.: Traumatic intrapelvic hemorrhage. An experimental study. J. Surg. Res., *9:*31, 1969.
8. Levine, J. I., and Crampton, R. S.: Major abdominal injuries associated with pelvic fractures. Surg. Gynecol. Obstet., *62:*223, 1963.
9. Peltier, L. F.: Complications associated with fractures of the pelvis. J. Bone Joint Surg., *47-A:*1060, 1965.
10. Rowe, C. R., and Lowell, J. D.: Prognosis of fractures of the acetabulum. J. Bone Joint Surg., *43-A:*30, 1961.
11. Quinby, W. C.: Fractures of the pelvis and other associated injuries in children. J. Pediatr. Surg., *1:*353, 1966.
12. Ring, E. J., et al.: Angiography in pelvic trauma. Surg. Gynecol. Obstet., *139:*375, 1974.
13. Reed, M. H.: Pelvic fractures in children. J. Can. Assoc. Radiol., *27:*255, 1976.
14. Barlow, B., Rottenberg, R. W., and Santulli, T. V.: Angiographic diagnosis and treatment of bleeding by selective embolization following pelvic fracture in children. J. Pediatr. Surg., *10:*939, 1975.
15. Margolies, M. N., et al.: Arteriography in the management of hemorrhage from pelvic fractures. N. Engl. J. Med., *287:*317, 1972.
16. Arnold, G. T.: A case of fracture of the pelvis with nipping of the small intestine between the fragments. Lancet, *I:*1157, 1907.

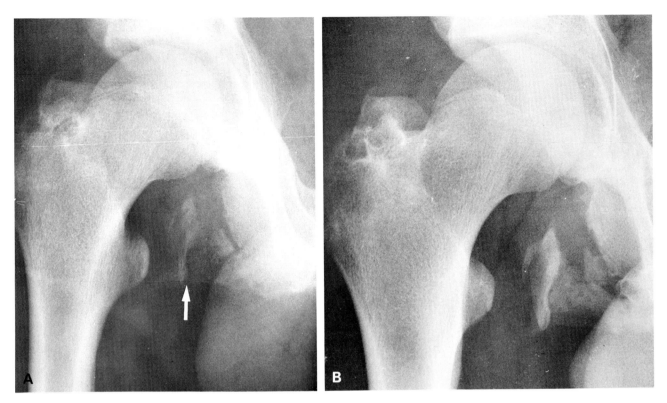

FIG. 15-35. *A,* Avulsion of ischial tuberosity with early bone formation (arrow). *B,* Seven weeks after the injury, extensive bone formation is evident. The symphysis was also separated in this case, and it is filling in with bone.

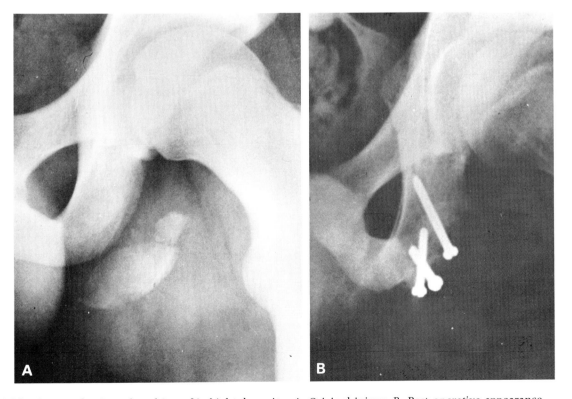

FIG. 15-36. Open reduction of avulsion of ischial tuberosity. *A,* Original injury. *B,* Post-operative appearance.

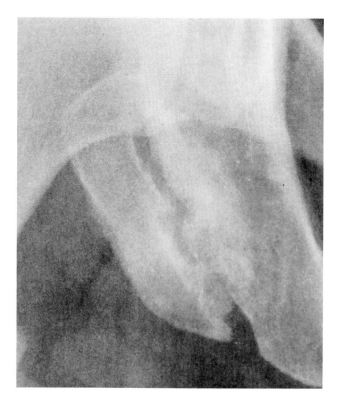

FIG. 15-37. Nonunion of ischial avulsion.

17. Lunt, H. R. W.: Entrapment of bowel within fractures of the pelvis. Injury, 2:221, 1970.

18. Everett, W. G.: Traumatic lumbar hernia. Injury, 4:345, 1972.

19. Pollen, A.: Fractures and Dislocations in Children. Baltimore, Williams & Wilkins, 1973.

20. Stewart, M. J., and Milford, L. W.: Fracture-dislocation of the hip. J. Bone Joint Surg., 36-A:315, 1954.

21. Watts, H.: Fractures of the pelvis in children. Orthop. Clin. North Am., 7:615, 1976.

22. Nerubay, J., Glancz, G., and Katznelson, A.: Fractures of the acetabulum. J. Trauma, 13:1050, 1973.

23. Judet, R., Judet, J., and Letournel, F.: Fractures of the acetabulum: classification and surgical approaches for open reduction. J. Bone Joint Surg., 46-A:1615, 1964.

24. Ljubosic, N. A.: Poraneni jamky kycelniho kloubu u deti. Acta Chir. Orthop. Traumatol. Cech., 34-5:393, 1967.

25. Jurkovskj, I. I.: Perelomy taza u detej. Diss. Kand. M., 1945.

26. Lansinger, O.: Fractures of the acetabulum. A clinical and experimental study. Acta Orthop. Scand. [Suppl.] 165, 1977.

27. Blair, W., and Hanson, C.: Traumatic closure of the triradiate cartilage. Report of a case. J. Bone Joint Surg., 61-A:144, 1979.

28. Rodrigues, K. F.: Injury of the acetabular epiphysis. Injury, 4:258, 1972.

29. Hallel, T., and Salvati, E. A.: Premature closure of the triradiate cartilage. A case report and animal experiment. Clin. Orthop., 124:278, 1977.

30. Fulkerson, J. P.: Arthrodesis for disabling hip pain in children and adolescents. Clin. Orthop., 128:296, 1977.

31. Hamsa, W. R.: Epiphyseal injuries about the hip joint. Clin. Orthop., 10:119, 1957.

32. Butler, J. E., and Eggert, A. W.: Fracture of the iliac crest apophysis: an unusual hip pointer. J. Sports Med. Phys. Fitness, 3:192, 1975.

33. Clancy, W. G., and Foltz, A. S.: Iliac apophysitis and stress fractures in adolescent runners. J. Sports Med. Phys. Fitness, 4:214, 1976.

34. Godshall, R. W., and Hansen, C. A.: Incomplete avulsion of a portion of the iliac epiphysis. An injury of young athletes. J. Bone Joint Surg., 55-A:1301, 1973.

35. Corlett, C. G.: Fracture of the anterior inferior spine of the ilium. Med. J. Aust., 2:682, 1927.

36. Gallagher, J. R.: Fracture of the anterior inferior spine of the ilium: sprinter's fracture. Ann. Surg., 102:86, 1935.

37. Hanke, H.: Zur Kenntnis der isolierten Abrissfraktur der interen Spina anterior ossis ilei. Arch. Orthop. Unfallchir., 31:377, 1932.

37a. Weitzner, I.: Fracture of the anterior superior spine of the ilium in one case, and anterior inferior in another case. A.J.R., 33:39, 1935.

38. Irving, M. H.: Exostosis formation after traumatic avulsion of the anterior inferior iliac spine. J. Bone Joint Surg., 46-B:720, 1964.

39. Milch, H.: Ischial apophysiolysis—a new syndrome. Clin. Orthop., 2:184, 1953.

40. Hamada, G., and Rida, A.: Ischial apophysiolysis (IAL). Clin. Orthop., 31:117, 1964.

41. Labuz, E. F.: Avulsion of the ischial tuberosity. J. Bone Joint Surg., 28:388, 1946.

42. McMaster, P. E.: Epiphysitis of the ischial tuberosity. J. Bone Joint Surg., 27:493, 1945.

43. DePalma, A. F., and Silberstein, C. E.: Avulsion fracture of the ischial tuberosity in siblings. Clin. Orthop., 38:120, 1965.

44. Martin, T. A., and Pipkin, G.: Treatment of avulsion of the ischial tuberosity. Clin. Orthop., 10:108, 1957.

45. Winkler, H., and Rapp, I. H.: Ununited epiphysis of the ischium. J. Bone Joint Surg., 29:234, 1947.

46. Schlonsky, J., and Oliz, M. L.: Functional disability following avulsion fracture of the ischial epiphysis. Report of two cases. J. Bone Joint Surg., 54-A:641, 1972.

16

Hip

Anatomy

The pertinent anatomy of the acetabulum is presented in Chapter 15, and aspects of proximal femoral development (especially the capital femur) are presented in Chapter 17. However, certain structures relate directly to the hip joint and the specific problems encountered in dislocation of the hip joint in the skeletally immature individual.

The capsule inserts along the chondro-osseous junction of the pelvis, making the acetabular labrum intra-articular. The femoral insertion is along the intertrochanteric margins, thus totally encapsulating the developing capital femur and femoral neck. This creates an enveloping "spherical" structure comprised of synovium and dense ligaments (Fig. 16-1).

The iliofemoral ligament, which may become a major obstacle to reduction, is somewhat triangular, resembles an inverted "Y," and is sometimes referred to as the Y-ligament of Bigelow. The apex of the ligament is in the markedly thickened longitudinal fibers of the capsule originating from the anteroinferior iliac spine and traversing the anterior aspect of the hip joint to attach to the anterior, inner trochanteric line (Fig. 16-2). As this fibrous band passes distally, it becomes broad and tends to separate into two bands. The iliofemoral ligament normally limits hyperextension and lateral rotation of the hip joint. The ligament is under maximum tension in extension, which also increases intra-articular pressure, especially if a hemarthrosis is present.

The capsule is torn either anteriorly or posteriorly, de-

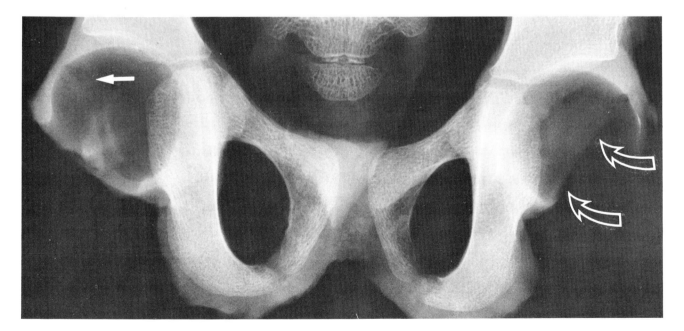

FIG. 16-1. Appearance of hip joints in a seven-year-old. The right hip capsule has been cut along the femoral insertion to emphasize contour and anterior extent of this structure. The solid arrow depicts the demarcation between labrum and capsule. Essentially, the capsule extends the hemispheric acetabulum to create an enveloping structure that is approximately three quarters of a sphere. The left hip capsule has been cut to emphasize the posterior intertrochanteric line (open arrows). This portion does not extend as far along the femoral neck as the anterior portion.

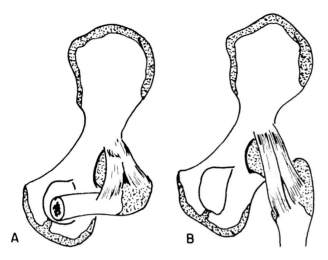

FIG. 16-2. Schematic of Y-ligament of Bigelow. *A,* In flexion the ligament relaxes. *B,* In extension the ligament is maximally taut.

pending on the direction of dislocation. It is likely that the tear will be closer to the pelvic attachment than the thicker femoral attachments. It often involves the midcourse of the ligament, as the actual ligamentous attachments into cartilage and bone are dense. Buttonholing through a capsular tear may impose restraints upon closed reduction and necessitate open reduction (Fig. 16-3). The Y-ligament may be taut in dislocation.

The iliopsoas tendon may slip behind the femoral head or acetabulum and cross the capsule, similar to congenital hip dislocation in the older child (Fig. 16-3). This dislocation may present a major impediment to closed reduction. Other muscles in the direct path of the dislocating femoral head may be stretched or partially torn. The external rotator muscle group (obturatorius externus and internus, piriformis and quadratus femoris) is either partially or completely torn, along with the posterior part of the capsule. The femoral head may occasionally push between the short external

rotators without tearing them. The gluteus maximus, medius, and minimus muscles are stretched and pushed backward by the femoral head, which usually lies deep to these muscles, similar to the distortion caused by a chronic congenital hip dislocation (Fig. 16-4).

The ligamentum capitis femoris limits displacement of the femoral head, no matter what the age of the patient. It generally has to rupture to allow complete anterior or posterior dislocation. Accordingly, any blood supply from the ligament into the femoral head will be impaired.

Incidence and Outcome

Individual experience with hip dislocation in children is usually limited.[1-5,5a,6-13] Epstein reported 75 dislocations in 74 patients over a span of 48 years.[14,15] These dislocations included 1 patient with bilateral dislocation, a 15-year-old girl who died 1 day after injury from fat embolism. They represented 9% of an overall series of 830 dislocations. Approximately 75% were male and 25% were female. The right and left hips were almost equally involved. There were 11 dislocations in the 2- to 4-year age group, 13 in the 5- to 7-year age group, 18 in the 8- to 12-year age group, and 33 in the 13- to 15-year age group. Of these dislocations, 67 were posterior and 8 were anterior; 4 had concurrent ipsilateral femoral fractures, and 1 was not recognized for 2½ months.

The Pennsylvania Orthopedic Society collected 51 cases of hip dislocation in skeletally immature patients: 41 were posterior, 8 anterior, and 2 central.[16,17] Of those patients, 9 had associated fractures of the acetabulum, femoral head, or greater trochanter; these particular concomitant injuries strongly influenced the prognosis. There were 5 additional patients who had associated ipsilateral tibial or femoral shaft

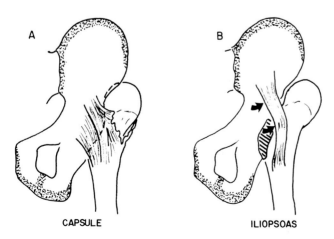

FIG. 16-3. *A,* Effect of buttonholing through the capsule. *B,* Effect of translocated iliopsoas tendon in preventing reduction. The structure marked by lines is the acetabulum.

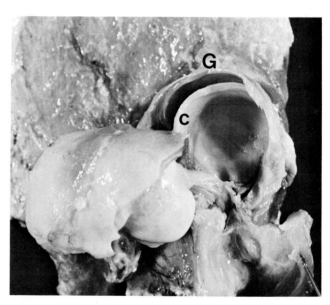

FIG. 16-4. Anatomy of chronic congenital hip dislocation in a ten-year-old. This distortion of capsule (C) and gluteus medius/minimus (G) may be seen in both acute traumatic dislocation and chronic, post-traumatic hip redislocation.

fractures. These aforementioned injuries did not influence the final results in 4 instances, but did delay diagnosis and treatment in 2 patients for 3 weeks and 6 months (the former going on to a normal hip and the latter an abnormal hip). The remaining 37 cases had no complicating associated lesions. The final results in their series showed 43 normal hips and 8 abnormal hips. However, they felt the predictive value was tentative, since only 18 of the 51 patients had attained skeletal maturity. By reviewing the literature, as well as their series, they felt that one third of the children had, or would have, abnormal hips or poor results by the time they reached skeletal maturity. Since patterns of ischemic necrosis complicating the closed treatment of congenital hip dysplasia may not cause significant deformity until the adolescent growth spurt, follow-up to skeletal maturation is imperative.[18]

Robertson and Peterson felt that if ischemic necrosis was not evident by 15 months after the injury, it probably would not develop.[19] Their series included 24 children, 1 of whom had bilateral hip dislocation, and another who died 2 days after the dislocation from other injuries. There were 23 posterior dislocations and 9 concomitant acetabular fractures. One child had an anterior dislocation; 2 children had recurrent posterior dislocations and both had concomitant posterior acetabular fractures. There were 5 children who suffered sciatic nerve injury.

Types of Dislocations. Traumatic dislocation of the hip may be classified according to the position of the displaced femoral head relative to the acetabulum (Fig. 16-5): (1) Posterior-iliac; the femoral head lies posterosuperiorly along the lateral aspect of the ilium. (2) Posterior-ischial; the femoral head is displaced posteroinferiorly and lies adjacent to the greater sciatic notch. (3) Anterior-obturator; the femoral head lies near the obturator membrane; the perineal type is an extremely inferiorly displaced form of anterior dislocation. (4) Anterior-pubic; the femoral head is displaced anterosuperiorly along the superior ramus of the pubic bone. (5) Central; there is a comminuted fracture of the central portion of the acetabulum with displacement of the femoral head and acetabular fragments into the pelvis. This is an unusual injury in a child. (6) Inferior dislocation with the femoral head lying directly inferior to the acetabulum.[20] (7) In rare instances a segment of the femoral head may remain; this is a rare type in children. (8) Dislocation of the hip in association with separation of the capital femoral epiphysis.[21] In such an injury the capital femur may remain in the joint while the neck "dislocates," or the capital femur may be totally extracapsular and variably separated from the displaced femoral neck.

Most posterior dislocations are of the iliac type, with the femur positioned between the sciatic notch and the acetabulum. High-iliac and ischial-posterior luxations are uncommon, particularly in children. On rare occasions both hips may be involved.[15,19] Bernhang reported bilateral traumatic dislocation of the hips in a 4-year-old boy (Fig. 16-6).[22]

Mechanism of Injury

The trauma sustained varies considerably.[23-29] One of the most striking observations is the benign nature of the injury that often causes the pediatric hip dislocation, in contrast to the significant force required to dislocate the adult hip. Trivial injury mechanisms become prevalent in the younger age groups (Fig. 16-7).

The immature acetabulum is largely pliable cartilage and joint laxity is common in younger children. Often no force is required to subluxate the hip to the rim, while little force is required to subsequently dislocate the hip completely. As age increases, greater portions of the acetabulum become osseous and there is a gradual lessening of joint laxity, such that more violent trauma is required to produce the same type of injury, and is more likely to create associated osseous damage to the acetabulum.

In Epstein's series, the majority of dislocations were due to relatively severe trauma.[15] About 60% were vehicular-related accidents; although 5 occurred during football. Of this series, 30% involved less severe trauma such as falling down stairs or tripping.

Diagnostic Features

In posterior-iliac dislocations, the deformity has a typical appearance. The involved lower limb is held in flexion, adduction, and internal rotation at the hip. There is both apparent and actual shortening of the limb. In posterior-ischial dislocation, abduction is more likely. The femoral head may be palpable in the gluteal region. The child generally is in severe pain and unable to stand or walk. Motion of the hip is painful and guarded by muscle spasm. The motions of extension, abduction, and external rotation are markedly restricted and painful. Flexion and internal rotation posturing of the hip are primarily produced by tension in the Y-ligament of Bigelow.

Because this injury is often sustained while sitting in a car with the hip flexed, evaluation of the femur, patella, and upper end of the tibia for concomitant injury must also be undertaken (Fig. 16-8).[30] Dislocation of the hip, even in children, may be missed if there is an ipsilateral femoral fracture. These are rare concomitant injuries, particularly in children.[31-33] Dehne and Immermann found that in 42 cases of dislocation of the hip with ipsilateral fracture of the femur, the dislocation was recognized at initial examination in only 15 cases.[34] In most cases, the diagnosis was not made until 4 to 6 weeks later.

Roentgenographic examination

Roentgenography discloses the specific type of dislocation (Figs. 16-9 to 16-13). It is imperative that adequate films be taken to rule out associated fractures, especially of the triradiate cartilage (see Chap. 15) or acetabular margin (Fig. 16-14). The hip region must be roentgenographed in any fracture of the femur following a severe injury to rule out the concomitance of hip dislocation and femoral shaft fracture.[33]

Barquet reported 6 retroacetabular dislocations.[1] He stressed the difficulty in diagnosing this particular dislocation pattern in children, since standard frontal roentgenograms may show a seemingly normal "concentric" projection of capital femoral physis and acetabulum. Other authors have also described this problem.[35-37] A true cross-table lateral view of the pelvis should demonstrate the posterior displacement.

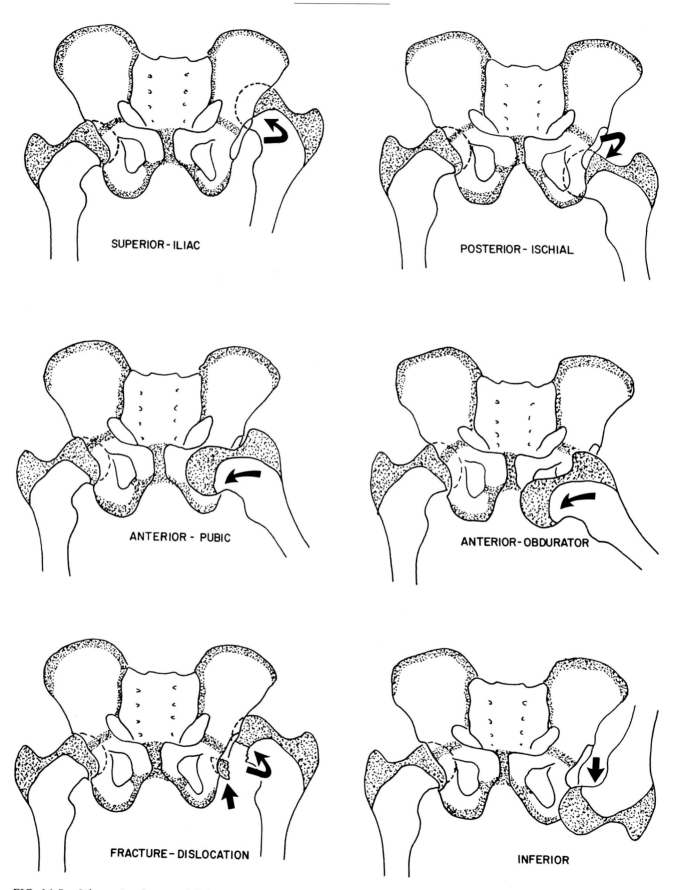

FIG. 16-5. Schematic of types of dislocation.

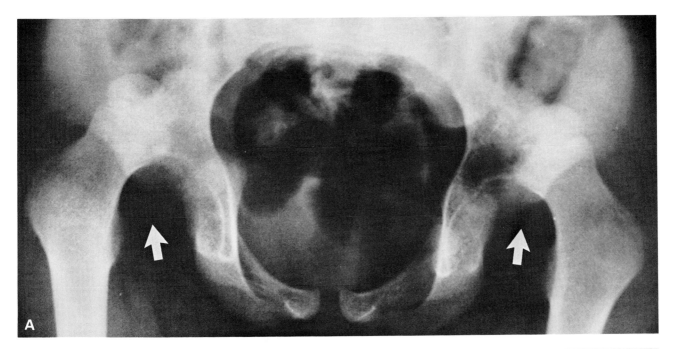

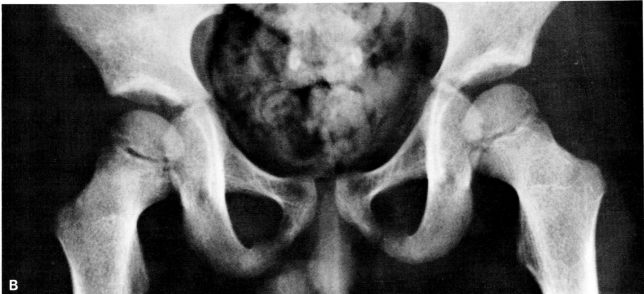

FIG. 16-6. *A,* Bilateral traumatic dislocation (arrows). *B,* Appearance after closed reduction.

Treatment

There is general agreement that early reduction within 24 hours is important in order to prevent undesirable sequelae such as ischemic necrosis. Closed reduction of uncomplicated, fresh, posterior dislocations is almost always possible, leaving open reduction for only a small number of neglected cases and the otherwise rare, irreducible, acute dislocations (usually due to some type of capsular or musculotendinous interposition).

The chief obstacle to reduction in posterior hip dislocation is the iliofemoral ligament. The following 3 common methods of closed reduction of posterior dislocations all utilize the principle of hip flexion, which causes the Y-ligament to relax and brings the femoral head adjacent to the acetabular margin near the capsular rent.[38]

(1) Gravity method of Stimson (Fig. 16-15). The patient is placed prone, with the lower limb hanging free from the end of the table. The pelvis is immobilized by pressing down on the sacrum and the greater trochanter. The knee is then flexed to 90° and pressure applied just below the bent knee. Gentle rocking or rotatory motions of the limb and direct pressure on the femoral head assist in the reduction. This method is the least forceful, and utilizes the weight of the limb to help the reduction. If necessary, a sandbag may be strapped to the leg to help relax tight muscles. However, if

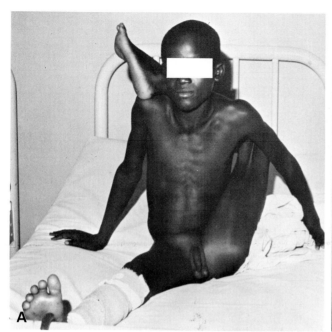
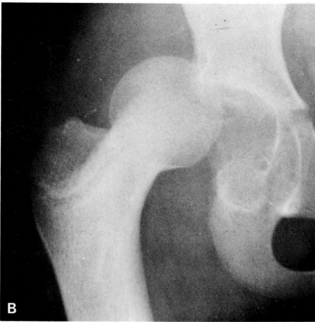

FIG. 16-7. *A,* Ten-year-old boy duplicating stunt with left leg that had resulted in right hip dislocation. No trauma was involved. *B,* Roentgenogram of hip of patient shown in *A*.

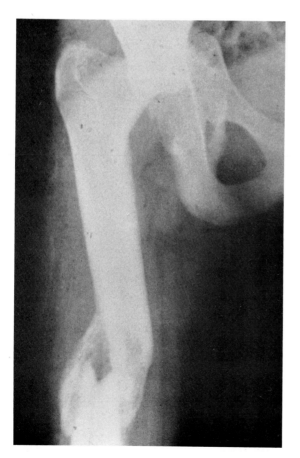

this is done under an adequate anesthesia with appropriate muscle-relaxing agents, excessive force is not necessary, and should be avoided to prevent complications such as iatrogenic slipped capital femoral epiphysis.

(2) Direct method of Allis (Fig. 16-16). The patient is placed in a supine position and the pelvis immobilized by pressing on the anterior superior spine. The hip and knee are both flexed to 90° with the thigh in slight adduction and medial rotation. With the forearm behind the knee, apply direct vertical traction, lifting the femoral head over the posterior rim of the acetabulum through the rent in the capsule

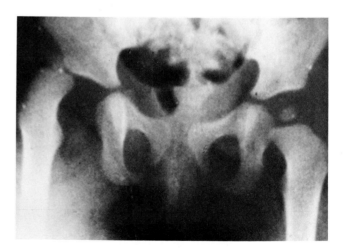

FIG. 16-8. Concomitant fracture of femur and dislocation of hip in 15-year-old girl. The dislocation was missed during the acute treatment.

FIG. 16-9. Posterior-iliac dislocation in a six-month-old infant. This injury is rare. In trauma, a fracture of the proximal femur is more likely. Often such dislocations in this age group are due to a septic process.

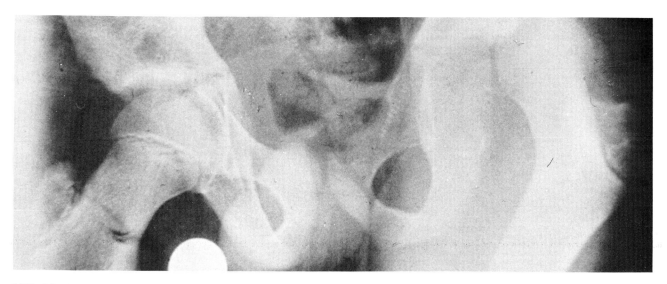

FIG. 16-10.   Posterosuperior dislocation in a 13-year-old.

into the acetabular socket. The hip and knee should then be gradually extended. Soft tissue resistance is occasionally encountered. This may be relaxed by increasing the degree of hip adduction and medial rotation. If the hip cannot be extended easily after the reduction, there probably is soft tissue interposition and another attempt at closed reduction should be undertaken before resorting to open reduction.

(3) Circumduction method of Bigelow (Fig. 16-17). The patient is placed supine and countertraction is applied. Adduct and internally rotate the thigh, flex the hip to 90° or more, and apply longitudinal traction in the line of the deformity. These motions convert an iliac to an ischial displacement by running the femoral head along the posterior margin of the acetabulum and causing increased relaxation in the Y-ligament. The femoral head is freed from the short

external rotators by gently rotating and rocking while traction is maintained. This allows levering of the femoral head into the acetabulum.

It is wise to use general anesthesia or a muscle relaxer, particularly in the older child. Attempts to reduce dislocation under analgesia, or a combination of analgesia and a drug such as diazepam, may not allow sufficient muscle relaxation for an easy reduction. Since most dislocations are posterior, attempts to reduce the hip without adequate relaxation could result in the femoral head being pushed backward against the posterior acetabular rim, comparable to the mechanism in chronic slipped capital femoral epiphysis (Fig. 16-18). Because of morphologic constraints, reduction of an anterior dislocation would not be as likely to cause such a displacement of the femoral head.

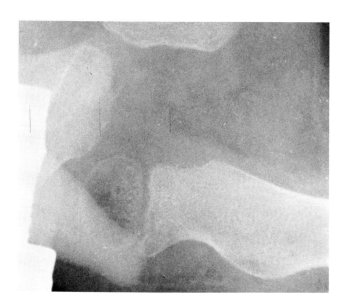

FIG. 16-11.   Posterior-ischial dislocation in a three-year-old.

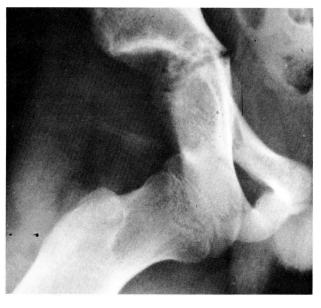

FIG. 16-12.   Posteroinferior dislocation in a seven-year-old.

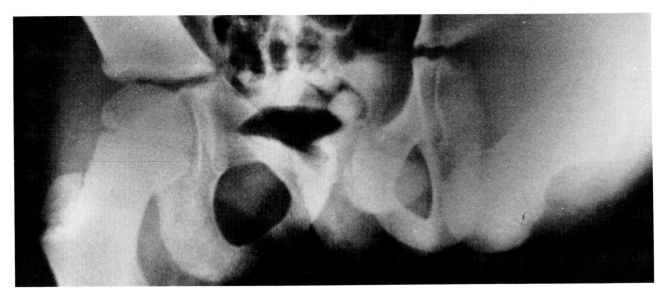

FIG. 16-13. Inferior dislocation in a ten-year-old.

Following reduction, roentgenograms are made to confirm the completeness of the reduction. Sometimes associated fractures of the margin of the acetabulum are not readily evident on pre-reduction films, but may become evident after reduction. Any widening of the joint space relative to the contralateral hip should make one suspicious of soft tissue or cartilage interposition and the need for displacement and reduction, or possibly even exploratory arthrotomy and excision of interposed tissue.[39-41] Possible impediments to closed reduction may be the piriformis tendon, an inverted labrum, or an osteocartilaginous fragment.

If closed reduction is unsuccessful, or if there are significant chondro-osseous acetabular fractures, open reduction may be necessary. A posterior or lateral approach is best to visualize the damaged areas. Large fragments should be se-

cured, but fixation pins or screws must not damage the triradiate cartilage. The capsular rent should be repaired.

Epstein performed open reductions in only four patients.[15] One was opened acutely and two others were done at two and seven days after injury and attempted closed reductions. Fair to good results were obtained because of structural damage, which limited non-operative reduction. Open reduction was tried unsuccessfully on the fourth patient ten months after a missed diagnosis.

Post-reduction

There is little agreement on immediate post-reduction treatment. Most surgeons use some sort of immobilization that lasts from a few days to about two months. This may be

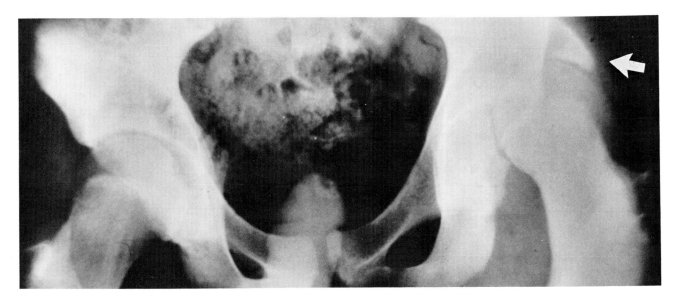

FIG. 16-14. Dislocation with acetabular lip fracture (arrow) in a 14-year-old. This was treated by open reduction.

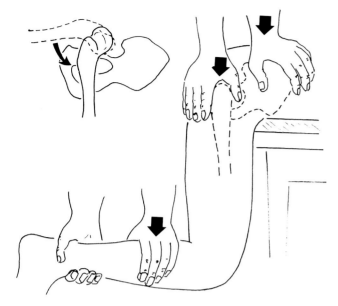

FIG. 16-15. Closed reduction. Method of Stimson.

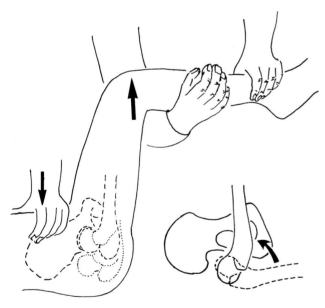

FIG. 16-16. Closed reduction. Method of Allis.

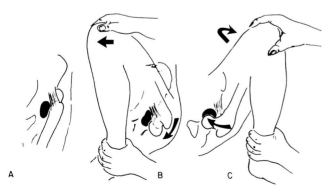

FIG. 16-17. Closed reduction. Circumduction method of Bigelow.

achieved by bed rest, traction, or spica cast. I recommend traction for one to three weeks in Russell's suspension with the hip flexed about 30° to relax the capsule. Three to six weeks of immobilization are probably sufficient to allow healing of capsular and soft tissue structures.

The presence of synovial irritation should be one of the guidelines to determine when the child can be allowed some protected activity. As long as acute synovial irritation or pain is present, the child should be in traction, and not in a cast. If symptoms of synovial irritation recur after the resumption of weightbearing, the patient should again be placed in traction, or at least in a non-weightbearing status.

It is difficult to assess the importance of the non-weightbearing period. Recommendations regarding the duration of this period range from a few days to three months.[41-44] A correlation between the period of non-weightbearing and the frequency of ischemic necrosis was proposed by Funk, but according to other authors there is no such correlation.[14,41,45] Hemmelbo recommended that weightbearing be avoided for two to three months, although most of the patients started weightbearing two to three weeks after release from traction.[46]

In children under the age of six, despite their excellent prognosis, it is advisable to prohibit weightbearing for at least a month, after which gradual resumption of activity may be permitted. Children over the age of six should be non-weightbearing for an additional period of time, probably three to four months. When persistent symptoms (e.g., synovitis) are present, this period should be prolonged further. However, it should be noted that almost all children resume full activities and full weightbearing *promptly* after removal of any restrictive device, regardless of advice to the contrary.

Fracture-Dislocation

Kelly described posterior dislocation of the hip with a portion of the femoral head remaining within the acetabulum.[47] This remaining fragment commonly possessed attachments of the retinacular layer as well as the ligamentum (capitis) femoris. He described 27 cases, the youngest being a 16-year-old male.[47] This injury is not generally associated with the immature skeleton, although it has been seen in young people (Fig. 16-19). Like the fracture of Tillaux, it is most likely to occur when the physis is undergoing closure. The best results follow closed reduction. Open reduction, particularly with excision of the medial head fragment (even though it is relatively non-weightbearing), had inferior results compared to either open reduction with internal fixation or closed reduction.

Epstein described a 6-year-old girl who underwent closed reduction.[15] At follow-up 13 years later, the fragment had reattached to the neck to form an exostotic mass that blocked full-flexion and adduction.

Traumatic Separation of the Capital Femur

The capital femur may be injured during a hip dislocation. The femoral head may remain within the confines of the acetabulum, with the femoral neck and greater trochanter

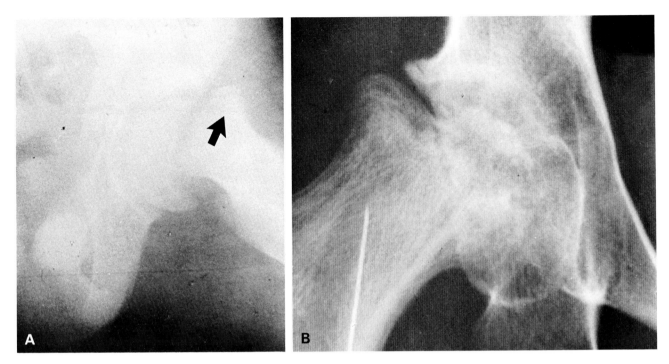

FIG. 16-18. *A,* Reduction of a posterosuperior dislocation in this patient resulted in an acute slipped capital femoral epiphysis (arrow). *B,* This hip dislocation was reduced closed. Several weeks later, the patient complained of thigh pain, but had no roentgenographic evaluation. Six months later, he was finally evaluated properly, and was found to have a severe chronic slip, which probably occurred early in the post-reduction period.

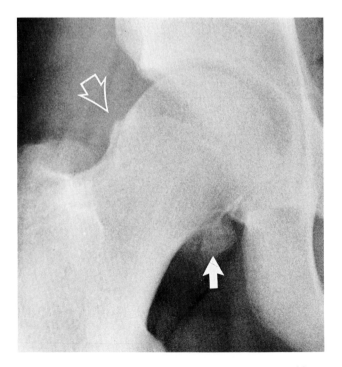

FIG. 16-19. Type IV fracture dislocation in 14-year-old resulting in a small, inferior fragment (solid arrow). This was not treated by open reduction. Five years later, the patient is skeletally mature and asymptomatic. A mild, slipped epiphysis may have accompanied this fracture/dislocation (open arrow).

displacing laterally. The capital femur may also be displaced from the acetabulum, as well as significantly separated from the femoral neck. A third possibility is displacement of the entire proximal femoral unit associated with a mild to moderate (incomplete) slip. The capital femur may also be displaced during reduction of a posterior dislocation (see Fig. 16-18). Such a capital femoral displacement, whether a part of the injury or a complication of the reduction, requires restoration of anatomy and pin fixation.

According to Mass, none of the patients with this injury had a good result.[21] The treatment of choice for this complication is reduction and internal fixation.

One patient had an isolated dislocation of the capital femoral epiphysis that was treated by open reduction and pinning. Another case, an 11-year-old, had a slipped capital femoral epiphysis and was treated by an open reduction, since the capital femoral segment was extra-articular.[19]

Results

Factors that influence results are as follows: (1) Age. In the birth to 5 year group there are usually no complications; whereas complications are evenly divided in the other two groups of 5 to 10 years and 10 to 15 years. The most frequent cause of an abnormal result is ischemic necrosis of the capital femur. (2) Severity of injury is of major significance from the standpoint of the prognosis. The increased severity of injury is also associated with an increase of concomitant fractures. (3) The correlation between delay in reduction and abnormal results in children is less significant than in adults, with the exception of the possible production of ischemic necrosis. (4) Although it seems logical to prohibit weightbearing for a 2- to 3-month period to provide adequate rest to the injured joint, there does not seem to be any correlation between the period of non-weightbearing and the final result. (5) The type of treatment, whether closed or operative reduction, does not affect the overall results. The 2 major factors that lead to ischemic necrosis are delay in reduction over 24 hours and severity of trauma.

Epstein described the results in 44 posterior dislocations, with an average follow-up of 78.6 months. Of these patients, 24 had excellent results and 11 had good results. There were 9 patients who had fair to poor results. These patients were all severely injured and usually had chondral or chondro-osseous injury that complicated the dislocation.

Complications

All patients must be followed regularly, both clinically and radiographically, to anticipate and document complications as early as possible. Follow-up can only be considered complete when the patients are skeletally mature.

Vascular changes

The most significant complication is vascular compromise eventuating in ischemic osseous changes (Fig. 16-20).[48-51] Fineschi reviewed approximately 150 cases, as well as his own 7 cases and found 16 complicated by avascular necrosis.[40] This figure concurs with that of the Pennsylvania Orthopedic Society; their ischemic necrosis incidence was only 4%.[17] Epstein reported a 6% incidence.[15]

Glass and Powell presented a study of 47 children who sustained traumatic hip dislocation before the age of 16; all dislocations were posterior.[23] The incidence of ischemic necrosis was approximately 20%. The average follow-up was 28 months, the shortest was 6 months and the longest 8 years. One child out of 26 under the age of 10 developed avascular necrosis. Of the 20 aged 10 or over, 5 were so affected. There was premature epiphyseal fusion in only 1 child.

Elmslie described avascular necrosis of the femoral head secondary to traumatic dislocation and termed it coxa plana.[52,53] Goldenberg described Perthes disease following hip dislocation; this most likely was ischemic necrosis comparable to other patients.[54] Undoubtedly, comparisons of avascular necrosis to Legg-Calvé-Perthes disease are not appropriate because one is a more chronic type of condition. However, the roentgenographic patterns are often similar in comparable age groups.

There seems to be a distinct age variation with regard to susceptibility to post-traumatic ischemic necrosis. This complication is almost unknown in children under 6 years of age, while in older children, the frequency is probably about 10%. The inference is sometimes cited that the young have some protection against the complication of ischemic necrosis. This is probably due to the anatomic particularities of the circulation and continuity of the proximal femoral epiphysis, as well as the relative positions of capsular insertion to blood vessels in the different age groups. This complication has also been attributed to changes in the function of the artery of the ligamentum capitis femoris, which is usually completely

disrupted. It seems more likely that the age-related differences relate to the volume of ossification within the capital femoral epiphyseal cartilage. The developing osseous centrum is a more vascular-dependent structure than unossified hyaline cartilage.[55,56] The greater the mass of bone at time of injury the more the normal vascular demand, such that it is less likely to withstand prolonged ischemia. Macro- and microvascular patterns also change significantly with age.[18]

The patient who sustains a posterior dislocation usually tears the capsule in the direction of the longitudinal fibers or transversely, and does not destroy the area where the blood supply, *per se*, courses. The capsular rent allows decompression, and therefore no buildup of hematoma under pressure in the joint. Furthermore, the intra-articular course of vessels should not be seriously compromised by this type of dislocation.

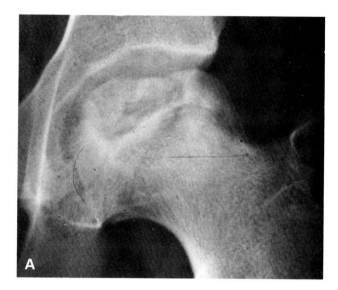

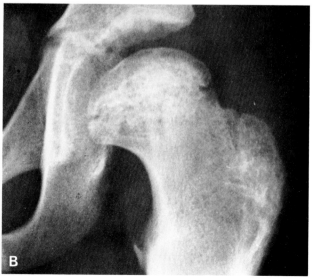

FIG. 16-20. *A,* Avascular necrosis with central collapse of femoral head following previous dislocation. *B,* Impaired development and premature physeal arrest following closed reduction.

In the case described by Haliburton, Brockenshire, and Barber, the authors were impressed by the fact that although necrosis was recognized radiographically 8 weeks after injury, within 5 months the proximal femoral epiphysis had regained its normal radiographic density.[57]

Of all the cases of ischemic necrosis reported in the literature, only 2 were first diagnosed more than 2 years after the injury. These cases were described by both Haliburton and Pearson; 1 of these was a neglected case in which the reduction took place a week after the dislocation.[44,57] Nevertheless, the final prognosis should be reserved until the patient reaches skeletal maturity, since unanticipated changes may occur during the adolescent growth spurt. As shown by Bucholz and Ogden, some of the subtle changes of ischemic necrosis that complicate congenital hip disease may not occur until the adolescent growth spurt, even though the vascular insult may have been rendered within the first few weeks to months of life.[18]

Once the patient has gotten over the phase of acute healing, usually 2 to 3 months after the injury, a baseline bone scan should be obtained to see if there is any decrease in blood supply to the affected femoral head. Radiographic review should continue until skeletal maturity to detect any problems, particularly long term changes in the femoral head, as some changes do not manifest until the growth spurt.

If ischemic (avascular) necrosis should occur, the first step should be non-weightbearing to try to prevent osseous collapse during the revascularization period. Osteotomy may also be beneficial (Fig. 16-21) as it may align the head in a more effective weightbearing position and enhance revascularization and venous outflow.

A common complication that is not stressed in the literature is the development of coxa magna, which occurred in 6 patients in one study.[23] This was probably caused by injury-induced hyperemia to the capital femur. Rather than the blood supply being damaged, it remained completely intact, and there was increased flow in response to the injury. If this causes acetabular-femoral incongruity, there may be a predisposition to subsequent osteoarthritis.

Recurrent dislocation

A less frequent complication is recurrent dislocation.[41,42,58-66] Choyce described 5 cases of recurrent dislocation.[48] Mauck and Anderson reported a 6-year-old male who had a subsequent dislocation 13 months after the initial injury.[26] Goldenberg reported a case, but Gaul questioned whether the hip had really been reduced.[54,67] Morton reported 5 cases of recurrent dislocation.[68] The report of the Pennsylvania Orthopedic Society mentions only 1 case.[17] With few exceptions, all children suffering the complication of recurrent dislocation appeared to be under 8 years of age at the time of injury. Interestingly, only 1 child went on to ischemic necrosis following recurrent dislocation.[42]

Of the cases, 2 had concurrent conditions that might have predisposed to the recurrence. One was a hypothyroid dwarf with 4 dislocations over a 5-year period.[41] The other had a congenital transverse hemimelia.[62] Recurrent dislocation may be relatively common due to the excessive ligamentous laxity normally found in children. This is even more common in children with predisposing conditions such as Down's syndrome or arthrochalasia.

An important causal factor in recurrent dislocation may be inadequate immobilization of the hip following reduction, with consequent incomplete healing of the capsule. Liebenberg and Dommisse felt that the mechanism in recurrent dislocation is incomplete healing of a posterior capsular defect, particularly if the reduction was delayed.[69] If this occurs, a false cavity with synovial lining develops and communicates with the true joint. Synovial fluid may flow freely between the two regions. Treatment should consist of excision of the pouch and repair of the capsular defect. The hip should be immobilized for 4 to 6 weeks with a hip spica cast to allow complete healing.

Simmons and Elder reported a case of a 5-year-old child who sustained a posterior dislocation of the hip.[70] On 2 subsequent occasions, 1 at 5 and the other at 7 months afterward, the femur redislocated as a result of minimal trauma. A third dislocation occurred 9 months after the original accident. Exploration revealed a large herniation of the posterior joint capsule deep and caudad to the piriformis tendon and capsular laxity with a large capsular tear deep to the quadratus femoris muscle. This was successfully closed without any significant problems.

The longest interval between recurrent dislocations was 7 years with 1½-years follow-up after the second dislocation. The average time between the initial and final dislocation was 2 years, and the shortest interval between dislocations was 1 month. On the basis of this, Simmons suggested that a minimal period of follow-up should be 2 years.[70]

Hip arthrography after the initial dislocation in a child has not been reported, but it may have some merit in determining which hips might redislocate by localizing a large defect in the joint capsule. If the results of arthrography suggest a capsular defect, a repair should then be undertaken. The operation should be done in such a way that the capsular tear or stretch is demonstrated and specifically repaired. Surgical exposure of the entire posterior capsule offers the best opportunity to exclude a discrete tear.

Acetabular fragments

A trapped intra-articular fragment is frequently not recognized until long after the reduction. Care should be taken to ensure that the intra-articular distances are equal after reduction, as this may give some early indication that soft tissue or cartilaginous interposition is present. If this occurs, it indicates a need for open reduction and removal of the tissue. However, an arthrogram may be performed prior to this and show the interposed tissue; however, this may not be easy in the acutely reduced child, as large tears in the capsule allow extravasation and puddling of dye, which make interpretation of the arthrogram difficult. CAT scans may be useful in delineating interposed cartilage fragments, even after reduction.

Osteoarthritis

It is essential to follow hip-injured children beyond skeletal maturity. Long term changes not evident in the early post-traumatic period may subsequently become significant osteoarthritis. Epstein reported 6 cases where that occurred.[15] Severe injuries in young children may lead to this complication even before they attain skeletal maturity.

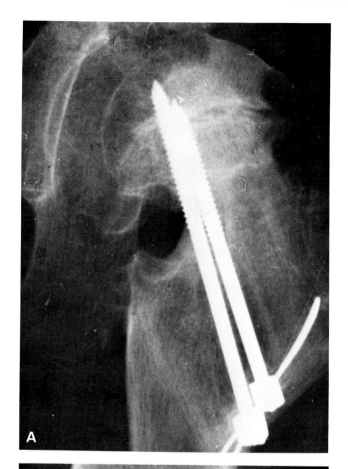

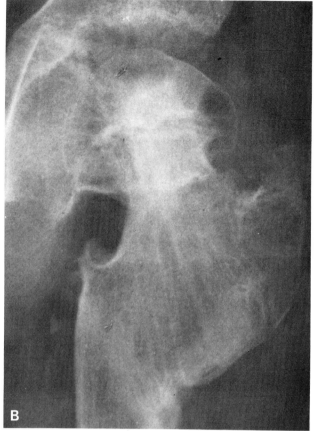

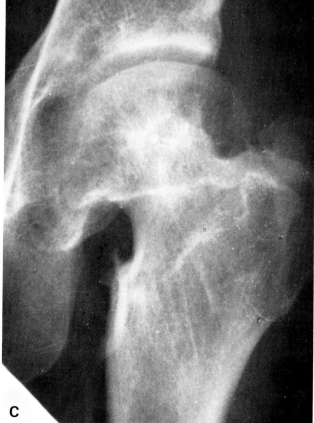

Fig. 16-21. *A,* Pain and collapse complicated this case of ischemic necrosis following closed reduction. An osteotomy was performed. *B,* Appearance six months later. *C,* Appearance two years later.

Osteochondrosis

Juan reported a case of an 8-year-old boy who developed osteochondrosis of the upper femoral epiphysis 3½ years after his original posterior dislocation;[71] Cros also reported a case with this complication.[72]

Myositis ossificans

Myositis ossificans is a rare complication, and is more likely in the patient with concomitant head injury. When it does occur, the process must be allowed to mature completely before any resection is attempted.

Neurologic deficiency[73]

Neurologic deficiency was the most frequent complication in Pearson's series.[44] Epstein reported 3 cases of neurologic deficiency in his series.[15] These all accompanied posterior dislocation and involved variable sensory or motor deficiency of the sciatic nerve. Although all experienced some degree of functional recovery, only 1 patient had complete recovery of nerve function in Pearson's series.[44] In Epstein's series, 2 patients had full recovery although 1 still had weakness in the great toe extensor 21 years after the injury.[15] The most important factor in producing a sciatic nerve injury in posterior dislocations may be the marked internal rotation of the hip that occurs at the time of dislocation.

Anterior Dislocation

Traumatic anterior dislocation of the hip joint is much less frequent, and probably constitutes less than 10% of all pediatric hip dislocations.[74] Anterior dislocations are usually simple extrusions of the femoral head through the front part of the joint capsule. The most important causal factor is forced abduction and external rotation.

Anterior and central dislocations are frequently caused by a direct blow to the greater trochanter. Anterior dislocation is more often sustained in a fall from a height, with the impact being a direct blow on the posterior aspect of the abducted and externally rotated thigh.

Anterior dislocations may be classified as pubic (superior) and obturator (inferior) (Fig. 16-22; also see Fig. 16-5). An avulsion fracture of the greater trochanter may accompany the dislocation (Fig. 16-22).

In anterior dislocations, the hip is held in abduction, external rotation, and some flexion. There is fullness in the region of the obturator foramen where the femoral head may be palpable. Motion of the hip is markedly restricted with almost no adduction and external rotation. It is difficult to palpate the greater trochanter.

In an uncomplicated anterior dislocation, prompt closed reduction generally gives a good result. Unlike posterior dislocations, there is not a good osseous fulcrum available to assist in the reduction. The iliofemoral ligament lies across the displaced femoral neck. The patient should be placed supine, the knee flexed to relax the hamstrings, and the hip adducted and brought into flexion (Fig. 16-23). The femoral head is gradually brought opposite the tear in the capsule through which it is levered into the acetabular socket. Longitudinal traction is then applied in the line of the axis of the femur, while concomitant lateral traction is applied at the level of the femoral head. The hip may be rotated medially as it is adducted to try to achieve reduction.

Failure of initial closed manipulation, which is extremely unusual, may be due to interposition of the torn capsule, a buttonhole lesion of the capsule, or iliopsoas interposition behind the femoral head.[75-77] In the case reported by Nerubay, there was interposition of the torn capsule and the iliopsoas and rectus femoris muscles.[78]

When the greater trochanter is avulsed (Fig. 16-22), open reduction is usually essential to restore morphology. This represents a type 3 or 4 growth mechanism injury. Smooth pins should be used, especially in the younger patient, and should be removed once healing occurs.

Of the 7 anterior dislocations in Epstein's series, the results were excellent in 6 cases and good in 1.[15] All cases had been reduced within 24 hours, and on the first attempt. Within 5 weeks 5 patients were fully weightbearing; the other 2 were delayed because of femoral and tibial fractures.

Acute occlusion of the femoral artery and venous occlusion have been described.[79-81] Nerubay reported a case of a 15-year-old boy who was injured in an automobile accident; he sustained an anterior dislocation of the hip, bilateral fractures of the pubic rami, and a fracture of the ischium.[78] At surgery, the cause for occlusion of the femoral artery with no distal pulses was evident; the femoral head was compressing the femoral artery against the inguinal ligament. The femoral vein had a 5-cm laceration. He developed severe ischemic necrosis 2 years after his injury and was treated with a total hip replacement (age 17). Bonnemaison and Henderson both observed cases of venous obstruction.[75,79] Chronic vascular complications (i.e., ischemic necrosis) of this mode of dislocation are rare. Ischemic necrosis of the femoral head after anterior dislocation was reported by Brav as 9% in 62 cases, although these patients were primarily adolescents and adults.[82]

Litton believed that ischemic necrosis was a rarity in anterior dislocation because the large vessels supplying blood to the femoral head were posterior.[77] Although damage to the posterior capsule is less likely in this injury, the fact that the femoral head is usually buttonholed through a piece of tight anterior capsule may cause direct pressure from the capsular rent, as well as the displaced iliopsoas, on some of the vessels. This may predispose to a greater risk of vascular injury if immediate reduction of the dislocation is not carried out. Bonnemaison showed that vascular complications were not as uncommon as described previously and felt that only the anterior epiphyseal vessels were damaged, while the lateral epiphyseal vascular supply was saved, accounting for the relatively low incidence of ischemic necrosis when the dislocation was promptly reduced.[79] None of the case reports, other than that of Nerubay, followed the patients through to skeletal maturity.

Periarticular calcification was present in Nerubay's case and was previously reported by Aggarwall in 6 of 7 unreduced anterior hip dislocations.[78,83] Brav found an incidence of 11% in 228 posterior dislocations, but none in the anterior type.[82]

Dall and Scudese both reported cases of recurrent anterior dislocation.[80,84]

Obstetric "Dislocation"

All presumed acute dislocations of the hip in the newborn are fractures across the entire proximal femoral metaphysis. This type of injury was produced easily in attempting acute dislocation of the hip in stillborns (see Chap. 17). Traumatic dislocation of the femoral head in the newborn is essentially nonexistent because the ligaments that reinforce the capsule are strong (although they can be hyperlax in the perinatal period because of the influence of maternal hormones). In cases of excessive trauma, as from energetic traction during delivery, epiphysiolysis or fracture of the femoral metaphysis may be produced. Elizalde reported two cases that he believed were true fracture-dislocations of the hip, but the roentgenograms indicated that the most likely diagnosis was a fracture through the transepiphyseal region.[85] In contrast to true congenital hip dysplasia, these injuries are painful to manipulate. These injuries are discussed in detail in Chapter 17.

Chronic Hip Pain

Choice of treatment for the patient with disabling hip pain consequent to complications of childhood hip dislocation is difficult, especially since available treatment modalities in-

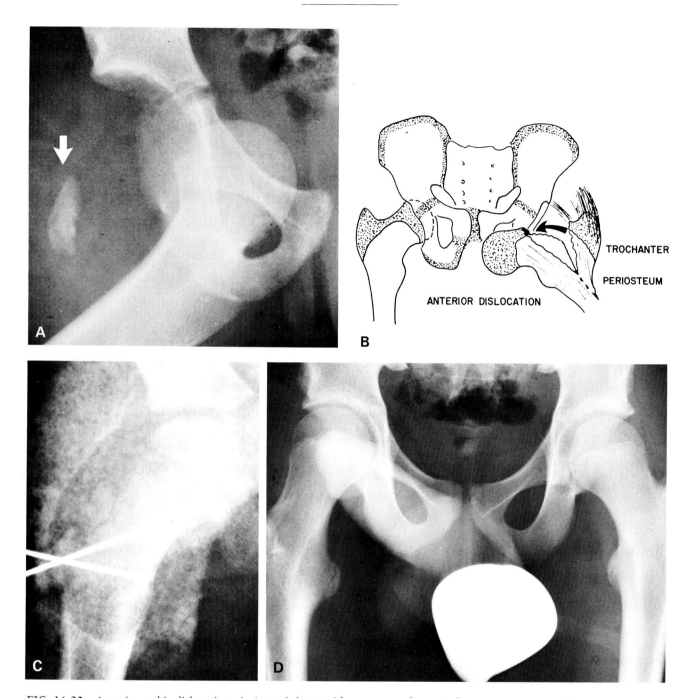

FIG. 16-22. Anterior-pubic dislocation. *A,* Acute injury, with greater trochanteric fragment (arrow). *B,* Schematic, showing how greater trochanter remained attached to periosteal sleeve and gluteal musculature. *C,* Open reduction. The capital femoral segment appeared denuded of the medial circumflex artery, especially posterosuperiorly. *D,* However, the greater trochanter underwent premature epiphysiodesis, leading to an elongated femoral neck and valgus at skeletal maturity (six years later). Most likely, the medial displacement of the main fragment disrupted the normal medial and lateral circumflex circulation to the greater trochanter. The capital femur exhibited no evidence of ischemic necrosis.

volve major risks and compromises.[86] Certainly, total joint replacement is not a reasonable initial alternative in a skeletally immature patient who is otherwise healthy. For the child sufficiently disabled to warrant surgical relief of hip pain, the options available are cup arthroplasty, endoprosthesis, pelvic or femoral osteotomy (see Fig. 16-21), or hip fusion (Fig. 16-24).

Fulkerson presented a long term comprehensive follow-up of hip fusions done for disabling hip pain in children; 3 of the patients had trauma and subsequently developed ischemic necrosis.[87] One of the significant findings of Fulkerson's study was that following hip fusion there was a tendency for the fused hips to progressively adduct after plaster removal. This was true of every hip fused in skeletally immature pa-

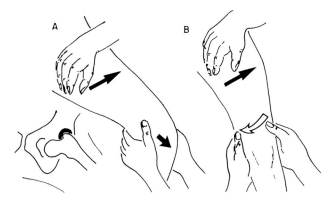

FIG. 16-23. Method of closed reduction of anterior dislocation.

tients. The average increase of adduction was 10°, usually occurring within 2 years after the initial fusion. Interestingly, the 1 patient whose hip was fused in significant abduction (15°) was somewhat less active than the others. The reasons for this adduction increase postoperatively have not been identified, but certainly growth at the trochanteric epiphysis and lateral capital epiphysis may contribute. In this series, the hips were fused in 20 to 40° of flexion, which may be allowable in a more active child, compared to the 45° of flexion considered optimal by Ahlbach and Lindahl.[87] Rotational alignment was not a problem and fusion near neutral rotation was generally accepted.

The results of adolescent hip fusions were satisfactory. Many of these children returned to vigorous physical activities and normal life-styles. Fusion of the hip certainly does not negate the possibility of subsequent conversion to a successful total hip arthroplasty.

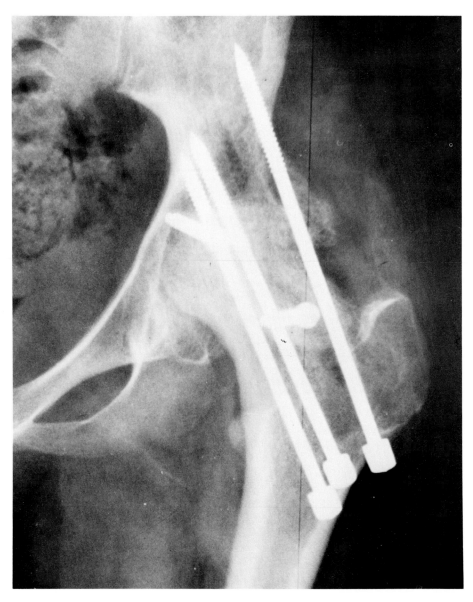

FIG. 16-24. Hip fusion for a dislocation complicated by avascular necrosis.

References

1. Barquet, A.: Traumatic hip dislocation in children. Acta Orthop. Scand., 50:549, 1979.

2. Clarke, H. O.: Traumatic dislocation of the hip joint in a child. Br. J. Surg., 16:690, 1929.

3. Glynn, P.: Two cases of traumatic dislocation of the hip in children. Lancet, 1:1093, 1932.

4. Haines, C.: Traumatic dislocation of the head of the femur in a child. J. Bone Joint Surg., 19:1126, 1937.

5. Hunter, G. A.: Posterior dislocation of fracture dislocation of the hip. J. Bone Joint Surg., 51-B:38, 1969.

5a. MacFarlane, I., and King, D.: Traumatic dislocation of the hip joint in children. Aust. N.Z. J. Surg., 46:226, 1976.

6. Meng, C. I.: Traumatic dislocation of the hip in childhood. Chin. Med. J., 48:736, 1954.

7. Murphy, D. P.: Traumatic luxation of the hip in childhood. J.A.M.A., 80:549, 1923.

8. Paus, B.: Traumatic dislocations of the hip. Acta Orthop. Scand., 21:99, 1951.

9. Piggot, J.: Traumatic dislocation of the hip in childhood. J. Bone Joint Surg., 41-B:209, 1959.

10. Platt, H.: Traumatic dislocation of the hip joint in a child. Lancet, 1:80, 1916.

11. Rocher, H. L., Rocher, C., and Cuzard, M.: Luxation traumatique de la hanche chez l'enfant. Bordeaux Chir., 8:255, 1937.

12. Tronzo, R. G.: Traumatic dislocation of the hip in children. A problem in anesthetic management. J.A.M.A., 176:526, 1961.

13. Wilson, D. W.: Traumatic dislocation of the hip in children. A report of four cases. J. Trauma, 6:739, 1966.

14. Epstein, H. C.: Traumatic dislocations of the hip. Clin. Orthop., 92:116, 1973.

15. Epstein, H. C.: Traumatic Dislocation of the Hip. Baltimore, Williams & Wilkins, 1980.

16. Pennsylvania Orthopedic Society: Traumatic dislocations of the hip joint in children. A report by the scientific research committee. J. Bone Joint Surg., 42-A:705, 1960.

17. Pennsylvania Orthopedic Society: Traumatic dislocation of the hip joint in children. A report by the scientific research committee. J. Bone Joint Surg., 50-A:79, 1968.

18. Bucholz, R. W., and Ogden, J. A.: Patterns of ischemic necrosis of the proximal femur in nonoperatively treated congenital hip disease. In The Hip. Vol. 6. St. Louis, C. V. Mosby, 1978.

19. Robertson, R. C., and Peterson, H. A.: Traumatic dislocation of the hip in children: review of Mayo Clinic series. In The Hip. Vol. 2. St. Louis, C. V. Mosby, 1974.

20. Sankarankutty, M.: Traumatic inferior dislocation of the hip (luxatio erecta) in a child. J. Bone Joint Surg., 49-B:145, 1967.

21. Mass, D. P., Spiegel, P. G., and Laros, G. S.: Dislocation of the hip with traumatic separation of the capital femoral epiphysis. Clin. Orthop., 146:184, 1980.

22. Bernhang, A. M.: Simultaneous bilateral traumatic dislocation of the hip in a child. J. Bone Joint Surg., 52-A:365, 1970.

23. Glass, A., and Powell, H. D. W.: Traumatic dislocation of the hip in children. J. Bone Joint Surg., 43-B:29, 1961.

24. Ingram, A., and Bachynski, B.: Fractures of the hip in children. J. Bone Joint Surg., 35-A:867, 1953.

25. Lugger, L. J.: Traumatische Huftverrenkung und gleichzeitiger Oberschenkelschaftbruch im Kindesalter. Zentralbl. Chir., 99:340, 1974.

26. Mauck, H. P., and Anderson, R. L.: Infracotyloid dislocation of the hip. J. Bone Joint Surg., 17:1011, 1935.

27. Mason, M. L.: Traumatic dislocation of the hip in childhood. J. Bone Joint Surg., 36-B:630, 1954.

28. Rinke, W., and Protze, J.: Offene traumatische Huftgelenksluxation und gleichseitige oberschenkelschaftfraktur im Kindesalter. Zentralbl. Chir., 101:177, 1976.

29. Schlonsky, J., and Miller, P. R.: Traumatic hip dislocations in children. J. Bone Joint Surg., 55-A:1057, 1973.

30. Lyddon, D. W., and Hartman, J. T.: Traumatic dislocation of the hip with ipsilateral femoral fracture. J. Bone Joint Surg., 53-A:1012, 1971.

31. Helal, B., and Skevus, X.: Unrecognized dislocation of the hip in fractures of the femoral shaft. J. Bone Joint Surg., 49-B:293, 1967.

32. Wadsworth, T. G.: Traumatic dislocation of the hip with fracture of the shaft of the ipsilateral femur. J. Bone Joint Surg., 43-B:47, 1961.

33. Wilson, J. C., Jr., and Aufranc, O. E.: Head-injured child with multiple fractures: reexamined at skeletal maturity. J.A.M.A., 217:1849, 1971.

34. Dehne, E., and Immermann, E. W.: Dislocation of the hip combined with fracture of the shaft of the femur on the same side. J. Bone Joint Surg., 33-A:734, 1954.

35. Chavette, J.: Luxation traumatique de la hanche chez l'enfant. Thesis, University of Lyon, 1968.

36. Fischer, L., and Imbert, J.: Luxation traumatique de la hanche retro-cotyloidienne chez l'enfant, sans displacement en hauteur. Lyon Med., 222:825, 1969.

37. Trillat, A., and Ringot, A.: Erreurs d'interpretation radiographique dans les fractures du cotyle avec luxation de la tete femorale. Lyon Chir., 46:472, 1951.

38. Tachdjian, M.: Pediatric Orthopedics. Philadelphia, W. B. Saunders, 1972.

39. Fernandez-Herrera, E.: Luxacion traumatica anterior de la cadera en la infancia. Bol. Med. Hosp. Infant Mex., 22:95, 1965.

40. Fineschi, G.: Die traumatische Huftverrenkung bei Kindern. Literaturubersicht und statistischer Beitrag von 7 Fallen. Arch. Orthop. Unfallchir., 48:225, 1956.

41. Funk, F. J.: Traumatic dislocation of the hip in children. Factors influencing prognosis and treatment. J. Bone Joint Surg., 44-A:1135, 1962.

42. Freeman, G. E., Jr.: Traumatic dislocation of the hip in children. J. Bone Joint Surg., 43-A:401, 1961.

43. Hovelius, L.: Traumatic dislocation of the hip in children. Acta Orthop. Scand., 45:746, 1974.

44. Pearson, D. E., and Mann, R. J.: Traumatic hip dislocation in children. Clin. Orthop., 92:189, 1973.

45. Piggot, J.: Traumatic dislocation of the hip in childhood. J. Bone Joint Surg., 43-B:38, 1961.

46. Hemmelbo, T.: Traumatic hip dislocation in childhood. Acta Orthop. Scand., 47:546, 1976.

47. Kelly, R. P., and Yarbrough, S. H., III: Posterior fracture-dislocation of the femoral head with retained head fragment. J. Trauma, 11:97, 1971.

48. Choyce, C. C.: Traumatic dislocation of the hip in childhood and relation of trauma to pseudocoxalgia. Br. J. Surg., 12:52, 1924.

49. Kleinberg, S.: Aseptic necrosis of the femoral head following traumatic dislocation. Report of two cases. Arch. Surg., 39:637, 1939.

50. Mutschler, H. M.: Sekundare Oberschenkelkopf-necrose nach traumatischer Ausrenkung des Huftgelenkes bei einem 14 Jahrigen. M. M. W., 86:258, 1939.

51. Quist-Hanssen, S.: Caput necrosis after traumatic dislocation of the hip in a 4-year-old boy. Acta Chir. Scand., 95:344, 1945.

52. Elmslie, R. C.: Pseudocoxalgia following traumatic dislocation of the hip in a boy aged four years. J. Orthop. Surg., 1:109, 1919.

53. Elmslie, R. C.: Traumatic dislocation of the hip in the child age seven with subsequent development of coxa plana. Proc. R. Soc. Med., 25:1100, 1932.

54. Goldenberg, R.: Traumatic dislocation of the hip followed by Perthes disease. J. Bone Joint Surg., 20:770, 1938.

55. Ogden, J. A.: Anatomic and histologic study of factors affecting development and evolution of avascular necrosis in congenital dislocation of the hip. In The Hip. Vol. 2. St. Louis, C. V. Mosby, 1974.

56. Ogden, J. A.: Changing patterns of proximal femoral vascularity. J. Bone Joint Surg., 56-A:941, 1974.

57. Haliburton, R. A., Brockenshire, F. A., and Barber, J. R.:

Avascular necrosis of the femoral capital epiphysis after traumatic dislocation of the hip in children. J. Bone Joint Surg., *43-B:*43, 1961.

58. Aufranc, O. E., Jones, W. N., and Harris, H. H.: Recurrent traumatic dislocation of the hip in a child. J.A.M.A., *190:*291, 1964.

59. Body, J.: Luxation recidivante de la hanche chez un garcon de 7 ans. Rev. Chir. [Orthop.], *55:*65, 1969.

60. Duytjes, F.: Recurrent dislocation of the hip joint in a boy. J. Bone Joint Surg., *45-B:*432, 1963.

61. Gula, D.: Recurrent traumatic dislocation of the hip in children. J. Am. Osteopathol. Assoc., *72:*32, 1972.

62. Hensley, C. D., and Schofield, G. W.: Recurrent dislocation of the hip. J. Bone Joint Surg., *51-A:*573, 1969.

63. Hohmann, D.: Rezidivierende traumatische Huftluxation beim Kind nach fehlerhafter Gipsfixation. Mschr. Unfallheilk., *67:*352, 1964.

64. Niloff, R., and Petrie, J. G.: Traumatic recurrent dislocation of the hip. Report of a case. Can. Med. Assoc. J., *62:*574, 1950.

65. Sullivan, C. R., Bickel, W. H., and Lipscomb, P. R.: Recurrent dislocation of the hip. J. Bone Joint Surg., *37-A:*1266, 1955.

66. Townsend, R. G., Edwards, G. E., and Bazant, F. J.: Post-traumatic recurrent dislocation of the hip without fracture. J. Bone Joint Surg., *51-B:*194, 1969.

67. Gaul, R. W.: Recurrent traumatic dislocation of the hip in children. Clin. Orthop., *90:*107, 1973.

68. Morton, K. S.: Traumatic dislocation of the hip in children. Can. J. Surg., *3:*67, 1959.

69. Liebenberg, F., and Dommisse, G. F.: Recurrent post-traumatic dislocation of the hip. J. Bone Joint Surg., *51-B:*632, 1969.

70. Simmons, R. L., and Elder, J. D.: Recurrent post-traumatic dislocation of the hip in children. South. Med. J., *65:*1463, 1972.

71. Juan, A. C.: Osteochondrosis of the upper femoral epiphysis following traumatic dislocation of the hip joint. J. Bone Joint Surg., *41-A:*1335, 1959.

72. Cros, A.: Osteochondrosis of the upper femoral epiphysis following traumatic dislocation of the hip joint. J. Bone Joint Surg., *41-A:*1335, 1959.

73. Kleiman, S. G., Stevens, J., Kolb, L., and Pankovich, A.: Late sciatic nerve palsy following posterior fracture-dislocation of the hip. J. Bone Joint Surg., *53-A:*781, 1971.

74. Hamada, G.: Unreduced anterior dislocation of the hip. J. Bone Joint Surg., *39-B:*471, 1957.

75. Henderson, R. S.: Traumatic anterior dislocation of the hip. J. Bone Joint Surg., *33-B:*602, 1951.

76. Katznelson, A. M.: Traumatic dislocation of the hip. J. Bone Joint Surg., *44-B:*129, 1962.

77. Litton, L. O.: Traumatic anterior dislocation of the hip in children. J. Bone Joint Surg., *40-B:*1419, 1958.

78. Nerubay, J.: Traumatic anterior dislocation of the hip joint with vascular damage. Clin. Orthop., *116:*129, 1976.

79. Bonnemaison, M. F. E., and Henderson, E. D.: Traumatic anterior dislocation of the hip with acute common femoral occlusion in a child. J. Bone Joint Surg., *50-A:*753, 1968.

80. Dall, D., MacNab, I., and Gross, A.: Recurrent anterior dislocation of the hip. J. Bone Joint Surg., *52-A:*574, 1970.

81. Hampson, W. G. J.: Venous obstruction by anterior dislocation of the hip joint. Injury, *4:*69, 1972.

82. Brav, E. M.: Traumatic dislocation of the hip. J. Bone Joint Surg., *44-A:*1115, 1962.

83. Aggarwall, N. D., and Singh, H.: Unreduced anterior dislocation of the hip. J. Bone Joint Surg., *49-B:*288, 1967.

84. Scudese, V. A.: Traumatic anterior hip redislocation. Clin. Orthop., *88:*60, 1972.

85. Elizalde, E. A.: Obstetrical dislocation of the hip associated with fracture of the femur. J. Bone Joint Surg., *28:*838, 1946.

86. Fairbank, H. A. T.: Case of pseudo-coxalgia following traumatic dislocation in a boy. Proc. R. Soc. Med. (Section of Orthopedics), *17:*40, 1924.

87. Fulkerson, J. P.: Arthrodesis for disabling hip pain in children and adolescents. Clin. Orthop., *128:*296, 1977.

17

Femur

Anatomy

Proximal femur

Development of the proximal femoral chondro-osseous epiphysis and physis is probably the most complex of all growth regions. Figures 17-1 to 17-3 illustrate several stages in the development of the proximal femur. Perhaps the two most important features are (1) the continuity of epiphyseal cartilage along the posterosuperior neck throughout postnatal development, and (2) the intracapsular course of the capital femoral blood vessels. Fortunately, significant growth mechanism injury secondary to direct trauma or selective vascular damage to the area is rare. However, when it does occur, complications assume great importance for subsequent development and hip and leg biomechanics.

Ossification usually begins in the capital femur by four to six months postnatally. This is a centrally located sphere of ossification that expands centrifugally, eventually conforming to the hemispheric shape of the articular surface by six to eight years, and forming a discrete subchondral (basal) plate following the capital femoral physeal contour. This ossification center is dependent upon an intact vascular supply, and any temporary or permanent decrease in blood flow, as in a femoral neck fracture, has variable effects upon the ability of capital femoral ossification to continue maturation.

Throughout development the capital femoral and trochanteric epiphyses have a cartilaginous continuity along the posterosuperior femoral neck (Fig. 17-4). Although this region becomes thin as the child grows, it is absolutely essential for normal latitudinal growth of the femoral neck (Fig. 17-5). Damage, as in a femoral neck fracture, may seriously impair the capacity of the neck to develop normally. The blood vessels course along the posterosuperior femoral neck; however, they have a variable intracartilaginous course, which makes them more susceptible to fracture if the injury to the subcapital or neck region propagates into the cartilage (Fig. 17-5).

Selective growth of the capital femoral and intertrochanteric physes leads to the establishment of a well-defined femoral neck (Fig. 17-6). The primary spongiosa initially formed during neck development is not completely oriented to biologic forces across the hip joint. However, the more responsive secondary spongiosa begins to form trabecular patterns oriented to compression and tension forces. This process becomes more prominent during adolescence. The area between these major osseous patterns is a potentially weak area known as Ward's triangle (see Fig. 17-2).

The development of the femoral neck brings about changes in the contour of the capital femoral physis. Initially the femoral neck is transversely directed (see Fig. 17-1), but during the first year it begins to exhibit preferential growth in the medial and middle sections. As these regions develop, the capital femoral physis becomes more medially (varus) and posteriorly oriented (Fig. 17-7), which may predispose to slipped capital femoral epiphysis (Fig. 17-8). Undulations and mammillary processes develop in the physis (see Fig. 17-1). These processes probably serve as a further "anchor" to prevent displacement due to biologic shear stresses.

The greater trochanter begins ossification at 5 to 7 years (Fig. 17-9) and is present first just above the trochanteric physis. With further development, ossification proceeds cephalad into the remainder of the epiphysis. This cartilaginous portion may be injured without any roentgenographic evidence. Epiphysiodesis occurs from 16 to 19 years, slightly later than the capital femoral region. The lesser trochanter does not ossify until adolescence, and fuses from 16 to 19 years.

Femoral diaphysis

The diaphysis is a long cylinder of heavy, compact, progressively osteon bone that is bowed anteriorly and laterally. The linea aspera is a sturdy, elevated ridge that extends along the posteromedial surface of the femoral shaft. This acts as a thickened buttress that provides strength and serves as a longitudinal muscular and fascial attachment. In normal stance, the femoral shaft inclines medially at an angle that varies from 3 to 15°, with an average of 10°. This tends to partially overcome the effect of the angle of inclination of the femoral neck by bringing the weightbearing articular surface of the knee closer to the center of gravity. Treatment methods for femoral shaft fractures should be directed at restoration of anterolateral bowing, even when the fragments are left overriding.

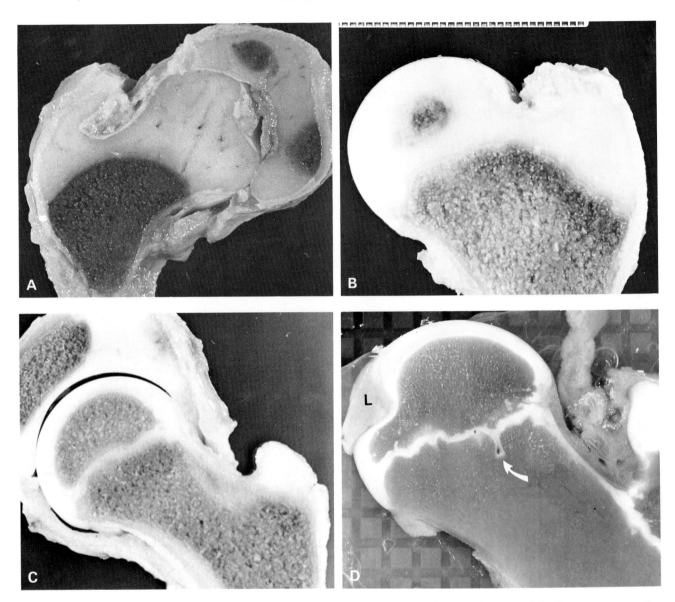

FIG. 17-1. Slab sections showing proximal femoral development. *A,* 2 months. Contiguous epiphysis encompasses the capital femur and greater trochanter. The intrinsic vascularity of the capital femoral cartilage is evident. *B,* 8 months. The capital femoral ossification center is developing, and the femoral neck (metaphysis) is beginning to form. *C,* 8 years. Undulations are just beginning to develop in the capital femoral physis. *D,* 12 years. Note the normal indentation of the ossification center at the site of attachment of the capital femoral ligament (L). The capital femoral physis is extensively undulated, and one elongated mammillary process is evident (arrow).

Distal femur

The epiphyseal ossification center of the distal femur is usually present at birth if the child is full-term. Expansion occurs relatively rapidly and fills both condylar regions (Fig. 17-10).[1] Irregularity of the margins of the epiphyseal ossification center is relatively common (Fig. 17-11), and should not be misconstrued as trauma. This is the largest and most actively growing epiphyseal-physeal unit in the body, contributing almost 70% of the length of the femur and 40% of the entire leg. It fuses with the metaphysis between 14 and 16 years of age in girls and 18 and 19 years of age in boys. The distal epiphysis includes the entire articular surface of the lower end of the femur, and serves as the origin of part of the gastrocnemius muscle.

The distal femoral metaphysis is the site of numerous developmental variations. Fibrous cortical defects have been recognized as normal variants. However, small pathologic fractures can sometimes occur in these defects. Another relatively common lesion is the avulsive cortical irregularity. Although usually benign in appearance, these radiologically apparent cortical erosions may sometimes be suggestive of destructive or infiltrative lesions.[2-6] The distal femoral metaphyseal "lesion" is almost exclusively observed on the posteromedial aspect of the femoral condyle, along the linea

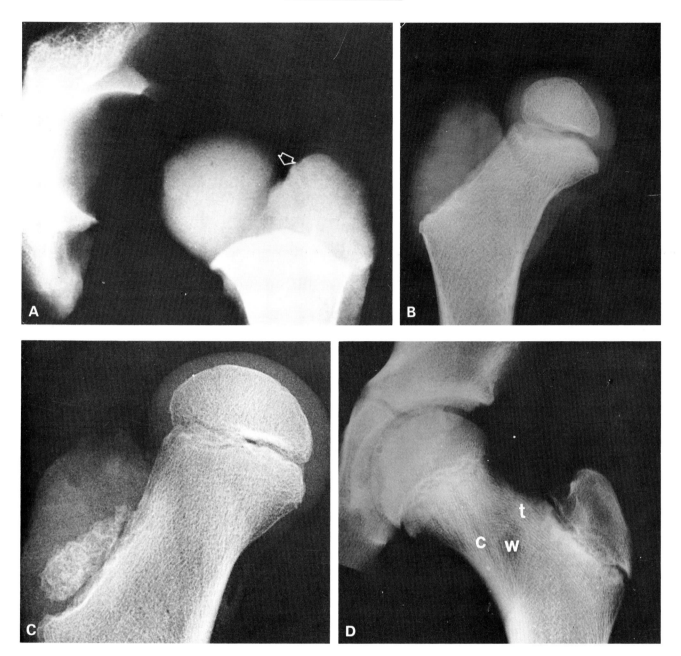

FIG. 17-2. Roentgenographic development of proximal femur. *A,* Neonate. The capital femur and greater trochanter are separated (arrow), even though a femoral neck is not roentgenographically definable. *B,* 3 years. There is no ossification in the trochanter, although the air/cartilage contrast technique has outlined a well-developed structure. *C,* 9 years. Trochanteric ossification is beginning near the physis. Note how the bulk of the trochanter is still unossified. *D,* 15 years. The capital femoral physis is undergoing physiologic epiphysiodesis, while the trochanteric physis is still functional. The compression responsive (c) and tensile responsive (t) trabeculae outline Ward's triangle (W).

aspera just above the adductor tubercle (Fig. 17-12). This portion of the medial ridge of the linea aspera is the site of insertion of a portion of the transverse fibers of the adductor magnus aponeurosis. Intense bone remodeling usually occurs continuously in this region during periods of rapid skeletal growth. The cortex of the bone is believed to be weakened by this constant remodeling, such that excessive mechanical stress produces micro-avulsions of the cortical bone. These micro-avulsions elicit a hypervascular and fi-broblastic response, which in turn stimulates osteoclastic activity and bone resorption. In this way, a cycle of fracture-resorption-fracture is established. The rapid appearance and subsequent regression of the lesion and its common occurrence in active, adolescent males suggest a mechanically induced lesion and may even represent a tension type of stress fracture. The inciting stimulus for the development of the lesion is believed to be the intense mechanical stress in the area of active bone remodeling.

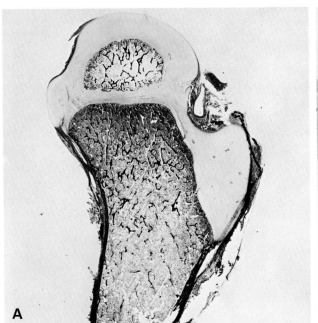

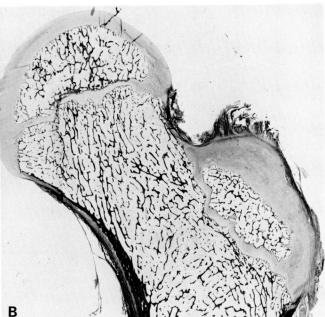

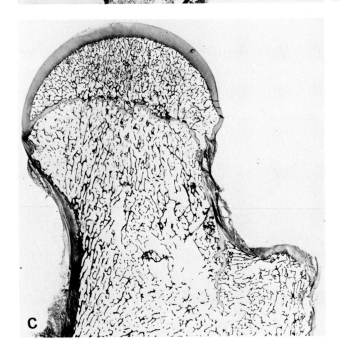

FIG. 17-3. Histologic development of proximal femur. *A,* 1 year. Note the transverse nature of the physis under the capital femur. The neck/trochanteric region is smooth. *B,* 9 years. Note the development of physeal undulations in both the capital femoral and trochanteric regions. *C,* 15 years. Closure is evident.

Proximal Femoral Injuries

Proximal femoral fractures are infrequent injuries in the immature skeleton.[7-38] These fractures are more common in boys, with the male to female ratio being approximately 3 to 2. Fractures can occur at any age; the highest incidence is between 11 and 12 years of age. Proximal femoral fractures may occur at birth and must be isolated diagnostically from congenital hip dysplasia.[39-44] The injury may also be seen in an abused infant. In young children and adolescents considerable violence is required to fracture the proximal femur; therefore, there are often accompanying injuries. In adoles-

cence, an acute injury represents one end of the spectrum of slipped capital femoral epiphysis. Pathologic fractures may occur in many diseased states, including renal osteodystrophy, hypothyroidism, juvenile rheumatoid arthritis, septic arthritis, and malignancies (Fig. 17-13).

There are several important differences between proximal femoral fractures in adults and children. Since the combined periosteal-perichondrial tube is much stronger, fractures are not always significantly displaced. Additionally, the presence of the cartilaginous intraepiphyseal bridge along the superior and posterior aspect of the neck tends to prevent displacement of the physis, unless this cartilage is also significantly disrupted, a factor that is impossible to discern with standard

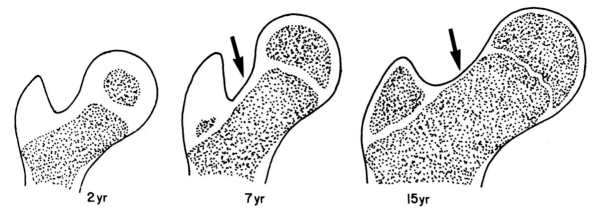

FIG. 17-4. A segment of physeal cartilage (arrows) exists along the posterosuperior femoral neck throughout most of development. This is necessary for widening of the femoral neck (also see Fig. 17-6).

roentgenographic techniques. A potential complication, ischemic necrosis, may affect, specifically or in combination, the epiphysis, the metaphysis, and the physis. The violence of the initial injury is generally blamed for the high incidence of ischemic necrosis in children (as high as 80 to 90% in some series, with an average of 40%). However, damage to the vessels along the intraepiphyseal cartilage may also be a factor.

Children tolerate cast immobilization. The chance of union is excellent in a child with an undisplaced fracture, as long as it remains undisplaced in the cast. *However, malunion of the developing femoral neck is a real hazard.* Other than the lateral condyle of the distal humerus, this fracture area seems to be the only one that carries a reasonable risk of nonunion in a young child. When a displaced or potentially unstable fracture is reduced and held only in a cast, coxa

vara may still occur. The hardness of a child's bone and the small size of the femoral neck limit acceptable fixation devices. Threaded pins or screws of small caliber should be used, but these must *not* cross the physis. When fracture-healing problems arise in a child, endoprosthetic replacement is not an available solution.

Classification

Proximal femoral fractures in children, as in adults, occur at different levels along the femoral neck (Fig. 17-14). However, because the femoral neck is actively elongating, certain types cannot occur at younger ages, and a given type may vary with age.

The type I injury pattern may assume several different patterns contingent upon both the age of the patient and the

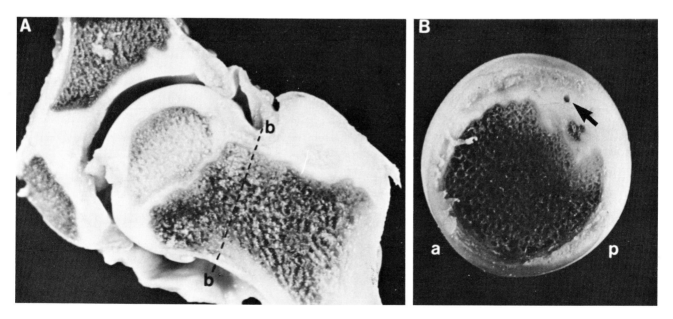

FIG. 17-5. The posterosuperior vessels may traverse along or through this neck (intraepiphyseal) cartilage. In childhood or adolescent femoral neck fractures, this vessel may be damaged, predisposing the bone to capital femoral ischemic necrosis. *A,* Section of hip from a seven-year-old. *B,* Transverse section (indicated by b—b in *A*). Note the vessel in the intraepiphyseal cartilage (arrow). The anterior and posterior sides are designated by a and p.

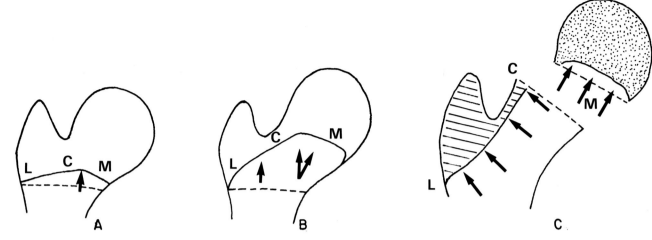

FIG. 17-6. Schematic of growth mechanisms of proximal femur. *A,* During the first few months of life, selectively greater growth rates occur in the intraepiphyseal region to begin contouring the physis (arrow). *B,* By one year, selective growth is such that the central region (C) is greater than the medial region (M), which in turn is greater than the lateral region (L). *C,* During childhood and adolescence, two major growth segments may be delineated: the capital femoral (stippled) and the trochanter-neck (lined) epiphyseal/physeal segments. The originally composite physis divides into three regions: greater trochanter (lateral), capital femoral (medial), and intraepiphyseal (central). These units must grow in an integrated fashion to develop the adult morphology. As is evident, the intraepiphyseal (central) physis contributes to femoral neck width and is clearly integrated with the capital femoral physis, which basically contributes to femoral neck length. Arrows indicate directions of growth.

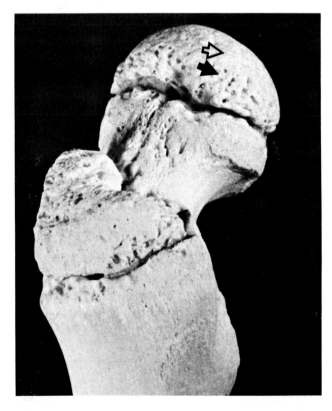

FIG. 17-7. The capital femoral physis normally has a slight posterior tilt (arrows), an anatomic factor which contributes to the natural "correction" of anteversion, but which may also predispose to slipped capital femoral epiphysis.

presence of any predisposing disease conditions such as a tumor or rickets (Fig. 17-14). During the neonatal period and the first year of life, the entire proximal femoral chondroepiphysis, including the capital femur, the intraepiphyseal region, and the greater trochanter traumatically separate as a contiguous unit. The lesser trochanter may also be included, depending upon the mechanism of injury. As shown subsequently, increased medial compression may cause localized type 5 injury with the potential for temporary or permanent growth arrest and a progressive traumatic coxa vara. As the femoral neck progressively develops, the fracture pattern changes and increasingly localizes just to the capital femoral region. The fracture line may extend from the intertrochanteric notch superiorly across the intraepiphyseal cartilage and along the capital femoral physis (type 3), or partially along the capital femoral physis, and finally into the metaphysis of the femoral neck (type 4). During adolescence, the fracture primarily involves the capital femoral physeal-metaphyseal interface crossing the remnants of the intraepiphyseal region. This type 3 injury is a true acute slipped capital femoral epiphysis.

Type II (transcervical) is a fracture through the midportion of the femoral neck. Type III is cervicotrochanteric, through the base of the femoral neck. Type IV is peritrochanteric, between the base of the femoral neck and the lesser trochanter.

In the younger child, limited development of the length of the neck affects the pattern of fracture, at least from the standpoint of defining types II, III, and IV. However, treatment is not significantly different in any, and the risks of complications such as ischemic necrosis and coxa vara are reasonably high in all types. It is important to remember that there is a variably thick cartilaginous continuity along the

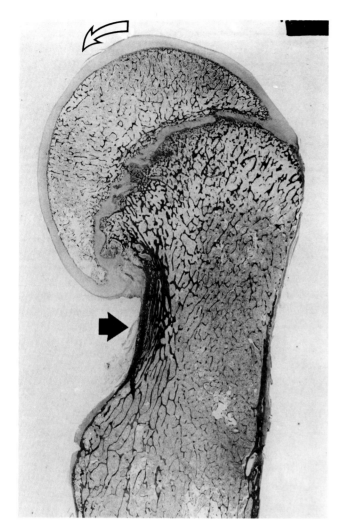

FIG. 17-8. Histologic appearance of posteriorly slipped capital femoral epiphysis (open arrow). Note the increased bone formation along the posterior femoral neck (solid arrow).

posterosuperior neck, and that the fracture undoubtedly propagates into and through this, essentially making types II, III, and IV each a type 4 growth mechanism injury, a type that mandates accurate anatomic reduction to prevent subsequent growth deformity.

Transepiphyseal injury (Type I)

Transepiphyseal fracture of the proximal femur of a young child is an infrequent lesion. Grassi described a case of traumatic separation (type 2 injury) of the upper femoral epiphysis in a two-year-old.[17] Transepiphyseal fractures are rarely associated with dislocation of the upper femoral epiphysis from the acetabulum.[28,45] Lesions of the proximal femur in patients with myelomeningocele were first described by Milgram.[25] With the exception of birth trauma, these children usually sustain multiple trauma.

This injury pattern is often difficult to diagnose (Figs. 17-15 to 17-17). The diagnosis must often be made as a clinical assumption, since roentgenographic corroboration is lacking. The distinction from congenital hip dislocation may

be difficult when the child is first seen, as roentgenograms show only upward and lateral displacement of the femoral shaft. A septic hip may also be difficult to distinguish from the traumatic lesion in child abuse, particularly since both children may be febrile.

Milgram obtained six post-mortem specimens from children who were dying from disease, presumably with no osseous involvement.[25] Manipulative epiphyseal separation was produced by simultaneously rotating and bending the specimens. Microscopically, the zone of dysjunction was variably through the hypertrophic cell layer. Haddenstein manipulated hips of newborn cadavers and found that the line of cleavage passed below the cartilage of the femoral head, not unlike my findings where the fracture occurred in the primary spongiosa (Fig. 17-18).[25]

Radiographically, the separation occurs at the physis and may or may not be associated with displacement of the neck of the shaft. In the lateral view, the neck of the femur is usually displaced forward in relation to the epiphysis, comparable to the type of external rotation that occurs in slipped capital femoral epiphysis. In some patients there may only be widening of the epiphyseal plate without significant displacement. Wide displacement is uncommon because the periosteal and perichondral attachments are usually intact. Displacement can occur only in certain ways because of the epiphyseal continuity along the posterosuperior surface of the neck. Furthermore, these are not true type 1 growth mechanism fractures, but more realistically represent type 3 injuries.

Arthrography described by Milgram shows placement of the cartilaginous epiphysis within the hip joint (Fig. 17-19).[25]

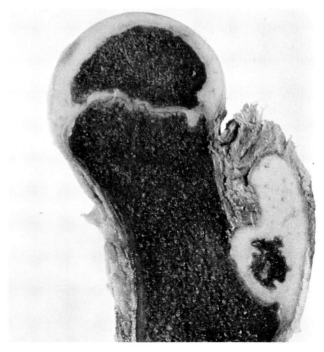

FIG. 17-9. Development of trochanteric ossification in an eight-year-old, showing irregular margins of secondary ossification and the extensive cartilaginous nature of the trochanteric epiphysis.

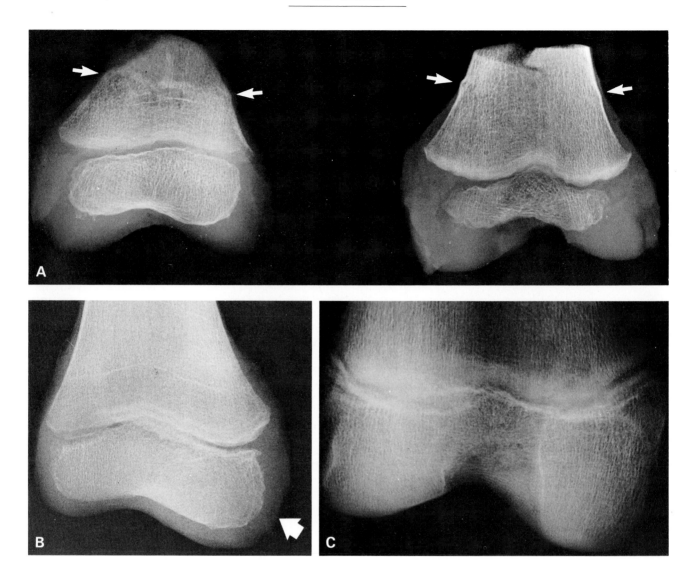

FIG. 17-10. Roentgenographic development of distal femur. *A*, Serial sections from a 3-year-old. This child was killed in an auto accident. Notice the torus fracture of the distal metaphysis (arrows). *B*, Note the irregular medial ossification (arrow) in this specimen from a 7-year-old. *C*, 15-year-old undergoing early stages of physiologic epiphysiodesis.

Treatment must be individualized. Whenever possible, conservative non-operative treatment should be instituted, with resultant deformities corrected at a later date. If the fracture line is undisplaced or minimally displaced less than one fourth, immobilize the hip in a spica cast with the affected side in moderate abduction, neutral extension, and mild internal rotation. If displaced more than one fourth, perform a gentle closed reduction under general anesthesia. In the older child, if displacement is significant and a manipulative reduction has to be undertaken, it may be necessary to internally fix the fracture with smooth K-wires that penetrate into the epiphysis and immobilize in a hip spica. Eight to ten weeks are usually required to achieve osseous union.

Prognosis of these lesions is frequently poor and must be emphasized to the parents. This may occur because of damage to the growth plate at the time of the injury, which may represent a localized type 5 injury, or by vascular injury that leads to ischemic necrosis. Each patient must be carefully followed by periodic roentgenograms for possible development of complications of ischemic necrosis, coxa vara,

or premature fusion of the physis. Premature fusion may occur even though there is no ossification center in the epiphysis at the time of the injury. The exact mechanism is unknown, but as Figure 17-17 points out, this is a real complication. Early treatment of the complications by appropriate osteotomy may salvage the hip. Using methods such as a fat or silicone interposition after resection of the osseous bridge in this particular region would not be easy and has not yet been reported.

Neonatal injury (Type I)

Proximal femoral fractures may occur during traumatic delivery and represent a relatively unique pattern of proximal injury (see Fig. 17-19). Most of these fractures are associated with complicated deliveries that involve breech or footling presentations. Michail described 2 cases of obstetric separation of the upper femoral epiphysis and described the appearance of the ossification center of the femoral head 15 days after birth, which was attributed to the consequences of

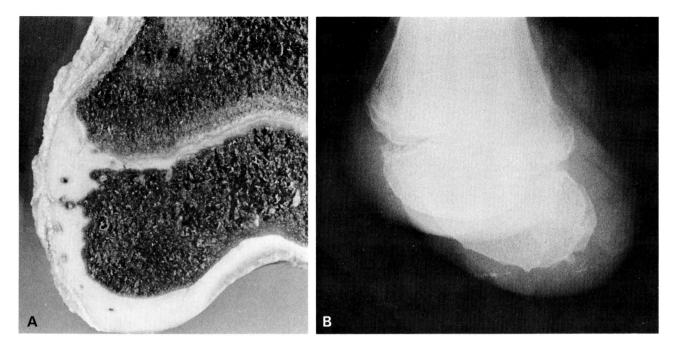

FIG. 17-11. *A,* Slab section showing irregularity of development of medial side of secondary ossification center. *B,* Roentgenogram showing similar irregularity along inferior region. These variations are normal.

the injury, and emphasized that "the existence of an obstetric (traumatic) dislocation of the hip has never been demonstrated."[46] Experiments in our Skeletal Development Laboratory have shown that an epiphysiolysis, *not* a dislocation, results (see Fig. 17-18).

Meier reported two cases of children with epiphysiolysis consequent to birth trauma.[24] One of these children died

several weeks later, and autopsy showed marked callus formation around the shaft with a fracture through the region just below the common growth plate separating the entire capital femur (including head and trochanter) away from the shaft.

The injury mechanism is usually hyperextension, abduction, and rotation during strong traction as the lower ex-

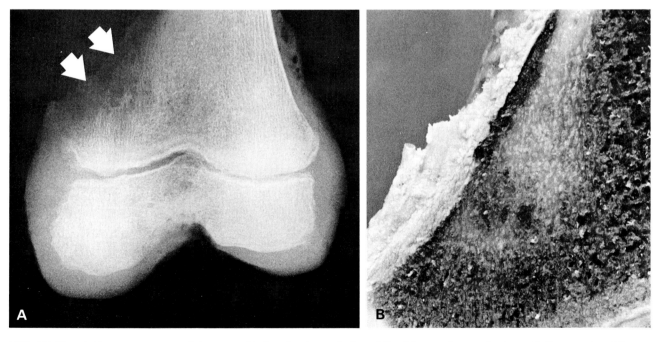

FIG. 17-12. *A,* Roentgenogram of six-year-old showing irregularity of distal femoral metaphysis medially at main adductor insertion (arrows). Compare this cortex to the lateral cortex. *B,* Sclerotic, irregular bone characteristic of this region.

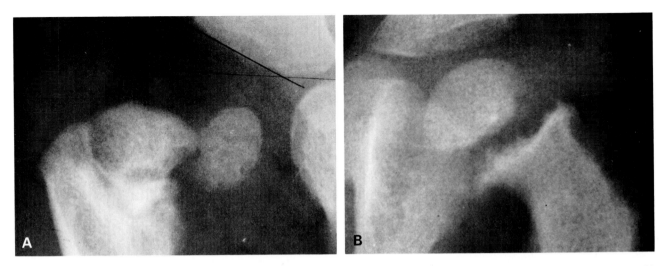

FIG. 17-13. Pathologic fractures of the proximal femur. *A,* Fracture causing coxa vara. This happened while the two-year-old boy was walking and proved to be caused by a metastatic neuroblastoma. *B,* Apparent slipped epiphysis with physeal widening in a three-year-old boy with renal rickets.

tremity is brought forward, particularly during a breech delivery. The separation generally occurs at or below the zone of cartilage hypertrophy of the growth plate (see Fig. 17-18). Crushing medially, propagation into the epiphysis, and splitting the physis were all noted experimentally, and certainly offer an explanation of type 5 growth mechanism injury that leads to eventual deformity.

The clinical symptoms are characteristic. The newborn

child lies with the limb in slight lateral rotation and adduction, avoiding and resisting movement. Swelling of the thigh is constant. The infant tends to keep the involved extremity in a position of flexion, abduction, and external rotation, and avoids and resists motion. Usually edema is in the inguinal crease, gluteal area, and proximal thigh. Considerable pain, often with crepitation, is elicited with passive motion, an important finding in distinguishing these fractures from

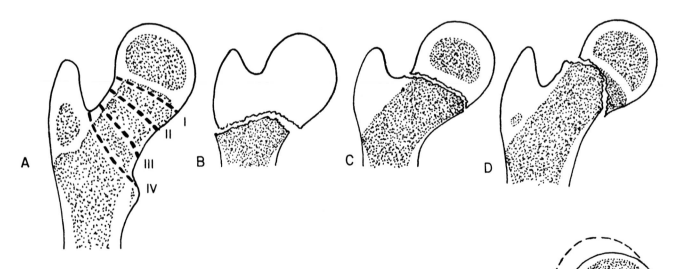

FIG. 17-14. *A,* Schematic of types of fracture of femoral neck. Type I is a transepiphyseal injury which is also a growth mechanism injury. In infancy it is classified as a type 1 injury. However, in the older child and the adolescent, the fracture splits the capital femoral and intraepiphyseal segments, and a type 3 injury occurs. In pathologic conditions (such as renal rickets), the presence of the metaphyseal fragment indicates a type 4 injury. Type II is a transcervical injury. Type III is a cervicotrochanteric injury. Type IV is a pertrochanteric injury. Figures *B* through *E* show age-related variations of type I neck fractures. *B,* Type 1 growth mechanism injury in an infant. *C,* Type 3 injury in a four-year-old. *D,* Type 3 injury in adolescent (acute slipped capital femoral epiphysis). *E,* Type 4 injury in a seven-year-old.

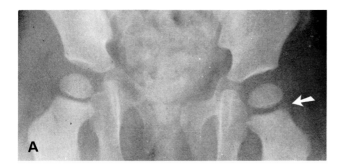

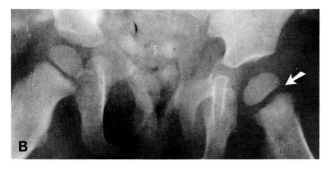

FIG. 17-15. Type 1 injury with widening of physis of left capital femur (arrows). *A,* AP view. *B,* Lateral view.

congenital hip disease, which is invariably pain free. Early diagnosis and prompt treatment are important for optimal patient care and may prevent serious sequelae.

Roentgenograms may show superolateral displacement of the upper end of the femur, which should not be confused with congenital dislocation of the hip. The displacement may often be slight and difficult to interpret. However, if the metaphysis appears to be significantly laterally displaced, yet there is a normal appearing acetabulum, one should be suspicious of a fracture. Since the femoral capital epiphysis is not ossified, this can be interpreted erroneously as a congenital hip dislocation. However, the secondary ossification center of the femoral head may appear early in response to the hyperemia. Arthrography may be useful (see Fig. 17-19). Later, the roentgenographic sign that gives irrefutable evidence of an obstetric fracture is ossification around the fracture site.

Pavlik advocated the use of Frejka pillow abduction splinting for this type of fracture as a means of keeping the leg in an acceptable position, as well as minimizing motion.[47]

Sequelae include severe coxa vara, heterotopic bone formation, ischemic necrosis, early fusion of the physis, and nonunion.

Acute slipped capital femoral epiphyseal injury (Type I)

This fracture is an acute traumatic separation of a previously normal epiphysis. However, the distinction between the acute and chronic conditions may be difficult. By definition, only those slips seen within three weeks of the onset of symptoms after definable trauma should be considered acute. Fahey and O'Brien described ten cases of acute slips.[48]

This injury may occur in children with pre-existent mild (chronic) slips or simply beginning symptoms (prodromal). Certainly, the femur undergoing changes that may predispose it to eventual slip can be acutely stressed to have a more significant displacement.[49-52] Acute slips of the proximal femoral epiphysis are characterized by abrupt onset of severe pain, limitation of motion, external rotation deformity, and the inability to bear weight on the affected limb in association with a specific traumatic event (Fig. 17-20).

The acute cases do not differ from the more common chronic type with regard to age, sex, or body build. Duration of prodromal symptoms of a dull ache or pain in the affected or ipsilateral knee range from 0 to 1 year, suggesting that acute slips do not necessarily occur in the early phase of epiphysiolysis. In fact, Barash showed a roentgenogram of a case taken 10 months prior to the time of acute slip that showed a definite early epiphysiolysis that had not been treated with prophylactic pinning.[53]

When symptoms have been present prior to the acute slipping, or when earlier roentgenograms have shown a mild slipping, there can be little doubt that trauma only precipitates acute or further displacement. Prodromal symptoms were recorded in all 10 patients reported by Fahey, and in 60 of 89 acute cases reported in the literature.[54] Lack of complaints, however, does not exclude the possibility of mild asymptomatic slipping. It may be difficult to ascertain the relative importance of trauma in an adolescent with no previous symptoms, especially when seen with acute displacement of the capital femoral epiphysis after a moderate to severe injury. Fahey believed that only 17 cases from the literature had trauma as the exclusive causal factor, and the majority of these cases occurred in the younger age group, rather than the characteristic slip group.[54] The trauma sustained was usually severe and associated injuries were frequently present. Of the reported cases, there were 8 with complete dislocations of the capital epiphysis from the acetabulum.

Fahey's report of acute slip involved one that occurred in the superior-posterior direction.[54] Howard's series had 3 cases of "valgus deformity."[51,55] Rothermel described a case of lateral slipping of the capital femoral epiphysis (epiphyseal coxa valga) and stated that 6 cases are described in the English literature.[51,55-58] It seems likely that this occurs in an older child in whom there is a thin remnant of cartilage along the posterior femoral neck that allows the capital femur to be pushed laterally as it is slipping posteriorly. Rothermel also felt that it tended to occur more frequently in patients with a horizontally disposed epiphyseal plate.[51] Wilson reported 2 superior-posterior slips.[58] Duncan and Kampner reported an anterior slip of the capital femoral epiphysis in a 9-year-old girl.[59,60] This case was complicated by a varus deformity, although clinically asymptomatic.

It is generally agreed that some form of closed reduction should be attempted in acute types of slipping, but closed reduction is not uniformly successful in securing reposition. In general, most cases may be treated with gentle traction and bed rest. In a few cases, manipulation and traction may be tried. The methods of Leadbetter or Whitman should be used cautiously.[61] Fahey felt the results of his ten cases supported the conviction that *gentle* manipulation was the preferred method of reduction, believing that the earlier closed reduction is attempted, the more likely it is to succeed in repositioning the head with minimal risk of vascular damage.[54] Others are of the opinion that acute manipulation

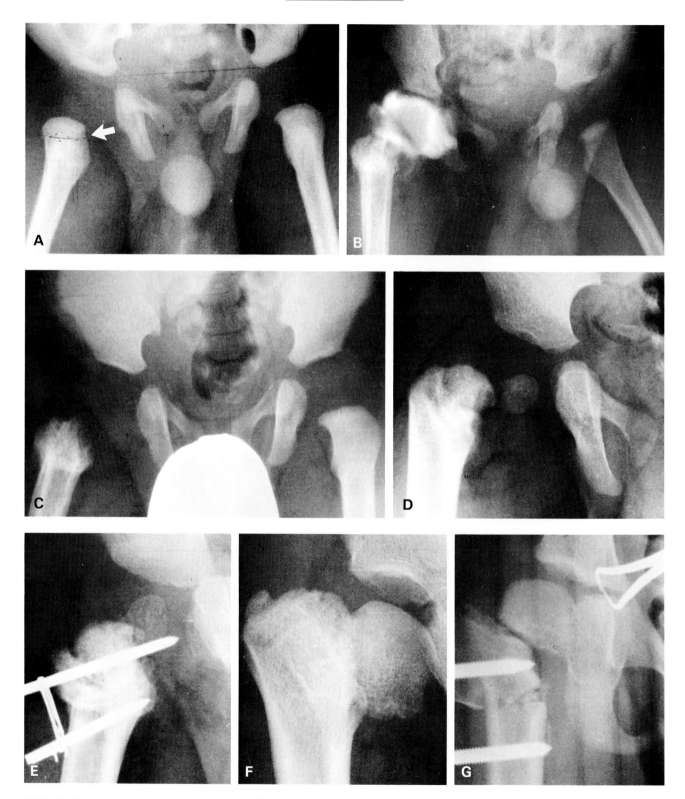

FIG. 17-16. *A,* Type I injury similar to that shown in Figure 17-15. Slight "joint widening" is evident (white arrow) due to lateral shift of metaphysis. The acetabular indices are symmetric. *B,* Arthrogram showing intact joint and lateral metaphyseal shift. *C,* Irregularity of metaphysis in this specimen three months after the injury suggests a potential problem. *D,* By eight months, coxa vara is becoming evident. Interestingly, the capital femoral ossification center is larger here than on the left side, suggesting a hyperemic rather than an ischemic state. *E,* This was treated by valgus osteotomy. *F,* However, the deformity recurred when the patient was five years old. *G,* He was treated again by a valgus osteotomy and greater trochanteric epiphysiodesis. The long term consequences will require continued follow-up treatment.

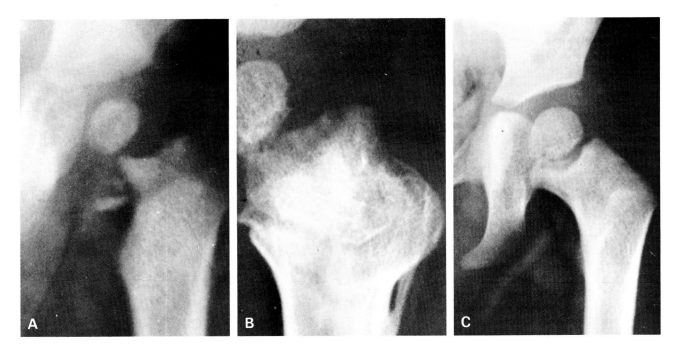

FIG. 17-17. *A,* Child abuse led to fracture of the proximal femur in this seven-month-old baby. *B,* Healing present at age nine months. *C,* Mild deformity and concavity of physeal/metaphyseal interface at age one year.

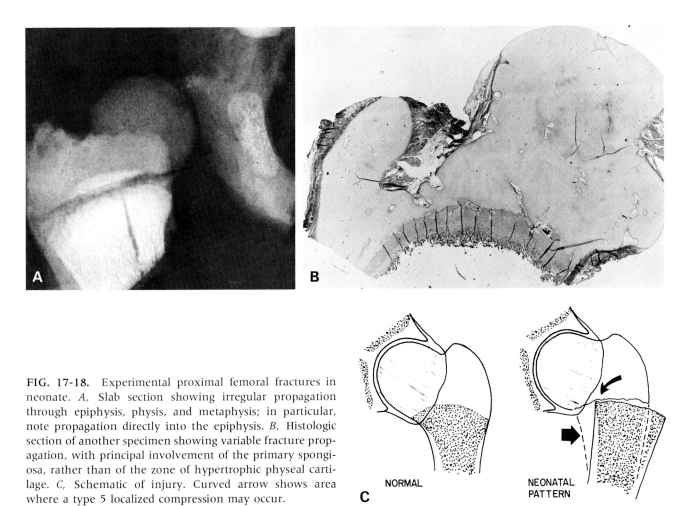

FIG. 17-18. Experimental proximal femoral fractures in neonate. *A,* Slab section showing irregular propagation through epiphysis, physis, and metaphysis; in particular, note propagation directly into the epiphysis. *B,* Histologic section of another specimen showing variable fracture propagation, with principal involvement of the primary spongiosa, rather than of the zone of hypertrophic physeal cartilage. *C,* Schematic of injury. Curved arrow shows area where a type 5 localized compression may occur.

NORMAL

NEONATAL PATTERN

C

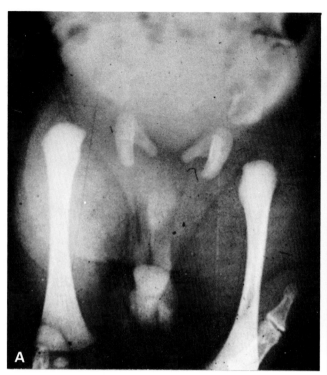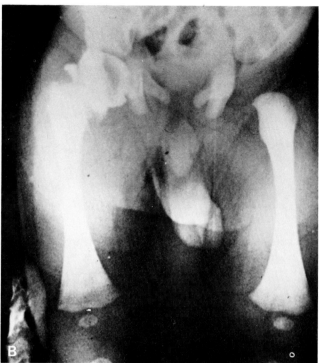

FIG. 17-19. *A,* This traumatic injury to the proximal femur occurred during birth. *B,* Arthrogram showing intact hip joint. This hip eventually developed normally.

predisposes to vascular injury, and recommend gradual reduction with traction. However, traction is usually carried out with the hip in extension, which is a position that increases joint pressure and may actually predispose to vascular problems in an acutely injured and possibly effused joint. When traction is used, even with derotation straps, the hip should be flexed at least 30°.

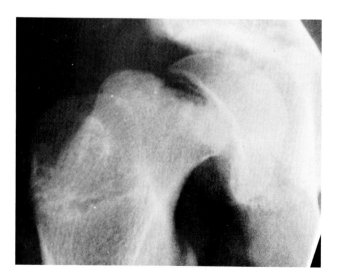

FIG. 17-20. Acute slipped capital femoral epiphysis following a fall. The patient had no prodromal symptoms. This was reduced over three days in traction (split Russell's with derotation strap), and subsequently pinned.

Closed reduction probably should not be attempted if more than two to three weeks have elapsed since the acute episode. Certainly, extra-articular fixation with threaded pins or some preferable method is indicated. The post-operative management consists of non-weightbearing for three to four months, followed by a gradual increase in weightbearing.

The only reported complication, other than ischemic necrosis, was a subtrochanteric fracture four weeks following pin removal. There are many who argue that pins should be removed routinely in order to avoid future difficulties, but this is an example of complication that can develop. Furthermore, biomechanical studies suggest that internal fixation devices reach peak efficacy at six months, and that surrounding bone actually begins to weaken after that as the bone "incorporates" the plate, pins, or screws into normal stress patterns. At Yale, in a large number of patients with chronic slip, this complication has been encountered only once. Furthermore, other methods of pinning the hip, such as the use of a bone peg, may be considered to avoid the necessity of removing the pins at a later date.

Femoral neck fractures (Types II, III, and IV)

In children, transcervical and basal fractures are the most frequent (Figs. 17-21 and 17-22). Ratliff reviewed 71 cases of femoral neck fractures of patients under 17 years of age.[29-31] The highest incidence appeared to be in the 11- to 13-year range. There were 2 transepiphyseal fractures (type I), 38 transcervical fractures (type II), 26 basal fractures (type III), and 4 intertrochanteric fractures (type IV). There were 21 undisplaced and 49 displaced fractures.

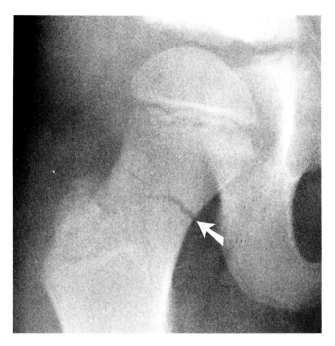

FIG. 17-21. Femoral neck fracture, type III injury pattern (arrow). Fracture was undisplaced and the child was treated with cast immobilization. The fracture appeared not to extend completely across the neck (metaphysis), thus decreasing likelihood of intraepiphyseal cartilage injury.

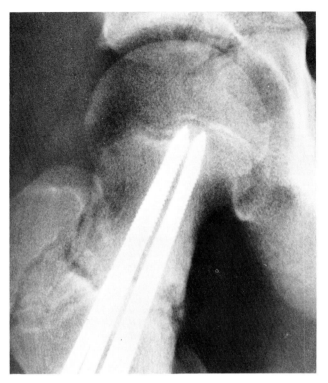

FIG. 17-22. Femoral neck fracture, type IV injury pattern. The pins are contained within the metaphysis.

Pathomechanics. Various muscle forces may lead to varus or valgus deformation of the proximal fragment (Fig. 17-23).[62] The iliopsoas tends to move the trochanteric area proximally, medially, anteriorly, and rotates it externally. The gluteus maximus moves the femur proximally, medially, posteriorly, and rotates it externally. The external rotators rotate the femur and shift it medially. The abductors pull the femoral shaft proximally and shift it medially. Thus, in theory, there are four muscular forces contributing to the upward pull; five forces contributing to the medial shift, and three forces contributing to external rotation. However, in practice there is no anteroposterior shift because the iliopsoas pulling anteriorly more or less neutralizes the opposite action of the gluteus maximus and external rotators. Therefore, after most fractures, the trochanteric area is pulled upward, rotated externally, and shifted medially. This displacement tends to take place regardless of the exact anatomic position of the fracture line.

The trochanteric area is pulled closer to the pelvis, creating an overall shortening of the lower extremity and a weakening of the abductors, resulting in the patient limping if left to heal in this position. The upper displacement of the trochanteric area is the result of muscular action upon the femur. This results not only in an upper displacement, but in a medial shift and an external rotation. Therefore, coxa vara is a three-dimensional deformity comprising elevation of the trochanter, external rotation of the femur, and shortening of the femoral neck. Muscular forces across the hip produce coxa vara in displaced fractures more often than in undisplaced fractures. Not only is the periosteum torn in the former, but the posterosuperior cartilaginous bridge must also be significantly damaged.

Diagnosis. The diagnosis is generally not difficult. There is a history of severe injury, following which the patient complains of sudden pain in the hip, and usually cannot stand or walk. However, greenstick or impacted fractures and stress fractures may allow some degree of weightbearing. The injured limb is usually held rigidly and in a varying degree of external rotation and slight adduction. It may be flexed to allow some relief of capsular distension. When the fracture is displaced, the patient is unable to move the hip actively. Actual shortening of 1 to 2 cm may be present. Generally, there is marked restriction of passive motion of the hip, par-

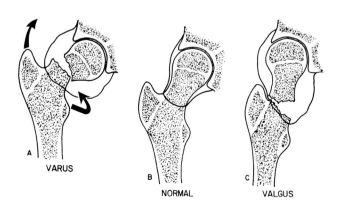

FIG. 17-23. Schematic of varus (most common) and valgus neck deformities in femoral neck fractures. The arrows in *A* show the major vectors of deforming force.

ticularly flexion, abduction, and internal rotation. The diagnosis is confirmed by roentgenograms, which should be made in both anteroposterior and lateral views. The direction of the fracture line, the degree of traumatic coxa vara, and the amount of posterior tilt should be noted, as well as whether the femoral head is retained in the acetabulum in its normal location (the distal fragment is usually displaced upward and anteriorly, or into slight external rotation).

It is important to remember that you only see the fracture through the osseous portion and the fracture may propagate further through the intraepiphyseal cartilage along the superior-posterior femoral neck.

Treatment. In undisplaced fractures, excellent results are generally, though not universally, achieved no matter how they are treated. Undisplaced fractures in children have some inherent stability, and the safest way to treat them is by hip spica. A 1½-hip spica cast with the leg held in internal rotation and abduction for 8 to 12 weeks is usually sufficient. It is imperative that the fracture be checked regularly for displacement. However, a spica cast cannot maintain hip stability in most instances when the hip itself is not intrinsically stable.

There is a temptation to treat undisplaced transcervical or cervicotrochanteric fractures non-operatively by immobilization in a 1 to 1½ spica. However, anatomic alignment may be lost and lead to displacement and a greater incidence of complications, particularly coxa vara. As a general rule, if Pauwel's angle is less than 40°, these fractures can be treated by spica cast with absolutely no weightbearing. A double hip spica may be necessary in a particularly active child. Frequent roentgenograms are necessary, and if any loss of position occurs, the fractures must be internally fixed.

In displaced fractures, the eventual risks of coxa vara and ischemic necrosis are high. Kay and Hall have argued that the hip should be aspirated to prevent tamponade of the vessels, although this has not been evaluated.[20] Manipulation under anesthesia generally corrects displacement, but this may be easily lost once the traction has been released. Initial reduction of a fracture may be obtained by counteracting muscle forces acting in the trochanteric area. As close to anatomic reduction as possible must be attained. Cast fixation after reduction does not completely neutralize the muscular forces, and displacement of the fracture fragments is almost certain. Most of these fractures must be treated with some type of internal fixation.

If Pauwel's angle is more than 40°, anatomic alignment is maintained by internal fixation with two small threaded pins, which should stop short of the epiphyseal plate. Again, a 1½-hip spica cast is applied to provide adequate immobilization. The importance of internal fixation in maintaining reduction when Pauwel's angle is greater than 40° cannot be overemphasized.

Although it has been stated that pinning in a young child may enhance the risk of ischemic change, there is no reason that the blood vessels should be damaged as long as the pins are kept within the femoral neck. Should ischemic changes occur, they are most likely caused by the original injury, rather than the surgical intervention.

The short neck in a young child sometimes makes fixation difficult. The best type of internal fixation is difficult because of the variety of methods reported and the differing anatomy. Certainly, large nails are to be condemned, as they

cause distraction of the fragments, are difficult to drive into the dense bone (compared to adult bone), and may lead to fragmentation and propagation of the fracture or premature epiphysiodesis. I agree with Rang in the use of threaded pin fixation with three or four pins, but stopping short of the capital femoral physis.[63] It is usually unnecessary to cross the growth plate, except in some high cervical fractures. In such a case, pins with an initial smooth shaft should be considered, and these pins should be removed as soon as possible to avoid interfering with subsequent, anticipated growth. If only one of the pins must cross the growth plate, it should be a smooth pin, and the other pins should be threaded. Threaded pins crossing the growth plate cause a higher rate of premature epiphysiodesis than using the same diameter, smooth fixation pins. A lag-screw, through a predrilled and tapped hole also offers a good method. However, it requires placing a large device, displacing much bone, and must *never* cross the physis.

Displaced transcervical and cervicotrochanteric fractures should be treated by gentle closed reduction followed by internal fixation with two or three threaded pins, although any pin crossing the plate should be smooth (Fig. 17-24). Age is not a factor in this suggested treatment modality. This should be followed by the use of a supplementary 1- to 1½-hip spica cast. If adequate reduction cannot be achieved, or if following reduction, particularly in transcervical fractures, Pauwel's angle still is greater than 50 to 60° with consequent high shearing stress, a primary subtrochanteric valgus osteotomy is recommended by some authors. However, in

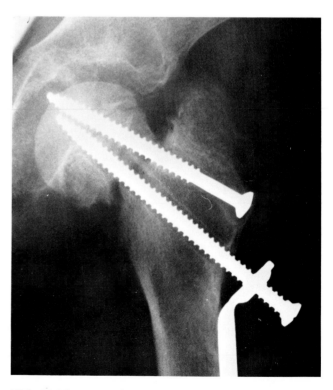

FIG. 17-24. Femoral neck fracture in an 11-year-old. This treatment is not acceptable. The screws have violated the trochanteric growth region, the capital femoral physis, and the joint, causing severe growth disturbance. Fixation pins should NOT cross the physis.

this situation, an anterior approach or extension of the exposure with direct visualization of the fracture may allow adequate reduction. If the capsule is opened, it should be opened anteriorly and great care taken not to place any retractors or instruments through the fracture line to the posterior region or around the neck for exposure, as these may damage the major circulatory systems to the femoral head.

Most intertrochanteric fractures can be reduced and held in skin traction. When callus is present at 3 to 4 weeks, a 1½-hip spica may be applied. The chief indication for internal fixation is irreducibility or inability to hold the fracture in traction because of concomitant injuries, particularly those involving the central nervous system. Open reduction is difficult, since these fractures are frequently comminuted. Ischemic necrosis does not carry the same potential risk as in higher neck fractures, and the tendency to varus deformity is more easily overcome than in proximal fractures. The only consistent late finding appears to be overgrowth.

Results. Canale and Bourland reviewed 61 fractures that included 5 transepiphyseal, 27 transcervical, 22 basilar, and 7 subtrochanteric.[10] Of these fractures, 55% had good results, 20% fair results, and 25% poor results. The use of Knowles' pin fixation appeared to reduce the complication of nonunion and coxa vara. Avascular (ischemic) necrosis caused most of the poor results. There were 26 patients who developed avascular necrosis; 13 developed coxa vara deformity; 4 had nonunion. Of 54 hips with adequate follow-up, 33 showed premature closure, an incidence of 62%. Canale and Bourland did not believe that subtrochanteric osteotomy was indicated as a reparative procedure, as recommended by Ratliff.[29-31]

McDougall observed equally good or bad results from either conservative or operative methods.[23] However, these statistics were misleading because all cervicotrochanteric fractures were treated conservatively by plaster casts, splint, or traction, whereas the transcervical fractures were, for the most part, treated by internal fixation.

Milgram described 14 cases of epiphysiolysis of the proximal femur in 11 patients aged 3 years or younger.[25] However, 10 of the 14 hips had significant underlying disease (4 associated with myelomeningocele and 6 secondary to battered-child syndrome). Of the remaining 4, a definite history of trauma was obtained in 2 patients. Of these patients, 9 were developing normally at the last follow-up, whereas 5 were developing significant varus deformity. However, of the 9 classified as normal, 2 were developing some varus. Avascular necrosis was definite in 2 patients and both had been treated by open reduction. Of the 4 severely displaced and 3 moderately displaced hips treated operatively, there was no definite incidence of avascular necrosis. Significant heterotopic bone deposition was seen in 6 patients and nonunion was seen in 4 patients. Premature growth plate closure was seen in 2 patients and suspected in 1.

Complications. There is a general agreement that there is a high incidence of complications independent of the therapeutic approach. In short, by a review of the pertinent literature, one may conclude that whatever the approach used, about 50% of the children with fractures of the femoral neck develop complications of varying degrees of severity.

The complications of proximal femoral fractures are as follows: (1) coxa vara, (2) avascular (ischemic) necrosis,

(3) delayed union, (4) nonunion, (5) leg-length inequality, and (6) epiphyseal slip. Ischemic necrosis has ranged from 16 to 45% in the various series. Coxa vara has been reported to range from 25 to 55%. Nonunion is approximately 10 to 33%. Of 189 cases reported in 5 large series, 60% developed one or more of these complications.[23,30,31,64,65] Thus, this fracture is one of the more challenging types of injury.

Jacob and Niemann described 20 cases of proximal femoral fractures.[19] Avascular necrosis occurred in 3 (15%), coxa vara in 30%, and delayed union and nonunion in 10%. Of those patients, 9 developed significant leg-length discrepancies. Their feeling was that intracapsular fractures should be treated with prompt open reduction and internal fixation with multiple pins; whereas extracapsular fractures should be treated with either open or closed methods.

Avascular (ischemic) necrosis is the major complication.[20,65] This complication developed in 30 patients (42%); in 26 patients the fragments had been displaced, and in 4 patients there was no displacement.[20] There were 32 patients who had transcervical fractures, 6 had basilar fractures, and in 1 the fracture level could not be adequately ascertained. Ischemic necrosis is usually apparent within a year after injury, although McDougall stated that radiographic signs of avascular necrosis may not be obvious for as long as 2 years after the injury.[23] Forbesca reviewed a series at the Hospital for Sick Children and found that 5 of 35 children developed ischemic necrosis and each of these had had manipulative reduction under anesthesia.[63]

Chong believed that the most important single prognostic factor was the degree of displacement at the time of injury.[13] He reported an incidence of avascular necrosis of 50%. In 2 patients, subtrochanteric osteotomy as a salvage procedure gave good results.

Weber stresses the importance of pressure exerted upon the blood vessels to the head by the hematoma formed within the capsule in a proximal femoral fracture, and that this may be a significant factor in reducing the blood supply.[66,67] He recommends that in every case of fracture of the femur the capsule should be promptly opened and the pressure alleviated.

The basic cause of necrosis is presumed to be damage to or occlusion (partial, temporary) of the anterior, posterosuperior, and posteroinferior vessels passing along the neck of the femur. It is not clear whether ischemia results from complete division of all vessels, kinking of those vessels that remain intact, or tamponade by hemarthrosis within the hip capsule (Figs. 17-25 and 17-26).

There appear to be 3 roentgenographic patterns of ischemic necrosis (Fig. 17-27). One is a total involvement of the epiphysis, physis, and metaphysis extending from the level of fracture. The second is anterolateral involvement, comparable to Legg-Calvé-Perthes disease, with presumed involvement of only the metaphysis and an intact and uninvolved epiphysis. The third type represents involvement of the anterior vessels from the lateral circumflex artery. In 7 patients, a uniform increase in density appeared in the femoral neck shortly after the fracture occurred, adequately outlined proximally by the epiphyseal plate and distally by the fracture line. In this group there was a striking incidence of premature fusion occurring at the upper femoral epiphyseal plate. McDougall also reported this particular type of avascular necrosis.[23]

The method of treatment seems to be a factor in the devel-

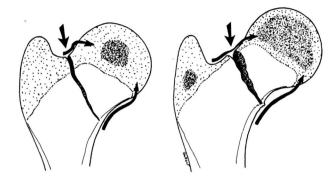

FIG. 17-25. Schematic of femoral neck fractures showing how fracture propagates into the intraepiphyseal cartilage and may attenuate the posterosuperior vessels, especially with varus deformation, yet leave the posteroinferior vessels relatively undamaged.

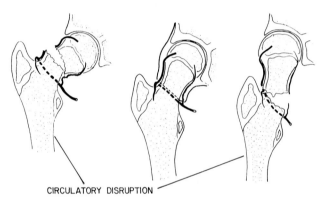

CIRCULATORY DISRUPTION

FIG. 17-26. Schematic of vascular disruption in varus and valgus injuries.

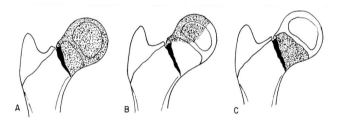

FIG. 17-27. Schematic of avascular necrosis patterns. *A,* Total involvement of capital femoral epiphysis, physis, and metaphysis (all vessels). *B,* Anterolateral involvement (probably of posterosuperior vessels). *C,* Metaphyseal involvement only.

opment of ischemic necrosis. Of fractures treated conservatively, 35% were complicated by this problem, as opposed to only 27% of those treated by internal fixation. Extreme abduction of the hip in the treatment of congenital dislocation of the hip (CDH) certainly decreases circulation, and it is significant that in many of the recommended conservative methods of casting, the fractured hip is forced into extreme positions to reduce the fracture. Following reduction, the affected hip should be brought into 30 to 40° of abduction

and moderate flexion to lessen mechanical impingement, as well as attenuation of vessels. Similarly, following internal fixation, the hip should not be immobilized in extreme positions.

This complication may occur following undisplaced as well as displaced fractures of the femoral neck in children. As reported by Durbin, it is possible that the extension of the fracture line through the cartilaginous bridge of the intraepiphyseal region results in damage to a major blood vessel[64] (see Fig. 17-4).

Transcervical fractures appear more likely to undergo necrosis than cervicotrochanteric fractures. Displaced transepiphyseal fractures have the poorest prognosis, with development of aseptic necrosis in 80%. The incidence of ischemic necrosis in those who are 10 years of age or younger is 21%, whereas in those over 10 years of age it is 47%.

According to Ratliff, fractures causing necrosis follow violent trauma and are often displaced transcervical or basal fractures.[31] Ratliff found 30 children with necrosis out of 70 (42%). Even intertrochanteric, nondisplaced fractures (type IV) can cause necrosis of the head.[31,64] The conclusion of most studies was that the violence of the injury, together with either the fracture of the neck or delayed reduction of a dislocation, are among the most important factors in the development of necrosis.

These children should have a bone scan 3 to 4 months after the injury heals, and have this repeated approximately 1 year after the injury occurred to assess any possible vascular damage or compromise.[68] A bone scan may be difficult to interpret because of the new bone formation from the healing fracture, as well as the changes consequent to injury and immobilization in the femoral head.[68] Certainly ischemia is present by a scan within the first few months, and probably always within a year, at which time you are also going to see gross radiographic changes. Radiographs should be obtained every 2 to 4 months during the first year. The first signs of ischemic necrosis are that the head does not become osteoporotic nor does it grow compared to the opposite side. The cartilage space widens. These signs are present long before gross fragmentation and deformity of the head, comparable to Legg-Calvé-Perthes disease.

If there is any suggestion of ischemic change, or if there seems to be a gradually appearing roentgenographic accompaniment, consideration should be given to premature epiphysiodesis of the greater trochanter to minimize the overgrowth and loss of the normal articulotrochanteric distance.

Premature fusion of the upper femoral epiphyseal plate is sometimes an early sign of avascular necrosis. Premature fusion of the upper femoral epiphyseal plate occurred in 11 patients; in 6 this followed ischemic necrosis. In 3 additional patients, premature fusion also occurred at the distal femoral epiphyseal plate.

Premature epiphyseal fusion results in total shortening of the lower limb and relative coxa vara. This may lead to a short neck and a weak lever arm for the hip abductor muscles, shortened leg, and limitation of abduction due to overgrowth of the greater trochanter. It would appear reasonable to implicate specific ischemia to selected regions of the growth plate with continued growth in other regions, similar to the avascular necrosis or ischemic necrosis encountered in the various patterns following closed and open treatment of CDH.[65,69]

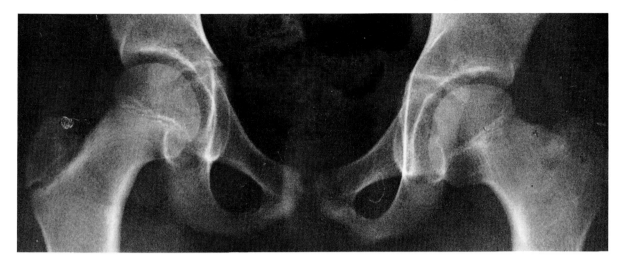

FIG. 17-28. A 12-year-old child presenting with leg-length inequality and limp. There was a left varus deformity due to a femoral neck fracture that occurred at 7 years of age (as a result of child abuse, old roentgenograms unavailable).

In contrast, increase in circulation consequent to the trauma may produce a coxa magna which is poorly covered if the acetabulum does not grow congruously. This is a good prognostic sign, as it implies more than adequate circulation, rather than ischemia.

Coxa vara is a common complication (Figs. 17-28 and 17-29).[70] Lam reported 23 instances in 75 fractures.[22] In 18 it developed in fractures during the immediate post-injury period, and in 5 as a late complication. It may be caused by several factors: (1) failure to reduce the fracture, (2) loss of alignment in the hip spica, either because of inadequate immobilization or delayed union, (3) ischemic necrosis and premature fusion of the capital femoral epiphyseal plate, in which instance relative discrepancy of growth between the capital femur and greater trochanter results in a progressive decrease in the neck-shaft angle. The clinical signs of coxa vara are prominence and elevation in the greater trochanter, shortening of the limb, decreased hip abduction, and gluteus medius limp. Treatment consists of subtrochanteric abduction (valgus) osteotomy.[71] If the capital femoral epiphyseal plate is prematurely fused, the relative varus deformity recurs with continued growth of the trochanter. It seems real-

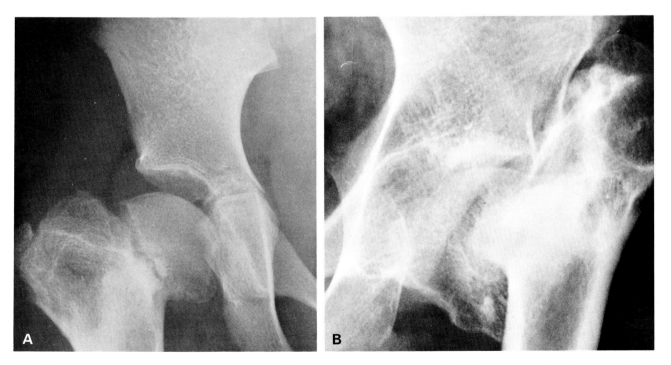

FIG. 17-29. *A,* Severe coxa vara and shortening of femoral neck. *B,* Severe proximal displacement of trochanter and shaft following an untreated femoral neck fracture.

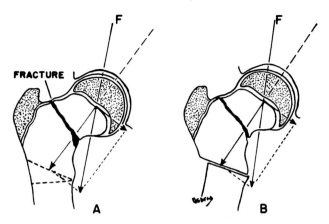

FIG. 17-30. *A,* Schematic of a femoral neck fracture left in varus, which probably predisposes the capital femoral epiphysis to slippage. *B,* Treatment by subtrochanteric osteotomy. Note the direction of the joint reaction force (F).

istic to consider a greater trochanteric epiphysiodesis at the time of the abduction osteotomy. The resultant leg-length discrepancy may require arrest of the contralateral distal femoral epiphysis at an appropriate age (or leg lengthening ipsilaterally).

Delayed union or nonunion usually develops in transcervical fractures; this occurs in about 85% of the cases with a Pauwel's angle greater than 60°, particularly when treated conservatively by cast immobilization. In those treated by internal fixation, the fracture fragments may be separated during insertion of trifin nails, or held apart by the threaded portion of a large pin such as a Knowles' pin. Nonunion should be treated by bone grafting and subtrochanteric abduction osteotomy aimed at converting the fracture angle from one of shearing or tensile stress to compression. In delayed union, abduction osteotomy alone is adequate, and it is not necessary to bone graft. In evaluating these patients prior to considering surgery, a bone scan again is indicated to make sure there is adequate blood supply to the proximal portion, particularly in the metaphysis.

Hoeksema stated that at least 4 cases of fracture of the neck and shaft of the same femur in children have been reported.[18,23,54] He reported a case in a 7-year-old boy who went on to have a repeat fracture of the neck of the femur 1 year after the Haggie pins were removed (these had been removed 4 months after the original injury). This is likely if the fracture is incompletely reduced, leaving an abnormal tensile strain area that will not heal well.

A rare complication of this type of coxa vara is the appearance of a slipped capital femoral epiphysis (Fig. 17-30). Jacob described 1 patient who apparently did develop a slipped capital femoral epiphysis; she had had bilateral involvement due to severe injury.[19]

Accompanying neural injuries may also contribute to growth deformity of the proximal femur (Fig. 17-31).

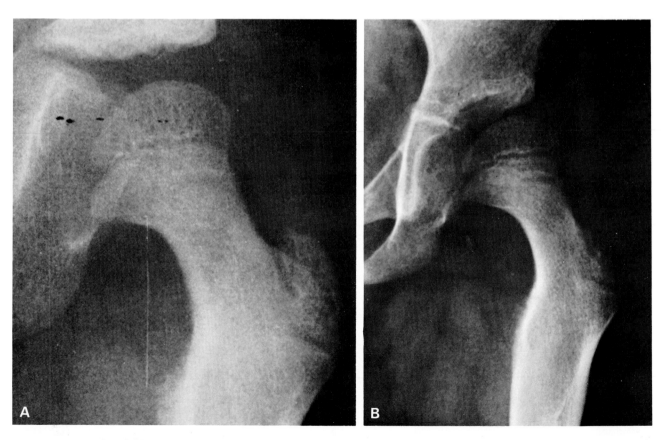

FIG. 17-31. *A,* This child sustained multiple pelvic and femoral shaft trauma 8 months before this roentgenogram. No neck fracture was evident then. However, the neck exhibits irregular development. *B,* 14 months after the injury, there was closure of the triradiate cartilage and further maldevelopment of the femoral neck.

Stress Fractures. Stress fractures of the femoral neck are most common in men in their early twenties. Wolfgang described a stress fracture of the femoral neck in a 10-year-old child.[72] Devas reported a stress fracture in a malnourished 14-year-old boy with multiple stress fractures.[73] Devas described 2 types of stress fractures of the femoral neck, the transverse type that appears as a small lucency in a superior part of the femoral neck and often becomes displaced. This is less likely in a child where there is still hyaline epiphyseal cartilage along the neck. The second is a compression type that appears as a haze of callus on the inferior aspect of the femoral neck associated with slight varus displacement and is more common in a young patient.

Trochanteric Injuries

Greater trochanter

Injuries to the greater trochanter generally occur as a result of muscular violence, a direct blow, or as part of a hip dislocation (Fig. 17-32). The greater trochanter may be avulsed by sudden contraction against resistance in the gluteus medius and minimus muscles. The fracture usually is undisplaced or minimally displaced. In more severe injury, the chondro-osseous fragment is retracted proximally, posteriorly, and medially.

Care must be taken not to interpret a small accessory ossification center at the tip of the greater trochanter as a fracture. This is a normal variation in the tip of the greater trochanter that appears between 7 to 10 years of age (Fig. 17-33).

Depending on the age of the patient at the time of this particular injury, part of the fracture most likely is through the intraepiphyseal cartilaginous continuity between the capital femur and greater trochanter. This may cause damage to the blood vessels along the posterosuperior femoral neck and lead to ischemic changes in the femoral head as a consequence of the injury. If the trochanter is avulsed from the lateral femoral metaphysis, an additional complication may be premature fusion of the physis with continued growth of the capital femur to create an elongated femoral neck (see Fig. 16-24).

Treatment should consist of immobilization of the hip in a spica cast with the hip in wide abduction to bring the greater trochanter into apposition with the upper end of the femoral shaft. The fracture will heal in about six weeks. With complete separation, the trochanter may have to be fixed with pins (see Fig. 16-24).

Lesser trochanter

Wilson reviewed 78 cases of this injury and also described an isolated fracture of the lesser trochanter that involved a 16-year-old boy who fell while high jumping.[74] Of the cases that he reviewed, 90% occurred in adolescents *following* the appearance of the ossification center in the lesser trochanter. Overwhelmingly, they were in boys. Most often they were associated with running or jumping. The lesser trochanter may be avulsed by the powerful contractions of the iliopsoas muscle against resistance. Only 2 of the cases were due to direct trauma.

There is usually pain along the inner side of the thigh associated with a limp. There is discomfort and frequent inability to flex the thigh, with deep-seated tenderness in the region of the lesser femoral trochanter and Scarpa's triangle. External rotation is a common finding. These findings are like those of slipped capital femoral epiphysis. Careful examination will reveal free passive motion in all directions, which helps differentiate this from a slipped epiphysis. The roentgenogram must be taken with the thigh in external rotation in order to rotate the lesser trochanter into an adequate view. Usually the lesser trochanter is avulsed and upwardly displaced, although not necessarily completely separated from the femur (Figs. 17-34 and 17-35).

The displaced fracture heals with little or no disability. Most of these fractures respond simply to bed rest and decreased activity. The patient should be kept in bed with the hip in flexion until comfortable, and then be allowed to ambulate with crutches and three-point partial weightbearing gait. Immobilization in a spica cast is not necessary. Open reduction is not usually indicated, although Wilson reported that 4% of his cases had undergone open reduction.[74]

Subtrochanteric Fractures

There has been little attention given to the management of children's subtrochanteric fractures. In most large series of femoral fractures these injuries have been grouped together with fractures of the proximal third of the femur. Daum published a report of 14 subtrochanteric fractures.[75] Ireland and Fisher found 20 cases among 150 femoral fracture cases.[76] These patients ranged from 2 to 15 years of age and their fractures were usually sustained by a direct blow from an automobile accident or athletic injuries. Of these children, 5 had severe head injuries with unconsciousness, and all of the fractures were displaced or compound. Approximately half showed some degree of comminution with overriding and anterior and varus angulation.

These fractures present unique management problems when they involve children.[75-77] This is due to the tendency of the short proximal fragment to displace into a flexed, abducted, and externally rotated position consequent to muscle forces (Figs. 17-36 and 17-37). Moreover, remodeling is not as extensive in this region, and malalignment may remain as a permanent deformity.

Treatment should consist of skeletal traction with a distal femoral (metaphyseal) pin. Skin traction will rarely be sufficient, except in a young child. The leg should be placed in 90°-90° traction. This counters both flexion and abduction of the proximal fragment. Use of less than 90° hip flexion makes alignment difficult. Frequent roentgenograms are necessary to be certain alignment is maintained.

Older patients with subtrochanteric fractures that cannot be adequately controlled by traction may be candidates for open reduction and internal fixation. The possibility or necessity of using open reduction increases, particularly if it is difficult to control the fracture due to head injury.[75] Choice of a fixation technique is difficult if the physes of the greater trochanter and capital femur are still functional. An intramedullary or Zickel nail is contraindicated, as it must traverse the portions of trochanteric and intraepiphyseal physes. The best method would be a compression plate and screw fixation, a method I routinely use for subtrochanteric

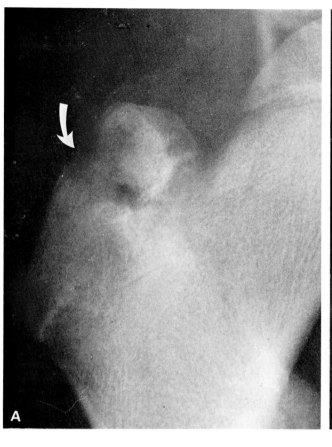

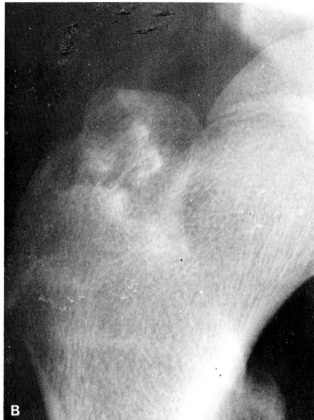

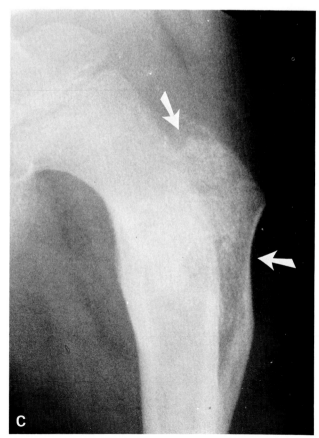

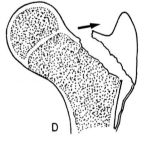

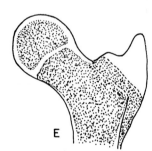

FIG. 17-32. *A,* Greater trochanteric fracture (arrow). *B,* Healing of fracture through trochanteric ossification center. *C,* Healed avulsion (arrows) of greater trochanter. *D-E,* Schematic of injury and the spontaneous repair shown in *C.*

osteotomy, for slipped capital femoral epiphysis, or femoral derotation. Again, care must be taken not to damage the trochanteric physis.

The average duration of traction immobilization was 9 weeks. There were no instances of fat embolism or serious complications of treatment. Regardless of the method of treatment, virtually all subtrochanteric fractures develop osseous union (Figs. 17-38 and 17-39). Overriding averaged 1 cm. Almost all fractures treated non-operatively healed with some anterior or varus angulation of the fracture apex. There were no significant rotational deformities. Of these patients, 18 were followed over a year and growth stimula-

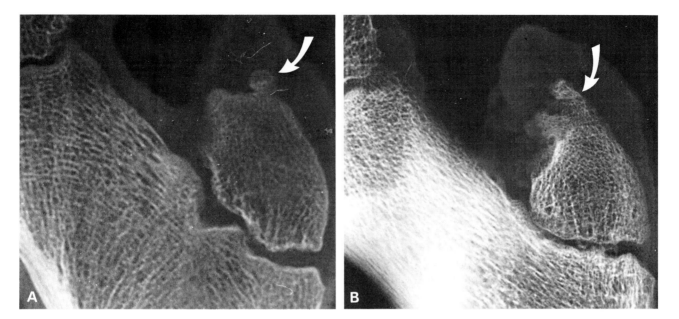

FIG. 17-33. Variations of greater trochanteric ossification. *A-B,* Roentgenograms showing extra ossification at tip of trochanter (arrows). These variations should not be misinterpreted as trauma.

tion of the affected extremity averaged 1 cm.[75] Improvement in angulation through growth and remodeling was also apparent. These compensatory changes in length and alignment were certainly most striking in the younger patients.

Mild anterior angulation and some varus or valgus alignment of the fractures frequently exist at union. In younger children, angular deformity corrects to a significant degree, while in older children, little change in alignment occurs with growth. In none of the children was this angulation or rotation at the fracture site a significant functional problem,

although there should be some concern for the child with increased varus and posterior direction of the growth plate that might increase susceptibility to slipped capital femoral epiphysis (see Fig. 17-30), particularly if this is an adolescent with a neck fracture as well as a subtrochanteric fracture.

Growth stimulation correcting leg-length inequality was better in children under 10 years of age, suggesting that a slight overriding of 10 to 15 mm might be acceptable. However, in teenage children there is little remodeling or compensation for shortening.

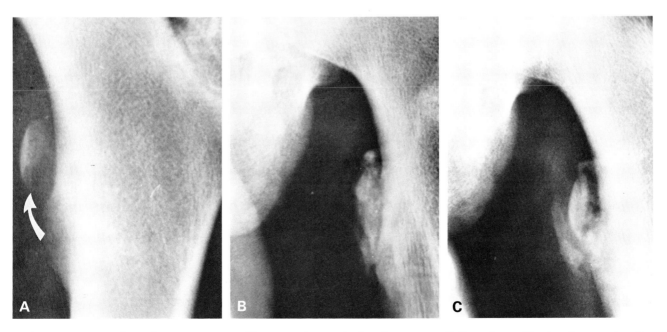

FIG. 17-34. *A,* Avulsion fracture (arrow) of lesser trochanter in female gymnast. *B,* Irregular ossification four weeks after injury. *C,* Follow-up one year later showing extensive bone formation.

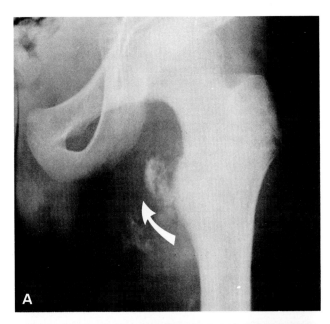

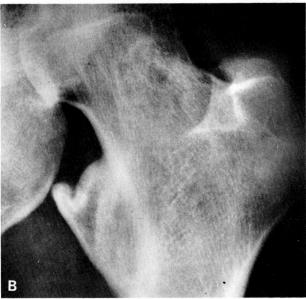

FIG. 17-35. *A*, Avulsion of lesser trochanter (arrow) in child with sensory neuropathy. *B*, Subsequent deformity at skeletal maturity.

Femoral Shaft Fractures

Shaft fractures of the femur are relatively frequent in children, and must be considered serious injuries because of the blood loss and potential shock accompanying the primary trauma. These fractures generally result from violent injuries, especially automobile accidents, and great care must be taken to rule out associated injuries as well as neurologic and vascular complications.[79-91]

Femoral shaft fractures in children may behave differently from similar fractures in adults. The important points to consider are: (1) early consolidation with considerable callus formation, (2) increased rate of longitudinal growth of the femur for approximately one year, and (3) spontaneous, but limited correction of axial deformity without corresponding rotational correction. Since femoral shaft fractures in children generally heal easily and satisfactorily, conservative (i.e., non-operative) treatment is almost always indicated.

The most frequent site of diaphyseal fracture is the middle third, where normal anterolateral bowing of the diaphysis is at its maximum. This is the area most commonly subjected to direct violence. Injuries less commonly involved are in the proximal third and least commonly are in the distal third. Greenstick fractures may occur, but are more common in the distal metaphysis. Fractures that result from obstetric trauma usually occur in the middle third of the shaft and are transverse (Fig. 17-40).

Classification

A torsional force produced by indirect violence results in a long, spiral (oblique) fracture, which is particularly common in the younger child (Fig. 17-41), whereas a transverse fracture is generally caused by direct trauma and is more frequent in the older child and adolescent (Fig. 17-42). When the direct force is severe, there may be comminution (Fig. 17-43). Segmental fractures are unusual because of differing stiffness throughout the developing femur.

Pathomechanics

The displacement of the fracture fragments depends on the breaking force, the pull of the attached muscles, and the force of gravity acting on the limb. As a rule, the distal fragment is laterally rotated consequent to outward rotation of the leg by the force of gravity. The severity of violence and the strong pull of muscles cause fracture fragments to be completely displaced with variable amounts of overriding. In fractures of the upper third of the femoral shaft, the proximal fragment is pulled into flexion by the iliopsoas, abduction by the gluteus medius and minimus, and external rotation by the short external rotators and gluteus maximus. The shorter the proximal fragment, the greater the degree of displacement. The distal fragment is drawn proximally by the hamstrings and quadriceps femoris muscles, and into adduction by the adductors. The distal fragment also falls posteriorly because of the force of gravity. Thus, the upper end of the distal fragment tends to lie posterior and medial to the proximal fragment, which is in flexion, abduction, and external rotation (Fig. 17-44). Displacement of fragments in a middle third fracture does not follow as regular a pattern. The tendency is for the proximal fragment to be in flexion and the distal fragment to be displaced forward. When the fracture level is in the upper half of the middle third, the proximal half may be abducted. When the break is in the lower half, it tends to abduct. However, displacements are not necessarily constant and depend on relative insertion and strength of muscles, factors that certainly change considerably as the child grows.

Diagnosis

A history of injury with resultant local pain, tenderness and swelling, inability to move the affected limb, deformity, shortening, abnormal mobility, lateral rolling of the limb distal to the level of fracture, and crepitus render the diagnosis

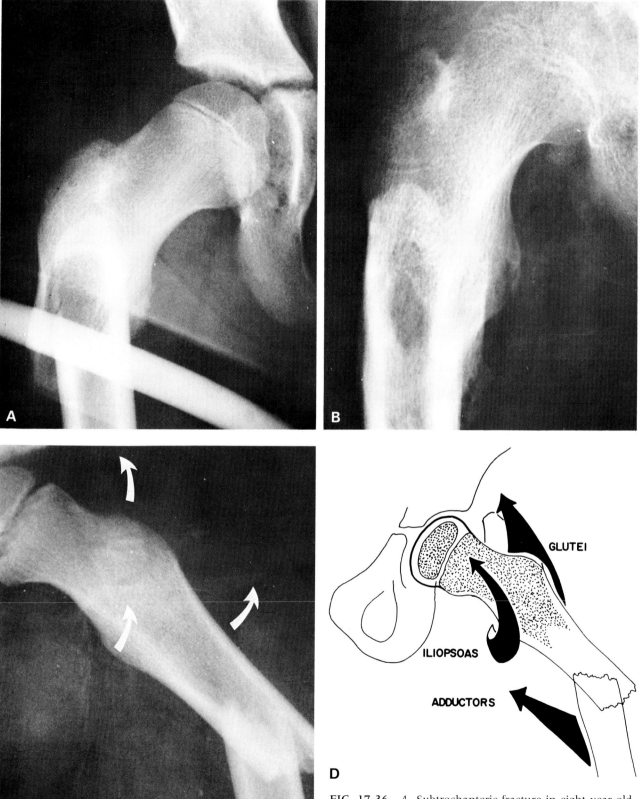

FIG. 17-36. *A,* Subtrochanteric fracture in eight-year-old. Overriding has been accentuated by varus and flexion of the proximal fragment. *B,* Final healed position. *C,* Abduction/flexion deformation due to subtrochanteric fracture. Arrows show deforming force vectors. *D,* Schematic of injury pattern.

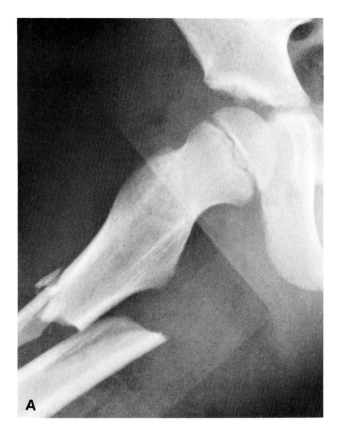

evident. The patient should be examined gently, so as not to inflict unnecessary pain. At that time the fracture is distinguished as being either open or closed. Neurovascular status in the lower limb should be carefully assessed and recorded, because injury to the femoral or popliteal vessels or the sciatic nerve, or both, may occur, especially from posterior displacement of the distal fragment of the fractures in the lower third of the shaft. Because femoral shaft fractures often result from major violence, it is imperative that the general condition of the patient be evaluated meticulously. The sensorium, blood pressure, and pulse must be observed. The patient should be carefully examined to detect any visceral damage to the abdominal, pelvic, and genitourinary area, any cranial injuries, or other fractures or hip dislocation.[92] The latter injury must be ruled out carefully with a good film of the hip joint, as it is embarrassing to finish treatment of a fracture of the femur and subsequently discover that the hip has been dislocated for the entire duration of traction.

Proper emergency care, such as initial gentle handling and adequate splinting of the fracture, is extremely important to prevent shock and further injury to soft parts. Any movement of the acutely injured limb is painful. An efficient means of immobilization is the Thomas splint, which must be suited to the size of the child.

While roentgenograms are necessary to determine the exact level and nature of the fracture, they should not be done until the patient has been properly immobilized on a Thomas splint or similar device and given adequate medication for relief of pain and muscle spasm.

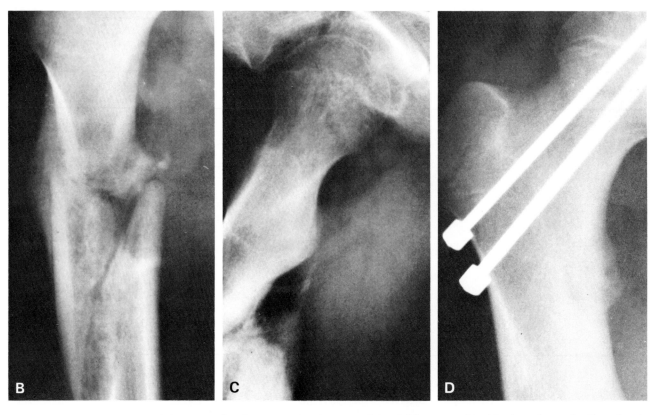

FIG. 17-37. *A,* Comminuted fracture. This fragmentation is unusual in children. *B,* This AP view shows healing that is apparently good. *C,* However, the lateral view shows residual flexion of the proximal fragment. *D,* Three years later this patient had a posterior slipped capital femoral epiphysis.

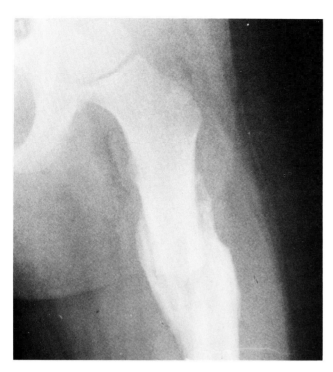

FIG. 17-38. Endosteal to subperiosteal callus healing, which is characteristic of these overriding fractures.

Treatment

Soft tissue injury inevitably accompanies a femoral shaft fracture. Excessive hemorrhaging with a blood loss of 500 ml or more is common. The sources of bleeding may be branches of the profunda femoris artery, which course around the posterior and lateral surfaces of the femoral shaft, the vessels of the richly vascular muscles that envelop the femur, or the medullary vessels of the bone. Occasionally the femoral artery may be torn (Fig. 17-45). If there is major damage to the femoral artery necessitating repair, this is one of the few instances where internal fixation is indicated in a child. This minimizes the tension of the suture line of the vascular anastomosis. However, a plate should be used rather than an intermedullary rod unless the patient is almost skeletally mature.

There is no routine treatment for displaced femoral fractures in children. A decision must be made as to what type of traction or fixation is indicated for the specific injury complex in a given individual. One must consider the age and weight of the patient in addition to local soft tissue trauma, the type and location of the femoral fracture, other injuries to the head, thorax, abdomen, or additional fractures of the same or opposite leg. Most physicians have their own favorite treatment.

Several principles that should be applied to the treatment of femoral shaft fractures in children are: (1) the simplest form of satisfactory treatment is the best, (2) if possible, the

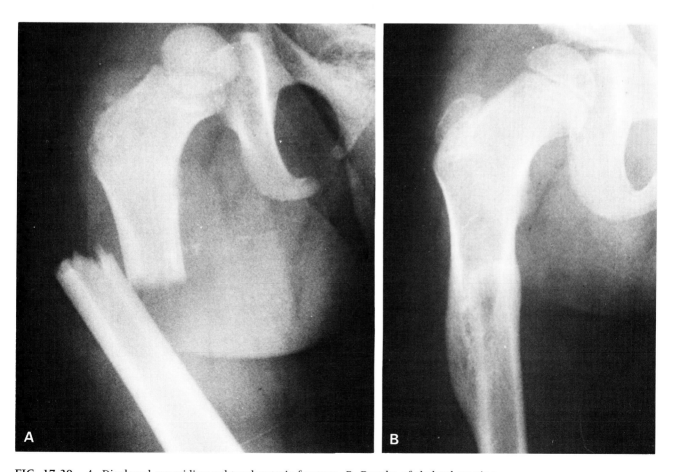

FIG. 17-39. *A,* Displaced overriding subtrochanteric fracture. *B,* Results of skeletal traction.

initial treatment should be the permanent treatment, (3) perfect anatomic reduction is not essential for perfect function, (4) the restoration of alignment (including rotation) is more important than the position of the fractured surfaces (i.e., overriding) with respect to one another, (5) the more growth remaining in the fractured femur, the more likelihood there is of restoration of normal osseous architecture as the bone remodels, (6) overtreatment is usually worse than undertreatment, (7) the injured limb should be immobilized in a Thomas splint before definitive therapy is begun, and (8) the hope that all deformities in children will correct themselves spontaneously is *no* excuse for leaving any deformity that could and should be corrected by simpler means and manipulation. Shortening of less than 2 cm, angulation of less than 20°, and absence of rotation are the major factors to seek in conservative treatment.

Several types of skin and skeletal traction have been used successfully and each has its advantages and advocates. The simplest, safest, and most effective method for a given child and a given fracture in a given age group should be the treatment of choice. Bryant's traction, properly applied and carefully watched, is ideal for children weighing less than 18 kg or under 2 years of age. For children weighing more, Russell's traction is probably the most frequently used with excellent results. However, frequent adjustments are needed.

Humberger advocates the use of proximal tibial 90°-90° traction with a skeletal pin.[93] However, because of knee pain and the difficulty in obtaining and maintaining length and alignment, its application is probably limited to children weighing less than 45 kg and under 10 years of age. A few physicians have expressed fear of stretching the cruciate ligaments and posterior capsule with this type of traction.

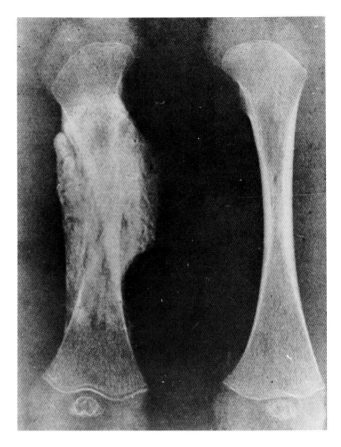

FIG. 17-40. Characteristic massive new bone in birth injury femoral shaft fracture. (Adapted from Truesdell[117]).

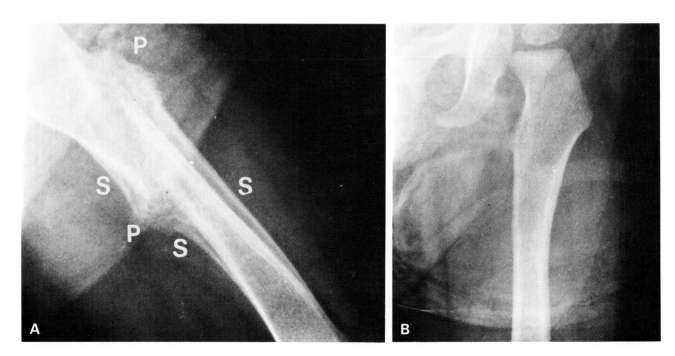

FIG. 17-41. *A,* Extensive subperiosteal new bone. Note the difference between the irregular proliferative callus bone (P) at the level of the fracture and the subperiosteal bone (S). This was caused by elevation of the periosteum due to dissecting hematoma and stripping during the injury. *B,* One year later, evidence of any of this callus is minimal consequent to remodeling.

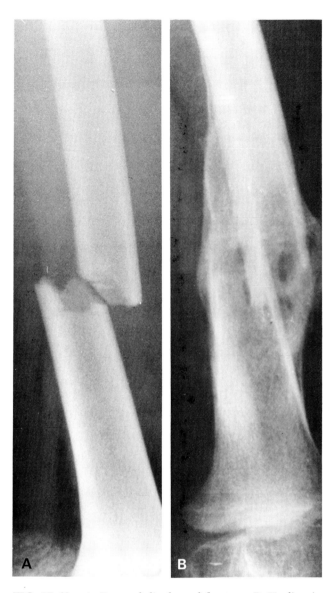

direction, 15° anteriorly, and 5° posteriorly. This requires frequent supervision of the fracture fragments and adjustment of traction. However, a child should not be subjected to frequent manipulations or unjustified trauma simply to correct minor angular displacement.

In infants and children up to 2 years of age Bryant's traction is probably efficient and satisfactory provided there is no spasticity and contracture of the hamstrings, and provided that the hips can be easily flexed to 90° with the knees in extension (Fig. 17-47). Traction should be applied to both legs. The legs should be wrapped from mid-thigh to the malleoli with padding (e.g., lambs wool, soft cotton) placed over the malleoli to prevent undue pressure. The same amount of weight should be applied to each leg, and should be sufficient to lift the infant's pelvis until the sacrum is just elevated from the mattress. One should be cautious not to overpull a small infant. The position of the fracture must be checked by periodic roentgenograms so that distraction of the fragments can be avoided. Medial bowing caused by an excessive pull of the hip abductors can be corrected by decreasing the amount of weight on the affected limb and increasing traction on the contralateral normal limb, thus tilt-

FIG. 17-42. *A,* Femoral diaphyseal fracture. *B,* Healing in skeletal traction.

Some patients do exhibit anterior subluxation of the tibia while in traction but this is difficult to assess accurately in young children who normally have increased laxity. Furthermore, the period of spica cast immobilization following traction should restore normal tautness to the ligaments. There is no strong evidence of instability in the knee in patients after removal from traction and thorough immobilization. Traction can be modified by using a cast around the lower leg to lessen movement of the pin. In the older child, consideration of a distal femoral pin should be undertaken, but care must be taken not to place it near or through the distal femoral epiphysis (Fig. 17-46).

It is recommended that fracture fragments be aligned as near a normal relationship as possible, and that angles that exceed the normal range by more than 5 to 10° not be accepted. The surgeon should strive for complete absence of rotational deformity and should try to achieve angular deformities that do not exceed 10° in the medial or lateral

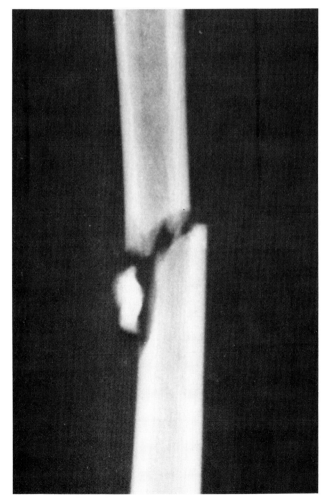

FIG. 17-43. Comminuted femoral diaphyseal fracture. This is not a common fracture pattern in children until adolescence.

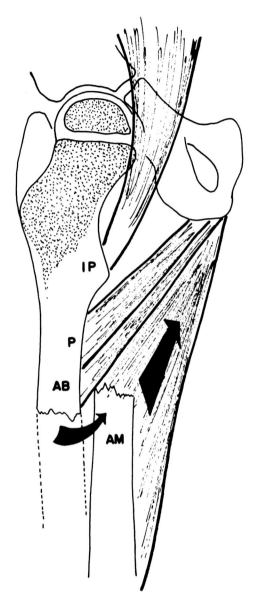

FIG. 17-44. Schematic of muscle pulls tending to deform a shaft fracture. Note the iliopsoas (IP); the pectineus (P); the adductor brevis (AB); and the adductor magnus (AM).

ing the pelvis and countering the pull of the hip abductors. The expectation that an osseous deformity in childhood will correct itself spontaneously with growth and remodeling is *not* an acceptable excuse for ignoring it, especially if correction can be obtained by simple means. Callus forms rapidly in infants and by 2 to 3 weeks from the time of trauma the tenderness over the callus will disappear and the fracture will probably be stable enough to allow removal from traction and placement in a 1- to 1½-inch hip spica for an additional 6 to 8 weeks.

This traction method should *not* be used in children over 2 years of age or those weighing over 25 pounds. The patient must be monitored closely for possible development of vascular and neurologic skin complications. Circulatory problems are the most serious. Blount pointed out that skin trac-

tion is not completely safe in children and that tight bandages and abnormal pressure can impair circulation and lead to Volkmann's ischemic contracture, even in the normal limb that is also being treated.[82,94] There are three basic degrees of circulatory insufficiency. The first is ischemic fibrosis of the muscles of the lower leg with patches of sensory loss. There is almost complete paralysis of the muscle distal to the knee, particularly the short toe flexors. The second degree of involvement is characterized by both the changes described above and by circumferential necrosis of the skin and underlying muscles in the calf. The third degree is the most severe form, in which the foot and ankle have gangrenous changes in addition to circumferential necrosis of the calf.

Nicholson and associates, in reviewing complications of Bryant's traction, attributed the vertical position of the lower extremities, the consequently increased hydrostatic pressure, the excessively tight leg wrapping, and the hyperextension of the knee as the factors contributing to decreased pulse pressure.[95]

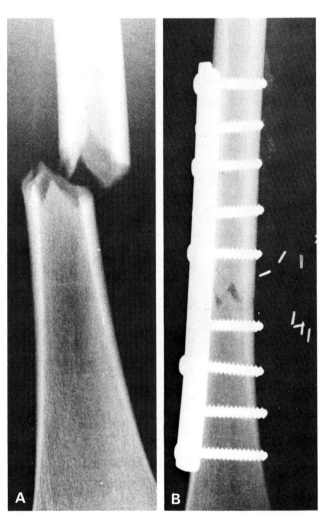

FIG. 17-45. *A,* Mildly displaced and distracted femoral shaft fracture in a 13-year-old. However, distal pulses were absent. *B,* A vascular repair was undertaken, coupled with plating of the femur.

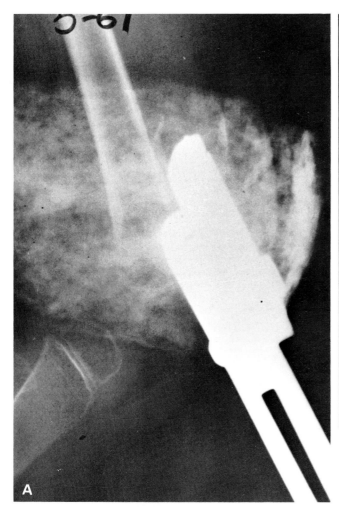

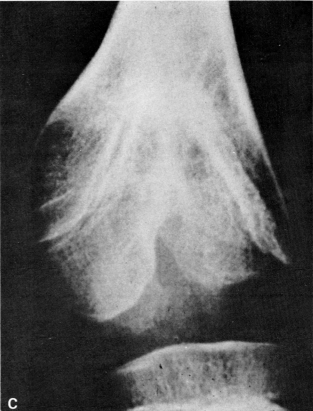

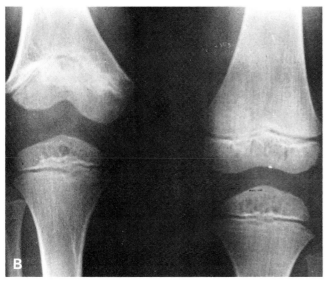

FIG. 17-46. Effect of traction pin being too close to growth plate. *A*, Placement of pin not readily evident. *B*, Central growth impairment one year later. *C*, Further central deformity four years later. Earlier recognition coupled with selective resection of this osseous bridge might have improved this deformity.

Ferry modified Bryant's traction by adapting the principle of Russell's traction.[96] The traction is applied using Russell's principle because less tightness is necessary in the wrapping. Further, by maintaining the knee in mild flexion, there is less likelihood of producing vascular or neurologic complications by overstretching these structures.

Dameron described treatment by closed reduction and immediate double cast spica immobilization as a preferred method for treating infants and young children.[84] The method is as follows: Under general anesthesia and aseptic conditions, a Kirschner wire is inserted immediately distal to the proximal tibial epiphysis on the affected side. A sterile Kirschner wire bow is attached and while longitudinal traction is applied the patient is gently transferred to the fracture table. The foot on the uninjured side is secured by strapping it to the foot piece of the fracture table. Traction is applied on the fractured thigh and normal leg while an assistant steadies the pelvis manually against the well-padded perineal post. The pull on the distal fragment should be in line with the proximal fragment. Ordinarily this is adequate to achieve reduction of oblique fractures. Roentgenograms are then made to determine the alignment of the fracture fragments. If there is any angulation, it is corrected by altering the direction of the traction forces.

A well-molded double hip spica cast is applied from the nipple line to include both feet, incorporating the Kirschner wire bow in the plaster. The patient is discharged on the following day. Immobilization in the cast is continued for 8 weeks. If the method is used for adolescents, an additional 2 to 4 weeks of immobilization may be necessary for solid bony union.

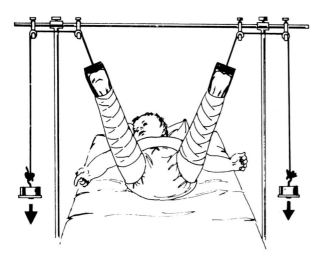

FIG. 17-47. Bryant's traction. Mild divarication may help in alignment.

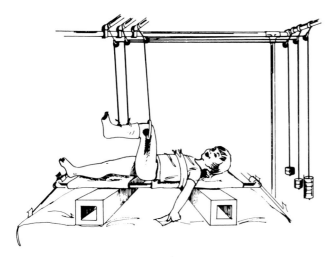

FIG. 17-48. 90°-90° skeletal traction with lower leg in cast.

Dameron and Thompson presented the end results in 53 patients treated by this method.[84] The average duration of follow-up was 6.9 years. They could not find any deformity, abnormality of gait, or limitation of hip and knee motion in any of their patients. The fractured leg was, on the average, $\frac{1}{16}$ inch longer than the normal leg. In only a few patients was the broken leg more than $\frac{1}{4}$ inch shorter than the normal leg, and in 5 patients the affected leg was more than $\frac{1}{4}$ inch longer. Complications of malunion, delayed union, nonunion, Volkmann's contracture, and gangrene were not encountered in any of their patients. They recommended this method as a safe, certain, comfortable, and economical method for treating femoral shaft fractures. The chief advantage of this method is that it decreases the duration of the hospital stay, which has obvious financial advantages. However in the older child, maintenance of reduction is sometimes difficult, requiring close supervision by repeated roentgenograms and wedging of the cast to correct angulation, should it occur.

For children over 2 years of age there are several types of traction available, namely: (1) skin traction, Russell, split Russell or Yale methods, (2) suspension skeletal traction with a Thomas splint and Pearson attachment, and (3) 90°-90° skeletal traction with a pin through the distal femur or the proximal tibia.[97-101] In general, traction is employed to maintain alignment until there is adequate callus for stability (i.e., the callus and fracture site are no longer tender and the femur moves as a unit on manipulation), and the leg can be effectively immobilized in a $1\frac{1}{2}$-hip spica cast.

Because of its effectiveness and simplicity, 90°-90° skeletal traction with a pin through the distal femur is frequently used (Fig. 17-48). Alignment of the fracture is easily achieved and maintained, as there is one line of traction and the pin through the distal femur provides good rotational control of the fracture fragments. The gastrocnemius, hamstring, and iliopsoas muscles are relaxed by the flexed position of the hip and knee, making alignment of the fracture fragments relatively easy.

Other advantages of 90°-90° traction are that it promotes dependent drainage; the thigh is readily accessible for clinical inspection of alignment with the use of portable roentgenographic equipment, and it facilitates change of dressings and wound inspection in infected or open fractures. A heavy threaded Steinmann pin or a large Kirschner wire is inserted 2 cm proximal to the adductor tubercle at the junction of the posterior third and anterior two thirds of the femoral shaft. Using this site, one should avoid injuring the physis or puncturing the suprapatellar pouch and knee joint. Pushing the skin slightly upward while drilling the wire through should prevent undue pressure on the skin while traction is applied. Sterile dressings are placed over the skin wounds and a traction bow of correct size is applied with the pin under tension. A light below-knee cast is applied with the ankle in a neutral position. This cast should be well-padded in the popliteal area and the dorsum of the foot and ankle to prevent pressure sores. Traction ropes suspend the lower leg in horizontal position with the knee in 90° of flexion. The weights are adjusted to counterbalance the weight of the leg, merely suspending the lower leg. An optional closed reduction of the fracture may be performed. Weights are placed by way of a rope on the traction bow with the hip in 90° of flexion, the traction forces acting vertically in line with the longitudinal axis of the femoral shaft.

Angulation and rotation are easily corrected by shifting the overhead traction in the appropriate direction. If additional external support is necessary in an unstable fracture, coaptation splints may be employed. Slings with 1 or 2 kg of traction can be applied over the fracture site to control lateral or anteroposterior angulation.

The position and alignment of the fracture fragments must be checked by periodic roentgenograms. Under no circumstances should one allow distraction of the fragments to take place. In children between 2 and 10 years of age, side-to-side apposition with 0.5 to 1 cm overriding is the ideal position, but it should not exceed 1.5 cm. In infants and adolescents, however, end-to-end apposition is desirable.

Traction is continued for 2 to 4 weeks until the callus is no longer tender on palpation and the femur moves as a unit. Adequate callus should also be visible on the roentgenograms. The patient is then placed in a $1\frac{1}{2}$-hip spica cast. The affected thigh should be in 10° of abduction or in neutral position with the opposite hip in moderate abduction to facilitate perineal hygiene. A common pitfall is to place the fractured thigh in marked abduction with resultant lateral bowing due to the pull of the strong adductors. It is always wise to extend the hip and knee gradually to 45° of flexion before applying the hip spica cast. The pin in the femur is removed and not incorporated in the cast.

Humberger and Eyring described a method of 90°-90° skeletal traction with the Kirschner wire inserted through the proximal tibia.[93] This method is not recommended because the Kirschner wire may injure the apophysis of the proximal tibial tubercle, either at the time of insertion or if it should migrate. Also, the wire in the proximal tibia does not provide direct control over the femur as does a wire through the distal femur.

Miller and Welch found 7 of 10 patients treated with 90°-90° traction and proximal tibial traction pin who exhibited subluxation (2 cases) or dislocation (5 cases).[100] Genu recurvatum developed in 1 case. Several patients had progressive knee pain and prolonged rehabilitation. They recommended distal femoral pin placement. However, this also has the potential for physeal damage (see Fig. 17-46).

Suspension traction is preferred by many orthopaedic surgeons for older children and adolescents. Skin traction is often unsatisfactory in the heavy child, and skeletal traction is applied with a Kirschner wire inserted through the distal femur (Fig. 17-49).

The thigh and leg are supported on a felt pad covered with stockinette and placed on the Thomas splint and Pearson attachment. With the hip in 35 to 40° of flexion, the Thomas splint is pushed up firmly against the ischial tuberosity and supported at both ends by sufficient weight to balance the limb. The traction ropes on the Thomas ring should pull cephalad to prevent the splint from sliding off the leg. The level of the Pearson attachment should be just above the knee joint level so that the knee can be flexed approximately 30° to relax the hamstrings. A traction rope with sufficient weight on the distal end of the Pearson attachment supports the weight of the leg. By careful adjustment of the weights, the limb can be counterbalanced so that it moves up and down with the patient without discomfort during nursing care. The foot of the bed is elevated so that the weight of the patient's body acts as countertraction.

In midshaft fractures, the tendency is toward posterior angulation. To prevent this and to restore the normal anterior bowing of the femur, the slings under the thigh should

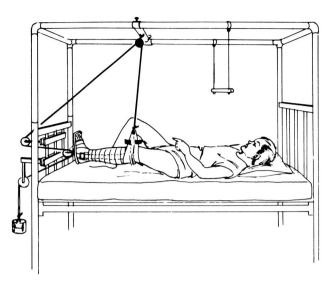

FIG. 17-50. Variation of Russell's skin traction applicable to femoral fractures in young children.

be taut and the knee should be in flexion to relax the gastrocnemius muscle. If there is persistent posterior angulation, a thick pad may be placed beneath the thigh at the fracture site, or a sling with direct overhead vertical pull at the appropriate level may be employed. Medial or lateral angulation may be corrected by aligning the distal fragment with the proximal one by shifting the position of the ends of the Pearson attachment, either proximally or distally on the Thomas splint, or by changing the direction of the pull, or both. Rotation is controlled by adjusting the suspension.

In about 3 to 4 weeks good callus is usually evident roentgenographically. Traction is removed and the fracture is immobilized in a 1½-hip spica cast for an additional 3 to 5 weeks, at which time the fracture will be solidly healed.

Mital and Cashman advocated use of skeletal traction for 2½ to 3½ weeks, followed by cast brace application and ambulation.[101a] They followed 28 children who had been treated with this method. Their ages ranged from 2 to 14 years. The average time for cast brace application was 20 days following traction, and the average time in the cast brace was 6½ weeks. No complications were encountered.

Russell's skin traction is preferred by some as an ideal method for treating femoral shaft fractures in older children (Fig. 17-50). The medial and lateral adhesive traction strips extend from the ankle to a point just below the knee and are attached with straps to a footplate with a pulley on its inferior surface. There should be two pulleys at the foot of the bed and one overhead. A well-padded sling is placed beneath the knee. The traction rope extends from the sling to the overhead pulley, which is distal to the knee joint, so that the rope is directed upward and distally at an angle of 25°, passing over the superior pulley attached to the end of the bed to which the skin traction straps are fixed and back again over the inferior pulley at the foot of the bed, where 2 to 5 kg of weight is suspended. The lower limb rests on 2 pillows arranged so that the knee is in 30° of flexion, the thigh is supported, and the foot clears the mattress. The foot of the bed is raised to provide countertraction. The vertical traction force is roughly equal to the amount of weight used, whereas the horizontal traction force is equal to approxi-

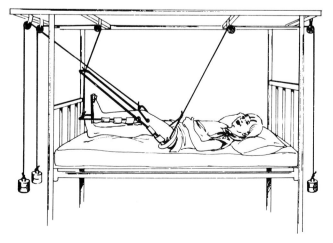

FIG. 17-49. Skeletal traction combined with splint.

mately twice the amount of weight. The vertical and horizontal forces create a parallellogram of forces with the resultant force in line with the long axis of the shaft of the femur.

Advocates of Russell's traction prefer it because of the ease with which it may be applied. The muscles are kept in balance, relatively less traction weight is required to overcome shortening and deformity, and the need for skeletal traction with its possible complications is eliminated. However, the disadvantages of this technique are: (1) the possible serious complication of peroneal nerve palsy with resultant foot drop due to pressure by the knee sling in the region of the common peroneal nerve; (2) the potential for development of posterior bowing at the fracture site due to lack of effective external support under the thigh (often it is necessary to apply an additional sling beneath the thigh with vertical traction to restore the normal anterior bowing of the femur); (3) the difficulty of nursing care and the necessity for careful vigil to ensure that correction traction is maintained; and (4) the child is initially in more pain than in 90°-90° traction.

Tachdjian employs split Russell's traction instead of the original Russell's traction with its 2:1 ratio of forces (Fig. 17-50). In split Russell's traction, skin traction is applied in the longitudinal axis of the limb and a balanced sling with a vertical force is placed under the distal femur or knee and suspended by weights to support the part and supply the necessary resolution of forces. External rotation of the leg is controlled with medial rotation traction straps.

Yale Method. For many years we have used a simple hip flexion-knee extension method for children up to 10 years of age (Fig. 17-51). The leg is placed in a Thomas splint. Skin traction is applied up to the fracture site. The splint is initially placed at 40 to 50°, but can be adjusted if further flexion deformity is present in the proximal fragment. Up to 5 kg of traction can be tolerated by this method. Rotation is initially controlled by allowing the leg to assume a natural, comfortable position. If necessary after a few days, rotation may be controlled by a derotation strap placed across the knee or by controlling the foot. However, our experience is that the child usually controls spontaneously as he or she begins to move about the bed with subsidence of swelling and pain.

Operative Methods. The operative treatment of femoral shaft fractures in children is generally considered unneces-

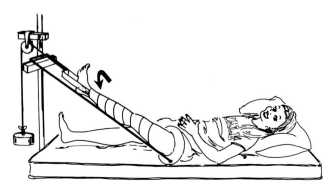

FIG. 17-51. Traction by Yale method.

sary and should be avoided as much as possible.[102-107] Perfect anatomic reduction of fracture fragments is less important in the child than in the adult, as most malunions correct with growth and remodeling, union occurs rapidly, pseudarthrosis is extremely rare, and there is a tendency to spontaneous correction of deformities.

Of 191 children in a series reported by Viljanto, et al., 45 (18%) were treated by surgery (18 by intramedullary nailing, 16 by other means of osteosynthesis, and 1 crushed extremity was treated by primary amputation).[107] No infections occurred. The mean longitudinal overgrowth of 9.8 mm did not differ significantly from that of 10.7 mm in conservatively (non-operative) treated patients. Interestingly, overgrowth was less in those treated by intramedullary nailing than those treated by other means of osteosynthesis.

Viljanto, et al., preferred intramedullary nailing.[107] They recommend it for transverse fractures that involve the middle third of the femoral shaft and pathologic fractures, and in patients in whom primary conservative treatment has not given an acceptable position. They also recommend it for blood vessel or nerve injuries together with shaft fractures and large soft tissue defects, as well as in multiple injuries of the same and other limbs or the unconscious or neurologically injured patient who creates difficulties for traction and casting. Mohan felt further indications for open reduction included muscle interposition and gross instability of the fracture.[88] Large soft tissue defects, multiple defects of the same or other limbs, unconsciousness, restlessness, and other difficulties that prevent traction and subsequent casting are additional potential indications for osteosynthesis.

However, osteosynthesis is contraindicated in most skeletally immature patients since it may damage the growth plate along the femoral neck (Fig. 17-52) and may also create distal problems. Raisch showed that intermedullary nailing may impinge against the distal epiphyseal plate, resulting in retarded growth of the extremity.[105] Contrary to this, Griessman and Kuntscher suggested that operative treatment by means of internal fixation did not cause any harmful reaction in children, and could therefore be carried out equally well in both children and adults.[87,103]

When there is an open fracture of the femur, the wound is thoroughly debrided of all foreign material, and any contused or damaged tissue is excised. After copious irrigation with saline solution the wound should be left open and the leg placed in 90°-90° skeletal traction, which increases spontaneous drainage. Appropriate antibiotics and tetanus antitoxin are administered. There is no justification for immediate internal fixation because the fracture is open and the bone ends are exposed. In a child, an open fracture does not ordinarily require a longer period of time to consolidate.

Results

No matter what the method of traction, these fractures generally heal well and rapidly in children. Roentgenographically evident callus formation occurs within 2 to 3 weeks in infants, 4 weeks in children, and 5 to 6 weeks in adolescents (Figs. 17-53 and 17-54). Such callus formation, accompanied by subsidence of pain, usually indicates that the patient is ready for a spica cast. Casting is necessary inasmuch as the callus is biologically plastic and may allow deformation if too much muscular activity is allowed, even in a spica cast. Cast removal should be based on clinical and

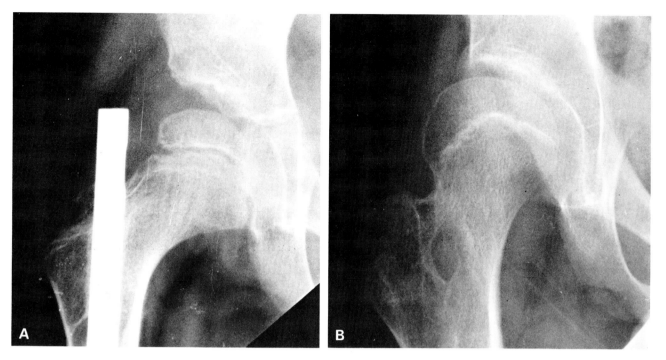

FIG. 17-52. *A,* K-rodding of subtrochanteric fracture. *B,* Subsequent growth deformity of proximal femoral neck with increased valgus of capital femur and premature epiphysiodesis of greater trochanteric physis.

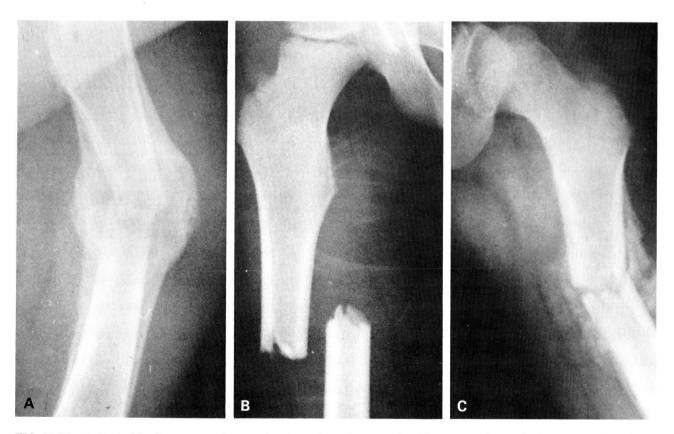

FIG. 17-53. *A,* Typical healing pattern shows subperiosteal new bone confined by a tissue plane, which is associated with the irregular callus around the actual fracture site, at which much of the periosteum presumably was disrupted. *B,* Displaced fracture. There is no way to determine the status of the periosteal sleeve. *C,* Early subperiosteal healing pattern of fracture shown in *B* indicates that the periosteal sleeve is reasonably intact.

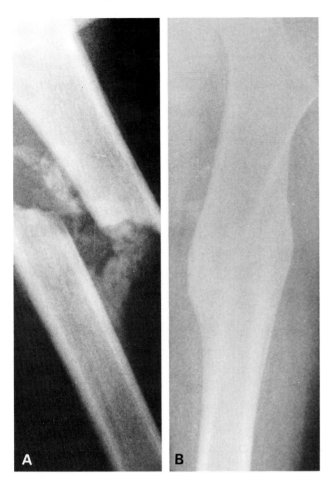

FIG. 17-54. *A,* Early subperiosteal to endosteal healing pattern. *B,* Final result.

roentgenographic appearance. The absence of pain on compression of the fracture site is an important sign. As a general rule, the amount of time (in weeks) for sufficient healing to begin protected activity out of the cast relates to the patient's age. A 10-year-old child takes about 10 weeks for adequate healing; a 16-year-old child takes about 16 weeks.

Functional recovery to pre-injury status is usually more rapid in children than in adults. However, they may limp for a long time afterward due to leg-length inequality and weak thigh musculature. This is often disturbing to relatives and parents, but an explanation of the reasons usually suffices to allay fears. Leg-length inequality, rotational differences, and muscular weakness are expected following these injuries. They are discussed in detail in the next section titled "Complications."

Complications

Leg-length inequality is the most frequent complication of femoral shaft fractures in childhood.[65,108-115] Growth acceleration following fractures occasionally results in significant leg-length inequality with a resulting limp, compensatory scoliosis, and back pain. Staheli studied 84 patients followed for 2 to 16 years following non-operative treatment of closed femoral shaft fractures.[116] Tibial length was not affected significantly by the femoral fractures. Among the 17 patients sustaining fracture during infancy, no late significant femoral inequality was observed. Among the children from 2 to 8 years of age, 25% showed significant inequality. Among the older children 8 to 12 years of age, significant late inequality was observed in 44%. Growth acceleration was less consistent in this age group and failures occurred because of excessive or insufficient overriding. Fractures in the proximal third and oblique-comminuted types were also associated with relatively greater growth acceleration. He did not find an active compensatory mechanism to equalize leg length.

Discrepancy in limb length following femoral shaft fractures may result from excessive overriding or distraction of the fragments or from stimulation of linear growth. These discrepancies usually stabilize within the first year and do not change significantly thereafter. While it has been taught that up to 3 cm of overriding may be accepted, approximately 1 cm is more realistic. However, in children under 2 years of age and adolescents, the normal growth stimulation is not as dramatic as in the midchildhood range. The infant and younger child heal rapidly; in adolescence there are fewer years of growth remaining to correct a deformity. Thus, in these two age groups, minimal overriding should be accepted.

The age of the child at the time of injury affects overall growth. Patients in midchildhood show more tendency to overgrowth compared to those in the younger or older groups. Fractures occurring in early childhood probably heal too quickly to manifest significant overgrowth, and those in late childhood occur at a time when growth potential is diminished. Furthermore, if relative adherence of the periosteum to the diaphysis is a normal physiologic control factor, this is also changing with age and is becoming more "adult" during adolescence, and the potential control and interplay between periosteal tension and growth rates at the physis are undoubtedly affected. Periosteal stripping without fracture can often promote overgrowth. Furthermore, greater amounts of initial fragment displacement may stimulate increased overgrowth.

The degree of overgrowth is unpredictable. Since Truesdell's original description, many authors have observed that the relative lengthening of the fractured femur averages approximately 1 cm.[117] The site of the fracture is not necessarily related to overgrowth, although several studies suggested increased likelihood of overgrowth from proximal third fractures. Similarly, the type of fracture is not clearly a factor (i.e., whether comminuted or not).

Barfod reported 117 patients with femoral fracture with a follow-up period ranging from 2 to 12 years.[109] Conservative treatment was used in 91 patients and osteosynthesis in 23. He felt that overgrowth of the injured limb following conservative treatment seemed to bear a direct relationship to the shortening observed at discharge. Of the fractures treated conservatively, 80% showed a normal length plus or minus 1 cm at follow-up. Following osteosynthesis, overgrowth occurred in every fracture as compared to the uninjured limb, with lengthening in excess of 1 cm in 20 of 23 cases.

Edvardsen studied 26 children and found that nearly two thirds of the patients had overgrown the femur 10 mm or more, that shortening of 15 to 20 mm at the fracture site was well compensated for by accelerated growth, that growth acceleration seemed to be taking place during the healing period, and that the difference at the end of healing was permanent.[111] Overgrowth seemed to be promoted by comminuted and long-oblique fractures and by overriding of the fracture ends.

According to most authors, the femoral fracture produces overgrowth for 1 to 2 years (3 at the most). The implication has been made that the longitudinal growth stimulus tends to continue as long as reconstruction itself takes place. Remodeling certainly can occur, but it appears that reactive longitudinal overgrowth has a limited time period.

Meals suggested that overgrowth might be due in part to the influence of handedness, (that is, cerebral control of the injured limb as judged by whether the fracture was ipsilateral or contralateral to the dominant hand).[114] When the fracture was on the same side as the dominant hand, the limb overgrew an average of 8 mm, compared with 14 mm when the fracture was on the side opposite the patient's dominant hand. The difference in his study was statistically significant.

Restoration of the normal anterolateral bow should be the goal, no matter what the treatment. Residual angulation at the time of casting may even worsen in a cast. Angular deformities should be minimal, even though 30° is often cited as an acceptable upper limit. The degree of remodeling and restoration of longitudinal alignment is unpredictable and less likely the closer the fracture is to the middle of the bone (see Figs. 17-55 and 17-56). The greatest amount of anticipated axial correction was purported by Nonnemann, according to whom axial deviation up to 30° tended to correct spontaneously.[118]

Lateral displacement completely corrected varus deformity on an average up to 40% and valgus deformity up to 60% of the initial angular defect. Ante and recurvatum could correct nearly 70% of any original deformity that was over 10°.[119] Viljanto, et al., found that as far as varus and valgus deformities, the greater the original angular deformity, the greater the number of degrees of correction. Overcorrection of this type of deformity did not occur. The normal femur is naturally curved in both the frontal and sagittal planes and creates difficulties in assessment, treatment, and measurement of post-healing angular deformities. Although slight angular deformities are of little consequence with regard to the end results of treatment, they are worth considering in a study of the phenomenon of remodeling.

Linear growth of long bone takes place at the epiphysis. Linear growth simply displaces angulation away from the physeal ends of the bone, instead of decreasing the angle. The remodeling of angular deformity is primarily that of decreasing the angle and is a response of normal endosteal and periosteal turnover to functional stresses in the femur. Remodeling and changes in alignment occur slowly, in contrast to stimulation in rate of growth of the fractured femur. Angular deformities occur more frequently in fractures of the proximal third, often with medial angulation, and correct themselves more slowly in the proximal third than those in the distal two thirds. Griffin, Anderson, and Green noted variable correction of bowing in different directions.[77] Barfod and Christensen felt that 25° of angulation or less in the diaphysis could be expected to undergo sufficient correction.[109]

Viljanto considers the relatively slow and limited correction of varus and valgus deformities the most significant

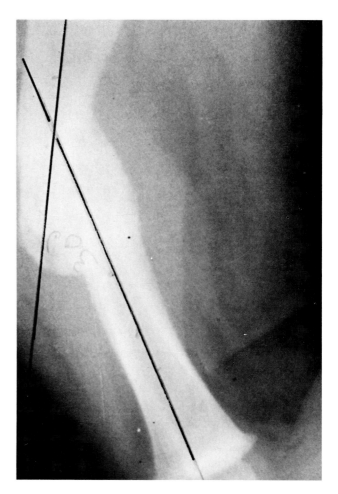

FIG. 17-55. Angular malunion in young child. This degree of deformity should not be accepted in children older than six to eight years of age.

finding in his study and feels he cannot agree with the concept that 25 or 30° should always be left as is, counting on them to correct spontaneously.[119] Ogden, et al., have shown that shaft fractures left with angular deformities have a possibility of long term complications such as slipped central femoral epiphysis (Fig. 17-57).[78] In both cases the capital femoral growth plate was placed in an abnormal position that probably increased susceptibility to shear forces. Miller did not report slipped epiphysis as a complication of femoral fractures, although he did describe several cases of coxa vara or posterior direction of the femoral head.[100] Kay and Hall mentioned premature closure of the growth plate in several cases of femoral neck fractures in children, but again did not mention slipped capital femoral epiphysis.[20]

Rotational deformity may occur with any of the traditional methods of treatment.[45] There is hardly any mention in the literature about rotational deformity. Vontobel is the only author who described rotational deformity in detail.[91] Late follow-up after femoral shaft fractures in the children in the series treated by traditional methods showed rotational deformities of 30° or more. Weber devised a method of treating children that is specifically directed at correcting rotational deformity.[67] The extent of correction of axial deviation in the frontal level was not significantly dependent on

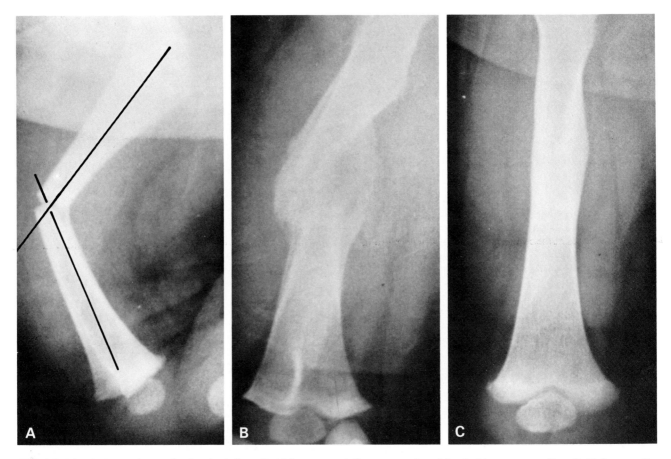

FIG. 17-56. *A,* Excessive malunion in infant. *B,* This was partially corrected and healed by excess callus. *C,* Eight months later, mild deformity was present. Significant angular deformities are likely to correct themselves in this young age group.

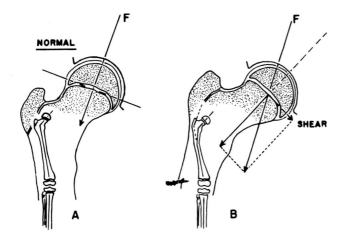

FIG. 17-57. Schematic of mechanism for slipped capital femoral epiphysis following femoral shaft fracture that healed with angular malunion of the diaphysis (compare to Fig. 17-37). Note the direction of the joint reaction force (F).

the patient's age at the time of fracture.[119] The long term effects and the possible relationship to adult-onset osteoarthritis are difficult to assess.

Damholt assessed quadriceps function following fractures of the femoral shaft in children.[120] Isometric as well as dynamic measurements revealed a significant reduction of strength in the affected leg. The literature is sparse with respect to elucidating muscle function following limb fractures, and this function is rarely used as a criterion for assessing the therapeutic results, particularly in children. The status of the muscles after femoral fractures has often been evaluated by measurements of circumference, but direct measurements of quadriceps function have not been carried out. A significant reduction of strength was most pronounced in children of the oldest age group. Damholt also showed that there was a tendency to greater reduction of strength the more distally the fracture was located. This factor should be taken into account during the rehabilitation of patients. Miller reported severe muscle function loss in a child sustaining ischemic fibrosis of the lower leg complicating femoral fracture.[121] Muscle herniation may also complicate healing as well as return of function (Fig. 17-58).

Refracture of the shaft of the femur is an infrequent complication. Saimon reviewed 21 patients ranging in age from 7 to 58 years and found that the incidence of refracture was highest in the 16 to 20 year range.[122] There was 1 patient in the 6 to 10 year range and 1 patient in the 11 to 15 year

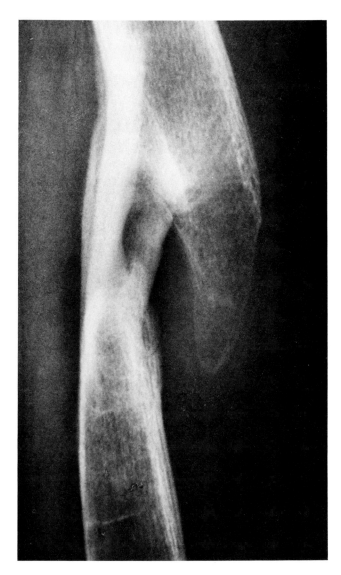

FIG. 17-58. Effect of muscular interposition with disruption of periosteal sleeve. The end of the proximal fragment cannot be remodeled effectively if it extends beyond this tissue.

range. He did not specifically break down the predisposing factors in the 2 children. He did feel that excessive emphasis on restoration of knee movement after cessation of splint or cast was a factor because of muscular tightness, particularly in the quadriceps. The amount of overriding of the fragments did not seem to be related in any way to the liability to refracture. Careful clinical assessment of the degree of union is important when considering discontinuation of bracing or casting. It is not sufficient just to palpate the callus gently to apply stress to the bone when it is painful. Firm pressure and strong stresses should be applied, for if the bone cannot stand up to this, it almost certainly will not stand up to the vigorous mobilization of the child. Radiologic criteria of adequate union is more difficult to define. In some cases refracture occurred despite the presence of a great deal of callus.[122] Therefore, the radiologic demonstration of warning cracks is obviously of great importance. The presence of such cracks

clearly indicates the need for further immobilization. All the cases sustaining refracture went on to complete healing.

Concomitant injury to the sciatic nerve does not affect the rate of fracture healing. However, the remainder of the bone may become excessively osteoporotic and susceptible to fracture following discontinuation of the cast (Fig. 17-59).

Bjerkreim and Benum reported seven cases of genu recurvatum as a late sequela after tibial traction for femoral shaft fracture. Unfortunately they were not able to obtain information regarding any early complications due to pin traction. They observed premature fusion of the anterior portion of the epiphyseal plate leading to tilting and reversal of the normal angle of the joint surface to the longitudinal axis of the tibia. Six of the patients eventually required corrective osteotomy. The anterior part of the growth plate can be damaged, as can that part under the tibial tuberosity if the traction wire is placed too close to the tibial tuberosity.[124] Only a small amount of damage need occur to the growth plate to lead to a small osseous bridge sufficient to cause a bowing deformity. Although it is expected that large deformities occur only with large growth slowdowns, it should be realized that even in cases such as type 6 injuries, a small peripheral osseous bridge can lead to a major angular deformity. Premature fusion of the proximal tibial epiphysis

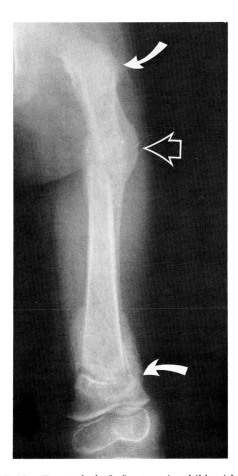

FIG. 17-59. Femoral shaft fracture in child with sciatic nerve injury. One week after removal of a spica cast, she sustained fractures proximal and distal (solid arrows) to the original fracture (open arrow).

has been observed following prolonged immobilization in tuberculosis of the hip.[112,125-128]

Miller and Welch described knee displacement while in traction as well as prolonged periods of rehabilitation secondary to knee symptoms.[100] It should be noted that this problem was present only in those patients treated with 90°-90° proximal tibial traction.

Premature arrest of growth in a lower extremity, especially in the epiphyses adjacent to the knee, has been described following direct trauma or insult to the epiphyseal plate after prolonged immobilization of the extremity for treatment of congenital hip dysplasia, slipped capital femoral epiphysis, chronic osteomyelitis, or pyarthrosis of the hip and occasionally following systemic abnormalities, such as scurvy, hypervitaminosis A, and homozygous thalassemia.[127-133] However, premature epiphyseal closure may complicate a fracture of the femoral shaft, including those fractures complicated by vascular insufficiency.

Hunter and Hensinger presented an 11-year-old with a comminuted spiral fracture of the femoral shaft.[134] There apparently were no neurovascular complaints or findings during treatments. During the year following the injury the child did not have good growth of the extremity, and the bones were osteoporotic. Growth arrest was occurring in all physes of the right lower extremity, with the exception of the distal fibular epiphysis; this included distal tibia, proximal tibia and fibula, distal femur, and proximal femur. This instance of multiple premature epiphyseal closure following a seemingly uncomplicated fracture of the femoral shaft appears to be unique, particularly since there was no detectable neurovascular injury to the affected extremity and no history or clinical evidence of direct trauma to the epiphyseal centers. Furthermore, the patient had no systemic illness and a total time of cast immobilization of 5½ months, which was considerably shorter than what has been reported in instances in which epiphyseal arrest was attributed to immobilization for 1 to 3 years. They felt that some generalized vascular or neural disturbance seemed to be the most reasonable explanation for the monomelic growth arrest.

Gillquist and Fraser both reported the problems of ipsilateral fracture of the femur and tibia or multiple fractures of a single leg.[85,86] These tended to occur in late adolescence and did not present a major problem as far as basic approaches to childhood fractures. In general, the femur does not cause as much trouble as the tibia, which carries a higher risk of pseudarthrosis, particularly as the patient gets older. Fat embolism and hypovolemia were found to contribute significantly to a high mortality rate in Gillquist's study.

Distal Femoral Metaphyseal Injuries

Distal femoral metaphyseal injuries are relatively common. The fracture line is usually transversely oriented. Torus (greenstick) fractures are frequent (Fig. 17-60) and must be treated carefully, since angular deformity may be introduced at the time of injury and not recognized during treatment, comparable to supracondylar humeral injuries. The fracture may also be complete, but undisplaced (Fig. 17-61). Again, beware of the degree of compression deformity of this fracture. The fracture may be displaced (Fig. 17-62), but this is a less common form of injury in this region.

The gastrocnemius is the chief deforming force in this re-

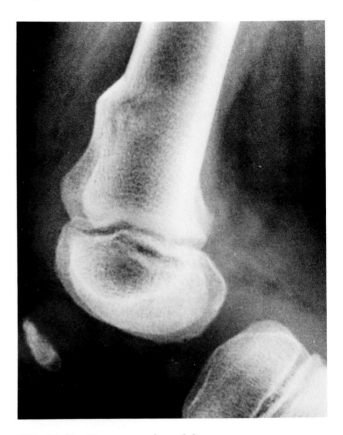

FIG. 17-60. Torus metaphyseal fracture.

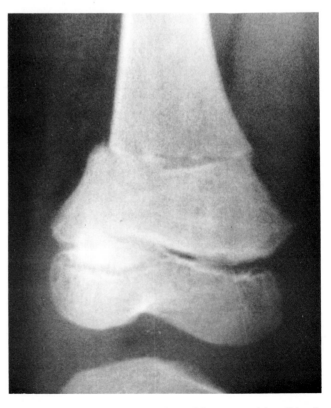

FIG. 17-61. Complete metaphyseal fracture, with mild valgus impaction. This should be corrected during treatment.

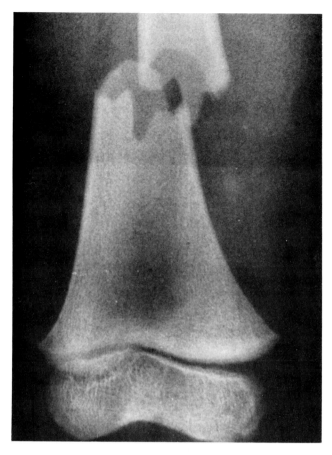

FIG. 17-62. Complete, partially displaced transverse fracture of diaphyseal/metaphyseal juncture.

gion. It arises from the posterior surface of the lower femur and pulls the distal fragment posteriorly into the popliteal space. The distal end of the proximal fragment is driven into, or may impinge upon, the vessels and nerves. Careful assessment of neurovascular function is essential immediately following injury and during care. The proximal fragment may also be driven forward into the quadriceps femoris muscle, and may cause significant damage to the vastus intermedius, with subsequent scarring and restriction of flexion and fibrosis.

In the displaced fracture, treatment should consist of manipulative reduction of any angular deformity followed by a long leg cast with 10 to 15° of knee flexion. The cast should be kept on for 3 to 4 weeks, at which time a cylinder cast may be applied to begin protected weightbearing. Knee stiffness is not a major concern in the young child. However, a hinged cast may be used to allow some knee motion in the adolescent.

In the undisplaced fracture the same type of casting may be used; however, frequent checks are necessary to be certain angular deformation due to the pull of the gastrocnemius does not occur. Mild knee and ankle flexion should relax this muscle. If the fracture is unstable, or if there is any neurovascular compromise, the patient should be placed in skin or skeletal traction.

These fractures usually heal rapidly and without any major complications. Angular deformity, especially in a varus or valgus plane, does not spontaneously correct, and requires correction during early treatment. Any permanent malunion may require a corrective osteotomy.

Distal Femoral Epiphyseal Injuries

These lesions are becoming less frequently encountered.[135-146] Originally termed "cartwheel" injuries due to the prevalent mechanism of injury of a child jumping onto large-wheeled wagons, the literature of the nineteenth century called attention to the high incidence of injuries in the distal femoral epiphysis caused principally by horse-drawn vehicles.[147] Boys attempting to jump on wagons frequently caught one of the lower limbs in the wheel spokes and sustained a hyperextension injury. Compound injury, amputation, and death were common sequelae. Certainly the frequency of this injury and its high complication rate have declined since that time. Automobile, bicycle, skateboard, go-kart, and athletic injuries have superseded the horse-drawn wagon as the leading causes of the fracture.

In the series described by Lombardo, the patients ranged in age from 1 month to 16 years 9 months, with a mean of 11 years and 3 months.[141] There were 28 males and 6 females. There is a relatively high incidence of bilaterality. Kaplan described a bilateral case.[139] In my series there were 4 cases.

Classification

Several patterns of growth mechanism injury may affect the distal femoral physis and epiphysis. Certainly, types 1 and 2 are relatively common. Types 3 and 4 may occur with a relatively significant frequency, and may be difficult to diagnose. Types 5 and 6 are infrequent. However, type 7 may be common as either an acute osteochondral fragment, or the more common chronic osteochondritis dessicans.

Type 1 injuries involve a fracture traversing the entire physeal-metaphyseal interface (Fig. 17-63). This necessitates the fracture following a contour that becomes increasingly undulated during adolescence. The direction of epiphyseal displacement varies: anterior, posterior (Fig. 17-64), varus, and valgus (Fig. 17-65). However, in some instances displacement may be minimal and may be indicated only by

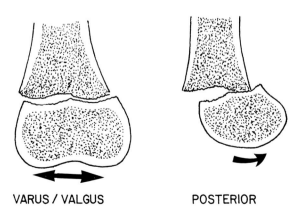

VARUS / VALGUS   POSTERIOR

FIG. 17-63. Schematic of type 1 growth mechanism injury patterns.

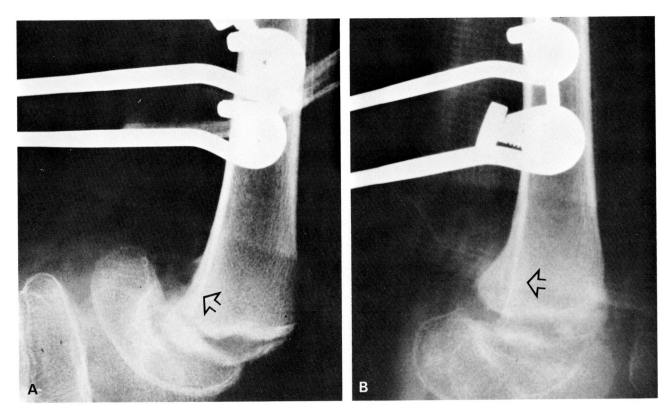

FIG. 17-64. *A,* Type 1 distal femoral physeal fracture with posterior displacement of epiphysis (hyperflexion injury). *B,* This was placed in skeletal traction and gradually reduced. The arrows indicate the direction of reduction.

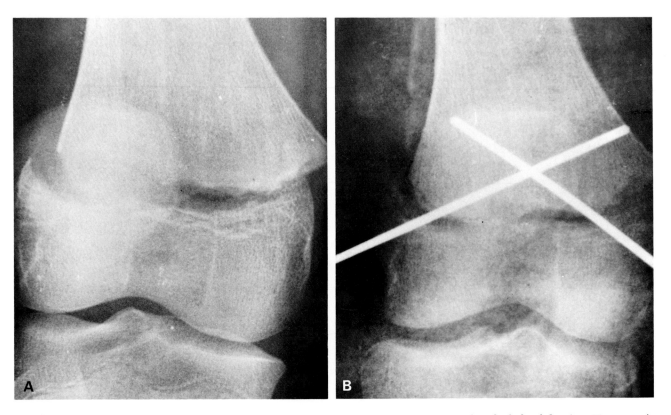

FIG. 17-65. *A,* Type 1 abduction injury. *B,* This was extremely unstable and was treated with skeletal fixation. However, it was not completely reduced. There is some residual valgus.

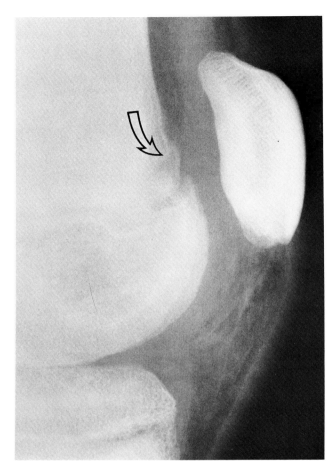

FIG. 17-66. Physeal fracture associated with mild anterior metaphyseal buckling (arrow) and hemarthrosis.

slight physeal widening or metaphyseal buckling (Fig. 17-66). In child abuse the distal femur is frequently injured. The only diagnostic finding may be small peripheral metaphyseal flake (Fig. 17-67).

Type 2 injury is probably the most common pattern (Fig. 17-68). Hyperextension injuries lead to anterior displacement of the epiphysis beneath the patella (Figs. 17-69 and 17-70). Varus or valgus deformations are associated with variable-sized metaphyseal fragments (Figs. 17-71 and 17-72).

Type 3 injuries may involve either medial or lateral condyle (Figs. 17-73 and 17-74). On rare occasions, the posterior condylar element may be involved. These injuries may be difficult to diagnose, and often require stress roentgenography (Fig. 17-75). Small pieces of the articular surface and subchondral bone may be fragmented and displaced into the joint (see Fig. 17-75).

Type 4 injuries may involve the medial or lateral condyle, or both (Fig. 17-76), or may occur in conjunction with a type 3 injury (Fig. 17-77). The fragment tends to displace proximally to a variable degree (Figs. 17-78 and 17-79). When both condyles are involved, the fragments are not only proximally displaced, but also split apart (Fig. 17-80). Similarly, types 3 and 4 injuries may occur concomitantly (Fig. 17-81). There is a high incidence of osseous bridge formation, especially in the smaller lesions (Fig. 17-82). In

other cases there is initial growth slowdown and irregularity in the secondary ossification center (Fig. 17-83).

Type 5 injuries are uncommon (Fig. 17-84) and more likely to occur in patients with other disorders such as myelomeningocele. Lombardo described a fracture of the proximal tibial metaphysis and diaphysis extending up as a type 4 injury into the proximal tibial epiphysis, but also leading to an initially unrecognized type 5 injury of the distal femur.[141]

Type 6 injuries may include glancing blows leading to destruction of a small peripheral segment (Fig. 17-85), which may lead to eventual formation of a physeal bridge. Other mechanisms such as burns, osteomyelitis, or irradiation may also contribute to this. Hyperextension injury may also damage areas where the capsule, periosteum, and perichondrium blend, creating formation of osteochondromata, which is a variation of a type 6 injury (Fig. 17-86).

Type 7 injuries involve fragments of the femoral condyles (Figs. 17-87 to 17-89). These may vary considerably in size.

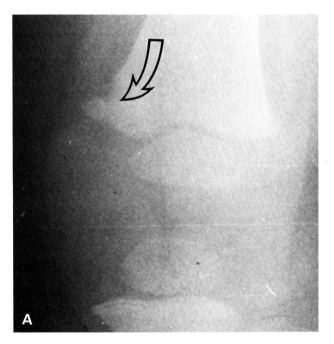

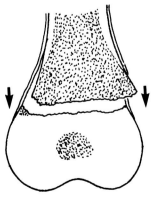

B   TYPE I - INFANCY

FIG. 17-67. *A,* Metaphyseal "beak" fracture (arrow) characteristic of type 1 physeal injury from child abuse. *B,* Schematic of this injury pattern.

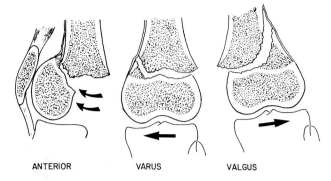

FIG. 17-68. Schematic of type 2 injury patterns.

ANTERIOR   VARUS   VALGUS

Pathomechanism

Distal femoral epiphyseal injuries may be grouped by 4 etiologic mechanisms: (1) abduction; (2) adduction; (3) hyperextension, which is where the distal end of the femoral shaft is driven posteriorly into the popliteal fossa, the periosteum of the posterior surface of the femur is torn, and the gastrocnemius is stretched (infrequent concomitant injuries include lacerations of the popliteal artery, peroneal nerve, tibial nerve, or both); and (4) hyperflexion, which is rare and caused by a direct blow to the femur driving the epiphysis posteriorly. All 4 basic mechanisms are accompanied by a variable degree of rotation.

Abduction Type. This type of injury is caused by a blow to the lateral side of the distal femur, frequently occurring in athletes, and is the same type of stress that causes medial soft tissue (especially meniscal and ligamentous) injuries in an older patient. The result is generally a type 2 physeal injury, in which the periosteum is ruptured on the medial side, and the distal femoral epiphysis is displaced laterally with a lateral fragment of the metaphysis. It is usually associated with some rotation. This fracture may reduce itself spontaneously and may be missed initially if the triangular piece of metaphyseal bone is small. One should carefully scrutinize the roentgenogram and take special abduction strain views to detect the lesion, if indicated.

Adduction Type. This type of injury is caused by a medial blow or an indirect injury. The epiphysis is medially displaced as a type 1 or 2 injury pattern. With the addition of a rotational component, a type 3 or 4 injury may occur.

Hyperextension Type. This type of injury was the most common variety in the past because of wagon wheel injuries, and is still seen in major vehicular accidents. The distal femoral epiphysis is displaced anteriorly by the hyperextension force and by the pull of the quadriceps muscle. The posterior periosteum is torn and the fibers of the gastrocnemius are stretched or partially torn. The triangular metaphyseal bone fragment and the intact periosteal hinge are anterior, although the latter structure is modified by syno-

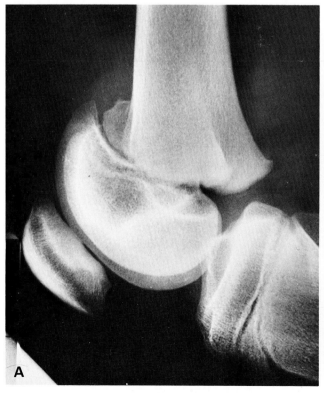
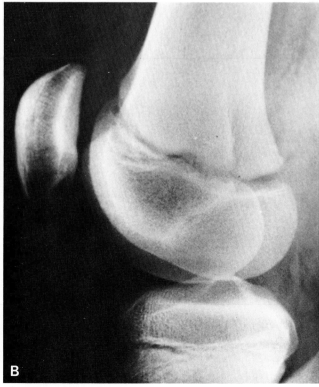

FIG. 17-69. *A,* Type 2 hyperextension injury. *B,* Appearance after closed reduction.

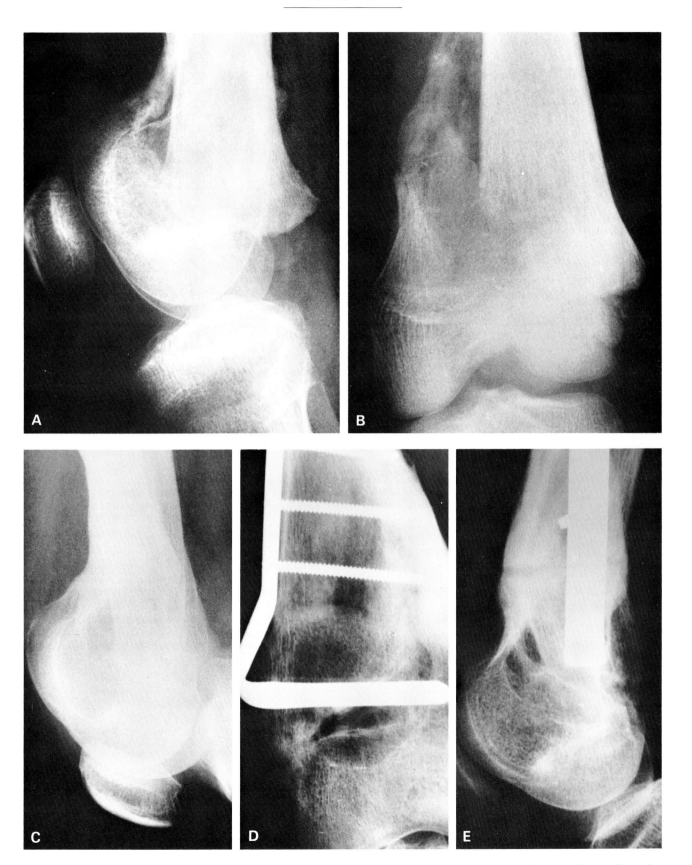

FIG. 17-70. Hyperextension deformity in boy with severe head injury. *A-B,* Reduction could not be done effectively. *C,* Appearance when the boy awoke from a coma four months after the injury occurred. *D-E,* A corrective osteotomy was done.

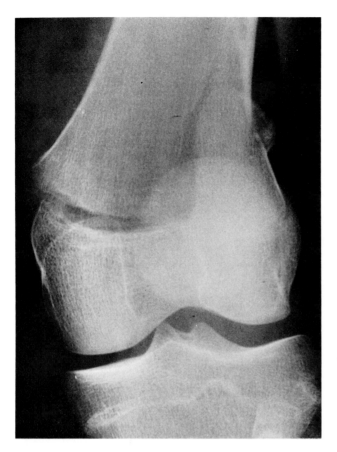

FIG. 17-71. Type 2 valgus injury with greenstick injury of lateral metaphyseal component.

vial extension into the suprapatellar pouch. The distal end of the femoral shaft is driven posteriorly and may injure structures in the popliteal region (Fig. 17-90).

Hyperflexion Type. Posterior displacement of the distal femoral epiphysis is rare, usually resulting from a forceful flexion injury caused by a direct blow to the distal femur.

Diagnosis

The usual history is violent injury with severe pain and inability to bear weight on the leg. The knee is markedly swollen and tense. There may be a true or reactive joint effusion, depending on where the fracture line propagates, and whether there is comminution with the joint, either through the intercondylar region or through the suprapatellar extension of the synovium and capsule. Neurovascular function must be examined.

These types of injury are particularly prone to spontaneous reduction. The diagnosis may only be suspected by a slightly widened growth plate or a fracture line extending into the metaphysis. Oblique projections are sometimes more revealing than stress roentgenograms.

Undisplaced types 1 and 2 epiphyseal fractures of the distal femur in the adolescent athlete may mimic injury to the knee ligaments. Roentgenographic examination with the knee under stress often reveals the diagnosis, thereby avoid-

ing unnecessary arthrotomy and indicating appropriate treatment at follow-up (see Fig. 17-75). Simpson and Fardon reported 3 cases that initially appeared to be pure ligamentous injuries until stress films were taken.[133] They noted that one type 3 injury had been misdiagnosed as a ligamentous disruption. Rogers and Jones described "clipping injury" fracture of the epiphysis in the adolescent football player as an occult lesion of the knee.[148] They described 7 cases of type 3 and 1 of type 2, all of which were confirmed either in the original film or with stress films.

Treatment

The position for immobilization is usually determined by the characteristics of the original displacement. If there is anterior displacement of the distal fragment, the patient is treated by reduction with traction in extension followed by gradual flexion and immobilization in flexion. With posterior displacement, the patient is treated by reduction (with traction) in gradual extension and immobilization and extension. Any medial or lateral displacement is corrected by traction and manipulation to correct the deformity. The patient is then maintained in 20 to 30° of flexion. Factors affecting the choice of treatment should include the ease of obtaining and maintaining reduction, the amount of swelling, the body habitus, and the presence of associated injuries.

Treatment may also include skeletal traction, traction followed by plaster immobilization, and immediate application of toe-to-groin cast. As pointed out by Bassett and Goldner, treatment of these injuries must be highly individualized.[136] In their treatment of the type 2 injuries, 12 of 24 patients were treated with open reductions and usually fixed by cross K-wires. Of the 5 type 3 patients, 3 were treated with open reduction and internal fixation, and 2 of the 3 type 4 injuries were treated with open reduction.

Abduction-type fractures are relatively simple to treat since there are no special problems of vascular injury or growth disturbance. To accomplish reduction the leg should be placed in longitudinal traction in extension and direct pressure should be used to push the laterally displaced epiphysis medially. The fracture may be held in a single-leg hip spica cast. The points of fixation in the cast should be well-padded. If only a leg cast is applied, the fracture may become displaced. Plaster immobilization is maintained for 4 to 6 weeks.

Hyperextension-type fractures present several problems of management; first, the potential injury to the popliteal vessels and nerves, and second, the difficulty of achieving and maintaining reduction since the plane of displacement and the plane of the knee joint motion are the same. There is lack of an adequate lever arm to grasp the distal fragment effectively. A closed reduction should always be attempted first, and if successful, followed by casting with a hip spica with the knee in 60 to 90° of flexion. Flexion is necessary to maintain anatomic reduction. However, swelling in the popliteal region may prevent use of much flexion; however, recurrence of anterior displacement is usually caused by immobilization with insufficient flexion. If necessary, Steinman pins may be used to traverse the distal femoral shaft. These particular injuries are often associated with major growth disturbances.

The posteriorly displaced distal femur (hyperflexion-type

fractures) must be reduced by pulling the distal epiphysis anteriorly. This fracture must be immobilized in complete extension, and at no time should the knee be immobilized in a position of semiflexion. Immobilization varies with a mean time of 7 weeks and a range from 3 to 16 weeks.

Type 3 injuries invariably require open reduction (Figs. 17-91 and 17-92). This should include an arthrotomy so that there can be completely accurate restoration of articular anatomy. Fixation, as much as possible, should be directed transversely across the epiphyseal ossification center fragments. Pins placed across the physis may be a factor in premature growth arrest (Fig. 17-93).

Type 4 fractures frequently require open reduction and internal fixation with smooth K-wires or screws (see Figs. 17-78, 17-80, and 17-93). An arthrotomy is an essential part of the procedure to gauge restoration of the articular surface and to remove any small fragments that could potentially form loose bodies.

Lee described a series of 26 patients from the Children's Hospital in Michigan.[140] There were 18 patients who were treated with closed reduction and no pin fixation, 2 were treated with closed reduction and percutaneous pin, 5 were treated with open reduction and internal fixation, and 1 patient was not treated with reduction because the fracture was undisplaced. The method of immobilization was a spica cast in 15 patients, a long leg cast in 10 patients, and 1 patient was treated with complete bed rest following fixation.

Results

These fractures generally heal rapidly. However, when they involve a child or adolescent with any remaining growth potential this region probably has the highest rate of complications. Most authors have indicated that 25 to 45% of patients demonstrate a growth disturbance. Fortunately, many patients are nearing skeletal maturity and do not exhibit major growth deformity as a consequence.

Prognosis based on the Salter-Harris classification alone is

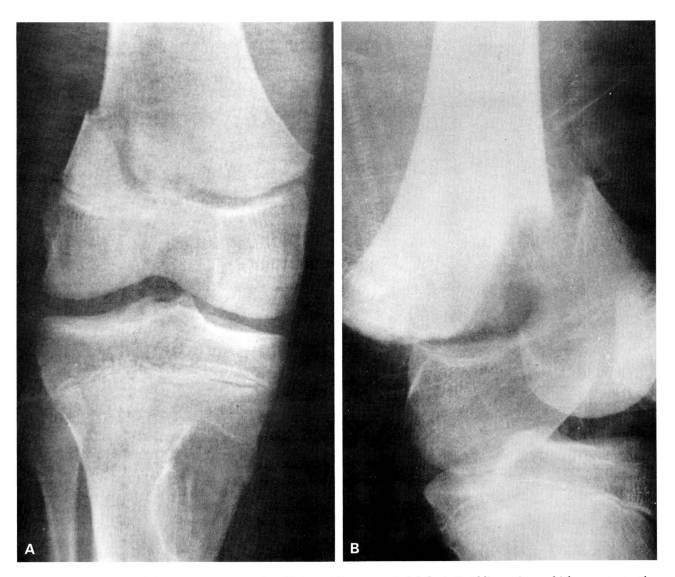

FIG. 17-72. *A,* Type 2 abduction injury. Note the tibial cyst (fibrous cortical defect). *B,* Oblique view, which accentuates the deformity.

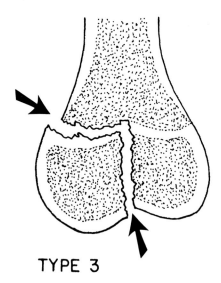

TYPE 3

FIG. 17-73. Schematic of type 3 injury.

not reliable. The development of deformity appears to be related to the degree of initial displacement of the fracture, the exactness of the reduction, the type of fracture, and the age of the patient.

Lee emphasized several findings.[140] First, correction may be lost while the patient is maintained in plaster. Second, type 4 fractures always require an open reduction. Third, orthoroentgenograms show that at least 90% of the patients with this type of injury have gradual shortening, which is in direct contrast to the recent study by Stephens and Louis who felt that growth disturbance was an all-or-none phenomenon.[146] Lee's study demonstrated that growth disturbance was present in nearly all epiphyseal fractures of the distal femur.[140]

Complications

The sequelae of this fracture include leg-length discrepancy, varus or valgus angulation, limitation of knee motion, and quadriceps atrophy. The primary problem is leg-length discrepancy, which may occur even in the absence of obvious premature epiphysiodesis because of a generalized slowdown (not complete arrest) of growth relative to the other distal femur. Lee has pointed out that it is imperative to follow these patients through to skeletal maturation in order to adequately document this type of complication, even when they appear to heal satisfactorily.[140]

Neer reported a 42% incidence of leg-length discrepancy.[101] Cassebaum showed a 25% incidence.[137] The combined series of Nicholson and Neer together showed 40% of patients with leg-length inequality.[95,101,142] Lombardo followed 34 fractures for an average of 4 years, finding a leg-length discrepancy of 2 cm or more.[141]

Lee followed several parameters, and evaluated growth disturbances for angular deformity and leg-length discrepancy. He measured them both clinically and roentgenographically and found that rotational deformity was not significant.[140] Of the 26 patients, 18 fit the criteria for his study and 16 demonstrated growth disturbances when compared to the normal side. These ranged between 5 mm and 6.2 cm. The mean shortening was 1.4 cm and the median was also 1.4 cm. Of the 2 patients who did not have growth disturbances evident on orthoroentgenograms, 1 had reached skeletal maturity with the epiphysis nearly closed at the time of injury, and the other had an opening wedge of osteotomy that may have corrected a leg-length discrepancy. In contrast to the evidence on the orthoroentgenograms, only 8 of the 18 showed a clinically measurable shortening. Of the 18 patients, 4 also had significant angular deformity.

The distal femoral epiphyseal growth plate contributes 70% of the longitudinal growth of the femur and 40% of the length of the lower extremity. Any injury that completely or partially arrests growth potential may lead to significant shortening or angular deformity of the extremity. The younger the child is at the time of injury, the greater the potential is for these undesirable complications. If one of these sequelae becomes evident with proper follow-up, appropriately timed epiphysiodesis or lengthening, as well as osteotomy or even resection of the bridge may serve to minimize the disability.

As shown in the anatomic section, the undulated contour of the growth plate and the mechanisms of injury, whether varus or valgus or anterior or posterior slip, introduce combined shearing-compression forces into the growth plate as it slides in certain directions. If a large metaphyseal fragment accompanies this, then it is less likely that problems will occur, as compared to shearing across the entire "transverse" plane of the epiphysis (Fig. 17-94).

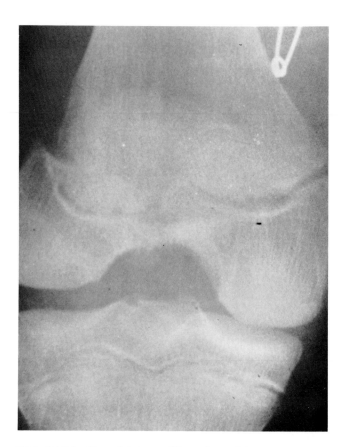

FIG. 17-74. Type 3 injury of lateral condyle.

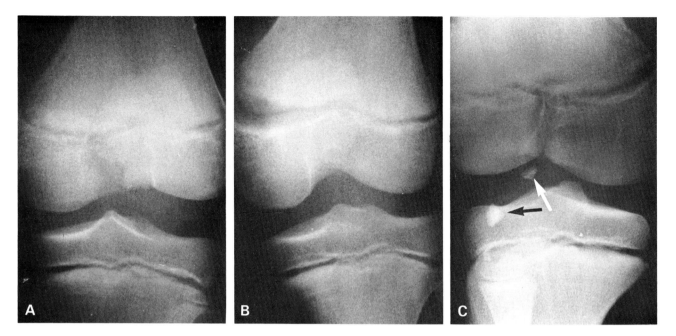

FIG. 17-75. Type 3 injury. *A,* Original film suggests fracture in notch. *B,* Stress roentgenogram elucidates physeal extension. *C,* Note the small, intra-articular osteochondral fragments (arrows) from the fracture margins.

The distal femoral epiphyseal cartilage plate is prone to growth disturbances not generally seen roentgenographically with equivalent injuries at other sites. This is specifically true of the type 2 injury and may relate to differences in the contour of this particular physis that predispose to certain kinds of injury through areas of the growth plate. Fortunately, epiphyseal injury to the distal femur often occurs at an age when little potential for major longitudinal growth remains. A direct crushing of the germinal cartilage cells or blood vessels seems to be the most logical explanation for this cessation of growth. Usually premature epiphysiodesis is evident within 6 months after the injury. The rapidity of the phenomenon indicates both a direct effect of the injury, as well as a gradual growth deceleration process.

A classic teaching is that the fracture line through the epiphyseal plate usually propagates through the zone of hypertrophy and provisional calcification. This becomes particularly marked in a plate like the distal femur where it is a binodal curve, rather than a clean transverse contour. If growth disturbance occurs on the tension side of the fracture, a late sequela would be angulation away from the angulation of the original injury. In fact, in Bright's work it was shown that there was a greater tendency to propagate the fracture line into the germinal zone on the tension side of the fracture rather than the compression side. Lee showed that a valgus injury might cause tension on the medial side of the distal femoral epiphysis with subsequent angulation into a varus position.[140] In 1 patient tension on the lateral side of the distal femoral epiphysis resulted in a subsequent valgus deformity, which was a later sequela to the fracture. The original treatment in traction was unsatisfactory and the patient was subsequently treated with closed reduction and

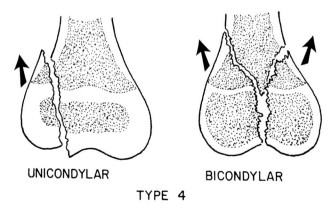

FIG. 17-76. Schematic of unicondylar type 4 injury (left), which can occur either medially or laterally. Schematic of bicondylar type 4 injury (right).

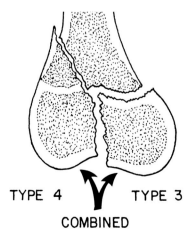

FIG. 17-77. Schematic of combined types 3 and 4.

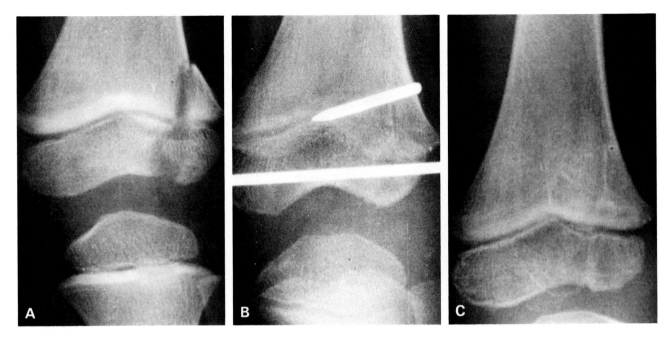

FIG. 17-78. *A*, Type 4 injury. *B*, Treatment by transversely directed pins. *C*, Appearance one year later.

percutaneous pinning. However, despite this the patient developed a progressive valgus deformity in the knee.

In looking at displacement versus growth disturbance, 8 nondisplaced fractures showed a mean limb-length discrepancy of approximately 5 mm, with a range of 0 to 1 cm, and no varus or valgus deformity. The displaced and reduced types included 8 patients with a mean length discrepancy of 8 mm and a range of 0 to 2.3 cm and 2 with varus-valgus deformity. Of the displaced and unreduced cases, the average length discrepancy was 2.52 cm and ranged from 0 to 7 cm and included 6 knees with varus-valgus deformity. Classifying these by type: patients with a type 1 injury had a 3 cm discrepancy; type 2 had 8 nondisplaced with a discrepancy of ½ cm and a range of 0 to 1 cm, while the displaced and reduced showed a discrepancy of 0.2 cm with a range of 0 to 0.3 cm, and the displaced and nonreduced showed a discrepancy of 2.5 cm with a range of 0 to 7 cm; of the type 3, the displaced and reduced showed a discrepancy of 0.9 cm with a range of 0.3 to 1.5 cm, and displaced and unreduced showed a discrepancy of 2.3 cm with a range of 1.7 to 3.5 cm; of the type 4, the displaced and reduced all showed limb-length inequality.[140]

Considering all types of fractures together with the correlation of the amount of the initial displacement and the amount of deformity that subsequently developed showed that the mean limb-length discrepancy was greater in the patients with fractures displaced more than one half the diameter of the bone. Of patients with this amount of displacement, 7 had an average discrepancy of 3.4 cm, while 12 with displacement of less had a mean discrepancy and deformity more closely related to the amount of displacement and quality of reduction than to the initial type of fracture. It cannot be assumed that the roentgenographic classification of the fracture has significant prognostic value in this region, except in the case of type 5 fractures. These observations are

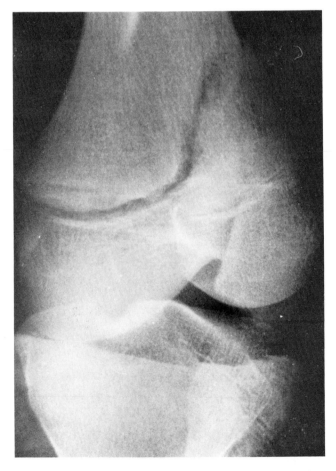

FIG. 17-79. Type 4 injury of medial condyle. This proved to be a combined lateral type 3 and medial type 4 injury.

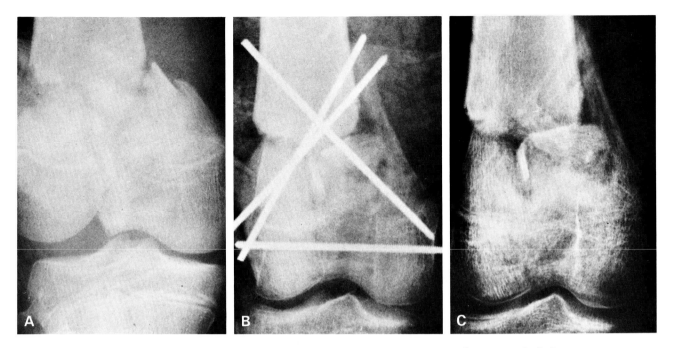

FIG. 17-80. *A,* Type 4 injury of both condyles. *B,* Open reduction. *C,* Appearance after removal of pins.

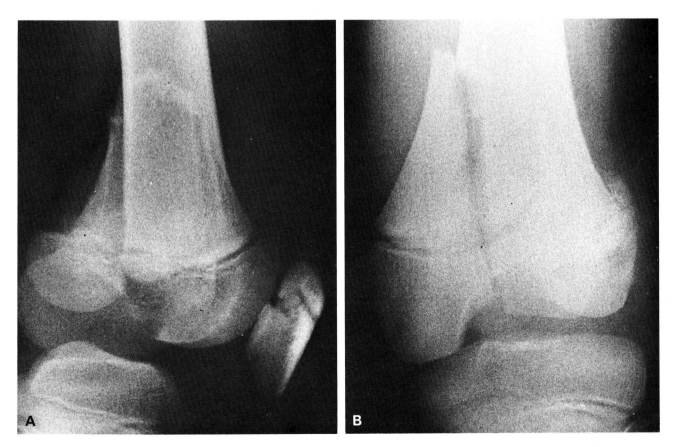

FIG. 17-81. *A-B,* Combination type 3 and type 4 injury of the distal femur. Also note the patellar fracture (see Fig. 17-93 for treatment of this case).

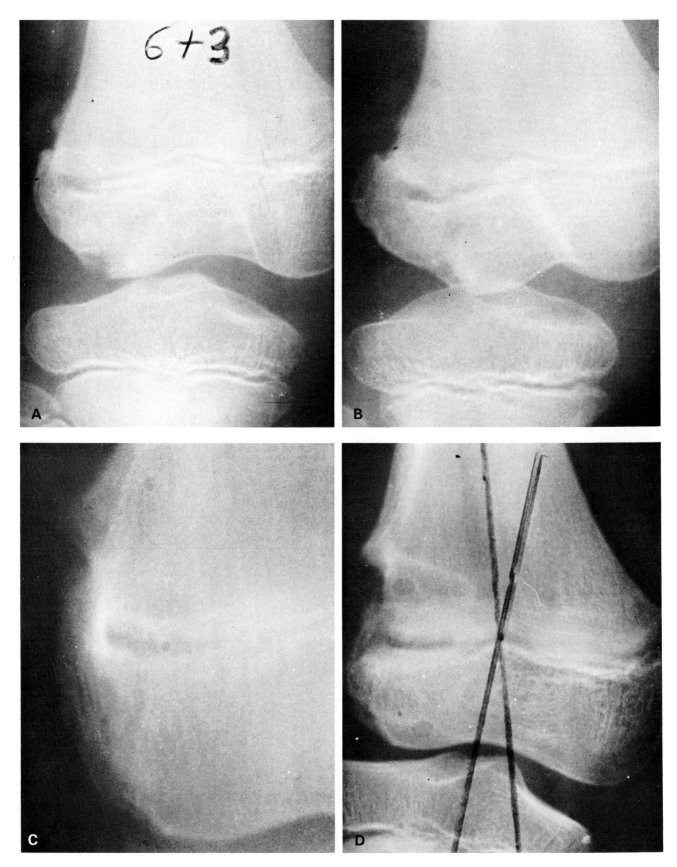

FIG. 17-82. *A,* Early bridge formation in peripheral type 4 injury. *B,* Appearance six months later. *C,* Tomogram of bridge. *D,* Resection and fat transplant.

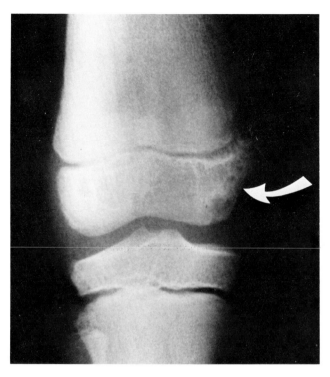

FIG. 17-83. Irregular development of right medial ossification center due to a type 4 injury.

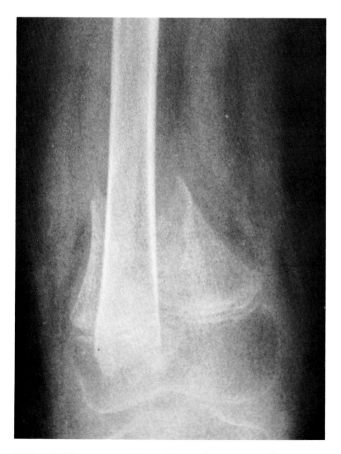

FIG. 17-84. Type 5 injury in myelomeningocele patient.

in general agreement with those of Neer, who stated that the greater the displacement of the fragments, the more likely it is that early closure will occur with the development of limb-length differences.[142] In the series of Lee, Pederson, and LaMont, 8 displaced, unreduced type 2 fractures (which are generally believed to be benign) resulted in an average limb-length discrepancy of 2.5 cm, indicating that some damage to the epiphyseal plate or its intrinsic blood supply must have occurred. Their study did not support Neer's concept that varus or valgus deformities of up to 20° tend to correct spontaneously provided 3 years of growth remain. Growth arrest, when it occurred, was usually present and permanent 12 to 18 months after injury.

Varus-valgus angular deformities may occur due to partial or complete unicondylar epiphysiodesis (Figs. 17-95 and 17-96). Treatment is dictated by the anticipated remaining growth. If less than one third of the *area* of the physis is involved, bridge resection may be attempted. Completion of the epiphysiodesis in the other condyle may also be done. Correction of angular deformity by osteotomy may also be necessary.

In 36%, varus or valgus deformity was measured by a difference of 5° or more from the normal and compared to the opposite uninvolved side in 33%. Reconstructive procedures, either osteotomy or epiphysiodesis, were required in 20%. Limitation of knee motion, ligament laxity, and quadriceps atrophy were also observed.[140]

There were 6 patients who underwent reconstructive procedures that included epiphysiodeses of the uninvolved femur. Of the 6, 1 also had a closing wedge femoral osteotomy for a valgus deformity of 22° consequent to a type 5 fracture. They felt that 2 patients would have benefited from epiphysiodesis earlier and that earlier and more aggressive reconstructive surgery would have benefited many of the patients.[140] Epiphysiodesis when the discrepancy exceeds 2 cm and consideration of osteotomy if there is a varus or valgus deformity greater than 10° could be considered a rough guideline. The failure of parents to bring a child back for the recommended follow-up appointments was the most common reason for gaps in adequate follow-up care.

The significance is that all patients with injuries to this region must be followed until the end of growth because an epiphyseal fracture at an early age that does not entirely close a growth plate can subsequently develop into a significant leg-length disturbance. Angulation can also occur as a late sequela without premature closure to the plate, and probably relates to subtle damage to a portion of the growth plate comparable to a type 5 injury. To alleviate the consequences of loss of correction in plaster, Lee recommended percutaneous pin fixation. Most authors feel that growth disturbance is an all-or-none phenomenon, and that if you can demonstrate that the epiphyseal plate is not closed immediately following injury, patients may be discharged from further follow-up. This is not an appropriate response to any epiphyseal injury, particularly in this region. Lee adequately documented that *nearly all patients have a growth disturbance,* and therefore, particularly the younger patient must be followed until the end of growth in order that appropriate surgical treatment can be performed.

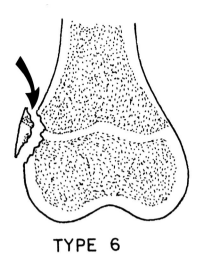

TYPE 6

FIG. 17-85. Schematic of type 6 injury to peripheral zone of Ranvier.

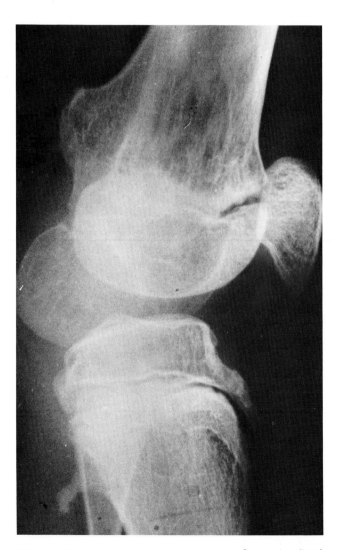

FIG. 17-86. Hyperextension type 6 injury of posterior distal femoral and proximal tibial physes, leading to formation of osteochondromata.

References

1. Caffey, J., Maddell, S. H., Royer, C., and Morales, P.: Ossification of the distal femoral epiphysis. J. Bone Joint Surg., 40-A:647, 1958.
2. Barnes, G. R., Jr., and Gwinn, J. L.: Distal irregularities of the femur simulating malignancy. A.J.R., 122:180, 1974.
3. Brower, A. C., Culver, J. E., and Keats, T. E.: Histologic nature of the cortical irregularity of the medial posterior distal femoral metaphysis in children. Radiology, 99:389, 1971.
4. Bufkin, W. J.: The avulsive cortical irregularity. A.J.R., 112:487, 1971.
5. Simon, H.: Medial distal metaphyseal femoral irregularity in children. Radiology, 90:258, 1968.
6. Young, D. W., Nogrady, M. B., Dunbar, J. S., and Wigelsworth, F. W.: Benign cortical irregularities in the distal femur of children. J. Can. Assoc. Radiol., 23:107, 1972.
7. Allende, G., and Lesama, L. G.: Fractures of the neck of the femur in children. J. Bone Joint Surg., 33-A:387, 1951.
8. Bonvallet, J. M.: Sur un cas exceptionnel de luxation traumatique de la hanche de l'enfant, associee à un décollement épiphysaire complet et a une fracture du noyau ciphalique. Rev. Chir. Orthop., 51:723, 1965.
9. Butler, J. E., and Cary, J. M.: Fracture of the femoral neck in a child. J.A.M.A., 218:398, 1971.
10. Canale, S. T., and Bourland, W. L.: Fracture of the neck and intertrochanteric region of the femur in children. J. Bone Joint Surg., 59-A:431, 1977.
11. Carrell, B., and Carrell, W. B.: Fracture in the neck of the femur in children with particular reference to aseptic necrosis. J. Bone Joint Surg., 23:225, 1941.
12. Chigot, P. L., and Vialas, M.: Fractures du col du femur chez l'enfant. Ann. Chir. Infant., 4:209, 1963.
13. Chong, K. C., Chacha, P. B., and Lee, B. T.: Fractures of the neck of the femur in childhood and adolescence. Injury, 7:111, 1975.
14. Dromer, H., and Penndorg, K.: Oberschenkelbruch im kindesalter. Ergebnisse einer mehrjarigen verlaufsbeobachtung. Chirurg., 38:284, 1967.
15. Fardon, D. F.: Fracture of the neck and shaft of the same femur. J. Bone Joint Surg., 52-A:797, 1970.
16. Feigenberg, Z., et al.: Fractures of the femoral neck in childhood. J. Trauma, 17:942, 1977.
17. Grassi, G., and Nigrisoli, P.: Traumatic separation of the upper femoral epiphysis in a child aged two. Ital. J. Orthop. Traumatol., 2:135, 1976.
18. Hoeksema, H. D., Olsen, C., and Rudy, R.: Fracture of femoral neck and shaft and repeat neck fracture in a child. J. Bone Joint Surg., 57-A:271, 1975.
19. Jacob, R., and Niemann, K.: Fractures of the hip in childhood. South. Med. J., 69:629, 1976.
20. Kay, S. P., and Hall, J. E.: Fracture of the femoral neck in children and its complications. Clin. Orthop., 80:53, 1971.
21. Kohli, S. B.: Fracture of the neck of the femur in children. J. Bone Joint Surg., 56-B:776, 1974.
22. Lam, S. F.: Fractures of the neck of the femur in children. J. Bone Joint Surg., 53-A:1165, 1976.
23. McDougall, A.: Fracture of the neck of the femur in childhood. J. Bone Joint Surg., 43-B:16, 1961.
24. Meier, A.: Geburtstraumatische epiphysenlosung am proximalen femurende. Arch. f. kinder., 116:267, 1939.
25. Milgram, J. W., and Lyne, E. D.: Epiphysiolysis of the proximal femur in very young children. Clin. Orthop., 110:146, 1975.
26. Miller, W. E.: Fracture of the hip in children from birth to adolescence. Clin. Orthop., 92:155, 1973.
27. Peltokallio, P., and Kurkipaa, M.: Fractures of the femoral neck in children. Ann. Chir. Gynaecol. Fenn. [Suppl.], 48:151, 1959.

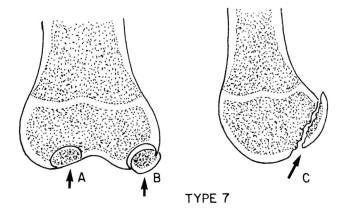

FIG. 17-87. Schematic of type 7 injury. *A,* Undisplaced. *B,* Displaced. *C,* Posterior involvement.

28. Pforringer, W., and Rosemeyer, B.: Fractures of the hip in children and adolescents. Acta Orthop. Scand., *51:*91, 1980.
29. Ratliff, A. H. C.: Fractures of the neck of the femur in children. J. Bone Joint Surg., *44-B:*528, 1962.
30. Ratliff, A. H. C.: Traumatic separation of the upper femoral epiphysis in young children. J. Bone Joint Surg., *50-B:*757, 1968.
31. Ratliff, A. H. C.: Fractures of the neck of the femur in children. Orthop. Clin. North Am., *5:*903, 1974.
32. Rigault, P., Iselin, F., Moureau, J., and Judet, J.: Fractures du col du femur chez l'enfant. Rev. Chir. Orthop., *52:*325, 1966.
33. Romer, K. H., and Reppin, G.: Zur Marknagelung kindlicher oberschenkelfrakturen. Zentralbl. Chir., *98:*170, 1973.
34. Rouiller, R., Griffe, J., and Crespy, G.: Epiphyseolyse femorale superieure apres fracture basicervicale. Resultat apres trois ans. Rev. Chir. Orthop., *57:*65, 1971.
35. Sonheim, K.: Fracture of the femoral neck in children. Acta Orthop. Scand., *43:*523, 1972.

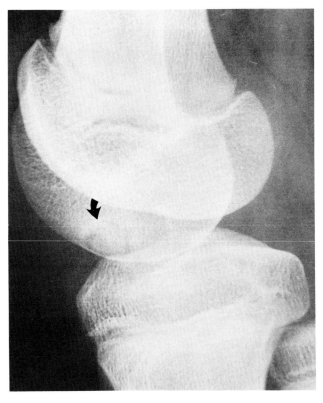

FIG. 17-89. Chronic type 7 injury. Note osteochondritis dissecans (arrow).

36. Weiner, D., and O'Dell, H.: Fractures of the hip in children. J. Trauma, *9:*62, 1969.
37. Wilson, J. C.: Fractures of the neck of the femur in children. J. Bone Joint Surg., *22:*531, 1940.
38. Zolczer, L., Kazar, G., Manoringer, J., and Nagy, E.: Fracture of the femoral neck in adolescents. Injury, *4:*41, 1973.
39. Lindseth, R. E., and Rosene, H. A.: Traumatic separation of the upper femoral epiphysis in a newborn infant. J. Bone Joint Surg., *53-A:*1641, 1971.
40. MacKenzie, I. G., Seddon, H. J., and Trevor, D.: Congenital dislocation of the hip. J. Bone Joint Surg., *42-B:*689, 1960.

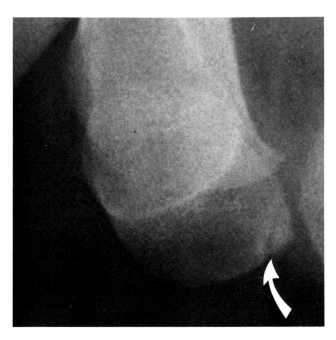

FIG. 17-88. Acute type 7 fracture of posterior femoral condyle (arrow).

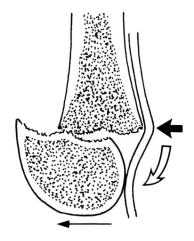

FIG. 17-90. Schematic of possible injury to popliteal artery as a result of posterior displacement of metaphysis.

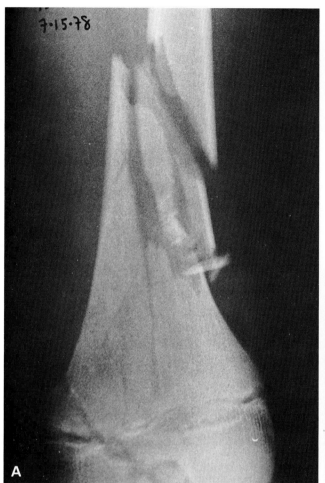

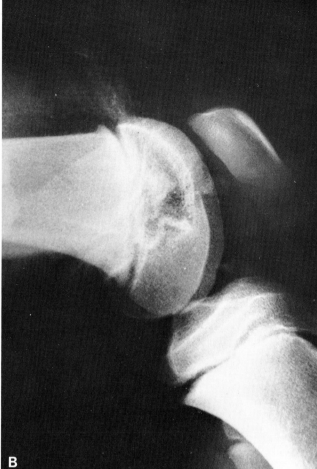

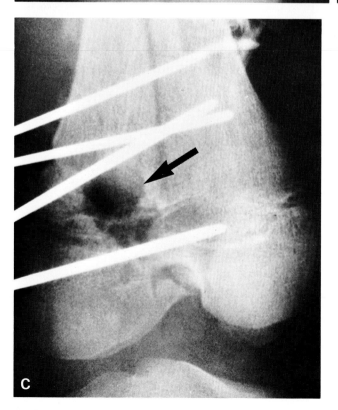

FIG. 17-91. *A-B,* Severe femoral shaft, physeal, and epiphyseal fractures. *C,* Treatment by multiple pin fixation. This figure shows a close-up view of the area of physeal damage, which was treated with a fat implant (arrow) at the time of injury, because it was anticipated that an osseous bridge would form without such treatment.

41. Mortens, J., and Christensen, P.: Traumatic separation of the upper femoral epiphysis as an obstetrical lesion. Acta Orthop. Scand., *34:*239, 1964.

42. Touzet, P., et al.: Les fractures du col du femur chez l'enfant. Rev. Chir. Orthop., *65:*341, 1979.

43. Towbin, R., and Crawford, A. H.: Neonatal traumatic proximal femoral epiphysiolysis. Pediatrics, *63:*456, 1979.

44. Weigel, K., and Conforty, B.: Die traumatische Epiphysen-ablosung am oberen Femurende beim Neugeborenen. Z. Orthop., *112:*1286, 1974.

45. Parvinen, T., Viljanto, J., Paananen, M., and Vilkki, P.: Torsion deformity after femoral fracture in children. Ann. Chir. Gynaecol. Fenn. [Suppl.], *62:*25, 1973.

46. Michail, J. P., Theodorou, S., Jouliaras, K., and Siatis, N.: Two cases of obstetrical separation (epiphysiolysis) of the upper femoral epiphysis. J. Bone Joint Surg., *40-B:*477, 1958.

47. Pavlik, A.: Treatment of obstetrical fractures of the femur. J. Bone Joint Surg., *21:*939, 1939.

48. Zoltan, J. D., Gilula, L. A., and Murphy, W. A.: Unilateral facet dislocation between the fifth lumbar and first sacral vertebrae. J. Bone Joint Surg., *61-A:*767, 1978.

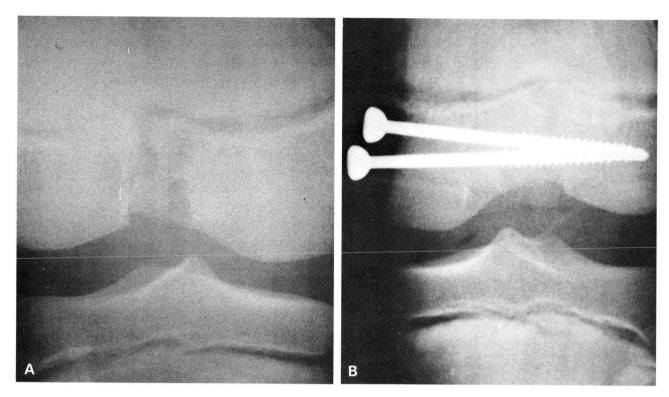

FIG. 17-92. *A,* Type 3 injury. *B,* Open reduction and fixation with transcondylar screws.

49. Chung, S. M., Batterman, S. C., and Brighton, C. T.: Shear strength of the human femoral capital epiphyseal plate. J. Bone Joint Surg., *58-A:*94, 1976.

50. Imhauser, G.: Zur pathogenese und therapie der jugendlichen huftkopflosung. Z. Orthop., *88:*3, 1957.

51. Rothermel, J. E.: Lateral slipping of the upper femoral epiphysis (epiphyseal coxa valga). Orthop. Rev., *8:*81, 1979.

52. Speer, D. P.: Experimental epiphyseolysis: an etiologic model of slipped capital femoral epiphysis. Trans. Orth. Res. Soc., *3:*47, 1978.

53. Barash, H. L., Galante, J. O., and Ray, R. D.: Acute slipped capital femoral epiphysis. Clin. Orthop., *79:*96, 1971.

54. Fahey, J. J., and O'Brien, E. T.: Acute slipped capital femoral epiphysis. J. Bone Joint Surg., *47-A:*1105, 1965.

55. Finch, A. D., and Roberts, W. M.: Epiphyseal coxa valga. J. Bone Joint Surg., *28:*869, 1946.

56. Meyer, L. C., Stelling, F. H., and Wise, F.: Slipped capital femoral epiphysis. South. Med. J., *50:*453, 1957.

57. Skinner, S. R., and Berkheimer, G. A.: Valgus slip of the capital femoral epiphysis. Clin. Orthop., *135:*90, 1978.

58. Wilson, P. D., Jacobs, B., and Schecter, L.: Slipped capital femoral epiphysis: an end result study. J. Bone Joint Surg., *47-A:*1128, 1965.

59. Duncan, J. W., and Lovell, W. W.: Anterior slip of the capital femoral epiphysis. Clin. Orthop., *110:*171, 1975.

60. Kampner, S. L., and Wissinger, H. A.: Anterior slipping of the capital femoral epiphysis. J. Bone Joint Surg., *54-A:*1531, 1972.

61. Leadbetter, G. W.: A treatment for fracture of the neck of the femur. J. Bone Joint Surg., *15:*931, 1933.

62. Jurkovskj, I. I.: Perilomy taza u detej. Diss. Kand. M., 1945.

63. Rang, M.: Children's Fractures. Philadelphia, J. B. Lippincott, 1974.

64. Durbin, F. C.: Avascular necrosis complicating undisplaced fractures of the neck of the femur in children. J. Bone Joint Surg., *41-B:*758, 1959.

65. Stougard, J.: Post-traumatic avascular necrosis of the femoral head in children. J. Bone Joint Surg., *51-B:*354, 1969.

66. Weber, B. G.: Zur Behandlung kindlicher Femurschaftbruche. Arch. Orthop. Unfallchir., *54:*713, 1963.

67. Weber, B. G.: Fractures of the femoral shaft in childhood. Injury, *1:*65, 1969.

68. Moss, C. M., Veith, F. J., Jason, R., and Rudavsky, A.: Screening isotope angiography in arterial trauma. Surgery, *86:*881, 1979.

69. Trueta, J.: The normal vascular anatomy of the human femoral head during growth. J. Bone Joint Surg., *39-B:*358, 1957.

70. DeLuca, F. N., and Keck, C.: Traumatic coxa vara. A case report of spontaneous correction in a child. Clin. Orthop., *116:*125, 1976.

71. Frost, H. M.: A simple method for achieving subtrochanteric valgus femoral osteotomy in infants and children. Clin. Orthop., *103:*18, 1974.

72. Wolfgang, G. L.: Stress fracture of the femoral neck in a patient with open capital femoral epiphyses. J. Bone Joint Surg., *59-A:*680, 1977.

73. Devas, M. B.: Stress fractures in children. J. Bone Joint Surg., *45-B:*528, 1963.

74. Wilson, M. J., Michele, A. A., and Jacobson, E. W.: Isolated fracture of the lesser trochanter. J. Bone Joint Surg., *21:*776, 1939.

75. Daum, R., Jungbluth, K. H., Metzger, E., and Hecker, W. C.: Subtrochantere und suprakondylare femurfrakturen im kindesalter, behandlung und ergebnisse. Chirurg., *40:*217, 1969.

76. Ireland, D. C. R., and Fisher, R. L.: Subtrochanteric fractures of the femur in children. Clin. Orthop., *110:*157, 1975.

77. Griffin, P. P., Anderson, M., and Green, W. T.: Fractures of the shaft of the femur in children. Orthop. Clin. North Am., *3:*213, 1972.

78. Ogden, J. A., Gossling, H. R., and Southwick, W. O.: Slipped capital femoral epiphysis following ipsilateral femoral fracture. Clin. Orthop., *110:*167, 1975.

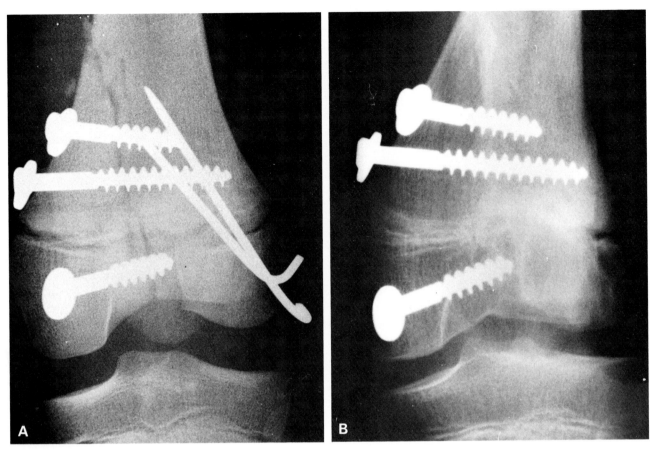

FIG. 17-93. *A*, Combined type 3 and 4 injury treated by pins (type 3 component) and screws (type 4 component). *B*, The type 3 injury led to growth arrest.

79. Allen, B. L., Kant, A. P., and Emery, F. E.: Displaced fractures of the femoral diaphysis in children. Definitive treatment in a double spica cast. J. Trauma, *17*:8, 1977.

80. Anderson, R. L.: Conservative treatment of fractures of the femur. J. Bone Joint Surg., *49-A*:1371, 1967.

81. Blomquist, E., and Rudstrom, P.: Uber Femurfrakturen bei Kindern unter besonderer Beruchsichtigung des gesteigerten Langenwachstums. Acta Chir. Scand., *88*:267, 1943.

82. Blount, W. P., Schaefer, A. A., and Fox, G. W.: Fractures of the femur in children. South. Med. J., *37*:481, 1944.

83. Burwell, H. N.: Fractures of the femoral shaft in children. Postgrad. Med. J., *45*:617, 1969.

84. Dameron, T. B., and Thompson, H. A.: Femoral-shaft fractures in children. J. Bone Joint Surg., *41-A*:1201, 1959.

85. Fraser, R. D., Hunter, G. A., and Waddell, J. P.: Ipsilateral fracture of the femur and tibia. J. Bone Joint Surg., *60-B*:510, 1978.

86. Gillquist, J., Reiger, A., Sjodahl, R., and Bylund, P.: Multiple fractures of a single leg. Acta Chir. Scand., *139*:167, 1973.

87. Griessman, H.: Die besonderheiten in Heilablauf der frakturen beim kinde. Med. Klin., *37*:299, 1941.

88. Mohan, K.: Fracture of the shaft of the femur in children. Int. Surg., *60*:282, 1975.

89. Pease, C. N.: Fractures of the femur in children. Surg. Clin. North Am., *37*:213, 1957.

90. Teutsch, W.: Nachuntersuchungsergebnisse kindlicher femur-schaftfrakturen. Zentralbl. Chir., *94*:1761, 1969.

91. Vontobel, V., Genton, N., and Schmid, R.: Die spatergebnisse der kindlichen dislozierten femurschaftfraktur. Helv. Chir. Acta, *28*:655, 1961.

92. Childress, H. M.: Concealed traumatic rupture of aorta in orthopedic patient. N. Y. State J. Med., *50*:1503, 1950.

93. Humberger, F. W., and Eyring, E. J.: Proximal tibial 90-90 traction in treatment of children with femoral shaft fractures. J. Bone Joint Surg., *51-A*:499, 1969.

94. Clark, M. W., D'Ambrosia, R. D. and Roberts, J. M.: Equinus contracture following Bryant's traction. Orthopedics, *1*:311, 1978.

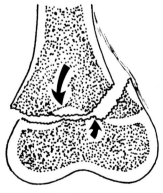

EFFECT OF UNDULATION

FIG. 17-94. Schematic of effect of undulation. Arrows show the central physeal area with a proximal fragment, which disrupts physeal continuity.

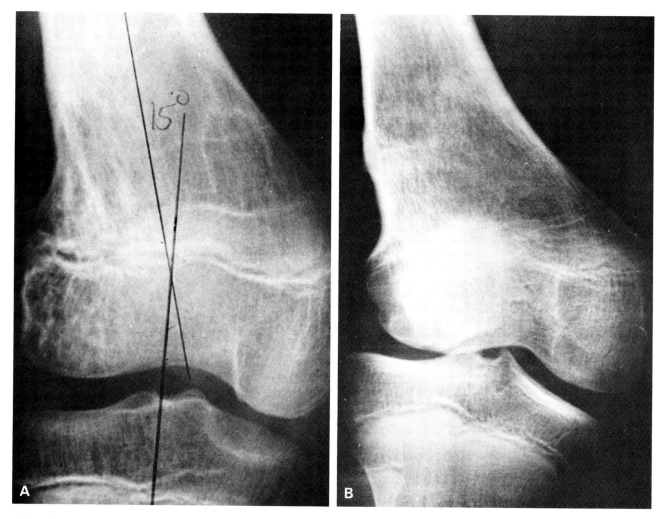

FIG. 17-95. *A,* Angular deformity due to premature closure of lateral physis. *B,* Progressive changes six months later.

95. Nicholson, J. T., Foster, R. M., and Heath, R. D.: Bryant's traction—a provocative cause of circulatory complications. J.A.M.A., *157:*415, 1955.

96. Ferry, A. M., and Edgar, M. S., Jr.: Modified Bryant's traction. J. Bone Joint Surg., *48-A:*533, 1966.

97. Burton, V., and Fordyce, A.: Immobilization of femoral shaft fractures in children aged 2-10 years. Injury, *4:*47, 1973.

98. Childress, H. M.: Distal femoral 90-90 traction for shaft fractures of the femur in children. Orthop. Rev., *8:*45, 1979.

99. Irani, R. N., Nicholson, J., and Chung, S. M. K.: Treatment of femoral fractures in children by immediate spica immobilization. J. Bone Joint Surg., *54-A:*1346, 1972.

100. Miller, P. R., and Welch, M. C.: The hazards of tibial pin replacement in 90-90 skeletal traction. Clin. Orthop., *135:*97, 1978.

101. Neer, C. S., II, and Cadman, E. F.: Treatment of fractures of the femoral shaft in children. J.A.M.A., *163:*634, 1957.

101a. Mital, M. A., and Cashman, W.: A fresh ambulatory approach to treatment of femoral shaft fractures in children—a comparison with traditional conservative methods. Presented at the annual meeting of the Eastern Orthopaedic Assoc., Oct. 1975.

102. Klems, H., and Weigert, M.: Stabile osteosynthese kindlicher oberschenkelfracturen. Indikation und Methode. Chirurg., *44:*511, 1973.

103. Kuntscher, G.: Die stabile osteosynthese bei der osteotomie. Chirurg., *14:*161, 1942.

104. Morita, S.: Surgical treatment of femur shaft fractures in children. Arch. Jpn. Surg., *36:*627, 1967.

105. Raisch, O.: Experimenteller beitrag zur frage der osteosynthese mit besonderd beruchsichtigung der marknagelung nach kuntscher. Beitr. Klin. Chir., *175:*548, 1944.

106. Thompson, S. A., and Mahoney, L. J.: Volkmann's ischemic contracture and its relationship to fracture of the femur. J. Bone Joint Surg., *33-B:*336, 1951.

107. Viljanto, J., Linna, M. I., Kiviluoto, H., and Paananen, M.: Indications and results of operative treatment of femoral shaft fractures in children. Acta Chir. Scand., *141:*366, 1975.

108. Aitken, A. P., Blackett, C. W., and Cincotti, J. J.: Overgrowth of the femoral shaft following fractures in childhood. J. Bone Joint Surg., *21:*334, 1939.

109. Barfod, B., and Christensen, J.: Fractures of the femoral shaft in children with special reference to subsequent overgrowth. Acta Chir. Scand., *116:*235, 1958.

110. David, V. C.: Shortening and compensatory overgrowth following fractures in children. Arch. Surg., *9:*438, 1924.

111. Edvardsen, P., and Syversen, G. M.: Overgrowth of the femur after fracture of the shaft in childhood. J. Bone Joint Surg., *58-B:*339, 1976.

112. Gill, G. G.: The cause of discrepancy in limb lengths following tuberculosis of the hip in children. J. Bone Joint Surg., *26:*272, 1944.

113. Greville, N. R., and Irvins, J. C.: Fractures of the femur in chil-

dren. An analysis of their effect on the subsequent length of both bones of the lower limb. Am. J. Surg., *93:*376, 1957.

114. Meals, R. A.: Overgrowth of the femur following fractures in children: influences of handedness. J. Bone Joint Surg., *61-A:*581, 1979.
115. Truesdell, E. D.: Inequality of lower extremities following fracture of the shaft of the femur in children. Ann. Surg., *74:*498, 1921.
116. Staheli, L. T.: Femoral and tibial growth following femoral shaft fracture in childhood. Clin. Orthop., *55:*159, 1967.
117. Truesdell, E.: Birth Fractures and Epiphyseal Dislocations. New York, Paul Harber, 1917.
118. Nonnemann, H. C.: Grenzen du Spontankorrektur fehlgeheilte. Frakturen bei Jugendlichen. Langenbecks Arch. Chir., *324:*78, 1969.
119. Viljanto, J., Kiviluoto, H., and Pannanen, M.: Remodeling after femoral shaft fracture in children. Acta Chir. Scand., *141:*360, 1975.
120. Damholt, B., and Zdravkovic, D.: Quadriceps function following fractures of the femoral shaft in children. Acta Orthop. Scand., *45:*756, 1974.
121. Miller, D. S., Martin, L., and Grossman, E.: Ischemic fibrosis of the lower extremity in children. Am. J. Surg., *84:*317, 1972.
122. Saimon, L. P.: Refracture of the shaft of the femur. J. Bone Joint Surg., *46-B:*32, 1964.
123. Bjerkriem, I., and Benum, P.: Genu recurvatum. A late complication of tibial wire traction in fractures of the femur in children. Acta Orthop. Scand., *46:*1012, 1975.
124. Dencker, H.: Wire traction complications associated with treatment of femoral shaft fractures. Acta Orthop. Scand., *35:*158, 1964.
125. Corlett, C. G.: Fracture of the anterior inferior spine of the ilium. Med. J. Aust., *2:*682, 1927.
126. Parke, W., Calvin, G. S., and Almond, A. H. G.: Premature epiphyseal fusion of the knee joint in tuberculosis disease of the hip. J. Bone Joint Surg., *31-B:*63, 1949.
127. Siebenmann, R.: Die osteomyelitis aus der sicht de pathologen. Z. Kinderchir., *8:*10, 1970.
128. Sissons, H. A.: Osteoporosis and epiphyseal arrest in joint tuberculosis. An account of histological changes in involved tissues. J. Bone Joint Surg., *34-B:*275, 1952.
129. Currarino, G., and Erlandson, M. E.: Premature fusion of epiphysis in Cooley's anemia. Radiology, *83:*656, 1964.
130. Botting, T. D. J., and Serase, W. H.: Premature epiphyseal fusion at the knee complicating prolonged immobilization for congenital dislocation of the hip. J. Bone Joint Surg., *47-B:*280, 1965.
131. Kestler, O. C.: Unclassified premature cessation of epiphyseal growth about the knee joint. J. Bone Joint Surg., *29:*788, 1947.
132. Ross, D.: Disturbance of longitudinal growth associated with prolonged disability of the lower extremity. J. Bone Joint Surg., *30-A:*103, 1948.
133. Simpson, W. C., Jr., and Fardon, D. F.: Obscure distal femoral epiphyseal injury. South. Med. J., *69:*1338, 1976.
134. Hunter, L. Y., and Hensinger, R. N.: Premature monomelic growth arrest following fracture of the femoral shaft. J. Bone Joint Surg., *60-A:*850, 1978.
135. Aitken, A. P., and Magill, H. K.: Fractures involving the distal femoral epiphyseal cartilage. J. Bone Joint Surg., *34-A:*96, 1952.
136. Bassett, F. H., III, and Goldner, J. L.: Fractures involving the distal femoral epiphyseal growth line. South. Med. J., *55:*545, 1962.
137. Cassebaum, W. H., and Patterson, A. H.: Fractures of the distal femoral epiphysis. Clin. Orthop., *41:*79, 1965.
138. Criswell, A. R., Hand, W. L., and Butler, J. E.: Abduction injuries of the distal femoral epiphysis. Clin. Orthop., *115:*189, 1976.
139. Kaplan, J. A., Sprague, S. B., and Benjamin, H. C.: Traumatic bilateral separation of the lower femoral epiphyses. J. Bone Joint Surg., *24:*200, 1942.
140. Lee, C. L., Pederson, H. E., and LaMont, R. L.: Fractures of the distal femoral epiphysis. Presented at the 44th meeting, American Academy of Orthopaedic Surgeons, Feb. 1977.
141. Lombardo, S. J., and Harvey, J. P., Jr.: Fractures of the distal femoral epiphyses. J. Bone Joint Surg., *59-A:*742, 1977.
142. Neer, C. S., II: Separation of the lower femoral epiphysis. Am. J. Surg., *99:*756, 1960.
143. Rehbein, F., and Hoffman, S.: Knochenvertetzungen in kindesalter. Arch. Klin. Chir., *304:*539, 1963.
144. Schneider, T.: Spatergebnisse der kuntschernagelung am junglichenden Knocher. Artzl. Wschr., *5:*846, 1950.
145. Sideman, S.: Traumatic separation of the lower femoral epiphysis. J. Bone Joint Surg., *25:*913, 1943.
146. Stephens, D. C., and Louis, D. S.: Traumatic separation of the distal femoral epiphyseal cartilage plate. J. Bone Joint Surg., *56-A:*1383, 1974.
147. Poland, J.: Traumatic Separation of the Epiphyses. London, Smith, Elder, and Co., 1898.
148. Rogers, L., Jones, S., David, A., et al.: "Clipping injury" fracture of the epiphysis in the adolescent football player: an occult lesion of the knee. A.J.R., *121:*69, 1974.

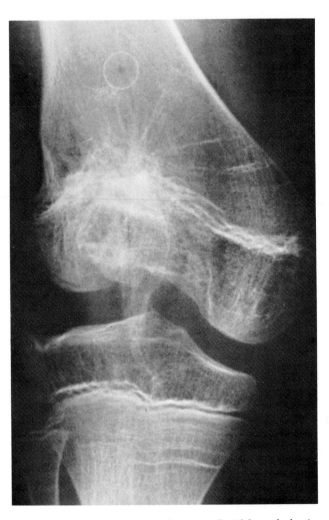

FIG. 17-96. Premature growth arrest of mid-lateral physis.

18

Knee

Anatomy

The developmental patterns of the distal femoral and proximal tibial epiphyses, two of the three chondro-osseous components of the knee, are described, respectively, in Chapters 17 and 19. The other major anatomic structures of the knee joint include the patella (including the quadriceps expansion and patellar tendon), the medial and lateral menisci, the component ligaments (collaterals and cruciates), and the capsule. Relative to acute knee injury, important structures external to the joint include the neurovascular tissues, accessory bones (e.g., fabella), and the popliteus tendon (although this is partially intra-articular).

The patella is a large sesamoid bone at the anterior aspect of the knee joint. With the exception of the medial and lateral articular surfaces, most of the patellar mass lies within the tendinous expansion of the quadriceps femoris muscle. The inferior pole, which is covered by a large fat pad and the synovial reflection, is extra-articular (Fig. 18-1). The patellar tendon is always separated from the knee joint by this retrotendinous fat pad. The tendon progressively blends into the patella and tibial tuberosity comparable to the cruciate attachments—fibrous to fibrocartilaginous to cartilaginous tissue. Sharpey's fibers that attach directly into bone are not present until late adolescence.

For the first few years the patella is completely cartilaginous and therefore radiolucent. Patellar ossification first becomes radiographically evident at two to three years; it normally develops from multiple small foci, although this is a transient phase (Fig. 18-2). Sometimes there is a distinct origin between the inferior and superior portions of the ossification center, which may be mistaken for a fracture. Ossification then expands toward the margins. During adolescence, the anterior, medial, and lateral cortical bone of the expanding ossification center becomes confluent with the fibrous tissue of the quadriceps tendon and creates a dense continuity between tendon and subchondral bone through Sharpey's fibers.

The developing patellar ossification is often irregular (Fig. 18-3), not unlike the expanding margins of the distal femoral epiphyseal ossification center. Because of this normal variability of marginal ossification, a diagnosis of osteochondrosis or osteochondritis of the patella, or even fracture,

solely on the basis of the roentgenographic appearance, must be made with caution.

Additional ossification centers may develop, particularly in the superolateral half of the bone. Accessory ossification centers, particularly those near the articular surfaces, may also be mistaken for osteochondritis. A separate ossification center at the inferior pole probably does not exist. Instead, one must consider Sinding-Larsen-Johansson syndrome, the patellar equivalent of Osgood-Schlatter disease.

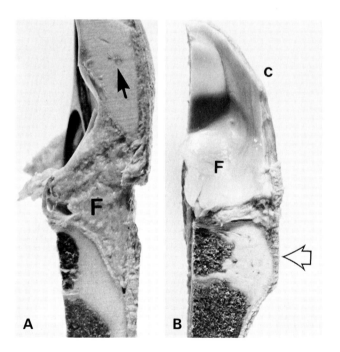

FIG. 18-1. *A*, Lateral, and, *B*, sagittal sections of patella, capsule, and proximal tibia from a six-year-old child. Cartilage occupies much of the mass of the patella. A small focus of ossification (solid arrow) is present. The retropatellar fat pad (F) covers much of the lower pole of the patella. The open arrow indicates the medial collateral ligament: note how it blends into the epiphyseal cartilage and the capsule (c).

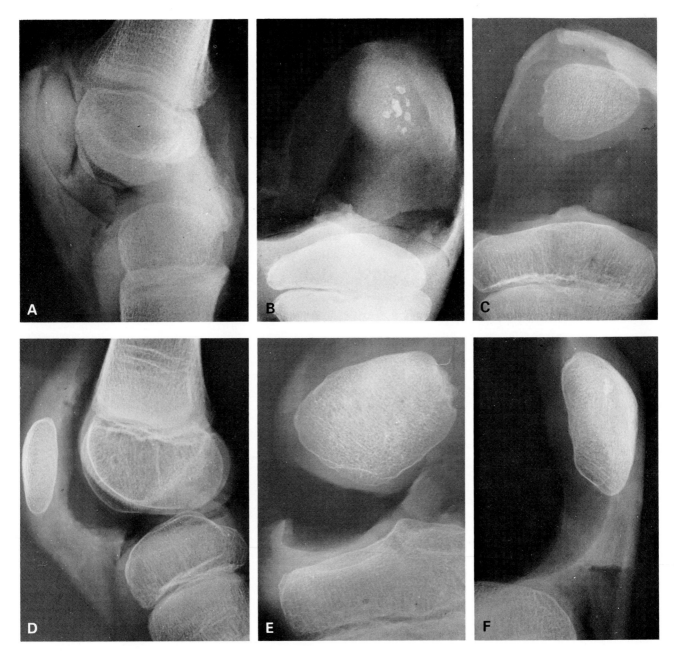

FIG. 18-2. Cadaver specimens showing progressive patellar development. *A,* At two years, no ossification is present. However, air/cartilage contrast outlines the patella, especially in the lateral view. *B,* Early ossification, shown here in a six-year-old, is often multifocal. *C-D,* Ossification then rapidly proceeds centrifugally to fill out the cartilaginous patella. *E-F,* During adolescence, patellar ossification will fill out all the cartilage, except for the articular region. Note the irregular development of the lateral side of the patella.

The bipartite patella (Fig. 18-4) is a developmental variation of ossification that often must be distinguished from a fracture.[1,2] Unfortunately, it is sometimes difficult to do this when evaluating an acute injury. Theoretically, a bipartite patella may be the result of either an ununited fracture or failure of primary and accessory ossification centers to fuse; the latter is the more likely explanation. Articular cartilage usually covers each fragment as well as the area over the roentgenographic discontinuity and generally shows minimal to no evidence of demarcation at the articular surface. In

the specimen shown in Figure 18-4, there were mild configurational differences compatible with the lesion, but no major defects in the articular surface. The tissue between these 2 ossification centers appeared to be both fibrous and fibrocartilaginous. There was no motion between the fragments. Ruggles reported an autopsy case of a 63-year-old man with bilateral involvement.[3] Even at that age, the patella was still bipartite with intervening fibrocartilage between the 2 osseous portions.

If a normal patella is sectioned transversely, the medial

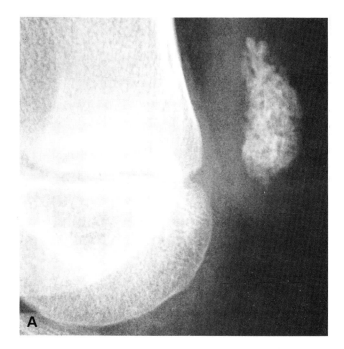

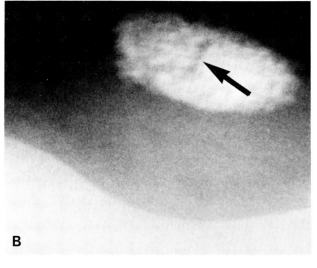

FIG. 18-3. *A,* Oblique and, *B,* transverse patellar views of six-year-old with knee pain following a direct blow to the patella. While the patella frequently exhibits a mottled, irregular appearance early during ossification, the transverse patellar view shows a definite fracture (arrow).

and lateral articular surfaces are approximately equal and subtend reasonably equivalent angles (Fig. 18-5). However, if the patella does not track properly (i.e., subluxates laterally), the "epiphyseal" and articular cartilage may gradually deform (plastic deformation) and the subsequently appearing ossification center then fills in the antecedent, deformed cartilaginous precursor. This eventually leads to the unequal osseous angles of the patellar articular surfaces characteristic of a chronically maltracking, subluxating, or dislocating patella.

The patella may be situated relatively high or low (patella alta and baja, respectively).[4] Normally, the distance from the lower pole of the patella to the tendinous insertion on the tuberosity should be 1.0 times the sagittal length of the patella (Fig. 18-6). More than 20% variation probably indicates an abnormal patellar position.[5,6] However, such measurements are not always realistic in the growing child. Depending upon age, there are significant amounts of epiphyseal cartilage at both the superior and inferior patellar poles and the tibial tuberosity, so that the sagittal length of the ossified patella and the distance from the patellar ossification center to the tibial tuberosity ossification center may be considerably different from the actual patellar and tendon lengths.

The formation of the coordinated menisco-ligamentous complex in the knee is well established in the 8-week embryo. From this common mesenchymal structure develop both cruciate ligaments and the fibrocartilaginous menisci. The menisci assume their characteristic gross shape during prenatal development. The only major postnatal changes are progressively decreased vascularity, morphologic growth commensurate with enlargement of the distal femur and proximal tibia, and accommodation of this growth to changing femorotibial contact (Fig. 18-7). The lateral meniscus tends to have more developmental variation, but at no time does it normally appear to have a discoid shape. Anterior extensions from both menisci to the anterior cruciate liga-

ment as well as to each other are a residual of their common origin. The transverse anterior ligament between the menisci tends to be overlooked and may be a source of some discomfort in children complaining of anterior knee pain. The more fixed medial meniscus possesses important peripheral capsular attachments, including the thickened medial capsular ligament and posteromedial capsular complex. The more mobile lateral meniscus has no attachment posterolaterally, particularly in the area of the popliteus tendon recess, and there may even be a communication from this region with the proximal tibiofibular joint. The menisco-femoral ligaments of Humphry and Wrisberg are variable, both as to size and presence.

The microscopic structure of the meniscus is related to weightbearing function. The collagen fiber alignment has been studied by polarized light microscopy as well as electron microscopy.[7-9] The majority of the fibers are arranged in circumferential fashion in the long axis of the meniscus. Other fibers traverse the circumferential ones in a radial direction. The radial fibers are located mainly on the surfaces of the meniscus, more on the tibial than the femoral side, and probably act as tie rods resisting longitudinal splitting. A few of the radial fibers change direction and run in a vertical fashion through the substance of the meniscus. These patterns undergo significant changing patterns as the child begins ambulation. How they change, particularly during adolescence, is currently under study.

Throughout most of development the cruciate ligaments blend into the epiphyseal cartilage of the distal femur (intercondylar notch) and proximal tibia (spines). This is a progressive transition of fibrous, fibrocartilaginous, and cartilaginous tissues. Only during late adolescence do the cruciate ligaments insert directly into the maturing ossification centers through the development of Sharpey's fibers. Most references suggest that the medial and lateral collateral ligaments attach primarily into the distal femoral epiphysis and

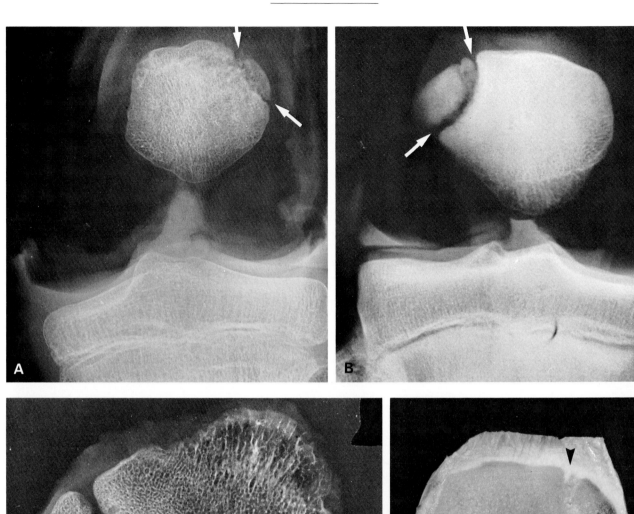

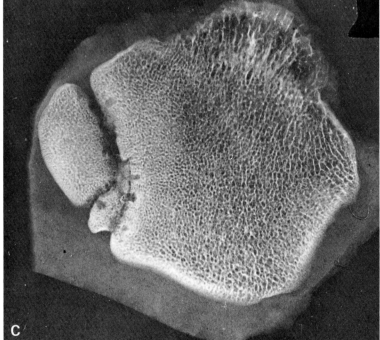

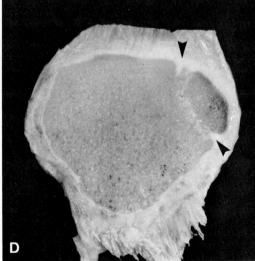

FIG. 18-4. *A,* Bipartite patella (arrows) from an 11-year-old. *B,* Bipartite patella (arrows) from a 14-year-old. *C,* Slab roentgenogram showing multiple accessory ossification in superolateral region. *D,* Slab section of bipartite patella (arrows).

proximal tibial metaphysis, an anatomic configuration that seems to make the distal femur more susceptible to epiphyseal-physeal injury. Certainly, the ligaments blend densely into the distal femoral epiphyseal perichondrium. However, dissection of over 30 pairs of skeletally immature knees shows that the deep collateral ligaments also *attach directly* into the proximal tibial epiphyseal perichondrium (Fig. 18-8). Some of the more superficial collateral fibers do continue onto the metaphysis, as does the pes anserinus. The classic

concept that the collateral ligaments have no tibial epiphyseal attachments is false.

The suprapatellar pouch normally extends a considerable distance under the quadriceps (Fig. 18-9). Developmental variations of the synovium (plicae) in this region may lead to compartmentalization of this pouch and chronic knee effusions. The posterior capsule has minimum redundancy. There are no normal communications from the posterior capsule to the popliteal space.

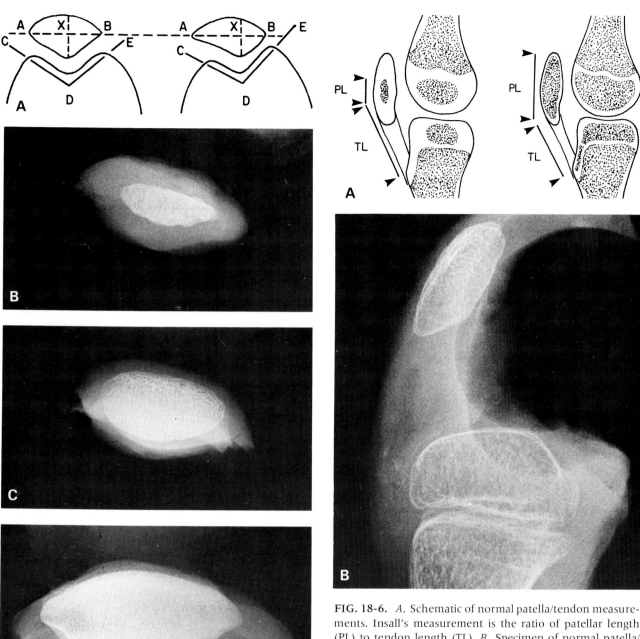

FIG. 18-5. *A,* Schematic sections of representative patellae showing, on the left, relatively equal medial and lateral segments. If deformation occurs (right), it happens first in the cartilage. Ossification then brings about progressive replacement of the deformed cartilage. Bone itself does not deform. *B-D,* Transverse patellar radiographs showing how the ossification center gradually fills out the cartilaginous patella, which has already developed characteristic contours (even though ossification does not necessarily mimic them). The articular surface faces down, and the lateral side is to the right, in each photograph.

FIG. 18-6. *A,* Schematic of normal patella/tendon measurements. Insall's measurement is the ratio of patellar length (PL) to tendon length (TL). *B,* Specimen of normal patella/tendon arrangements in an eight-year-old showing the problems of measurement, even in a cadaver. The tuberosity, in particular, is not well defined.

Radiographic Examination

When evaluating an injury, the patella is best seen in either the lateral or sunrise projections. In the anteroposterior view, because of the normal position of the patella overlying the distal femoral metaphysis and epiphysis, much of the patella is obscured. However, this view is often the only way to adequately establish a bipartite patella.

Since the epiphyseal regions of the younger child contain more radiolucent cartilage than during the adolescent period, the evaluation of suspected internal derangement of the knee becomes more difficult. Only a thin piece of sub-

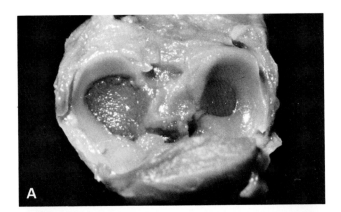

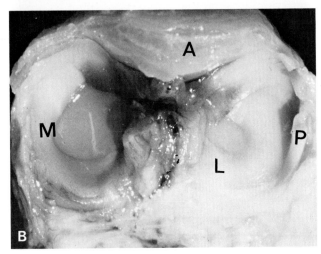

FIG. 18-7. Progressive postnatal development of the menisci. *A,* 1 year. *B,* 11 years. Note the medial (M) and lateral (L) sides, the popliteal tendon recess (P), and the anterior side (A).

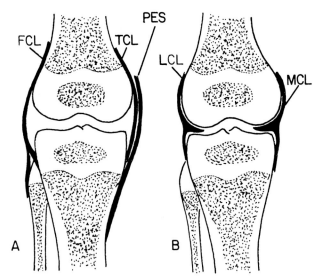

FIG. 18-8. Schematic of, *A,* superficial, and, *B,* deep collateral ligament attachments. Note the fibular collateral ligament (FCL); the pes anserinus (PES); the tibial collateral ligament (TCL); the deep lateral collateral ligament (LCL); the deep medial collateral ligament (MCL). The collateral ligaments attach to the epiphyseal perichondrium of the proximal tibia, not the metaphysis.

ture of the distal femoral or proximal tibial epiphysis in children.[11,12] Dislocation is usually accompanied by major disruptions of the soft tissues and ligaments, and frequently by neurovascular damage, which must be accurately diagnosed so that appropriate and adequate repairs may be instituted. The complications of ischemia or gangrene, which may worsen with growth and increasing functional demands, are usually preventable if initial diagnosis and treatment are adequate.[13]

chondral bone may be associated with a larger, cartilaginous fragment in a disease like osteochondritis dissecans or an acute osteochondral fracture. If the knee is placed in the usual diagnostic positions, especially the sunrise or tangential view, portions of the anterior proximal tibia or tibial tuberosity ossification centers may be projected in a manner suggestive of an osteochondral fragment (Fig. 18-10). In actuality, such an apparent lucency is the physis of the tuberosity, which parallels the roentgenographic beam in this particular view.[10]

Children normally have a greater degree of ligamentous laxity than adults. This makes possible phenomena such as "vacuum arthrography," which is due to cavitation of gas from joint fluid. Such cavitation may outline all or part of the joint and should not be misinterpreted as a loose body or chondro-osseous fracture (Fig. 18-11).

Knee Dislocation

Complete dislocation of the knee is an infrequent injury in children, since the massive trauma usually necessary to produce dislocation in an adult is more likely to cause a frac-

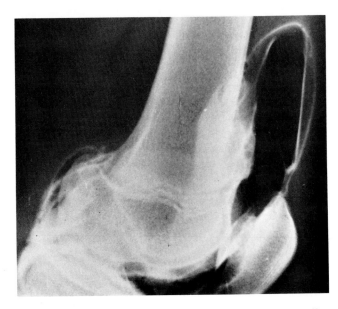

FIG. 18-9. Arthrogram showing extent of suprapatellar pouch.

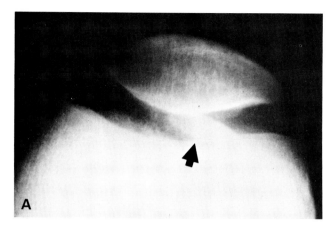

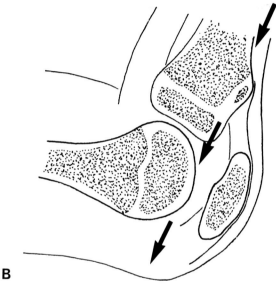

FIG. 18-10. *A,* Transverse patellar views in children with suspected injuries or loose bodies must be evaluated carefully, as normal anatomy may appear "suspicious." This "loose body" (arrow) was the ossification center of the tibial tuberosity. *B,* Schematic showing path of X-ray beam through tuberosity.

This type of dislocation usually does well if reduced immediately (closed reduction). If there is a well-defined area of capsular laxity after the child goes through a subsequent period of development, such an area may be explored and a formal repair undertaken. However, when these procedures are done, care must be taken to restore the normal anatomic relationships and not damage any cartilage, either residual hyaline cartilage along the epiphyseal margins or growth plate *per se.* The pes anserinus attaches along the medial metaphysis of the proximal tibia, and during reflection for a pes repair it must be elevated away with the periosteum, with which it is confluent and reflected proximally. Such a procedure might damage the physeal periphery (zone of Ranvier) and lead to a localized osseous bridge and angular growth deformity of either the main tibial or tuberosity physes. The sutures could be placed through portions of the tibial tuberosity and might also cause premature closure of this region.

Adequately documented follow-up of children below 10 or 11 with this injury is rare.[11] Since the large percentage of adolescents and adults do well *without* any open repair, surgery should not be undertaken except under well-defined circumstances in children.

Figure 18-12 shows a 14-year-old boy who was struck by a car and sustained a dislocation accompanied by a type 3A fibular epiphyseal fracture. He was treated initially with a closed reduction. However, the concomitant epiphyseal fracture of the fibula did not reduce. Several days later the lateral side of the knee was explored and the fibular fracture reduced. The lateral collateral ligament was repaired where it directly avulsed from the femoral epiphysis. There was no repair of the medial collateral ligament. Follow-up 5 years later showed a knee that was sufficiently functional to allow him to play competitive football (running back).

The collateral circulation about the knee is poor, at least from the standpoint of being able to sustain functional activity, particularly the vigorous activity of a young child or adolescent (Fig. 18-13). The artery is variably fixed to the femur at the adductor hiatus and tibia by a fibrous arch. Within the popliteal region, the artery gives rise to the geniculate branches, which are the medial and lateral superior and inferior genicular arteries and the middle genicular artery. Although these arteries eventually anastomose with the branches of the anterior tibial recurrent artery, they are small and may not provide adequate blood supply to maintain the *functional* needs of the lower leg musculature of an active child or adolescent, even though resting circulatory demands may be adequately met. An acute popliteal artery injury, particularly one associated with concomitant damage to some of the smaller vessels, hardly allows time for compensatory hypertrophy of collateral circulatory patterns. In some cases, the viability of the musculature and skeleton, even at rest, will not be adequately provided by an acute circulatory deficiency, which may lead to Volkmann's ischemia in the lower leg.

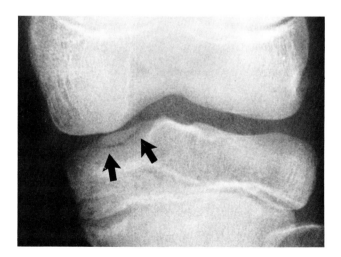

FIG. 18-11. Seven-year-old boy being evaluated for knee trauma. The radiolucent line (arrows) was first interpreted as an osteochondral fracture of the medial tibial plateau. However, this proved to be a thin layer of gas, present because of "cavitation," that was outlining a portion of the medial femoral condyle.

Green and Allen analyzed 245 knee dislocations in patients of varying ages and found that the popliteal artery was injured in almost one third, whether the dislocation was anterior or posterior.[14] They emphasized that vascular repair must be completed within 6 to 8 hours *from the time of injury* in order to avoid either amputation or the subsequent chronic ischemic problems of *relative functional insufficiency*. Of the patients not treated within that sharply defined time period, 86% went on to amputation and two thirds of the remaining 14% had chronic ischemic changes.

The posterior tibialis and dorsalis pedis pulses should be evaluated thoroughly in any child with knee dislocation. If they are not normal, the dislocation must be reduced as quickly as possible and circulation immediately re-evaluated. If, at this point, the circulation is still not normal, the popliteal artery should be explored. Arteriography gives little additional information, since the location of the lesion should be obvious. However, intimal damage may be more easily diagnosed by arteriography. If performed, arteriography must not prolong the time interval between injury and completion of the surgical anastomosis beyond the aforementioned 6- to 8-hour period.

In Green's study, even if the artery was repaired beyond 8 hours, many of these patients required eventual amputation of their leg. Spasm often is implicated as a cause of poor peripheral circulation after trauma, but does not appear to be the primary cause of vascular insufficiency with this particular injury. If there is gross clinical insufficiency, most likely the artery is significantly injured, rather than simply in spasm. If spasm is noted during surgical exploration, this will usually be associated with an intimal tear and thrombosis. An arteriotomy is necessary to determine the true extent of the intimal damage, and the damaged segment must be resected and replaced by an end-to-end anastomosis, a venous graft, or an artificial graft. Every attempt should be made in a child or an adolescent to use direct anastomosis or an autogenous vein, rather than an artificial vascular graft.

At no time during any attempt at vascular repair should an extensive reconstruction of the knee ligaments be undertaken, as this only increases the swelling, tissue damage, and potential for further damage to the collateral circulation. At the time of arterial repair, reasonably complete fasciotomy is recommended because of the marked increase in muscular compartment swelling after restoration of the circulation. Resection of a segment of the fibula has been advocated in adults for complete decompression, but is contraindicated in the skeletally immature patient.

Patellar Dislocation

These injuries are relatively common if the entire spectrum of acute and chronic subluxation and dislocation is considered. However, true acute dislocation of the patella is an infrequent injury in a skeletally immature individual. Predisposing disorders include Down's syndrome, muscular dystrophy, arthrogryposis, or other neuromuscular abnormalities. More frequently, chronic subluxation mimics actual dislocation.

Acute lateral dislocation is usually caused by either a direct blow to the medial side of the patella, or twisting, violent muscular contractions when the knee is placed in a valgus stress. The dislocation may be complete or incomplete, with the patella sitting on the lateral edge of the condyle (Fig. 18-14). Lateral displacement must be accompanied by a variable degree of soft tissue injury to the medial patellar

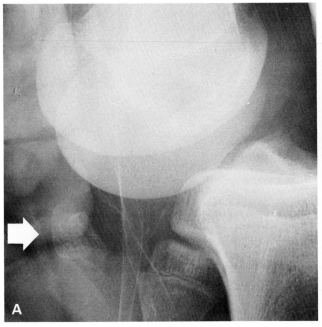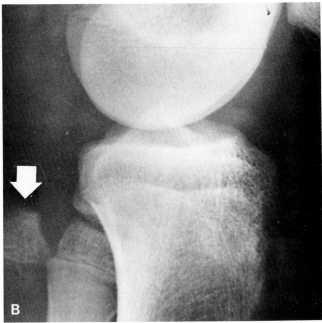

FIG. 18-12. Knee dislocation in a 14-year-old. *A,* Acute injury. The arrow indicates a concomitant type 3 fibular injury. *B,* Initial reduction was successful. However, the concomitant type 3 fracture of the proximal fibular epiphysis did not reduce (arrow). Several days later, this fracture was reduced surgically, and at the same time the fibular collateral ligament was reattached to the femoral condyle (the ligament avulsed along with a small segment of epiphyseal cartilage).

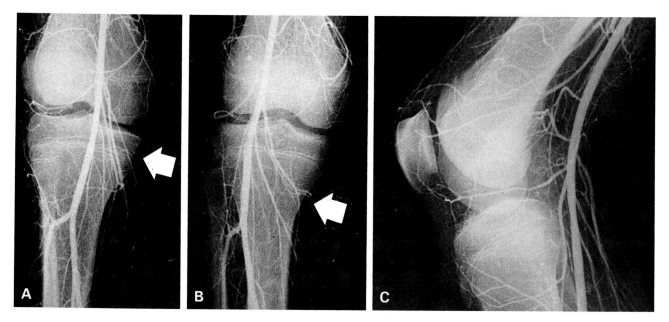

FIG. 18-13. *A,* Oblique, *B,* anterior, and, *C,* lateral views of femoral artery injection of 14-year-old male cadaver. Collateral circulation is more extensive along the medial side (arrows). However, most collaterals are transversely directed, and longitudinal communications are small. These probably allow sufficient resting flow, but may not be able to meet functional demands, especially as the child grows.

retinaculum. There also may be hemorrhage into the joint. In the reparative phase, there may be contracture in the iliotibial band and further lateralization, which accentuates the tendency for the patella to chronically subluxate following acute dislocation. In rare instances, the patella may be displaced medially.

The laterally displaced patella often reduces spontaneously, or a bystander may push it back (sometimes inadvertently). The orthopaedic surgeon rarely has the benefit of seeing the patella in the dislocated state. The knee is maintained in some flexion with a definite limitation toward full extension. Unless the patient presents with the patella dislocated, diagnosis must be on an historical basis, and is often difficult to distinguish from chronic subluxation.

Ordinarily, reduction of acute dislocation is easy. The hip is flexed to relax the rectus femoris, while the knee is gradually extended and the patella pushed medially into its normal position. General anesthetic is rarely necessary. After reduction there is usually some effusion in the knee joint, but aspiration is not necessary unless the swelling is painful. Since the patella does not redislocate easily, the knee should be radiographed following reduction, with good views to ascertain whether there are any obvious osteochondral fractures from either the condyles or patella (Fig. 18-15). It may not be possible to obtain a complete roentgenographic examination at the time of acute injury and reduction, as a sunrise view may be distinctly uncomfortable. The limb should be immobilized in a cylinder cast. The evaluation

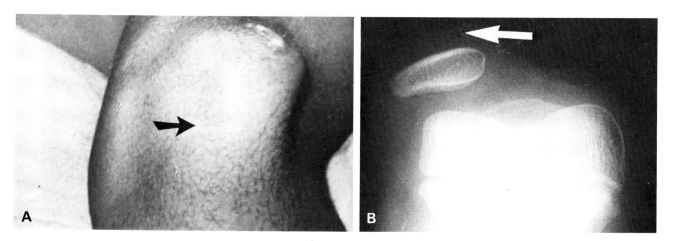

FIG. 18-14. *A,* Acute patellar dislocation (arrow) in a 12-year-old. *B,* Roentgenogram of dislocated patella (arrow) in an 8-year-old. The patella is locked on the lateral femoral condyle.

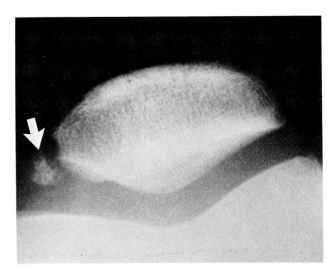

FIG. 18-15. Fracture of lateral margin (arrow) of patella following acute dislocation.

procedure should be repeated in the subsequent recovery phase after return of sufficient motion to allow adequate positioning for roentgenographic examination.

McManus reviewed 55 cases and felt that the majority of children with acute dislocation of the patella demonstrate roentgenographic signs of a pre-existent patellofemoral dysplasia, strongly suggesting that the majority of acute dislocations occur in knees with some abnormality.[15] Acute dislocations simply add damage to the dysplasia and result in the knee becoming symptomatic. In this study, 1 child in 6 developed recurrent dislocation, 2 children in 6 had minor symptoms, and the remainder were asymptomatic.

Surgical intervention is indicated only in the rare patient who exhibits some major degree of concomitant soft injury to the knee, or when there is displacement of the patella into the joint, or in the patient with a chronically subluxating or dislocating patella. In the latter instance, surgery is more effective if done electively after the knee has recovered from the acute injury.

Intra-articular dislocation

Intra-articular dislocation of the patella with rotation around the transverse axis is an unusual injury in children.[16-18] This disorder appears to be more common in boys than in girls, with the average age of reported patients being 16 years and an age range of 7 to 64. An explanation for the high incidence of the lesion in skeletally immature individuals is that the soft tissue attachments to the patella are more lax, mobility is greater, and with direct trauma to the flexed knee, the soft tissues can be stripped relatively easily from the chondro-osseous patella. In the adult, the same type of injury would most likely cause a fracture.

There are basically two types of intra-articular dislocations. The most common type involves the superior pole of the patella being torn loose from the quadriceps mechanism so that it lodges into the femoral intercondylar notch with its articular surface directed toward the tibia (Fig. 18-16). In the other type, which is a rare type, the inferior pole is separated

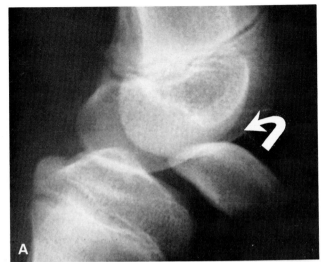

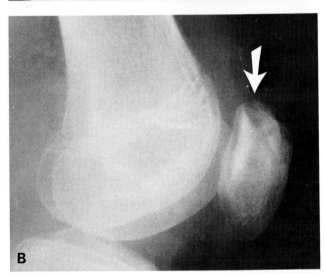

FIG. 18-16. *A,* Lateral roentgenogram of intra-articular dislocation (arrow) of the patella. *B,* Post-reduction film showing some osteoporosis of proximal pole where a quadriceps avulsion had occurred (arrow).

from the patella tendon and pushed posteriorly into the joint where it wedges with the articular surface facing proximally.

The mechanism of injury is probably more complex than a simple fall on the flexed knee. A direct blow probably initially engages the patella in the intercondylar notch, but the actual dissection of the patella from the extensor mechanism undoubtedly occurs when the quadriceps contracts strongly from the blow. The failure is partially at the chondro-osseous junction.

Additional associated lesions should be sought in either type of intra-articular dislocation. The quadriceps tendon may be ruptured completely or partially torn from the tibial tuberosity. Tears of the cruciates and collateral ligaments may also occur.

Closed reduction is generally not effective. Open reduction should be the primary procedure, if only to inspect the extent of injury and repair of soft tissue as well as chondro-osseous damage.

Chronic Subluxation-Dislocation

Chronic subluxation of the patella is a common knee disorder, especially in adolescent girls. A significant number of subluxations and recurrent dislocations of the patella in the young child or adolescent are associated with a congenital or developmental deficiency of the extensor mechanism. Such deficiencies of the extensor mechanism may be divided into three categories: (1) abnormalities of patellofemoral configuration, (2) deficiencies of the supporting muscles or guiding mechanism, and (3) malalignment of the extremity relative to knee mechanics. Often deficiencies in more than one category contribute to patellar instability. Wiberg and Baumgartal have described different types of patellae based upon relative degrees of sloping of the medial and lateral articular facets in the sunrise view.[6]

Certainly, the combination of low profile of the femoral sulcus and relative deficiencies of the lateral condyle and patellar facet predispose to patellofemoral instability. Weakness of the anteromedial retinaculum, dystrophy or weakness of the vastus medialis obliquus muscle, and hypermobility of the patella due to poor muscle tone also constitute predisposing factors. Genu recurvatum may cause laxity of the extensor mechanism. Patella alta and tightness of the lateral retinaculum also allow the patella to subluxate or dislocate. A wide variety of other structural abnormalities of the lower extremity may influence patellar tracking; these can include femoral and tibial torsion, and even foot mechanics. Because of such abnormalities, subluxation may often occur without any significant trauma.

Symptoms are vague. Chronic patellar instability is frequently confused with meniscal injury, and should be considered in all patients with nonspecific knee complaints. Limited use of the knee in these painful stages may lead to chondromalacia. The patella may also forcefully reduce if it has been partially displaced onto the lateral condyle and cause injury to either the medial patellar articular surface or intercondylar region of the medial femoral condyle. Diagnosis is usually by history, as the patella is rarely completely displaced. Maltracking may be evident on physical examination.

Roentgenograms show patellar deformation and a less prominent lateral condyle (Fig. 18-17). Radiographic diagnosis is sometimes subtle and difficult in young children or adolescents. AP views are not particularly remarkable. A lateral view taken with the knee at 30° to assess certain relationships has resulted in the concept of the line of Blumensaat.[6] Insall and Salvati also described length of patella to length of tendon.[19] *However, all these assessments require a reasonably completely ossified patella and tibial tuberosity or they become inaccurate.* Similarly, tangential views, such as the Hughston view, require almost complete ossification of the femoral condyles, as well as the patella, in order to create totally accurate lines.

Treatment should be immobilization when the patient is acutely symptomatic, and a rigorous exercise program subsequently. Operative correction, if at all possible, should be deferred until skeletal maturation is achieved. Transplantation of the tibial tuberosity medially in order to effect a better biomechanical axis of the patellofemoral joint is frequently advocated for chronic patellar subluxation. However, use in children who have not yet attained skeletal maturity may be associated with the development of growth abnormalities and, in particular, premature epiphysiodesis of the anterior portion of the proximal tibial physis.

Rosenthal and Levine studied the effects of tibial tubercle transplantation in skeletally immature children (16 patients with 24 transplantations).[20] Many of these children had neuromuscular disorders; cerebral palsy was the disorder most commonly seen. There were 6 patients who had recurrent lateral dislocation of the patella. The procedures were performed when the children were between 7 and 11 years of age. All were treated by the Bosworth and Thompson method of transplanting the whole tibial tubercle and its epiphysis as a block. Of the patients, 3 sustained a fracture through the operative site. Growth continued in the contiguous proximal tibial epiphysis in many of these cases with resultant further distal "migration" of the transplanted tuberosity. *In all cases, the tibial tuberosity epiphysis failed to develop completely normally after transplantation.*

Collateral Ligaments

Ligament injury must be considered in the differential diagnosis of any child sustaining knee trauma, even though fractures or physeal injuries are more common. Injury to the ligaments of the knee in children less than 14 years old is unusual, presumably because the resiliency and strength of the ligaments are greater than those of the physis and bone.[21] Another factor is the degree of laxity around a joint, which is dramatic in young children, but becomes progressively less as physeal closure is approached.[22]

The incidence of significant disruption of ligaments about the knee joint in the older child or adolescent is on the increase. Reasons probably relate to more vigorous participation in athletic activities, but may also result from increased awareness of the possibility of both ligamentous as well as intra-articular lesions in this age group. The belief that open epiphyseal plates yield before supporting ligaments is not always true. Certainly when the child is undergoing physiologic epiphysiodesis in adolescence, the ligaments do increase their propensity to failure.

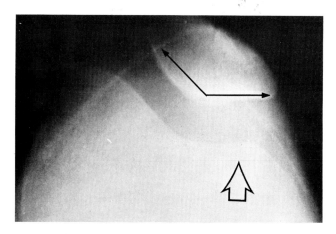

FIG. 18-17. Transverse patellar roentgenogram of patient with chronic subluxation of the patella showing deficient lateral femoral condyle (open arrow) and increased acclivity of the medial patella (small arrows).

Both medial and lateral collateral ligament injuries in children are infrequent, with most stresses that normally produce such soft tissue injuries in older adolescents or young adults instead causing epiphyseal fracture, primarily of the distal femur. Knee ligament injuries are also rare because of the intrinsic resiliency of the ligaments. Hyperlaxity is common in children, although it decreases with increasing age. Also, the relative mode of failure of the ligament versus the growth plate and bone requires much more force.

Few patients less than 14 years old with knee ligament injuries have been reported, and of those, only 2 were discussed in any detail.[23-27] Hyndman described 15 cases of acute knee ligament injuries in children between the ages of 9 and 15.[28] The youngest child reported was a 4-year-old boy who sustained an isolated traumatic rupture of the medial collateral ligament. The site of the rupture was the exact midportion, rather than the origin or insertion of the medial collateral ligament.[29] O'Donoghue described a 6-year-old girl in a series of 82 patients; she was the only patient in his series less than 15 years of age.[25]

Bradley described 6 patients with tears of the medial collateral ligament; their ages ranged from 6 to 11 years.[30] Follow-up of 7 months to 13 years showed normal results in 3, good results in 2, and fair results in 1 patient. Of those patients, 3 also had an injury in the anterior cruciate ligament or an avulsion injury to the anterior tibial spine. The tears described by Bradley occurred in the superficial medial collateral ligament near its tibial insertion or in the midportion. From the manner of attachment of the superficial parts of that ligament to the femur, one could predict that tears near that attachment would be unlikely. In 4 of the 6 patients, disruption of the deep part of the ligament also occurred toward the tibial side.

Clanton reported a well-studied series of 9 skeletally immature patients. Despite initial thorough physical and roentgenographic evaluations, the full extent of the lesions was determined only during surgery in 7 of the 9 patients. The intercondylar eminence of the tibia was avulsed in 5 patients, 4 of whom had associated collateral ligament injuries and a positive anterior drawer sign. This association in children must be emphasized. While Meyers and McKeever noted no associated collateral ligament injuries in children with tibial spine avulsions, Zaricznyj described 1 case and Hyndman and Brown described 7 cases of concomitant collateral-cruciate damage.[9,32,33]

Numerous factors are involved in the site of ligament failure, including the histologic structure, attachment into bone or cartilage, and the degree of chondro-osseous maturation in the epiphysis and physeal anatomy.[6,34,35] The rate of strain has been shown to be important, as well as the site and direction of application of force related to the position of the knee when the strain is applied.[34,36] The relationship of the attachment of the collateral ligaments and joint capsule to the epiphyseal growth plate and the fact that the ligaments appear to be stronger than the growth plate, at least to tensile strain, may influence the site of injury.

Since ligament disruptions are uncommon in children, one must be aware of their potential existence when examining an injured knee. The initial examination must be undertaken carefully, as this probably will be the examination leading to major decisions for or against surgery. Medication is usually appropriate in order to assure relaxation. After standard history, physical examination, and roentgenograms, several other diagnostic alternatives are available to fully delineate the lesion. Aspiration of the knee may allow a more thorough examination, especially when a local anesthetic is instilled. Stress roentgenograms may occasionally be obtained; examination under anesthesia may help; arthroscopy is another useful tool.

Examination must include the entire knee. The medial structures should be tested with the knee both in extension and 30° of flexion (Fig. 18-18). The examination should in-

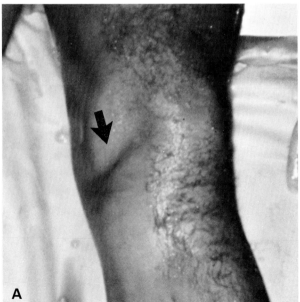
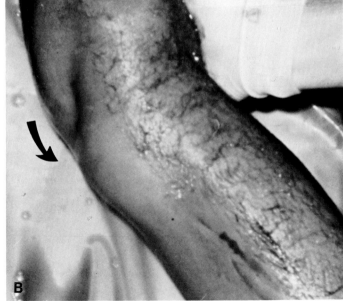

FIG. 18-18. A 16-year-old boy injured in a motorcycle accident. *A,* "Dimpling" of medial joint line (arrow). *B,* Valgus stress (arrow) opened the joint.

clude a thorough check for rotatory instability. The anterior drawer sign must be sought with the knee tested in neutral, internal, and external rotation. This sign is best elicited by having the patient lie supine with the knee flexed to 90°. The foot should be on the table to minimize dependent stretch in the cruciates, as happens when the knee hangs over the side of the table. Instability of the lateral side is less common, but can be more disabling. This compartment tends to be capable of a greater amount of physiologic widening, and comparison should be made with the contralateral uninjured side.

Kennedy cites 15 adolescents ranging in age from 12 to 18 with both clinical and radiologic instability of the knee sufficient to warrant surgical intervention.[6] Only 2 cases occurred in organized football. However, in a comparable series of 22 adolescents, a greater incidence occurred during organized sports, 18 of 22 (10 during football). Kennedy presents detailed discussions of the injured adolescent knee and particularly discusses a method of classification which involves: (1) one-plane instabilities, (2) rotatory instabilities, and (3) combined instabilities.[6]

Occasionally, combinations of epiphyseal separation and ligamentous disruption may be encountered (Fig. 18-19). Kennedy reported a 14-year-old who suffered a type 3 physeal injury as well as avulsion of the anterior cruciate ligament from the tibial spine.[37] Reduction of the epiphyseal plate injury alone would not have controlled the existing instability. The physician must be extremely alert when epiphyseal separations are diagnosed in the adolescent, as ligamentous damage may accompany the chondro-osseous lesion.

Stress radiography may help to rule out potential ligament injury. If a fracture is obvious, then it is less unlikely that there is concomitant collateral ligament injury (Fig. 18-20). Smith described 2 patients who almost underwent operative intervention for a torn medial collateral ligament, and in each case stress films of the knee showed that the cause of

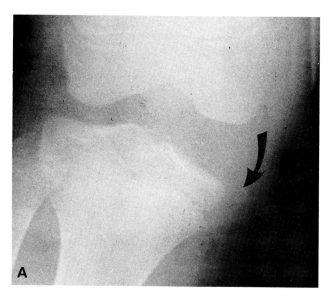

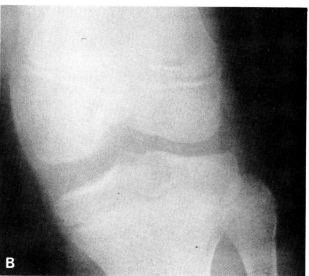

FIG. 18-20.   Patient with medial joint injury and avulsion of tibial spine. Stress films of both knees showed widening of the medial joint space (arrow) of the right knee, *A*, compared to the normal knee, *B*.

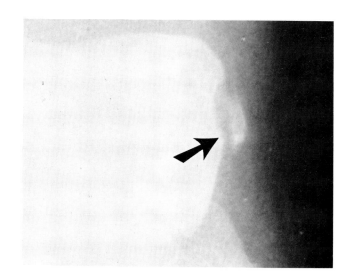

FIG. 18-19.   Avulsion of deep portion of lateral collateral ligament has included an osteochondral fragment (arrow) from the epiphysis. This is the site of collateral ligament attachment, not the metaphysis.

the valgus instability was, in fact, a distal femoral growth plate injury, which had spontaneously and completely reduced, rather than any damage to the ligaments. However, if the stress only opens the joint, then an isolated injury is more probable. Look for peripheral disruption of the secondary ossification center, which may be an extremely small fragment.

Stress roentgenograms of a relaxed patient allow acceptable initial evaluation of potential acute instability. Although Kennedy has published guidelines for limits of medial side widening, they are primarily for skeletally mature individuals, and great care must be taken in using these guidelines for children, inasmuch as the normal width of the joint space is greater due to incomplete ossification of the entire epiphysis.[6]

The following are aids in selecting conservative treatment: (1) The knee should be stable in extension. (2) There should be no anteromedial rotatory instability. (3) There should be a definite end point where resistance is met as valgus forces are applied, suggesting that a substantial percentage of the fibers remain intact. (4) The prognosis is more favorable if ligamentous tenderness is either at the femoral origin or tibial insertion rather than the joint line (midligament). Conservative treatment should be plaster immobilization with the knee in approximately 30 to 40° of flexion. This should be non-weightbearing for 6 to 8 weeks.

Although treatment tends to be conservative in the skeletally immature individual, there are certain indications for surgical repair even in the adolescent patient. Such surgical treatment is complex, depending upon the particular pattern of instability, and the reader is referred to Kennedy's excellent review of the subject for recommended surgical repairs for specific anatomic lesions.[6]

The best method of treatment of knee ligament injuries in children has not been adequately defined. Unfortunately, documented studies of ligament healing in children (or skeletally immature animals) compared to adults have not been reported. In Clanton's study, despite primary surgical repair followed by 6 weeks of cast immobilization, some degree of ligament laxity persisted, suggesting such injuries in children are analogous to adult ligament injuries in this respect.[31] Although some degree of objective knee ligament laxity may persist, this may not be associated with subjective symptoms of instability.

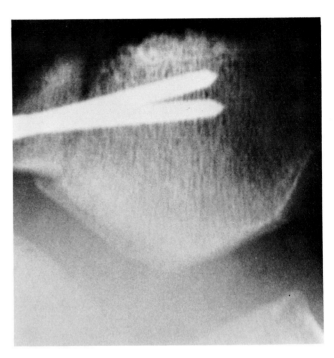

FIG. 18-21. Fracture of medial patella following direct injury in a 16-year-old. The fragment was fixed with 2 pins, but the joint was not accurately restored. Significant chondromalacia was present 5 years later.

Cruciate Ligaments

The youngest person to sustain an avulsion of the attachment of the posterior cruciate ligament was an 11-year-old boy.[38,39] He also had a tear of the posterior capsule and peripheral detachment of the medial meniscus. Based on experiments, two mechanisms of injury to the posterior cruciate ligament have been postulated by Kennedy.[37,40,41] The first is a forceful posterior displacement of the flexed tibia on the femur, and the second a hyperextension injury of the knee. As the knee hyperextends 30°, the more the posterior capsule and ligament tear. Pure cruciate ligament injuries are rare in children.[34] The tibial spine usually fails at the chondro-osseous transition (see Chap. 19).

Patellar Fractures

Fractures of the patella are unusual in children and must be adequately differentiated from normal developmental variations such as bipartite patella.[42,43] Lateral marginal fractures may also be produced when a direct blow is applied to the periphery, rather than the center of the bone (Fig. 18-21). A direct blow may crush the patella against the femoral condyles and cause a stellate, comminuted fracture, which is more likely in an adolescent than a younger child, in whom the resiliency of the primarily cartilaginous patella protects from major injury. A sudden, powerful contraction of the quadriceps mechanism may cause fracture.

Diebold found that only 1% of patellar fractures involved patients under 15 years of age, a fact more recently corroborated by Senst.[44,45] The youngest case reported is in a 2-year-old child. It is common for the diagnosis to be missed or delayed significantly, especially if the patella is not ossified or minimally ossified. Ronget and Hallopeau both reported cases in which the diagnosis was not made until several months after fracture.[46,47]

The mechanisms of injury are a direct blow to the patella, sudden acute flexion, or a combination of both. Previous injury to the knee with compromised quadriceps mechanism and function may also be a predisposing factor in certain kinds of neuromuscular disease (e.g., cerebral palsy). These fractures often occur in children who take part in activities that require forceful extension of the knee with the quadriceps contracting against resistance. There is an association of this type of injury with high jumping.[48-50] Interestingly, in Houghton's series, the injury always involved the "take off" leg with no direct trauma to the knee occurring in any case.[51]

Roentgenograms disclose the fracture best in the lateral projection (Figs. 18-22 and 18-23). In rare instances, the patellar tendon may be avulsed from the tibial tuberosity, rather than a fracture of the patella itself (Fig. 18-24).

In a child, treatment of the transversely fractured patella should follow the same principles as in an adult. Undisplaced or minimally displaced fractures should be treated by immobilization of the knee in extension in a cylinder cast. Avulsion fractures with significant separation of the fragments require open reduction and repair of the torn medial and lateral quadriceps expansions. Circumferential wiring through the soft tissue, rather than the patella, *per se*, is probably indicated so as not to disrupt further normal growth patterns in the patella (Fig. 18-25). Furthermore,

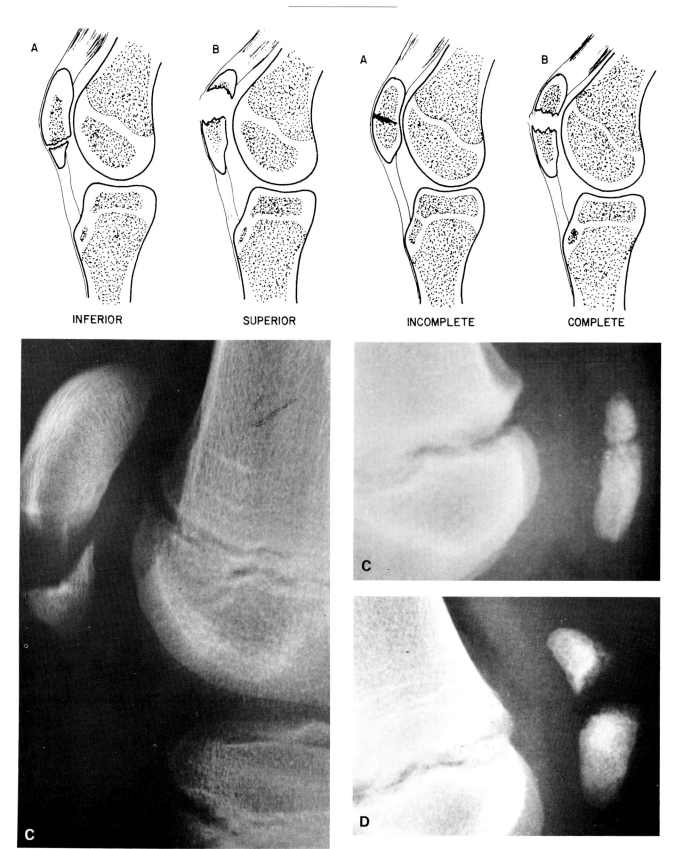

FIG. 18-22. Schematics of patellar fracture showing involvement of, *A,* the inferior pole and, *B,* the superior pole. *C,* Displaced fracture of the inferior pole.

FIG. 18-23. *A-B,* Schematics of incomplete and complete fractures of midportion of patella. *C,* Undisplaced fracture of patella. *D,* Displaced fracture which was treated by open reduction.

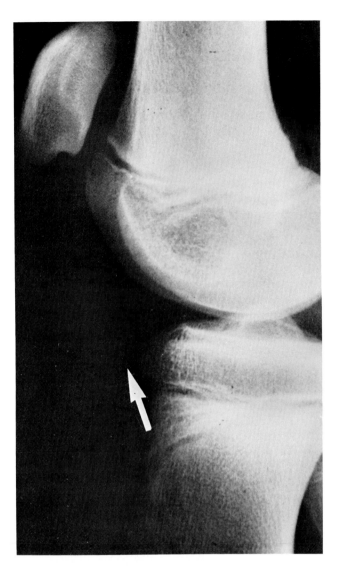

FIG. 18-24. Avulsion of patellar tendon from tibial tuberosity (arrow), leading to acute patella alta.

because of the thickness of the hyaline cartilage and articular cartilage, there may be an incomplete separation of the inferior (cartilaginous) portion of the patella, even though it appears separated in the osseous portion, and a compression type of wiring of the superficial region will often be sufficient to restore normal anatomy and not cause gaping at the articular surface.

Belman reported a case of transverse fracture of the patella in an 11-year-old boy who sustained a direct blow to the knee.[52] When surgically incised, the patellar fragments were found to be incompletely separated because the thick segment of retropatellar articular cartilage and hyaline cartilage was still intact and served as a hinge. The fragments were approximated using absorbable sutures.

Failure to diagnose and adequately treat these injuries may result in an established nonunion between the superior and inferior fragments (Fig. 18-26), although there may be sufficient intrinsic healing of the quadriceps expansion to stabilize the degree of separation of the fragments.

Stress fracture

Devas demonstrated three cases of stress fractures of the patella: in two, there was a crack along the lateral side;[53] the other case was a transverse fracture. These injuries occurred during vigorous athletic activity. Devas believed that stress fractures were seldom severe enough to require operative treatment. However, there may be significant problems associated with the articular surface of the patella that one must look for and evaluate thoroughly before stating that this will be a normal joint.

Sleeve fracture

Houghton described a patellar injury pattern that is unique to children—the sleeve fracture (Fig. 18-27)—and drew attention to the fact that the diagnosis may be missed because the distal osseous fragment may be sufficiently small to be minimally detectable radiographically.[51] An extensive sleeve of cartilage may be pulled from the main body of the osseous patella together with an osseous fragment from the distal pole. When the patellar tendon disrupts in children, it usually does so at either the upper or lower pole, rather than interstitially.[54] Although avulsion of the tibial tuberosity has been reported,[55] avulsion of the lower pole of the patella is more usual and rarely a fracture of the body of the patella may occur. These cases tend to occur in children participating in sporting activities that require vigorous extension of the knee.

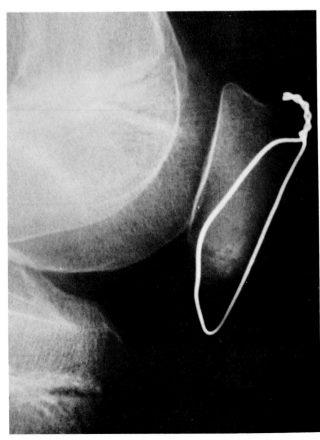

FIG. 18-25. Circumferential wiring of patellar fracture.

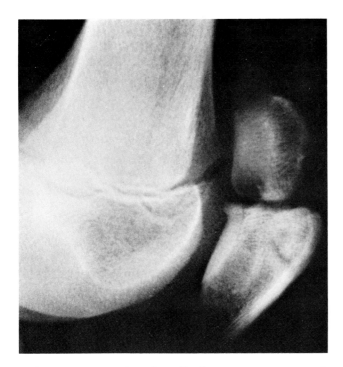

FIG. 18-26. Nonunion of patellar fracture. However, quadriceps function was still good because the soft tissues were intact. The fragments move as a unit from flexion to extension.

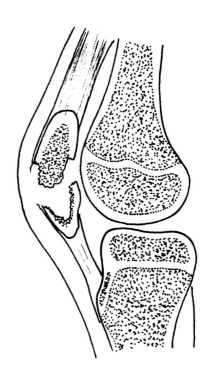

A

The diagnosis is suggested by the absence of a direct blow to the knee with a sudden giving way, severe pain in the knee, and an inability to bear weight. On examination there is a tense knee effusion and active extension of the knee is not possible. The patella is often high riding on the affected side and a palpable gap can frequently be felt in the extension mechanism of the distal pole of the patella. This is a particularly valuable clinical sign, since the fragment of avulsed bone may be so small as to not be detectable radiographically. The radiograph usually corroborates the effusion and high-riding patella, and often shows the fragmentation of the patella.

The avulsed patellar fragment always includes an important "sleeve" of cartilage, which must be accurately reduced in order to reestablish the articular surface of the patella. Houghton also recommends the importance of wire fixation, stating that the failure of a case reported by Betto and Wilson did not give satisfactory results because the fixation was not rigid and damage to the nutrient vessels led to avascular necrosis of the patella.[51] Conservative treatment with extension or hyperextension is likely to lead to marked deformity of the patella with elongation of the patella (Fig. 18-28) and restriction of eventual knee movement. Rigid fixation also allows more rapid rehabilitation.

Sinding-Larsen-Johansson Disease

This syndrome is comparable to partial separation of the tibial tuberosity (Osgood-Schlatter disease), affecting the patella either at the attachment of the patellar ligament inferiorly or the quadriceps confluence superiorly.[56-58] The pa-

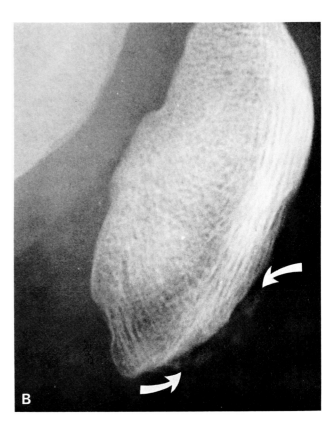

B

FIG. 18-27. *A,* Schematic of sleeve fracture of patella. *B,* Sleeve fracture in ten-year-old. This close-up view shows new bone formation (arrows) at chondro-osseous separation interface.

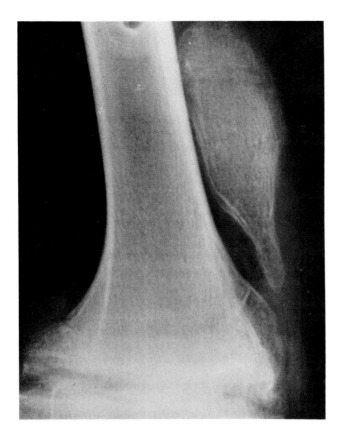

FIG. 18-28. Attenuation of inferior pole of patella following chronic damage in a child with congenital sensory neuropathy.

tient is usually an active boy in the 10- to 14-age group who complains of pain in the knee accompanied by a limp. Bilateral symptoms are less common. As in Osgood-Schlatter disease, there may be bilateral involvement radiographically, but only unilateral symptoms. Examination shows tenderness and occasional swelling located at the inferior or superior pole of the patella.

Wolf found an incidence of 3% in his series of 100 patients, all normal children, although this appears to be high.[59] The type of trauma is more consistent with a fatigue or stress type of fracture and possible disturbance of normal ossification patterns due to abnormal stress.

Radiographs may reveal fragmentation at the superior or inferior pole, or there may be extension cephalad to the anterior-inferior surface of the patella (Figs. 18-29 and 18-30). The inferior pole may develop an over-enlarged appearance comparable to the deformity seen in the tibial tuberosity. As in Osgood-Schlatter disease, the roentgenographic appearance is not necessarily related to the severity of the symptoms (Fig. 18-31).

Sinding-Larsen-Johansson disease is a traction lesion. Like any traction epiphysitis, treatment should be directed at the various symptoms, as well as the possible affect on the future relationship of the patella to the femoral condyles. This condition must be treated with rest for a sustained period of up to 12 weeks using a cylinder cast. The problem may persist to the end of skeletal maturity and may lead to irregular development of the lower or upper pole of the patella and may even be associated with the development of a "loose body,"

although this is usually connected by fibrous or fibrocartilaginous tissue. The disease tends to be self-limited, but may remain insidiously active during skeletal growth. Since the involved area is non-articular and separated from the joint by the fat pad, joint changes other than associated immobilization chondromalacia are unlikely.

Association with neuromuscular disorders

Rosenthal and Levine, who reported on 88 patients with spastic cerebral palsy, found 10 instances of variable fragmentation of the distal pole of the patella.[20] In addition, 12 knees, including the uninvolved ones, exhibited changes in the tibial tuberosity compatible with Osgood-Schlatter disease. Excessive tension in the quadriceps mechanism, usually in the presence of a significant flexion contracture, appeared to be the cause of the lesions. Of the fragmented patellae, 4 healed after hamstring release and correction of the flexion deformity. The association between fragmentation of the distal pole of the patella and cerebral palsy was further emphasized by Kaye and Freiberger, who described fragmentation of the patella in 7 patients ranging in age from

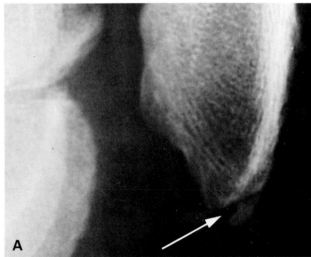

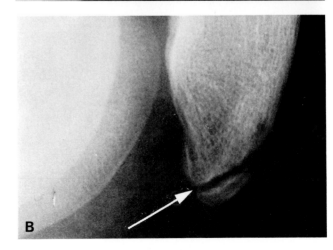

FIG. 18-29. Sinding-Larsen-Johansson disease (arrows) in, *A,* a 9-year-old and, *B,* a 13-year-old.

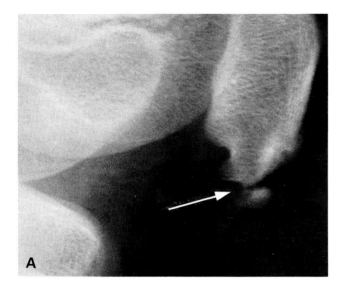

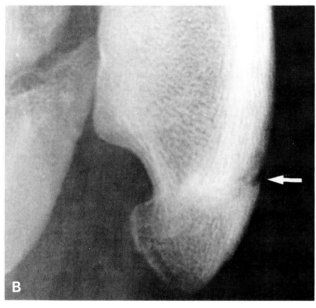

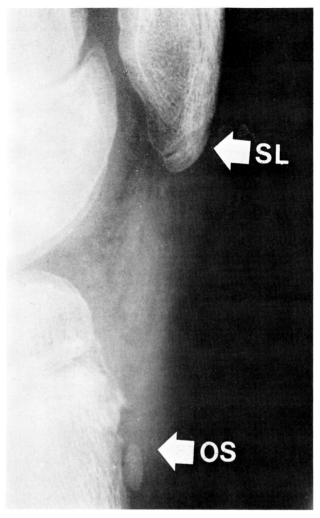

FIG. 18-31.   Healing case of Sinding-Larsen-Johansson disease (SL) in a child who subsequently complained of tibial tuberosity pain compatible with Osgood-Schlatter disease (OS).

FIG. 18-30.   *A*, Sinding-Larsen-Johansson disease (arrow). Appearance at time of acute onset of symptoms. *B*, Six months later (including nine weeks of cast immobilization), the lesion has fused to the patellar ossification center (arrow).

7 to 15.[60] Their cases seem to differ slightly from the more classic cases of Sinding-Larsen-Johannson disease. They felt that the patellar fragmentation was traumatic with the flexion contractures and spasticity causing abnormal stresses at the knee joint resulting in repeated minor trauma.

Rosenthal and Levine supported Chandler's contention that the elongation of the patellar tendon and the secondarily high position of the patella seen in spastic patients represented adaptive changes caused by prolonged increased tension during the phases of rapid growth, particularly in the presence of the knee flexion contracture.[20] In their study of the results of surgical advancement of the insertion of the patella tendon in patients with cerebral palsy, Roberts and Adams found one spontaneous fracture of the patella in a patient who had not sustained any trauma and proposed that overactivity of the quadriceps had caused the avulsion fracture.[61] If the tension in the extensor mechanism in a growing child is prolonged and of sufficient grade, a high-riding patella or stress fragmentation of the distal pole of the patella or tibial tuberosity may occur, especially in the presence of a knee flexion contracture. Perry and co-workers showed that the quadriceps force required to stabilize the flexed knee during stance in children with cerebral palsy was proportional to the angle of the knee flexion and that for each degree of flexion, the required force increased an average of 6%.[62] Therefore, a flexion contracture of 30° may cause forces of 210% of body weight.

Fabellar Fracture

Dashefsky reported a case of a 13-year-old boy who was struck over the knee during a soccer game and sustained a fracture through the sesamoid bone behind the knee.[63] This is an unusual cause for pain, but one that might be sought in a knee that proves difficult to diagnose and is associated with considerable posterior pain beyond obvious physical signs.

Osteochondral Fractures

Osteochondral fractures of the medial or lateral femoral condylar articular surfaces may be caused by a direct blow or rapid lateral subluxation or dislocation of the patella, often accompanied by spontaneous reduction.[64-67] These injuries may also involve the medial surface of the intercondylar notch, although this is commonly the site of a chronic, possibly developmental lesion, osteochondritis dissecans. The fracture fragment may be visualized as a loose body, although it is not always easy to visualize this in young children.

Kennedy divides these fractures into two types: exogenous, in which the condyle strikes an external, direct shearing force, and endogenous, in which there is a twisting injury with contact between the tibia and the condyle that causes the lesion.[6] He also includes an additional case in which, because of patellar dislocation or subluxation, there is a fracture of the lateral femoral condyle. The exogenous lesion tends to result from direct shearing trauma, while the endogenous lesion tends to result from a combination of rotatory and compression forces. In the adult, a compressive or rotatory force appears to be dissipated through the tide mark between calcified and uncalcified cartilage where the subchondral bone is not involved. In contrast, in the adolescent, the subchondral bone is penetrated and an osteochondral fracture results.

Diagnosis of these particular injuries is sometimes difficult (Fig. 18-32). Nonstandard projections can be misleading and may suggest the diagnosis of a loose body, when in reality the tibial tuberosity is visualized (see Fig. 18-10). Since the epiphyseal regions of the young child contain more radiolucent cartilage than during adolescence, the evaluation of suspected internal derangement of the knee is even more difficult. Chronic osteochondral fragmentation (osteochondritis dissecans) is more common than a meniscal tear in these age groups.

The knee should be aspirated. The presence of fat globules suggests intra-articular fracture through the subchondral plate. Treatment should consist of arthrotomy (Fig. 18-33), removal of the loose fragment, and shaving of the sites of origin, or reinsertion and fixation by small pins if a large fragment is found, particularly one that involves a joint surface.

Kennedy feels strongly that treatment of osteochondral fractures in the knee joint is operative, and that the inability to determine with certainty the size of the dislodged fragments pre-operatively, the unexpectedly large weightbearing donor area often discovered at operation, and the subsequent internal derangements of the knee resulting from ignored fragments warrant this approach.[6] At arthrotomy, replacement is indicated if the fragment or fragments are fresh, if the osseous components are sizable, and if the host area is weightbearing and surgically accessible. A period of delay as limited as 10 days between the accident and surgery may compromise the result, because the area begins to fill in with fibrous and fibrocartilaginous tissue requiring trimming of the fragments or curetting to achieve a reasonably precise

fit. Fixation pins should not be left protruding into the joint, as they may provoke a synovitis, pannus formation, and joint stiffness.

Osteochondritis Dissecans

Kennedy prefers to differentiate osteochondral fractures from osteochondritis dissecans. He feels that the two entities are totally unrelated.[6] The exact cause of this lesion is not known.[68] However, it may represent a combination of ischemic disease as proposed by Olsson's studies of similar lesions in other animals (see Chap. 4). Osteochondritis dissecans is seen frequently in children during the growth spurt, and particularly in children who are taller than average (Figs. 18-34 and 18-35).

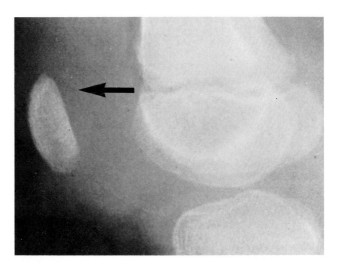

FIG. 18-32. Elevation of patella by chondral fragment in a four-year-old. The radiolucent fragment was locked between the patella and the intercondylar notch (arrow).

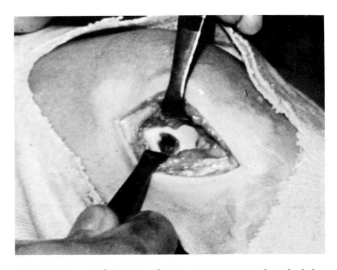

FIG. 18-33. Arthrotomy showing acute osteochondral defect of lateral condyle in an 11-year-old following a fall from a bicycle.

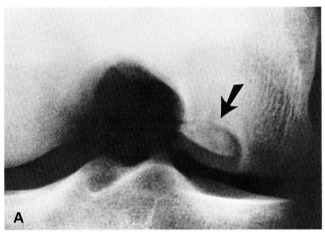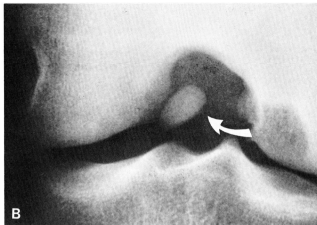

FIG. 18-34. *A,* Anteroposterior view showing undisplaced osteochondritis (arrow). *B,* One week later the patient fell during a basketball game, and the fragment displaced (arrow). It was subsequently removed.

Green and Banks suggest that the disease starts when both subchondral bone and contiguous trabecular bone die.[68] The cartilage remains healthy because of synovial nutrition, but the necrotic bone is gradually replaced and resorbed. This may cause loss of support of the cartilage with subsequent softening and degeneration. Trauma, a relatively common occurrence in adolescence, may then disrupt the region and transform the lesion into a displaced fragment.

Landells stated that injured human articular cartilage tends to tear along the junction of calcified and uncalcified cartilage, leaving the osteochondral junction undisturbed.[69] However, the child and adolescent have less calcified carti-

lage, so that tangential forces, whether normal repetition or acute trauma, are directed to the subchondral region. As in other areas of the epiphyseal-physeal cartilage, the normal failure mode is through bone, not the more resilient cartilage.

Theories invoking trauma have suggested that there was an impingement between the tibial spine on the lateral (intercondylar) aspect of the medial condyle.[70] This was further supported clinically and experimentally by Smillie.[71] The initial fracture that these authors proposed was a subchondral fracture with intact articular cartilage overlying the infarcted bone, with subsequent normal use leading to eventual mo-

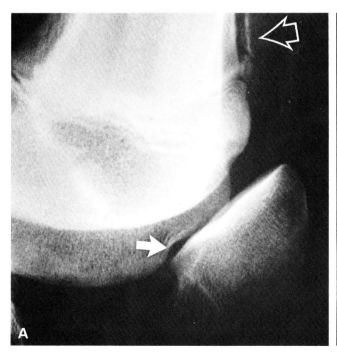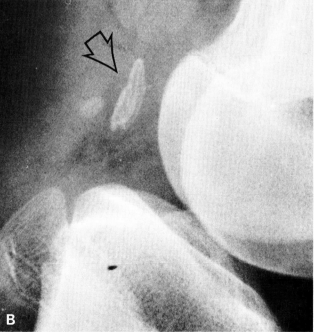

FIG. 18-35. *A,* Initial presentation of adolescent with knee pain and loose body in suprapatellar pouch (open arrow). The original lesion site has healed (solid arrow). *B,* One month later, the loose body has lodged in a posterior capsular recess (arrow).

tion of the fragment in its bed and final propagation of the fracture through the articular surface. The fact that Berndt was not able to accomplish this fracture experimentally in human cadavers does not necessarily rule out the proposed mechanism as a cause, particularly since these studies were carried out in adult cadavers, and the relationship of articular cartilage, hyaline cartilage, and epiphyseal ossification in the developing knee may allow different anatomic and biomechanic mechanisms.[71] Forces transmitted through the patella have also been postulated to cause subchondral fractures eventuating in the dissecans lesion of the medial femoral condyle. Support for this theory has come from the experimental work of Aicroth.[72]

In contrast, some people have strongly suggested ischemia to that area of the developing ossification center, with the development of ischemic necrosis and isolation of a necrotic fragment of bone unable to totally and completely bear weight in a proper fashion. Several authors have suggested that a separate ossification center may exist for that position of the medial femoral condyle typically involved with the dissecans lesion, and that roentgenographic visualization is no more than a representation of this normal variation in epiphyseal growth and development.[6,71] This is probably not totally true, but it may be that there is irregularity of ossification in this region that makes certain children more susceptible. Olsson was able to show that irregularities in the development of the cartilage with thickening of the cartilage in the area eventually formed a dessicans lesion.[73]

Treatment for the younger patient with a nondetached fragment should be conservative, often with no more than restriction of symptom-producing activities. The older patient with a detached fragment is treated best by arthrotomy with excision of the fragment and removal of joint debris (Fig. 18-35). Larger fragments that involve weightbearing areas should be replaced and fixed. In either case, the subchondral bone at the base of the defect should be drilled to stimulate a fibroblastic-fibrocartilaginous response.

Osteochondritis Dissecans of the Patella

Prior to the report by Edwards and Bentley, osteochondritis of the patella had been described in 34 patients, with 7 cases showing bilateral involvement.[74] These cases involved varying nonmarginal areas of medial and lateral articular facets, with the medial articular facet being involved more often (Fig. 18-36). They also tend to involve the inferior, rather than the superior, half of the patella. The possibility that ischemic necrosis was a major causal factor in these, as opposed to other types of osteochondritis, was proposed by Smillie who felt that these fragments did not have a blood supply, whereas osteochondral fractures did.[71] However, according to Scapinelli, the patellar blood supply primarily enters the lower pole and proceeds upward.[75] Thus, if this lesion were related to defects of blood supply, one would expect more lesions in the upper rather than the lower pole. Other authors feel that trauma is a predisposing factor.

Flexion of the knee under load usually duplicates the symptoms, suggesting that repetitive stress on the patellar surface may be an important causal factor.

The indication for operating is a loose osteochondral fragment that is either partially or completely detached from the

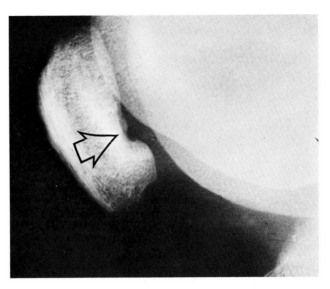

FIG. 18-36. Osteochondritis of the patella (arrow) in a 13-year-old girl with bilateral involvement.

articular surface. Excision of the affected area with drilling of the subchondral bone usually gives good results.

Open Knee Injuries

Lacerations around the knee joint should be treated with a high degree of suspicion for the possibility of penetration of an object into the knee joint.[22] However, lacerations around the patellar tendon may not necessarily be in the knee joint (Fig. 18-37). Instead, they may be totally in the fat pad around the patellar tendon, and therefore extra-synovial (extra-articular). In any suspicious case of penetration into the knee joint a diagnosis should be made as accurately as possible, since the joint should be debrided and irrigated adequately to prevent the possibility of infection and serious secondary changes. If the joint has been penetrated by the laceration, there frequently is air within the joint (Fig. 18-38). However, there may be the appearance of an air arthrogram due to an associated osteochondral fracture with bleeding and fat from the underlying epiphyseal ossification center filling the joint with a hemarthrosis and creating sufficient radio-contrast to allow visualization and seeming involvement of the knee.

The correct diagnosis of retained foreign bodies accompanying small wounds about the knee demands a high index of suspicion. Since recurrent falls and knee wounds are a common occurrence in children, especially in the 4- to 8-year range, parents often defer medical advice thinking that the pain and swelling will subside and that nothing could have entered the deep tissues or joint. Biologic structures (e.g., thorns, wood) may penetrate the skin and even the joint, but may come out as the child gets up from the ground.[76-78] If the patient or parent attempts to remove them, small pieces may break off and remain within the joint. Unfortunately most of these objects are radiolucent. If they remain in the joint they may serve as a mechanical or chemical irritant, and create a foreign-body reaction or even pyarthrosis.

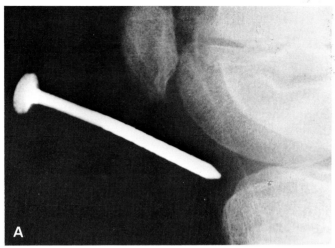 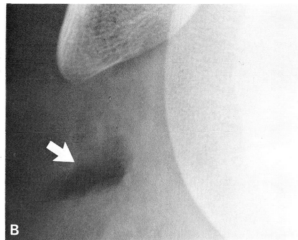

FIG. 18-37. *A,* Nail seemingly penetrating into joint. However, this was embedded totally in the fat pad, and was therefore extra-articular. *B,* Laceration with gas (arrow) in fat pad. Again, this was an extra-articular injury.

Any child presenting with a history suggestive of penetration of a foreign object into the knee may only exhibit painful range of motion and joint swelling. Elevation of temperature, white blood counts, or sedimentation rate may be absent. If routine roentgenograms are negative, xerography may be helpful.

History and clinical examination may be entirely negative. Following local wound care, tetanus therapy, and antibiotics (if indicated), roentgenograms are mandatory. A knowledge of synovial recesses and suprapatellar pouch anatomy of the knee enables one to determine if a foreign body may be lying in or communicating with the intra-articular space. Once recognized, the intra-articular foreign body *must be* removed (Fig. 18-39). The desire to avoid a general anesthetic, to avoid a scar on the knee, or fear of not being able to locate a foreign body should not be contraindications, especially if one considers the potential damage to articular surfaces that may occur if the foreign body is left within the joint.

Potential problems with intra-articular foreign bodies also include septic arthritis and osteomyelitis (Fig. 18-40), me-

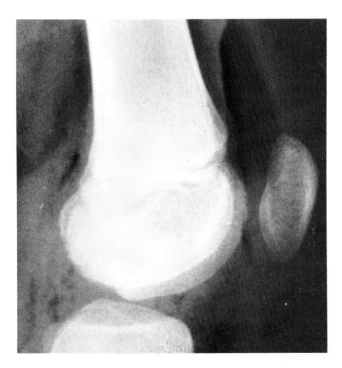

FIG. 18-38. Compound knee injury associated with a relatively small external wound. However, intra-articular gas made the injury to the joint obvious.

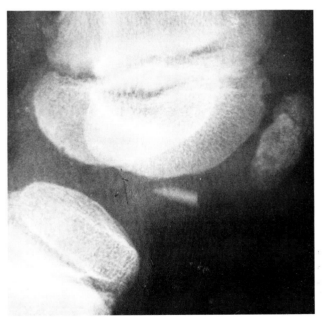

FIG. 18-39. This child fell on a piece of glass. Allegedly, the glass was completely pulled from the wound by the ambulance attendant, leaving a 4-mm laceration. However, the roentgenogram shows an obvious intra-articular fragment of lead-containing glass.

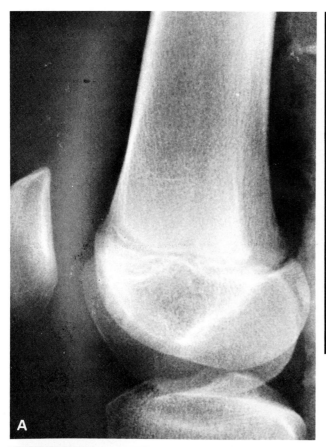

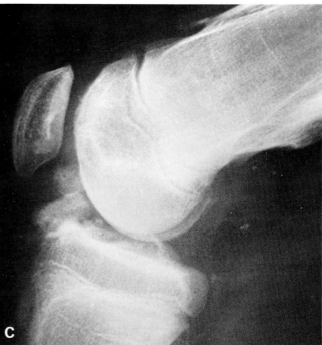

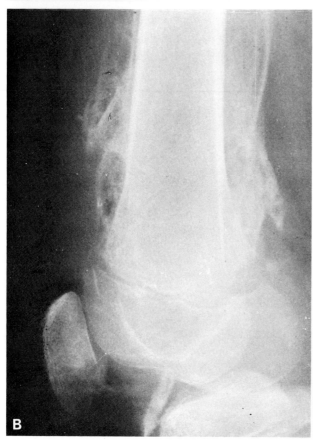

FIG. 18-40. *A*, This 11-year-old was stabbed in the knee but not treated until 48 hours after the injury, at which time presenting symptoms included pain and fever. Arthrotomy was performed immediately. *B*, Within 3 weeks, extensive heterotopic bone was evident, both in the capsule and subperiosteally. *C*, 6 months later, remodeling has made the reactive bone much less evident.

chanical trauma to the articular cartilage, epiphyseal plate trauma, and growth disturbance as a result of the effects of any of the preceding on the epiphyseal plate. As alluded to in earlier chapters, articular cartilage lacerations heal poorly and sometimes not at all, and may initiate early secondary arthritic changes.

Menisco-Synovial Plications (Plica Syndrome)

Variable folds of the synovial membrane may occasionally be found extending from the upper tibial fringe at the infrapatellar fat pad to the undersurface of the suprapatellar synovial plications.[79] Such a plica may sometimes snap back and forth over the condyle as the knee goes from full extension to full flexion, symptomatically duplicating the problems of a torn anterior horn of the meniscus. Other plica may involve the suprapatellar pouch (Fig. 18-41). Most synovial folds are constantly being tensed and relaxed during joint movement. They contain a large portion of elastic fibers to facilitate changing shape and length and may be detached easily consequent to trauma. A knee that clicks approaching full extension is a well-known clinical entity, especially in the adolescent patient. Although the multiple causes of clicking knees are not considered in this discussion, those produced by the shelf or medial plica are associated with the palpable tensed cords slipping medially over the anterior edge of the femoral condyle.

Children with plica are often asymptomatic, but occasionally may have discomfort, effusion, and pain and may require arthrotomy. Arthroscopy and arthrotomy may also reveal the band that is tense by flexing the joint. A tight band can be treated by division or excision, as necessary.

Meniscus Injuries

Meniscus injuries are unusual in young children, but become increasingly prevalent in adolescence (Fig. 18-42). Traumatic rupture of a previously intact normal medial meniscus in a child below the age of 10 is rare.[80-88] Saddawi described a meniscal tear in a young child.[89] Smillie stated that his youngest patient was a 3-year-old girl.[71] Ritchie felt that the lower age limit was between 10 and 15 years.[90] Fairbank felt that internal derangements of the knees in adolescents and children, particularly torn menisci, usually occurred only in congenitally abnormal menisci.[70] Volk described a tear of the medial meniscus in a 5-year-old boy.[91] Abrams reported 3 cases of medial meniscus tears in children aged 5, 10, and 12 and 2 children with lateral meniscus tears aged 9 and 12.[92] Schlonsky reported lateral meniscus tears in 3 patients aged 4, 6, and 7.[93] Only 1 of these represented a tear in a discoid lateral meniscus, which is one of the most common meniscal problems during childhood.

Ritchie described 39 meniscectomies.[90] These included tears in normal menisci (7 medial and 6 lateral), 9 cases of discoid menisci (all lateral), 10 cases of cystic menisci (again, all lateral), and 7 patients in whom apparently normal menisci were found and treated with meniscectomy. All children were 14 years of age or younger with the lower limit being 4. However, for the tears in otherwise normal menisci, the age range was 10 to 14. Ritchie felt that meniscus lesions were rare in children and concluded that the lateral meniscus was the prime site for such lesions in children.

Zaman and Leonard reported the results of meniscectomy in 59 knees of 49 children.[94] In 10 children menisci had been removed from both knees, and in 2 knees both menisci had been removed. The average age at surgery was 13 years. The average length of follow-up was 7½ years. They found 3 definable groups at follow-up. In group 1 the children were symptom-free as young adults; this included 25 knees, 21 of which had a definite abnormality of the meniscus. Group 2 included those with symptoms present only during sporting activity; there were 11 knees in this group, and there was no clear relationship between the symptoms and the abnormality of the meniscus. In group 3 there were symptoms on normal activity; there were 23 patients in this group and 16 had *no* abnormality of the meniscus when it was removed. They stressed that in one-third of all cases the menisci had been found to be *normal* at the time of operation. Despite such a finding the meniscus was removed in each case. They stressed that the results showed meniscectomy in children was *not* a benign procedure, particularly in view of the fact that long term radiologic changes were present in 43 of the knees, and only 42 were symptom-free at follow-up. Only 27% had normal radiographs at follow-up. The results in girls were worse than in boys. *A definite relationship existed between poor results and the removal of normal menisci.* They recommended that every child have arthroscopy before arthrotomy. If a normal meniscus is found, *it should not be*

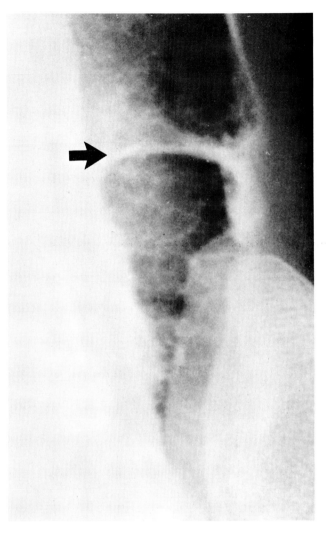

FIG. 18-41. Plica (arrow) extending across the suprapatellar pouch. This caused chronic synovitis and knee effusions for two years.

removed; other sources of joint derangement such as chondromalacia, patellar subluxation, or plica syndrome must be sought.

Fowler reviewed 117 adolescents under 17 years of age who underwent meniscectomy.[95] This study included 77 boys and 40 girls. There were 56% that were medial; the bucket-handle tear was noted 30% of the time and posterior horn tears occurred 19% of the time. Discoid menisci comprised only 9% of the group. Of the meniscectomies, 15% were peripheral detachments and 15% were described as hypermobile or normal. This group of almost 30% of the patients perhaps could have had the tear repaired, or had a meniscus removed for questionable reasons.

Derangements occur in the adolescent meniscus and can cause problems typical of any older age group. A recent review of patients undergoing meniscectomy prior to the age of 17 shows 60% having some type of difficulty up to 9 years after surgery.[6,95] The meniscus is an important primary stabilizer and weight transmitter in the knee and there should be extremely well-defined indications for its removal, particularly in an adolescent or younger patient.

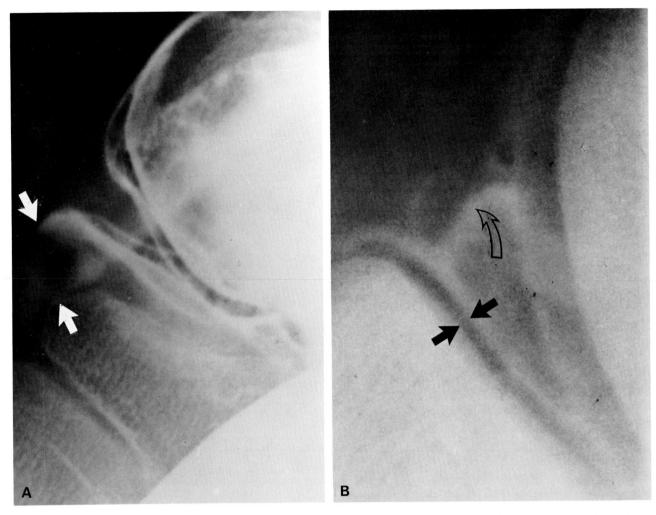

FIG. 18-42. *A,* Normal medial meniscus in a 9-year-old with intermittent locking of the knee. Note the width of the epiphyseal cartilage (arrows). *B,* Torn medial meniscus in a 12-year-old (open arrow). Note narrowing of epiphyseal cartilage (black arrows) compared to younger child shown in *A.*

The surgeon must render an accurate diagnosis. He has to rule out lesions that mimic meniscal tear, confirm the tear with arthrography or arthroscopy, and then if possible define the type and extent of the tear along with other predisposing causal factors.[96-98] Only when all information is available should any consideration of surgical removal be undertaken. Lesions that must be differentiated from a torn meniscus include patellofemoral derangement, chondral and osteochondral lesions, synovial disorders, and inflammations of tendon and fat, attachments and adjacent bone lesions such as osteochondromata, giant cell tumors, and cysts.

Excision is certainly not the treatment of choice for all torn menisci. Patients with small tears and with tears not causing any block to movement appear to do better with non-operative treatment. The important contributions made by the meniscus to knee stability and load transmission must not be forgotten. When the meniscal tear causes abnormal mechanics, operative treatment is warranted. Increasing evidence demonstrates that partial meniscectomy, when possible, may be the procedure of choice. In adults, the concepts of meniscal preservation and partial meniscectomy are gaining acceptance due to the decreased incidence of subsequent degenerative joint disease and the maintenance of joint stability.[51,99-105] In children and adolescents every effort should be made to preserve peripherally detached menisci by careful reattachment.

Discoid Lateral Meniscus

Smillie reported only 29 cases of congenital discoid menisci in a series of 1300 meniscectomies.[71] The cause of discoid meniscus and the mechanism of the clicking sound that it produces have only been partially explained. One of the most persistent symptoms of a discoid meniscus is a loud clicking sound produced by flexion and extension of the knee joint. The true incidence of this anomaly is difficult to determine since many progress into adult life without symptoms (Fig. 18-43). Discoid menisci become torn more frequently than their normal lateral counterparts.[106]

Some people believe that the discoid meniscus is caused by the arrest of development of the meniscus *in utero.* Smillie felt that this was simply a reflection of persistence of the

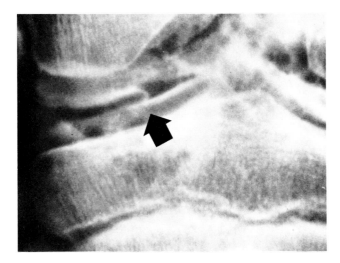

FIG. 18-43. Arthrogram showing discoid lateral meniscus (arrow).

normal fetal state of development from a cartilaginous disc. He felt that there were three types: the primitive, the intermediate, and the infantile.[71]

Kaplan studied human fetal material, stillborns, premature, and full-term infants, and conclusively demonstrated that the menisci did not, in any phase of development, normally assume a discoid shape and concluded that the discoid meniscus was a definite pathologic entity.[107] He also observed that human discoid menisci were hypermobile since they lacked the normal attachment posteriorly and that the meniscofemoral ligament represented the only posterior attachment. This may also allow sufficient abnormal motion to cause the snapping sensation.

In an embryologic note, Ross reviewed the literature and stated that the occurrence of discoid cartilage was due to the persistence of a fetal state.[108] However, others have failed to show any embryologic evidence suggesting that undifferentiated middle mesenchyme normally goes on to form a complete disc of fibrocartilage, the central portion of which is later absorbed to produce the adult semilunar form.

Heplin, in an extensive embryologic study, came to the conclusion that at no time in the development of the human fetus do the lateral or medial menisci assume a discoid form.[108] He also did an extensive comparative study that included various primates and did not find any structures that could be termed a congenital discoid meniscus, although in several animals the lateral meniscus was circular. He also found that at operation on individuals with discoid menisci, there was no attachment at the posterior horn to the tibial plateau. Instead of this attachment there was a continuous Wrisberg's ligament or meniscofemoral ligament that formed a link between the posterior horn in the meniscus and the medial condyle of the femur, a situation that was a normal arrangement observed in all animals except man. He further felt that the discoid form developed gradually after birth as a result of abnormal motion of the lateral meniscus. The hypertrophied meniscus actually varied in shape, but has been termed discoid.

Nathan emphasized the importance of mechanical factors in association with failure of the posterior horn of the discoid meniscus to attach to the lateral intercondylar tubercle of

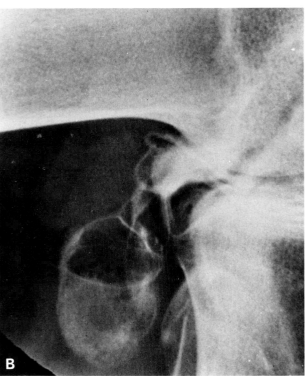

FIG. 18-44. *A,* Popliteal cyst (arrow) in an 8-year-old girl who underwent three previous cyst excisions. While unusual in children, the arthrogram demonstrated continuity between cyst and joint, but no meniscal damage was evident. *B,* Arthrogram in a 14-year-old with chronic knee effusion. No meniscal tears were evident. The cyst was excised and the posterior capsular tear repaired; the symptoms were completely relieved and effusions ended.

the tibia, resulting in abnormal motility, compression, and deformation into the discoid shape.[109] With continued stress, the meniscus interferes with normal knee mechanics.

The mere presence of such an anomaly is *not* a sufficient indication for excision, nor are symptoms such as a clicking knee. As with traumatized menisci, there should be a significant reason for removing a discoid meniscus. Chronic locking of the knee, chronic joint effusion, or chronic pain should be indications.

Popliteal Cysts

These cysts are often found in children, but are usually believed to represent non-articular lesions stemming from bursal enlargement in the popliteal fossa. Figure 18-44 shows a recurrent cyst in an 8-year-old girl with joint laxity. Repeated surgical excisions had been followed by recurrences. Following the arthrogram, the posterior capsular communication was exposed and repaired. She has not had any subsequent recurrence.

Charcot Knee

In children with a sensory neuropathy, no matter what the underlying neurologic deficiency, chronic changes may result from seemingly normal use because of the inability to perceive pain in the knee region. Figure 18-45 shows the knee in a 13-year-old boy with congenital sensory neuropa-

thy, but intact motor function. He developed lateralization of the femur on the tibia following a type of fracture through the medial condyle. This led to further destructive changes and eventually necessitated knee arthrodesis.

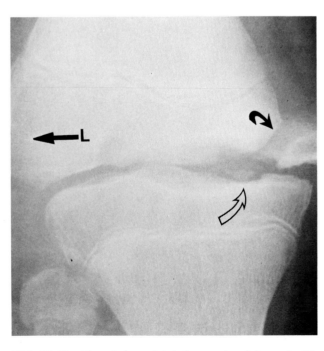

FIG. 18-45. Chronic knee joint changes in adolescent with congenital sensory neuropathy. A type 7 osteochondral fracture (curved arrow) of the medial femoral condyle has allowed lateralization (L) of the distal femur. The medial collateral ligament was intact. A loose body is evident (open arrow).

References

1. George, G. R.: Bilateral bipartite patella. Br. J. Surg., *22*:555, 1935.
2. Oetteking, B.: Anomalous patellae. Anat. Rec., *23*:269, 1922.
3. Ruggles, G.: Bilateral bipartite patellae. Br. J. Surg., *22*:555, 1935.
4. Lanscourt, J. E., and Cristini, J. A.: Patella alta and patella infera. J. Bone Joint Surg., *57-A*:1112, 1975.
5. Cross, M. J., and Waldrop, J.: The patellar index as a guide to the understanding and diagnosis of patellofemoral instability. Clin. Orthop., *110*:174, 1975.
6. Kennedy, J. C. (ed.): The Injured Adolescent Knee. Baltimore, Williams & Wilkins, 1979.
7. Bullough, P. G., Muneura, L., Murphy, J., and Weinstein, A. M.: The strength of the menisci of the knee as it relates to their fine structure. J. Bone Joint Surg., *52-B*:564, 1970.
8. Cameron, H. U., and MacNab, I.: The structure of the meniscus of the human knee joint. Clin. Orthop., *89*:215, 1972.
9. Inorre, H., Isomaki, A. M., and Oka, M.: Scanning electron microscopic studies. Acta Rheum. Scand., *17*:187, 1971.
10. Ogden, J. A., Albright, J. A., and Ettelson, D. M.: An apparent loose body in the knee. Clin. Orthop., *103*:33, 1974.
11. DeLee, J. C.: Complete dislocation of the knee in a nine-year-old. Contemp. Orthop., *1(6)*:29, 1979.
12. Gartland, J. J., and Brenner, J. H.: Traumatic dislocations in the lower extremity in children. Orthop. Clin. North Am., *7*:687, 1976.
13. Dart, C. H., Jr., and Braitman, H. E.: Popliteal injury following fracture of dislocation at the knee. Diagnosis and management. Arch. Surg., *112*:969, 1977.1575.
14. Green, N. E., and Allen, B. L.: Vascular injuries associated with dislocation of the knee. J. Bone Joint Surg., *59-A*:236, 1977.
15. McManus, F., Rang, M., and Heslin, D. J.: Acute dislocation of the patella in children. A natural history. Clin. Orthop., *139*:88, 1979.
16. Brady, T. A., and Russell, D.: Interarticular horizontal dislocation of the patella. J. Bone Joint Surg., *47-A*:1393, 1965.
17. Donelson, R. G., and Tomaiuoli, M.: Intra-articular dislocation of the patella. J. Bone Joint Surg., *61-A*:615, 1979.
18. Frangakis, E. K.: Intra-articular dislocation of the patella. A case report. J. Bone Joint Surg., *56-A*:423, 1974.
19. Insall, J., and Salvati, E.: Patella position in the normal knee joint. Radiology, *101*:101, 1971.
20. Rosenthal, R. K., and Levine, D. B.: Fragmentation of the distal pole of the patella in spastic cerebral palsy. J. Bone Joint Surg., *59-A*:934, 1977.
21. Rang, M.: Children's Fractures. Philadelphia, J. B. Lippincott, 1974.
22. Wolfgang, G. L.: Intraarticular foreign body of the knee. Problems of recognition and treatment. Orthop. Rev., *6*:79, 1977.
23. Abbott, L. C., Saunders, J. B., Bost, F. C., and Anderson, C. E.: Injuries to ligaments of the knee joint. J. Bone Joint Surg., *26*:503, 1944.
24. Fetto, J. F., and Marshall, J. L.: Medial collateral ligament injuries of the knee: a rationale for treatment. Clin. Orthop., *132*:206, 1978.
25. O'Donoghue, D. H.: An analysis of end results of surgical treatment of major injuries to the ligaments of the knee. J. Bone Joint Surg., *37-A*:1, 1955.
26. Palmar, I.: On the injuries to the ligaments of the knee joint. A clinical study. Acta Chir. Scand., [Suppl.] 53, 1938.
27. Shelton, M. L., Neer, C. S., II, and Grantham, S. A.: Occult

knee ligament ruptures associated with fractures. J. Trauma, 11:853, 1971.

28. Hyndman, J. C., and Brown, D. C. S.: Major ligament injuries of the knee in children. Presented at the Canadian Orthopaedic Association, Vancouver, B.C., 1978.

29. Joseph, K. N., and Pogrund, H.: Traumatic rupture of the medial ligament of the knee in a four-year-old boy. J. Bone Joint Surg., 60-A:402, 1978.

30. Bradley, G. W., Shives, T. C., and Samuelson, K. M.: Ligament injuries in the knees of children. J. Bone Joint Surg., 61-A:588, 1979.

31. Clanton, T. O., DeLee, J. C., Sanders, B., and Neidre, A.: Knee ligament injuries in children. J. Bone Joint Surg., 61-A:1195, 1979.

32. Meyers, M. H., and McKeever, F. M.: Fracture of the intercondylar eminence of the tibia. J. Bone Joint Surg., 41-A:209, 1959.

33. Zaricznyj, B.: Avulsion fracture of the tibial eminence: treatment by open reduction and pinning. J. Bone Joint Surg., 59-A:1111, 1977.

34. Noyes, F. A., and Grood, E. S.: The strength of the anterior cruciate ligament in humans and rhesus monkeys. Age-related and species-related changes. J. Bone Joint Surg., 58-A:1074, 1976.

35. Tipton, C. M., Matthes, R. D., and Martin, R. K.: Influence of age and sex on the strength of bone-ligament junctions in knee joints of rats. J. Bone Joint Surg., 60-A:230, 1978.

36. Crowninshield, R. D., and Pope, M. H.: The strength and failure characteristics of rat medial collateral ligaments. J. Trauma, 16:99, 1976.

37. Kennedy, J. C., and Grainger, R. W.: The posterior cruciate ligament. J. Trauma, 7:367, 1976.

38. Mayer, P. J., and Micheli, L. J.: Avulsion of the femoral attachment of the posterior cruciate ligament in an eleven-year-old boy. J. Bone Joint Surg., 61-A:431, 1979.

39. Sanders, W. E., Wilkins, K. E., and Neidre, A.: Acute insufficiency of the posterior cruciate ligament in children. J. Bone Joint Surg., 62-A:129, 1980.

40. Kennedy, J. C., Hawkins, R. J., Willis, R. B., and Danylchuk, K. D.: Tension studies of human knee ligaments. Yield point, ultimate failure, and disruption of the cruciate and tibial collateral ligaments. J. Bone Joint Surg., 58-A:350, 1976.

41. Noyes, F. R., DeLucas, J. L., and Torrik, P. J.: Biomechanics of anterior cruciate ligament failure: an analysis of strain-rate sensitivity and mechanisms of failure in primates. J. Bone Joint Surg., 56-A:236, 1974.

42. Bensahel, H., and Spring, R.: Les fractures de la rotule de l'enfant. J. Chir. (Paris), 99:45, 1970.

43. Springorum, P. W.: Meniskuslasionen bei Jugendlichen. Zentralbl. Chir., 39:1581, 1979.

44. Diebold, O.: Uber Kniescheibenbruche im Kindesalter. Arch. Klin. Chir., 14:664, 1927.

45. Senst, W., and Nowak, W.: Behandlungsergebnisse der Patellafrakturen. Deutsche Gesundheit., 23:433, 1968.

46. Hallopeau, P.: Des certaines Fractures de la Rotule chez l'enfant. J. Med. Paris, 42:927, 1923.

47. Ronget, D.: Deux Cas de Fractures de la Rotule meconnues chez l'enfant. Rev. Chir. [Orthop.], 16:248, 1929.

48. Blazina, M. E., et al.: Jumper's knee. Orthop. Clin. North Am., 4:665, 1973.

49. Sugiura, Y., and Kaneko, F.: Rupture of the patella ligament with avulsion fracture of the lower pole of the patella—a case report. Orthop. Surg., (Tokyo), 23:384, 1972.

50. Weigert, M.: Spontanruptur des Kniescheibenbandes bei Hochspringern. Z. Orthop., 104:429, 1968.

51. Houghton, G. R., and Ackroyd, C. E.: Sleeve fractures of the patella in children. J. Bone Joint Surg., 61-B:165, 1979.

52. Belman, D. A. J., and Nevaiser, R. J.: Transverse fracture of the patella in a child. J. Trauma, 13:917, 1973.

53. Devas, M. B.: Stress fractures of the patella. J. Bone Joint Surg., 42-B:71, 1960.

54. Peterson, L., and Stener, B.: Distal disinsertion of the patellar ligament combined with avulsion fractures at the medial and lateral margins of the patella. Acta Orthop. Scand., 47:680, 1976.

55. Holstein, A., Lewis, G. B., and Schultz, R.: Heterotopic ossification of patellar tendon. Bull. Hosp. Joint Dis., 25:191, 1964.

56. Johansson, S.: En forut icke beskriven sjukdom i patella. Hygiea, 84:161, 1922.

57. Medlar, R. C., and Lyne, E. D.: Sinding-Larsen-Johansson disease. J. Bone Joint Surg., 60-A:1113, 1978.

58. Sinding-Larsen, M. F.: A hitherto unknown affection of the patella. Acta Radiol., 1:171, 1921.

59. Wolf, J.: Larsen-Johansson disease of the patella. Seven new case reports. Its relationship to other forms of osteochondritis. Use of male sex hormones as a new form of treatment. Br. J. Surg., 23:335, 1950.

60. Kaye, J. J., and Freiberger, R. H.: Fragmentation of the lower pole of the patella in spastic lower extremities. Radiology, 101:97, 1971.

61. Roberts, W. M., and Adams, J. P.: The patellar-advancement operation in cerebral palsy. J. Bone Joint Surg., 35-A:958, 1953.

62. Perry, J., Antonelli, D., and Ford, W.: Analysis of knee joint forces during flexed knee stance. J. Bone Joint Surg., 57-A:961, 1975.

63. Dashefsky, J. H.: Fracture of the fabella. J. Bone Joint Surg., 59-A:698, 1977.

64. Ahstrom, J. P.: Osteochondral fracture in the knee joint associated with hypermobility and dislocation of the patella. J. Bone Joint Surg., 47-A:1491, 1965.

65. Bailey, W. H., and Blundell, G. E.: An unusual abnormality affecting both knee joints in a child. J. Bone Joint Surg., 56-A:814, 1974.

66. Coleman, H. M.: Recurrent osteochondral fractures of the patella. J. Bone Joint Surg., 30-B:153, 1948.

67. Rosenberg, N. J.: Osteochondral fractures of the lateral femoral condyle. J. Bone Joint Surg., 46-A:1013, 1964.

68. Green, W. T., and Banks, H. H.: Osteochondritis dissecans in children. J. Bone Joint Surg., 35-A:26, 1953.

69. Landells, J. W.: The reaction of injured human articular cartilage. J. Bone Joint Surg., 39-B:548, 1957.

70. Fairbank, H. A. T.: Internal derangement of the knee in children and adolescents. Proc. R. Soc. Med., 30:427, 1936.

71. Smillie, I. S.: Injuries of the Knee Joint. 4th Ed. New York, Churchill Livingstone, 1970.

72. Aicroth, P.: Osteochondritis dissecans of the knee. A clinical survey. J. Bone Joint Surg., 53-B:440, 1971.

73. Olsson, S. E.: Osteochondros hos hund. Patologi, rontgendiagnostik och klinik. Sv. Vet., 29:577, 1977.

74. Edwards, D. H., and Bentley, G.: Osteochondritis dissecans patellae. J. Bone Joint Surg., 59-B:58, 1977.

75. Scapinelli, R.: Blood supply of the human patella. J. Bone Joint Surg., 49-B:56, 1967.

76. Kahn, B.: Foreign body (palm thorn) in knee joint. Clin. Orthop., 135:104, 1978.

77. Karshner, R. G., and Hanafee, W.: Palm thorns as a cause of joint effusion in children. Radiology, 60:592, 1953.

78. Sugarman, M., et al.: Plant thorn synovitis. Arthritis Rheum., 20:1125, 1977.

79. Harty, M., and Joyce, J. J., III: Synovial folds in the knee joint. Orthop. Rev., 6:91, 1977.

80. Barucha, E.: Meniskurisse bei kinder. Z. Orthop., 102:430, 1967.

81. Baryluk, K., Oblonczek, G., and Zolmowski, J.: Kriegelenk meniskusverletzungen im kindesalter mit Berucksiontigung der Nachuntersuchungen. Arch. Orthop. Unfallchir., 87:65, 1977.

82. Bhadurt, T., and Glass, A.: Menisectomy in children. Injury, 3:176, 1972.

83. Cotta, H.: Kindlicher Meniscusschaden. Hefte Unfallheilkd., 128:59, 1976.

84. Schettler, G.: Beitrag zum Meniskusschaden im Kindesalter. Z. Orthop., 110:443, 1972.

85. Schulitz, K. P.: Meniscusverletzungen im Kindes-und Jugen-dalter. Arch. Orthop. Unfallchir., 76:195, 1973.

86. Smith, L.: A concealed injury to the knee. J. Bone Joint Surg., 44-A:1659, 1962.

87. Spalding, C. B.: Patellar fracture in child two years old. Int. Clin., 4:245, 1918.

88. Vahvanen, V., and Aalto, K.: Menisectomy in children. Acta Orthop. Scand., 50:791, 1979.

89. Saddawi, N. D., and Hoffman, B. K.: Tear of the attachment of a normal medial meniscus of the knee in a four-year-old child. J. Bone Joint Surg., 52-A:809, 1970.

90. Ritchie, D. M.: Menisectomy in children. Aust. N. Z. J. Surg., 35:239, 1965.

91. Volk, H., and Smith, F. M.: "Bucket-handle" tear of the medial meniscus in a five-year-old boy. J. Bone Joint Surg., 35-A:234, 1953.

92. Abrams, R. C.: Meniscus lesions of the knee in young children. J. Bone Joint Surg., 35-A:194, 1957.

93. Schlonsky, J., and Eyring, E. J.: Lateral meniscus tears in young children. Clin. Orthop., 97:117, 1973.

94. Zaman, M., and Leonard, M. A.: Menisectomy in children: a study of fifty-nine cases. J. Bone Joint Surg., 60-B:436, 1978.

95. Fowler, P. J., and Brock, R. M.: Meniscal lesions in the adolescent. Presented at the annual meeting. American Academy of Orthopaedic Surgeons, Las Vegas, Nev., 1977.

96. Dalinka, M. K., Brennan, R. E., and Canino, C.: Double contrast knee arthrography in children. Clin. Orthop., 125:88, 1977.

97. Moes, C. A. F., and Munn, J. D.: The value of knee arthrography in children. J. Can. Assoc. Radiol., 16:226, 1965.

98. Stenstrom, B.: Diagnostic arthrography of traumatic lesions of the knee joint in children. Ann. Radiol., 18:391, 1975.

99. Appel, H.: Late results after meniscectomy in the knee joint. A clinical and roentgenologic follow-up investigation. Acta Orthop. Scand. [Suppl.], 133, 1970.

100. Cargill, A. O., and Jackson, J. P.: Bucket handle tear of the medial meniscus. A case for conservative surgery. J. Bone Joint Surg., 58-A:248, 1976.

101. Hsieh, H. H., and Walker, P. S.: Stabilizing mechanisms of the loaded and unloaded knee joint. J. Bone Joint Surg., 58-A:87, 1976.

102. Krause, W. R., Pope, M. H., Johnson, R. J., and Wilder, D. G.: Mechanical changes in the knee after meniscectomy. J. Bone Joint Surg., 58-A:599, 1976.

103. McGinty, J. B., Geuss, L. F., and Marvin, R. A.: Partial or total meniscectomy. A comparative analysis. J. Bone Joint Surg., 59-A:763, 1977.

104. Oretrop, N., Alm, A., Ekstrom, H., and Gillquist, J.: Immediate effects of meniscectomy on the knee joint. The effects of tensile load on knee joint ligaments in dogs. Acta Orthop. Scand., 49:407, 1978.

105. Price, C. T., and Allen, W. C.: Ligament repair in the knee with preservation of the meniscus. J. Bone Joint Surg., 60-A:61, 1978.

106. Hall, F. M.: Arthrography of the discoid lateral meniscus. A. J. R., 128:993, 1977.

107. Kaplan, E. B.: Discoid lateral meniscus of the knee joint. J. Bone Joint Surg., 39-A:77, 1957.

108. Ross, J. K., Tough, I. C. K., and English, T. A.: Congenital discoid cartilage. Report of a case of discoid medial cartilage, with an embryological note. J. Bone Joint Surg., 40-B:262, 1958.

109. Nathan, P. A., and Cole, S. C.: Discoid meniscus. Clin. Orthop., 64:107, 1969.

19

Tibia and Fibula

Anatomy

Proximal tibia

The proximal tibia epiphysis usually forms a secondary ossification center during the first to third postnatal months. This centrally located ossification process progressively expands in response to both biologic growth and knee biomechanics (Fig. 19-1). If significant genu varum, a relatively normal state for the neonate, persists beyond the development of active ambulation, the secondary center may exhibit irregular marginal ossification, particularly at the medial side. Although this area may appear "damaged" in the child presenting with knee trauma, such ossification patterns usually represent biologic variation (Fig. 19-2). The ossification center is slightly conical centrally as it extends toward the tibial spines and becomes more prominent in late childhood and adolescence (Fig. 19-2C), commensurate with increasing susceptibility to avulsion fractures of the tibial spines.

Throughout development the plane of the articular surface (plateau) normally tilts backwards about 15 to 20° (Fig. 19-3). Accordingly, special angled views may be necessary to rule out intra-articular extension of fractures, although this may only be helpful during adolescence when the ossification center is sufficiently developed to have extensive subchondral bone associated with each plateau. During the reduction of proximal tibial epiphyseal fractures, consideration must be given to this retrograde tilt. Failure to restore this angle leaves the tibia in relative recurvatum and may have an adverse effect on subsequent development, especially if the injury occurs in a young child (Fig. 19-4).

Both the lateral and medial collateral ligaments are firmly attached into portions of the distal femoral epiphysis, such that various stresses applied to the knee are partially dissipated through the distal femoral epiphysis and physis. The fibular collateral ligament has some attachment directly into the tibial epiphysis, but primarily attaches to the proximal fibular epiphysis, with some fibers spreading out over the lateral side of the tibial epiphysis and metaphysis.[1] It is usually taught that the medial collateral ligament has only a small area of attachment directly into the epiphysis, with the major portion of the ligament attached directly into the me-

taphysis under the pes anserinus, and that such an anatomic structure protects the proximal tibia from major epiphyseal injuries. *This is not true.* As shown in Figure 19-5, there are dense attachments of the ligaments and capsule into the epiphyseal perichondrium both medially and laterally. In the last stages of postnatal development the ligaments attach directly into the periosteum and the expanded epiphyseal ossification center. It is more likely that the overall anatomic configuration of the proximal tibial physis, muscular attachments (e.g., gastrocnemius, biceps, medial hamstrings), and angular moment arms are the important factors in the relative failure rates of distal femoral and proximal tibial physes.

The combination of epiphyses and external (collateral) and internal (cruciate) ligaments creates a moment arm such that when angular or rotatory stress is applied to the lower leg, maximum strains occur at the end of this composite unit—the distal femoral physis. Thus, the more important factor is strain dissipation throughout the chondro-osseous and ligamentous complex, rather than any discrete anatomic attachments of the ligaments to the tibia, fibula, and femur.

Tibial tuberosity

The tibial tuberosity (tubercle) initially develops as a morphologically discrete anterior cartilaginous extension of the proximal tibial epiphysis at about 12 to 15 fetal weeks, at which time there is a concomitant ingrowth of fibrovascular tissue from the zone of Ranvier (Fig. 19-6). By the end of fetal development a well-defined tuberosity is present, although it is still approximately level with the main tibial physis and epiphysis. Distal "migration" is primarily a postnatal phenomenon.

The tuberosity initially does not have a typical growth plate. Several months postnatally a histologically defined physis appears, but this is modified by the replacement of cell columns with constantly changing amounts of fibrocartilage. The physis underlying this tuberosity is initially comprised almost completely of fibrocartilage, rather than the columnar, hypertrophic cellular structure that usually characterizes the growth zone.[1,2] This cellular arrangement may be found in the tuberosity of other animals and is postulated to be a cytoarchitectural modification to resist normal tensile

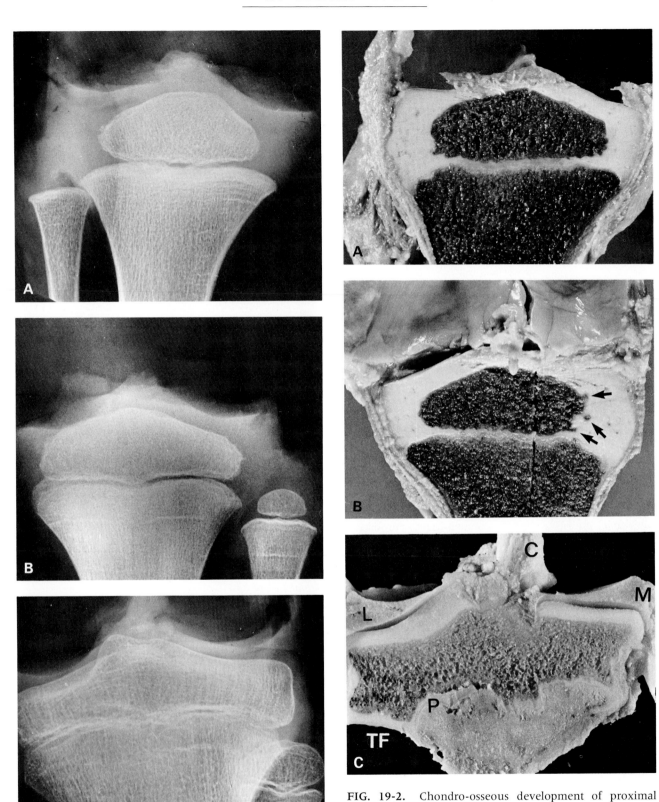

FIG. 19-1. Roentgenographic development of proximal tibia. *A*, 2 years. *B*, 5 years. *C*, 11 years.

FIG. 19-2. Chondro-osseous development of proximal tibia. *A*, Smooth contours in a 6-year-old. *B*, Irregular medial ossification (arrows) in another 6-year-old. *C*, Posterior slab from a 12-year-old showing how tibial spine bone may extend to, or beyond, the articular limits and, perhaps, predispose the tibial spine to avulsion. Note: cruciate ligament (C); lateral meniscus (L); medial meniscus (M); physis (P); proximal tibiofibular joint (TF).

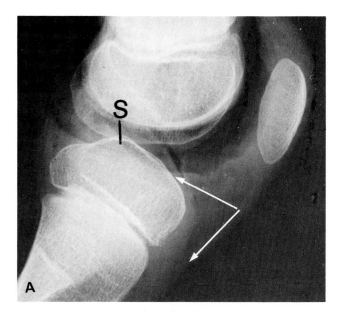

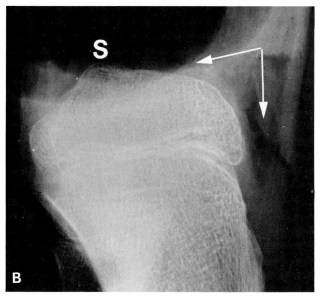

FIG. 19-3. Lateral roentgenographic appearance of proximal tibia. A, Seven years. B, Ten years. Note the retrograde tilt of the tibial articular regions (arrows). Also note how the tibial spine (S) extends beyond the articular planes.

stresses imparted by the quadriceps muscles through the patellar tendon. Near the junction with the proximal tibial physis the cells begin to exhibit some columnar formation (Fig. 19-7).

By 7 to 9 years the tuberosity develops a secondary center of ossification, usually in the most distal region (Figs. 19-8 and 19-9). This gradually enlarges and extends toward the secondary ossification center of the tibia. During adolescence, these two centers are separated by a small cartilaginous bridge, but they eventually coalesce. Concomitant with the osseous maturation that occurs within the cartilage of the tuberosity, the growth plate exhibits a progressive change from fibrocartilage to columnar physeal cartilage,

with gradual extension of the cell columns from the proximal tibial physis toward the tip of the tuberosity, which always retains a fibrocartilaginous tissue mode.

The fibrocartilaginous nature of the tuberosity physis, especially distally, appears to be a biologic response to the imparted tensile stresses. As the tuberosity undergoes progressive secondary ossification, normal tensile stresses are more often dissipated through the entire composite proximal tibial-tuberosity ossification center, rather than the tuberosity, and the histologic structure changes to that more characteristic of a physis.

Coincident with the age-range of susceptibility to Osgood-Schlatter disease, there are major changes in the histologic structure of the distal epiphysis. The cells in the region of the eventual secondary ossification center begin to hypertrophy. Subsequently, ossification begins within this hypertrophic cellular mass. At this point in development these cellular changes anticipatory to and including actual secondary ossification introduce biomechanically responsive tissue changes that may predispose the anterior portion of the tuberosity ossification to failure if excessive tensile stresses are applied. Bone is more likely to fail in tension, although cartilage is more resistant to tension. Major or repetitive stress increases may cause failure of small chondro-osseous areas that normally are subjected to constant tension. These small regions of the pre-ossification center may be avulsed to create, with subsequent maturation of the tissue modes, roentgenographically evident Osgood-Schlatter disease. However, while this anterior failure pattern is occurring, the underlying portions of the distal tuberosity epiphyseal and physeal cartilage remain intact and in close apposition to the metaphysis.

The final step is physiologic epiphysiodesis. The tuberosity epiphyseal center fuses with the main proximal tibial center at 15 years old. The tuberosity physis closes from 13 to 15 years in girls and 15 to 19 years in boys. Like the process in other regions, there are regional modifications. The physis under the proximal tibia closes first, starting centrally and proceeding centrifugally. The region under the tuberosity appears to be the last to close (Fig. 19-10), proceeding in a proximodistal direction along the tuberosity. Therefore, a situation similar to the distal tibia exists. Just as the fracture of Tillaux may occur because of different rates of physiologic epiphysiodesis distally, similar limited failure of the proximal tuberosity may occur. Initial failure in a tuberosity fracture commences at the distal tip of the tuberosity physis and propagates proximally.

During most of the development the patellar tendon has primary attachment into the more distal regions of the tuberosity, as well as adjoining metaphysis. However, with relative distal displacement of the tuberosity during skeletal growth and maturation, the patellar tendon develops a more extensive and proximal insertion on the anterior surface of the tuberosity.

Proximal fibula

The proximal fibula articulates with the tibial epiphysis (Fig. 19-11). The primary functions of the proximal tibiofibular joint appear to be: (1) dissipation of torsional stresses applied at the ankle; (2) dissipation of lateral tibial bending moments; and (3) tensile rather than compressive weight-bearing.

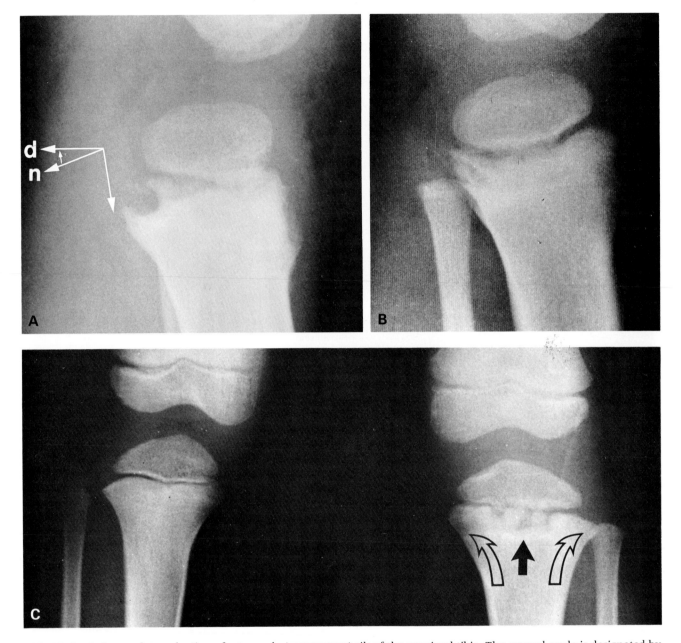

FIG. 19-4. *A,* Incomplete reduction of retrograde (recurvatum) tilt of the proximal tibia. The normal angle is designated by (n) and the deformed angle by (d). Follow-up examination 16 months later showed slowed growth, probably because of an unrecognized type 5 injury. *B,* Lateral view of injured proximal tibia with slowed down central growth, but continued peripheral (latitudinal) development. There has been some correction of the genu recurvatum. *C,* Normal (left) and damaged (right) proximal tibias in AP plane. Again, note the centrally located growth impairment (solid arrow) and more normal latitudinal growth (open arrows) in the damaged tibia.

Some of the collateral ligaments of the proximal tibiofibular joint insert into the epiphysis (specifically, into the perichondrium throughout most of development). This further stabilizes the anatomy of the region and decreases the probability of fracture or displacement. A major factor in stability of the proximal tibiofibular joint is the fibular collateral ligament. With the knee in extension, this ligament holds the fibula tautly in its normal position. With increasing flexion, the ligament becomes relaxed and permits increasing anteroposterior subluxation. In many young children, normal joint laxity permits significant subluxation, even in extension.

There are two basic anatomic types of proximal tibiofibular joints.[1,3] The first is a horizontal articular surface (usually circular and planar) that articulates with a similar planar surface on the tibial epiphysis (Fig. 19-12). These articular surfaces are under and behind a projection of the lateral edge of the tibial epiphysis that provides some anterior stability and prevents significant forward displacement of the fibula. The second type is oblique. These articular surfaces

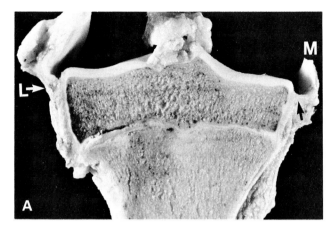

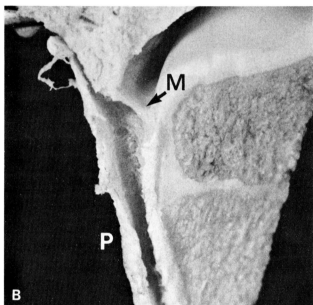

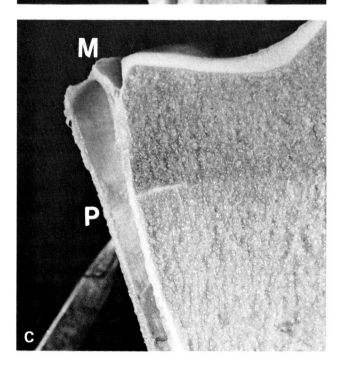

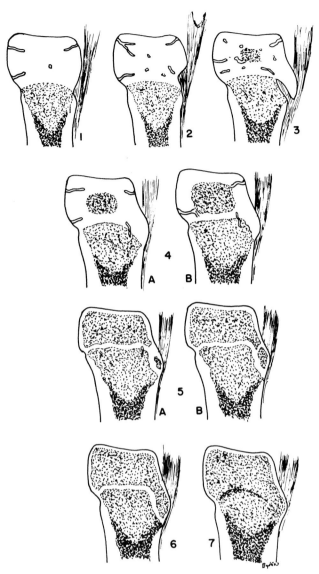

FIG. 19-6.   Schematic of development of tibial tuberosity. *1–3*, Prenatal development. *4–7*, Postnatal development.

FIG. 19-5.   Attachments of capsule and ligaments **directly** into the proximal tibial epiphysis. *A,* Section from a 14-year-old showing deep medial (M) and lateral (L) collateral ligament attachments into the cartilaginous portion of the epiphysis (specifically, the perichondrium), and **not** into the metaphysis. *B,* Section from a 6-year-old showing attachments of medial collateral ligament (M) into the epiphyseal perichondrium. In contrast, the pes anserinus (P) attaches to the metaphyseal/diaphyseal regions. *C,* Similar appearance of medial collateral ligament/meniscus complex and pes anserinus in a 15-year-old. However, due to expansion of the secondary ossification center, the medial collateral ligament now attaches into periosteum rather than perichondrium. The physis is almost completely closed. Note the textural differences between the epiphyseal and the metaphyseal bone.

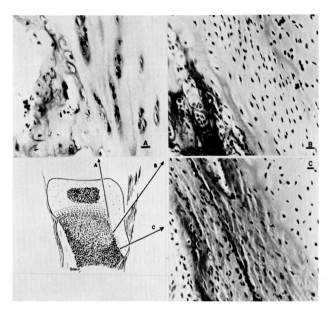

FIG. 19-7. Variable appearance of the physeal cartilage of the tibial tuberosity in childhood. *A,* Modified columnar cartilage. *B,* Fibrocartilage. *C,* Fibrous tissue.

allows a greater degree of rotation before disruption. The horizontal type is associated with increased rotatory mobility and increased joint surface area. The oblique type is associated with less rotatory mobility and less joint surface area, and therefore is more susceptible to displacement.

The proximal fibular epiphysis begins secondary ossification at 2 to 4 years. There are no significant variations that mimic fracture patterns, and the protected location makes injury to the epiphysis among the rarest of all epiphyseal injuries. The lateral collateral ligament and biceps tendon attachments may lead to avulsion of a portion of the proximal fibula (type 3 or 4 injury). Physeal closure occurs at 15 years in boys and 14 years in girls.

Tibiofibular shafts

The metaphyseal regions undergo typical changes comparable to other long bones (Fig. 19-13). However, the tibial diaphysis must undergo major changes that lead to the thickened cortex characteristic of this bone. This requires extensive remodeling to create biomechanically responsive Haversian systems (Fig. 19-14). Different fracture patterns relate to the degree of development and maturation of this cortical remodeling system. The toddler's fracture of the proximal tibial metaphysis shortly after inception of weight-bearing is a classic example of this.

Distal tibia

The secondary ossification center of the distal tibial epiphysis generally appears during the second year. The medial malleolus ossifies as a downward prolongation from this main center, generally about 7 years in girls and 8 years in boys (Figs. 19-15 and 19-16). By 14 to 15 years, the entire

are more variable in area, configuration, and inclination. The more oblique the joint, the less the overall amount of articular surface. These latter joint configurations are more often associated with disruption (subluxation or dislocation).

The biomechanics of fibular rotation necessary to accommodate ankle motion are such that the more horizontal joint

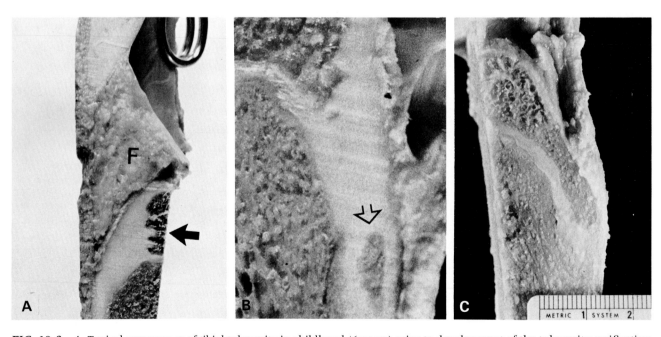

FIG. 19-8. *A,* Typical appearance of tibial tuberosity in childhood (6 years) prior to development of the tuberosity ossification center. The proximal tibial epiphyseal ossification center is present (arrow). Also note the large fat pad (F) behind the patellar tendon. *B,* The ossification center initially appears in the distal portion (arrow) of the tibial tuberosity. *C,* Appearance of fused proximal tibial and tuberosity centers in a 12-year-old.

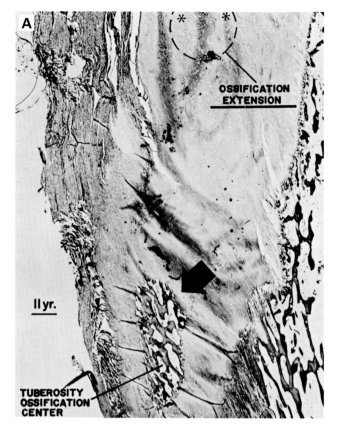

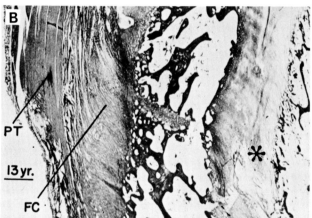

FIG. 19-9. *A,* Histologic appearance of early tuberosity ossification center (arrow) at 11 years. Extension of ossification (*) from the main tibial ossification center is evident. *B,* Subsequent development, at 13 years, showing how patellar tendon (PT) grades into the ossification center. Fibrocartilage (FC) blends from the tendon into the tuberosity ossification center. The histologic appearance of this is similar to the appearance of the fibrocartilage between the tuberosity and metaphysis (*).

distal epiphysis, including the malleolus, is ossified and from 16 to 18 years it unites to the metaphysis.

The initial physeal contour is transverse. However, an anteromedial undulation develops within the first 18 to 24 months (see Figs. 19-16*B* and 19-18*B*). This structural change

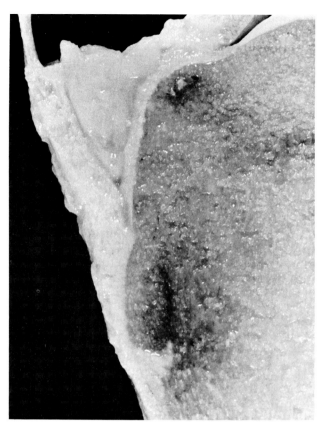

FIG. 19-10. Closure of tibial tuberosity. The last area to close is the fibrous tissue and fibrocartilage at the distal end, a factor that may predispose the tuberosity to fracture in late adolescence.

effectively divides the distal tibial epiphysis into lateral and medial areas, and may have a significant effect upon fracture patterns.

The medial malleolus may occasionally develop a separate center of ossification comparable to the one sometimes found in the tip of the greater trochanter (Fig. 19-17). The incidence and significance of accessory centers of ossification in the foot have been well investigated (see Chap. 20), but

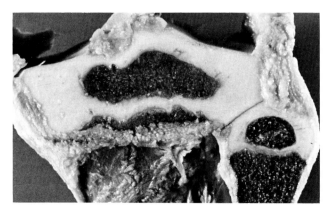

FIG. 19-11. Proximal tibiofibular relationships in a six-year-old.

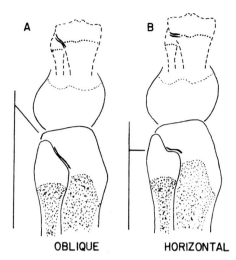

FIG. 19-12. Two basic types of proximal tibiofibular joint. *A*, Oblique. *B*, Horizontal.

similar variations in the malleolar regions have received little attention. Most reports include one or two cases and imply that such centers are infrequent. In contrast, Powell and Hoed described accessory ossification centers of the medial malleolus as being present in 14% of the children studied, and concluded that an accessory center of ossification of the medial malleolus, and, to a lesser extent, the lateral malleolus, is probably a relatively common developmental variation.[4,5] Their figures may be relatively low, as these variations are generally found only when evaluating trauma to the ankle.

Bilateral accessory centers may be found in some children. Histologically there is a bipolar physis between the secondary and accessory centers. Most appear to fuse to the main distal tibial ossification center during adolescence, although they may infrequently remain as a radiologically, but not anatomically separate entity into adult life. Since these accessory centers are found most often in the evaluation of acute trauma, they may be mistaken for fractures. The

smooth appearance should obviate this diagnosis. However, fractures can and do occur through this region (a type 7 growth mechanism injury), so that an acutely symptomatic patient with an irregularity in this region, rather than a smooth-bordered ossification, should be considered and treated as a fracture patient.

Closure of the distal tibial physis shows a fairly characteristic pattern. Epiphysiodesis initially involves the medial portion, including the aforementioned undulation. The lateral portion begins fusion later (Fig. 19-16). The distal tibial growth plate closes from medial to lateral over a 1½-year period between 13 to 18 years of age. If the ligaments remain intact during a severe external rotation stress to the adolescent ankle, a fracture can occur through the unfused lateral portion of the distal growth plate and cause a fracture of Tillaux or triplane fracture.

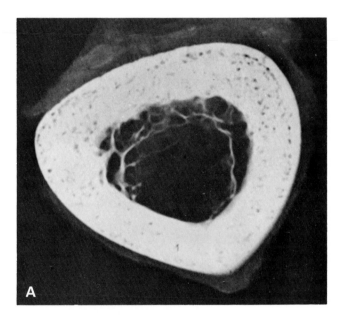

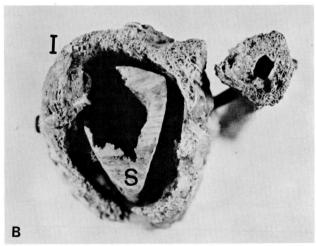

FIG. 19-14. *A*, The dense, thickened, triangular-shaped cortex is characteristic of the tibial diaphysis. *B*, Osteomyelitis specimen showing dense tibial diaphyseal cortex, which has formed a sequestrum (S), and an involucrum (I), or new surrounding cortex.

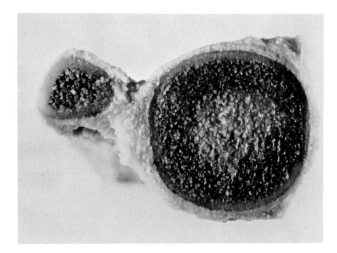

FIG. 19-13. Typical appearance of cross section of proximal tibia and fibula at the metaphyseal level.

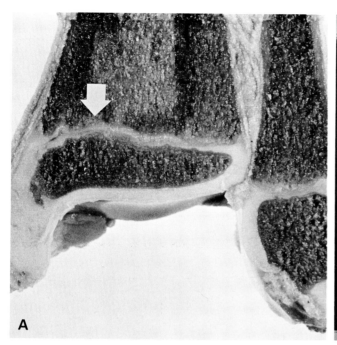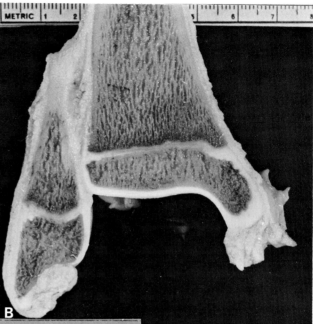

FIG. 19-15. Gross appearance of the distal tibia and fibula at, *A*, 6 years and, *B*, 11 years. Note how the fibular physis is level with the tibial articular surface. Also note the medial undulation in *A* (arrow).

Distal fibula

The distal fibula develops an ossification center during the second to third years. The distal fibular epiphysis may also exhibit irregular ossification at the tip and show significant undulation of the physis (Fig. 19-18). Both factors may lead to a mistaken diagnosis of fracture.

Syndesmosis

The ankle is stabilized by the anterior and posterior tibiofibular ligaments and the distal continuation of the interosseous membrane. The distal tibia and fibula have a mobile articulation that allows fibular rotation during ankle dorsiflexion-plantarflexion. The apposed tibial and fibular epiphyseal contours curve slightly to create a small joint (Fig. 19-19). The synovium extends into this joint to the level of the tibial physis, above which the syndesmosis is present. The distal tibiofibular relationships are such that the distal fibular physis is usually level with either the tibial articular surface or the lower limits of the tibial ossification center (Fig. 19-15).

Tibial Spine Injuries

Avulsion of the anterior tibial spine is an unusual injury in children.[6-11] Bicycle, automobile, and athletic injuries appear to be the main causes.

The anterior cruciate ligament attaches to the base of the anterior spine, as well as to a slip of the anterior horn of the medial meniscus. The ligament does not attach completely onto the tibial spine, but also attaches anterior and lateral to it.[12,13] This attachment may be stressed by a force that would probably lead to an isolated tear of the anterior cruciate liga-ment in an adult. However, in most children, the incompletely ossified tibial spine, compared to the ligament and its dense chondral (perichondral) attachments, is the weakest point to excessive tensile stress, so failure usually occurs through the cancellous bone immediately beneath the subchondral plate.[12]

Jones and Smith pointed out that not all fractures of the tibial spine are the result of cruciate ligament avulsion, as initially proposed by Pringle.[14,15] Kennedy and co-workers found only 2 cases of bone avulsion in 50 patients with specific anterior cruciate ligament injury.[16] However, more recent studies strongly suggest that the chondro-osseous fragment of the skeletally immature patient has some of the anterior cruciate ligament attached to it.

Classification

Based upon a review of 70 fractures, 47 of which involved children, Meyers and McKeever presented a concise classification scheme that related closely to recommended treatment modalities (Fig. 19-20).[8] In their classification, type 1 is minimal displacement of the fragment from the remainder of the proximal tibial ossification center. Type 2 is displacement (angular elevation) of the anterior one third to one half of the avulsed fragment, which produces a beak-like appearance on the lateral roentgenogram. Type 3 is complete separation of the avulsed segment from the remainder of the ossification center with no bone-to-bone apposition. Types 1 and 2 accounted for 80% of the cases. Of 14 patients with type 3 injuries, 10 were children.[8] Zaricznyj further classified type 3 into A and B categories, A having the fragment aligned relatively normally, albeit displaced, and B having the fragment angulated.[11] An additional type 4 lesion was a comminuted fracture. All these types represent variations of a type 7 growth mechanism injury (see Chap. 4).

Diagnosis

It is essential to obtain AP and lateral roentgenograms to adequately visualize the degree of displacement of the fragment (Figs. 19-21 to 19-23). Furthermore, a special AP view paralleling the normal posterior tilt of the proximal tibial articular surface may help visualize minimally displaced fractures. Since these injuries are intra-articular, there may be a significant hemarthrosis.

Garcia and Neer reported a series of 42 tibial spine fractures in patients ranging from 7 to 60 years old.[7] Only 6 had a positive anterior drawer sign, and *all* had concomitant collateral ligament tears. Clanton agreed that a positive anterior drawer sign in the presence of avulsion of the tibial spine was most likely indicative of an associated tear of the collateral ligament. Other authors did not report anterior instability in cases of pure tibial spine avulsion.[9,11]

Treatment

According to Borch-Madsen, closed reduction by hyperextension was first proposed by Clark.[6] Bakalim used this method in 10 cases, reporting fair to good results in 7 of 8 patients with adequate follow-up.[17] None of the children had any evidence of shortening of the anterior cruciate ligament, but a number of them did complain of slight anteroposterior instability. Smillie believed that closed reduction with hyperextension could be accomplished only if the fragment was large.[18]

Since the intercondylar space is wide, there can be no direct apposition of the surfaces of the femoral condyles against the tibial fragment to provide compression. However, the large infrapatellar fat pad (see Fig. 19-8) may act as a space-occupying, elastic cushion pushing against the fragment in hyperextension. In contrast, Meyers and McKeever

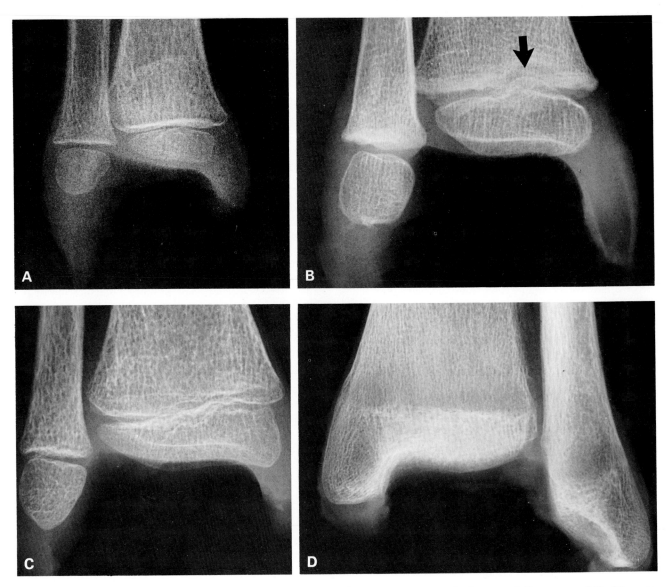

FIG. 19-16. Roentgenographic appearance of distal tibia and fibula at, *A,* 3 years; *B,* 4 years; *C,* 7 years; and *D,* 15 years. Again, note the development of the medial undulation *B* (arrow). In *D,* note that the physeal remnant is less evident medially. This medial to lateral closure pattern is undoubtedly a factor in distal tibial fracture patterns.

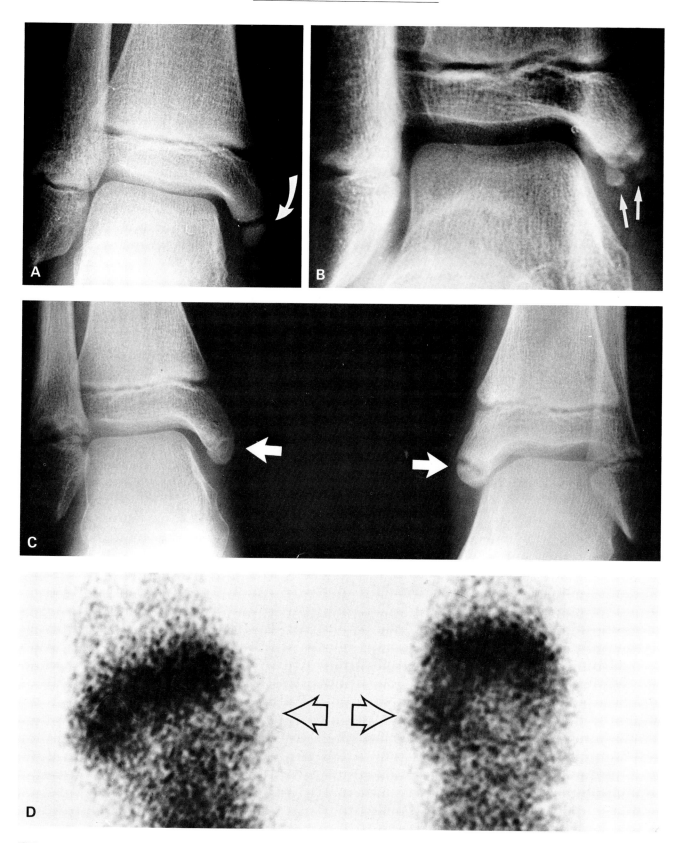

FIG. 19-17. *A,* Accessory ossification (arrow) at medial malleolar tip. *B,* Variation showing multifocal ossification (arrows). *C,* Patient with bilateral involvement (arrows). The center has coalesced on the right (where there is also a distal fibular fracture), but it is still open on the left. *D,* Bone scan of the patient shown in *C* shows increased uptake (arrows), suggesting these lesions may be injured.

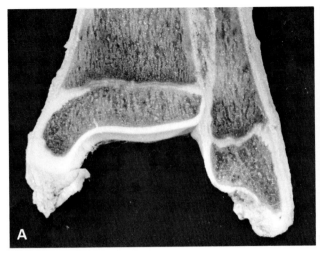
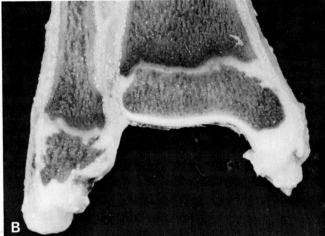

FIG. 19-18. *A*, Undulated contour of the distal fibular physis contrasted with the transverse contour of the distal tibia. *B*, Irregular contour of distal fibula. The distal tibia is also undulated and shows the characteristic medial "rise."

recommended cast immobilization with the knee in 20% of flexion, without any manipulation, for all type 1 and 2 fractures.[9] They felt that hyperextension did not improve the roentgenographic appearance in any of their patients, and it worsened the situation in one (converting a type 2 fracture to a type 3 fracture).

Most type 1 and 2 fractures of the intercondylar region of the proximal tibia do not require arthrotomy and open reduction in the child or adolescent. Excellent results, without any residual instability, may be anticipated from protective immobilization in mild flexion (no more than 20°). Follow-up roentgenograms should be taken within 10 days to be certain that the fragment does not displace. The cast should be maintained for 6 to 8 weeks. The foot should be included

in the cast to discourage walking and possible rotatory stresses that might displace the fragment.

In contrast, type 3 injuries treated by closed reduction have a high incidence of poor results, characterized by locking, chronic effusion, loss of normal range of motion, moderate pain, and complaints of intermittent collapse with strenuous activity (Fig. 19-24). When the fragment is completely separated from the underlying epiphyseal ossification center, arthrotomy, open reduction, and internal fixation are recommended. The best reduction, even with the knee open, was evident at 20° of flexion. The fragment should be placed back in anatomic position and retained by sutures that may be placed in the anterior cruciate ligament, the edges of the fragment, and the edge of the anterior horn of

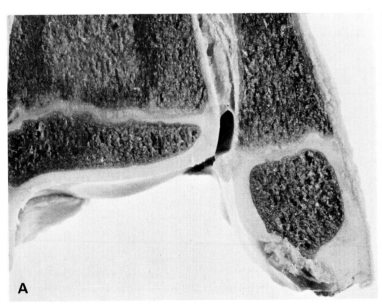
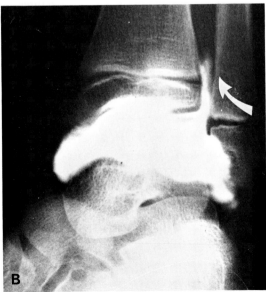

FIG. 19-19. *A*, Extension of synovial recess between tibia and fibula. The syndesmosis stops approximately at the level of the tibial physis. The lateral side of the tibia forms an articular surface juxtaposed to the fibula. *B*, Arthrogram showing this extension toward the proximal tibiofibular joint (arrow).

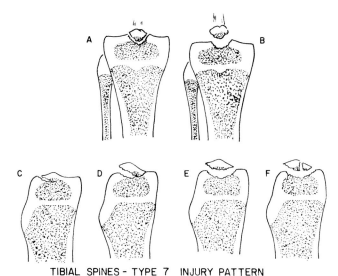

TIBIAL SPINES - TYPE 7 INJURY PATTERN

FIG. 19-20. Classification of types of injury to the tibial spine. These are type 7 growth mechanism injuries (see Chap. 4). *A-B,* Anterior views showing undisplaced and displaced patterns. *C,* Incomplete injury, which is still intact posteriorly. *D,* Complete fracture, which is hinged posteriorly but still undisplaced. *E,* Displaced fragment. *F,* Comminuted fragment.

the medial meniscus. Metallic internal fixation should be avoided. Removing the fragment or the anterior cruciate ligament is not indicated. Zaricznyj found that portions of the anterior horn of either medial or lateral meniscus blocked reduction, but that they could be easily retracted to effect reduction of the spine to anatomic position.[11] He also described a method of pin fixation, introducing them retrograde through the anterior epiphysis (avoiding the patellar tendon). The pins were removed two to three months later.

Results

If the type 3 fragment is not reduced and stabilized, chronic complaints may be expected from the presence of a large intra-articular fragment with, at most, a fibrous nonunion (Fig. 19-24). However, be wary of the radiographic appearance (Fig. 19-25). Apparent nonunion may not be so, and arthrography or arthroscopy should help delineate a need for further operative procedures. Further, since the anterior cruciate ligament contains significant blood vessels, the avulsed fragment may receive sufficient nourishment to "enlarge" considerably. Such an enlarged fragment may significantly impair normal joint mechanics.

Proximal Tibial Epiphyseal Injuries

Although other epiphyseal injuries are reasonably common during childhood, injury of the proximal tibial epiphysis is infrequent and probably constitutes less than 1% of all epiphyseal injuries.[19-31] In 1 series, the average age was 14.2 years and only 1 patient was less than 10 years old at the time of injury.[28]

One of the major factors controlling susceptibility to injury is the anatomic structure of the proximal tibia and the anterior downward extension of the tibial tuberosity. This arrangement appears capable of preventing posterior displacement of the epiphysis relative to the metaphysis and diaphysis. Proximal tibial growth mechanism injury usually occurs either as a varus, a valgus, or a posterior (or combined) displacement of the metaphyseal unit.

It is imperative to adequately evaluate the circulatory status in the region of the knee as well as distal to the knee, since there is significant incidence of injury to the popliteal artery with this particular type of fracture (Fig. 19-26). The problems of ischemic complications and basic approaches to concomitant vascular injuries are discussed in Chapters 7 and 18.

Classification

Virtually all types of growth mechanism injuries may affect the proximal tibia. Type 7 injuries are essentially confined to the tibial spines, but types 1 through 6 may affect the proximal tibial and tibial tuberosity epiphyses and physes (Figs. 19-27 and 19-28).

Most injuries to this region appear to be type 2 with posterolateral or posteromedial displacement of the metaphyseal portion (Fig. 19-29; also see Fig. 19-26). Most type 2 injuries exhibit a typical posterior displacement of the metaphysis with the proximal-distal fracture relationships essentially being in recurvatum. The proximal tibial epiphysis retains its normal relationship to the distal femoral epiphysis, and the tibial shaft is displaced posteriorly with concomitant medial or lateral displacement. Because of the anatomy of the tuberosity, it is rare for a fracture to be associated with anterior displacement of the distal fragment (Fig. 19-30).

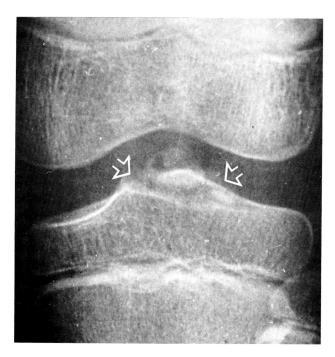

FIG. 19-21. Undisplaced tibial spine fracture (arrows) in a 12-year-old.

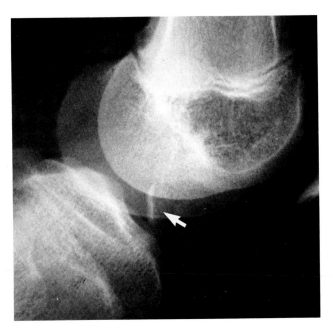

FIG. 19-22. Anteriorly displaced fragment (arrow) in a 14-year-old.

Type 1 injuries are the next most common (Fig. 19-31). They are often difficult to diagnose because of minimal displacement. Because of stresses imparted by flexion contractures, the proximal tibia is frequently involved with type 1 fractures in children with neuromuscular disorders such as myelomeningocele and cerebral palsy (Fig. 19-32), especially when vigorous physical therapy is undertaken to overcome postoperative contractures (see Chap. 8).

Type 3 injuries are less common (Fig. 19-33). The detached epiphyseal fragment is usually unstable and may be significantly displaced. Type 4 injuries are also uncommon (see Fig. 19-28). It is sometimes difficult to diagnose type 4 fractures in younger children when they occur in the unossified portion (see Fig. 19-38). Type 5 injuries can be seen in association with proximal tibial and tibial tuberosity fractures, and may be the result of crushing in that region (see Fig. 19-4).[32,33]

Propagation of the fracture force sometimes leads to a concomitant fracture of the fibular metaphysis or diaphysis (Fig. 19-34).

Diagnosis

Clinical evaluation is important when diagnosing injuries to the proximal tibial epiphysis. Neurovascular status must be evaluated initially and re-evaluated at appropriate intervals. There is usually a high incidence of damage to the popliteal artery (see Fig. 19-26), and it is imperative that this complication be recognized. Absence of major distal pulses should be sought and use of a Doppler may be beneficial. Because of collateral circulation through the geniculate vessels, capillary filling may seem adequate; but such flow may be insufficient for the active, growing child. Damage to the major nerves in the popliteal region is not as frequent. However, when the proximal fibula is also fractured, the peroneal nerve or one of its initial branches may be injured.

In some of these injuries, especially when they occur during adolescence, it may be necessary to do a roentgenographic stress test to find if there is a type 1 or 2 lesion, particularly if there is minimal displacement. In a series of 39 fractures of the proximal tibial epiphyseal cartilage, stress roentgenograms were essential to make the diagnosis in 3 patients.[28] On direct clinical examination, if there is marked instability of the medial side of the knee in an adolescent (particularly in a football player with a history of being tackled or clipped), roentgenograms should be taken in both a relaxed position as well as under stress to distinguish between opening of the joint (ligament injury or laxity) versus opening of a physeal fracture.

Treatment

Closed reduction should be performed initially in all type 2 fractures and the lower limb should be immobilized for a period of 4 to 6 weeks. It is important to get as accurate an anatomic reduction as possible, remembering that the direction of the proximal tibial articular surfaces is angled slightly downward posteriorly relative to the longitudinal axis of the

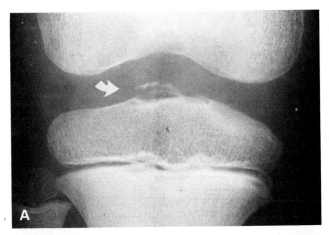

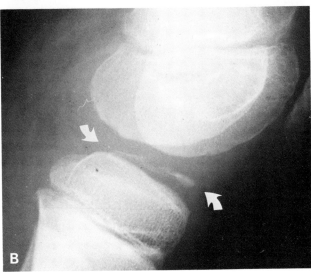

FIG. 19-23. *A-B,* Avulsion of large fragment (arrows), best evident in the lateral view (*B*).

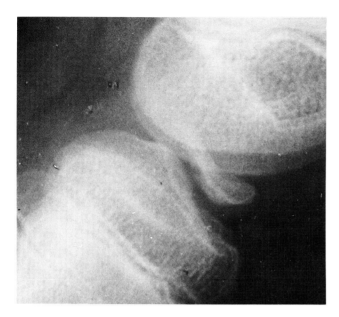

FIG. 19-24. Overgrowth of fragment treated initially by closed reduction. The patient was asymptomatic, but had moderate anterior instability.

shaft. Trying to align the joint surface or epiphysis perpendicular to the shaft may result in a functional recurvatum that may not correct spontaneously with growth, especially if there is a type 5 component (see Fig. 19-4). A mild degree of posterior displacement of the metaphysis may be acceptable. An alternative is placement in skeletal traction with gradual correction of deformity (Fig. 19-35).

Many reports agree on the problem of instability of these fractures, even the type 2 injuries, and the difficulty experienced in maintaining the initial reduction. If it is not possible to affect an adequate reduction, some type of skeletal fixation performed either surgically or percutaneously under fluoroscopy (image-intensification) should be attempted (Fig. 19-36). If there is a large metaphyseal fragment, it may be possible to transfix the two portions of the metaphysis to stabilize the fracture, thus avoiding crossing the physis or epiphysis with wires. The wires should be removed as soon as possible after fracture healing.

Type 3 injuries require open reduction, precise anatomic replacement, and internal fixation with either a malleolar-type compression screw or a transepiphyseal bolt (Fig. 19-37). Similar operative procedures are also indicated in type 4 fractures, even when the fragments are minimally displaced, in order to minimize risks of premature epiphysiodesis (Fig. 19-38).

Results

The results of adequate treatment of this type of fracture are generally good. The majority do not involve the joint, thus knee joint mechanics are good. However, an increase in varus, valgus, or recurvatum may alter mechanics and eventually predispose to joint degeneration. Of 28 fractures in 27 patients with an average follow-up of 7.1 years, there were satisfactory results in 24.[28] Unsatisfactory results in the other 4 patients were due to chronic neurovascular insufficiency, growth disturbance, or traumatic arthritis.

Growth complications

The first complication is the possibility of a localized or complete injury to the proximal physis, which leads to leg-length inequality or angular deformity (Figs. 19-39 to 19-41). Since many of these injuries occur during adolescence, at a time when the child is going through the final phases of growth, major growth deformities are fortunately uncommon. However, younger children have sufficient growth capacity to manifest significant deformities, especially during the pre-adolescent growth spurt (see Fig. 19-4). These children must be followed closely for any evidence of premature growth arrest, so that the physician can be aware of the potential angle of deformity, deficiency of length, and the best methods of correction, as many of these children may eventually require osteotomy, resection of an osseous bridge, or leg-length equalization for improvement.

Premature growth arrest with resultant varus, valgus, or recurvatum deformity frequently accompanies type 3 and 4 injuries, as well as some type 2 injuries. The parents must be warned about this possibility.

While Shelton and Canale mention only 4 unsatisfactory results, it is interesting to note that 7 of the final 28 fractures had a longitudinal growth disturbance of 1 cm or more, representing a 25% incidence of growth retardation.[28] All patients with a growth disturbance had fractures that would be classified as type 1 or 2. Interestingly, no significant longitu-

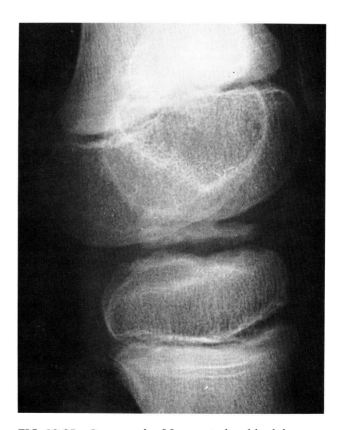

FIG. 19-25. Overgrowth of fragment placed back by open reduction at time of initial injury. A second exploration of the knee revealed that the fragment had healed solidly through fibrous interposition, even though the roentgenogram suggested nonunion.

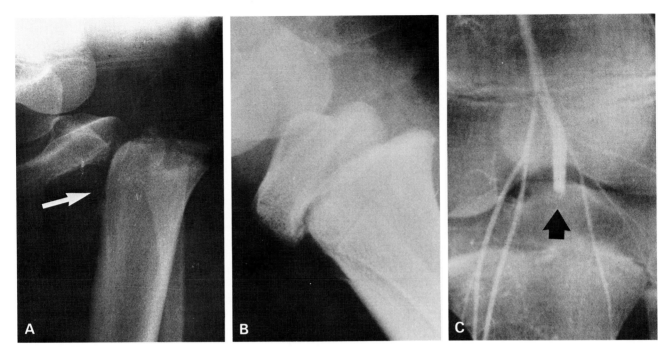

FIG. 19-26. *A,* Anterior displacement of the proximal tibial epiphysis, with corresponding posterior displacement (arrow) of metaphysis. *B,* Initial reduction (closed reduction), which failed to restore distal circulation. *C,* Arteriogram showing complete disruption of the popliteal artery (arrow).

dinal growth disturbances were associated with type 3 or 4 fractures. Only 1 patient had a symptomatic unsatisfactory angular deformity of more than 7°, compared to the uninjured extremity. Although 8 patients had angular discrepancies of 5 to 7°, angular discrepancies of less than 5° were disregarded. Therefore, longitudinal and angular changes consequent to this injury pattern are probably common, but because of the incidence of injury close to the end of skeletal growth, major changes are rare.

The other immediate complications are anterior compartment syndrome, peroneal nerve palsy, and associated ligamentous, meniscal, patellar tendon, and joint capsule injuries. All contribute to the biomechanics of fracture of this particular epiphysis, and all must be treated as indicated.

Vascular complications

The most important complication to recognize in the initial or subsequent evaluations is vascular injury.[34] Two patients in one series required surgery.[28] Curry reported a case in which the proximal tibial epiphysis was anteriorly displaced; the vascular injury was not recognized and the patient subsequently developed gangrene.[23]

Because of the posterior displacement of the distal fragment, there may be impingement, occlusion, intraluminal damage, or variable transection of the popliteal artery. The distal fragment is closely attached to the posterior distal femur and proximal tibia, which renders minimal flexibility during displacement. Further, the distal fragment may directly impinge on the vessel, leading to any of the various types of vascular injury previously discussed in Chapter 7. Most reported cases of proximal tibial injuries associated with vascular damage are hyperextension injuries. Careful

evaluation must be undertaken at frequent intervals to assess the possibility of vascular damage, either as an acute or more insidious chronic problem.

Arteriography is an excellent means of evaluating these injuries (see Fig. 19-26). If damage is found, appropriate repair must be undertaken rapidly. At the same time the frac-

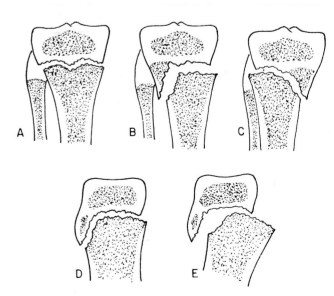

FIG. 19-27. Schematic of, *A,* type 1 and, *B-C,* type 2 injuries. *D* and *E* show undisplaced and displaced fractures. The metaphysis usually displaces posteriorly, with additional varus or valgus angulation.

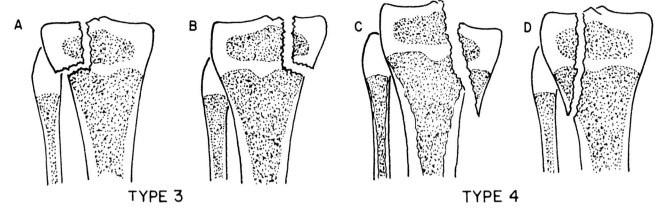

TYPE 3   TYPE 4

FIG. 19-28. Schematic of type 3 and type 4 proximal tibial injuries.

ture should be stabilized by some type of skeletal fixation so as not to jeopardize the vascular repair. Bovill appears to be the first to report the use of arteriography to evaluate damage to the popliteal vessels with this injury.[34] His case was a compound fracture with both posterior and superior displacement of the metaphysis relative to the epiphysis. The initial films showed complete lack of filling of the normal vascular beds of the metaphyseal part of the fracture fragment and the epiphyseal plate. Interestingly, this defect was still present in an arteriogram taken three months after the injury, which demonstrated that there was increased blood supply to the vascular beds about the knee both in the distal femur and proximal tibia, yet not in the metaphyseal fragment. The normal vascular bed was not altered in the small portion of the plate to which a triangular fragment of the metaphysis had remained attached. A subsequent arteriogram three years after injury showed persistent complete

occlusion of the popliteal artery with filling by collateralization. An end-to-end anastomosis of both the artery and vein had been done at the time of injury. The pulse had decreased during the post-operative course over a several week period, and became nonpalpable by six weeks. No attempt was made to re-explore because of the amount of collateral circulation; however, this probably should not have been accepted. In view of the current state of vascular repair, re-exploration should be undertaken to create a functioning artery, particularly in a child. Although Bovill did not describe any vascular insufficiency three years post-injury, the child was only ten and had not gone through her growth spurt. With the anticipated increased functional demands of adolescence there might be a problem with increased functional demand, such as the ischemia commonly associated with activity, but not with rest, in people with progressive adult-onset vascular occlusion.

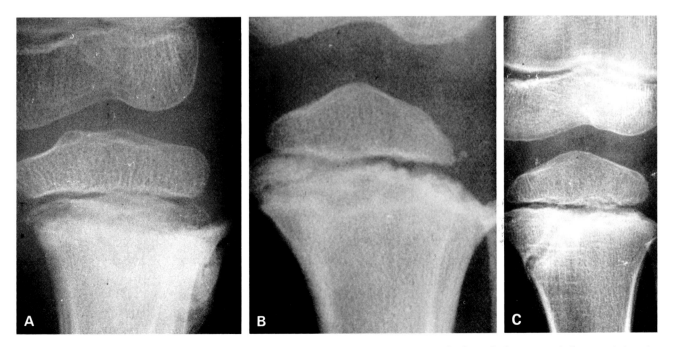

FIG. 19-29. *A,* Lateral type 2 injury with extensive subperiosteal new bone along the lateral tibia. *B,* Medial type 2 injury in a three-year-old. *C,* Medial type 2 injury in a five-year-old.

Tibial Tuberosity Injuries

Avulsion fractures of the tuberosity commonly occur in boys between the ages of 14 and 16.[26,35-39] The distal ligamentous expansion of the insertion of the quadriceps mechanism spreads out like a fan as it approximates the proximal tibial surface. The apophysis of the tuberosity is located within this tendinous expansion. Because of the diffuse insertion of the quadriceps mechanism, and its confluence with more distal soft tissues such as periosteum and pes anserinus, it is rare for the tibial tuberosity to be completely avulsed. Partial avulsion is more frequent and probably represents the majority of cases of Osgood-Schlatter disease, particularly when it is of a more chronic nature.

Acute fracture of the tibial tuberosity is a relatively rare injury, if based upon reported cases. Borch-Madsen described a boy who fell and sustained fractures of both tibial tuberosities that propagated into the knee, which led to concomitant tibial spine fracture-avulsions.[6] Deliyannis described a similar lesion in brothers, each with the onset of injury at about the same chronologic age.[36] Hand et al. reported 7 cases;[37] I and my co-workers recently reported 11 cases, including 1 with simultaneous bilateral injuries.[38]

Classification

Watson-Jones first classified tuberosity injuries into three types. This elementary classification scheme did not suggest propagation into the knee joint, it failed to discuss the problems of such intra-articular extension, it made no mention of the possibility of fragmentation of the avulsed regions, and it did not emphasize degrees of separation of the avulsed portions. Accordingly, the following types and subtypes of injury were proposed (Fig. 19-42).[38]

In type 1 only the more distal portions of the tuberosity are injured. The simplest injury pattern (1A) is a fracture through the tuberosity ossification center with mild anterior displacement of the fragment. Based on operative observations it would seem likely that the soft tissue components are incompletely separated, so that this injury is relatively stable. In the other subtype (1B), the fragment is separated from the metaphysis and may or may not also be separated from the rest of the secondary ossification center. Concomitant soft tissue injury and disruption of continuity are more likely. This type of injury may need open reduction.

The type 2 injury appears to involve the cartilage junction between the two secondary ossification centers, and usually leads to the avulsion of the distal (tuberosity) center. This is probably the failure mode of adolescence, which is analogous to Osgood-Schlatter disease in the earlier age group. The only difference is the tissue level involved. Type 2 injuries involve separation of the entire tuberosity ossification center with variable propagation into the main proximal tibial ossification center. The tuberosity segment may fracture (usually a compression-impaction type of injury) at the junction of the main tibial and tuberosity ossification centers, or propagate through a variable-sized anterior portion of the proximal tibial ossification center. However, there is minimal separation of the two portions of the proximal tibia. Soft tissue disruption is again contingent upon the maximum degree of separation, which may not always be evident in the roentgenogram taken in the emergency room when

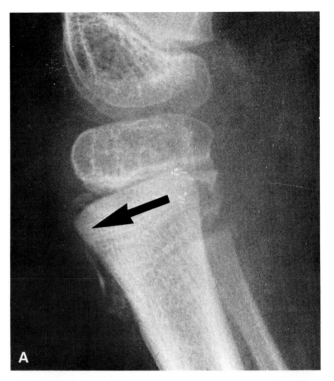

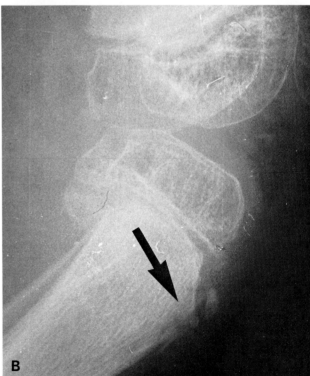

FIG. 19-30. Unusual patterns of posterior displacement of epiphysis and anterior displacement of metaphysis (arrows). *A*, Mild displacement. *B*, The tibial tuberosity ossification center appears to be in its normal place, suggesting some separation between the tibial epiphysis and tuberosity. The children in both *A* and *B* had neuromuscular disorders, which may have been a factor in this unusual displacement pattern.

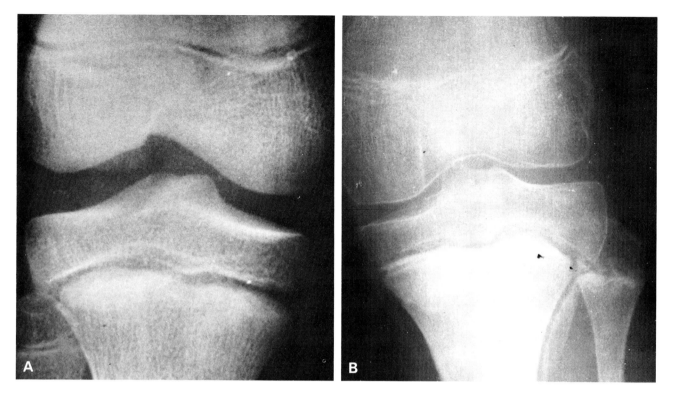

FIG. 19-31. *A*, Type 1 injury showing mild widening of the physis. *B*, Minimal widening of physis was not detected initially, but three weeks later, extensive subperiosteal new bone was present.

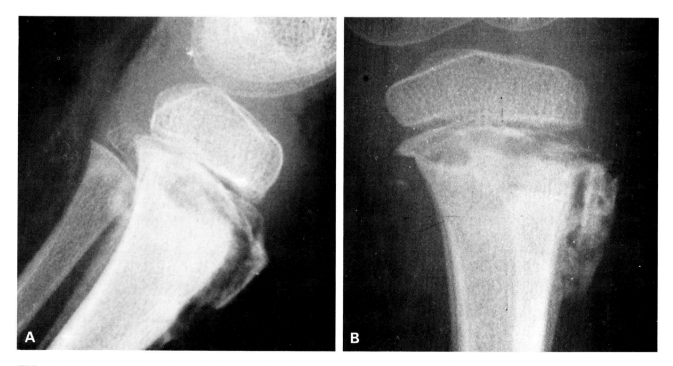

FIG. 19-32. Type 1 injury of epiphysis and tuberosity in a myelomeningocele patient. *A*, Lateral view. *B*, AP view.

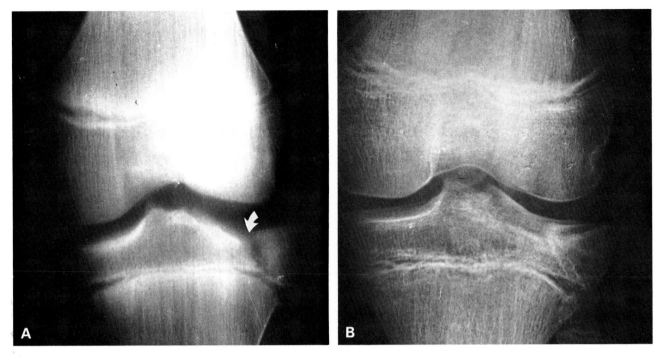

FIG. 19-33. *A,* Type 3 injury (arrow) of lateral epiphysis. *B,* Appearance six months after open reduction and transepiphyseal pin fixation.

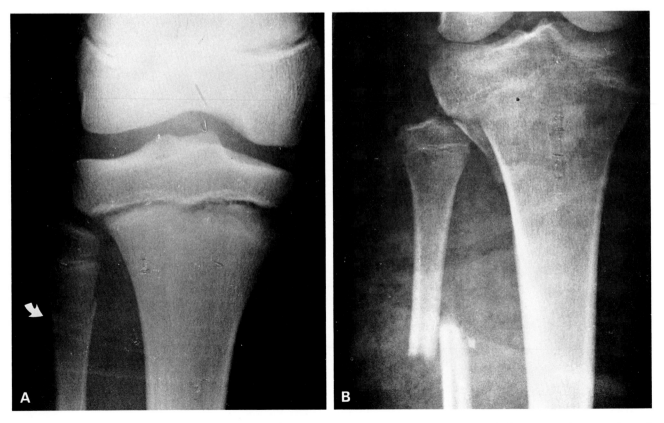

FIG. 19-34. *A,* Type 1 tibial injury with fracture of fibular metaphysis (arrow). *B,* Type 2 tibial injury with posterolateral metaphyseal fragment and concomitant diaphyseal fibular fracture.

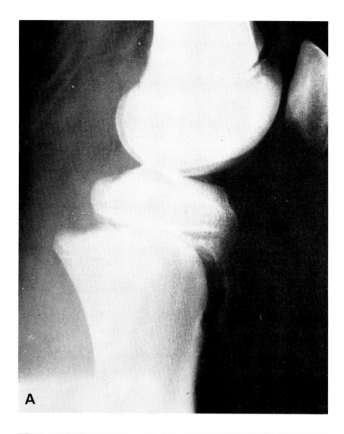

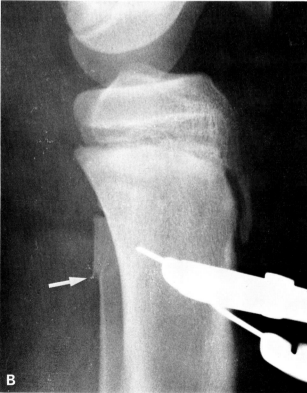

the knee is extended. Type 2 injuries almost invariably require anatomic reduction by open methods.

In type 3 injuries there is significant separation of the fragments as well as propagation into the knee joint, which leads to disruption of the articular surface under the anterior attachments of the medial or lateral menisci. However, fracture propagation may go into the anterior fat pad instead, so that there is minimal involvement of the articular surface. The displaced fragment may be unitary (3A) or comminuted (3B). Open reduction is necessary to restore joint surface contiguity. In type 3A injuries some of the soft tissue extensions onto the metaphysis may be intact, especially in the region of the pes anserinus.

Fragmentation and angulation in types 2 and 3 also probably occur in or near the region of cartilage that intervenes between the two ossification centers.

The comminution evident in types 2B and 3B is significant in that the anatomically more distal fragment becomes more proximally displaced, which leads to proximal displacement of the patella (i.e., traumatic patella alta). Such proximal patellar displacement may also occur, albeit to a lesser degree, in types 1B, 2A, and 3A. Since idiopathic patella alta is associated with subluxation and chondromalacia, restoration of the pre-injury anatomy would seem indicated to avoid these potential complications.

Concomitant disease

Osgood-Schlatter disease was described in the contralateral knee by Deliyannis,[36] and in the ipsilateral knee in 1 of the patients in Hand's series.[37] Our series had ipsilateral involvement in 2 knees (asymptomatic prior to injury), and

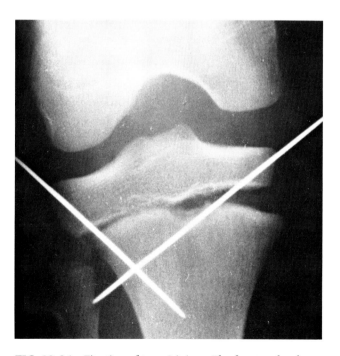

FIG. 19-35. *A,* Posteriorly displaced type 1 injury. *B,* The patient was placed in skeletal traction with correction of the displacement over a three-day period. Also note the fibular fracture (arrow).

FIG. 19-36. Fixation of type 1 injury. The fracture has been incompletely reduced. This should not have been accepted, since it left the leg in mild valgus, and spontaneous correction may not occur. Accurate anatomic reduction should be the end-point of any open procedure.

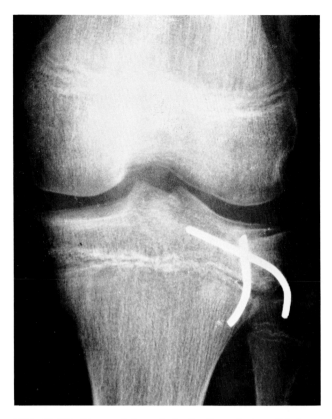

FIG. 19-37. Transepiphyseal pin fixation of a type 3 injury. This method avoids possible physeal damage.

contralateral involvement in 6 patients, all of whom had experienced symptoms 2 to 26 months prior to injury, but had never experienced similar symptoms in the knee with the acute tuberosity fracture.[38]

Pathomechanics

Tibial tuberosity ossification develops as a tongue-shaped downward protrusion of the proximal tibial epiphysis onto the anterior proximal tibial surface, or as a separate center of ossification that fuses with the main body of the epiphysis at the age of 16, and eventually fuses to the tibial metaphysis around the age of 18. Complete or partial avulsions, either acute or chronic, may occur in either type of anatomic arrangement. Recent studies implicate the second anatomic arrangement as the prevailing one, although the first would appear to be the one in which there has been early fusion of the tuberosity and proximal tibial centers.[2,38] As shown in Figures 19-8 and 19-9, a bipolar growth plate may exist between the 2 centers (i.e., those of the proximal tibia as well as the tuberosity).

The mechanism of injury appears to be violent active extension or passive flexion of the knee with the quadriceps rigidly contracted. The pre-existence of Osgood-Schlatter disease has been noted by several authors. This may imply increased susceptibility to injury since the area has already shown mild tension failure.

The data from our cases support the contention that this is an angular, distal to proximal avulsion of the tuberosity.[38] This is probably due to sudden, unexpected contraction in the quadriceps while the knee is being flexed (frequently forcibly). The increased tensile force is too much for the tuberosity to resist, and failure occurs.

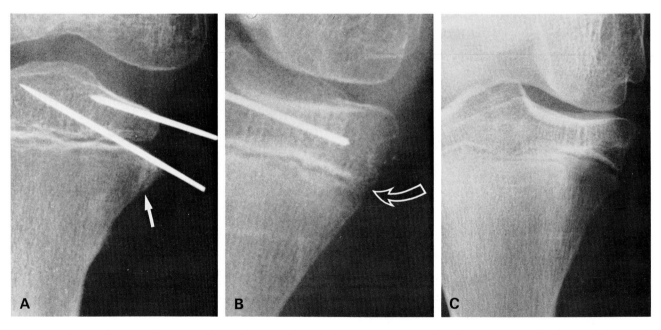

FIG. 19-38. *A,* Fixation of type 4 injury. This growth mechanism pattern was barely evident on the basis of the small metaphyseal fragment (arrow). The epiphyseal extension into the cartilage was not evident roentgenographically. *B,* The upper pin migrated into the epiphysis. Pin ends should be bent 90° to prevent such a complication. Unfortunately, a peripheral bony bridge formed (arrow). *C,* This was subsequently resected and replaced by fat (Langenskiöld procedure) with no evidence of reformation of the bridge 17 months later.

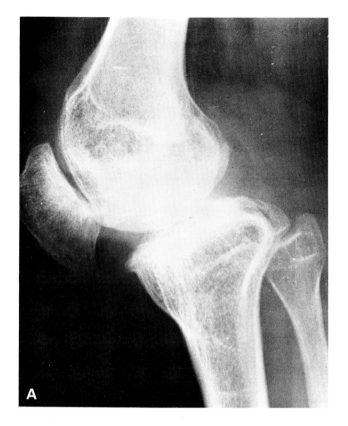

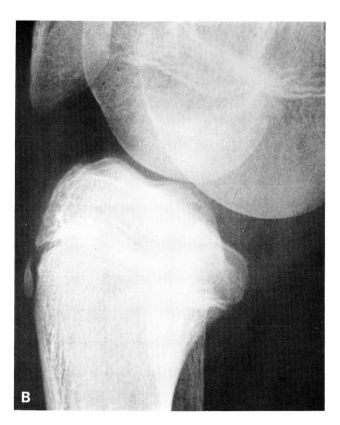

FIG. 19-39. Growth arrest. *A,* Genu recurvatum deformity due to anterior displacement and subsequent closure. *B,* Increased posterior angulation due to posterior osseous bridge.

Interestingly, like the Tillaux fracture of the distal tibia, the tuberosity fracture tends to be associated with adolescents who are going through physiologic epiphysiodesis. This certainly is in the patient's favor, inasmuch as it lessens the risk of growth abnormality, particularly genu recurvatum, consequent to premature growth arrest. In any case, prognosis must be guarded because of the potential for premature closure of the anterior portion of the tuberosity or proximal tibial physis and subsequent recurvatum. The proximal tibial physis may be subjected to compression (type 5 injury), particularly if the mechanism is one of hyperextension and violent contracture of the quadriceps.

Diagnosis

Pain and swelling about the anterior part of the proximal end of the tibia with an inability to extend the knee against force or gravity are common findings. In fractures with extension of the fracture into the proximal epiphysis there is usually an associated hemarthrosis in the knee.

Roentgenography is essential for definitive diagnosis (Figs. 19-43 to 19-47). This may require oblique views that adequately visualize the tuberosity ossification center.

Treatment

Treatment generally depends upon the degree of displacement and must be directed at anatomic correction. In cases where the tuberosity is still partially attached, manipulative reduction is essential to restore anatomic integrity and evaluate the presence of herniated tissue. Watson-Jones emphasized closed reduction for these fractures whenever possible, and minimized the consequences of extension proximally into the joint.[38] If closed methods are used initially, the patient must be roentgenographed at appropriate intervals to be certain that the distal fragment does not displace significantly.

With rare exception, type 1B and all type 2 and 3 injuries should be subjected to open reduction with accurate anatomic restoration of tibial surface congruity, repair of any peripheral meniscal tears, and appropriate fixation of the fragments (Figs. 19-45*C,* 19-46*B,* and 19-47*B*). Although screws are the most common method used, fragmentation may limit their effectiveness. Staples and wire may also be used; the latter in a manner analogous to fixation of an olecranon fracture.

Cases may be treated by open reduction with screw fixation through the tuberosity into the metaphysis. This method of fixation would not be ideal to use in the young child with this type of injury. Tension band wiring with additional suture fixation of the fragment to the pes anserinus and periosteum is recommended in young patients.

A large periosteal flap may be reflected along with the tuberosity at the time of injury.[38] This facilitates surgical repair in that it can be easily resutured to its original position. In fact, it can be densely attached to the pes anserinus to make a strong fixation, a factor to be taken advantage of in order to minimize the use of internal metallic fixation. In two cases the periosteum was also herniated behind the tibial tuberosity, which prevented adequate closed reduction.[38] In case of displacement, it is essential to do an open reduction to explore the area and remove any herniated tissue, a

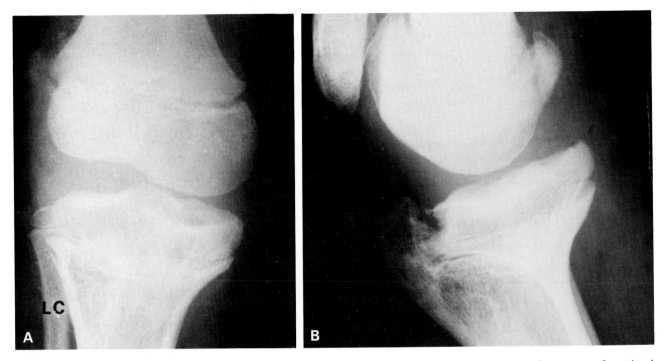

FIG. 19-40. *A,* AP and, *B,* lateral views in boy with unilateral sensory neuropathy. Growth arrest involving most of proximal tibia (this probably represents a chronic type 5 growth mechanism injury). In *B,* also note the posterior condylar fracture of the distal femur.

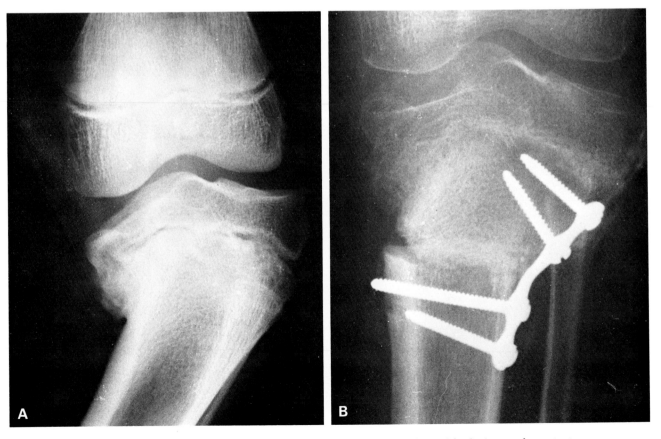

FIG. 19-41. *A,* Medial growth arrest with severe varus deformity. *B,* Correction with closing wedge osteotomy.

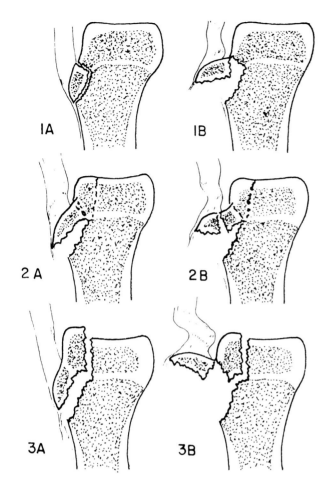

FIG. 19-42. Schematic of patterns of tibial tuberosity fracture. See text for details of the three types.

factor that has been described as a mechanism of injury in valgus deformity consequent to proximal tibial fractures.

The knee joint should be explored in appropriate type 2 and all type 3 injuries. Any intra-articular damage, especially to the menisci, should be repaired.

Results

The results of treatment of this injury are generally excellent. Since the growth plate is in the final stages of closure, premature growth arrest rarely occurs. Adequate quadriceps rehabilitation is essential for a good result.

Complications

None of the previous authors reported actual complications, although they suggested genu recurvatum as a potential complication.[36,37] In my study premature epiphysiodesis was found in only one patient, and in this case the entire physis, both proximal tibia as well as tuberosity, was involved, which was probably due to a neuropathic joint (myelomeningocele) rather than specific tuberosity physeal damage.[38]

Another complication of this injury is failure of fixation. By isometric contracture, the quadriceps may pull the tuberosity off again and cause extensive ectopic bone formation (Fig. 19-48). This ectopic bone may be resected, and the tendon reattached. In this case a compression clamp was applied to transverse pins in the patella and metaphysis to hold the patella in an anatomic position while the tendon healed to bone.

Osgood-Schlatter Disease

Osgood-Schlatter disease may be defined as a partial separation of large or small fragments of the chondrous or

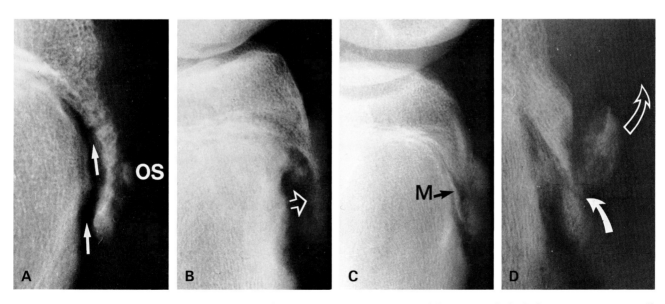

FIG. 19-43. Type 1 injury pattern. A, Avulsion of entire tuberosity up to part of the proximal tibial physis (arrows). A small Osgood-Schlatter's ossicle is present (OS). B, Displaced fracture of entire tuberosity, with separation from proximal tibia (arrow). C, Variation of pattern, with fracture through the metaphysis, leaving the metaphyseal subchondral plate (M) attached to the tibial tuberosity. D, Fracture of anterior portions of ossification center (open arrow), an acute analogue of Osgood-Schlatter disease. The fracture may extend posteriorly through the ossification center (solid arrow).

chondro-osseous tubercle, along with variable areas of patellar tendon disruption.[2,40] It is generally assumed that chronic, repetitive trauma is associated with its cause, although other proposed causes have included vascular damage, systemic disease, and endocrinopathy.[41] Intense trauma may also cause the injury.

Pathomechanics

Ehrenborg purported that the cause of Osgood-Schlatter disease was traumatic and the causal mechanism was avulsion of some of the patellar ligament with consequent detachment of fragments of cartilage or bone from a portion of

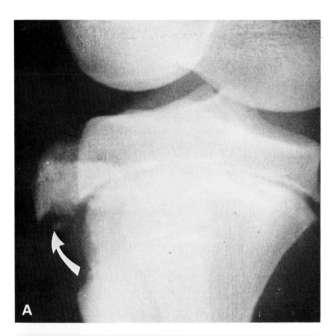

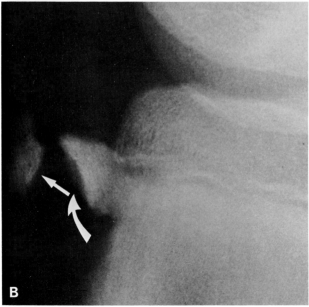

FIG. 19-44. Type 2 injury pattern. *A*, Avulsion and displacement (arrow) of tuberosity. *B*, Fragmentation (arrows).

the tibial tuberosity.[2] Willner believed that increased obliquity of the angle of the patellar tendon from patella down to the insertion was a causative (predisposing) factor.[2] This would be similar to the anatomy in children who tend to laterally subluxate the patella.

Cole and Uhry reported on microscopic studies of sections removed from the area of the tibial tubercle during surgical procedures.[2] These sections showed hemorrhage, clotting, invasion of fibroblasts and connective tissue, as well as other features of nonunion and increased vascularity. Figure 19-47 shows one of the most complete specimens available. The posterior portion of the patellar tendon between the ossicle and tuberosity was frayed and in varying stages of repair. The ossicles contained viable bone with fibrocartilage at the periphery, similar to that shown in the normal situation (see Fig. 19-9).

Osgood-Schlatter disease most likely results from a portion of the ossification center of the tuberosity being pulled away from the tuberosity (Figs. 19-49 and 19-50). This may also occur when the cartilage cells are hypertrophic (pre-ossification) phase, a time when they are not roentgeno-graphically evident. Once pulled away, the cartilage or bone may continue to grow and enlarge. However, because of chronic motion, the intervening area may become fibrous, essentially creating a localized nonunion.

Treatment

Since chronic stress with formation of a localized nonunion is significant, the first treatment should be discontinuation of programmed sports activities and immobilization with a splint. If the disease becomes more chronic or painful, then rigid immobilization in a cylinder cast should be used. Patients and their parents must be made aware of the probable traumatic cause, and the possibility of recurrence following muscle rehabilitation. Graduated quadriceps strengthening is important after cast removal.

Since this disorder represents a healing fracture, which is a process that requires inflammation as part of the normal biologic response, do not use steroids.[42] Nonunions are generally painful; therefore, the fracture should be treated with a method that promotes healing, rather than steroids, which discourage healing.

Children rarely complain because of prominence of the tuberosity; however, they do complain about the restriction of activities forced upon them because of pain and discomfort. It is well recognized that Osgood-Schlatter disease is a self-limited condition, and as a rule amenable to conservative management. It is only in rare instances that tendon enlargement about the epiphysis is continuously troublesome and persistent in symptoms such that operative treatment is indicated.

Operative intervention should be used in patients only after the following conditions are met: (1) The patient has had repeated attacks of severe pain with tenderness, functional disability, and deformity. (2) Even after conservative treatment with cast or splint immobilization, the symptoms have returned. (3) The child has reached sufficient development in adolescence to justify a surgical procedure. This has been used in the past to justify major procedures of resection. However, these children should not be operated on until there is an established fragment(s) and evident nonunion. If a localized procedure (resection of the fragment) is

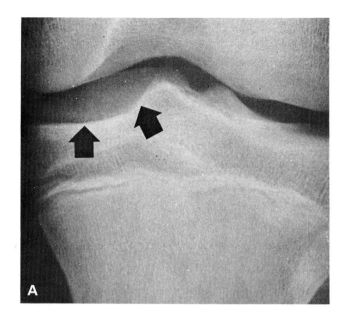

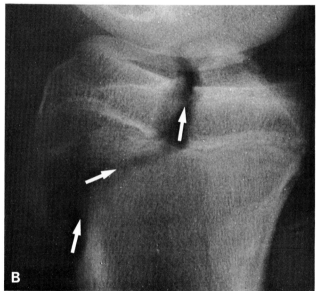

FIG. 19-45. Type 3 injury. *A,* Note appearance of tuberosity obscuring the medial joint (arrows). *B,* Lateral view, showing extension of fracture (arrows) through middle of proximal tibia.

used, then it is possible to operate on children who have not yet attained skeletal maturity.

Ferciot recommended surgical treatment of anterior tibial epiphysitis and described a surgical exposure of splitting the patellar tendon.[43] I do not recommend this procedure, but instead prefer a lateral approach with release of the lateral retinaculum along the patellar tendon and patella, and elevation of the patellar tendon from the tuberosity to expose the area of nonunion (i.e., the ossicles, which should be excised).

The primary operative approach should be removal of the nonunion fragment(s), decreasing lateralizing tensile stress, and explaining to both patients and their parents pre-operatively that the prominence of the tuberosity will remain

post-operatively.[44] Attempts to remove large portions of the tuberosity are contraindicated and may lead to complications of healing, as well as problems in knee-joint mechanics.[45-47]

Proximal Tibiofibular Subluxation and Dislocation

Injuries to the proximal tibiofibular joint, whether acutely symptomatic subluxations or obvious dislocations, have been considered infrequent, if not rare, injuries.[48] However, they are probably more common than appreciated. In a recent large series and review of the literature, one of the major findings was how these injuries escaped recognition because of lack of familiarity.[3]

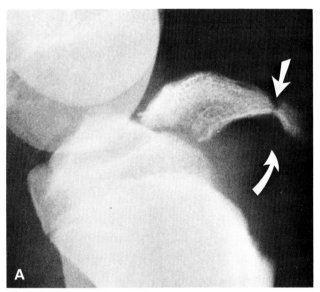

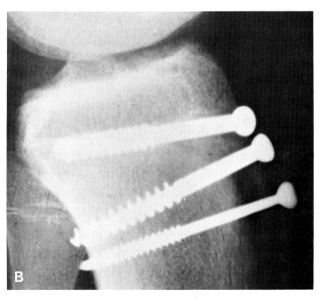

FIG. 19-46. Type 3 injury. *A,* Upward displacement (curved arrow), with fragmentation of distal end (straight arrow). *B,* Operative reduction.

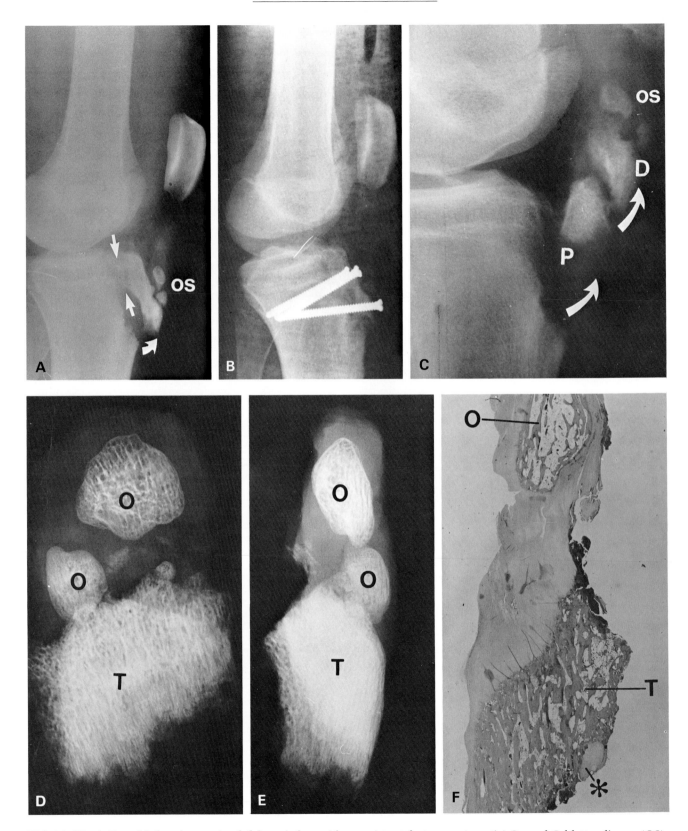

FIG. 19-47. *A,* Type 3 injury (arrows) to left knee in boy with preexistent (but asymptomatic) Osgood-Schlatter disease (OS). *B,* Operative reduction. *C,* Type 3 injury to right knee in same patient. Note Osgood-Schlatter ossicles (OS). Also note how the distal fragment (D) has been pulled more proximally than the proximal fragment (P). *D-E,* AP and lateral roentgenograms of fragment removed from right knee. Note the tuberosity (T) and Osgood-Schlatter ossicles (O). *F,* Histologic section showing Osgood-Schlatter ossicle (O) and distal tibial tuberosity (T), with fragments of closing tuberosity physis (*).

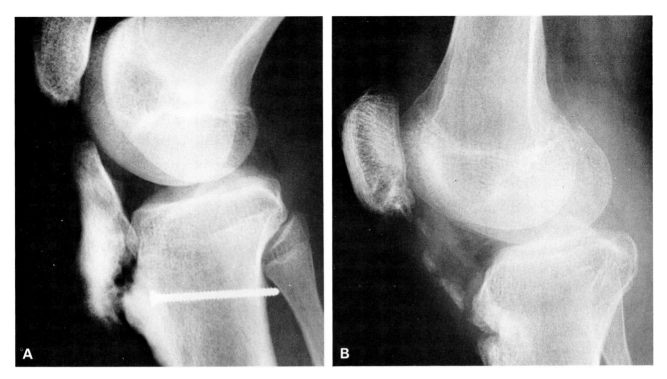

FIG. 19-48. *A,* Despite initial operative reduction, the tuberosity avulsed again and displaced proximally, causing ectopic bone formation, nonunion, and limited knee function. *B,* This was resected and the patellar tendon reattached.

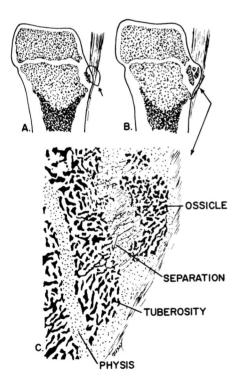

FIG. 19-49. Schematic of development of Osgood-Schlatter disease. *A,* Normal. *B,* Involved, with fragmentation of ossification center. *C,* Higher-power view showing how ossicle pulls away from the main tuberosity ossification center. The region of separation fills in with fibrous and fibrocartilaginous tissue.

Classification

Several types of instability or disruption of the proximal tibiofibular joint are possible. These can be classified as (1) subluxation, (2) anterolateral dislocation, (3) posteromedial dislocation, and (4) superior dislocation (Fig. 19-51).

Idiopathic subluxation of the proximal end of the fibula, which is best defined as excessive symptomatic anteroposterior motion without complete displacement, appears to be a self-limited condition of youth with decreasing symptoms as the patient approaches skeletal maturity.[49] Anterolateral dislocation is the most common injury;[3] posterior dislocation is infrequent; superior dislocation is usually an accompaniment of tibial fracture, and may be considered analogous to the forearm Monteggia injury.

Diagnosis

Patients with subluxation usually complain of pain along the lateral side of the knee and lower limb. This is a chronic type of complaint, although it may acutely follow certain kinds of athletic events or twisting injuries. Transient parasthesia of the peroneal nerve may also occur during periods of hyperactivity. The injury can be elicited by direct pressure over the fibular head, which pushes it either forward or medially (Fig. 19-52). It is frequently a concomitant finding in children with multiple joint hypermobility, and may also be present in disease conditions such as muscular dystrophy or Ehlers-Danlos syndrome.

The isolated anterolateral proximal fibular dislocation may be discerned by clinical examination, which will reveal a mass lateral to the tibia (Fig. 19-53). The dislocation is usually evident roentgenographically, although direct pressure

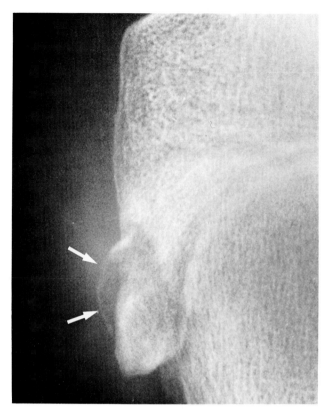

FIG. 19-50. Early development of Osgood-Schlatter disease, showing separation of anterior subchondral bone (arrows) from the tuberosity ossification center.

to accentuate the deformity, as described for subluxation, is sometimes necessary. Unfortunately, the diagnosis is initially missed in about one third of the cases.

Pathomechanics

Most of these dislocations occur during athletic activity, especially during violent twisting exercises. Some may also be associated with other skeletal injury, particularly fractures of the proximal tibial region.

Treatment

In subluxation, subsidence of the symptoms generally follows rest. If not, the pain usually responds well to cylinder cast immobilization. Sometimes the foot may have to be included to prevent ankle motion, since such motion may cause mild rotation at the proximal fibula and accentuate any synovitis.

Most patients with dislocation can be treated with closed reduction, particularly when the diagnosis is made acutely. The knee should be flexed 90 to 110°, the foot externally rotated, and direct pressure applied to the fibular head. Once reduction has been attained, which usually is evident by a loud snapping sensation, the patient should be immobilized for approximately 3 weeks. The joint is stable in extension, a factor that is evident in anatomic dissections in which it was impossible to displace the fibula anteriorly unless the knee was flexed 70 to 80° The foot should be included to limit fibular rotation secondary to angular motion.

Two surgical approaches are used to alleviate these complications: resection of the proximal end of the fibula and arthrodesis of the joint (Figs. 19-53 and 19-54). Arthrodesis of the proximal tibiofibular joint is complicated by a pro-

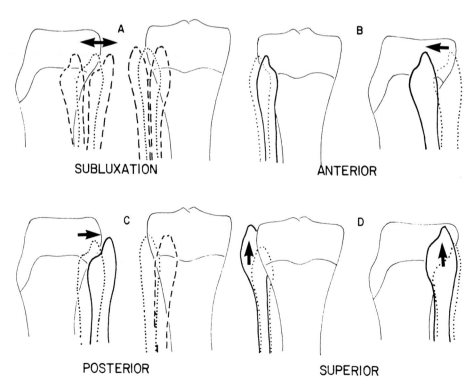

FIG. 19-51. Schematic of four patterns of proximal tibiofibular injury. See text for details.

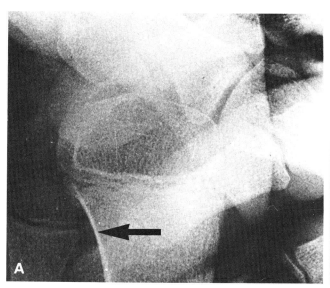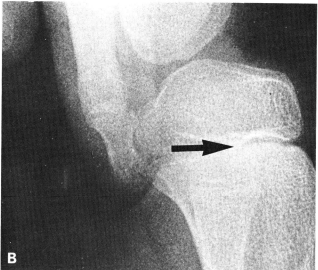

FIG. 19-52. Anterior subluxation of the proximal fibula in seven-year-old with chronic pain over lateral region of knee. *A,* Anterior stress (arrow) pushed the fibula backwards. *B,* Posterior stress (arrow) duplicated the pain by displacing the fibula anteriorly.

longed period of fusion, as well as by eventual development of pain and instability in the ankle. Those patients treated with arthrodesis had uniformly poor results. In contrast, four patients treated by resection of the fibular head had uneventful recoveries, and none has ever experienced the ankle pain and instability that occurred in the patients with arthrodesis. Resection of the proximal end of the fibula was associated with significantly more satisfactory results in long term follow-up. However, this is not an operation to be undertaken lightly in a child still in an active growth phase, although it is possible to use it in children approaching skeletal maturity. Resection of the proximal end of the fibula might lead to cephalad migration of the tibia, as has been described by Hsu in taking out complete portions of the distal fibula for subtalar arthrodesis.[50]

Results

Most cases respond satisfactorily to closed reduction, but only if carried out within the first week following injury. Several of the dislocations developed into either a chronic subluxation or arthritis of the proximal tibiofibular joint, although the latter was not a frequent complication in children. Unfortunately many of these patients developed symptoms of "insecurity" after the injury, although this is more common in adults than in children.

Wong reported an unusual case of proximal rather than distal tibiofibular synostosis following trauma.[51] However, other than the acute injury, neither patient seemed to have any chronic problems.

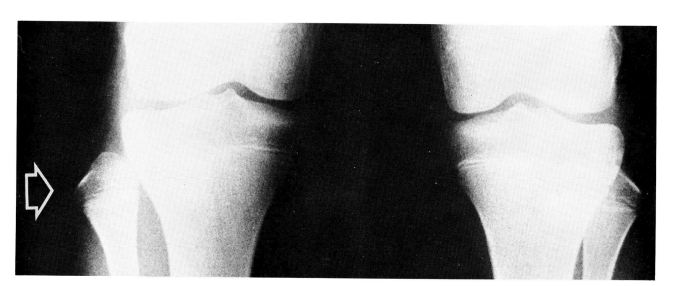

FIG. 19-53. Anterolateral dislocation (arrow).

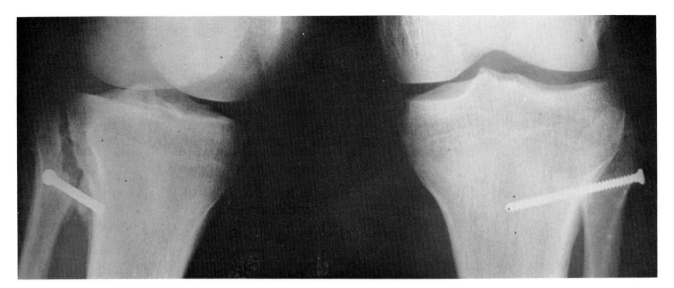

FIG. 19-54. Displacement in a 17-year-old who originally injured his knee at age 14 while jumping. The displacement was fused, but a nonunion developed.

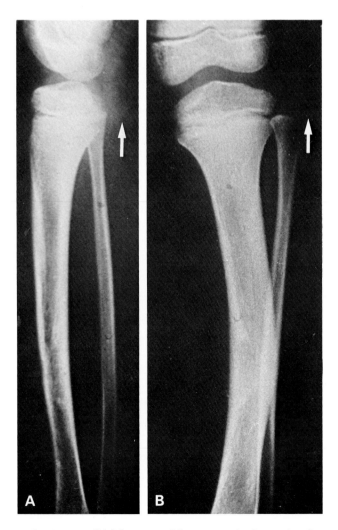

FIG. 19-55. Tibial fracture with unrecognized superior disruption (arrows) of proximal tibiofibular joint.

Posterior dislocation

Posteromedial dislocations are more unstable after initial reduction and frequently require surgical repair. This injury is usually the result of a severe blow directly to the knee, such as that inflicted by a car bumper; the proximal part of the fibula is pushed posteriorly and medially. Severe disruption of the anterior and posterior capsular ligaments of the tibiofibular joint, along with a significant tear of part of the fibular collateral ligament, allows the biceps to draw the unsupported proximal part of the fibula posteriorly.

In view of the poor results of the few reported cases that were treated conservatively, a posterior dislocation probably should be treated by open reduction, capsulorrhaphy, and fibular collateral ligament repair with temporary internal fixation below the joint.

Superior dislocation

Superior dislocations are rare and usually associated with fractures of the tibia. One patient had a fracture during the first year of life that had been allowed to heal with 1 to 2 cm overriding; the patient was seen at the age of seven because of a lateral ''mass'' that proved to be the dislocated fibular head (Fig. 19-55).

Figure 19-56 shows a 12-year-old boy who sustained multiple trauma (including a severe fracture of the pelvis). He had an unstable tibial fracture with no evidence of a fibular fracture. It was impossible to control his fracture, which proved difficult to reduce at the time of open reduction even when compression fixation was used. It was necessary to reduce a superior displacement of the proximal fibula, which was the cause of the failure, in order to attain reduction. This was difficult since he was seen two weeks post-injury. This type of injury is similar to a Monteggia injury in the forearm.

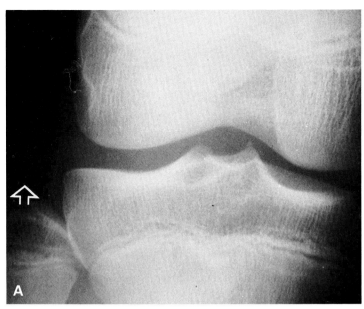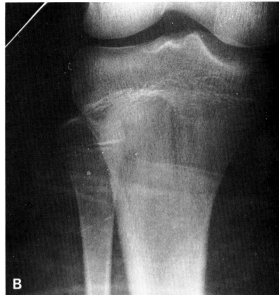

FIG. 19-56. A 12-year-old boy with multiple injuries. *A,* The proximal fibula was displaced superiorly (arrow) concomitant with a tibial fracture (see Fig. 19-71). *B,* At the time of plating of the unstable tibial fracture, the proximal fibula was reduced (closed reduction).

Proximal Fibular Injuries

Injuries specifically involving the proximal fibular physis and epiphysis are rare (Fig. 19-57) and may be associated with significant soft tissue injury to the knee. The peroneal (fibular) nerve may be injured and must be carefully assessed clinically. If the nerve is injured, decompression may be necessary.

Because the biceps is a strong muscle these fractures may displace, even if treated in a cast. Displacement of a type 1 or 2 injury should be treated by open reduction, as should any type 3 or 4 injury. If the fracture involves the articular surface of the proximal tibiofibular joint, long term degenerative changes may occur. Such joint pain should be treated by resection of the proximal fibula, not by arthrodesis.

Proximal Metaphyseal Injuries

Fractures of the proximal metaphysis or upper diaphysis are relatively common in children and generally occur when children are between 3 and 6 years of age. Toddler's fractures may also involve this area (Fig. 19-58). Direct violence is a less common cause of fracture in this region than in the diaphysis.

The distal fragment is angulated laterally, but there does not seem to be any significant loss of apposition. Fragments do not usually override. The fibula frequently escapes injury, although it occasionally may sustain a greenstick fracture that may not be appreciated at the time of the original injury.

Classification

The primary injury patterns are torus (compression) fractures and incomplete tension-failure fractures (Figs. 19-59 and 19-60). Displaced, complete fractures are more common in the older child or adolescent (Fig. 19-61).

Diagnosis

Roentgenographic diagnosis should include oblique views, or even fluoroscopy, which may allow a better appreciation of any acute valgus deformation, thereby permitting a better

FIG. 19-57. Type 3 fracture of the proximal fibula (arrow). This fracture complicated an acute knee dislocation (see Fig. 18-12), and was treated by open reduction.

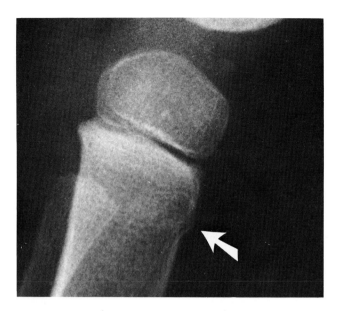

FIG. 19-58. Toddler's fracture of the proximal metaphysis. The child had been limping for several days. Minimal buckling was evident (arrow), as shown on this lateral roentgenogram.

approach to treatment (e.g., complete the greenstick component of the medial side). Magnification views may better reveal minimal cortical buckling.

Diagnosis is not always easy. These children may limp or even refuse to bear weight on the involved extremity. Examination may reveal a tender area over the proximal tibia.

Treatment

Treatment must consist of correction of any lateral (valgus) angulation by manipulative reduction and immobiliza-

tion in a long-leg cast for 4 to 6 weeks. If it is not possible to easily reduce the fracture, then the greenstick component should be completed by bending the leg toward the angulation and slightly overcorrecting the deformity, just as in a fracture of the radius and ulna. Failure to do so may result in a recurrence of the deformity while in plaster.

Displaced fractures in older children and adolescents should be reduced. As long as the normal longitudinal axial relationships of proximal and distal fragments are maintained, mild displacement may be accepted.

Reduction should be checked at weekly intervals for the first 3 weeks to be certain that reduction is not lost.

Results

Fractures of the tibial shaft in children are not generally associated with major complications. This has led to the concept that when the metaphysis is involved, the injury is relatively innocuous. However, these injuries may lead to significant valgus deformity with subsequent skeletal growth (Fig. 19-62). The mechanisms of this deformity are not completely understood, particularly when associated with minimal displacement of the fracture.[52]

Cozen reported 4 cases with relatively minor fractures of the proximal tibial metaphysis that subsequently went on to major valgus deformities.[53,54] In two of his cases there was no displacement at the time the patients were seen in the emergency room. None of the patients were allowed out of plaster early and there was no radiographic evidence of malfunction in the epiphyseal plate.

In children it is well known that after certain fractures of long bones, more than the normal growth in length of the involved bone may occur. This longitudinal overgrowth is not dependent on any shortening due to overriding of the fracture fragments and may occur without significant displacement of the fragment. The overgrowth is somewhat variable from patient to patient. Certainly the pattern in the tibia following injury to the metaphysis has not been estab-

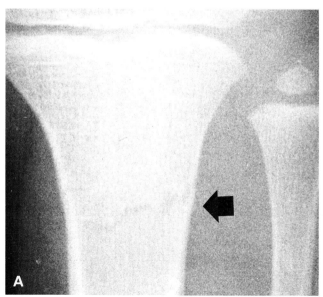
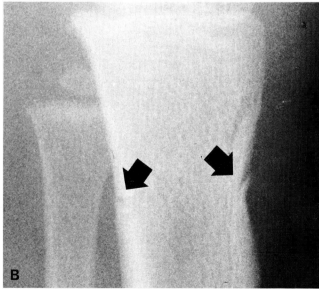

FIG. 19-59. *A,* Undisplaced proximal fracture. *B,* Lateral view, in which mild recurvatum (arrows) is evident.

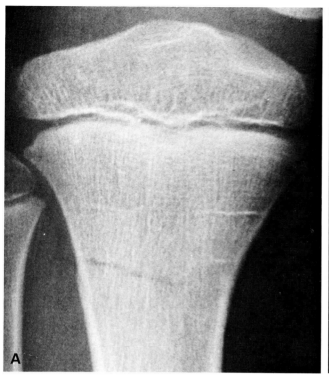

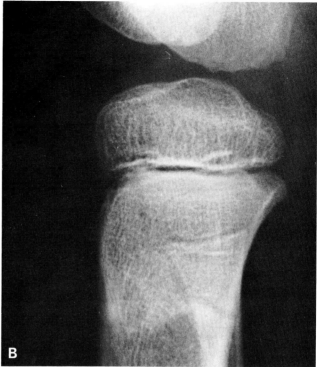

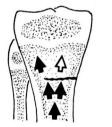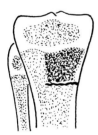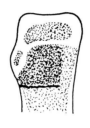

C CIRCULATORY CHANGE (TRANSIENT)

FIG. 19-60. *A,* Undisplaced fracture. *B,* Two weeks later, extensive sclerosis is present, suggesting temporary impairment of metaphyseal vascular supply. *C,* Schematic of injury.

lished as clearly as that of the femur, although tibial overgrowth has been reported after fracture, osteotomy, removal of bone graft, and osteomyelitis.[55] When an increase in growth occurs after a fracture, it continues for at least 6 months and the greatest gain is in the first few months.

Valgus deformity is a limited phenomenon that leads to an initial angulation that is subsequently stabilized. The deformity usually develops within 5 months, depending upon skeletal age, implying that the deformity occurs rapidly (Fig. 19-62C). Subsequently, further angular deformity (progression) is unlikely. In reviewing many cases described in the literature, it appears that when there is an acute angulation it can probably be related to the time of fracture and subsequent early healing phase. There is usually no further angular deformity, and it begins to dissipate toward the diaphysis by continued longitudinal growth and physeal realignment.

Jackson and Cozen described 10 patients with valgus deformity.[56] The earliest deformity was observed at 10 to 11 weeks, but more commonly it was not seen for 20 to 40 weeks after the injury. All the tibial fractures were undisplaced except for some angulation. Of the 10 fractures, 8

were greenstick and 2 were complete. The fibula was fractured in 3 and intact in 7 of the patients. The angular apex appeared to occur at the fracture site. In no instance was there any evidence of injury to the proximal epiphyseal plate, either initially or during subsequent follow-up. The amount of valgus deformity ranged from 5 to 25° more than normal. Of the 10 children, 8 had overgrowth of the involved tibia of 1.3 cm or more, and in each of these there was more than 15° of genu valgus. The 2 patients with the mildest deformities had less than 1.3 cm of overgrowth in the fractured tibia.

Overgrowth is usually such that the medial side is longer than the lateral side (Fig. 19-62C). The discrepancy in growth may also result from the fibula exerting a tethering effect laterally, while the medial side becomes hyperemic in response to the fracture.

A potential stimulus to overgrowth is vascular response that leads to unequal growth between the medial and lateral tibia and fibula.[57,58] If the stimulus to growth is greater in the medial tibia than in either the lateral side or the fibula, then a valgus deformity can occur.

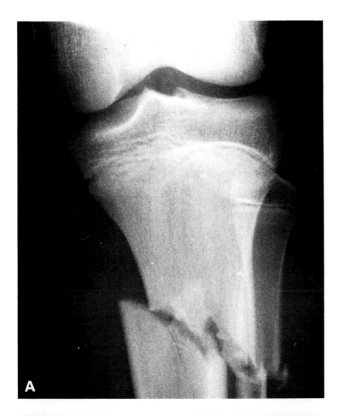

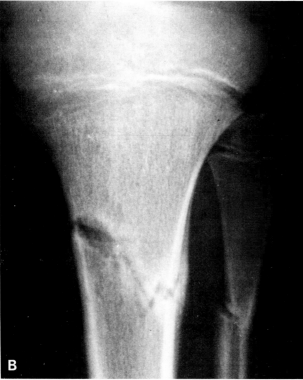

FIG. 19-61. *A,* Displaced metaphyseal fractures of tibia and fibula. *B,* Four weeks later, subperiosteal bone is present laterally, where the periosteum is intact. However, medially, where the periosteum was disrupted, there is no evidence of callus. A slight valgus is present between the proximal and distal fragments.

Bovill's case was interesting in that the particular pattern of revascularization of the metaphysis showed a slight delay in certain areas relative to others; this may be a factor in the overgrowth and valgus that occur in metaphyseal fractures.[34]

Cadaver arteriography (see Fig. 18-13) showed increased primary and collateral geniculate vascularity to the medial proximal tibia compared to the lateral proximal tibia. This implies that any increased vascularity probably brings a greater flow medially, thus stimulating endochondral ossification on a relatively temporary basis. This seems the most likely explanation for the medial overgrowth, which is self-limited.

Taylor felt that the deformity occurred because of temporary stimulation of the tibial epiphysis and physis concomitant with a tethering effect from the fibula, which did not experience the same response in an isolated fracture.[59] Certainly this deformity has been observed following fractures, but it has also occurred at the proximal tibial metaphysis consequent to surgery and osteomyelitis. Valgus rarely occurs when the tibia and fibula are *both* fractured.

Another possible cause of the deformity might be the restraining influence of the iliotibial band (Fig. 19-63), which certainly has been described as a deforming power in poliomyelitis.[60] Its influence on healing fractures may be similar, although this is hypothetical.

The possibility of a mild retardation of growth at the lateral side of the tibial physis must also be considered, since these fractures usually involve cortical breaks in the medial cortex that may or may not extend all the way across the transverse diameter of the shaft (Fig. 19-64, *A-B*). It is possible that the lateral physis absorbs more of the compression and has a temporary type 5 injury (Fig. 19-64C). This complication has been described by Morton, who reported two cases in which the anterior portion of the upper tibial epiphysis and physis closed prematurely as a complication of tibial shaft fracture.[33] In both cases the patients developed progressive hyperextension deformities. Interestingly, both these children sustained fractures in the lower third of the tibia. Smillie also reported a similar case.[18]

Weber reported a case of genu valgus following a fracture of the upper tibial metaphysis due to interposition of a flap of fibrous tissue consisting of the pes anserinus and the periosteum avulsed from the lower fragment (Fig. 19-65).[61] The ensuing biomechanical disturbance induced bowing of the shaft and asymmetrical growth at both ends of the bone. He described four cases of established deformity at the distal end that allowed some restoration of the normal biomechanics of weightbearing.[61] He also reported two cases of fresh fracture that were successfully treated by surgical clearance of the fibrous tissue from the gap. In this type of injury, a valgus force opens a fracture gap at the level of the lower border to the pes anserinus which, together with some periosteum, can be detached from the lower fragment, slip into the gap, and stay there. The residual deformity after manipulation, plaster fixation, and rapid healing of the fracture is minimal, and in the ordinary course of events would correct with growth. Weber feels that the following sequence leads to persistent valgus deformity: the medial structures and their normal force transmission are interrupted, particularly on the lower fragments, such that they respond more to the lateral courses of the iliotibial band and fascia lata. Once the deformity of the shaft is present, the proximal tibial physis seems to produce metaphyseal bone asymmetrically. How-

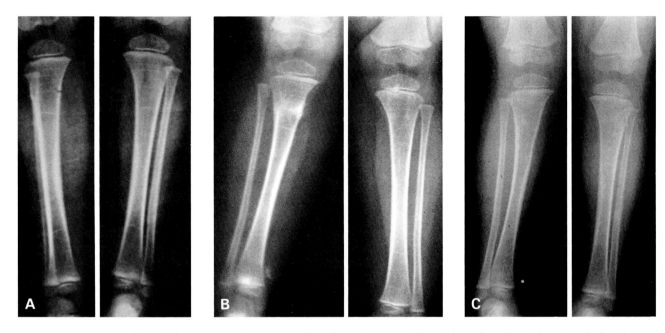

FIG. 19-62. *A,* Metaphyseal fracture in a three-year-old. This involved medial and lateral cortices. No valgus deformity was evident. *B,* Appearance eight weeks after injury. Valgus deformity is already present, and the medial physis-to-physis distance is 2 mm greater on the right than on the left. *C,* Eight months later, the medial side of the tibial shaft is 5 mm longer than the contralateral medial side, while the lateral measurements are equal, suggesting selective medial longitudinal overgrowth.

ever, this mechanism cannot happen in every case, especially in the undisplaced torus fractures in infants and small children.

Prevention of the deformity is problematic. It may be possible to immobilize these fractures in slight varus anticipating the propensity to valgus. However, the exact incidence of this complication is unknown and it may be that an over-reduction, in anticipation, could lead to loss of the normal valgus angle.

The deformity may develop regularly despite acceptable reduction and rapid consolidation (see Fig. 19-62), and often requires secondary treatment to correct the valgus and overgrowth.[53] Correction of the deformity, once it is recognized, since it is progressive only in its initial phase, may often be accomplished by means of a long-leg brace. A valgus-knee

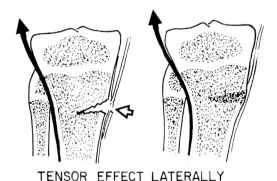

TENSOR EFFECT LATERALLY

FIG. 19-63. The iliotibial band may accentuate medial opening of the fracture by progressively pulling on the fragment distal to the fracture.

orthosis may be appropriate to accelerate correction. Jackson and Cozen treated three patients with long-leg braces for one year with spontaneous correction, four patients were treated with lifts in the shoes, and one patient underwent two osteotomies.[56] However, once it is well established and appears to be stable, corrective osteotomy may have to be considered. It should be noted that if osteotomy is undertaken, there may be a similar deformity consequent to this. Medial epiphysiodesis or stapling is not appropriate unless there is an osseous bar or cartilaginous growth arrest.

Diaphyseal Injuries

Injuries to this region vary considerably with both the age of the child and the mechanism of injury. They may occur following either a direct blow or a rotational, twisting force that is applied to the foot and subsequently transmitted along the tibial shaft. The developing infant and young child have not evolved the dense mid- and distal-third cortical thickening and density characteristic of an adult tibia, and this region seems more susceptible to injury as a child is going through early phases of learning to walk.

In infants and children, the typical injury is a spiral tibial fracture with an intact fibula. Between 3 and 6 years of age, a torsional stress similarly applied usually causes a spiral fracture of the tibia with or without a fracture of the fibula, but more likely may propagate proximally, which leads to a fracture through the proximal fibular metaphysis. This may be a greenstick fracture. As the child gets older (5 to 10 years), a more common injury is a simple transverse fracture, again with or without displacement and with or without injury to the fibula. This usually is due to direct trauma. In adolescence, athletic injuries result in more characteristic

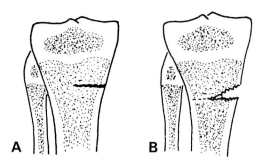

MEDIAL TENSILE / LATERAL COMPRESSIVE
FAILURE

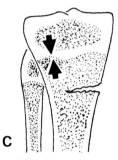

LATERAL TYPE 5

FIG. 19-64. *A-B,* Schematics of medial failure in tension and lateral failure in compression. *C,* Schematic of lateral type 5 growth mechanism injury. Temporary growth slow-down might be a cause of medial overgrowth, especially if the lateral cortex is intact.

fractures in the junction of the middle and distal third of the tibia and fibula, frequently with the formation of a butterfly fragment. Ordinarily, the fracture fragments are held together by the thick periosteal sleeve and displacement is minimal; most of these are rotational stresses rather than direct blows, and there is usually intrinsic stability through the fibula. Open surgical reduction is generally contraindicated, although there are situations when it is beneficial.

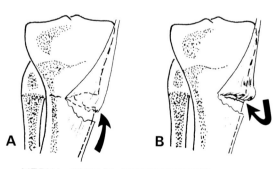

MEDIAL TISSUE INTERPOSITION

FIG. 19-65. Schematic of mechanism of soft tissue interposition (especially portions of the pes anserinus) according to Weber.[112] *A,* Fracture gap at the time of injury. The periosteum is torn. *B,* As the fracture gap closes, a portion of the disrupted periosteum is trapped.

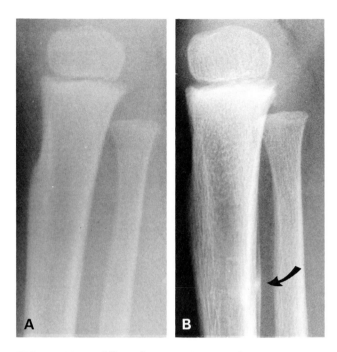

FIG. 19-66. Toddler's fracture. *A,* Normal roentgenogram three days after onset of limping. No fracture is evident. *B,* Two weeks later, posterior callus is present (arrow).

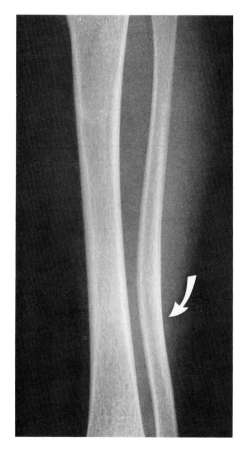

FIG. 19-67. Another variation of toddler's fracture is greenstick bowing of the fibula, with no evidence of tibial injury.

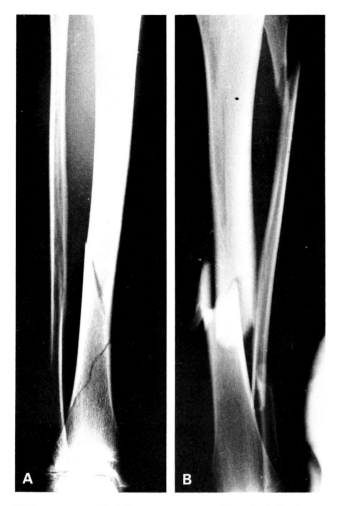

FIG. 19-68. Typical fracture patterns of the tibial diaphysis. *A,* Spiral fracture. *B,* Relatively oblique injury, with concomitant double fracture of the fibula. Notice that the distal tibial fragment is in valgus, whereas the midfibular fragment is in varus. These both must be corrected during treatment.

Delayed healing, as in a comparable adult injury, is not a significant problem, even in the adolescent approaching skeletal maturity.

Infant

Fracture of the tibia with an intact fibula in infancy and early childhood is usually produced by torsional force, as when the child twists in or falls from the crib, or when the child is first learning to walk (Fig. 19-66). The resiliency of the fibula makes it less susceptible to disruptive injury. Further, since this is a torsional stress, the fibula is uniquely adapted through its usual joint mechanism proximally and syndesmosis distally to resist just this type of stress. The tibia may be intact, but the fibula may be plastically deformed (Fig. 19-67). This must be carefully assessed in deciding upon treatment, since an apparent adequate reduction may be displaced by the intrinsic "spring" in the fibula.

Usually the child is irritable, cries frequently, refuses to walk or bear weight on the affected lower limb, or walks with an antalgic limp. Examination shows no obvious de-

formity, especially if there is minimal displacement. However, with palpation of the extremity, the area can be localized reasonably well. There is a tendency to evaluate the hip or foot in this situation; however, the tibia should not be overlooked. The fracture may not always be evident at the time of the original injury, and may not be obvious clinically until 10 to 14 days later when there is beginning callus formation or a palpable thickening of the tibia (Fig. 19-66). At this time roentgenograms will easily disclose the subperiosteal new bone formation. Even at this point, the hairline fracture may or may not be visualized. Care must be taken not to over-interpret the films as showing other lesions such as osteomyelitis, eosinophilic granuloma, acute leukemia, or some other neoplastic lesion. Child abuse must sometimes be included in the differential diagnosis.

Treatment should consist of immobilization in a long-leg cast for 3 weeks. Treatment must often be based upon an empiric diagnosis, but a child suspected of having a "toddler's fracture" should be treated with a cast. The child should be allowed to stand in the cast when comfortable, because this will help stimulate bone remodeling necessary to decrease risk of stress failure in the cortical bone.

Older child

As the child grows, and the midshaft tibial diaphysis progressively develops the characteristic thickening, fracture patterns change and there is a greater tendency to fragmentation. Spiral fracture patterns are relatively common (Fig. 19-68). The concomitant fibular response varies. There may be bowing, simple fracture, multiple fractures, or disruption of proximal or distal tibiofibular relationships. Posterior displacement is also common (Fig. 19-69).

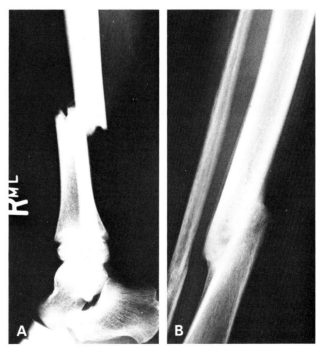

FIG. 19-69. *A,* Posterior displacement of proximal fragment. *B,* Since the periosteum is intact posteriorly, callus fills the gap.

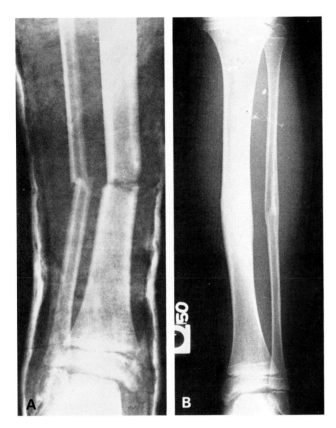

FIG. 19-70. Angular deformities. *A,* Initial treatment showed valgus deformity. *B,* The cast was wedged, correcting most of the deformity.

Fractures of the tibia and fibula in older children and adolescents should be treated by closed reduction whenever possible, correcting both angular and rotational malalignment (Fig. 19-70). The limb must be immobilized in a long-leg cast with the knee flexed to approximately 90°. Flexion is necessary to control rotation as well as to prevent, or at least discourage, the child from bearing weight. The child should be immobilized for at least 6 weeks; the last 2 weeks of which may be accompanied by partial weightbearing.

In adolescence, unstable midshaft fractures may be difficult to hold and may require some sort of pins and plaster technique, or even open reduction with appropriate skeletal fixation (Fig. 19-71).

Results

Stanford reported a study of 234 tibial shaft fractures that included 79 children with adequate follow-up. The average healing for 61 closed fractures was 3.26 months; 18 open fractures were also followed. Of the open fractures that were internally fixed, 2 were infected; 1 healed (with the infection arrested) in 11 months and the other in 24 months. The average rate of healing of open fractures, not including the 2 that became infected, was 3.14 months. The average healing rate of open fractures in children, most of whom were adolescents, was 5.47 months. The longest healing rates were in those fractures that occurred in the distal third of the tibial shaft. The next longest healing rate was in fractures located in the proximal third of the tibial shaft, and the most favora-

ble healing rate was in midshaft fractures. Segmental fractures exhibited a slow rate of healing.

Complications

Angular malunion in the varus and valgus planes may disrupt normal knee-ankle mechanics and must be restored to parallel relationships. If chronic pain occurs, corrective osteotomy may be necessary. Anteroposterior angular malunion may be less of a problem, although knee-ankle relationships may be affected. If the fracture is in the midshaft, spontaneous correction may not occur, although new bone will form anteriorly (Fig. 19-72). Interestingly, although the deformity of the midshaft may remain, the physes usually realign to the normal axial response patterns.

Compound injuries, especially with loss of some bone, may require subsequent bone grafting (Fig. 19-73). However, this should be done only after the soft tissue injury is healed and there is no evidence of complicating osseous or soft tissue infection. Quantitative bacteriology should be used to determine appropriate timing.

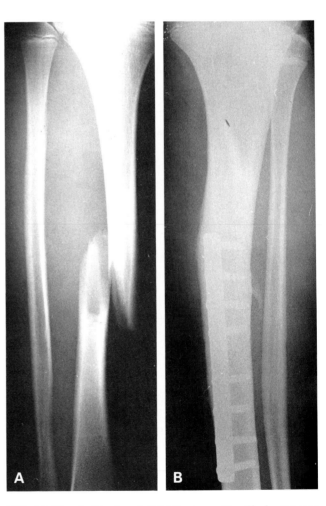

FIG. 19-71. *A,* Displaced tibial fracture. The fibula appears intact. However, a proximal tibiofibular dislocation was present (also see Fig. 19-56). *B,* This was treated by open reduction of tibia, with closed reduction of fibular dislocation.

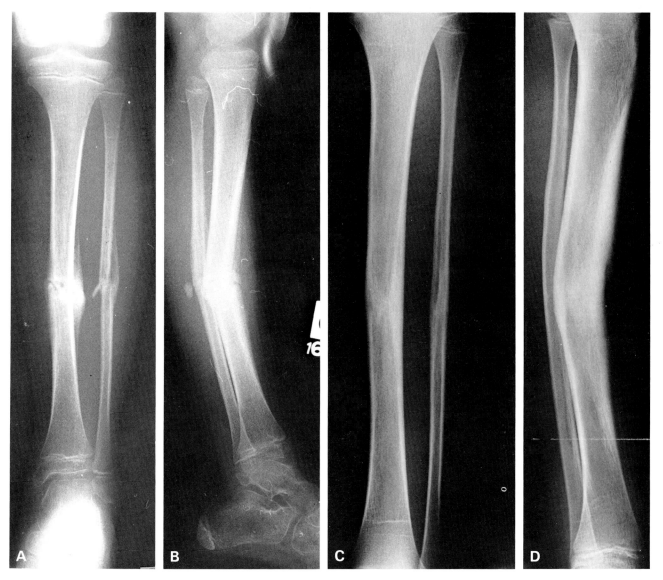

FIG. 19-72. *A-B*, Tibiofibular fractures in child with head injury and severe spasticity. The recurvatum recurred each time closed reduction was attempted. *C-D*, 30 months later, remodeling is complete in the anterior plane, and the recurvatum has improved at the fracture site.

Synostosis formation is extremely rare following children's tibiofibular injuries (Fig. 19-74).[62] The cause is unclear, especially in the type of case shown in Figure 19-74 where a seemingly simple tibial fracture occurred. Resection may be attempted, but only after the lesion has fully matured.

Pseudarthrosis may also occur in children, although it is rare (Fig. 19-75). Bone grafting is the recommended method of treatment.

Distal Metaphyseal Injuries

The distal metaphysis may sustain injury patterns of varying severity, similar to the proximal region. Toddler's fractures may be difficult to diagnose (Fig. 19-76) and should be treated presumptively if symptoms (i.e., limping) warrant it.

Classification

Because of the differences in cortical macro- and microstructure in grading from the thick diaphysis to the thinner metaphysis, greenstick fractures are relatively common (Fig. 19-77). More complete fractures may occur, although the thick tibial periosteum and the tendency of the fibula to plastically deform limits major displacement (Fig. 19-78).

Treatment

In a greenstick fracture or a variably displaced, complete fracture, any angular deformity must be corrected, especially in the varus-valgus plane. Partial to complete displacement requires closed or open reduction (Fig. 19-79). Some intrinsic stability remains because portions of the periosteum are intact.

Results

These injuries generally heal without any significant deformity and with complete restoration of function.

Distal Epiphyseal and Physeal Injuries

The ankle is a true mortise joint essentially moving in only one plane from plantar to dorsiflexion. The lateral malleolus allows minimal rotation to accommodate the changing width of the talar dome. The anatomy and limited joint motion render the distal tibial epiphysis particularly vulnerable to crushing and twisting injuries. The growth plate is more likely to fail than the ligaments during the years of skeletal development. Injuries are commonly caused by indirect violence, with the fixed foot being forced into eversion, inversion, plantarflexion, external rotation, or dorsiflexion. Fractures may also be sustained by direct violence, with the usual history being that the child was in an automobile accident, fell from a height, or was engaged in contact sports.

Distal tibial injuries are more frequent in boys, with the usual age being between 11 and 15 years. Fractures involving the lower tibial epiphyseal plate constitute approximately 10% of all physeal injuries.[63-80]

These injuries may also be relatively common in children with neurologic disorders such as myelomeningocele (Figs. 19-80 and 19-81; see Chap. 7). Unfortunately they are usually pain-free. Swelling of the ankle, redness, or a fever of unknown origin must make one suspicious of this injury pattern. Stern described bilateral distal tibial and fibular epiphyseal separations in patients with spina bifida.[81] These separations are fairly common due to the Charcot-type joints that are present. They must be recognized early so that adequate immobilization and protection can be undertaken. Otherwise the child continues to walk on the fracture, introducing frequent displacement, excessive callus formation, and possibly impairing further growth.

Classification

Fractures of the distal tibia vary considerably in their anatomy, and may include types 1 through 7 growth mechanism injuries.

Type 2 injuries are the most common (Figs. 19-82 to 19-88). The metaphyseal fragment may be medial, lateral, or posterior, contingent upon the deforming mechanism. Accompanying fibular fractures are common and usually involve the metaphysis. Since the region of fibular metaphyseal fracture contains higher amounts of thin cortical bone and is not directly weightbearing (compression-responsive), this fracture may result in a severe greenstick buckling with 90° bends (Fig. 19-89). The point where the fracture changes angulation and propagates from physis into metaphysis is a critical area. If compression forces summate here, there may be a localized area of physeal damage (type 5 pattern), leading to the premature growth arrest (Fig. 19-

90). In severely displaced posterior type 2 injuries, the periosteum may be stripped from the anterior surface and pulled into the fracture gap. Reduction may only lock this tissue into the gap (Fig. 19-91).

Types 3 and 4 injuries of the medial malleolus (Figs. 19-92 and 19-93) are also relatively common injuries and must be treated with proper respect for both disruption of ankle mechanics (including articular surface), as well as premature growth arrest and osseous bridging. Type 3 injuries can be deceiving, especially when there is incomplete ossification of the malleolar region in a young child. Sometimes oblique views of an apparent type 3 injury reveal a small metaphyseal flake, which makes the injury a type 4. Both fracture patterns usually require open reduction and accurate restoration of anatomy. The roentgenogram may not show the true extent of cartilage injury, which may propagate transversely beyond the osseous limits, not unlike a sleeve-

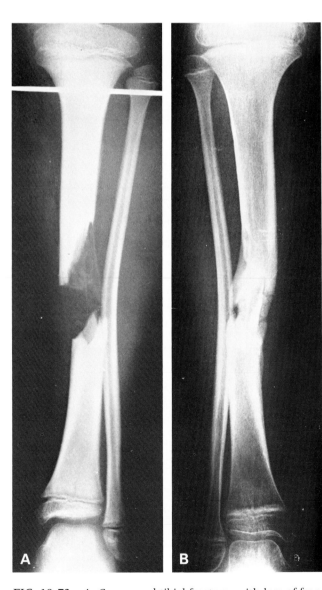

FIG. 19-73. *A,* Compound tibial fracture, with loss of fragment. *B,* This was treated by a bone graft after secondary wound healing.

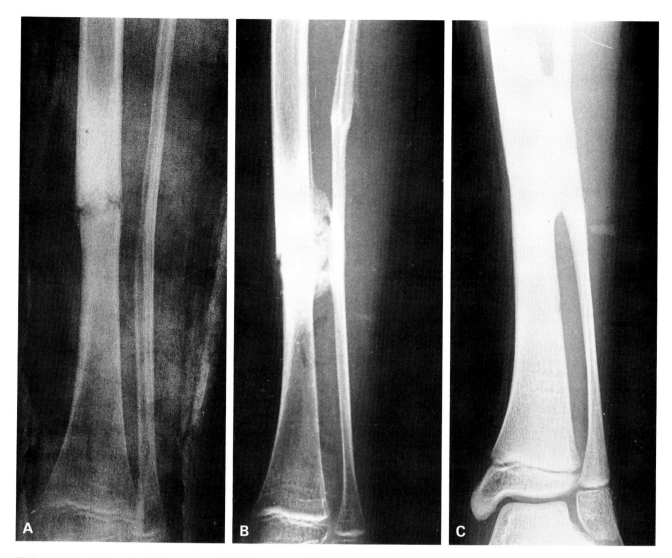

FIG. 19-74. *A,* Seemingly innocuous tibial fracture and bowed (greenstick) fibular injury. *B-C,* Progressive development of a tibiofibular synostosis, a rare complication in children.

fracture of the patella. Fixation methods should respect the degree of remaining function of the physis (Figs. 19-94 and 19-95). In type 3 injuries, transversely oriented pins may fix the malleolus to the remainder of the tibial epiphyseal ossification center. In type 4 injuries, transversely oriented pins may be placed metaphysis-to-metaphysis and epiphysis-to-epiphysis, thereby avoiding the physis and lessening the risk of premature growth arrest.

Type 1 injuries are most likely in children with myelodysplasia or comparable neuropathies associated with a Charcot-like joint (see Fig. 19-80). They are also common in young children, especially in syndromes such as child abuse. However, in the latter situation, variable amounts of transversely oriented metaphyseal bone may be included with the epiphyseal fragment (Figs. 19-96 and 19-97). These fractures may be minimally displaced and hard to diagnose roentgenographically. However, rotation may also occur, which makes the diagnosis more obvious (Fig. 19-98).

Because of the adduction and internal rotation (supination) injury mechanism present in many of these injuries,

localized type 5 compression growth mechanism damage may occur. This is difficult to ascertain at the time of the original injury, but must be sought by adequate long term follow-up to skeletal maturity.

Type 6 injuries (Fig. 19-99) may be more common than fully appreciated. A common mechanism of injury is catching an ankle in the spokes of a bicycle wheel. The attendant injury may be closed or open. This injury is an avulsion or compression of the periphery of the physis, and specifically the zone of Ranvier, and carries a reasonably high incidence of peripheral osseous bridge formation.

Type 7 injuries may occur. These involve the extension of the epiphyseal secondary ossification center into the malleolar region (Figs. 19-100 to 19-103). However, separation may occur at the junction between ossified and non-ossified regions, which may be difficult to diagnose in the young child.

Types 1 and 2 growth mechanism injuries involving either the tibia or fibula have good prognoses. However, with more extensive injuries, such as types 3 and 4 with displacement, there is a high incidence of growth deformity with localized premature epiphysiodesis and osseous bridging. Aitken observed that many of these injuries occurred in children nearing skeletal maturity, so that premature ossification is not a major consequence.[19-21]

Rotational Fractures. This is an infrequent pattern of a type 1 injury. Broock and Nevelos each described rotational displacement of the distal tibial growth plate.[82,83] The ankle mortise is essentially rotated as a unit (Fig. 19-104). No ligamentous injury appears necessary for this rotation to occur, although some of the periosteal-perichondral attachments must, of necessity, be detached. The fibula is not fractured, but is rotated with the tibial epiphysis. The foot and ankle are externally rotated approximately 45°, even though roentgenograms seem to show 90° of rotation. Undoubtedly because of anatomy, the syndesmosis is minimally disrupted. Broock duplicated the injury using an amputation specimen and found that 45° of external rotation accomplished the same radiographic appearance.[82] The periosteum and perichondrium had to be excised and the growth plate transsected transversely; however, the interosseous ligament did not have to be disrupted. The fibula was simply carried posteriorly behind the tibia by the attached ligaments of the fibula to the calcaneus. It is possible to reduce this injury by closed means.

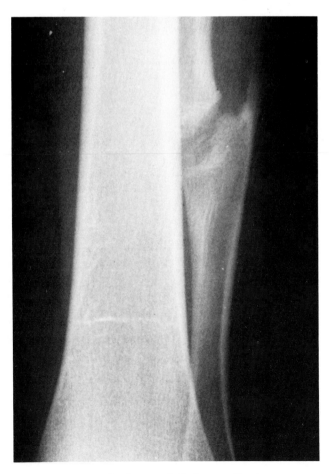

FIG. 19-75. Pseudarthrosis of fibula complicating an open fibular fracture.

Fracture of Tillaux. The fracture of Tillaux is a type 3 injury involving a variably-sized portion of the anterolateral tibial epiphysis (Fig. 19-105). This segment may be extruded anteriorly. In actuality, the fracture attributed to Tillaux was first described by Sir Astley Cooper.[84] This may or may not be accompanied by a posterior metaphyseal fragment (making it a triplane fracture).

Kleiger reviewed 8 cases seen in children undergoing skeletal closure; he also showed an interesting roentgenogram from a section of the distal end of the tibia from a 13-year-old girl that showed trabecula crossing the middle third of the epiphyseal plate but with remnants of the subchondral plate remaining in the lateral third (Fig. 19-106), which suggested that this anatomic factor was significant in the fracture pattern.[85]

There is a normal contour change toward the more medial portion of the epiphysis. This upward bump is about 1 cm from the middle margin and may protect the propagation of a fracture, particularly in the child undergoing closure, since this area is fused to the metaphysis. Closure of the distal tibial epiphysis proceeds in an asymmetric manner, closing first the middle portion, then on the medial side, and finally on the lateral portion, a process that takes about 1½ years to complete.

It is generally agreed that lateral rotation is responsible for the injury. The fracture line is vertical and extends from the distal articular surface upward (Figs. 19-107 to 19-109). The displaced fragment may be small or large. It is believed that the injury is produced by avulsion of the lateral portion of the tibial epiphysis by the inferior tibiofibular ligaments during lateral rotation of the foot and ankle. However, since there are no direct ligamentous attachments to this region, it seems more likely that as the foot is externally rotated, the talus applies a compression-torque stress that propagates a crack through the articular surface up to the growth plate, which then shears. On the basis of stress roentgenograms, it appeared that displacement of the epiphyseal fragment is produced by the pull of the tibiofibular ligaments. An operation corroborates that the lateral fragment is detached from the remainder of the epiphysis, but may be partially attached to the anterior-inferior tibiofibular ligament.

Triplane Fractures. The triplane fracture occurs across the transverse, sagittal, and coronal planes. When this occurs, the fracture lines cross the articular surface epiphyseal ossification center, physis, and metaphysis and create a type 4 growth mechanism injury. The principal displaced fragment may be either lateral (more common) or medial (Figs. 19-110 to 19-112). Lateral injury usually results from an external rotation mechanism and medial injury is caused by adduction and direct compression. The importance of defining the triplane nature of these fractures, which may look like a type 3 injury in the AP plane and a type 2 injury in the lateral plane, is the unusual anatomy of the fragment, the large amount of articular surface, and the potential for growth deformity. However, the latter is not a major problem since most of these injuries occur near skeletal maturity.

Marmor observed that at open reduction the fracture usually had three parts; the fragments were (1) the tibial shaft, (2) an anterolateral epiphyseal fragment, and (3) the combination of the remainder of the epiphysis and attached posterometaphyseal fragment.[86] Lynn reported two cases that required open reduction and internal fixation; he gave

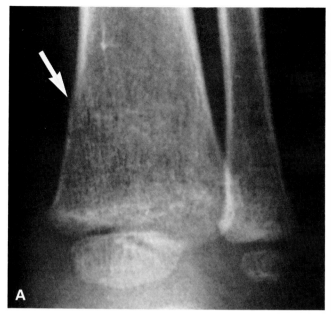
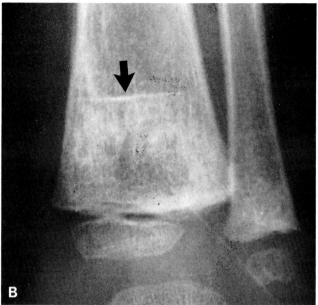

FIG. 19-76. *A,* Toddler's fracture of the distal tibial metaphysis. Minimal trabecular compression is evident (arrow). *B,* Two weeks later, a sclerotic line (arrow) demarcates the trabecular injury, and mottled sclerotic bone indicates temporary cutoff of the nutrient artery.

these lesions the name of triplane fractures, a term that Rang and Cooperman subsequently adopted.[87] Torg reported a fracture with the same anatomy and emphatically stated that this fracture was unstable and required open reduction.[88]

Cooperman, et al., did an excellent study of triplane fractures;[89] they surveyed 15 children with an average age of 13 years. There were 13 who were treated by closed reduction and 2 who were treated by open reduction. In the 5 cases in which tomography was used to determine the three-dimensional configuration of the fracture, two- rather than three-fragment fractures were consistently found. A medial fragment included the tibial shaft, the medial malleolus, and the anteromedial part of the epiphysis together with a piece of posterior metaphysis with attached fibula.

In Cooperman's study, three patients had premature closure of the epiphyseal plate, but none had significant shortening or angulation, probably due to the age of the patients at the time of injury. Nearly all patients with this type of injury were nearing the end of skeletal growth. Three addi-

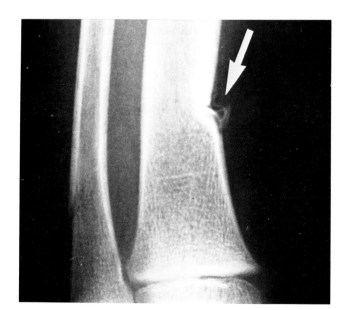

FIG. 19-77. Compression failure (arrow) of distal metaphysis.

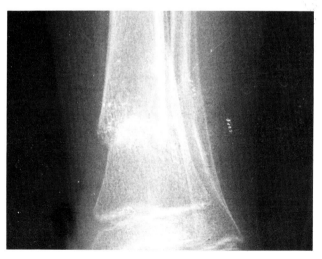

FIG. 19-78. Transverse, valgus deformed fracture, with bowing of the distal fibula. This was incompletely reduced, leaving excessive valgus, which will not correct spontaneously. Note the extensive subperiosteal new bone along the lateral sides of the tibia and the fibula.

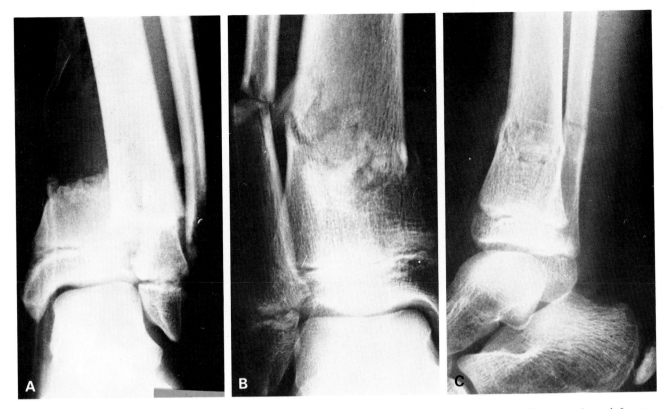

FIG. 19-79. Comminuted, open fracture of the distal tibia. *A,* Original injury. *B-C,* Post-reduction. The wound was left open following debridement and irrigation. The fracture healed without complication, although wound cultures at the initial debridement grew multiple flora, including many gram-negative organisms from pond mud that had been introduced. Wound healing was delayed and several irrigations and dressing changes under anesthesia were required to cleanse the bone adequately. With such aggressive treatment, and intravenous antibiotics, there was no complicating osteomyelitis.

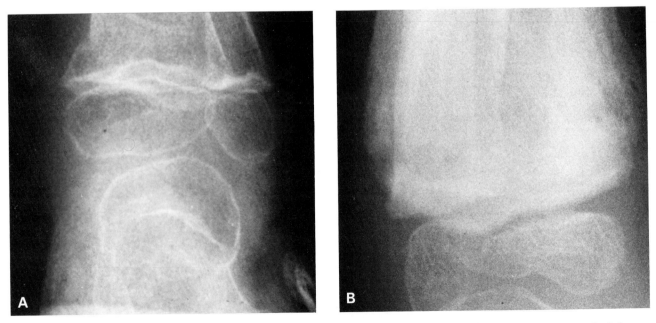

FIG. 19-80. Myelomeningocele patient who underwent a soft tissue clubfoot release. *A,* Two weeks after removal of plaster, a crushing, type 2 injury occurred. *B,* The patient was placed in her brace only, and allowed to bear weight. Eight weeks later, massive bone formation is present along the distal metaphysis due to chronic epiphysiolysis.

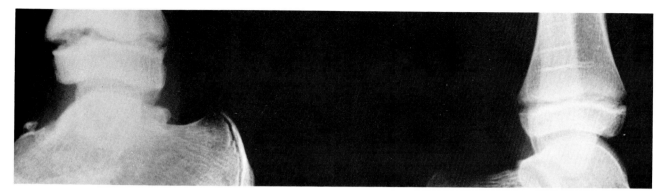

FIG. 19-81. Lateral view of chronic epiphyseal damage in patient with unilateral sensory neuropathy.

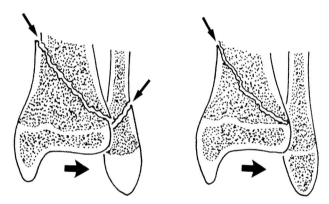

TYPE 2
SUPINATION - EXTERNAL ROTATION

FIG. 19-82. Schematic of type 2 injury with a large, medially based metaphyseal fragment. The fibula may or may not be fractured. The mechanism of injury appears to be combined supination and external rotation.

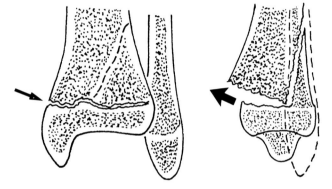

TYPE 2
SUPINATION - PLANTAR FLEXION

FIG. 19-84. Schematic of type 2 injury with posteriorly-based metaphyseal fracture. The mechanism of injury appears to be supination and plantar flexion.

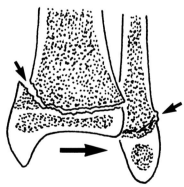

TYPE 2
SUPINATION-EXTERNAL ROTATION

FIG. 19-83. Schematic of type 2 injury with small medial metaphyseal fragment and compression failure of fibular metaphysis.

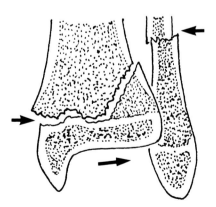

TYPE 2
PRONATION - EVERSION

FIG. 19-85. Schematic of type 2 injury with a laterally-based metaphyseal fragment. The mechanism of injury appears to be pronation-eversion.

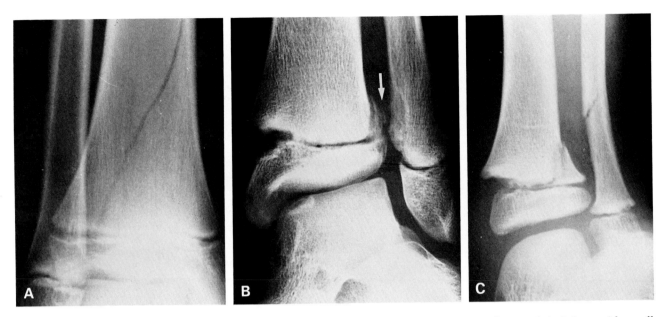

FIG. 19-86. *A,* Undisplaced type 2 fracture with large metaphyseal fragment. *B,* More characteristic injury with small posterolateral metaphyseal fragment (arrow) and lateral displacement of intact fibula. *C,* Eversion injury causing fracture propagation across the fibular diaphyseal-metaphyseal junction.

tional patients had external rotation deformities, and one also had joint incongruity. These complications are potentially serious and may lead to early degenerative arthritis. They were the result of incomplete reduction of the fracture.

Tomograms showed these injuries were external rotation deformities that required internal rotation to narrow the gap. An associated fibular fracture can complicate the closed

reduction, particularly if this is a greenstick fracture, which may prevent closed reduction by maintaining the angular deformity and result in shortening of the attached tibial fragment. On the basis of their series, Cooperman believed that the majority of the triplane fractures had no free anterolateral epiphyseal fragments, and therefore were two- and not three-part fractures.

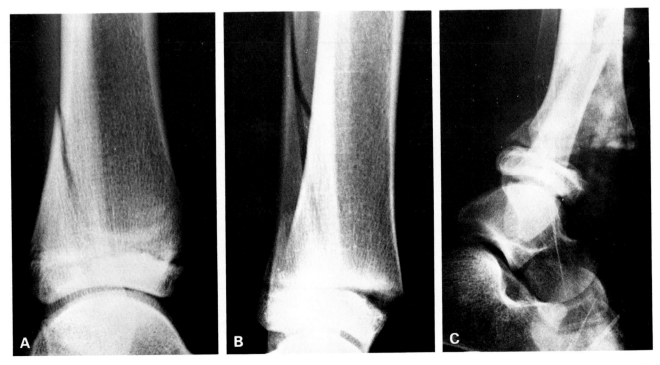

FIG. 19-87. Lateral views showing characteristic posterior location of the metaphyseal fragment. *A,* Undisplaced. *B,* Mild displacement with fibular fracture. *C,* Severe posterior displacement with fibular fracture.

Pathomechanisms

Carothers and Crenshaw reviewed 54 distal tibial epiphyseal injuries.[90] These cases were derived from a series of over 1400 ankle fractures and represented approximately 4% of all ankle fractures seen at the Campbell Clinic. They classified the injuries into abduction, external rotation, plantar flexion, axial compression, and adduction injuries. Adduction injuries appeared to be more commonly associated with complications than abduction or external rotation type injuries, which were more commonly associated with fractures through the epiphysis (type 3 and type 4 injuries).

Carothers showed experimentally that the force exerted through bone in compression is many times greater and probably more destructive than that which can be exerted through shear.[90] There is a greater tendency for compression to be applied in an adduction rather than abduction injury. In external rotation or abduction injuries, a large element of shear force causes a transverse fracture through the weak point, carrying the intact epiphysis past the vertical lateral border of the tibial metaphysis and propagating toward and possibly through the fibula. In adduction injuries, however, the medial border of the talus, after epiphyseal separation or fracture of the fibula, still exerts a compressive force through the tibial epiphysis, as its medial migration is blocked by the medial malleolus.[91]

The Lauge-Hansen studies demonstrated that two factors are important relative to ankle injuries: (1) position of the foot at the moment of impact, and (2) direction of the deforming force. Dias and Tachdjian have effectively applied these guidelines to distal epiphyseal fractures.[67] Four basic mechanisms have to be considered. In each, the first term represents the fixed position of the foot at the time of injury, and the second is the direction of the deforming force transmitted across the ankle joint.

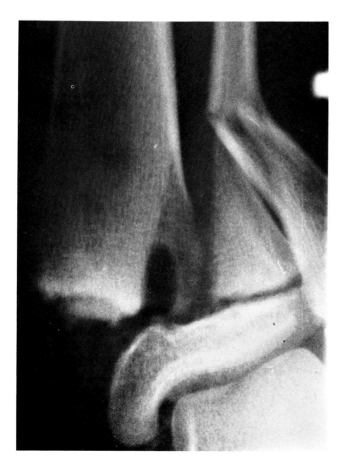

FIG. 19-88. Note how the posterolateral fragment "folds out" from the rest of the tibia.

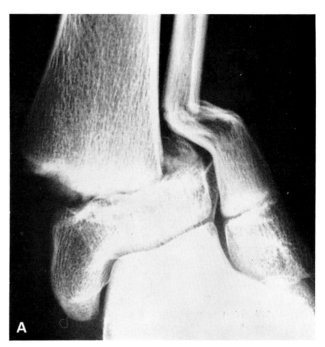

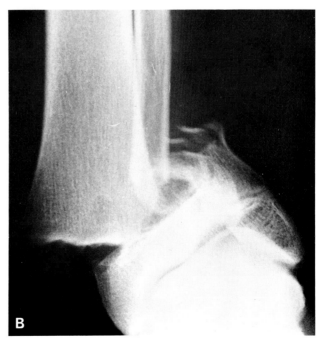

FIG. 19-89. Pronation-eversion injury may cause severe, multiple angulation deformation of the fibula by, *A,* greenstick, or, *B,* complete cortical failure.

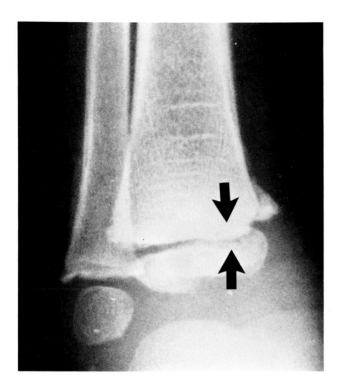

FIG. 19-90. Type 2 injury in a two-year-old. The medial area (arrows) represents potential type 5 injury that subsequently may form an osseous bridge.

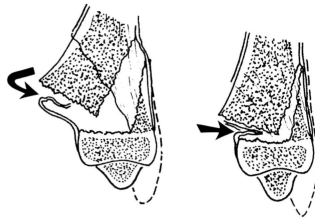

A   PERIOSTEAL HERNIATION

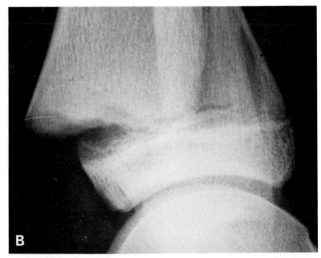

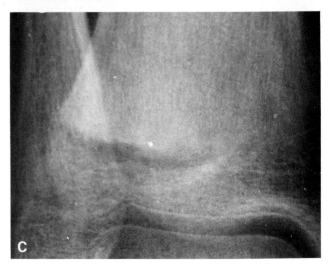

FIG. 19-91. *A*, Schematic of anterior periosteum being stripped from the metaphysis and pulled into the fracture gap. Reduction "locks" the periosteal flap into the fracture. *B*, Roentgenogram of posterior type 2 injury treated by closed reduction. *C*, AP view of this injury ten weeks later shows an anteromedial gap that has probably failed to fill in with bone because of herniated periosteum.

Supination-Inversion. In the mild injury pattern, traction by the lateral ligaments results in separation of the distal fibula (type 1 or 2 injury). Less frequently there is disruption of the lateral collateral ligaments or a type 7 fracture of the tip of the lateral malleolus. In contrast, the distal tibia does not fail. However, if the inversion force either persists or is of a greater force, the talus, which acts as a wedge, will cause a type 3 or 4 injury of the distal tibia.

Adduction injuries appear in approximately 15% of the cases and are characterized by medial displacement of either part or all of the distal tibial epiphysis. These injuries can include type 3 or 4 fractures of the medial malleolus and may or may not be accompanied by injury to the lateral malleolus, particularly a fracture through the shaft of the fibula. Adduction injuries are associated with a much higher incidence of growth deformity, and affected children are usually younger. In a series of 7 patients reported by Crenshaw, the median age was 9½ years.[92] In these injuries, the talus is forcibly adducted after separation of the lower fibular epiphysis or fracture of the distal fibula. The medial border of the upper surface of the talus impinges on the medial half of the lower end of the tibia and exerts a crushing force at this point. The interarticular shearing force causes a fracture that extends from the joint surface to the zone of hypertrophic cartilage cells of the physis, and then either along the physis or into the metaphysis, creating a type 3 or 4 physeal injury. Displacement of the medial malleolus and adjacent medial epiphyseal fragment may be slight to moderate. The germinal layer of the physis may be crushed by the mechanism and its compressive force. Occasionally an adduction injury displaces the entire distal tibial epiphysis medially with a

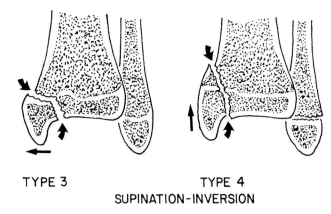

TYPE 3   TYPE 4
SUPINATION-INVERSION

FIG. 19-92. Schematic of type 3 and type 4 growth mechanism injuries of the medial malleolar region. The mechanism of these injuries appears to be supination and inversion.

medial metaphyseal fragment attached to it, as in a type 2 injury. The shearing force rarely splits the epiphysis completely to create a large type 4 injury.

Supination-Plantarflexion. With the foot in supination the posteriorly directed force creates a type 2 fracture of the distal tibia, although a type 1 pattern may occur in the younger child. Concomitant fibular injury does not usually occur. Plantarflexion injuries occur in approximately 12% of the cases. These injuries are distinguished by a variable posterior displacement of the entire distal tibial epiphysis, usually without a concomitant fracture of the fibula and an associated posterior metaphyseal tibial fragment. Again, this does not appear to be associated with a significant amount of deformity post-injury.

Supination-External Rotation. In its mild form this is a type 2 injury of the distal tibia characterized by a long spiral

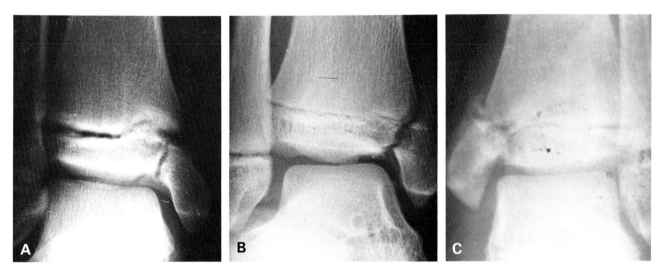

FIG. 19-93. *A*, Type 3 fracture of medial malleolus. *B*, Type 4 injury. *C*, Type 4 injury of medial malleolus with type 1 injury of distal fibula.

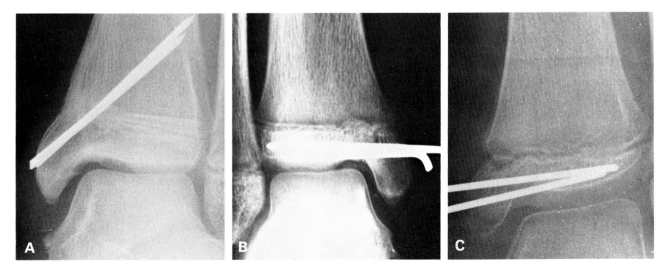

FIG. 19-94. Methods of fixation. *A*, Pins across physis. This should be avoided, if possible. Premature epiphysiodesis is evident. *B-C*, Type 3 and type 4 injuries treated by transepiphyseal pinning.

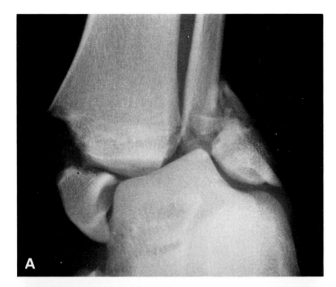

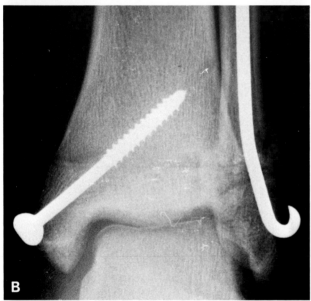

FIG. 19-95. *A,* Type 3 medial malleolar injury during physeal closure in adolescence. *B,* Open reduction. Since the physes are undergoing final stages of physiologic epiphysiodesis, fixation devices may be placed across them.

fracture starting laterally at the distal tibial zone of Ranvier. The metaphyseal fragment is primarily posterior. In the more severe type a similar tibial fracture is present, but a fibular metaphyseal fracture is characteristically found.

External rotation injuries are the second most common form, accounting for approximately 25% of the cases. They are characterized by posterolateral displacement of the entire distal tibial epiphysis and they are almost always accompanied by a posterior metaphyseal fragment from the tibia. The fracture of the fibula may be buckled (torus), but more often it is a transverse or oblique type of injury. Posterior displacement varies from 10 to 90% of the width of the metaphysis, and the epiphysis is usually accompanied in each instance by a posterior or posterolateral metaphyseal fragment. Again, this does not appear to be associated with

major problems of the ankle. Posterior displacement may vary and is generally associated with an oblique fracture of the distal fibular shaft.

Pronation-Eversion-External Rotation. These abduction injuries are the most frequent, occurring in 40% of the cases. This mechanism causes concomitant tibial and fibular fractures. A type 2 tibial fracture with a lateral (posterolateral) metaphyseal fragment is the most common pattern. There is lateral displacement of the entire distal tibial epiphysis. The fibular fracture is usually metaphyseal, and often 4 to 7 cm from the physis.

In this particular injury the fracture does not usually involve the distal fibular epiphyseal plate. The degree of lateral displacement varies, but is never extreme since it is checked by the fibula (unless that is also fractured). The entire distal tibial ankle mortise moves as a unit. It is frequently accompanied by a fragment of the lateral metaphysis, but is rarely associated with a major growth deformity. Prognosis for future growth is usually excellent, as the germinal layer is not damaged. However, there may be a crush (type 5) injury where the fracture propagates into the metaphysis.

Axial compression injuries and those caused by direct violence are associated with some posterior or posteromedial displacement, or a direct blow to the ankle. Again, these are not usually associated with major problems.

Treatment

Definitive treatment must usually be predicated upon the specific fracture type, as well as the reactive swelling that develops soon after injury and makes closed reduction difficult. A well-padded compression dressing and posterior splint should be applied before diagnostic roentgenograms are made. Gentle closed reduction should be carried out under a general anesthetic, as relaxation of muscles and absence of pain are essential to any minimally traumatic manipulation. The knee should be flexed to 90° and the foot plantarflexed to relax the gastrocnemius-soleus group of muscles. Overcorrection and forcible manipulation should be avoided.

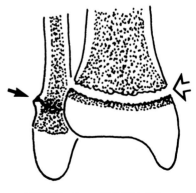

TYPE I - INFANCY

FIG. 19-96. Schematic of type 1 injury in infancy. Because of relative failure patterns, the fracture is more likely to leave a thin, transverse segment of metaphyseal bone.

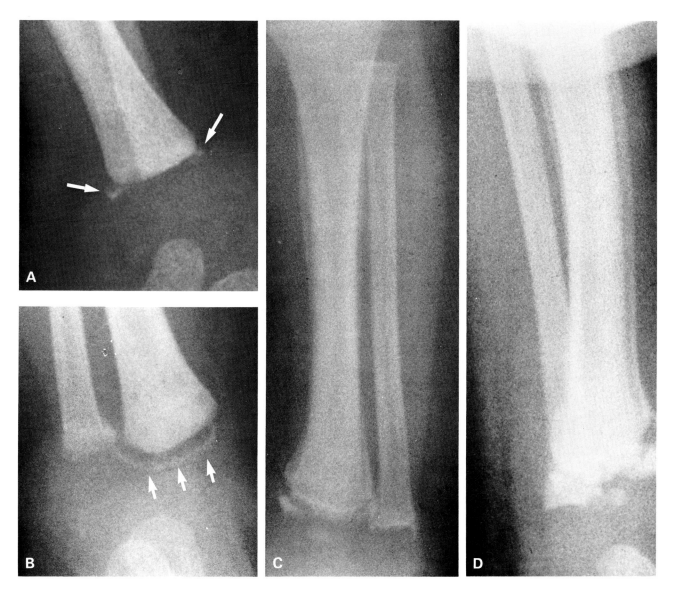

FIG. 19-97. Injury to the distal tibia in the infant tends to be a variation of a type 1 injury, with, *A*, small peripheral metaphyseal fragments (arrows) or, *B*, a transverse subchondral fragment (arrows). *C*, Subperiosteal bone may form along the entire shaft because of the loose periosteal attachments. *D*, A crushing fracture may also be present and will require long term follow-up. These injury patterns are characteristic of child abuse.

Accurate reposition of the displaced epiphyses at the expense of forced or repeated manipulation or operative intervention is not indicated, since spontaneous realignment of the ankle can occur late in the growing child, particularly if in the plane of motion of the ankle joint. Growth deformity at the ankle can be predicted reasonably well at the time of injury because it usually occurs in the adduction group and is accompanied by roentgenograms that demonstrate disruption of the epiphysis and physis. Many of the factors responsible for the high incidence of permanent damage probably result from the addition of a compression force through the medial side of the physis. There is evidence that massive displacement of the epiphyses results in clinically discernible disturbance of growth, or in subsequent defects in the ossification of the adjacent metaphysis.

In type 3 and 4 fractures accurate anatomic reduction is necessary. If this cannot be achieved by closed methods, open surgical reduction should be performed and smooth K-wires or a transepiphyseal fixation device should be used (see Fig. 19-94).

In the displaced type 3 and 4 injuries of the tibia, open reduction should be done to try to prevent cross-union between metaphysis and epiphysis, and to restore the congruity of the ankle mortise and articular surface. Obviously it is not possible to improve the prognosis for growth of the damaged epiphysis by surgical treatment, and it is conceivable that the surgical approach might cause further damage to the growth center. Nevertheless, the effective restoration of congruity to the ankle joint, which can be reliably achieved by open operation, is sufficient reason for recommending

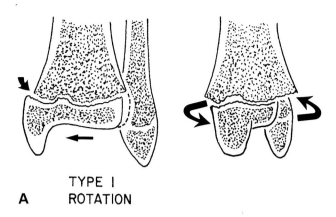

TYPE I
A ROTATION

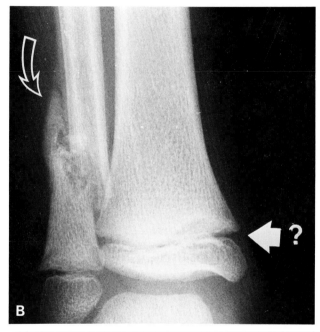

B

FIG. 19-98. *A,* Schematic of type 1 injury in an older child. This injury may be significantly rotated (see Fig. 19-104). *B,* Rotatory displacement of fibular metaphyseal fracture (open arrow). The tibial physis was tender on examination, but a fracture was not evident roentgenographically (arrow). This presumed type 1 injury pattern must be based primarily on clinical suspicion. The patient must be protected for three to four weeks with a non-weightbearing cast.

open reduction in these cases. The complications of shortening or bone deformity are not nearly as important as permanent disruption of the articular surfaces of the ankle.

Stampfel reported 16 open reductions with excellent results.[93] These reductions were primarily carried out for type 3 and 4 disruptions. In many cases cancellous screws were placed across the epiphyseal ossification center and not across the growth plate. In instances where a large type 4 fragment led to a large metaphyseal fragment, the screws were all placed in the metaphysis. This allowed good compression of the epiphyseal fragment; however, in type 3 injuries it was necessary to place the screw across the epiphyseal ossification center.

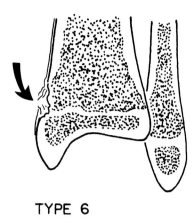

TYPE 6

FIG. 19-99. Schematic of type 6 injury to peripheral physis with disrupted zone of Ranvier and periosteal-perichondrial transition. This may predispose the injury to peripheral osseous bridge formation.

Type 6 injuries, which are usually acquired by catching the ankle in the spoked wheel of a bicycle, often result in an open injury. Definitive treatment must be directed at the wound to prevent osteomyelitis. The fracture itself does not require treatment. However, long term observation is essential to rule out subsequent formation of an osseous bridge, which can be resected if it creates a significant deformity.

Type 7 injuries do not generally involve a major weightbearing region. Closed reduction with the foot cast in mild adduction-inversion should be sufficient.

Results

Goldberg stressed that injury to the distal tibial epiphysis is becoming increasingly common with the stress on competitive athletics and greater overall participation in athletics.[94] Of 237 fractures, 184 were followed an average of 28 months following injury. Goldberg identified 3 groups according to the risks of developing shortening of the leg, angular deformity of the bone, or incongruity of the joint. The low-risk group consisted of 89 patients, only 6.7% of whom had complications. This group included all type 1 and type 2 fibular fractures, all type 1 tibial fractures, type 3 and type 4 tibial fractures with less than 2 mm of displacement, and epiphyseal avulsion injuries. In contrast, the high-risk group

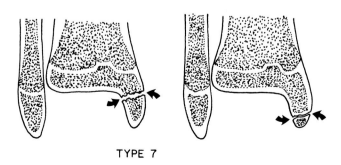

TYPE 7

FIG. 19-100. Schematic of type 7 injuries involving the medial malleolus. These do not involve weightbearing areas.

Pathomechanisms

Carothers and Crenshaw reviewed 54 distal tibial epiphyseal injuries.[90] These cases were derived from a series of over 1400 ankle fractures and represented approximately 4% of all ankle fractures seen at the Campbell Clinic. They classified the injuries into abduction, external rotation, plantar flexion, axial compression, and adduction injuries. Adduction injuries appeared to be more commonly associated with complications than abduction or external rotation type injuries, which were more commonly associated with fractures through the epiphysis (type 3 and type 4 injuries).

Carothers showed experimentally that the force exerted through bone in compression is many times greater and probably more destructive than that which can be exerted through shear.[90] There is a greater tendency for compression to be applied in an adduction rather than abduction injury. In external rotation or abduction injuries, a large element of shear force causes a transverse fracture through the weak point, carrying the intact epiphysis past the vertical lateral border of the tibial metaphysis and propagating toward and possibly through the fibula. In adduction injuries, however, the medial border of the talus, after epiphyseal separation or fracture of the fibula, still exerts a compressive force through the tibial epiphysis, as its medial migration is blocked by the medial malleolus.[91]

The Lauge-Hansen studies demonstrated that two factors are important relative to ankle injuries: (1) position of the foot at the moment of impact, and (2) direction of the deforming force. Dias and Tachdjian have effectively applied these guidelines to distal epiphyseal fractures.[67] Four basic mechanisms have to be considered. In each, the first term represents the fixed position of the foot at the time of injury, and the second is the direction of the deforming force transmitted across the ankle joint.

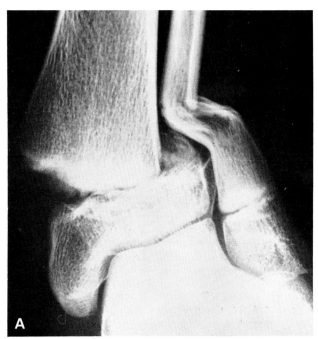

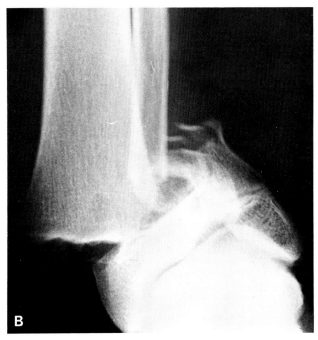

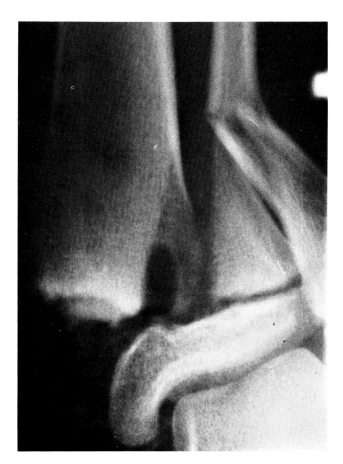

FIG. 19-88.   Note how the posterolateral fragment "folds out" from the rest of the tibia.

FIG. 19-89.   Pronation-eversion injury may cause severe, multiple angulation deformation of the fibula by, *A,* greenstick, or, *B,* complete cortical failure.

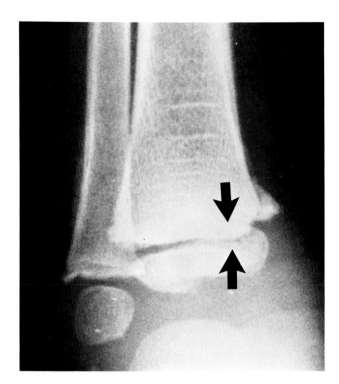

FIG. 19-90. Type 2 injury in a two-year-old. The medial area (arrows) represents potential type 5 injury that subsequently may form an osseous bridge.

Supination-Inversion. In the mild injury pattern, traction by the lateral ligaments results in separation of the distal fibula (type 1 or 2 injury). Less frequently there is disruption of the lateral collateral ligaments or a type 7 fracture of the tip of the lateral malleolus. In contrast, the distal tibia does not fail. However, if the inversion force either persists or is of a greater force, the talus, which acts as a wedge, will cause a type 3 or 4 injury of the distal tibia.

Adduction injuries appear in approximately 15% of the cases and are characterized by medial displacement of either part or all of the distal tibial epiphysis. These injuries can include type 3 or 4 fractures of the medial malleolus and may or may not be accompanied by injury to the lateral malleolus, particularly a fracture through the shaft of the fibula. Adduction injuries are associated with a much higher incidence of growth deformity, and affected children are usually younger. In a series of 7 patients reported by Crenshaw, the median age was 9½ years.[92] In these injuries, the talus is forcibly adducted after separation of the lower fibular epiphysis or fracture of the distal fibula. The medial border of the upper surface of the talus impinges on the medial half of the lower end of the tibia and exerts a crushing force at this point. The interarticular shearing force causes a fracture that extends from the joint surface to the zone of hypertrophic cartilage cells of the physis, and then either along the physis or into the metaphysis, creating a type 3 or 4 physeal injury. Displacement of the medial malleolus and adjacent medial epiphyseal fragment may be slight to moderate. The germinal layer of the physis may be crushed by the mechanism and its compressive force. Occasionally an adduction injury displaces the entire distal tibial epiphysis medially with a

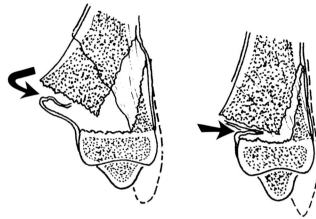

A PERIOSTEAL HERNIATION

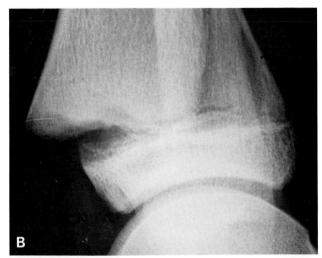

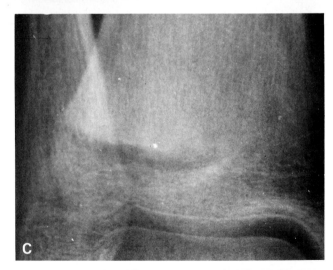

FIG. 19-91. A, Schematic of anterior periosteum being stripped from the metaphysis and pulled into the fracture gap. Reduction "locks" the periosteal flap into the fracture. B, Roentgenogram of posterior type 2 injury treated by closed reduction. C, AP view of this injury ten weeks later shows an anteromedial gap that has probably failed to fill in with bone because of herniated periosteum.

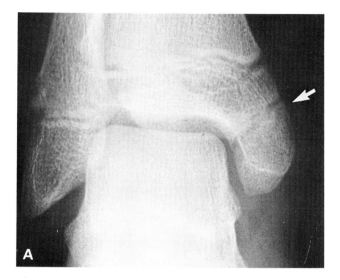

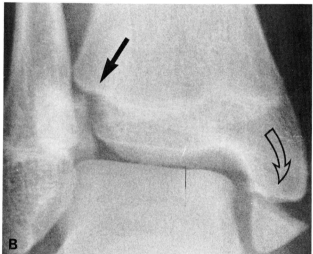

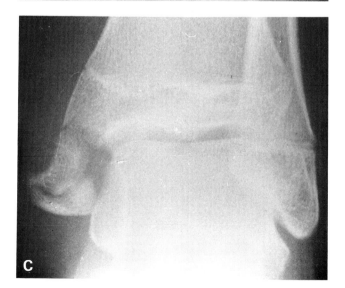

FIG. 19-101. Type 7 injuries of medial malleolus. *A,* Undisplaced. *B,* Mild displacement (open arrow), with concomitant fracture of Tillaux (solid arrow). *C,* Displaced, rotated and comminuted.

consisted of 28 patients, 32% of whom developed complications. This group included type 3 and type 4 tibial fractures with 2 mm or more displacement, juvenile Tillaux fractures, triplane fractures, and comminuted tibial epiphyseal fractures (type 5). The third, unpredictable group was made up of 66 patients, 16.7% of whom had complications, and included only type 2 tibial fractures. The incidence and types of complications certainly correlated well with the type of fracture, the severity of displacement or comminution, and the adequacy of the reduction.

Guiliani felt that each of these injuries was associated with some degree of deformity, claiming that the commonest deformity was a discrepancy in leg length and that varus and valgus deformity appeared as late complications.[95] Hohman also concurred with this high incidence of complications, whereas other authors have stated that growth deformity usually occurs only following adduction-type fractures.[71,90,96,97] Johnson felt that growth deformity could occur consequent to injuries other than adduction injuries.[98]

Complications

The most significant complication is growth arrest with or without the formation of an osseous bridge (Figs. 19-113 to 19-117). Growth arrest is most likely to develop after an adduction injury as a result of crushing of the germinal layer of the physis.[99] However, it is not always easy to predict whether this will occur. In types 3 and 4 fractures the medial part of the tibial physis may fuse, whereas the lateral portion may continue to grow, which leads to varus deformity at the ankle. The younger the patient, the worse the deformity. Premature growth arrest of the entire distal tibial epiphysis results in shortening of the tibia.

Langenskiöld showed that complications of traumatic premature closure are understressed, and that when they do occur care must be taken to assess the distal fibula, as it might require epiphysiodesis so as not to result in a few millimeters of overgrowth of the fibula that might affect joint mechanics.[100] He subsequently was able to treat some of these injuries with resection of the premature epiphysiodesis.

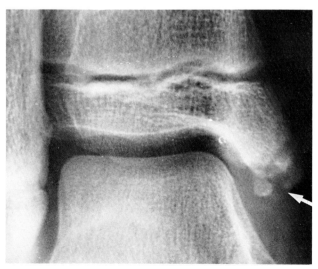

FIG. 19-102. Multifocal accessory ossification, with possible fracture (arrow).

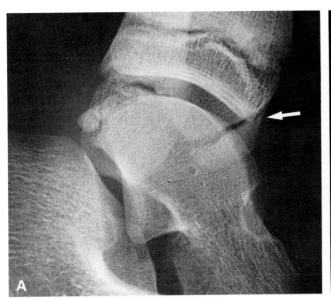 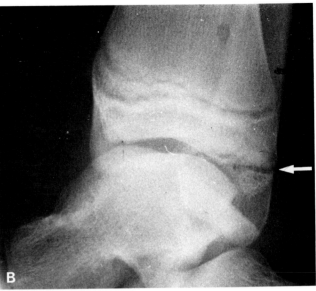

FIG. 19-103. Type 7 injuries of, *A,* anterior and, *B,* posterior tibial epiphysis.

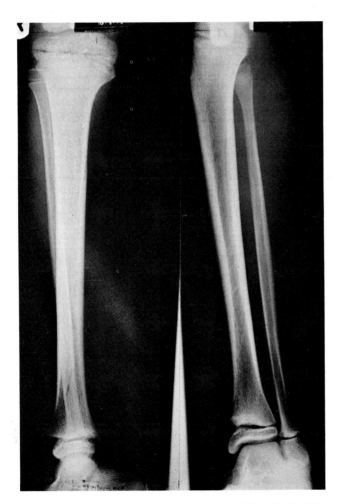

FIG. 19-104. Type 1 rotational injury of the distal tibia. Compare proximal and distal ends.

If the distal tibial physis does close prematurely, overgrowth of the distal fibula may block normal heel valgus and cause pain (Fig. 19-118). It is essential that epiphysiodesis be performed on the distal fibula to prevent such overgrowth.

King injected sodium diatrizoate (Hypaque) into the peroneal tendon sheath and showed that in rheumatoid patients with significant amounts of lateral pain there was a block in the flow of contrast medium in the sheath at the

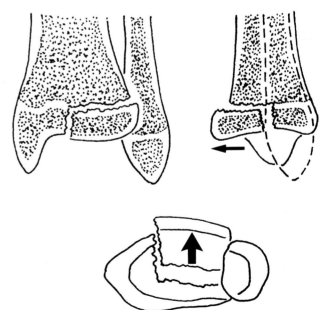

TYPE 3 - FRACTURE OF TILLAUX

FIG. 19-105. Schematic of fracture of Tillaux, a type 3 injury of the anterolateral tibial epiphysis.

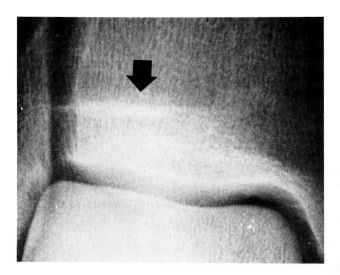

FIG. 19-106. Adolescent distal tibia, showing complete closure and remodeling medially, and residual physeal subchondral bone laterally (arrow).

tip of the lateral malleolus due to calcaneofibular weight-bearing impingement.[101] The pain was completely stopped by excising the tip of the lateral malleolus.

Robertson and Siffert and Arkin described osteochondritis as a complication following a bimalleolar fracture with a crush injury of the lateral half of the epiphysis.[102,103] Robertson's case did not sustain a fracture, but merely a "sprain." The patient was 3-years-old at the time of injury, and a roentgenogram failed to diagnose a type 2 fracture. The roentgenogram probably could not totally rule it out if it was a pure epiphyseal displacement and reduction; however, 4 months later when roentgenograms were taken there was flattening and sclerosis of the distal tibial physis, particularly laterally.

Tibiofibular synostosis has also been reported as a rare complication of a distal tibial epiphyseal injury.[104] This undoubtedly results from periosteal disruptions and subsequent ectopic bone formation between the metaphyses just above the syndesmosis.

Distal Fibular Injuries

Most often the distal fibular metaphysis or physis fails concomitant with an abduction or adduction injury of the distal tibia. However, the distal fibular physis may fail, albeit infrequently, as a solitary injury.

The patterns include failure through the physis as a type 1 or 2 growth mechanism injury (Figs. 19-119 to 19-122). This often occurs just as the physis is undergoing normal closure, comparable to the fracture of Tillaux of the distal tibia. Type 7 injuries of the distal portion of the secondary ossification may occur, but these should not be confused with normal accessory ossification centers at the tip (Fig. 19-123).

The pathomechanics usually involve an abduction-eversion injury, which forces the talus and calcaneus against the fibular epiphysis. Since the physis is at the tibial articular level, transversely directed forces summate in the physis. Adduction injury mechanisms may occur, but are probably much less frequent.

Diagnosis is difficult because displacement is usually minimal. Comparison to the opposite side may help. However, direct palpation with elucidation of tenderness directly over the physis is the most accurate sign, even when the roentgenogram appears normal.

Since these are generally undisplaced, simple cast immobilization with the ankle in neutral is all that is necessary. The cast should be maintained for 3 to 4 weeks. If the region is still tender, a full 6 weeks of immobilization may be necessary. If there is any displacement, it should be reduced as anatomically as possible by closed manipulation. Pin fixation is rarely necessary.

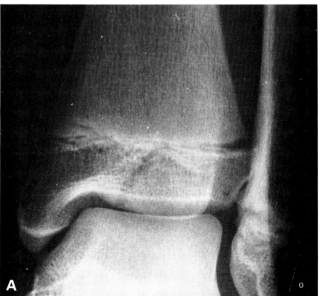

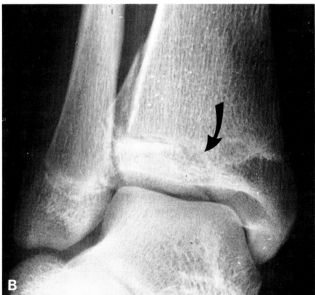

FIG. 19-107. *A,* Type 3 injury of lateral tibia (Tillaux fracture). *B,* Comparable type 4 injury (arrow).

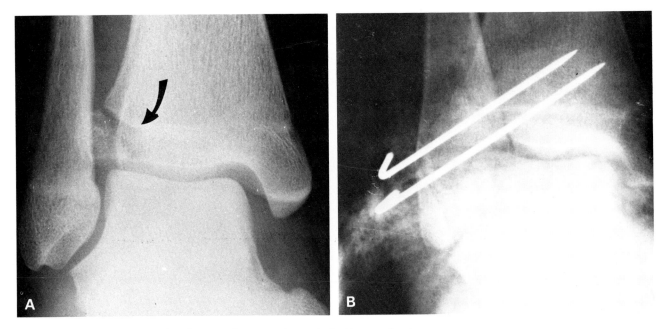

FIG. 19-108. *A,* Small, displaced type 3 fragment (arrow). *B,* Open reduction.

Sometimes these injuries are not recognized as chondro-osseous fractures, but dismissed as an ankle "sprain." Continued use, despite discomfort, in an active child with a normal valgus posture to the hindfoot may create a chronic epiphysiolysis. The boy shown in Figure 19-122 had twisted his ankle 6 months before the roentgenogram was taken. He had chronic swelling and pain over the lateral malleolus, but had continued unrestricted activity without any definitive treatment. A bone scan showed marked uptake of technetium (see Fig. 19-17), and a biopsy was performed because of the lytic appearance of the metaphysis adjacent to the physis. During the operation chronic inflammation, cartilage, and epiphyseal mobility were evident. A histologic study revealed irregular islands of growth cartilage that included some growing into the trabecular bone of the metaphyseal cortex. A diagnosis of epiphyseal nonunion was made and the boy was treated for 8 weeks in a short-leg cast; after the cast was removed there was roentgenographic and clinical healing. Whether this will predispose the boy, who is 13 but small relative to parents and siblings, to growth disruption in the fibula is unknown, but must remain a distinct possibility because of the prolonged, repetitive trauma.

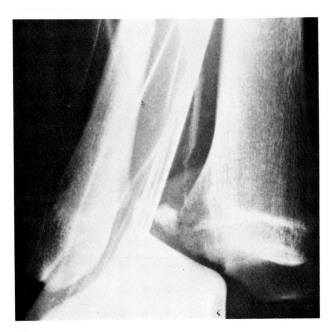

FIG. 19-109. Severe displacement and disruption of syndesmosis with a Tillaux fracture.

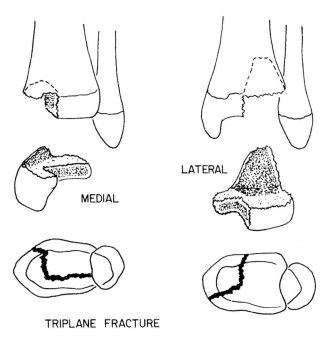

FIG. 19-110. Schematic of medial and lateral triplane fractures.

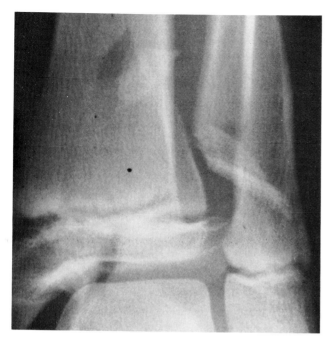

FIG. 19-111. Mortise view showing a triplane fracture. This fracture is a three part injury with a lateral type 4 fragment and a medial type 3 fragment. This is an infrequent injury pattern.

Tibiofibular Ligament Injuries

Tibiofibular ligament injuries are unusual in children.[105] The injury mechanisms that normally would produce these injuries in adults cause disruption of the ligaments around the tibiofibular syndesmosis and subsequent fracture of the fibula above the level of the syndesmosis in children. However, this same valgus strain applied to a child's ankle usually results in epiphyseal disruption of the distal fibula or tibia, rather than a ligament injury. There may be a fracture

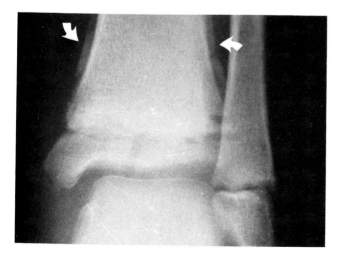

FIG. 19-112. This apparent type 3 Tillaux fracture was actually a triplane injury, as evidenced by the subsequent development of subperiosteal new bone formation (arrows).

through the distal fibular metaphysis, which in essence is intra-articular because of the extent of the capsular reflection up to the region of the syndemosis to cover the tibial lateral articular surface and the modification of the lateral malleolus in the metaphyseal region (see the section titled "Anatomy" in this chapter).

In late childhood and adolescence acute inversion injuries may lead to chronic lateral ligament and capsular attenuation or disruption. This must be considered in children who participate in intensely competitive sports programs, such as gymnastics, where acute and chronic inversion injuries are relatively common. Ankle arthrography may be helpful in delineating capsular damage (Fig. 19-124). However, soft tissue repairs, especially those emphasizing peroneal tendon placement through the distal fibula, should be deferred until skeletal maturity. Theoretically, if the tendon is directed through the epiphysis, tensile stress might increase in the open fibular physis during subsequent inversion and pull off the epiphysis.

Arthrodesis of the Ankle

Because of significant fracture involving the articular surface and major growth deformity, arthrodesis may be necessary in some instances for a painful ankle joint, even prior to skeletal maturity.[106] In such instances a method proposed by Chuinard and Peterson is applicable to use particularly in children with functioning physes (Fig. 19-125).[107] Most procedures for ankle fusion utilize bone grafts that transgress the epiphyseal line and thus have limited applicability during the growth period. Several authors have employed central bone grafts and stated that growth arrest does not occur when the graft passes through the epiphyseal plate at or near the central region. In contrast, Turner described gross deformities with extra-articular arthrodesis crossing the growth plate at the ankle.[108] The graft essentially is the anterior placement of a full-thickness iliac bone graft impacted between the denuded surfaces of the tibial epiphysis and the talar ossification center.

Tendon Injuries

Like ligament injuries, tendon injuries around the ankle are rare. In a large series, Ralston reported only 1 child with tendon injuries. The patient was 14 years of age and had struck his midtendon; a week later, while engaged in an athletic activity, he suffered an acute onset of pain and had a distinct and obvious rupture.[109] Treatment should initially be conservative with the ankle casted in plantar flexion. The reparative capacity of the child's tendon is much greater than the adult's.

Peroneal Tendon Dislocations

Dislocation of the peroneal tendons appears to be encountered more often with the increased popularity of athletics, particularly certain athletic endeavors that tend to stress the lateral side of the ankle mechanism.[110] Increased impetus toward competitive gymnastics, in particular, and some of the exercise routines that increase stress on the lateral and

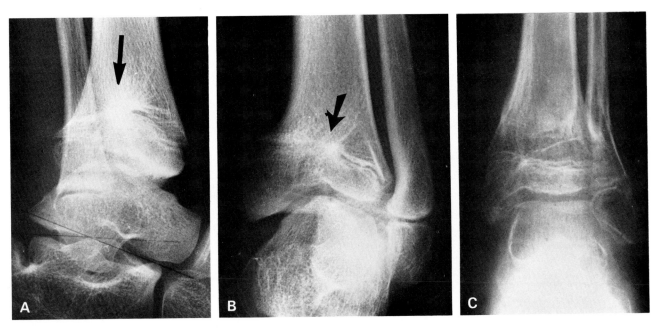

FIG. 19-113. *A-B,* Localized bridge formation (arrows). *C,* Osteotomy without resection of bridge.

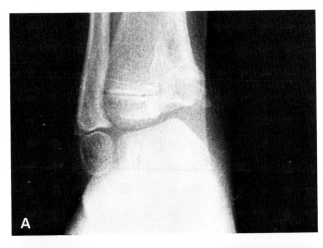

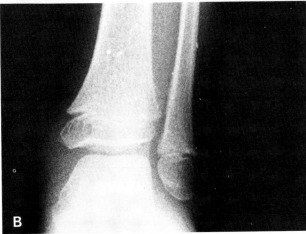

FIG. 19-114. Examples of severe, *A,* and moderate, *B,* growth arrest after medial malleolar fracture.

medial ankle ligaments are associated with an increasing incidence of injuries.

The peroneal muscles originate from the lateral surface of the fibula and the inner muscular septa and end distally in strong tendons. The tendon of the peroneus longus inserts into the lateral surface of the medial cuneiform bone and the base of the first metatarsal; that of the peroneus brevis muscle attaches into the base of the fifth metatarsal. These tendons lie close together in a tendon sheath in a groove behind the lateral malleolus. The tendon of the peroneus longus lies superficial to that of the brevis. A short distance proximal to the lateral malleolus the tendon sheath is reinforced by a fibrous band, the superior peroneal retinaculum, which extends from the posterior margin of the fibula to the calcaneus. This retinaculum constitutes the lateral boundary of the tunnel in which the tendons run behind the lateral malleolus. The mobility of the tendons and the depth of the fossa in which they lie vary.

Instances of recurrent dislocation of the peroneal tendon are infrequent, but often disabling. However, there is no instability of the ankle or subtalar joint, and the patient will often admit to noticing a so-called "pop" in the ankle. In acute anterior dislocation of the peroneal tendons, they go from their normal position and ride on the lateral malleolus. Usually this occurs in patients with a predisposing anatomic abnormality with the groove in the fibula serving as a pulley for the tendons being absent or lax. Zoellner gives a good review of the anatomy and its variations and how it affects potential occurrence of this disorder.[111]

Physical examination will reveal bow-stringing or easily dislocatable peroneal tendons and a shallow peroneal groove. Interestingly, I encountered an additional variation in which the muscle belly of the peroneus longus extended down through the superior peroneal retinaculum down to the tip of the lateral malleolus; this was obviously inflamed and created symptoms analogous to and indistinguishable from those of recurrent dislocation of the peroneal.

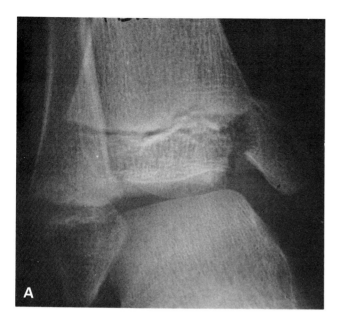

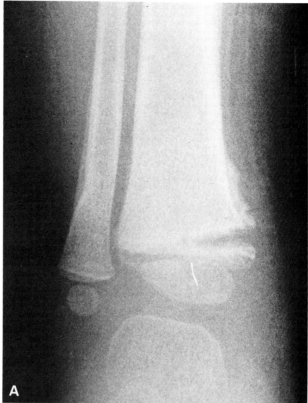

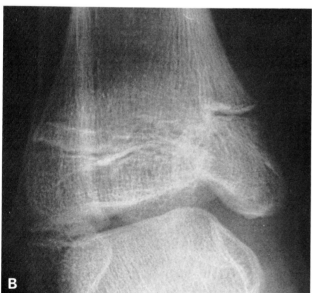

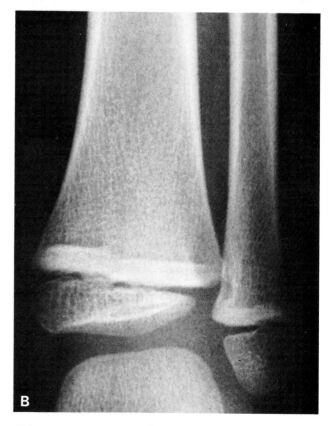

FIG. 19-115. *A,* Type 3 medial malleolar fracture. This was treated by closed "reduction." *B,* Osseous bridge formation eight months later.

Acute dislocation is manifest as a painful ankle with swelling behind the lateral malleolus. The retromalleolar region is tender, and often one or both tendons can be felt to be moving under the skin onto the malleolus. Although the tendons may reduce spontaneously, redislocation may be provoked by active pronation of the foot and dorsiflexion of the ankle. Recurrent dislocation is characterized by pain and instability at the ankle, and the peroneal tendons can be felt to be displacing over the ankle.

Mounier-Kuhn, after operating on 40 patients, established the following varieties of dislocation: (1) rupture of the superior peroneal retinaculum, including avulsion of the retinaculum from the fibula. (2) Interposition of one or both tendons between the lateral malleolus and the retinaculum

FIG. 19-116. *A,* Seemingly innocuous type 2 fracture in a two-year-old. *B,* One year later, a central bony bridge is forming.

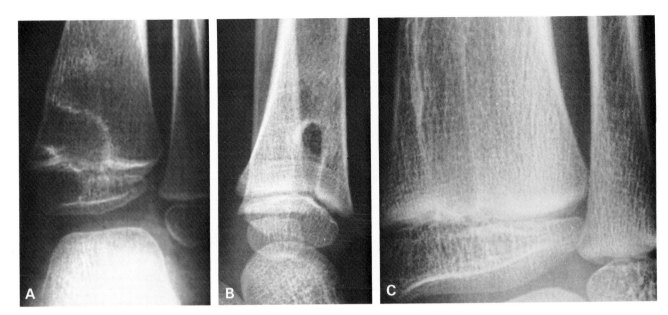

FIG. 19-117. (Patient shown in Figure 19-116). *A-B,* The bridge was resected through a metaphyseal window and filled with fat. *C,* 38 months later, the bridge has not reformed.

with this ligament remaining intact.[111] In this case, the tendons may have forced themselves between the retinaculum and the periosteum, or between the bone and periosteum of the lateral malleolus. (3) When the retinaculum is inserted too far forward on the fibula, dislocation or subluxation of the tendons readily occurs. As a result of this anomaly, the retinaculum may be stretched, displacing the tendons to the anterolateral surface.

Acute dislocation should be treated conservatively with repositioning of the tendons and fixation of the ankle in slight plantar flexion by means of a below-knee plaster cast. Treatment with an elastic bandage is inadequate. For recur-

rent dislocation, surgical treatment is preferred. Numerous techniques have been described for surgical treatment of the lesion; some were directed at substitution or suturing of the superior peroneal retinaculum. Ellis Jones took a strip of Achilles tendon, leaving one end attached to the calcaneus and passed it through a hole drilled in the lateral malleolus; he then fixed it to the malleolus. The retinaculum may also be replaced by strips in the fascia lata or skin. The tendon sheath can be sutured more tightly to the posterior edge of the lateral malleolus.

Zoellner and Clancy reported a method of fixing recurrent dislocation of the peroneal tendon by making a groove in the fibula.[111] However, operations to deepen the fossa should not be used in children until skeletal maturity has been reached, as the suggested operation may cause damage to the distal fibular physis and lead to eccentric growth arrest, or may predispose to physeal disruption with subsequent inversion injury.

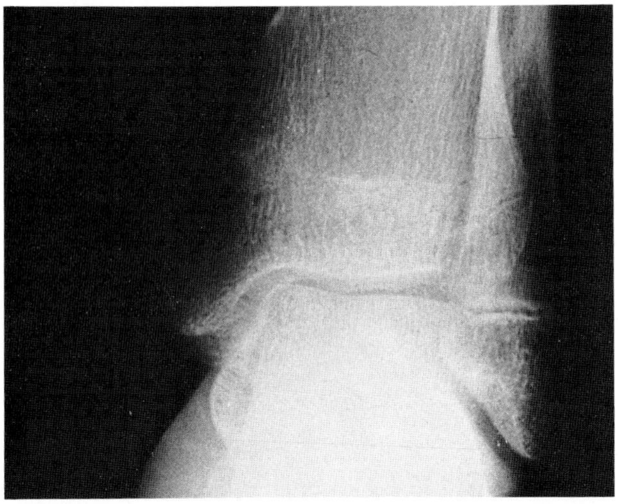

FIG. 19-118. Fracture of the distal tibia has led to premature closure of the physis. The distal fibula is still open and could cause mild overgrowth. Epiphysiodesis should be undertaken.

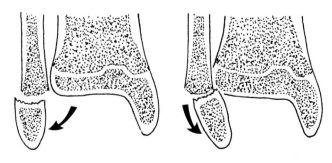

TYPE I - FIBULA

FIG. 19-119. Schematic of type 1 fibular physeal failure patterns in abduction and adduction.

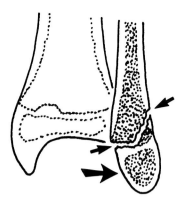

A   TYPE 2 - FIBULA

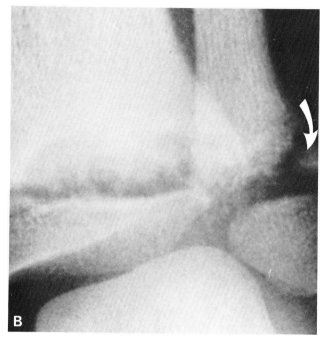

FIG. 19-120. *A,* Schematic of type 2 injury pattern of the distal fibula. *B,* Roentgenogram of patient presenting with lateral ankle pain. A type 2 fibular growth mechanism injury (arrow) is evident. However, the tibial physis is widened. Subsequent evaluation showed dietary, hypocalcemic rickets.

References

1. Ogden, J. A.: The anatomy and function of the proximal tibiofibular joint. Clin. Orthop., *101:*186, 1974.
2. Ogden, J. A., and Southwick, W. O.: Osgood-Schlatter's disease and tibial tuberosity development. Clin. Orthop., *116:*180, 1976.
3. Ogden, J. A.: Subluxation and dislocation of the proximal tibiofibular joint. J. Bone Joint Surg., *56-A:*145, 1974.
4. Hoed, D. D.: A separate centre of ossification for the tip of the internal malleolus. Br. J. Radiol., *30:*67, 1925.
5. Powell, H. D. W.: Extra centre of ossification for the medial malleolus in children. J. Bone Joint Surg., *43-B:*107, 1961.
6. Borch-Madsen, P.: On symmetrical bilateral fracture of the tuberositas tibiae and eminentia intercondyloides. Acta Orthop. Scand., *24:*44, 1954.
7. Garcia, A., and Neer, C. S. II: Isolated fractures of the intercondylar eminence of the tibia. Am. J. Surg., *95:*593, 1958.
8. Meyers, M. H., and McKeever, F. M.: Fracture of the intercondylar eminence of the tibia. J. Bone Joint Surg., *41-A:*209, 1959.
9. Meyers, M. H., and McKeever, F. M.: Fracture of the intercondylar eminence of the tibia. J. Bone Joint Surg., *52-A:*1677, 1970.
10. Roth, P.: Fracture of the spine of the tibia. J. Bone Joint Surg., *29:*509, 1928.
11. Zaricznyj, B.: Avulsion fracture of the tibial eminence: treatment by open reduction and pinning. J. Bone Joint Surg., *59-A:*1111, 1977.
12. Girgis, F. B., Marshall, J. L., and Al Monajem, A. R. S.: The cruciate ligaments of the knee joint. Anatomical, functional and experimental analysis. Clin. Orthop., *106:*216, 1975.
13. Horne, J. G., and Parsons, C. J.: The anterior cruciate ligament: its anatomy and a new method of reconstruction. Can. J. Surg., *20:*214, 1977.
14. Jones, R., and Smith, S. A.: On rupture of the crucial ligaments of the knee, and on fractures of the spine of the tibia. Br. J. Surg., *1:*70, 1913.
15. Pringle, J. A.: Avulsion of the spine of the tibia. Ann. Surg., *46:*169, 1907.
16. Kennedy, J. C., Weinberg, H. W., and Wilson, A. S.: The anatomy and function of the anterior cruciate ligament. As determined by clinical and morphological studies. J. Bone Joint Surg., *56-A:*223, 1974.
17. Bakalim, G., and Wilppula, E.: Closed treatment of fracture of the tibial spines. Injury, *5:*210, 1974.
18. Smillie, I. S.: Injuries of the Knee Joint. 4th Ed. New York, Churchill Livingstone, 1970.
19. Aitken, A. P.: The end results of the fractured distal tibial epiphysis. J. Bone Joint Surg., *18:*685, 1936.
20. Aitken, A. P., and Ingersoll, R. E.: Fractures of proximal tibial epiphyseal cartilage. J. Bone Joint Surg., *38-A:*787, 1956.
21. Aitken, A. P.: Fractures of the proximal tibial epiphyseal cartilage. Clin. Orthop., *41:*92, 1965.
22. Cahill, B. R.: Stress fracture of the proximal tibial epiphysis. Am. J. Sports Med., *5:*86, 1977.
23. Curry, G. J., and Bishop, D. L.: Diastasis of the superior tibial complicated by gangrene. J. Bone Joint Surg., *19:*1093, 1937.
24. Gibson, A.: Separation of the upper epiphysis of the tibia. Ann. Surg., *77:*485, 1923.
25. Kaplan, E. B.: Avulsion fracture of proximal tibial epiphysis. Bull. Hosp. Joint Dis., *24:*119, 1963.
26. Nolan, R. A., et al.: Tibial epiphyseal injuries. Contemp. Orthop., *1:*11, 1978.
27. Schlatter, C.: Verletzungen des schnabelformigen fortsatzes der oberen tibiaepiphyse. Beitr. Klin. Chir., *38:*874, 1903.
28. Shelton, W. R., and Canale, S. T.: Fractures of the tibia through the proximal tibial epiphyseal cartilage. J. Bone Joint Surg., *61-A:*167, 1979.
29. Silberman, W. W., and Murphy, J. L.: Avulsion fracture of the proximal tibial epiphysis. J. Trauma, *6:*592, 1966.
30. von Stubenbauch, L.: Uber dei traumatische (subcutane) Epiphysenlosung am oberen Tibiaende. Arch. f. Klin. Chir., *164:*621, 1931.
31. Welch, P. H., and Wynne, G. F.: Proximal tibial epiphyseal fracture separation. J. Bone Joint Surg., *45-A:*782, 1963.
32. Kestler, D. C.: Unclassified premature cessation of epiphyseal growth about the knee joint. J. Bone Joint Surg., *29:*788, 1947.
33. Morton, K. S., and Starr, D. E.: Closure of the anterior portion of the upper tibial epiphysis as a complication of tibial-shaft fracture. J. Bone Joint Surg., *46-A:*570, 1964.
34. Bovill, E. G.: Arteriographic visualization of the juxta-epiphyseal vascular bed following epiphyseal separation. J. Bone Joint Surg., *45-A:*1260, 1963.

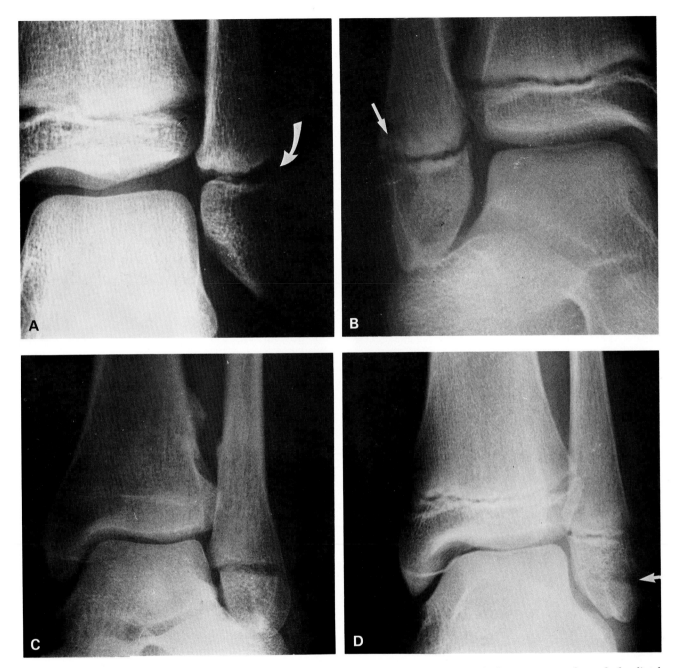

FIG. 19-121. *A,* Type 1 fracture of distal fibula (arrow). *B,* Type 2 injury (arrow) of distal fibula. *C,* Fracture through the distal fibula just after closure (comparable to Tillaux injury). *D,* Type 7 injury (arrow).

35. Cancelmo, R. P.: Isolated fracture of anterior tibial tubercle. A.J.R., *87:*1064, 1962.

36. Deliyannis, S. N.: Avulsion of the tibial tuberosity. Report of two cases. Injury, *4:*431, 1973.

37. Hand, W. L., Hand, C. R., and Dunn, A. W.: Avulsion fractures of the tibial tubercle. J. Bone Joint Surg., *53-A:*1579, 1971.

38. Ogden, J. A., Tross, R. B., and Murphy, M. J.: Fractures of the tibial tuberosity in the adolescents. J. Bone Joint Surg., *62-A:*205, 1980.

39. Osmond Clarke, H.: Discussion on fracture of the tibia involving the knee-joint. Proc. R. Soc. Med., *28:*1035, 1935.

40. Osgood, R. B.: Lesions of the tibial tubercle occurring during adolescence, Boston Med. Surg. J., *148:*114, 1903.

41. D'Ambrosia, R. D., and MacDonald, G. L.: Pitfalls in the diag-

nosis of Osgood-Schlatter disease. Clin. Orthop., *110:*206, 1975.

42. Rostron, P. K. M., and Calver, R. F.: Subcutaneous atrophy following methylprednisolone injection in Osgood-Schlatter's epiphysis. J. Bone Joint Surg., *61-A:*627, 1979.

43. Ferciot, C. F.: Surgical management of anterior tibial epiphysis. Clin. Orthop., *5:*204, 1955.

44. Mital, M., and Matza, R. A.: The unresolved Osgood-Schlatter's condition. Orthop. Trans., *2:*71, 1978.

45. Fielding, J. W., Liebler, W. A., and Tambakis, A.: The effect of a tibial-tubercle transplant in children on the growth of the upper tibial epiphysis. J. Bone Joint Surg., *42-A:*1426, 1960.

46. Thomson, J. E. M.: Operative treatment of osteochondritis of the tibial tubercle. J. Bone Joint Surg., *38-A:*142, 1956.

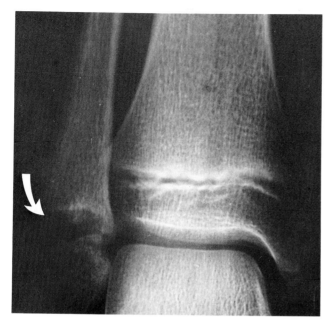

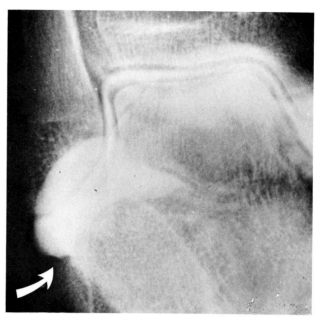

FIG. 19-122. Chronic widening of distal fibula in a boy whose ankle was swollen and painful for six months after an injury (arrow). This proved to be a localized cartilaginous dysplasia (also see Fig. 19-17C).

FIG. 19-124. Ankle arthrogram showing pooling of dye laterally (arrow) at site of chronic lateral disruption and chronic inversion.

47. Wall, J. J.: Compartment syndrome as a complication of the Hauser procedure. J. Bone Joint Surg., 61-A:185, 1979.
48. Agoropoulos, Z., Papachristou, G., Velikas, E., and Wretos, S.: Isolierte traumatische Dislokation des oberen Tibia-Fibular Gelenks. Chirurg., 47:149, 1976.
49. Ogden, J. A.: Subluxation of the proximal tibiofibular joint. Clin. Orthop., 101:192, 1974.
50. Hsu, L. C. S., O'Brien, J. P., Yau, A. C. M. C., and Hodgson, A. R.: Valgus deformity of the ankle in children with fibular pseudarthrosis. J. Bone Joint Surg., 56-A:503, 1974.
51. Wong, D., and Weiner, D. S.: Proximal tibiofibular synostosis. Clin. Orthop., 135:45, 1978.
52. Salter, R. B., and Best, T.: The pathogenesis and prevention of valgus deformity following fractures of the proximal metaphyseal region of the tibia in children. J. Bone Joint Surg., 55-A:1324, 1973.
53. Cozen, L.: Fracture of the proximal portion of the tibia in children followed by valgus deformity. Surg. Gynecol. Obstet., 97:183, 1953.
54. Cozen, L.: Knock knee deformity after fracture of the proximal tibia in children. Orthopedics, 1:230, 1959.
55. Steel, H., Sandrow, R., and Sullivan, P.: Complications of tibial osteotomy in children for genu varum or valgum. J. Bone Joint Surg., 53-A:1629, 1971.
56. Jackson, D. W., and Cozen, L.: Genu valgum as a complication of proximal tibial metaphyseal fractures in children. J. Bone Joint Surg., 53-A:1571, 1971.

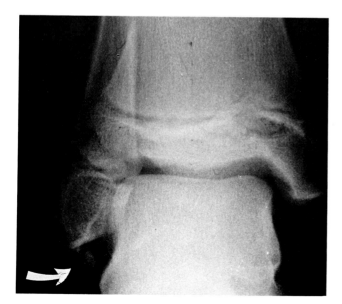

FIG. 19-123. Type 7 injury (arrow) of distal end of fibular epiphysis.

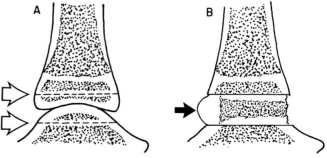

FIG. 19-125. Schematic of arthrodesis technique for the skeletally immature patient. This method allows continued growth in the distal tibial physis. A, Open arrows indicate levels of parallel cuts to expose subchondral trabecular bone. B, Iliac crest graft in place.

57. Morgan, J. D.: Blood supply of growing rabbit's tibia. J. Bone Joint Surg., *41-B:*185, 1959.

58. Wray, J. B., and Lynch, C. J.: The vascular response to fracture of the tibia in the rat. J. Bone Joint Surg., *41-A:*1143, 1959.

59. Taylor, S. L.: Tibial overgrowth: a cause of genu valgum. J. Bone Joint Surg., *45-A:*659, 1963.

60. Irwin, C. E.: The iliotibial band. J. Bone Joint Surg., *31-A:*141, 1949.

61. Weber, B. G.: Fibrous interposition causing valgus deformity after fracture of the upper tibial metaphysis in children. J. Bone Joint Surg., *59-B:*290, 1977.

62. Grobelski, M.: Congenital tibiofibular synostosis. Chir. Narzadow Ruchu Ortop. Pol., *30:*1, 1965.

63. Bartl, R.: Die traumatische Epiphysenlosung am distalen Ende des Schiebeines und des Wadeneines. Hefte Unfallheilkd., *54:*228, 1957.

64. Bishop, P. A.: Fractures and epiphyseal separation fractures of the ankle. A.J.R., *28:*49, 1932.

65. Cameron, H. U.: A radiologic sign of lateral subluxation of the distal tibial epiphysis. J. Trauma, *15:*1030, 1975.

66. Chironi, P.: Considerazioni sulla frattura isolata de margine esterno dell epifisi tibiale inferiore. Minerva Ortop., *6:*123, 1955.

67. Dias, L. S., and Tachdjian, M. J.: Physeal injuries of the ankle in children. Clin. Orthop., *136:*230, 1978.

68. Dingeman, R. D., and Shaver, G. B., Jr.: Operative treatment of displaced Salter-Harris III distal tibial fractures. Clin. Orthop., *135:*101, 1978.

69. Duhaime, M., Gauthier, B., Labelle, P., and Simoneau, R.: Traumatismes épiphysaires de l'extrémite distale du tibia. Union Med. Can., *101:*1827, 1972.

70. Frain, P.: Les décollements epiphysaires de l'extrémite inférieure de tibia. J. Chir. (Paris), *91:*113, 1966.

71. Hohmann, G.: Zur Korrektur frischer und veratteter Falle von Verletzung der distalen Tibiaepiphyse. Arch. Orthop. Unfallchir., *45:*395, 1952.

72. Kleiger, B., and Barton, J.: Epiphyseal ankle fractures. Bull. Hosp. Joint Dis., *25:*240, 1964.

73. Kleiger, B.: The mechanism of ankle injuries. J. Bone Joint Surg., *38-A:*59, 1956.

74. Kump, W. L.: Vertical fractures of the distal tibial epiphysis. A.J.R., *97:*676, 1966.

75. Lauge, N.: Fractures of the ankle: analytic historic survey as basis of new experimental, roentgenologic, and clinical investigations. Arch. Surg., *56:*259, 1948.

76. Lovell, E. S.: An unusual rotatory injury of the ankle. J. Bone Joint Surg., *50-A:*163, 1968.

77. McWilliams, D. J.: Fracture of fibular aspect of lower tibial epiphysis. Ulster Med. J., *31:*185, 1962.

78. Mandell, J.: Isolated fractures of the posterior tibial lip at the ankle as demonstrated by an additional projection, the ''poor'' lateral view. Radiology, *101:*319, 1971.

79. Paleari, G. L.: Sul meccanismo di poduzione dei distacchi antero-esterni dell' epifisi distale della tibia. Arch. Orthop., *73:*1146, 1960.

80. Spiegel, P. G., Cooperman, D. R., and Laros, G. S.: Epiphyseal fractures of the distal ends of the tibia and fibula. J. Bone Joint Surg., *60-A:*1046, 1978.

81. Stern, M. B., Grant, S. S., and Isaacson, A. S.: Bilateral distal tibial and fibular epiphyseal separation associated with spina bifida. Clin. Orthop., *50:*191, 1967.

82. Broock, G. J., and Greer, R. B.: Traumatic rotational displacements of the distal tibial growth plate. J. Bone Joint Surg., *52-A:*1666, 1970.

83. Nevelos, A. B., and Colton, C. L.: Rotational displacement of the lower tibial epiphysis due to trauma. J. Bone Joint Surg., *59-B:*331, 1977.

84. Molster, A., Soreide, O., Solhaug, J. H., and Raugstad, T. S.: Fractures of the lateral part of the distal tibial epiphysis (Tillaux or Kleiger fracture). Injury, *8:*260, 1976,

85. Kleiger, B., and Mankin, H. J.: Fracture of the lateral portion of the distal tibial epiphysis. J. Bone Joint Surg., *46-A:*25, 1964.

86. Marmor, L.: An unusual fracture of the tibial epiphysis. Clin. Orthop., *73:*132, 1970.

87. Lynn, M. D.: The triplane distal tibial epiphyseal fracture. Clin. Orthop., *86:*187, 1972.

88. Torg, J. S., and Ruggiero, R. A.: Comminuted epiphyseal fracture of the distal tibia. Clin. Orthop., *110:*215, 1975.

89. Cooperman, D. R., Spiegel, P. G., and Laros, G. S.: Tibial fractures involving the ankle in children. The so-called triplane epiphyseal fracture. J. Bone Joint Surg., *60-A:*1040, 1978.

90. Carothers, C. O., and Crenshaw, A. H.: Clinical significance of a classification of epiphyseal injuries at the ankle. Am. J. Surg., *89:*879, 1955.

91. Ashhurst, A. P. C., and Bromer, R. S.: Classification and mechanism of fractures of the leg bones involving the ankle. Arch. Surg., *4:*51, 1922.

92. Crenshaw, A. H.: Injuries of the distal tibial epiphysis. Clin. Orthop., *41:*98, 1965.

93. Stampfel, O., Zoch, G., Scholz, R., and Ferlic, P.: Ergbnisse der operativen Behandlung von Verletzunger der distalen Tibia epiphyse. Arch. Orthop. Unfallchir., *84:*211, 1976.

94. Goldberg, V. M., and Aadalen, R.: Distal tibial epiphyseal injuries: the role of athletics in 53 cases. Am. J. Sports Med., *6:*263, 1978.

95. Giuliani, K.: Spatzustande nach traumatische-mechanishen Schadigungen der Epiphyse am distalen Tibiaende. Arch. Orthop. Unfallchir., *45:*386, 1952.

96. Burrows, H. J.: Brockman's operation for talipes varus resulting from defective tibial growth. Proc. R. Soc. Med., *30:*207, 1973.

97. McFarland, B.: Traumatic arrest of epiphyseal growth at the lower end of the tibia. Br. J. Surg., *19:*78, 1931.

98. Johnson, E. W., and Fahl, J. C.: Fractures involving the distal epiphysis of the tibia and fibula in children. Am. J. Surg., *93:*778, 1957.

99. Gill, G., and Abbott, L.: Varus deformity of ankle following injury to distal epiphyseal cartilage of tibia in growing children. Surg. Gynecol. Obstet., *72:*659, 1941.

100. Langenskiöld, A.: Traumatic premature closure of the distal tibial epiphyseal plate. Acta Orthop. Scand., *38:*520, 1967.

101. King, J., Burke, D., and Freeman, M. A. R.: The incidence of pain in the rheumatoid hindfoot and the significance of calcaneofibular impingement. Int. Orthop., *2:*255, 1978.

102. Robertson, D. E.: Post-traumatic osteochondritis of the lower tibial epiphysis. J. Bone Joint Surg., *46-B:*212, 1964.

103. Siffert, R. S., and Arkin, A. M.: Post-traumatic aseptic necrosis of the distal tibial epiphysis. J. Bone Joint Surg., *32-A:*691, 1950.

104. McMaster, J. H., and Scranton, P. F., Jr.: Tibiofibular synostosis—a cause of ankle disability. Clin. Orthop., *3:*172, 1975.

105. Monk, C. J. E.: Injuries of the tibia-fibular ligaments. J. Bone Joint Surg., *51-B:*330, 1969.

106. Hatt, R. N.: The central bone graft in joint arthrodesis. J. Bone Joint Surg., *22:*394, 1940.

107. Chuinard, E. G., and Petersen, R. E.: Distraction-compression bone-graft arthrodesis of the ankle. J. Bone Joint Surg., *45-A:*481, 1963.

108. Turner, H.: Deformities of the foot associated with arthrodesis of the ankle joint performed in early childhood. J. Bone Joint Surg., *16:*423, 1934.

109. Ralston, E. L., and Schmidt, E. R.: Repair of the ruptured Achilles tendon. J. Trauma, *11:*15, 1971.

110. Wobbes, T.: Dislocation of the peroneal tendons. Arch. Chir. Neerl., *27:*209, 1975.

111. Zoellner, G., and Clancy, W.: Recurrent dislocation of the peroneal tendon. J. Bone Joint Surg., *61-A:*292, 1979.

112. Weber, B. G., Brunner, C., and Freuler, F.: Die Frakturenbehandlung bei Kindern und Jugendlichen. Berlin, Springer-Verlag, 1978.

20

Foot

Anatomy

Despite relatively rapid postnatal osseous maturation rates, the foot is not well ossified at birth; there is extensive retention of much of the cartilaginous model, especially in the tarsal region. As the child grows, the tarsals gradually enlarge the primary ossification centers. However, not until the child approaches skeletal maturity will the tarsal osseous contours, especially those of the calcaneus and talus, assume the characteristic mature (adult) contours on which many measurements, such as Bohler's angle, are based (Figs. 20-1 and 20-2).

The calcaneus develops a physis and secondary center of ossification posteriorly (Fig. 20-3). This may be the site of trauma as well as developmental problems such as Sever's disease, although increasingly such osteochondroses are considered to be caused by trauma. Ossification of this secondary center may be irregular and should not be mistaken for a fracture. A secondary epiphyseal ossification center develops at the proximal end of the first metatarsal; however, a pseudoepiphysis occasionally may be formed at the distal end (Fig. 20-4). The other 4 metatarsals (2 through 5) develop secondary ossification centers distally. In addition, the fifth metatarsal develops a secondary ossification center at the proximal, lateral portion, where the peroneus brevis inserts (Fig. 20-5). This small secondary center, which becomes increasingly evident between 9 and 14 years, often is confused with an avulsion fracture. The middle phalanges may lack secondary ossification centers (Fig. 20-5).

Tarsal ossification centers develop earlier than corresponding centers in the hand; calcaneal and talar primary ossification are present at birth. The cuboid appears shortly thereafter. The lateral cuneiform appears within the first year. The tarsal navicula is the last to appear. All centers are generally present by 3 to 4 years. Secondary centers appear in the metatarsal and phalangeal epiphyses by 5 years. Secondary ossification of the calcaneal apophysis, which appears between 6 and 10 years, is often multicentric, a factor that must be considered in ruling out a fracture (which would be analogous to a type 3 or 4 injury in a longitudinal bone). The physeal-metaphyseal juncture is undulated in response to the tensile compressive and shearing forces generated in this area during normal activity. Union with the body of the calcaneus occurs between 15 and 18 years.

During development the foot is characterized by a large number of normal anatomic variations and ossification patterns that may be difficult to distinguish from fractures. These anatomic variations may be discrete accessory bones or simple extensions of the primary ossification components. As many as 22% of all children have at least one of these structural variations.[1] The most important, as well as most common, accessory bones are the accessory navicula (accessory hallux) and the os trigonum. These two are discussed in more detail because of their potential association with skeletal trauma. Additional accessory bones are illustrated schematically in Figure 20-6. In addition to these variations, trauma may also render a tarsal coalition symptomatic, although symptoms may commence without obvious antecedent trauma. Most commonly coalitions involve the calcaneonavicular and talocalcaneal regions. Special views may be necessary to rule out such congenital deformities as causes of persistent pain following inversion or eversion injuries.

The tarsal navicular may develop a secondary center that does not become radiographically evident until 12 years or later, and does not always unite with the primary ossification center. It may persist as a separate accessory center and be associated with problems of a spastic flatfoot, which often becomes symptomatic at the time of injury. The accessory tarsal navicula, which is also referred to as the prehallux or os tibiale externum, may be present in 10% of the population. It is located at the medial side of the navicula and extends proximally along the head of the talus. A separate center of ossification develops, but during adolescence this usually coalesces with the primary center of ossification of the navicular (Fig. 20-7). The posterior tibial tendon partially or completely attaches to this accessory bone, which may interfere with normal longitudinal arch mechanics. Trauma to the foot may render this anatomic variant symptomatic. Treatment should be conservative and directed at support beneath the longitudinal arch with either a scaphoid pad or molded short-leg cast. Prolonged symptoms eventually may necessitate surgical excision and redirection of the posterior tibial tendon (Kidner procedure).

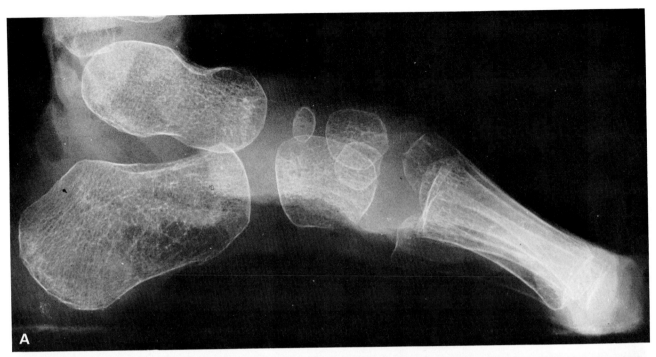

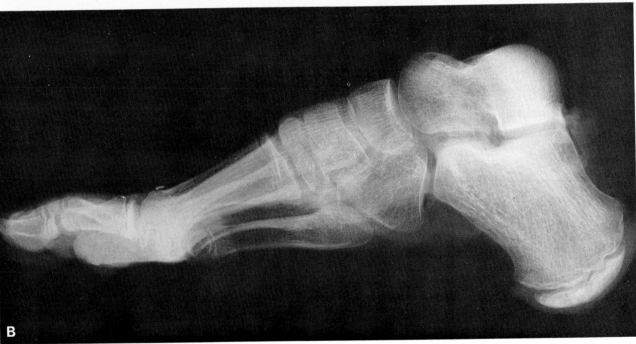

FIG. 20-1. Lateral roentgenograms of feet from cadavers aged, *A*, 3 and, *B*, 11 years. Only in the latter stages of maturation does the calcaneus begin to develop contours allowing measurement of Bohler's angle.

The os trigonum extends from the posterior aspect of the talus, adjacent to the groove for the flexor hallucis longus. Between 8 and 11 years a separate center of ossification may appear (Figs. 20-8 and 20-9), which eventually fuses to the main body of the talus. The connecting, radiolucent cartilage may be misinterpreted as a fracture. The os trigonum may impinge directly against the posterior tibial epiphysis, especially when the ankle is in maximum plantarflexion, and may sustain a fracture. Similar to the Tillaux fracture of the

distal tibia, this fracture occurs most often during the period of fusion to the body of the talus. The os trigonum may persist as a separate ossicle.

The metatarsals and phalanges also may exhibit accessory ossification, as well as irregular appearances of the secondary ossification centers (bifid centers are common) and the development of pseudoepiphyses (see Fig. 20-5). The great toe occasionally may be triphalangeal. The fifth toe may have only two phalanges, and the middle phalanx may lack

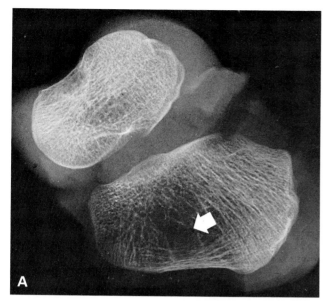

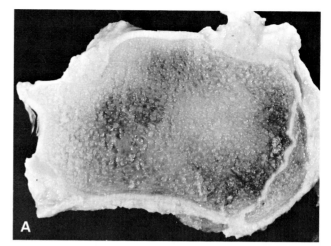

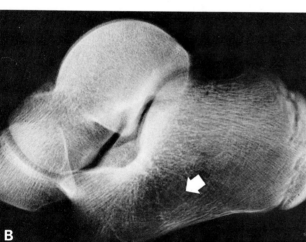

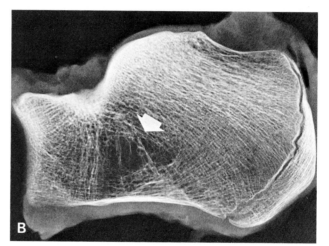

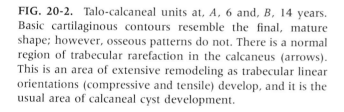

FIG. 20-2.   Talo-calcaneal units at, *A*, 6 and, *B*, 14 years. Basic cartilaginous contours resemble the final, mature shape; however, osseous patterns do not. There is a normal region of trabecular rarefaction in the calcaneus (arrows). This is an area of extensive remodeling as trabecular linear orientations (compressive and tensile) develop, and it is the usual area of calcaneal cyst development.

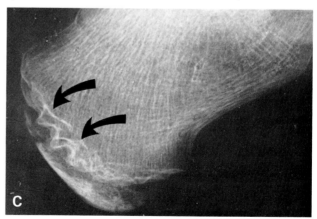

an epiphysis. There is considerable structural variation in the epiphyseal ossification centers, which may be discoid, conical, or even fissured.[1] The sesamoids under the first metatarsal-phalangeal joint may be bipartite (Fig. 20-10).

The sinus tarsi is located at the lateral side of the tarsus just below the distal fibular epiphysis. This region is the entry point for much of the blood supply of the talus and the calcaneus and should be minimally disturbed in any surgical procedure (Fig. 20-11). The child has a more flexible blood supply to the talus, which is supplied by branches from the anterior tibial, perforating peroneal, and posterior tibial arteries. The lateral artery of the sinus tarsi is a branch of the perforating peroneal artery; the artery of the medial tarsal

FIG. 20-3.   *A*, Slab section of calcaneus from a 13-year-old showing variation in physeal contour and secondary ossification center configuration. *B*, Roentgenogram of morphologic slab. Arrow indicates normal area of trabecular thinning surrounded by tensile and compressive trabecular patterns. Also in this area, unicameral bone cysts form. *C*, The junction between the calcaneal "metaphysis" and physis gradually forms undulations (arrows) that aid it in resisting the various compressive, tensile, and shearing forces associated with normal childhood and adolescent activity.

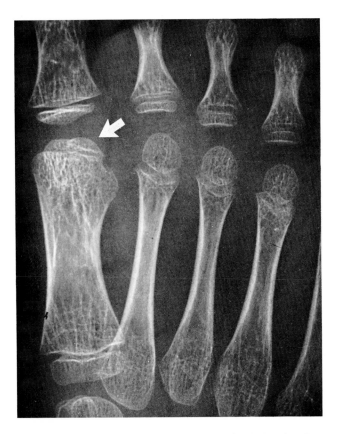

FIG. 20-4. Development of pseudoepiphysis in the first metatarsal (arrow).

canal is a branch of the posterior tibial artery. These branches form an anastomotic sling in the subtalar region and supply the head, neck, and much of the body of the talus. The posterior tibial artery also gives off small branches that enter the region of the posterior tubercle to supply a portion of the body. The anterior tibial artery gives off small branches that enter the superior surface of the head and neck. Although the process of formation of the primary talar ossification center is dependent on a functioning vascular supply, in the child there appears to be less dominance on a single system with retrograde flow from the neck into the body compared to the adult, and avascular (ischemic) necrosis is a rare complication following talar fractures.

The calcaneus eventually develops a cortical shell, except in the posterior region where the secondary center of ossification appears. This shell surrounds a complicated trabecular network that continually remodels during growth in response to dynamic weightbearing stresses, especially in the posterior region, which correspond to the metaphysis of a long bone. The young child has a cartilaginous cortex that imparts an additional protective resiliency to the bone and makes calcaneal fractures infrequent. Only during the second decade does the subchondral plate extend out to the previous cartilage contours and landmarks such as Bohler's tuber-joint angle become significant. Because of the extensive remodeling and osteolysis in the primary ossification center, calcaneal cysts may occur.[2] These cysts may occur with pathologic fractures following minor trauma. Similar cysts have also been described in the talus.[3]

The rates of growth and maturation of the skeletal components of the foot exhibit not only the expected sex differences, but also accelerated development when compared to

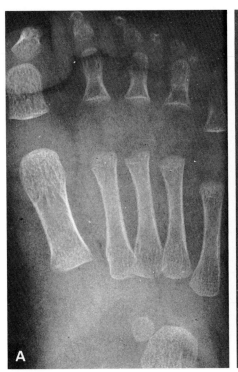 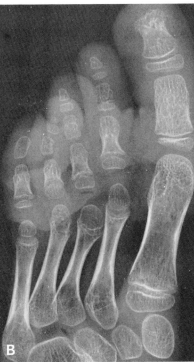 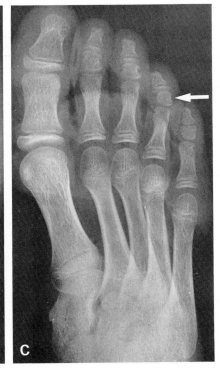

FIG. 20-5. Sequential metatarsal-phalangeal maturation at, *A,* 7 months, *B,* 4 years, and, *C,* 11 years. Note the lack of secondary ossification centers in the middle phalanges (arrow).

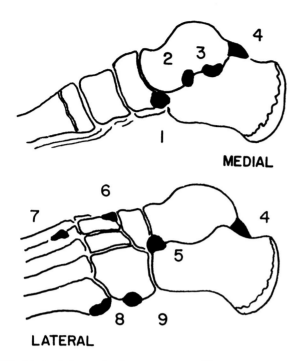

FIG. 20-6. Schematic of accessory tarsal bones. *1*, Os tibiale externum (10%); *2*, Os sustentaculi (5%); *3*, Talus secundarius; *4*, Os trigonum (13%); *5*, Calcaneus secundarius; *6*, Os intercuneiforme; *7*, Os intermetatarseum (9%); *8*, Os vesalianum; and *9*, Os fibular (10%). (Percentages are approximate number of people who have each accessory bone.)

the corresponding rates of maturation of the longitudinal bones of the arm and leg. At the ages of 1 year in girls and 1½ years in boys, the foot has already achieved almost 50% of its mature length. In contrast, the femur and tibia do not reach 50% of their mature length until 3 years before comparable physeal closure in the long bones.[4] Thus, factors that might disturb growth and the ultimate length of the foot or an individual bone would be proportionally less in the older child than they might be for similar growth mechanism injuries to the femur or tibia. Therefore, the extent of longitudinal growth in the metatarsals and phalanges that might correct malalignment is not comparable to the major long bones. Longitudinal growth patterns should not be counted upon to correct significant malalignment, particularly when the complication may have an effect upon the normal weightbearing capacity of the foot.

Injuries

Other than phalangeal and proximal fifth metatarsal fractures, injuries to the chondro-osseous components of the child's foot are uncommon. Flexibility and resiliency render the foot relatively immune to major skeletal injury. Forces of indirect violence usually are transmitted more proximally to the tibia and fibula.

The majority of significant foot fractures result from direct violence, such as a crush or a fall. Soft tissue injury is the usual concomitant and more significant result of trauma, so

initial treatment must be directed toward the swelling and associated cutaneous, muscular, neural, or vascular problems. Potential circulatory and neurologic complications always must be thoroughly evaluated during the first few days following trauma. Compression dressings and elevation comprise the initial treatment for most of these injuries. Definitive fracture treatment may have to be rendered several days later when the status of the underlying soft tissue injury has been assessed adequately and found compatible with manipulation, reduction, and immobilization of the fracture(s).

Fractures of the foot vary in extent and location, and are contingent upon the direction and severity of the external forces responsible for the injury. It is essential to consider not only the type of fracture or dislocation, but also the mechanism and direction of the forces producing the injury. Such knowledge enhances appropriate reduction techniques, and may lessen the manipulations necessary to accomplish anatomic restoration. Preservation of soft tissues, particularly the ligaments essential to long term function of the longitudinal and transverse arches, is just as important as actual fracture reduction in restoring complete function to the injured foot. Fractures involving a joint surface carry a worse prognosis compared to non-articular fractures, particularly when the tarsal bones are involved.

Talus

The talus is fractured infrequently in the child.[5-8,8a,8b] The most common injury is a vertical fracture through the talar neck (Fig. 20-12). This is usually associated with minimal displacement and may be treated by immobilization in a

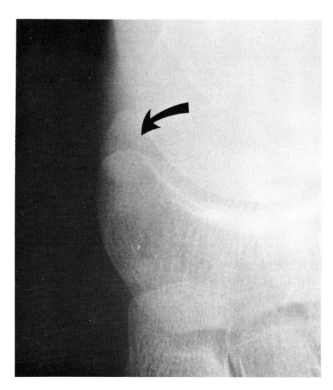

FIG. 20-7. Accessory navicula. Note the secondary ossification center (arrow).

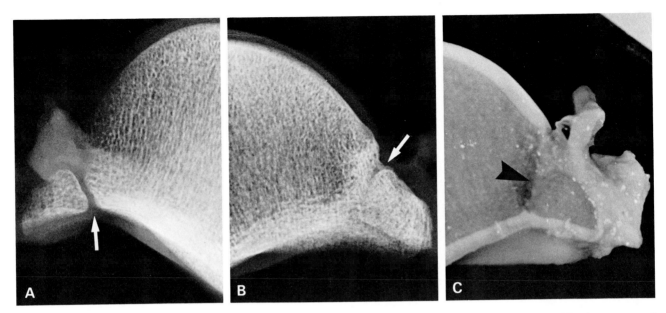

FIG. 20-8. Os trigonum. *A*, Roentgenogram of talar specimen from a 12-year-old showing accessory ossification separated from main talar ossification center by a cartilaginous bridge (arrow). *B*, Roentgenogram of specimen from a 14-year-old showing consolidation of the accessory and main talar ossification centers (arrow). *C*, Slab section of specimen shown in *B*, showing consolidation (arrow).

non-weightbearing cast, once soft tissue swelling has subsided. If the head of the talus is superiorly displaced, relative to the body, a closed reduction should be attempted and the foot immobilized in plantarflexion to avoid recurrence of the deformity. If the reduction is not stable, then the fragments may be transfixed with K-wires, either by percutaneous pinning under an image intensifier or open reduction. In the latter instance, dissection should be minimal to lessen risk of potential or further vascular damage.

Although collapsing ischemic (avascular) necrosis rarely appears in children, overall talar ossification center development may be temporarily or permanently impaired, depending on the amount of ischemia. In the older child (over 10 years), ischemic necrosis becomes an increasingly probable complication because of the rapid osseous maturation of the hindpart of the foot.[9] A technetium bone scan may allow early diagnosis of this complication and should be considered in any patient as part of the routine follow-up after

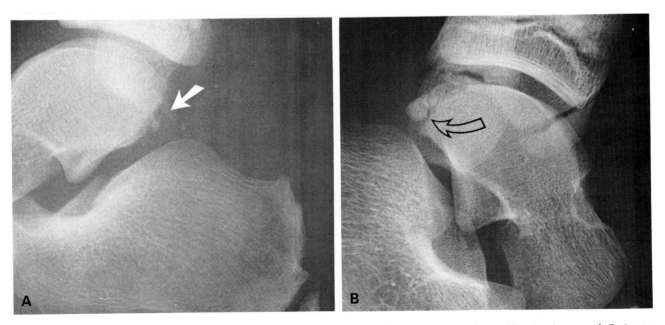

FIG. 20-9. *A*, Early development of os trigonum. Irregularity (arrow) of such posterior talar ossification is normal. *B*, Acute fracture (arrow) through posterior portion of talus, a rare injury that must be distinguished from the os trigonum. Also notice the ossification variation of the medial malleolus, which should not be mistaken for a fracture.

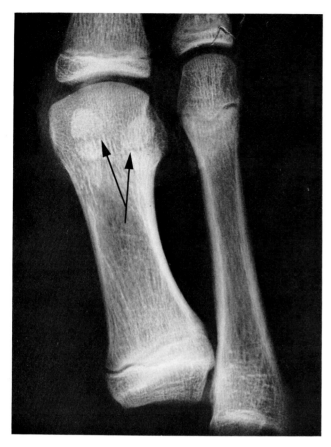

FIG. 20-10. Bipartite sesamoids (arrows). This is usually a normal structural variation, not a fracture.

allowing for adequate healing and remodeling (at least 2 to 3 months). If roentgenographic changes or bone scan suggest ischemic necrosis, the child or adolescent may be protected with a patellar tendon bearing brace for at least 9 to 12 months following the injury. As in Legg-Calvé-Perthes disease, the critical period is not that of actual vascular insult, but subsequently when dead bone is being replaced and initial reactive trabecular patterns are more randomly oriented, not stress oriented as they would be with normal, progressive trabecular maturation.

Inversion and eversion injuries may cause chondral or osteochondral fractures of the medial or lateral wall of the talus (Fig. 20-13), which are ligamentous avulsion fractures. Persistent pain around a malleolus, especially the lateral malleolus, warrants close examination with oblique radiographs that adequately visualize the region between the talus and malleolus. Since these fragments may be completely cartilaginous they may not be visible until many months after the injury when they subsequently ossify with reactive bone. Even if the injury is only suspected and not demonstrated radiologically the child should be immobilized in a short-leg cast for 3 to 4 weeks to enhance healing of the associated ligamentous injury. If there is persistent pain with ankle motion following such treatment, excision of the fragment may be necessary.

Chronic, excessive plantarflexion and dorsiflexion of the ankle, as occur in certain competitive sports such as gymnastics, may cause disruption of the anterolateral ligaments

or "impingement" syndrome (Fig. 20-14). The accepted cause of this lesion is chronic, repetitive contact between the anterior tibial articular surface and the talar neck.

A less frequent fracture is an osteochondral fragment from the talar dome (Fig. 20-15).[10] This may affect either the medial or lateral margin, although the lateral side is affected more frequently.[7] The mechanism of injury is uncertain; however, direct compression associated with failure of the collateral ligaments appears to be the most likely cause (inversion or inversion-dorsiflexion injury). Lateral lesions are morphologically shallow and more likely to become displaced into the joint, thereby causing chronic symptoms. Medial lesions are usually deeper but tend to be less symptomatic. The diagnosis requires an adequate mortise view, since the region of injury may lie behind a malleolus on a routine anteroposterior view. This fracture must be treated with non-weightbearing cast immobilization, followed by protected weightbearing in a patellar tendon bearing cast or cast-brace. Excision of the fragment and curettage may be necessary if symptoms persist after adequate conservative treatment. Further, the fragment may be rotated 180° at the time of initial injury. Should this occur, open reduction is indicated.

Calcaneus

Although relatively uncommon, fractures of the calcaneus are probably the most frequently encountered tarsal injuries in children.[11] Schofield and Zayre each described 1 child in their extensive series of calcaneal fractures, whereas Essex-

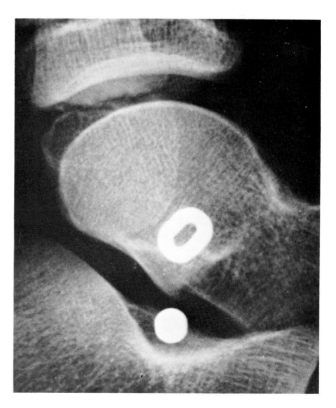

FIG. 20-11. BB pellet in sinus tarsi. This must be approached with caution, as extensive dissection could disrupt much of the normal vascular supply to this region.

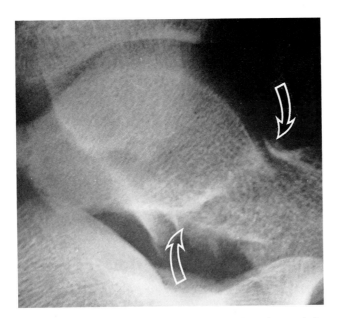

FIG. 20-12. Mildly displaced fracture of the talar neck in a 10-year-old.

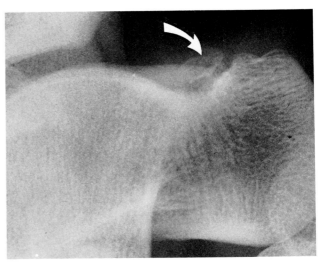

FIG. 20-14. Fracture of the anterior talus (arrow) due to chronic impingement between anterior tibia and talar neck in a 14-year-old world class gymnast.

Lopresti found 12 young patients in 241 cases.[12-14] Thomas, who selectively described the injury in children, reported 6 cases.[15] In all reports the children were older and ranged in age from 6 to 18 years, however, most of them were over 10 years old. However, Matteri described 3 children all less than 3 years old with calcaneal fractures consequent to relatively minor trauma, and stressed the difficulty in making a roentgenographic diagnosis in these children.[16] Buchanan described a stress fracture of the posterior calcaneus in a young child.[17] Calcaneal stress fractures have also been described in children.[8]

Most calcaneal fractures follow a significant fall or vehicular accident. Consequently, extensive soft tissue swelling is just as common in children as adults. However, if a young child refuses to bear weight or limps, the calcaneus should be examined closely, as a stress fracture may have occurred (Fig. 20-16) and, depending upon the degree of primary ossification, is extremely difficult to diagnose.[17,18]

Roentgenographic evaluation should be done in any child with heel or foot pain with or without a history of trauma. Such pain may be the first symptom of a systemic disease such as leukemia (Fig. 20-17), or a more localized process such as Sever's disease (Fig. 20-18). There is some support that Sever's disease is a response to repetitive trauma.

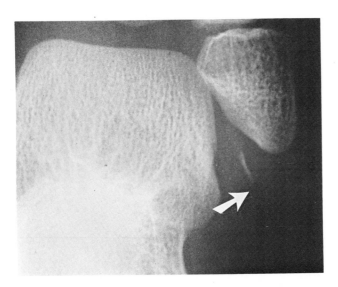

FIG. 20-13. Avulsion fracture from the side of the talus (arrow). As in other areas, the trabecular bone adjacent to ligamentous attachments is much more likely to fail than the ligament itself during an acute inversion injury in a child.

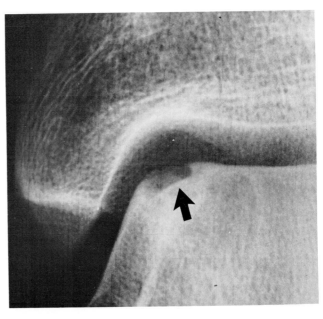

FIG. 20-15. Osteochondral fracture (arrow) of medial talar dome. The fragment is displaced posteriorly. However, ankle motion was not restricted.

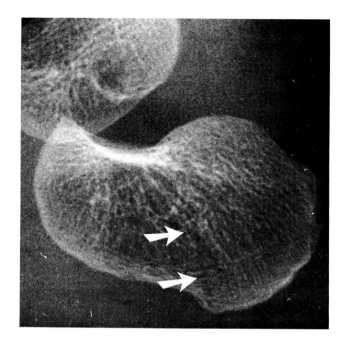

FIG. 20-16.   Linear lucency (arrows) in two-year-old boy with limp. This fracture was not evident until the third week following the onset of symptoms.

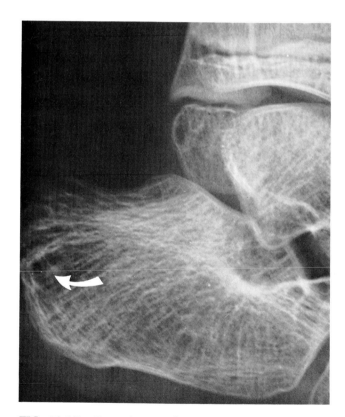

FIG. 20-17.   Extensive rarefaction (arrow) of trabecular bone and microfractures in "metaphysis" of a boy whose presenting symptoms were ankle and heel pain. These changes were secondary to leukemic expansion within the marrow space of the actively growing region associated with the calcaneal physis.

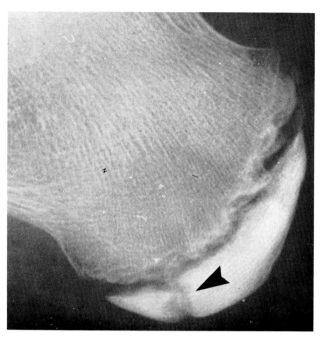

FIG. 20-18.   Sever's disease. Note the sclerotic appearance of the secondary ossification center. This ossification center frequently has an area of incomplete ossification (arrow). Also note the extensive undulation of this particular physis, which is almost uniquely subjected to weightbearing compression forces along with tensile forces from the plantar muscles (inferiorly) and the Achilles tendon (superiorly).

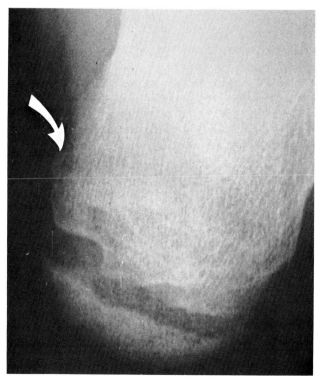

FIG. 20-19.   Type 1 calcaneal fracture (arrow) of the postero-lateral margin.

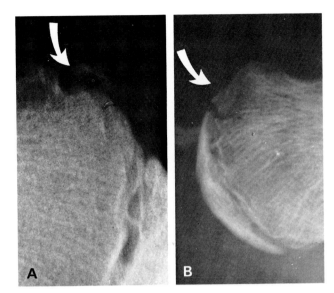

FIG. 20-20. Type 2 calcaneal injuries. *A*, Avulsion of small portion of subchondral bone (arrow) near anterior tendon insertion. *B*, "Beak" fracture of posterosuperior calcaneus (arrow).

There are several classification schemes for calcaneal fractures. The classification of Rowe is summarized in Table 20-1.[19] Representative cases are shown in Figures 20-19 through 20-24. Most fractures involve the posterior non-articulating portion of the calcaneus (type 3) and tuberosity (type 1). Less frequently, the tendo-Achillis insertion may be

TABLE 20-1. *Calcaneal Fracture Patterns**

Type 1

Fracture of the tuberosity.
Fracture of the sustentaculum tali.
Fracture of the anterior process.

Type 2

"Beak" fracture.
Avulsion fracture of the tendo-Achillis insertion.

Type 3

Oblique fracture in the posterior portion not involving the subtalar joint; corresponds to a metaphyseal fracture of a longitudinal bone.

Type 4

Fracture involving the subtalar region with or without actual articular involvement.

Type 5

Central depression with varying degrees of comminution.

Type 6

Involvement of the secondary ossification center.

* Modified from Rowe.[19]

avulsed (type 2). Involvement of the subtalar joint (type 4) is infrequent. Because of the resilient nature of developing bone and cartilage in the subtalar region, fragment depression in a type 5 injury appears unusual in children. Type 6 injuries involve major injury to the epiphysis, usually of a compression nature at the heel (Fig. 20-24).

Initial treatment should be directed toward the soft tissue swelling, which is usually extensive. The foot and ankle should be immobilized in a well-padded compression dressing and the leg elevated for 2 to 3 days. A cast should not be applied until the bulk of the swelling has subsided, at which time the intrinsic stability of the fracture can be better evaluated. Significant displacement is not common in children (the extensive surrounding cartilage, perichondrium, and periosteum help maintain intrinsic stability), so excessive manipulation is usually unnecessary. However, manual molding while the cast is being applied may improve fragment positions. When casted, the foot should be kept in neutral or mild dorsiflexion. However, in types 2 and 3, if this position causes fragment distraction or a tendency for the proximal fragment to drift into equinus relative to the rest of the foot (e.g., type 3), it may be necessary to initially use plantarflexion. Further, failure to wait for soft tissue swelling to subside may limit ability to bring the foot out of plantarflexion to neutral. In children there is rarely any indication for open reduction. These fractures should heal sufficiently within 4 to 6 weeks to allow cast removal and early range of motion. However, weightbearing should not be allowed for 8 to 12 weeks, especially if the subtalar joint or tendo-Achillis insertion is involved.

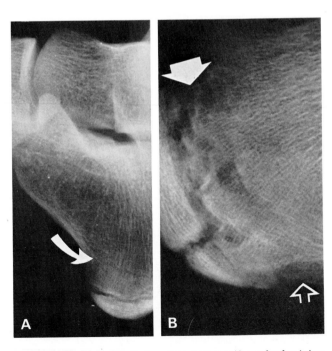

FIG. 20-21. Type 3 injuries not involving the subtalar joint. These are analogous to metaphyseal fractures. *A*, Undisplaced linear fracture (arrow). *B*, Crushing injury to heel has caused fragmentation (solid arrow), and new subperiosteal bone formation (open arrow). The calcaneal secondary ossification center exhibits a normal gap, not an extension of the fracture.

These particular injuries should not be confused with Kohler's disease, a possibly traumatic osteochondrosis often found during the evaluation of a painful foot. Like other tarsal injuries, these fractures are generally accompanied by extensive soft tissue swelling, especially on the dorsum of the foot.

Tarsometatarsal region

Fracture-dislocation of Lisfranc's joint is probably the most common major dislocation, and is usually seen in the older child following violent trauma.[20] Rarely is the injury just a dislocation of the metatarsals. There usually are accompanying fractures that most often involve the second metatarsal, which extends more proximally than the other four (Figs. 20-27 and 20-28). Closed reduction usually requires a general anesthetic and K-wire fixation to maintain the reduction. Varus or valgus deformity must be corrected.

Viability of the skin and soft tissue must be observed closely. Decompression of the dorsum of the foot may be necessary. Extensive soft tissue injury, particularly involving disruption of major vessels, may require amputation (Fig. 20-29).

Metatarsals

Probably the most common injury to the developing foot is an avulsion fracture of the proximal, lateral fifth metatarsal. This is usually caused by a strong inversion force or sudden twisting of the foot associated with an abnormal muscle pull or strain in the peroneus brevis attachments and causes avulsion of a portion of the cartilage and bone. This region normally develops a small secondary center of ossification that easily may be misinterpreted as a fracture. Several types of fractures may occur, all of which involve some of this growth apparatus (Fig. 20-30). First, the entire chondroosseous epiphysis may be avulsed from the metaphysis, although the degree of separation is usually minimal. Second, the fracture may extend into the metaphysis with varying degrees of comminution. Third, the developing secondary

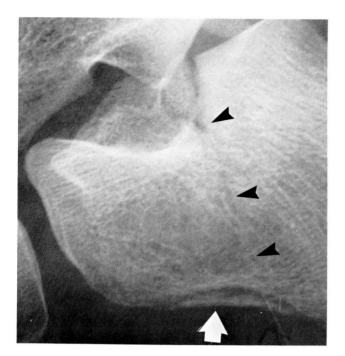

FIG. 20-22. Type 4 calcaneal injury with involvement of subtalar joint. Three weeks after injury, the fracture line is evident (black arrows) and subperiosteal new bone is present inferiorly (white arrow) where the fracture extended to the inferior cortex.

Other tarsal bones

The remainder of the tarsus appears relatively free of injury, except when accompanying extensive fracture-dislocations of the tarsometatarsal junction. The tarsal navicular may be injured (Fig. 20-25), but rarely displaced. Percutaneous fixation with K-wires may be necessary to keep the fragments aligned. The tarsal navicular may also be the site of a more localized, trauma-related process (Fig. 20-26).

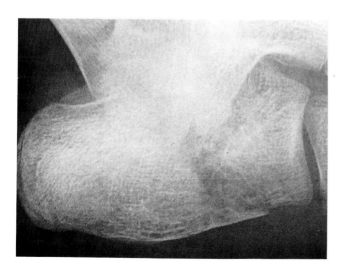

FIG. 20-23. Type 5 calcaneal injury with moderate widening of the subtalar fracture site and depression of central fragments.

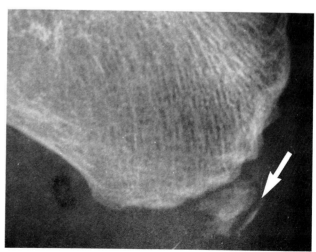

FIG. 20-24. Irregular ossification in calcaneal epiphysis (arrow) following fall with impact directly on the heel. This is a type 6 injury.

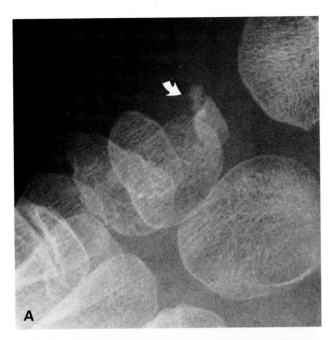

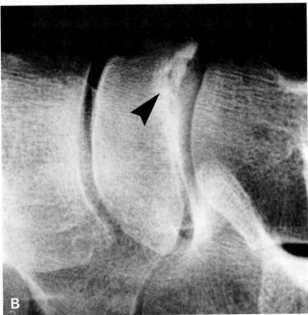

FIG. 20-25. *A*, 6-year-old with pain over the dorsum following a fall. This roentgenographic appearance is usually termed Kohler's disease (arrow). *B*, 11-year-old with tenderness over the navicula (arrow). She had activity-related discomfort, particularly with jumping.

ossification center or the pre-ossification center may be split and a portion distracted along with the tendon.

Treatment of all types should consist of immobilization in a short-leg walking cast for 3 to 4 weeks. Open reduction is rarely indicated since significant distraction of the avulsed portion is infrequent. Growth deformities are unusual. However, overgrowth may occur and cause enlargement of this region. This may cause discomfort in shoes and the patient may benefit from excisional surgery. Nonunion of this fracture is infrequent.

Solitary fractures of the metatarsal diaphyses are usually undisplaced. Most often the first and fifth metatarsals are involved (Fig. 20-31). Less commonly the second or third metatarsal may be injured. However, when the latter is involved it is more often a stress fracture. Such a possibility should be considered in any child who complains of persistent pain along the longitudinal arch. Since these fractures may not be visible using routine roentgenographic techniques, a bone scan should be considered. When multiple metatarsal fractures are present, the first metatarsal is fractured proximally and the remaining metatarsals are fractured distally (Fig. 20-32). The distal fractures usually involve the metaphysis, rather than the growth plate. The metatarsal heads are malaligned, exhibiting increased valgus and plantarward deviation. Correction of these angular displacements is extremely important. When multiple fractures are present there may be a concomitant dislocation of at least one tarsometatarsal joint. There may also be widening of the space between the first and second proximal metatarsals.

Because of the strong interosseous membranes and ligaments between the metatarsals, displacements are unusual except between the first and second metatarsals. However, most exhibit angular displacement relative to the midpart of the foot. These varus or valgus malalignments must be corrected during reduction. When the majority of the fractures involve the distal metatarsal heads they should be reduced as accurately as possible to correct plantar displacement. Further, the transverse ligaments between the distal first and second metatarsals may be disrupted. Re-approximation of this region by closed reduction and a well-molded cast is essential to prevent a splayfoot and functional loss of the transverse and longitudinal arches. Malunion of the distal metatarsals is rare. As soft tissue swelling subsides radiographs should be repeated at appropriate intervals to be certain the reduction is maintained. Proper alignment is necessary because growth and remodeling may not be sufficient to correct angular (plantarflexion) deformity and abnormal weight distribution. Traction with the use of percutaneous pins may be necessary to prevent plantarflexion of the injured distal metatarsals.

The first metatarsal may be injured proximally, either in the metaphysis or at the proximal growth plate (Fig. 20-33).[21] If there is damage to the physis, shortening of the medial side of the foot and deficiency of the longitudinal arch may occur. Because of the locations of the physes at the proximal end of the first and distal ends of the second through fifth metatarsals, trauma may affect rates of growth differentially, either by direct injury or relative response to the increased blood flow caused by the injury.

There is no recognized correlation between injury to the metatarsal heads and appearance of Freiberg's disease.[22] Occasionally small osteochondral fragments may be fractured from the rest of the distal metatarsal. These fragments may require open reduction if there is significant joint involvement.

Phalanges

Dislocation of the metatarsal-phalangeal joint is unusual in children. More likely, there is a fracture through the proximal phalangeal growth plate. These fractures are relatively common injuries, especially to the first toe (Figs. 20-34 to

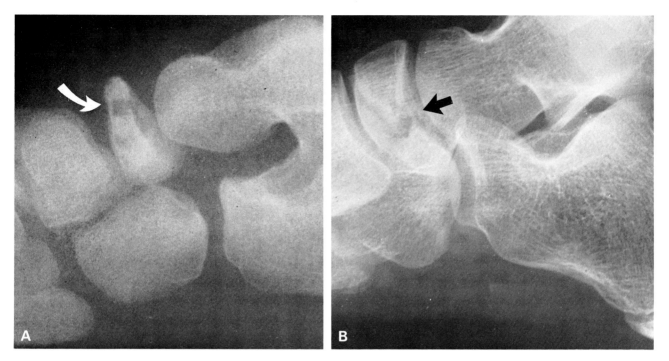

FIG. 20-26. *A*, Navicular fracture (arrow) sustained by this 5-year-old in a fall from a skateboard. *B*, Navicular fracture (arrow) in a 12-year-old. This followed a crushing type of injury.

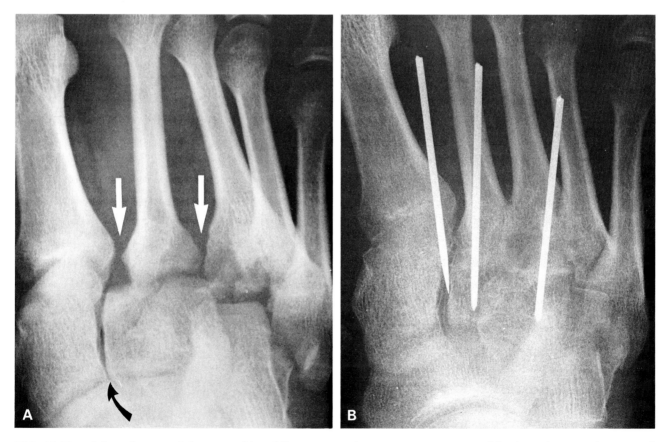

FIG. 20-27. Lisfranc fracture-dislocation of foot following a crushing injury in a 14-year-old girl. *A*, The second metatarsal was fractured as well as being separated from the first and third metatarsals (white arrows). The soft tissue disruption also separated the first 2 cuneiforms (black arrow). *B*, She was treated by closed reduction and percutaneous pinning.

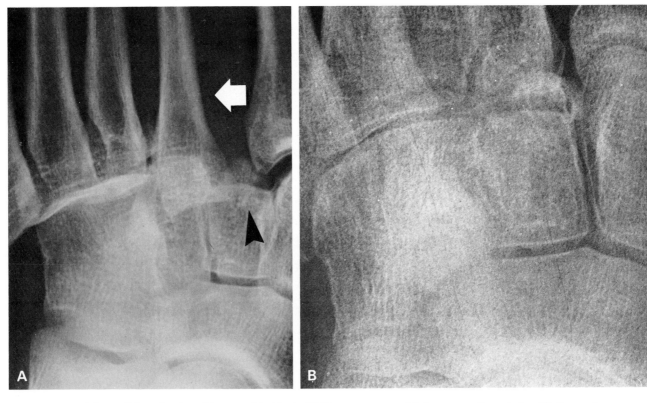

FIG. 20-28. Lisfranc dislocation in a 15-year-old girl. *A,* All 5 tarsometatarsal joints were disrupted, with the major separation being between the first and second (white arrow). A small fragment of the second metatarsal remained (black arrow). *B,* Appearance 6 months later (treatment was by closed reduction).

20-37). Type 3 epiphyseal injuries are common and may require open reduction if significantly displaced. Sometimes only a small portion of the epiphyseal ossification center is involved (type 7). Damage may be seemingly innocuous, but may crush regions of the physis (type 5) and cause subsequent growth deformity (Fig. 20-35). Physeal injuries may also involve the more distal phalangeal epiphyses.

The usual mechanism of injury of the lateral four toes is crushing. When the first toe is injured, a crushing force may also be implicated. It is common for the first toe to be angulated by fixation relative to the rest of the foot, an accident pattern that often occurs when a table leg or similar object is jammed against the first toe or between the toes of the barefooted child.

Fractures of the lateral four toes seldom require more than symptomatic treatment. Most can be adequately treated by taping the injured toe to adjacent, uninjured toes. Cotton, lamb's wool, or some other suitable material should be placed between the toes to prevent maceration.

Fractures of the first toe require close observation and accurate reduction. Malalignment may affect the normal weightbearing axes of the foot. The deformity should be reduced anatomically, especially if the joint is involved. Open reduction should be considered if a large type 3 fragment is present. Skeletal traction may be necessary to maintain reduction. Varus or valgus malalignment should be avoided.

Fractures of the proximal phalanx of the great toe are associated with a higher incidence of osteomyelitis than might be expected routinely. The crushing nature of the injury probably causes small breaks in the skin that allow bacterial penetration. Such injuries must be watched closely for this complication. A course of prophylactic antibiotics for 10 days is warranted. If the complication still occurs, adequate drainage and debridement are essential to prevent chronic osteomyelitis.

Puncture wounds

The barefoot child or adolescent frequently sustains a penetrating wound to the foot or toes (Fig. 20-38). Although skin penetration may appear insignificant, these wounds require adequate debridement, tetanus toxoid, and a broad-spectrum antibiotic. Many children present several days later, and may not even recall a specific injury. The penetration may extend to the periosteum or even to the cortical bone, and may eventually lead to osteomyelitis. Many of these infections are caused by gram-negative rather than gram-positive microorganisms. Early diagnosis of osteomyelitis prior to roentgenographic changes (which may take 7 to 10 days to appear) can be done with osseous scans utilizing technetium or gallium, or even using the newer technique of labeled-leukocytes. Osteomyelitis should be treated with adequate debridement, although this may not be sufficient to arrest osseous destruction in the child presenting several days after an obvious penetrating wound and soft tissue infection (Fig. 20-39).

Although *Pseudomonas aeruginosa* is an unusual causative agent of hematogenous osteomyelitis in children, it is a rela-

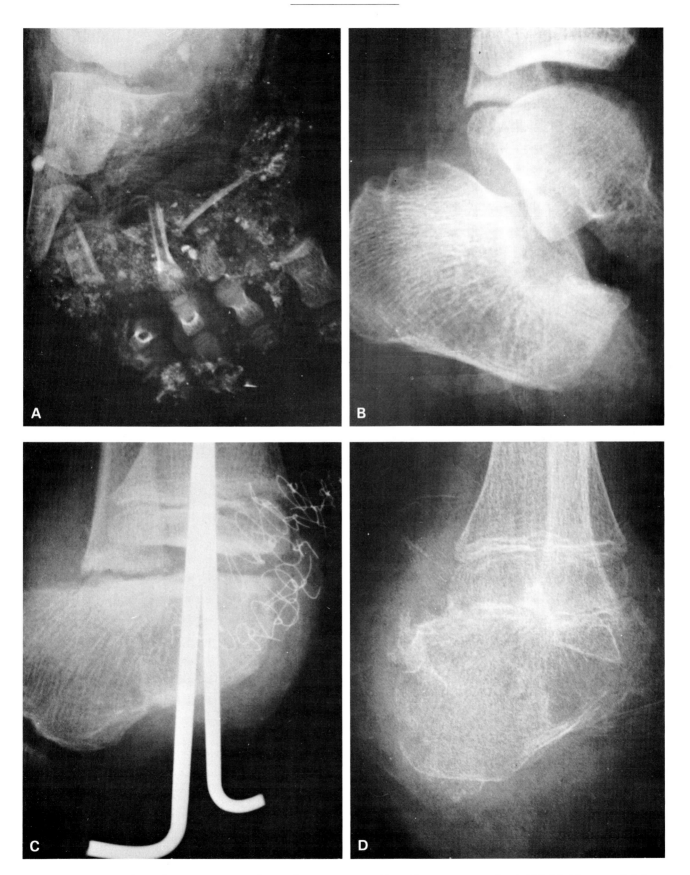

FIG. 20-29. *A*, Crush-avulsion injury secondary to lawn mower accident. *B*, Appearance after initial debridement. *C*, Subsequent treatment to fuse calcaneus to distal tibial ossification center. *D*, Final result.

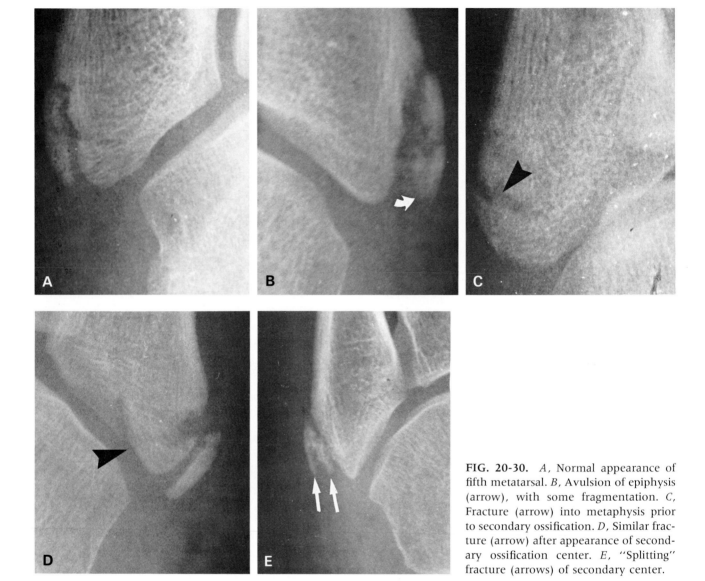

FIG. 20-30. *A*, Normal appearance of fifth metatarsal. *B*, Avulsion of epiphysis (arrow), with some fragmentation. *C*, Fracture (arrow) into metaphysis prior to secondary ossification. *D*, Similar fracture (arrow) after appearance of secondary ossification center. *E*, "Splitting" fracture (arrows) of secondary center.

tively common cause of foot infections following puncture wounds.[23] These microorganisms are found in soil and may be normal inhabitants of the skin. Therefore, they may be reasonably expected to cause infection if the skin barrier is broached.

The typical history appears to be a patient with an onset of local pain and swelling 2 to 5 days following a puncture wound and initial or subsequent therapy that usually consists of cleansing, elevation, soaks, tetanus toxoid, and perhaps one of several antibiotics, either broad-spectrum or antistaphylococcal. Roentgenograms show no bone changes initially. There usually is partial resolution of the inflammation with the initial therapeutic regimen, but symptoms and signs of infection either return or do not fully subside. If cultures from spontaneous drainage or from the surgical drainage incision reveal Pseudomonas, they may be considered a contaminant, particularly if the culture shows a mixture of organisms. There is usually persistence of symptoms and subsequent roentgenograms demonstrate osseous changes between 8 and 21 days after injury. These changes

lead to specific bacteriologic diagnosis because of the indications for aspiration or surgical drainage. A more aggressive therapeutic course is then instituted, but the infection is relatively advanced by this stage. Johanson reported an average delay before diagnosis of 3 weeks from the time of onset of symptoms.[9] In Brand's series, the average delay from injury to diagnosis was 23 days.[23] The results are generally good with surgical drainage and various antibiotic regimens. None of the reports has sufficiently long term follow-up to determine whether antibiotics alone had been effective. However, the combination of antibiotics with surgical drainage and debridement has been effective. It is commonly thought that osteomyelitis, particularly from gram-negative organisms, is difficult to cure and prone to recur. This is not as likely in children, especially when they are treated aggressively and early in the course of the disease.

Early diagnosis is aided by a high index of suspicion, especially if the object was long enough to have penetrated to the bone. Atypical osteomyelitis of the foot in children, particularly caused by *Pseudomonas aeruginosa,* should be suspected

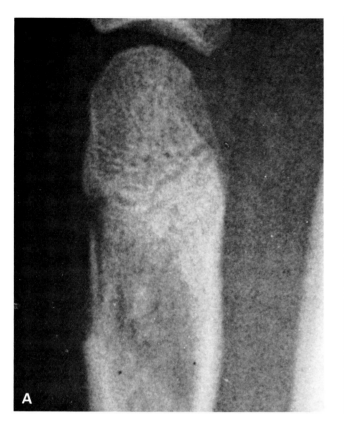

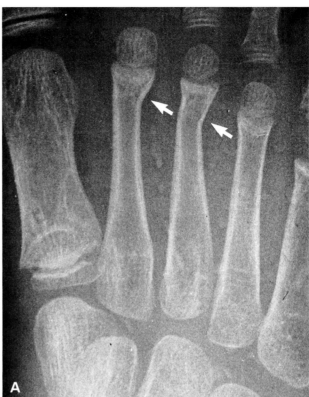

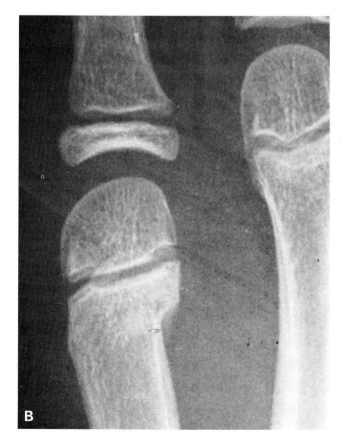

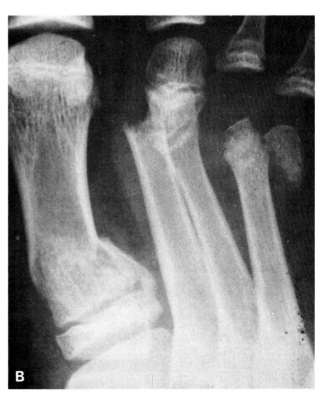

FIG. 20-31. *A*, Fracture of distal metaphysis of fifth metatarsal. *B*, Compression fracture of fifth metatarsal metaphysis.

FIG. 20-32. *A*, Greenstick fractures (arrows) of second and third metatarsals. *B*, Fractures of proximal first metatarsal and distal second and third metatarsals.

when any puncture wound has occurred and the symptoms and signs of infection do not abate within 2 to 4 days after beginning therapy. Specific bacteriologic diagnosis by culture of fluid from spontaneous drainage, aspiration, surgical incision, and adequate debridement are essential. Carbenicillin or a combination of carbenicillin and gentamycin are the antibiotics of choice in the case of pseudomonas osteomyelitis, depending on sensitivity studies. The length of antibiotic therapy varies from case to case, but significant bone involvement is generally an indication for parenteral therapy.

Despite treatment, premature epiphysiodesis of the proximal phalanx of the first toe may occur (Fig. 20-40). If the child is young, significant shortening of the toe may occur. The infection involves the peripheral growth regions (zone of Ranvier), which are intracapsular in this epiphyseal-physeal unit (Fig. 20-39D). This leads to progressive epiphysiodesis as extensive peripheral osseous bridges form.

Painful foot

Foot pain that occurs following childhood injury may result from rendering a congenital defect symptomatic. Tarsal coalitions particularly must be ruled out in children with painful flatfeet. These most commonly are calcaneonavicular and talocalcaneal. As these coalitions mature, resilience lessens. Cartilaginous or fibrocartilaginous bars are reasonably flexible, whereas osseous maturation decreasingly removes motion and increases the likelihood of trauma-induced pain or even fracture.

An accessory hallux may also become symptomatic following trauma, which is often relatively innocuous in these particular patients. Initial treatment should be immobilization followed by the use of a scaphoid pad to lessen stress in the midfoot. If symptoms recur frequently, the prehallux should be exised and the tendon reattached (Kidner procedure).

References

1. Caffey, J.: Pediatric X-ray Diagnosis. 6th Ed. Chicago, Yearbook Medical Publishers, 1972.
2. Garceau, G. J., and Gregory, C. F.: Solitary unicameral bone cysts. J. Bone Joint Surg., 36-A:267, 1954.
3. Ogden, J. A., and Griswold, D. M.: Solitary cyst of the talus. J. Bone Joint Surg., 54-A:1309, 1972.
4. Tachdjian, M.: Pediatric Orthopaedics. Philadelphia, W. B. Saunders, 1972.
5. Davidson, A. M., Steele, H. D., MacKenzie, D. A., and Penny, J. A.: A review of twenty-one cases of transchondral fracture of the talus. J. Trauma, 7:378, 1967.
6. Mindell, E. R., Cisek, E. E., Kartalian, G., and Dziob, J. A.: Late results of injuries to the talus. J. Bone Joint Surg., 45-A:221, 1963.
7. Scharling, M.: Osteochondritis dissecans of the talus. Acta Orthop. Scand., 49:89, 1978.
8. Stein, R. E., and Stelling, F. H.: Stress fracture of the calcaneus in a child with cerebral palsy. J. Bone Joint Surg., 59-A:131, 1977.
8a. Pathi, K.: Fracture of the neck of the talus in children. J. Indian Med. Assoc., 63:157, 1974.
8b. Spak, I.: Fractures of the talus in children. Acta Chir. Scand., 107:553, 1954.

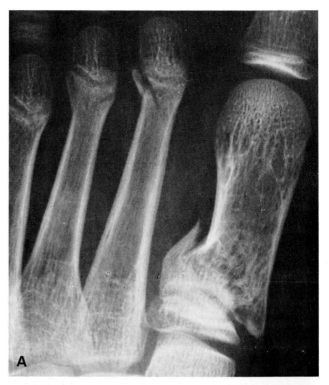

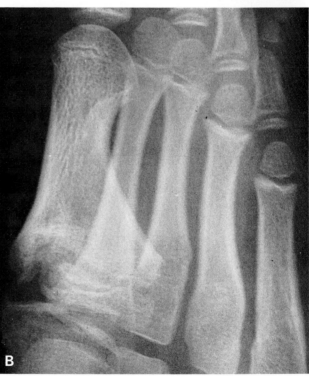

FIG. 20-33. *A*, Type 2 physeal injury of proximal first metatarsal, with concomitant fracture of distal second metatarsal. This barefoot girl fell off a skateboard. *B*, Three years later, the physis is assuming an irregular appearance suggestive of a type 5 injury. The fracture still has not remodeled extensively, and irregularity of the physis now confirms some growth arrest, especially centrally. The first metatarsal is shorter than the other four.

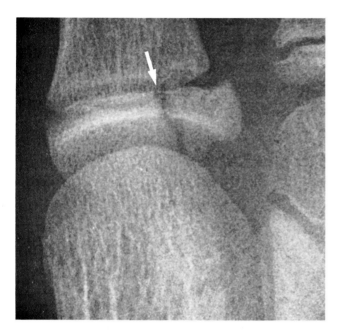

FIG. 20-34.   Type 3 injury of the phalangeal epiphysis (arrow).

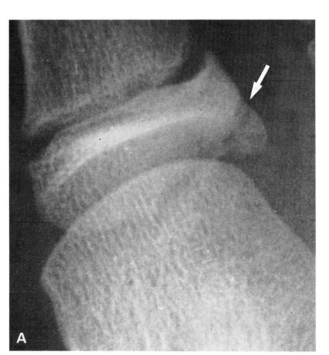

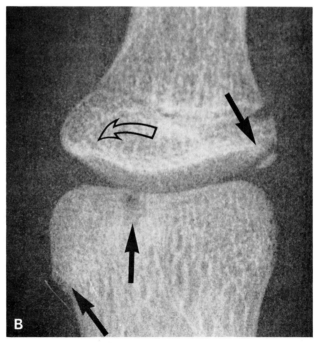

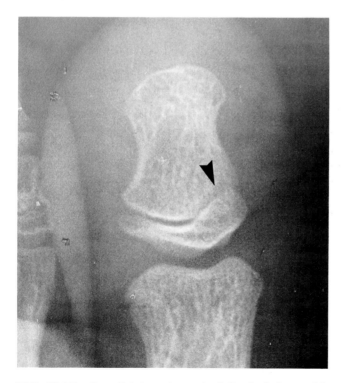

FIG. 20-35.   Type 5 injury (arrow) of distal phalanx with growth slowdown on the medial side.

FIG. 20-36.   Type 7 avulsion injuries of secondary ossification center of first toe. *A*, Proximal phalanx (arrow). *B*, Distal phalanx. As the toe was forced into varus (open arrow) the fracture ''propagated'' obliquely (solid arrows) across the joint to involve the medial proximal phalanx.

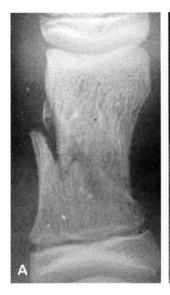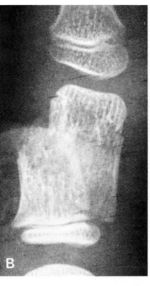

FIG. 20-37. *A*, Shaft fracture with mild angulation. *B*, Moderate angular deformity accompanying a shaft fracture. This must be corrected, since there is not enough longitudinal growth to restore longitudinal alignment.

9. Johanson, P. H.: Pseudomonas infections of the foot following puncture wounds. J.A.M.A., *204:*262, 1968.
10. Canale, S. T., and Belding, R. H.: Osteochondral lesions of the talus. J. Bone Joint Surg., 62-A:97, 1980.
11. Tomaschewski, H. K.: Ergebnisse der Behandlung des post-traumatischen Fehlwuchses des Fusses bei Kindern und Jugendlichen. Beitr. Orthop. Traumatol., *22:*90, 1975.
12. Essex-Lopresti, P.: The mechanism, reduction, technique and results in fractures of the os calcis. Br. J. Surg., *39:*395, 1952.
13. Schofield, R. O.: Fractures of the os calcis. J. Bone Joint Surg., *18:*566, 1936.
14. Zayre, M.: Fracture of the calcaneus. A review of 110 fractures. Acta Orthop. Scand., *40:*530, 1969.
15. Thomas, H. M.: Calcaneal fracture in childhood. Br. J. Surg., *56:*664, 1969.
16. Matteri, R., and Frymoyer, J.: Fracture of the calcaneus in young children. J. Bone Joint Surg., 55-A:1091, 1973.
17. Buchanan, J., and Greer, R. B., III: Stress fractures in the calcaneus of a child. Clin. Orthop., *135:*119, 1978.
18. Stephens, N. A.: Fracture-dislocation of the talus in childhood. Br. J. Surg., *43:*600, 1956.
19. Rowe, C. R., Sakellarides, H. T., Freeman, P. A., and Sorbie, C.: Fractures of the os calcis. J.A.M.A., *184:*920, 1963.
20. Aitken, A. P., and Poulson, D.: Dislocations of the tarsometatarsal joint. J. Bone Joint Surg., 45-A:246, 1963.
21. Trafton, P. G.: Epiphyseal fracture of the base of the first metatarsal: A case report. Orthopedics, *2:*256, 1979.
22. Harrison, M.: Fractures of the metatarsal head. Can. J. Surg., *11:*511, 1968.
23. Brand, R. A., and Black, H.: Pseudomonas osteomyelitis following puncture wounds in children. J. Bone Joint Surg., 56-A:1637, 1974.

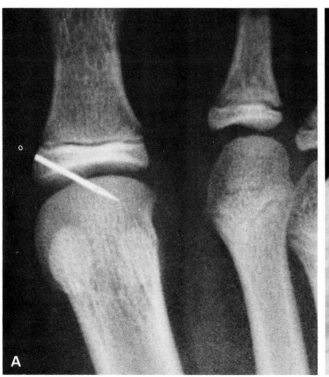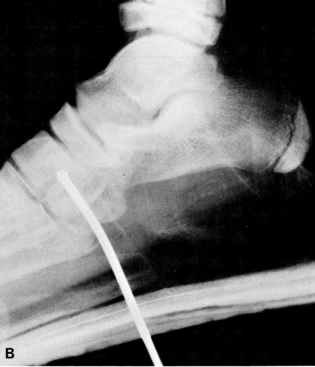

FIG. 20-38. *A*, Puncture wound from needle that broke and was left in the joint. *B*, Roentgenogram of patient showing a toy axle that penetrated through the shoe and into the foot.

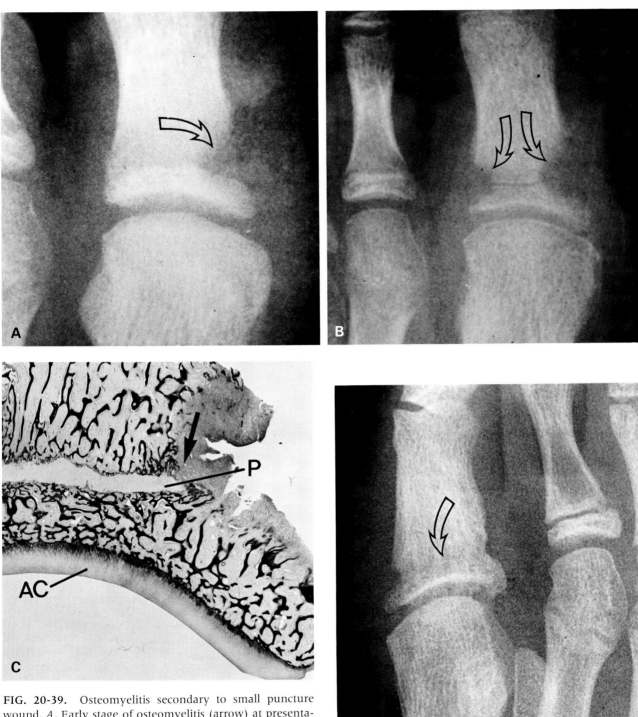

FIG. 20-39. Osteomyelitis secondary to small puncture wound. *A*, Early stage of osteomyelitis (arrow) at presentation three weeks after original injury. *B*, Despite debridement, further destruction (arrows) continued. *C*, Surgical specimen showing peripheral destruction of physis (arrow). Note the articular cartilage (AC), and the physis (P).

FIG. 20-40. Premature closure (arrow) of physis of proximal phalanx following infection of a puncture wound.

Appendix I
Joint Range of Motion

In the evaluation of children injured in accidents, it is often necessary to define ranges of motion at the initial assessment and their improvement, or lack thereof, with time. This serves as a basis for disability assessment, although one might question the relevance of such schemes as those used routinely in adults. The handbook published by The American Academy of Orthopaedic Surgeons is probably the best known source book.[1] However, this basically refers to joint motion in adults. Amplitudes of joint motion, coupled with joint laxity, certainly seem to differ in children, although little information exists about the influence of aging on the ranges of motion.[2-4] Boone and Azen have recently published a study of joint motion in boys, specifically addressing the comparison of changing patterns with increasing age.[5] The "young" group, which included 53 subjects, ranged from 18 months to 19 years. These data are partially reproduced in Table I-1.

In particular, their study showed that boys 12 years of age or younger had a greater degree of shoulder extension, ankle flexion, and foot eversion. The youngest group, comprised of individuals 5 years old or less, exhibited greater forearm supination and pronation; greater flexion, radial and ulnar deviation of the wrist; greater abduction, adduction and internal and external rotation of the hip; and greater inversion of the foot. However, this youngest group had less hip extension and was unable to assume zero starting positions (full extension) for hip and knee flexion. Children in the 6- to 12-year range had slightly more horizontal shoulder, elbow, and wrist extension capacity.

Increasing rigidity of connective tissue, particularly as it involves muscles and tendons, becomes a factor associated with increasing age, so temporal changes in joint laxity and motion might be expected.[6]

Amplitudes of motion for left and right joints were consistently similar.[5] Therefore, the motions of the joints of a patient's "healthy" limb may routinely be used for comparison to the injured side.

Unfortunately, the data provided by Boone and Azen only concern male patients. Comparable studies for developing females are necessary. Further, studies of specific subgroups would be important. Do changes in laxity accompany the (pre)adolescent growth spurt?

TABLE I-1. *Comparison of Estimated Ranges of Motion (In Degrees)*

Joint	AAOS Averages*	Boone-Azen Study†
Shoulder		
Horizontal flexion	135	141
Horizontal extension	—	47
Neutral abduction	170	185
Forward flexion	158	168
Backward extension	53	67
Inward rotation	70	70
Outward rotation	90	108
Elbow		
Flexion	146	145
Extension	0	1
Forearm		
Pronation	71	77
Supination	84	83
Wrist		
Flexion	73	77
Extension	71	76
Radial deviation	19	22
Ulnar deviation	33	37
Hip		
Beginning position flexion	—	30
Flexion	113	123
Extension	28	7
Abduction	48	52
Adduction	31	28
Internal rotation	45	50
External rotation	45	50
Knee		
Beginning position flexion	—	21
Flexion	134	144
Ankle		
Plantar flexion	48	58
Dorsiflexion	18	13
Forefoot		
Inversion	33	37
Eversion	18	22

*Primarily in adults.
†Range mean in children (age range 18 months to 19 years).

References

1. American Academy of Orthopaedic Surgeons: Joint Motion: Measuring and Recording. Chicago, AAOS, 1965.
2. Coon, V., Donato, G., Houser, C., and Bleck, E. E.: Normal ranges of hip motion in infants six weeks, three months and six months of age. Clin. Orthop., *110:*256, 1975.
3. Davies, D. V.: Aging changes in joints. *In* Structural Aspects of Aging. Edited by G. H. Bourne. New York, Hafner, 1961, pp. 23–27.
4. Smahel, Z.: Joint motion of the child's hand. Acta Chir. Plast., *17:*113, 1975.
5. Boone, D. C., and Azen, S. P.: Normal range of motion of joints in male subjects. J. Bone Joint Surg., *61-A:*756, 1979.
6. Hall, D. A.: The Aging of Connective Tissue. London, Academic Press, 1976, p. 62.

Appendix II

Analysis of Longitudinal Discrepancy

The surgical improvement or correction of longitudinal arm or leg discrepancies prior to chondro-osseous maturity must rely upon a reasonably accurate prediction of the remaining growth in both the involved and uninvolved bones, as well as an understanding of the pathomechanism of the discrepancy. Further, one must ascertain whether the difference is static or changing. The successful treatment of limb-length discrepancy depends on an accurate assessment of the limb length over a period of time, knowledge of the cosmetic and functional deficits anticipated, and a proper perspective of the various treatment modalities. The pattern of growth of the femur and tibia must be determined. For most congenitally short limbs the growth of the two extremities tends to be proportionate. Traumatic shortening is more variable, and may increase dramatically during the adolescent growth spurt. For prediction and treatment, the pattern of growth is as important as the absolute difference between the two extremities at any point in time.

Serial measurements at yearly intervals usually determine whether the growth is proportionate or variable. Roentgenographic estimation of limb lengths is more accurate and reproducible than clinical measurements. Full-length scanograms provide the most accurate reproductions (see Chap. 3 for technique).

Each patient has different overall functional requirements, and must be evaluated individually. The patient's functional evaluation, the amount of pelvic obliquity, the gait pattern, the sensory and motor function of the extremity, and the stability of range and motion of the joints are the most important factors. Cosmetic factors relate to the sex of the patient, the overall predicted height, the proportions of the trunks-legs-arms, and the social disadvantages of being short. Full-length photographs with cutouts to lengthen and shorten the extremities give some idea of the cosmetic results of treatment. Using this technique, major body image distortion can be avoided, such as a shortening procedure in someone with long arms, which might produce an anthropoid appearance.

The bases for growth prediction were introduced by Todd, who formalized the concept of skeletal maturation, and by Gill and Abbott, who emphasized that growth, aging, and maturation are three different, but related processes.[1,2] Concepts were further refined by the skeletal aging methods of Greulich and Pyle and the growth studies of Anderson and Green who correlated the lengths (growth rates) of the femur and tibia of boys and girls with their skeletal ages (Fig. II-1), and introduced a graph showing anticipated remaining distal femoral and proximal tibial growth (Fig. II-2).[3-6]

Fries determined a method for straight-line equations derived from the standard charts of growth remaining at normal epiphyses.[7] These equations offer a quick means of calculation, based on the Green and Anderson growth charts.[5,6]

More recently, Moseley has introduced a straight-line graphic analysis method for evaluating leg-length discrepancies (Fig. II-3).[8] This is based on two important concepts. The first is that leg growth can be represented graphically by a straight line. The second is that a nomogram relating leg lengths to skeletal age can provide a mechanism for considering the child's growth percentile and the relationship to overall leg-length discrepancy.

The first concept is a simple mathematical manipulation comparable to plotting exponential growth data against a logarithmic scale. Accordingly, the growth of the short leg is represented by a straight line that lies below that of the normal leg, which may have a different slope. The leg-length discrepancy at any given skeletal age is represented by the distance between the two parallel, converging, or diverging lines. The percentage of inhibition of growth in the shorter leg is represented by the difference in slope of the two lines (the slope of the normal leg is arbitrarily defined as 100%).

The second concept is related to the implication of Anderson and Green that a child's growth percentile should be considered in leg-lengthening predictions. In Moseley's straight-line graphic method, the nomogram represents an attempt to accomplish this.

It is widely accepted that skeletal age is a more appropriate

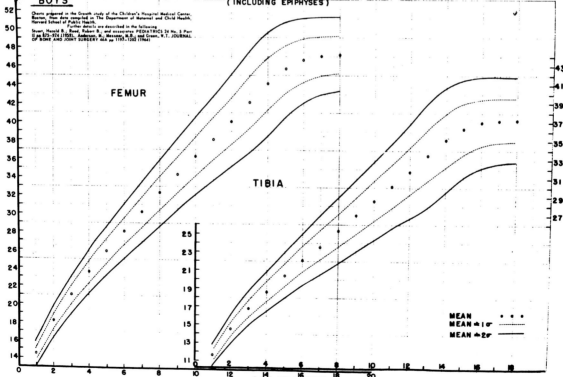

FIG. II-1. Green-Anderson growth rate graphs for the femur and tibia. Plotting length versus skeletal age over time allows one to ascertain the slope of growth versus the normal growth curve and standard deviations. *A*, Chart for girls. *B*, Chart for boys.

criterion than chronologic age in the study of growth. However, assessment of skeletal maturity by the method of Greulich and Pyle is difficult in cases in which the ossification centers appear in a different order and enlarge at different relative rates than that described in their Atlas, and it is virtually impossible in some skeletal dysplasias in which ossification is grossly disrupted. These problems are discussed in detail in Chapter 3. There is also an unavoidable error of technique, since the standards of comparisons are as much as 14 months apart at some ages. The question of accuracy has been approached by others who have developed more rigorous techniques for the knee, hand, and wrist.[9,10] However, these methods have not been correlated with leg-length data; therefore the applicability of the leg-length problems cannot be fully assessed.

Growth of the normal leg is represented by a straight line, by definition. However, this method also depends upon the implicit assumption that the growth line of the short leg will also be straight. This assumption is false in legs recently afflicted with poliomyelitis, where the growth rate is known to vary, but would appear true in cases of congenital short legs and legs with polio after resolution of the acute phase of the disease.[11] In leg-length deformity consequent to femoral shaft fractures in children there may be considerable variations in the first year or two after injury that must also be considered, although rarely are there sufficient differences in leg length to warrant any surgical procedures. Similarly, growth slowdown, rather than growth cessation, following physeal injuries is not as predictable and may not follow a straight line. Finally, the late appearance of a peripheral osseous block will affect both the length as well as the angulation of an extremity. This may not appear until the child enters the adolescent growth spurt, at which point a rapid change in the slope of the line may result. The final problem is angulation, which is not adequately factored into either method. Furthermore, resection of an osseous bridge and possible pickup of growth rate are also not predictable by this method.

Figure II-4 shows the initial steps for using the Moseley graph for the depiction of growth to date. At the time of each assessment, 3 parameters have to be obtained. These are: (a) the length of the (normal) leg measured by scanogram from the most superior part of the capital femoral ossification center to the inferior part of the distal tibial ossification center, (b) the comparable length of the short leg, and (c) the radiologic estimate of the skeletal age. In the rare instance where one is dealing with congenital hemihypertrophy or fracture overgrowth, the longer leg is the abnormal one, and should be plotted comparable to the short leg, but above the normal line, rather than below. The point for

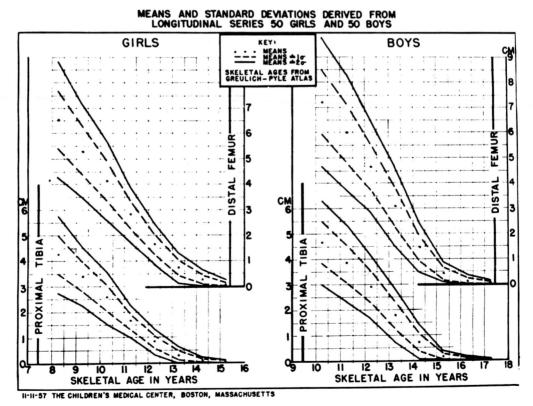

GROWTH REMAINING IN NORMAL DISTAL FEMUR AND PROXIMAL TIBIA FOLLOWING CONSECUTIVE SKELETAL AGE LEVELS

MEANS AND STANDARD DEVIATIONS DERIVED FROM LONGITUDINAL SERIES 50 GIRLS AND 50 BOYS

11-11-57 THE CHILDREN'S MEDICAL CENTER, BOSTON, MASSACHUSETTS

FIG. II-2.   Growth remaining graph for use with the Green-Anderson charts shown in Figure II-1. When the probable difference at maturity has been predicted, this graph may be used to determine which physis or physes to surgically epiphysiodese, and when to do so.

the normal leg is placed at the appropriate point (1). A vertical line is drawn through the point just plotted, extending into the skeletal age area for either girl or boy, as the case may be (2). Place the point for the short leg on the vertical line at the appropriate length (3). Plot the point for skeletal age on that vertical line where it crosses the appropriate line in the skeletal age area (4). Interpolating between 2 skeletal age lines is often necessary. For example, the vertical line crosses the skeletal ages at 4, 5, and 6 for both boys and girls. Points are depicted for a girl of 4½ years and a boy of 6 years (skeletal ages). Plot successive sets of points in the same fashion (5). Each of the child's assessments will then be represented by a vertical line on which the 3 points for that particular visit are plotted. Draw the straight line that best fits the points previously plotted for successive lengths of the short leg (6). This is the growth line of the short leg. The leg-length discrepancy at any given time is represented by the vertical distance between the 2 growth lines (7), and the growth inhibition is represented by the difference in slope between the 2 lines, taking the slope of the normal leg line as 100%.

Figure II-5 depicts the steps in predicting future growth to skeletal maturity. Extend the growth line of the short leg to the right of the graph (1). Draw the horizontal line that best fits the points plotted in the skeletal age area (2). Due to the inaccuracy inherent in estimating skeletal age, these points often do not closely approximate a straight line. The horizontal straight line should be drawn so that the total of the distance of points lying above the line is equal to the total for

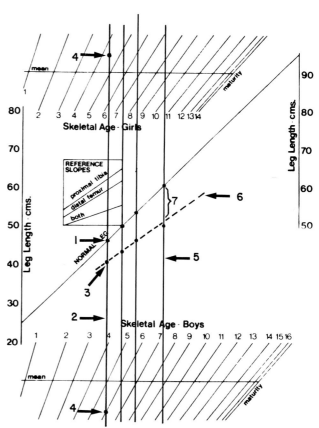

FIG. II-4. Steps for plotting lengths of normal and involved leg and skeletal age on successive visits. See text for details.

points lying below the line. This can also be put on a computer to accurately plot the most likely slope. At the point at which that horizontal line meets the sloping line, draw a vertical straight line that intersects the growth line of the normal and short leg (3). These points of intersection provide the prediction of the anticipated leg lengths and discrepancy at skeletal maturity (4).

Figure II-6 considers the steps for timing and the effects of leg lengthening. The new growth line for the lengthened leg should be drawn exactly parallel to the previous line of the short leg (1), but displaced upward by an amount exactly equal to the increase in length achieved (2). The short leg should be lengthened by an amount equal to the *anticipated discrepancy* at maturity, and not by the amount of the present discrepancy. If there is a significant growth inhibition in the short leg, one must lengthen the short leg longer than the long leg, anticipating that because of the difference in growth rates, this overcorrection will be equalized by maturity. The growth of a leg that has undergone surgical lengthening thereafter follows a straight line of the same slope that is displaced upward on the graph by an amount equal to the lengthening achieved.

Following surgical lengthening, the projection of the growth line as the line of unchanged slope ignores the possibility that a surgical procedure on the diaphysis or metaphysis might stimulate the physis (physes) of that bone, thereby changing rates of growth (i.e., slope). There does not appear to be any way of confidently predicting whether or not such

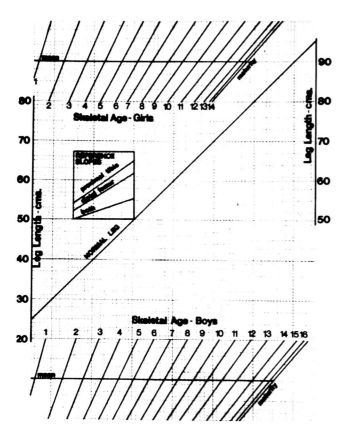

FIG. II-3. Moseley graph for depicting leg growth parameters and predicting timing of various surgical procedures.

an effect will occur, or the amount of additional length that it might contribute. Clinical experience and previous reports suggest that the stimulation is temporary, and when present is minimal and usually beneficial to the clinical situation, since it adds length to a leg that needs lengthening.

Figure II-7 plots the timing of surgical epiphysiodesis. At the point representing cessation of growth of the short leg, having taken into account the effect of a lengthening procedure, if necessary, draw a line to the left parallel to the particular reference slope for the proposed surgery until it intersects the growth line of the long leg (1). The point at which this line meets the growth line of the long leg indicates the point at which the surgery should be done (2). Note that this point is defined not in terms of the calendar or skeletal age, but in terms of the length of the long leg. The time that it will take for the child to reach that point cannot be stated exactly, but can be estimated by dropping a vertical line from that point to meet the horizontal line for the skeletal age (3). This will be an appropriate estimate for surgery.

After surgical epiphysiodesis, the slope of the longer leg will be altered, such that it should intersect the line of the shorter leg at skeletal maturity. The straight line of decreased slope following epiphysiodesis equals the percentage contribution that the fused growth plate would otherwise have made to the total growth of the extremity. Because the contributions of the proximal tibial and distal femoral epiphyseal plates are approximately 28 and 37%, respectively, of the

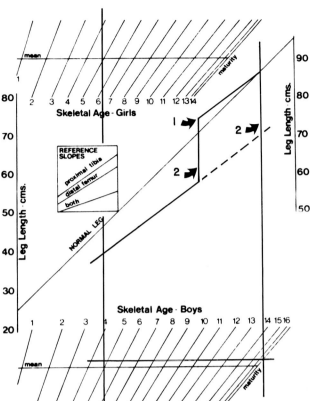

FIG. II-6. Steps for planning leg lengthening prior to chondro-osseous maturity. Note that the leg is overlengthened, and then equilibrates. See text for details.

total growth of the leg, one can predict the amount of inhibition introduced by epiphysiodesis. The growth line of the leg, which has undergone tibial, femoral, or combined epiphysiodesis will, thereafter, have a slope of 72, 63, or 35%, respectively.

Some epiphyseal plates appear to continue growing for a limited period of time after epiphysiodesis. In some cases up to 5 mm will be added to the bone before the fusion is complete. How often this occurs is difficult to assess, because the amount in question is close to the standard error of the measuring technique. It would seem reasonable that this effect would be minimized if the epiphysiodesis is accompanied routinely by curetting the growth plate to the greatest extent possible.

Another assumption has been made in Moseley's data, namely that the individual child remains in the same growth percentile with respect to each determined skeletal age. This assumption is open to question even for normal children, but the inaccuracy for individual skeletal age estimates makes it difficult to test. Neither the straight-line graph nor other methods provide an accurate quantitative means that account for such factors as varying nutrition and levels of activity, which may influence the rate of leg growth from year to year. The skeletal age nomogram is based on the assumption that the lengths of the lower extremities of all children of a certain skeletal age are the same proportion of the leg lengths of those individuals when they reach adulthood, regardless of the growth percentiles or chronologic

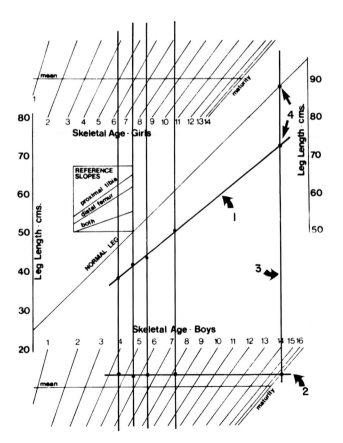

FIG. II-5. Steps for plotting anticipated leg lengths and overall discrepancy at chondro-osseous maturity. See text for details.

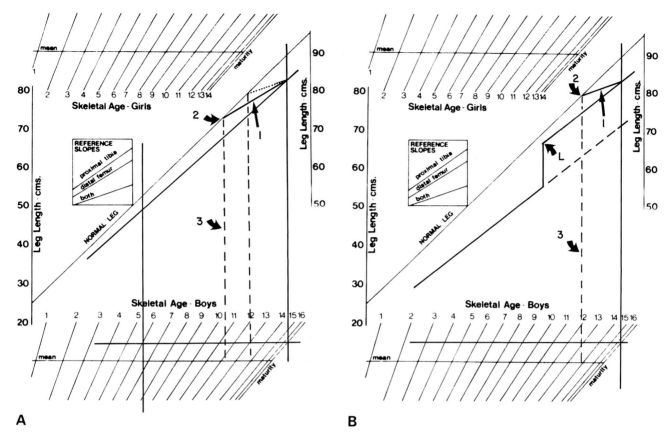

FIG. II-7. Steps for planning surgical arrest of physeal growth to equalize leg lengths. *A,* Surgical epiphysiodesis of the distal femur (solid line) or both proximal tibia and distal femur (dotted line). *B,* Surgical epiphysiodesis of both distal femur and proximal tibia after leg lengthening (L). See text for details.

ages. It is unlikely that this assumption is true for children of different races, or with markedly dissimilar habits. There do not appear to be satisfactory data describing the patterns of growth in children of other than the white race, and the surgeon must recognize this as a possible source of error in applying the straight-line graph or the growth-remaining method.

Minor discrepancies of 0 to 3 cm can usually be treated without surgery. Discrepancies of 1 to 1.5 cm usually require no treatment at all. Gross reported that 50% of patients with over 2 cm of shortening felt that they were unbalanced.[12] Only 10% of his patients felt a need to wear a lift if the discrepancy was 1.5 cm, increasing to 35% if the discrepancy was 2 cm, and 45% if the discrepancy was 3 cm. Generally, when using a shoe lift, the entire discrepancy does not need to be corrected. Usually $\frac{1}{2}$ to 1 cm residual discrepancy causes no functional problems, and makes the orthosis more attractive. Furthermore, patients with footdrop, weakness of hip flexion, and knee extension are often improved functionally with 1 to 2 cm of shortening, which facilitates clearance of the lower extremity during the swing phase of gait.

Discrepancies of 3 to 6 cm produce more significant deformities and functional disturbance. If the estimated final discrepancy is between 3 and 6 cm, shortening of the long extremity by epiphysiodesis is the safest means of achieving limb-length equality. Epiphysiodesis has good reliability when carefully conceived and performed.[13] Absolute equal-

ity of the limbs may not be a realistic goal due to scatter in the growth prediction table; therefore, if an error is made, it is usually better to undercorrect the short limb than to overcorrect the normal extremity. Reducing the discrepancy to a centimeter or less is an appropriate goal for the majority of patients.

In considering surgical epiphysiodesis, the principle is to slow down the growth of the contralateral bone(s) to allow the shorter traumatized bone(s) to equilibrate. Accuracy therefore rests on the ability to predict not only the amount that the long leg will be slowed down, but also the ability of the short leg to catch up. Is the growth arrest in the physis secondary to trauma incomplete or complete? If incomplete, is this a longitudinal slowdown or an angulation abnormality? If the growth arrest is complete, one can reasonably predict the loss. However, if the growth arrest is incomplete, it is sometimes difficult to accurately predict how much growth may still occur in the involved side, especially when the child begins the (pre)adolescent growth spurt.

Controversy regarding the most efficacious treatment method may be seen with leg-length discrepancies greater than 6 cm. Leg lengthening should be considered, primarily for the extremity that has good motor and sensory function, good stability, and functional range of motion of the involved joints. Limb lengthening may cause some loss of function or stability of the adjacent joints, and some decrease in motor strength. If these are already compromised preoperatively, it may not be advisable to lengthen the extremity. Age also appears to be a factor, since the results are best when lengthening is delayed until the adolescent period. Multiple methods for leg lengthening may be found in a symposium on equalization of leg length.[14-22] In any lengthening procedure the aim is to increase the length of the leg by that amount which will result in equal (or relatively equal) lengths at maturity, rather than by the current discrepancy when the patient is initially evaluated, as that may change.

The general categories for leg lengthening are one-stage lengthening or gradual lengthening. The one-stage lengthening described by Cauchoix must be limited to approximately 15% of the length of the femur to prevent neurologic and vascular complications.[15] He also reported a reasonably high incidence of nonunion (15%) and infection (8%). Although the method described by Herron also had a significant rate of nonunion, neurologic, and vascular complications, the infection rate was decreased.[20] One-stage lengthening has the advantage of preserving hip and knee motion in achieving the total lengthening at one time.

Staged femoral lengthening described by Eyring is safer as far as vascular and neurologic complications are concerned, but has a high incidence of fracture (14 of 22 cases) after the procedure.[17] In addition, staged femoral lengthening has the disadvantage of repeated hospitalization and operations. Additional problems noted by Manning and Coleman include some loss of motor strength and hip and knee motion with femoral lengthening, and equinus contractures with tibial lengthenings.[16,22]

Wagner offers a technical advance in instrumentation that appears to allow progressive distraction while the osseous components are held rigidly fixed.[18] This method appears to offer the advantage of allowing continued joint motion while protecting the neurologic and vascular structures from rapid stretch. The technical problems of infection, varus angulation, nonunion and refracture, plating, and removal of the plates still have not been completely solved by this method. In addition, the safe limits of lengthening without damage to the adjacent joints and motor function of the leg have not been completely established, nor has the efficacy of repeated lengthenings of the same bone or ipsilateral femoral and tibial lengthening.

Ultimately, the goal might be to influence the rate of growth of the epiphysis directly. Means such as electrical stimulation or mechanical distraction described by Sledge, Fishbane and Riley may someday find clinical usefulness; they have been used to some extent in Italy and Russia.[23,24] However, they still remain experimental.

References

1. Todd, T. W.: Atlas of Skeletal Maturation. St. Louis, C. V. Mosby, 1937.
2. Gill, G. G., and Abbott, L. C.: Practical method of predicting growth of the femur and tibia in a child. Arch. Surg., 45:286, 1942.
3. Greulich, W. W., and Pyle, S. I.: Radiographic Atlas of Skeletal Development of the Hand and Wrist. Stanford, Stanford University Press, 1959.
4. Green, W. T., and Anderson, M.: The problem of unequal leg lengths. Pediatr. Clin. North Am., 2:1137, 1955.
5. Green, W. T., and Anderson, M.: Epiphyseal arrest for the correction of discrepancies in length of the lower extremities. J. Bone Joint Surg., 39-A:853, 1957.
6. Green, W. T., Wyatt, G. M., and Anderson, M.: Orthoroentgenography as a method of measuring the bones of the lower extremities. Clin. Orthop., 61:110, 1968.
7. Fries, I. B.: Growth following epiphyseal arrest. A simple method of calculation. Clin. Orthop., 114:216, 1976.
8. Moseley, C. F.: A straight-line graph for leg-length discrepancies. Clin. Orthop., 136:33, 1978.
9. Roche, A. F., Wainer, H., and Thessen, D.: Skeletal Maturity. The Knee Joint as a Biological Indicator. New York, Plenum Publishing, 1975.
10. Tanner, J. M., et al.: Assessment of Skeletal Maturity and Prediction of Adult Height (TW2 Method). New York, Academic Press, 1975.
11. Stinchfield, A. J., Reidy, J. A., and Barr, J. S.: Prediction of unequal growth of the lower extremities in anterior poliomyelitis. J. Bone Joint Surg., 31A:478, 1949.
12. Gross, R. H.: Leg length discrepancy: how much is too much? Orthopedics, 1:307, 1978.
13. Stephens, D. C., Herrick, W., and MacEwen, G. D.: Epiphysiodesis of limb length inequality: results and indications. Clin. Orthop., 136:41, 1978.
14. Bianco, A. J., Jr.: Femoral shortening. Clin. Orthop., 136:49, 1978.
15. Cauchoix, J., and Morel, G.: One stage femoral lengthening. Clin. Orthop., 136:66, 1978.
16. Coleman, S. S., and Stevens, P. M.: Tibial lengthening. Clin. Orthop., 136:92, 1978.
17. Eyring, E. J.: Staged femoral lengthening. Clin. Orthop., 136:83, 1978.
18. Wagner, H.: Operative lengthening of the femur. Clin. Orthop., 136:125, 1978.
19. Winquist, R. A., Hansen, S. T., Jr., and Pearson, R. E.: Closed intramedullary shortening of the femur. Clin. Orthop., 136:54, 1978.
20. Herron, L. D., Amstutz, H. C., and Sakai, D. N.: One stage femoral lengthening in the adult. Clin. Orthop., 136:74, 1978.
21. Liedberg, E., and Persson, B. M.: Technical aspects of midshaft femoral shortening with Kuntscher nailing. Clin. Orthop., 136:62, 1978.
22. Manning, C.: Leg lengthening. Clin. Orthop., 136:105, 1978.
23. Fishbane, B. M., and Riley, L. H.: Continuous transphyseal traction: experimental observations. Clin. Orthop., 136:120, 1978.
24. Sledge, C. B., and Noble, J.: Experimental limb lengthening by epiphyseal distraction. Clin. Orthop., 136:111, 1978.

Index

Page numbers in *italics* indicate figures; page numbers followed by "t" indicate tables.